FROM MELANOCYTES TO MELANOMA

FROM MELANOCYTES TO MELANOMA

THE PROGRESSION TO MALIGNANCY

Edited by

VINCENT J. HEARING, PhD

Laboratory of Cell Biology
National Cancer Institute
National Institutes of Health
Bethesda, MD

STANLEY P. L. LEONG, MD

Department of Surgery
University of California, San Francisco, School of Medicine
San Francisco, CA

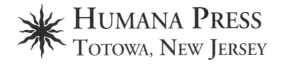

HUMANA PRESS
TOTOWA, NEW JERSEY

© 2006 Humana Press Inc.
999 Riverview Drive, Suite 208
Totowa, New Jersey 07512
www.humanapress.com

Production Editor: Amy Thau

Cover design by Patricia F. Cleary

Cover Illustration: Fig. 2, Chapter 11, "Genetic Progression From Melanocyte to Malignant Melanoma," by Boris C. Bastian (background image). Foreground images (top to bottom):Fig. 2Ca, Chapter 21, "Optical Imaging Analysis of Atypical Nevi and Melanoma," by Amanda Pfaff Smith and Dorothea Becker; Fig. 4, Chapter 18, "Pigmentation, DNA Repair, and Candidate Genes: *The Risk of Cutaneous Malignant Melanoma in a Mediterranean Population*," by Maria Teresa Landi; and Fig. 2, Chapter 26, "Role of Melanoma Inhibitory Activity in Early Development of Malignant Melanoma," by Anja-Katrin Bosserhoff.

For additional copies, pricing for bulk purchases, and/or information about other Humana titles, contact Humana at the above address or at any of the following numbers: Tel.: 973-256-1699; Fax: 973-256-8341, E-mail: orders@humanapr.com; or visit our Website: www.humanapress.com

Printed in the United States of America. 10 9 8 7 6 5 4 3 2 1
eISBN: 1-59259-994-X
Library of Congress Cataloging-in-Publication Data

From melanocytes to melanoma: the progression to malignancy / edited by Vincent J. Hearing, Stanley P.L. Leong.
 p. ; cm.
 Includes bibliographical references and index.
 ISBN 1-58829-459-5 (alk. paper)
 1. Melanoma. 2. Cell transformation. 3. Melanocytes.
 [DNLM: 1. Melanoma--physiopathology. 2. Cell Transformation, Neoplastic.
3. Melanocytes--physiology. 4. Melanoma--therapy. QZ 200 F931 2006] I.
Hearing, Vincent J. II. Leong, Stanley P. L.
 RC280.M37F76 2006
 616.99'477--dc22
                                       2005010788

PREFACE

The normal precursor of malignant melanoma is the melanocyte, a cell of neural crest origin. In their embryological state, neural crest cells are unique in that they dissociate from the notochord on days 10–14 and migrate out, or "metastasize," to numerous sites of the body as their new "homes." These cells are known as "argentaffin cells" and include the melanocytes. Of interest is that melanocytes can also accumulate abnormally in clusters as nevi and thereafter reside in the lower stratum of the epithelium just above the level of the dermis (and occasionally in the dermis). The most important function of these melanocytes either singularly or in clusters is to manufacture melanin, a pigmented biopolymer that is distributed throughout the skin to protect the host from the damage of ultraviolet radiation. Indeed, the amount of pigmentation sets the background of racial groups in human beings. It is estimated that the number of melanocytes in the body is relatively constant between different racial groups, although the production of melanin varies dramatically from one race to the other. Melanocytes in lightly colored skin make the least amount of melanin, whereas melanocytes in darker skin make larger amounts of melanin, which provides significantly greater protection against the direct ultraviolet radiation at the equator and its subsequent photocarcinogenesis.

It is in the transformation and mutation of these melanocytes that melanoma cells are derived. Approximately 95% of the time, melanoma can be traced to a pre-existing nevus, but about 5% of the time, the original site may not be determined because melanoma presents as metastatic melanoma. Although melanoma is a potentially incurable disease, especially in its late stage, the overall incidence of melanoma is relatively low compared with other types of cancer. Of special interest is the incidence of cutaneous melanoma, which is dramatically lower in the more heavily pigmented populations, such as blacks and Asians. The mechanisms of melanogenesis have been studied, but are still not fully understood. It is our hope that *From Melanocytes to Melanoma: The Progression to Malignancy* presents all available evidence to date in order to establish a scholarly record of what is known about the progression of changes from melanocytes to melanoma. The intriguing differences between the lighter and darker skinned racial groups with respect to the different incidences of melanoma need to be explained. Patients with xeroderma pigmentosum (XP), a multigenic, multiallelic, autosomal recessive disease, have more than a 1000-fold increased risk of cutaneous melanoma. Thus, XP deserves special attention, since mechanisms responsible for the genesis of melanoma in these patients can be understood and applied to melanoma in general. One important goal of these studies is to understand the molecular mechanisms involved in melanogenesis and in malignant transformation of melanocytes. Potential therapeutic maneuvers may then be developed to either block these steps or use relevant specific molecules of melanogenesis as targets of attack.

From Melanocytes to Melanoma: The Progression to Malignancy is divided into three parts, with Part I addressing the basic biology of melanocytes and the molecular mechanisms involved in the development, migration, and differentiation of melanoblasts to melanocytes. Part II is devoted to elucidating processes involved in the transformation of melanocytes to malignant melanoma. Finally, Part III focuses on mechanisms involved in the further progression of primary melanomas into invasive and metastatic melanomas. We hope that by studying the molecular signals involved in these processes, we will be able to develop model systems by which we can trace the molecular mechanisms involved in the malignant transformation of melanocytes to malignant melanoma.

From Melanocytes to Melanoma: The Progression to Malignancy will be a valuable reference for all biologists and basic scientists who are interested in the biology of pigment cells, as well as to pathologists, dermatologists, surgeons, and medical oncologists who are interested in the diagnosis and treatment of melanoma.

Vincent J. Hearing, PhD
Stanley P. L. Leong, MD

ACKNOWLEDGMENT

This work was supported in part by a grant from the Llumar (UV) Window Film (www.windowfilm.com).

CONTENTS

CONTRIBUTORS

ZALFA A. ABDEL-MALEK • *Department of Dermatology, University of Cincinnati College of Medicine, Cincinnati, OH*

NEIL A. ACCORTT • *Biostatistics and Bioinformatics Unit, Comprehensive Cancer Center, University of Alabama at Birmingham, Birmingham, AL*

NATALIE G. AHN • *Department of Chemistry and Biochemistry, Howard Hughes Medical Institute, University of Colorado, Boulder, CO*

HEINZ ARNHEITER • *Mammalian Development Section, National Institute of Neurological Disorders and Stroke, National Institutes of Health, Bethesda, MD*

MENASHE BAR-ELI • *Department of Cancer Biology, University of Texas M. D. Anderson Cancer Center, Houston, TX*

BORIS C. BASTIAN • *Departments of Dermatology and Pathology, University of California, San Francisco, CA*

DOROTHEA BECKER • *Department of Pathology, University of Pittsburgh School of Medicine, Pittsburgh, PA*

YAACOV BEN-DAVID • *Molecular and Cellular Biology, Sunnybrook and Women's College Health Sciences Center and Toronto Sunnybrook Regional Cancer Centre; Department of Medical Biophysics, University of Toronto, Toronto, Canada*

DOROTHY C. BENNETT • *Department of Basic Medical Sciences, St. George's Hospital Medical School, London, UK*

PABLO LÓPEZ BERGAMI • *Department of Oncological Sciences, Mount Sinai School of Medicine, New York, NY*

KAPIL BHARTI • *Mammalian Development Section, National Institute of Neurological Disorders and Stroke, National Institutes of Health, Bethesda, MD*

ANINDITA BHOUMIK • *Department of Oncological Sciences, Mount Sinai School of Medicine, New York, NY*

KEREN BISMUTH • *Mammalian Development Section, National Institute of Neurological Disorders and Stroke, National Institutes of Health, Bethesda, MD*

ERNEST BORDEN • *Taussig Cancer Center, Cleveland Clinic Foundation, Cleveland, OH*

ANJA-KATRIN BOSSERHOFF • *Institute of Pathology, University of Regensburg, Regensburg, Germany*

GLEN M. BOYLE • *Melanoma Genomics Group, Queensland Institute of Medical Research, Brisbane, Australia*

DAHU CHEN • *Department of Pathology, Huffington Center on Aging, Baylor College of Medicine, Houston, TX*

KEVIN G. CHEN • *Laboratory of Cell Biology, National Cancer Institute, National Institutes of Health, Bethesda, MD*

LYNDA CHIN • *Department of Medical Oncology, Dana-Farber Cancer Institute, and the Department of Dermatology, Harvard Medical School, Boston, MA*

JAMES E. CLEAVER • *Auerback Melanoma Laboratory, Department of Dermatology, University of California, San Francisco, CA*

ANTHONY L. COOK • *Melanogenix Group, Institute for Molecular Bioscience, The University of Queensland, Brisbane, Australia*

A. NEIL CROWSON • *Departments of Dermatology, Pathology, and Surgery, University of Oklahoma College of Medicine, Tulsa, OK*

TAMAS CSERMELY • *Mammalian Development Section, National Institute of Neurological Disorders and Stroke, National Institutes of Health, Bethesda, MD*

DAVID E. ELDER • *Division of Anatomic Pathology, Hospital of the University of Pennsylvania, University of Pennsylvania Health System, Philadelphia, PA*

DONG FANG • *Program of Tumor Biology, The Wistar Institute, Philadelphia, PA*

EREZ FEIGE • *Department of Pediatric Oncology and Melanoma Program in Medical Oncology, Dana-Farber Cancer Institute, Harvard Medical School, Boston, MA*

DAVID E. FISHER • *Department of Pediatric Oncology and Melanoma Program in Medical Oncology, Dana-Farber Cancer Institute, Harvard Medical School, Boston, MA*

MICHAEL M. GOTTESMAN • *Laboratory of Cell Biology, National Cancer Institute, National Institutes of Health, Bethesda, MD*

ADÈLE C. GREEN • *Division of Population Studies and Human Genetics, Queensland Institute of Medical Research, Brisbane, Queensland, Australia*

RISHAB K. GUPTA • *Department of Immunodiagnosis and Protein Biochemistry, John Wayne Cancer Institute, St. John's Health Center, Santa Monica, CA*

RUTH HALABAN • *Department of Dermatology, Yale University School of Medicine, New Haven, CT*

VINCENT J. HEARING • *Laboratory of Cell Biology, National Cancer Institute, National Institutes of Health, Bethesda, MD*

MARY J. C. HENDRIX • *Cancer Biology and Epigenomics Program, Children's Memorial Research Center, Feinberg School of Medicine, Northwestern University, Chicago, IL*

MEENHARD HERLYN • *Program of Tumor Biology, The Wistar Institute, Philadelphia, PA*

ANGELA R. HESS • *Cancer Biology and Epigenomics Program, Children's Memorial Research Center, Feinberg School of Medicine, Northwestern University, Chicago, IL*

DAVE S. B. HOON • *Department of Molecular Oncology, John Wayne Cancer Institute, Santa Monica, CA*

LING HOU • *Mammalian Development Section, National Institute of Neurological Disorders and Stroke, National Institutes of Health, Bethesda, MD*

ANA LUISA KADEKARO • *Department of Dermatology, University of Cincinnati College of Medicine, Cincinnati, OH*

PETER A. KANETSKY • *Center for Clinical Epidemiology and Biostatistics, University of Pennsylvania, Philadelphia, PA*

MOHAMMED KASHANI-SABET • *Auerback Melanoma Research Laboratory, University of California at San Francisco, San Francisco, CA*

JULIAN A. KIM • *Taussig Cancer Center, Cleveland Clinic Foundation, Cleveland, OH*

MARIA TERESA LANDI • *Division of Cancer Epidemiology and Genetics, Genetic Epidemiology Branch, National Cancer Institute, Bethesda, MD*

J. HELEN LEONARD • *Queensland Radium Institute Research Unit, Queensland Institute of Medical Research, Brisbane, Australia*

STANLEY P. L. LEONG • *Department of Surgery, University of California, San Francisco, School of Medicine, San Francisco, CA*

QIUSHI LIN • *Huffington Center on Aging, Department of Pathology, Baylor College of Medicine, Houston, TX*

WENFANG LIU • *Mammalian Development Section, National Institute of Neurological Disorders and Stroke, National Institutes of Health, Bethesda, MD*

CYNTHIA MAGRO • *Division of Dermatopathology, Department of Pathology, Ohio State University, College of Medicine and Public Health, Columbus, OH*

STEVE R. MARTINEZ • *Department of Molecular Oncology, John Wayne Cancer Institute, Santa Monica, CA*

ANA M. MCELRATH-GARZA • *Department of Immunodiagnosis and Protein Biochemistry, John Wayne Cancer Institute, St. John's Health Center, Santa Monica, CA*

ESTELA E. MEDRANO • *Huffington Center on Aging, Department of Molecular and Cellular Biology, and Department of Pathology, Baylor College of Medicine, Houston, TX*

I. SAIRA MIAN • *Life Sciences Division, Lawrence Berkeley National Laboratory, Berkeley, CA*

MARTIN C. MIHM, JR. • *Departments of Dermatology and Pathology, Harvard Medical School, Boston, MA*

DONALD L. MORTON • *Department of Surgical Oncology, John Wayne Cancer Institute, St. John's Health Center, Santa Monica, CA*

HIDEKI MURAKAMI • *Mammalian Development Section, National Institute of Neurological Disorders and Stroke, National Institutes of Health, Bethesda, MD*

MINH-THANH T. NGUYEN • *Mammalian Development Section, National Institute of Neurological Disorders and Stroke, National Institutes of Health, Bethesda, MD*

BRIAN J. PAK • *Molecular and Cellular Biology, Sunnybrook and Women's College Health Sciences Centre and Toronto Sunnybrook Regional Cancer Centre, Toronto, Canada*

PETER G. PARSONS • *Melanoma Genomics Group, Queensland Institute of Medical Research, Brisbane, Australia*

WILLIAM J. PAVAN • *Genetic Disease Research Branch, National Human Genome Research Institute, National Institutes of Health, Bethesda, MD*

LAURA L. POLING • *Department of Pediatric Oncology and Melanoma Program in Medical Oncology, Dana-Farber Cancer Institute, Harvard Medical School, Boston, MA*

TIMOTHY R. REBBECK • *Center for Clinical Epidemiology and Biostatistics, University of Pennsylvania, Philadelphia, PA*

JON REED • *Department of Pathology, Baylor College of Medicine, Houston, TX*

KATHERYN A. RESING • *Department of Chemistry and Biochemistry, University of Colorado, Boulder, CO*

HEIKE RÖCKMANN • *Skin Cancer Unit at the German Cancer Research Center, Heidelberg, Germany*

ZE'EV RONAI • *Department of Oncological Sciences, Mount Sinai School of Medicine, New York, NY*

DIRK SCHADENDORF • *Skin Cancer Unit at the German Cancer Research Center, Heidelberg, Germany*

ELISABETH A. SEFTOR • *Cancer Biology and Epigenomics Program, Children's Memorial Research Center, Feinberg School of Medicine, Northwestern University, Chicago, IL*

RICHARD E. B. SEFTOR • *Cancer Biology and Epigenomics Program, Children's Memorial Research Center, Feinberg School of Medicine, Northwestern University, Chicago, IL*

NORMAN E. SHARPLESS • *Department of Medicine and Genetics, The University of North Carolina School of Medicine, Chapel Hill, NC*

DEBRA L. SILVER • *Genetic Disease Research Branch, National Human Genome Research Institute, National Institutes of Health, Bethesda, MD*

SUSAN SKUNTZ • *Mammalian Development Section, National Institute of Neurological Disorders and Stroke, National Institutes of Health, Bethesda, MD*

AMANDA PFAFF SMITH • *Department of Pathology, University of Pittsburgh, School of Medicine, Pittsburgh, PA*

SENG-JAW SOONG • *Biostatistics and Bioinformatics Unit, Comprehensive Cancer Center, University of Alabama at Birmingham, Birmingham, AL*

RICHARD A. STURM • *Melanogenix Group, Institute for Molecular Bioscience, The University of Queensland, Brisbane, Australia*

HIROYA TAKEUCHI • *Department of Molecular Oncology, John Wayne Cancer Institute, Santa Monica, CA*

CARMEN TELLEZ • *Department of Cancer Biology, University of Texas M. D. Anderson Cancer Center, Houston, TX*

MICHAEL WEGNER • *Institut für Biochemie, Universität Erlangen-Nürnberg, Erlangen, Germany*

QINGYI WEI • *Department of Epidemiology, University of Texas M. D. Anderson Cancer Center, Houston, TX*

CLAUDIA WELLBROCK • *Signal Transduction Team, Cell and Molecular Biology Section, The Institute of Cancer Research, London, UK*

DAVID C. WHITEMAN • *Division of Population Studies and Human Genetics, Queensland Institute of Medical Research, Brisbane, Queensland, Australia*

YUJI YAMAGUCHI • *Laboratory of Cell Biology, National Cancer Institute, National Institutes of Health, Bethesda, MD*

LIST OF COLOR PLATES

I MELANOCYTE DEVELOPMENT AND FUNCTION

1

The Origin and Development of Neural Crest-Derived Melanocytes

Debra L. Silver and William J. Pavan

CONTENTS

Summary

Melanocytes are specified from pluripotent neural crest cells that delaminate from the developing neural tube and overlying ectoderm early in development. As a subset of these neural crest cells migrate along the dorsal–lateral path, they begin to differentiate into melanocyte precursors (called melanoblasts). While the melanoblasts continue to differentiate, the population expands through proliferation and prosurvival processes. Melanoblasts eventually migrate through the dermis, into the epidermis, and, in mice and humans, into hair follicles, in which they produce melanin. Several classes of proteins, including transcription factors, extracellular ligands, transmembrane receptors, and intracellular signaling molecules regulate these processes. The genes that are currently implicated in melanocyte development and their relationship with each other will be discussed in this chapter.

Key Words: Neural crest; melanocyte.

INTRODUCTION

Melanocytes are pigment-producing cells that populate the integument, inner ear, and eyes of vertebrate organisms. Arising entirely from pluripotent neural crest cells, melanocytes undergo complex developmental processes that can be divided into several stages based on location and marker expression (Fig. 1). First is the initial specification of the neural crest cells, followed by their emigration from the neuroepithelium. Next, a subset of this population is specified as melanocyte precursors (termed melanoblasts), and expands and migrates along a dorsal–lateral path beneath the ectoderm. As development progresses, the melanoblasts simultaneously differentiate, proliferate, and migrate extensive distances throughout the embryo until finally populating the entire organism.

From: *From Melanocytes to Melanoma: The Progression to Malignancy*
Edited by: V. J. Hearing and S. P. L. Leong © Humana Press Inc., Totowa, NJ

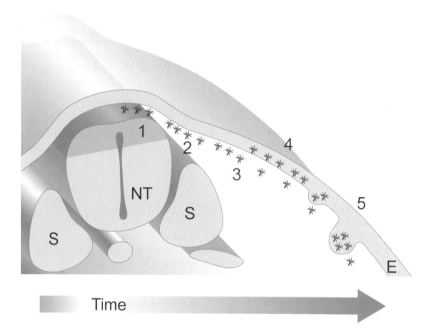

Fig. 1. Cartoon depicting stages of melanocyte specification and migration. The neural crest population is induced from dorsal edges of the neural tube (dark shading), and undergoes an epithelial to mesenchymal transition into the migration staging area (**1**). A subset of neural crest cells is specified as melanoblast precursors and migrate dorsal-laterally beneath the ectoderm (early migration) (**2**). The melanoblasts migrate through the dermis and then into the epidermis (mid migration) (**3**). The melanoblasts migrate within the epidermis and become incorporated into developing hair follicles (late migration) (**4**). The melanoblasts continue to populate the epidermis and hair follicles, eventually becoming melanocytes that produce pigment (**5**). NT, neural tube; S, somite; E, ectoderm.

The neural crest cells initially form as the neural tube is closing: at 8 d of gestation in mice and at 22 d in humans. Neural crest cells develop in a rostral to caudal direction from the neuroepithelium at the lateral edges of the neural folds and the junction with the ectoderm. Remarkably, neural crest cells differentiate into many distinct cell types that are dramatically different in function and location in the adult vertebrate. For example, in addition to melanocytes, other neural crest derivatives include the neurons and glial cells of the entire peripheral and enteric nervous systems, as well as craniofacial tissues and cardiac cells. These cell types develop in distinct and consistent spatial and temporal patterns, and are identifiable by their pattern of migration, by lineage specific markers, and by intrinsic cell characteristics, such as pigment production.

Before their emigration from the neuroepithelium, the neural crest cells are specified within the dorsal neural tube, as evidenced from expression of markers including *Wingless/INT-related (Wnt) 1 and 3*, *Paired box transcription factor (Pax3)*, *Foxd3*, and in chick and *Xenopus* only, *Slug* (Table 1 and Fig. 1, no. 1) *(1–9)*. The specified neural crest population then undergoes an epithelial to mesenchymal transition, migrates out from the neuroepithelium as individual cells and into a region called the migration staging area, located dorsal to the neural tube and underneath the ectoderm. At this stage the premigratory neural crest cells are multipotent and express pan-neural crest markers: SRY box containing transcription factor (*Sox10*), *Sox9*, and, in mice, *Snai2 (10–12)*. In support of this theory, single neural crest cells that are marked by dye injections in mouse dorsal neural tubes give rise to multiple lineages *(13)*. In addition, individual neural crest cells in culture form mixed colonies of differentiated cells *(14,15)*.

After the neural crest cells leave the migration staging area, they migrate either ventrally or dorsal-laterally away from the neural tube (Fig. 1, no. 2). In mice, these migratory events appear to occur simultaneously, whereas, in chick, dorsal–lateral migration of melanoblasts appears to be delayed 1 d compared with ventral neural crest migration *(16,17)*. The ventrally migrating cells follow a path between the somites and neural tube, and eventually give rise to the peripheral nervous system and some endocrine cells. The dorsal-laterally migrating cells follow a path between the dermamyotome and ectoderm and eventually become melanocytes. Analysis in chick and mice suggests that melanocytes migrate primarily along the somite boundaries but may show some mixing along the midline and anterior–posterior axes *(18)*. Because melanoblasts are the only neural crest derivative thought to migrate along the dorsal–lateral pathway, the presence of neural crest-derived cells in this pathway has also been used as one characteristic trait to identify melanoblasts. Nonmelanoblasts that migrate along the dorsal–lateral pathway may be eliminated through selective cell death, because nonmelanocyte neuronal lineages have been observed along this pathway but undergo apoptosis before melanoblast migration *(19)*.

In vivo expression data support two theories regarding when neural crest cells are specified to the melanocyte lineage. Melanocyte markers, such as *Kit* and *microphthalmia associated basic helix-loop-helix leucine zipper transcription factor* (*Mitf*), are expressed in the migration staging area, followed soon after by expression of *dopachrome-tautomerase* (*Dct*) (Table 1) *(20–22)*. This suggests that the neural crest cells are predestined to become melanocytes before migration along the dorsal–lateral pathway and therefore select the migratory path because they are specified. Alternatively, the presence of extrinsic factors in the environment through which the cells migrate may contribute to the specification of melanocytes. In support of this latter theory, adhesion molecules, including *Ephrin-B* (*EphB*), extracellular matrix (ECM) proteins, and cadherins, show reduced expression in melanoblasts and the surrounding cells when the melanoblasts initiate their migration *(22–28)*. It may be that the expression of some melanocyte-specific genes is required to promote their initial spatiotemporal migration, and expression of additional genes is necessary for cells to continue to migrate.

In vitro culture experiments also provide conflicting evidence regarding when cells are committed to becoming melanocytes. Luo and colleagues have demonstrated that cultured quail neural crest cells expressing *Kit* (which marks melanoblasts in the migration staging area) always give rise to clones that contain only melanocytes *(29)*. However, experiments from Dunn and Pavan demonstrate that descendants of retrovirally infected *Dct*-positive melanoblasts in culture give rise to neural crest derivatives other than melanoblasts, the majority of which are smooth muscle cells *(166)*. Further analysis is necessary to clarify the multipotent nature of melanoblasts at this stage, because these conflicting results could be attributed to different species and culture conditions.

As melanoblasts migrate, the population expands by actively dividing and simultaneously inhibiting apoptosis *(19,30)*. They migrate extensive distances through the dermis, eventually cross the basement membrane, and then enter the epidermis (Fig. 1, no. 3,4). Mosaic analysis of melanoblasts in mice sought to uncouple the processes of migration and proliferation and suggests that melanoblasts undergo periods of high proliferation, then extensive migration into the epidermis without proliferation, then a second phase of proliferation, followed by migration to a final destination *(31)*. The *Kit* signal-transduction pathway is required for melanoblast expansion, survival, and migration *(32)*, whereas the endothelin receptor B *(Ednrb)* pathway functions primarily in neural crest cell proliferation *(33)* and perhaps migration *(34–36)*. Melanoblast specification and proliferation also may be regulated by several transcription factors, including *Foxd3, Sox9, Sox10, Pax3, Snai2,* transcription factor activator protein *Ap2α, Tcfap2α,* and *Mitf (1,2,11,12,21,37,38)*. In avian species, melanoblasts migrate into feather buds, whereas, in mice and humans, the melanoblasts gain entry into hair follicles (Fig. 1, no. 5), in which both *Kit ligand (Kitl)* and *Adamts20* are expressed *(20,22,39)*. Once in the hair follicle, the melanoblasts begin to produce pigment and function as fully differentiated melanocytes; they transfer pigment to the keratinocytes of the developing hair shaft, resulting in hair pigmentation.

Our current understanding of melanoblast development is based largely on in vivo studies of classical coat color mouse mutants, quail and chick transplantation experiments, and, more recently, rats, zebrafish, and *Xenopus*. The forward genetic screen is a valuable tool for the identification of novel genes that function in melanocyte development. DNA arrays, *in situ* hybridization, and antibody staining are complementary approaches to identify genes that are expressed in melanocytes *(40)*. Melanocyte development and the genetic pathways that govern it can also be explored using neural crest cultures. The melanocyte population can be targeted in these cultures using the RCAS-TVA system *(41)* and can be targeted in vivo using Cre-Lox technology *(42,43)*. Thus, these combined in vitro and in vivo approaches have helped to elucidate the molecular mechanism of melanocyte migration, proliferation, and differentiation. Together, these studies have revealed roles for transcription factors, adhesion molecules, and signaling pathways in different aspects of melanocyte development. In this chapter, we will provide an overview of the main molecules currently implicated as critical for melanocyte development (Table 1 and Fig. 2).

CELL SIGNALING AND ADHESION

The *Wnt/β-catenin*-signaling pathway is essential for neural crest induction and, subsequently, for melanocyte development. In addition, components of this pathway are expressed in melanoma and may be associated with progression of the disease *(44–47)* (Table 1). Signaling through this pathway provides a mechanism for extracellular signals to be directly transduced to transcriptional activation of targets. After Wnt binding to its receptor (Frizzled), β-catenin accumulates, enters the nucleus, and subsequently interacts with members of the lymphoid enhancer-binding factor (LEF)-1/T-cell specific (TCF) family of transcription factors, which then modulate transcription of target genes *(48)*. A subset of Wnt and Frizzled family members is expressed in spatiotemporal patterns consistent with the timing of neural crest induction. The extracellular ligands, *Wnt1* and *Wnt3,* are expressed in the dorsal part of the neural tube *(3,4,7,9)*, and β-catenin is expressed in both premigratory neural crest and in migrating neural crest in chick *(25)*. *Wnt6* is expressed in the chick ectoderm *(49)*, and, in zebrafish, *Wnt8* is also expressed in a spatiotemporal pattern consistent with neural crest induction *(50)*.

Studies in several model organisms suggest that components of the *Wnt/β-catenin*-signaling pathway are required for induction of melanocyte fate. In chick, *Wnt6* is required for neural crest induction *(49)*. E11.5-d-old mouse embryos that are null for both *Wnt1* and *Wnt3* exhibit a marked reduction in melanoblasts *(3)*. Furthermore, when

Table 1
Genes Functioning in Melanocyte Development[a]

Protein family	Gene symbol	Gene name	Expression pattern	Proposed function	Associated diseases (OMIM No)	Role in melanoma tumors/cell lines
Cell signaling and adhesion	Wnts	Wingless-related MMTV integration site	Dorsal NT (2,4,7,9)	Induction, proliferation. differentiation (3,4,37,41,50)	WNT3: Tetra Amelia (#273395) (169)	WNT5A: increased expression (44)
	Catnβ	β-catenin premigratory,	Mostly ubiquitous, proliferation, and migratory Mb (25)	Induction, differentiation (3,49–55)	Various cancers	Increased expression (45)
	Lef1βTcf	Lymphoid enhancer binding factor 1 (HMG/TCF)/ T-cell specific (HMG/TCF) transcription factor	Hair follicles, skin, mostly ubiquitous (1,70)	Induction, differentiation (50,53,54)	NA	Increased expression (46)
	Cdh	Type I (no. 5) and Type II (no. 5) Cadherins	Mb, Mc, dermis, epidermis (24,27,57,58)	All stages of migration (26,59)	E-CDH: various cancers, P-CDH:HJMD (#601553) (58,61)	Dynamic expression (58,61)
	Integrin, collagen. laminin. lectin. fibronectin	Membrane and secreted proteins	ECM between ectoderm and dermatome (22,23,62–64)	Early migration	various cancers	Integrinβ1: increased expression (65)

(continued)

Table 1 (*Continued*)
Genes Functioning in Melanocyte Development[a]

Protein family	Gene symbol	Gene name	Expression pattern	Proposed function	Associated diseases (OMIM No)	Role in melanoma tumors/cell lines
	Adamts20	Disintegrin-like and metalloprotease (reprolysin type) with thrombospondin type 1 motif, 20	Skin, hair follicles (39)	Late migration (39,66)	NA	NA
Signaling through growth factors and receptors	*Efnb*	Ephrin B (extracellular ligand)	Epithelium, Mb (74)	Early migration (28,74–76)	NA	NA
	EphB	Ephrin B receptor (tyrosine kinase)	Mb (128)	Early migration (28,74–76)	NA	EPHA1,2: increased expression (77,78) EPHB6: decreased expression (79)
	BMPs2 and *4*	Bone Morphogenetic Protein (extracellular ligand)	Dorsal NT, dorsal surface ectoderm, hair follicle (4,80,81)	Promotes/inhibits Mb specification (4,82,83)	NA	NA
	Ednrb	Endothelin receptor B (G protein-coupled receptor)	Mb (34,84)	Proliferation, survival, mid-migration (35,92–96)	WSIV (#277580), HSCR (#142623), ABCD (#600501) (87,90,91)	Increased/decreased expression (86)
	Edn3	Endothelin 3 (extracellular ligand)	Skin (36,85)	Proliferation, survival, mid-migration (21,33,36,94)	WSIV (#277580), HSCR (#142623), CCHS (#209880) (88,89)	NA

Gene	Name	Expression domain	Function	Disease	Expression change
Kit	Kit oncogene (receptor tyrosine kinase)	Premigratory and postmigratory Mb (21,22,100,101)	Migration, proliferation, survival (23,30,93,100, 102–104)	Piebaldism (#172800) (97)	Decreased expression (98,99)
Kitl	Kit ligand (extracellular ligand)	Dorsal and epithelial dermatome, dermis (20,22,101)	Migration, proliferation, survival (21,105,106)	NA	NA

Transcription factors

Gene	Name	Expression domain	Function	Disease	Expression change
Foxd3	Forkhead box D3 (Forkhead)	Dorsal NT, premigratory NC, early pan-NC, (1,5,109)	NC induction inhibits Mb specification? (105,109–111)	NA	NA
Sox9	SRY-box-containing gene 9 (HMG box)	Pan-NC, Mb (12)	Induction, differentiation (12,37,112,113)	CMPD (#114290) (171)	NA
Sox10	SRY-box-containing gene 10 (HMG box)	Early pan-NC, premigratory and postmigratory, Mb (11,37,114–119)	Early survival, proliferation, differentiation (37,115,117,119,120)	WSIV (#277580) (11,124)	Increased expression (125,126)
Pax3	Paired box gene 3 (HOX domain)	Dorsal NT, premigratory and postmigratory pan-NC (2,127)	Early specification, proliferation, survival (128,129)	WSI, II, III, (#193500, #193510, #148820) (134–136)	Increased expression (132,133)
Snai2/Slug	Snail homolog gene 2 (Zn finger)	Dorsal NT, pan-NC (6,8,10,138)	Induction (37,138–140)	WSII (#193510), Piebaldism (#172800) (139)	Increased expression (137)
Tcfap2α	Transcription factor AP-2, α (AP-2)	Premigratory and postmigratory NC (38,141)	Differentiation (38,141–144)	NA	Decreased expression (47,145,146)

(continued)

Table 1 (*Continued*)
Genes Functioning in Melanocyte Development[a]

Protein family	Gene symbol	Gene name	Expression pattern	Proposed function	Associated diseases (OMIM No)	Role in melanoma tumors/cell lines
	Mitf	Microphthalmia-associated (bHLH)	Premigratory and postmigratory Mb, Mc (*148*)	Differentiation, survival (*128,149–161*)	WSIIA (#193510) (*162*)	Increased expression (*125,163,164*)

[a]Genes are organized according to the section they were mentioned in the text. For simplicity, mouse nomenclature is used for gene symbols.
NT, neural tube; NC, neural crest; Mb, Melanoblast; Mc, Melanocyte; OMIM, Online Mendelian Inheritance in Man; NA, not applicable; WS, Waardenburg Syndrome; HSCR, Hirschprung's Disease; ABCD, Albinism, Black lock, Cell Migration Disorder of the Gut and Deafness; CCHS, Central Congenital Hypoventilation Syndrome; CMPD, Campomelic Dysplasia; bHLH, Basic Helix-Loop-Helix; MMTV, Mammary Tumor Virus; HJMD, Congenital Hypotrichosis with Juvenile Macular Dystrophy.

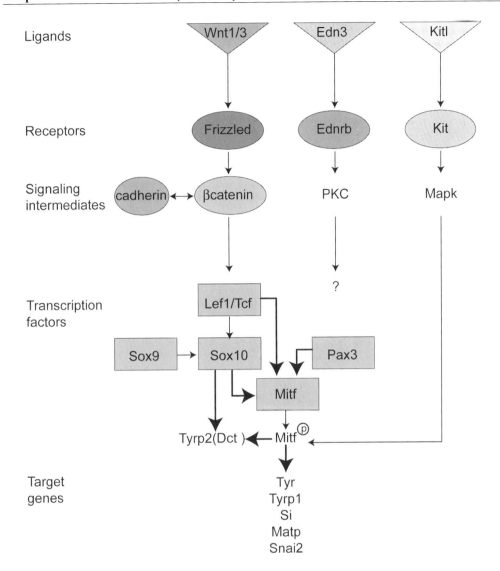

Fig. 2. Schematic representing the genetic relationships between genes functioning in melano-cyte development. Extracellular ligands are indicated with triangles, receptors and signaling intermediates are indicated with ovals, and transcription factors are indicated with rectangles. Heavy arrows indicate relationships in which direct transcriptional activation has been shown.

β-catenin is eliminated specifically in neural crest cells, these mice lack both melano-blasts and sensory neurons (51). Similarly, Lewis et al. showed that depletion of *Wnt8* in zebrafish results in an absence of neural crest derivatives, including pigment cells *(50)*. In addition, inhibition of Wnt signaling at later stages using overexpression of a truncated form of *Tcf* causes significantly reduced expression of the pigment cell marker, *Mitf*, but with no effect on other neural crest markers, such as *Sox10 (50)*.

In vivo and in vitro studies also indicate that the *Wnt/β-catenin*-signaling pathway is sufficient for melanoblast development. Overexpression of *β-catenin* in zebrafish pro-motes melanoblast formation and reduces formation of neurons and glia *(52)*. In *Xeno-*

pus, injection of Wnt1 causes an expansion of *Slug* and *Sox10* expression, whereas injection of GSK-3β, a Wnt antagonist, prevents their expression, consistent with a role for Wnt signaling in induction of early melanoblast markers *(37)*. Similarly, expression of *Wnt1* in cultured mouse neural crest cells and treatment of cultured chick neural crest with Wnt3a promotes the differentiation and expansion of melanoblasts *(4,41)*. Interestingly, there is a highly conserved binding site for the LEF transcription factor in the *Mitf* promoter *(53,54)*. Together, these studies indicate that *Wnt/β-catenin* signaling may promote both melanoblast induction and melanoblast differentiation.

Somewhat paradoxically, however, *β-catenin* is also sufficient for formation of other neural crest derivatives, such as sensory neurons, that are induced from pluripotent neural crest before melanocyte induction. Mice that express a constitutively active form of *β-catenin* specifically in neural crest cells have ectopic sensory neurons at the expense of other neural crest derivatives, including melanoblasts *(55)*. It seems the temporal and spatial responses to Wnt1 and Wnt3a *(166)*, and perhaps cell-restricted expression of Wnt inhibitors *(4)* could explain how this pathway promotes sensory neuron and melanoblast induction.

In addition to signaling through the *Wnt* pathway, *β-catenin* also functions in a cell adhesion pathway downstream of cadherins. Because cadherins are required for cell migration of many cell types *(56)*, it has been proposed that a regulated switching of expression of cadherins promotes melanoblast migration first into the dermis and then into the epidermis and hair follicles. The cadherins, composed of type I (N, E, and P-Cdh) and type II (Cdh5–Cdh12 in mice), have a dynamic expression pattern during melanocyte induction. In early mouse embryos, cadherin 6 is expressed in the neural folds and neural crest cells both before and after their delamination *(57)*. In avian species, neural crest precursors express high levels of type II *cadherin 6B* and low levels of *N-cadherin*, but once they migrate from the epithelium, *cadherin 7* becomes the predominant family member expressed in migrating neural crest derivatives *(25,58)*.

Immunohistochemical studies in mice indicate that as the melanoblasts migrate throughout the embryo (Fig. 1, no. 2–5), expression of E-cadherin and P-cadherin is upregulated and their expression pattern is identical with that of surrounding cells *(27)*. This is consistent with the formation of cell–cell contacts between similar cadherin molecules. In E11.5-d embryos, the melanoblasts are present in the dermis but express neither cadherin. E-cadherin expression is dramatically upregulated in the melanoblasts by E13.5, just before when the melanoblasts invade the epidermis. Epidermal melanoblasts express high levels of E-cadherin and low levels of P-cadherin, although those that eventually enter the hair follicle exclusively express P-cadherin. N-cadherin is expressed in the melanoblasts that remain in the dermal layer (and is also a marker in melanoblast cell lines) *(24,27)*.

In vivo studies indicate a role for cadherins in melanoblast migration. Overexpression of *N-cadherin* and *cadherin 7* in chick inhibits migration of *Mitf*-positive cells out of the neural tube *(26)*. However, no pigmentation defects have been attributed to mice with loss of function mutations in *P-cadherin (59)*, and homozygous null mutants in *E-cadherin* are embryonic lethal, thus, a role for this protein in pigmentation has not been addressed using these knockout mice *(60)*. Because expression of different cadherins may also be associated with melanoma progression, further analyses of this family of proteins may elucidate their role in both development and disease *(58,61)* (Table 1).

Adhesion to the ECM also may influence the timing of neural crest emigration from the neural tube, and the differentiation and migratory path chosen by melanoblasts. ECM proteins such as collagen, fibronectin, and laminin are expressed in the premigratory neural crest cells of chick and between the ectoderm and dermatome during neural crest emigration in mice and chick (22,23,62). Interestingly, expression of peanut agglutinin lectin and chondroitin-6-sulfate in the dorsal–lateral path decreases as cells migrate along this pathway (63) (Fig. 1, no. 1,2), suggesting that these molecules may regulate the timing of melanoblast migration, although this has not been functionally proven. In addition, melanocytes have been reported to express integrins α-2, α-3, and α-5, which bind ECM proteins; however, it is not known whether other integrins are also expressed (64). Although integrins have been associated with the progression of melanoma (65) (Table 1), further studies are needed to define the spatial and temporal distribution of ECM components and their binding partners and to elucidate their requirement in melanoblast migration and disease.

A role for ECM proteases in melanocyte development was recently revealed with the cloning of the *Adamts20* metalloprotease (39). *Adamts20* is expressed in cells adjacent to the migratory melanoblasts, in a pattern that precedes melanoblast migration (39). This expression pattern along with the observation that it is enriched in hair follicles, suggests that *Adamts20* may be required for melanocytes to migrate into hair follicles (Fig. 1, no. 4,5).

Adamts20 is mutated in *belted* mice, a classic coat color mutant that lacks pigment only in a belt-like region of the trunk (39). Grafting experiments support the hypothesis that *Adamts20* acts in the ectoderm to promote melanocyte development. In 1964, Mayer and Maltby grafted ectoderm and underlying mesoderm from regions of the presumptive belt of *belted* embryos onto chick coelom and found that grafts from belted regions displayed melanocytes in the grafted skin, but fewer pigmented hairs than those from unbelted regions (66). When Schaible performed similar experiments using older chick hosts, he obtained significantly more pigmented hairs (167). However, because some grafts contained white hairs, these results are not completely incongruous and the difference in results may be caused by the age of hosts and mouse stocks used. Although *Adamts20* is expressed throughout the embryo, belted mutants only have defects in a localized region of the trunk. The nature of this pattern is unknown, however, it may be a result of redundancies with other metalloproteases, such as *Adam17*, which is expressed in mouse hair shafts (67).

Consistent with a role in melanoblast migration, *Adamts20* is homologous to a *Caenorhabditis elegans* gene, *gon-1*, which is required for cell migration in embryos (68,69). In addition to ECM proteins, extracellular ligands, such as kitl, endothelin 3 (Edn3), or EphB, are also substrates for regulation by proteases. Thus, *Adamts20* may promote melanoblast migration into the hair follicles by modifying the ECM and/or ligands secreted by the skin, and this could help generate a migratory path and/or activate chemoattractants. Related to this developmental function, metalloproteases have been implicated in cancer metastasis and ADAMTS20 is enriched in cancer lines (70) (Table 1), although its expression in melanoma cell lines has not yet been reported.

SIGNALING THROUGH GROWTH FACTORS AND RECEPTORS

Melanoblasts migrate over very long distances throughout the embryo, while continuing to expand and promote their own survival, suggesting that melanoblast development is highly dynamic and likely to require rapid activation of signaling pathways. The stereotypical melanoblast migration throughout the embryos is reminiscent of chemoattractant-guided axon guidance. In fact, the presence of a long distance attractive cue in the dermis for melanoblast induction and migration has been proposed *(71–73)*. In support of this, dermis grafted distally on one side of the chick neural tube induces specific and early migration of melanoblasts toward the graft *(73)*. The precise molecules and signaling pathways responsible for this induction are not definitive, however, there are several candidates.

Evidence supports a role for the EphB receptor tyrosine kinase pathway in both promoting and inhibiting melanoblast migration. In chick, EphB receptors are expressed in melanoblasts *(28)*, and ephrin-B ligands (Efnb) are expressed along the dorsal–lateral pathway before and after melanoblast migration *(74)* (Fig. 1, no. 1,2). Because Efnb inhibit neural crest migration in vitro, it was suggested that this pathway acts as a repulsive cue for melanoblast migration *(74)*. However, recent studies showed that addition of Efnb to chick trunk neural crest explants also results in precocious migration of early neural crest, suggesting that ephrin signaling also promotes melanoblast migration *(28)*. Santiago et al. also showed that melanoblast migration is prevented when EphB signaling is blocked in vivo in chick embryos. However, neural crest migration is unaffected in mice null for either *Efnb2* or for both *EphB2* and *EphB3*, suggesting that there may be redundant genes that regulate the timing and location of melanoblast migration in mice *(75,76)*. Because ephrin receptors are expressed in melanoma samples *(44,77–79)* (Table 1), further studies of this pathway may have important developmental and clinical applications.

Another family of proteins that can both promote and inhibit melanoblast induction are the bone morphogenetic proteins (BMPs)/transforming growth factor-β growth factors. In chick, BMP-4 expression in the neural tube decreases as melanocytes initiate their migration *(4)*. In mice, *BMP-2* is expressed in the surface ectoderm of E8.5 embryos and *BMP-4* is expressed in hair follicles of E16.5 to 19.5 embryos *(80,81)*. In vitro experiments indicate that these proteins inhibit melanocyte development. Neural tube cultures treated with BMP-4 have reduced numbers of melanocytes but increased numbers of neurons and glia *(4)*, and chick cranial cultures treated with both FGF2 and BMP-2, also have reduced pigment cell production *(82)*. However, independent experiments have shown that treatment of quail neural crest cultures with BMP-2 can increase expression of the melanocyte-specific gene, tyrosinase *(83)*. These findings suggest that BMPs affect melanocyte development in a complex manner, depending on the family member, the stage of development, and the model organism and experimental approach used for the assay.

Ednrb and one of its ligands, endothelin-3 (Edn3), are expressed in patterns consistent with a requirement in melanocyte development. In mice, *Ednrb* is expressed in melanoblasts, albeit at low levels throughout their development *(34)*. In avian species, two isoforms, *Ednrb1* and *Ednrb2*, are expressed in complementary expression patterns during melanoblast development *(84)*. During both mouse and chick development, *Edn3* is expressed in the skin *(36,85)*. In addition, changes in *EDNRB* expression are associated with melanoma *(86)*. Mutations in both *EDNRB* and *EDN3* are associated with Waardenburg Syndrome (WS)IV, Hirschprung disease (HSCR), and ABCD syndromes *(87–91)* (Table 1).

Embryonic analysis of *Ednrb* mutants indicates that this signaling pathway is required for melanocyte development. *Ednrb^{sl}/Ednrb^{sl}* E10.5 embryos display reduced numbers

of *Dct*-positive melanoblasts, suggesting that Ednrb is involved in expansion of melanoblasts as opposed to specification *(92)*. Elegant studies in which the *Ednrb* gene was
inducibly eliminated in mice showed that it is required between E10 and E12.5 *(35)*.
Further analyses indicate that E10 to E11-d-old *Ednrb^lacZ* heterozygous and homozygous embryos contain melanoblasts in the trunk region where skin is unpigmented in
postnatal animals, but fewer *Dct*-positive cells in E11.5-d-old embryos *(34)*. Similar to
this phenotype, melanoblasts are absent from the trunk of younger *Edn3 ^ls/Edn3 ^ls*
embryos but repopulate these regions during migration into the epidermis *(93)* (Fig. 1,
no. 3,4). Together, these results suggest that Ednrb signaling is required primarily for
proliferation of melanocytes, and possibly for their migration.

Numerous in vitro studies of melanocytes in culture strongly support a role for Edn3
in their survival, proliferation, and differentiation *(21,33,36,94,168)*. Because the in
vivo data do not indicate a role for Endothelin signaling in melanoblast survival and
differentiation, it is likely that this pathway is partially redundant with other signaling
pathways. One possible candidate that is also required for melanocyte development is
Kit, because the *Ednrb*- and *Kit*-signaling pathways exhibit genetic interactions in vivo
and in vitro *(94–96,168)*.

The Kit receptor tyrosine kinase is expressed throughout mouse development. In
humans, *KIT* expression is downregulated in melanoma and *KIT* mutations are associated with human Piebaldism *(97–99)* (Table 1). *Kit* is expressed in premigratory melanoblasts in the migration staging area, and continues as the melanoblasts migrate through
the dermis and into the epidermis *(21,22,100,101)*. *In situ* hybridization and immunohistochemical studies indicate that *Kitl* (also called steel factor) is expressed initially in the
dermamyotome, then in the dermis and in hair follicles before melanocyte invasion, but
in lower levels in the ventral paths of neural crest *(20,22,101)*.

Consistent with these expression patterns, mouse mutations in the receptor (*KitW*) and
ligand (*Kitl^Sl*) are hypopigmented, indicating their requirement for melanocyte development *(102)*. The spatiotemporal regulation of Kit signaling is likely to be important
because *Kit^sash/Kit^sash* embryos which contain a mutation in the regulatory domain of *Kit*,
display ectopic *Kit* in defined regions in which *Kitl* is normally expressed *(100)*, and
resulting mice have regionalized hypopigmentation.

Embryonic analyses of mouse mutants indicate that the pathway is required throughout melanocyte development for survival, proliferation, and migration. Comparative
analysis of mice homozygous for a *Kitl* null allele, *Sl*, and mice homozygous for a *Kitl*
allele, *Sld*, which eliminates only the membrane form of *Kitl,* suggests that the soluble
form of the ligand is essential for early migration and/or survival along the dorsal–lateral
pathway, whereas the membrane form is required for early melanoblast survival in the
dermis *(22)* (Fig. 1, no. 1,2). *Kit^W/Kit^W* and *Kit^wv* heterozygous and homozygous embryos
have an overall decreased density of melanoblasts but relatively normal distribution, and
these phenotypes are exacerbated in older embryos *(30,103)*, indicating that Kit signaling regulates melanoblast survival and/or proliferation but not later melanoblast migration throughout the embryo.

Additional studies corroborate roles for Kit signaling in later stages of melanocyte
development. Nishikawa et al. and Yoshida et al. showed that injection of Kit antibodies
into pregnant mice at three different stages of development causes three different patterns of melanocyte density and pigmentation in embryos and adults *(93,104)*. From
these experiments, the authors conclude that Kit signaling is required for melanoblast
migration from the dermis into the epidermis, for melanocyte proliferation and survival

in the epidermis, but not for late melanoblast migration into hair follicles (Fig. 1, no. 3–5). This last point is questioned by experiments from Jordan and Jackson, who show that exogenous Kitl can promote migration of melanocytes into hair follicles using skin explants (105). The Kit-dependent migration of melanoblasts into the epidermis may be caused by its activation of E-cadherin expression, because transgenic mice that ectopically express *Kitl* in epidermal keratinocytes have increased expression of E-cadherin in epidermal melanocytes postnatally (27) but not in dermal melanoblasts embryonically (106). In vitro studies also indicate that Kit signaling promotes melano-blast proliferation because treatment of neural crest cultures with Kitl causes an increased number of *Dct*-positive cells (21). Together, these results suggest that Kit signaling is required for multiple aspects of melanocyte development but its role is complex.

Some studies have helped to distinguish the roles of Kit signaling in the varied processes of survival, proliferation, and migration. Analysis in zebrafish of *kit* alleles that distinctly affect first melanocyte survival and then migration, clearly suggests that Kit signaling promotes both of these processes and that these functions are distinguish-able (107). To separate the role for Kit in survival and migration in mice, *Nf1* mice, which have increased melanoblast survival, were crossed to *Kit* mutant mice. In double mutant embryos, melanoblasts failed to leave the migration staging area, suggesting that Kit functions in early migration, in addition to its role in melanoblast survival (108). Further in vivo and in vitro analyses will be useful to clarify the exact mechanism of Kit signaling in melanocyte development.

TRANSCRIPTION FACTOR NETWORKS AND CELL SPECIFICATION

The transcription factor, *Foxd3*, is important for formation of many neural crest derivatives but may inhibit melanoblast induction. In chick, mouse, and *Xenopus*, *Foxd3* is expressed in the dorsal neural tube, in premigratory neural crest, and in neural crest cell derivatives, with the exception of melanoblasts (1,5,109). In *Xenopus* embryos, a dominant negative *Foxd3* inhibits neural crest cell differentiation and overexpression of *Foxd3* induces expression of neural crest markers (110). However, an independent group has shown that *Foxd3* overexpression in *Xenopus* prevents neural crest formation (109), indicating that Foxd3 may be dosage sensitive and its function in neural crest induction is not straightforward.

In vivo and in vitro evidence suggests a specific role for *Foxd3* in repression of melanoblast development. *Foxd3* depletion in chick embryos and in neural crest cell cultures causes melanocytes to form at the expense of neurons and glia, whereas *Foxd3* overexpression in embryos prevents melanoblast formation in vitro (5). Overexpression of a tagged form of *Foxd3* in chick neural tube prevents neural crest cells from migrating along the dorsal–lateral pathway beneath the epidermis (1) (Fig. 1, no. 1–3). Because *Foxd3*-null mice are early embryonic lethal, its role in mouse neural crest and melano-blast development has not yet been assessed (111).

Two members of the SRY-box-containing transcription factor family have significant roles in melanocyte development. *Sox9* is expressed in *Xenopus* progenitor neural crest cells, coincident with *Sox10* expression (12). Depletion of *Sox9* in *Xenopus* results in a loss of neural crest progenitors and *Sox10* expression, whereas *Sox9* injection expands *Sox10* expression (12,37). When *Sox9-GFP* is ectopically expressed in the chick neural tube, green fluorescent protein is detectable in glial cell lineages and cells migrating dorsolaterally, but not in neuronal lineages. In these chick embryos, the presumptive melanoblasts migrate early, suggesting that *Sox9* also promotes induction of the melano-blasts *(112)* (Fig. 1, no. 2,3). These studies implicate *Sox9* in melanocyte development, however, *Sox9* knockout mice are embryonic lethal *(113)* so a role for *Sox9* in mouse pigmentation has not yet been addressed.

Sox10 is a close relative of *Sox9* and is expressed in a pattern consistent with its requirement for melanocyte development. *Sox10* expression in premigratory neural crest stem cells and derivatives including dorsal root, sympathetic and enteric ganglia, and peripheral glia has been detected in humans, mice, chick, zebrafish, and *Xenopus* *(11,37,114–119)*. *Sox10* is expressed in melanoblasts before, during and at the completion of their migration *(119)*, however, the levels of *Sox10* expression may decrease during melanoblast development in vivo (W. Pavan, unpublished observation).

Studies of *Sox10* mouse mutants suggest that it is required for both specification and survival of melanoblasts. $Sox10^{Dom}$ mice have an insertional mutation in *Sox10*, render-ing it either nonfunctional or possibly dominant negative *(119)*. $Sox10^{LacZ}$ mice harbor a *β-galactosidase* gene replacing *Sox10* coding regions *(115)*. Heterozygous mice of both genotypes exhibit hypopigmentation of the ventrum and megacolon because of lack of melanocytes and enteric ganglia, respectively, whereas homozygous mice are embry-onic lethal. The hypopigmentation phenotype can be attributed in part to defects in differentiation, because $Sox10^{Dom}$/+ embryos transiently lose expression of *Dct* but have only a slightly reduced population of melanoblasts, as indicated by *Kit* expression *(115,120)*. In E10.5 $Sox10^{Dom}$ homozygous embryos, the neural crest cells also undergo apoptosis, as indicated by increased terminal deoxynucleotidyl transferase biotin-dUTP NICK END labeling (TUNEL) staining *(119)*. Consistent with studies in the mouse, analysis of the colorless *Sox10* zebrafish mutant also reveals a role for *Sox10* in neural crest survival and migration, and in pigment cell differentiation *(117)*.

Studies in *Xenopus* and in cultured cells suggest that *Sox10* is sufficient for melano-cyte differentiation. Overexpression of *Sox10* in *Xenopus* causes ectopic pigment cells *(37)*. Interestingly, these studies also showed that *Sox10* expression is dependent on *Wnt*, *Slug*, and *Sox9*, indicating that *Sox10* may be a downstream target of these molecules. Sox10 transactivates expression of melanocyte genes, including *Mitf* and *Dct (11,120–123)*. Further analyses of Sox10 function have important clinical implications because *SOX10* mutations are associated with WSIV *(11,124)*, and *SOX10* expression may be associated with melanoma *(125,126)* (Table 1).

A transcription factor that has been demonstrated to cooperate with Sox10 in melano-cyte development is the paired homeodomain transcription factor 3 (*Pax3*). In mouse and zebrafish, *Pax3* is expressed in the dorsal neural tube and in migrating neural crest cells *(2,127)*. Similar to *Sox10* mutants, $Pax3^{Sp}$/+ mice are semidominant and hypopigmented on their ventrum, whereas homozygous mutant mice are embryonic lethal *(128)*. $Pax3^{Sp}$/$Pax3^{Sp}$ embryos, thought to contain a loss-of-function *Pax3* allele, have reduced num-bers of melanoblasts emigrating from the neural tube and in the trunk but normal distri-bution of melanocytes overall *(128,129)*. These findings suggest that Pax3 may function in early expansion of the melanocyte population but not migration. Interestingly, transplantation of neural tubes from mice containing $Pax3^{Sp}$ and *LacZ* driven by a *Wnt1* promoter into chick embryos demonstrates rescue of mutant neural crest migration defects *(129)*. This indicates that this Pax3 defect is nonautonomous to the neural crest cells. However, intrinsic functions of Pax3 in melanocytes are also likely, because Pax3 transactivates the melanogenic enzyme, *Tyrp1 (130)*, and acts synergistically with *Sox10* to activate *Mitf (123,131)* and *Ret (121)*. Because PAX3 is expressed in human melanoma *(132,133)* and is mutated in WSI, II, and III *(134–136)* (Table 1), further studies of Pax3 function will elucidate its role in development and disease.

Members of the Snail family of transcription factors, which includes *Slug* and *Snail,* are required for development of several neural crest derivatives, including melanocytes, and are expressed in melanoma samples *(137)* (Table 1). In *Xenopus*, chick, and zebrafish, *Slug* and *Snail* are early markers for premigratory and postmigratory neural crest *(6,8)*. In contrast, in mice, *Snai2* (also called *Slug*) expression is evident only in migratory neural crest *(10,138)*.

In vivo experiments suggest that this family of proteins is both necessary and sufficient for melanoblast formation. *Snai2^{lacZ}/Snai2^{lacZ}* and *Snai2^{Δ1}/Snai2^{Δ1}* mice, which contain loss-of-function alleles of *Snail2*, exhibit a low penetrance of hypopigmentation at their extremities and on their head, and exhibit dominant genetic interactions with *Kit* mutants *(10,139)*. In Xenopus, *Slug* depletion inhibits *Sox10* expression *(37)* and *Slug* overexpression results in ectopic melanoblasts *(140)*. Because Mitf has been shown to activate the *Slug* promoter in vitro, this suggests that *Mitf* acts upstream of *Slug (139)*. However, the precise role of *Slug* in the transcriptional hierarchy of melanocyte development needs further clarification. Because this family of proteins also act as repressors of E-cadherin expression, which is expressed in epidermal melanoblasts, this may be one mechanism by which Slug/Snail2 regulates melanocyte development.

Recent studies have indicated that the *Tcfap2α* (transcription factor activator protein [AP]-2, α) transcription factor family is also required for melanocyte development. In mice and zebrafish, *Tcfap2α* is expressed in the neural ectoderm and lateral edges of the neural fold, in premigratory neural crest and in migratory neural crest derivatives *(38,141)*. Zebrafish mutants in *Tcfap2α (mont blanc)* exhibit defects in neural crest development and specifically in pigment cell differentiation *(38,142,143)*. Mice lacking *Tcfap2α* only in the neural crest lineage have belly spots similar to those seen in *Sox10* and *Pax3* mutants *(144)*. Interestingly, a decrease in AP-2 expression may be associated with metastatic progression of melanoma, indicating that the transcription factor may negatively regulate migration *(47,145,146)* (Table 1). The precise function of AP-2 in development and cancer requires further study.

The earliest known marker of specified melanoblasts is microphthalmia-associated transcription factor (*Mitf-M*). There are multiple isoforms of *Mitf* that are likely transcribed by different promoters because they are expressed in different cell types *(147)*. Expression of *Mitf* is evident in dorsal neural tubes of E10-d-old mouse embryos, when the neural crest begins to emigrate, and in migratory melanoblasts throughout their development *(148)*.

In vivo studies have suggested that *Mitf* is necessary for melanocyte survival and differentiation. *Mitf^{mi}/+* mice are hypopigmented on their ventral side and *Mitf^{mi}/Mitf^{mi}* mice lack any pigmentation *(128,149)*. *Mitf^{mi}/+* mouse embryos of all ages have reduced numbers of melanoblasts and sparse distribution in the trunk region that is approximate to the region of hypopigmentation in affected adults.

Mitf has been proposed to be a master regulator of melanoblast fate, primarily because it is sufficient to direct melanocyte fate in transformed fibroblasts and fish embryonic stem cells *(150,151)*. In addition, misexpression of *Mitf* in zebrafish results in ectopic melanocytes *(152)*. Indeed, in vitro and in vivo studies in mice suggest that *Mitf* is upstream of the melanocyte-specific genes, *Tyr, Melastatin, Tyrp1, Dct, Si, Matp, Melan-a*, and *Slug (139,153–157)*, as well as other genes not specific to melanocytes, such as *bcl-2 (158)*.

Analysis of the *Mitf* promoter and in vivo experiments suggest that *Mitf* expression is regulated by a complex series of transcription factors and signaling pathways, including *Sox10*, *Pax3*, *CREB*, and *Lef1* (which is activated by WNT/β-catenin signaling) *(54)*. Mitf can cooperate with Sox10 to transactivate expression of melanocyte specific genes, such as *Dct (122,159)*. Consistent with such synergistic interactions, *Sox10^{Dom}* and *Mitf^{mi}* double heterozygotes exhibit dramatically increased hypopigmentation *(123)*. Experiments in zebrafish have led to the proposal that *Mitf* is the only relevant target gene of Sox10 that is needed for melanoblast development *(160)*. However, this relationship has not been established in mice. Interestingly, Mitf also synergizes with LEF-1 to activate expression of *Dct* and its own promoter, indicating that regulation of *Mitf* levels is tightly regulated *(161)*. *MITF* haploinsufficiency is associated with the human disease, WSII *(162)*, and *MITF* is expressed in primary melanoma *(125,163,164)* (Table 1). Future studies of *Mitf* will contribute to an understanding of both melanocyte development and disease.

CONCLUSIONS AND PERSPECTIVES

One theme that emerges from the genetic analysis of melanocyte development is that the same molecules function throughout melanocyte development from the initial induction of neural crest to the subsequent differentiation, migration, and expansion of the melanoblast population. Many of the genes have pleiotropic effects, promoting not only melanoblast induction but also the earlier induction and specification of dramatically different neural crest subtypes. It remains to be determined how the functions of such genes are regulated through protein interactions, and how the dynamic spatiotemporal expression patterns are modulated. In fact, in many cases, the mechanism by which many of these proteins affect melanoblast development and communicate with each other is not yet clear. For example, it is often not straightforward to assign which molecules act intrinsically or noncell autonomously by signaling from surrounding cells, as has been found with Ednrb signaling *(168)*.

Defects in neural crest cell migration, proliferation, and/or differentiation can result in genetic disorders, such as Hirschsprung disease (reduced enteric ganglia); WS (reduced melanocytes and hypopigmentation); and a number of cancers, including melanoma (melanocyte tumor). Melanoma is a malignant cancer caused by overproliferation of melanocytes in adults, is highly metastatic, and is the most deadly of all forms of skin cancer. Interestingly, many of the genes expressed in either melanoma cell lines or melanoma tumors are required specifically during melanocyte development (Table 1) and similar categories of genes are expressed in metastatic melanoma and in migratory neural crest cells *(23,125,165)*. This indicates that studies of neural crest cell development may provide insight into the genetic causes of cancer and its progression.

REFERENCES

1. Dottori, M., M.K. Gross, P. Labosky, and M. Goulding. 2001. The winged-helix transcription factor Foxd3 suppresses interneuron differentiation and promotes neural crest cell fate. Development 128:4127–4138.
2. Goulding, M.D., G. Chalepakis, U. Deutsch, J.R. Erselius, and P. Gruss. 1991. Pax-3, a novel murine DNA binding protein expressed during early neurogenesis. Embo J 10:1135–1147.
3. Ikeya, M., S.M. Lee, J.E. Johnson, A.P. McMahon, and S. Takada. 1997. Wnt signalling required for expansion of neural crest and CNS progenitors. Nature 389:966–970.
4. Jin, E.J., C.A. Erickson, S. Takada, and L.W. Burrus. 2001. Wnt and BMP signaling govern lineage segregation of melanocytes in the avian embryo. Dev Biol 233:22–37.

5. Kos, R., M.V. Reedy, R.L. Johnson, and C.A. Erickson. 2001. The winged-helix transcription factor FoxD3 is important for establishing the neural crest lineage and repressing melanogenesis in avian embryos. Development 128:1467–1479.

6. Locascio, A., M. Manzanares, M.J. Blanco, and M.A. Nieto. 2002. Modularity and reshuffling of Snail and Slug expression during vertebrate evolution. Proc Natl Acad Sci U S A 99:16841–16846.

7. Roelink, H., and R. Nusse. 1991. Expression of two members of the Wnt family during mouse development—restricted temporal and spatial patterns in the developing neural tube. Genes Dev 5:381–388.

8. Sechrist, J., M.A. Nieto, R.T. Zamanian, and M. Bronner-Fraser. 1995. Regulative response of the cranial neural tube after neural fold ablation: spatiotemporal nature of neural crest regeneration and up-regulation of Slug. Development 121:4103–4115.

9. Wilkinson, D.G., J.A. Bailes, and A.P. McMahon. 1987. Expression of the proto-oncogene int-1 is restricted to specific neural cells in the developing mouse embryo. Cell 50:79–88.

10. Jiang, R., Y. Lan, C.R. Norton, J.P. Sundberg, and T. Gridley. 1998. The Slug gene is not essential for mesoderm or neural crest development in mice. Dev Biol 198:277–285.

11. Mollaaghababa, R., and W.J. Pavan. 2003. The importance of having your SOX on: role of SOX10 in the development of neural crest-derived melanocytes and glia. Oncogene 22:3024–3034.

12. Spokony, R.F., Y. Aoki, N. Saint-Germain, E. Magner-Fink, and J.P. Saint-Jeannet. 2002. The transcription factor Sox9 is required for cranial neural crest development in Xenopus. Development 129:421–432.

13. Serbedzija, G.N., M. Bronner-Fraser, and S.E. Fraser. 1994. Developmental potential of trunk neural crest cells in the mouse. Development 120:1709–1718.

14. Sieber-Blum, M. 1989. Commitment of neural crest cells to the sensory neuron lineage. Science 243:1608–1611.

15. Stemple, D.L., and D.J. Anderson. 1992. Isolation of a stem cell for neurons and glia from the mammalian neural crest. Cell 71:973–985.

16. Serbedzija, G.N., M. Bronner-Fraser, and S.E. Fraser. 1989. A vital dye analysis of the timing and pathways of avian trunk neural crest cell migration. Development 106:809–816.

17. Serbedzija, G.N., S.E. Fraser, and M. Bronner-Fraser. 1990. Pathways of trunk neural crest cell migration in the mouse embryo as revealed by vital dye labelling. Development 108:605–612.

18. Yip, J.W. 1986. Migratory patterns of sympathetic ganglioblasts and other neural crest derivatives in chick embryos. J Neurosci 6:3465–3473.

19. Wakamatsu, Y., M. Mochii, K.S. Vogel, and J.A. Weston. 1998. Avian neural crest-derived neurogenic precursors undergo apoptosis on the lateral migration pathway. Development 125:4205–4213.

20. Matsui, Y., K.M. Zsebo, and B.L. Hogan. 1990. Embryonic expression of a haematopoietic growth factor encoded by the Sl locus and the ligand for c-kit. Nature 347:667–669.

21. Opdecamp, K., A. Nakayama, M.T. Nguyen, C.A. Hodgkinson, W.J. Pavan, and H. Arnheiter. 1997. Melanocyte development in vivo and in neural crest cell cultures: crucial dependence on the Mitf basic-helix-loop-helix-zipper transcription factor. Development 124:2377–2386.

22. Wehrle-Haller, B., and J.A. Weston. 1995. Soluble and cell-bound forms of steel factor activity play distinct roles in melanocyte precursor dispersal and survival on the lateral neural crest migration pathway. Development 121:731–742.

23. Gammill, L.S., and M. Bronner-Fraser. 2002. Genomic analysis of neural crest induction. Development 129:5731–5741.

24. Jouneau, A., Y.Q. Yu, M. Pasdar, and L. Larue. 2000. Plasticity of cadherin-catenin expression in the melanocyte lineage. Pigment Cell Res 13:260–272.

25. Nakagawa, S., and M. Takeichi. 1995. Neural crest cell-cell adhesion controlled by sequential and subpopulation-specific expression of novel cadherins. Development 121:1321–1332.

26. Nakagawa, S., and M. Takeichi. 1998. Neural crest emigration from the neural tube depends on regulated cadherin expression. Development 125:2963–2971.

27. Nishimura, E.K., H. Yoshida, T. Kunisada, and S.I. Nishikawa. 1999. Regulation of E- and P-cadherin expression correlated with melanocyte migration and diversification. Dev Biol 215:155–166.

28. Santiago, A., and C.A. Erickson. 2002. Ephrin-B ligands play a dual role in the control of neural crest cell migration. Development 129:3621–3632.

29. Luo, R., J. Gao, B. Wehrle-Haller, and P.D. Henion. 2003. Molecular identification of distinct neurogenic and melanogenic neural crest sublineages. Development 130:321–330.

30. Mackenzie, M.A., S.A. Jordan, P.S. Budd, and I.J. Jackson. 1997. Activation of the receptor tyrosine kinase Kit is required for the proliferation of melanoblasts in the mouse embryo. Dev Biol 192:99–107.

31. Wilkie, A.L., S.A. Jordan, and I.J. Jackson. 2002. Neural crest progenitors of the melanocyte lineage: coat colour patterns revisited. Development 129:3349–3357.

32. Wehrle-Haller, B. 2003. The role of Kit-ligand in melanocyte development and epidermal homeostasis. Pigment Cell Res 16:287–296.

33. Lahav, R., C. Ziller, E. Dupin, and N.M. Le Douarin. 1996. Endothelin 3 promotes neural crest cell proliferation and mediates a vast increase in melanocyte number in culture. Proc Natl Acad Sci U S A 93:3892–3897.

34. Lee, H.O., J.M. Levorse, and M.K. Shin. 2003. The endothelin receptor-B is required for the migration of neural crest-derived melanocyte and enteric neuron precursors. Dev Biol 259:162–175.

35. Shin, M.K., J.M. Levorse, R.S. Ingram, and S.M. Tilghman. 1999. The temporal requirement for endothelin receptor-B signalling during neural crest development. Nature 402:496–501.

36. Reid, K., A.M. Turnley, G.D. Maxwell, Y. Kurihara, H. Kurihara, P.F. Bartlett, and M. Murphy. 1996. Multiple roles for endothelin in melanocyte development: regulation of progenitor number and stimulation of differentiation. Development 122:3911–3919.

37. Aoki, Y., N. Saint-Germain, M. Gyda, E. Magner-Fink, Y.H. Lee, C. Credidio, and J.P. Saint-Jeannet. 2003. Sox10 regulates the development of neural crest-derived melanocytes in Xenopus. Dev Biol 259:19–33.

38. Knight, R.D., S. Nair, S.S. Nelson, A. Afshar, Y. Javidan, R. Geisler, G.J. Rauch, and T.F. Schilling. 2003. lockjaw encodes a zebrafish tfap2a required for early neural crest development. Development 130:5755–5768.

39. Rao, C., D. Foernzler, S.K. Loftus, S. Liu, J.D. McPherson, K.A. Jungers, S.S. Apte, W.J. Pavan, and D.R. Beier. 2003. A defect in a novel ADAMTS family member is the cause of the belted white-spotting mutation. Development 130:4665–4672.

40. Loftus, S.K., and W.J. Pavan. 2000. The use of expression profiling to study pigment cell biology and dysfunction. Pigment Cell Res 13:141–146.

41. Dunn, K.J., B.O. Williams, Y. Li, and W.J. Pavan. 2000. Neural crest-directed gene transfer demonstrates Wnt1 role in melanocyte expansion and differentiation during mouse development. Proc Natl Acad Sci U S A 97:10050–10055.

42. Delmas, V., S. Martinozzi, Y. Bourgeois, M. Holzenberger, and L. Larue. 2003. Cre-mediated recombination in the skin melanocyte lineage. Genesis 36:73–80.

43. Guyonneau, L., A. Rossier, C. Richard, E. Hummler, and F. Beermann. 2002. Expression of Cre recombinase in pigment cells. Pigment Cell Res 15:305–309.

44. Bittner, M., P. Meltzer, Y. Chen, Y. Jiang, E. Seftor, M. Hendrix, M. Radmacher, R. Simon, Z. Yakhini, A. Ben-Dor, N. Sampas, E. Dougherty, E. Wang, F. Marincola, C. Gooden, J. Lueders, A. Glatfelter, P. Pollock, J. Carpten, E. Gillanders, D. Leja, K. Dietrich, C. Beaudry, M. Berens, D. Alberts, and V. Sondak. 2000. Molecular classification of cutaneous malignant melanoma by gene expression profiling. Nature 406:536–540.

45. Kageshita, T., C.V. Hamby, T. Ishihara, K. Matsumoto, T. Saida, and T. Ono. 2001. Loss of beta-catenin expression associated with disease progression in malignant melanoma. Br J Dermatol 145:210–216.

46. Murakami, T., S. Toda, M. Fujimoto, M. Ohtsuki, H.R. Byers, T. Etoh, and H. Nakagawa. 2001. Constitutive activation of Wnt/beta-catenin signaling pathway in migration-active melanoma cells: role of LEF-1 in melanoma with increased metastatic potential. Biochem Biophys Res Commun 288:8–15.

47. Poser, I., and A.K. Bosserhoff. 2004. Transcription factors involved in development and progression of malignant melanoma. Histol Histopathol 19:173–188.

48. Nelson, W.J., and R. Nusse. 2004. Convergence of Wnt, beta-catenin, and cadherin pathways. Science 303:1483–1487.

49. Garcia-Castro, M.I., C. Marcelle, and M. Bronner-Fraser. 2002. Ectodermal Wnt function as a neural crest inducer. Science 297:848–851.

50. Lewis, J.L., J. Bonner, M. Modrell, J.W. Ragland, R.T. Moon, R.I. Dorsky, and D.W. Raible. 2004. Reiterated Wnt signaling during zebrafish neural crest development. Development 131:1299–1308.

51. Hari, L., V. Brault, M. Kleber, H.Y. Lee, F. Ille, R. Leimeroth, C. Paratore, U. Suter, R. Kemler, and L. Sommer. 2002. Lineage-specific requirements of beta-catenin in neural crest development. J Cell Biol 159:867–880.

52. Dorsky, R.I., R.T. Moon, and D.W. Raible. 1998. Control of neural crest cell fate by the Wnt signalling pathway. Nature 396:370–373.

53. Dorsky, R.I., D.W. Raible, and R.T. Moon. 2000. Direct regulation of nacre, a zebrafish MITF homolog required for pigment cell formation, by the Wnt pathway. Genes Dev 14:158–162.

54. Takeda, K., K. Yasumoto, R. Takada, S. Takada, K. Watanabe, T. Udono, H. Saito, K. Takahashi, and S. Shibahara. 2000. Induction of melanocyte-specific microphthalmia-associated transcription factor by Wnt-3a. J Biol Chem 275:14013–14016.

55. Lee, H.Y., M. Kleber, L. Hari, V. Brault, U. Suter, M.M. Taketo, R. Kemler, and L. Sommer. 2004. Instructive role of Wnt/beta-catenin in sensory fate specification in neural crest stem cells. Science 303:1020–1023.

56. Tepass, U., K. Truong, D. Godt, M. Ikura, and M. Peifer. 2000. Cadherins in embryonic and neural morphogenesis. Nat Rev Mol Cell Biol 1:91–100.

57. Watari, N., Y. Kameda, M. Takeichi, and O. Chisaka. 2001. Hoxa3 regulates integration of glossopharyngeal nerve precursor cells. Dev Biol 240:15–31.

58. Pla, P., R. Moore, O.G. Morali, S. Grille, S. Martinozzi, V. Delmas, and L. Larue. 2001. Cadherins in neural crest cell development and transformation. J Cell Physiol 189:121–132.

59. Radice, G.L., H. Rayburn, H. Matsunami, K.A. Knudsen, M. Takeichi, and R.O. Hynes. 1997. Developmental defects in mouse embryos lacking N-cadherin. Dev Biol 181:64–78.

60. Riethmacher, D., V. Brinkmann, and C. Birchmeier. 1995. A targeted mutation in the mouse E-cadherin gene results in defective preimplantation development. Proc Natl Acad Sci U S A 92:855–859.

61. Sanders, D.S., K. Blessing, G.A. Hassan, R. Bruton, J.R. Marsden, and J. Jankowski. 1999. Alterations in cadherin and catenin expression during the biological progression of melanocytic tumours. Mol Pathol 52:151–157.

62. Perris, R., and D. Perissinotto. 2000. Role of the extracellular matrix during neural crest cell migration. Mech Dev 95:3–21.

63. Oakley, R.A., C.J. Lasky, C.A. Erickson, and K.W. Tosney. 1994. Glycoconjugates mark a transient barrier to neural crest migration in the chicken embryo. Development 120:103–114.

64. Morelli, J.G., J.J. Yohn, T. Zekman, and D.A. Norris. 1993. Melanocyte movement in vitro: role of matrix proteins and integrin receptors. J Invest Dermatol 101:605–608.

65. Pasco, S., L. Ramont, F.X. Maquart, and J.C. Monboisse. 2004. Control of melanoma progression by various matrikines from basement membrane macromolecules. Crit Rev Oncol Hematol 49:221–233.

66. Mayer, T.C., and E.L. Maltby. 1964. An Experimental Investigation of Pattern Development in Lethal Spotting and Belted Mouse Embryos. Dev Biol 22:269–286.

67. Peschon, J.J., J.L. Slack, P. Reddy, K.L. Stocking, S.W. Sunnarborg, D.C. Lee, W.E. Russell, B.J. Castner, R.S. Johnson, J.N. Fitzner, R.W. Boyce, N. Nelson, C.J. Kozlosky, M.F. Wolfson, C.T. Rauch, D.P. Cerretti, R.J. Paxton, C.J. March, and R.A. Black. 1998. An essential role for ectodomain shedding in mammalian development. Science 282:1281–1284.

68. Blelloch, R., S.S. Anna-Arriola, D. Gao, Y. Li, J. Hodgkin, and J. Kimble. 1999. The gon-1 gene is required for gonadal morphogenesis in Caenorhabditis elegans. Dev Biol 216:382–393.

69. Blelloch, R., C. Newman, and J. Kimble. 1999. Control of cell migration during Caenorhabditis elegans development. Curr Opin Cell Biol 11:608–613.

70. Llamazares, M., S. Cal, V. Quesada, and C. Lopez-Otin. 2003. Identification and characterization of ADAMTS-20 defines a novel subfamily of metalloproteinases-disintegrins with multiple thrombospondin-1 repeats and a unique GON domain. J Biol Chem 278:13382–13389.

71. Erickson, C.A., T.D. Duong, and K.W. Tosney. 1992. Descriptive and experimental analysis of the dispersion of neural crest cells along the dorsolateral path and their entry into ectoderm in the chick embryo. Dev Biol 151:251–272.

72. Ideta, R., T. Soma, M. Tsunenaga, and O. Ifuku. 2002. Cultured human dermal papilla cells secrete a chemotactic factor for melanocytes. J Dermatol Sci 28:48–59.

73. Tosney, K.W. 2004. Long-distance cue from emerging dermis stimulates neural crest melanoblast migration. Dev Dyn 229:99–108.

74. Wang, H.U., and D.J. Anderson. 1997. Eph family transmembrane ligands can mediate repulsive guidance of trunk neural crest migration and motor axon outgrowth. Neuron 18:383–396.

75. Wang, H.U., Z.F. Chen, and D.J. Anderson. 1998. Molecular distinction and angiogenic interaction between embryonic arteries and veins revealed by ephrin-B2 and its receptor Eph-B4. Cell 93:741–753.

76. Williams, S.E., F. Mann, L. Erskine, T. Sakurai, S. Wei, D.J. Rossi, N.W. Gale, C.E. Holt, C.A. Mason, and M. Henkemeyer. 2003. Ephrin-B2 and EphB1 mediate retinal axon divergence at the optic chiasm. Neuron 39:919–935.

77. Easty, D.J., M. Herlyn, and D.C. Bennett. 1995. Abnormal protein tyrosine kinase gene expression during melanoma progression and metastasis. Int J Cancer 60:129–136.

78. Easty, D.J., S.P. Hill, M.Y. Hsu, M.E. Fallowfield, V.A. Florenes, M. Herlyn, and D.C. Bennett. 1999. Up-regulation of ephrin-A1 during melanoma progression. Int J Cancer 84:494–501.

79. Hafner, C., F. Bataille, S. Meyer, B. Becker, A. Roesch, M. Landthaler, and T. Vogt. 2003. Loss of EphB6 expression in metastatic melanoma. Int J Oncol 23:1553–1559.

80. Coucouvanis, E., and G.R. Martin. 1999. BMP signaling plays a role in visceral endoderm differentiation and cavitation in the early mouse embryo. Development 126:535–546.

81. Petiot, A., F.J. Conti, R. Grose, J.M. Revest, K.M. Hodivala-Dilke, and C. Dickson. 2003. A crucial role for Fgfr2-IIIb signalling in epidermal development and hair follicle patterning. Development 130:5493–5501.

82. Abzhanov, A., E. Tzahor, A.B. Lassar, and C.J. Tabin. 2003. Dissimilar regulation of cell differentiation in mesencephalic (cranial) and sacral (trunk) neural crest cells in vitro. Development 130:4567–4579.

83. Bilodeau, M.L., J.D. Greulich, R.L. Hullinger, C. Bertolotto, R. Ballotti, and O.M. Andrisani. 2001. BMP-2 stimulates tyrosinase gene expression and melanogenesis in differentiated melanocytes. Pigment Cell Res 14:328–336.

84. Nataf, V., L. Lecoin, A. Eichmann, and N.M. Le Douarin. 1996. Endothelin-B receptor is expressed by neural crest cells in the avian embryo. Proc Natl Acad Sci U S A 93:9645–9650.

85. Nataf, V., A. Amemiya, M. Yanagisawa, and N.M. Le Douarin. 1998. The expression pattern of endothelin 3 in the avian embryo. Mech Dev 73:217–220.

86. Eberle, J., S. Weitmann, O. Thieck, H. Pech, M. Paul, and C.E. Orfanos. 1999. Downregulation of endothelin B receptor in human melanoma cell lines parallel to differentiation genes. J Invest Dermatol 112:925–932.

87. Attie, T., M. Till, A. Pelet, J. Amiel, P. Edery, L. Boutrand, A. Munnich, and S. Lyonnet. 1995. Mutation of the endothelin-receptor B gene in Waardenburg-Hirschsprung disease. Hum Mol Genet 4:2407–2409.

88. Bidaud, C., R. Salomon, G. Van Camp, A. Pelet, T. Attie, C. Eng, M. Bonduelle, J. Amiel, C. Nihoul-Fekete, P.J. Willems, A. Munnich, and S. Lyonnet. 1997. Endothelin-3 gene mutations in isolated and syndromic Hirschsprung disease. Eur J Hum Genet 5:247–251.

89. Edery, P., T. Attie, J. Amiel, A. Pelet, C. Eng, R.M. Hofstra, H. Martelli, C. Bidaud, A. Munnich, and S. Lyonnet. 1996. Mutation of the endothelin-3 gene in the Waardenburg-Hirschsprung disease (Shah-Waardenburg syndrome). Nat Genet 12:442–444.

90. Puffenberger, E.G., K. Hosoda, S.S. Washington, K. Nakao, D. deWit, M. Yanagisawa, and A. Chakravart. 1994. A missense mutation of the endothelin-B receptor gene in multigenic Hirschsprung's disease. Cell 79:1257–1266.

91. Verheij, J.B., J. Kunze, J. Osinga, A.J. van Essen, and R.M. Hofstra. 2002. ABCD syndrome is caused by a homozygous mutation in the EDNRB gene. Am J Med Genet 108:223–225.

92. Pavan, W.J., and S.M. Tilghman. 1994. Piebald lethal (sl) acts early to disrupt the development of neural crest-derived melanocytes. Proc Natl Acad Sci U S A 91:7159–7163.

93. Yoshida, H., T. Kunisada, M. Kusakabe, S. Nishikawa, and S.I. Nishikawa. 1996. Distinct stages of melanocyte differentiation revealed by anlaysis of nonuniform pigmentation patterns. Development 122:1207–1214.

94. Opdecamp, K., L. Kos, H. Arnheiter, and W.J. Pavan. 1998. Endothelin signalling in the development of neural crest-derived melanocytes. Biochem Cell Biol 76:1093–1099.

95. Hou, L., J.J. Panthier, and H. Arnheiter. 2000. Signaling and transcriptional regulation in the neural crest-derived melanocyte lineage: interactions between KIT and MITF. Development 127:5379–5389.

96. Rhim, H., K.J. Dunn, A. Aronzon, S. Mac, M. Cheng, M.L. Lamoreux, S.M. Tilghman, and W.J. Pavan. 2000. Spatially restricted hypopigmentation associated with an Ednrbs-modifying locus on mouse chromosome 10. Genome Res 10:17–29.

97. Giebel, L.B., and R.A. Spritz. 1991. Mutation of the KIT (mast/stem cell growth factor receptor) protooncogene in human piebaldism. Proc Natl Acad Sci U S A 88:8696–8699.

98. Luca, M.R., and M. Bar-Eli. 1998. Molecular changes in human melanoma metastasis. Histol Histopathol 13:1225–1231.

99. Winnepenninckx, V., R. De Vos, M. Stas, and J.J. van den Oord. 2003. New phenotypical and ultrastructural findings in spindle cell (desmoplastic/neurotropic) melanoma. Appl Immunohistochem Mol Morphol 11:319–325.

100. Duttlinger, R., K. Manova, T.Y. Chu, C. Gyssler, A.D. Zelenetz, R.F. Bachvarova, and P. Besmer. 1993. W-sash affects positive and negative elements controlling c-kit expression: ectopic c-kit expression at sites of kit-ligand expression affects melanogenesis. Development 118:705–717.

101. Wehrle-Haller, B., and J.A. Weston. 1999. Altered cell-surface targeting of stem cell factor causes loss of melanocyte precursors in Steel17H mutant mice. Dev Biol 210:71–86.

102. Geissler, E.N., M.A. Ryan, and D.E. Housman. 1988. The dominant-white spotting (W) locus of the mouse encodes the c-kit proto-oncogene. Cell 55:185–192.

103. Cable, J., I.J. Jackson, and K.P. Steel. 1995. Mutations at the W locus affect survival of neural crest-derived melanocytes in the mouse. Mech Dev 50:139–150.

104. Nishikawa, S., M. Kusakabe, K. Yoshinaga, M. Ogawa, S. Hayashi, T. Kunisada, T. Era, and T. Sakakura. 1991. In utero manipulation of coat color formation by a monoclonal anti-c-kit antibody: two distinct waves of c-kit-dependency during melanocyte development. Embo J 10:2111–2118.

105. Jordan, S.A., and I.J. Jackson. 2000. MGF (KIT ligand) is a chemokinetic factor for melanoblast migration into hair follicles. Dev Biol 225:424–436.

106. Kunisada, T., H. Yamazaki, T. Hirobe, S. Kamei, M. Omoteno, H. Tagaya, H. Hemmi, U. Koshimizu, T. Nakamura, and S.I. Hayashi. 2000. Keratinocyte expression of transgenic hepatocyte growth factor affects melanocyte development, leading to dermal melanocytosis. Mech Dev 94:67–78.

107. Rawls, J.F., and S.L. Johnson. 2003. Temporal and molecular separation of the kit receptor tyrosine kinase's roles in zebrafish melanocyte migration and survival. Dev Biol 262:152–161.

108. Wehrle-Haller, B., M. Meller, and J.A. Weston. 2001. Analysis of melanocyte precursors in Nf1 mutants reveals that MGF/KIT signaling promotes directed cell migration independent of its function in cell survival. Dev Biol 232:471–483.

109. Pohl, B.S., and W. Knochel. 2001. Overexpression of the transcriptional repressor FoxD3 prevents neural crest formation in Xenopus embryos. Mech Dev 103:93–106.

110. Sasai, N., K. Mizuseki, and Y. Sasai. 2001. Requirement of FoxD3-class signaling for neural crest determination in Xenopus. Development 128:2525–2536.

111. Hanna, L.A., R.K. Foreman, I.A. Tarasenko, D.S. Kessler, and P.A. Labosky. 2002. Requirement for Foxd3 in maintaining pluripotent cells of the early mouse embryo. Genes Dev 16:2650–2661.

112. Cheung, M., and J. Briscoe. 2003. Neural crest development is regulated by the transcription factor Sox9. Development 130:5681–5693.

113. Akiyama, H., M.C. Chaboissier, J.F. Martin, A. Schedl, and B. de Crombrugghe. 2002. The transcription factor Sox9 has essential roles in successive steps of the chondrocyte differentiation pathway and is required for expression of Sox5 and Sox6. Genes Dev 16:2813–2828.

114. Bondurand, N., A. Kobetz, V. Pingault, N. Lemort, F. Encha-Razavi, G. Couly, D.E. Goerich, M. Wegner, M. Abitbol, and M. Goossens. 1998. Expression of the SOX10 gene during human development. FEBS Lett 432:168–172.

115. Britsch, S., D.E. Goerich, D. Riethmacher, R.I. Peirano, M. Rossner, K.A. Nave, C. Birchmeier, and M. Wegner. 2001. The transcription factor Sox10 is a key regulator of peripheral glial development. Genes Dev 15:66–78.

116. Cheng, Y., M. Cheung, M.M. Abu-Elmagd, A. Orme, and P.J. Scotting. 2000. Chick sox10, a transcription factor expressed in both early neural crest cells and central nervous system. Brain Res Dev Brain Res 121:233–241.

117. Dutton, K.A., A. Pauliny, S.S. Lopes, S. Elworthy, T.J. Carney, J. Rauch, R. Geisler, P. Haffter, and R.N. Kelsh. 2001. Zebrafish colourless encodes sox10 and specifies non-ectomesenchymal neural crest fates. Development 128:4113–4125.

118. Kuhlbrodt, K., B. Herbarth, E. Sock, I. Hermans-Borgmeyer, and M. Wegner. 1998. Sox10, a novel transcriptional modulator in glial cells. J Neurosci 18:237–250.

119. Southard-Smith, E.M., L. Kos, and W.J. Pavan. 1998. Sox10 mutation disrupts neural crest development in Dom Hirschsprung mouse model. Nat Genet 18:60–64.

120. Potterf, S.B., R. Mollaaghababa, L. Hou, E.M. Southard-Smith, T.J. Hornyak, H. Arnheiter, and W.J. Pavan. 2001. Analysis of SOX10 function in neural crest-derived melanocyte development: SOX10-dependent transcriptional control of dopachrome tautomerase. Dev Biol 237:245–257.

121. Lang, D., F. Chen, R. Milewski, J. Li, M.M. Lu, and J.A. Epstein. 2000. Pax3 is required for enteric ganglia formation and functions with Sox10 to modulate expression of c-ret. J Clin Invest 106:963–971.

122. Ludwig, A., S. Rehberg, and M. Wegner. 2004. Melanocyte-specific expression of dopachrome tautomerase is dependent on synergistic gene activation by the Sox10 and Mitf transcription factors. FEBS Lett 556:236–244.

123. Potterf, S.B., M. Furumura, K.J. Dunn, H. Arnheiter, and W.J. Pavan. 2000. Transcription factor hierarchy in Waardenburg syndrome: regulation of MITF expression by SOX10 and PAX3. Hum Genet 107:1–6.

124. Pingault, V., N. Bondurand, K. Kuhlbrodt, D.E. Goerich, M.O. Prehu, A. Puliti, B. Herbarth, I. Hermans-Borgmeyer, E. Legius, G. Matthijs, J. Amiel, S. Lyonnet, I. Ceccherini, G. Romeo, J.C. Smith, A.P. Read, M. Wegner, and M. Goossens. 1998. SOX10 mutations in patients with Waardenburg-Hirschsprung disease. Nat Genet 18:171–173.

125. Segal, N.H., P. Pavlidis, W.S. Noble, C.R. Antonescu, A. Viale, U.V. Wesley, K. Busam, H. Gallardo, D. DeSantis, M.F. Brennan, C. Cordon-Cardo, J.D. Wolchok, and A.N. Houghton. 2003. Classification of clear-cell sarcoma as a subtype of melanoma by genomic profiling. J Clin Oncol 21:1775–1781.

126. Tani, M., N. Shindo-Okada, Y. Hashimoto, T. Shiroishi, S. Takenoshita, Y. Nagamachi, and J. Yokota. 1997. Isolation of a novel Sry-related gene that is expressed in high-metastatic K-1735 murine melanoma cells. Genomics 39:30–37.

127. Seo, H.C., B.O. Saetre, B. Havik, S. Ellingsen, and A. Fjose. 1998. The zebrafish Pax3 and Pax7 homologues are highly conserved, encode multiple isoforms and show dynamic segment-like expression in the developing brain. Mech Dev 70:49–63.

128. Hornyak, T.J., D.J. Hayes, L.Y. Chiu, and E.B. Ziff. 2001. Transcription factors in melanocyte development: distinct roles for Pax-3 and Mitf. Mech Dev 101:47–59.

129. Serbedzija, G.N., and A.P. McMahon. 1997. Analysis of neural crest cell migration in Splotch mice using a neural crest-specific LacZ reporter. Dev Biol 185:139–147.

130. Galibert, M.D., U. Yavuzer, T.J. Dexter, and C.R. Goding. 1999. Pax3 and regulation of the melanocyte-specific tyrosinase-related protein-1 promoter. J Biol Chem 274:26894–26900.

131. Watanabe, A., K. Takeda, B. Ploplis, and M. Tachibana. 1998. Epistatic relationship between Waardenburg syndrome genes MITF and PAX3. Nat Genet 18:283–286.

132. Scholl, F.A., J. Kamarashev, O.V. Murmann, R. Geertsen, R. Dummer, and B.W. Schafer. 2001. PAX3 is expressed in human melanomas and contributes to tumor cell survival. Cancer Res 61:823–826.

133. Vachtenheim, J., and H. Novotna. 1999. Expression of genes for microphthalmia isoforms, Pax3 and MSG1, in human melanomas. Cell Mol Biol (Noisy-le-grand) 45:1075–1082.

134. Hoth, C.F., A. Milunsky, N. Lipsky, R. Sheffer, S.K. Clarren, and C.T. Baldwin. 1993. Mutations in the paired domain of the human PAX3 gene cause Klein-Waardenburg syndrome (WS-III) as well as Waardenburg syndrome type I (WS-I). Am J Hum Genet 52:455–462.

135. Pasteris, N.G., B.J. Trask, S. Sheldon, and J.L. Gorski. 1993. Discordant phenotype of two overlapping deletions involving the PAX3 gene in chromosome 2q35. Hum Mol Genet 2:953–959.

136. Tassabehji, M., A.P. Read, V.E. Newton, M. Patton, P. Gruss, R. Harris, and T. Strachan. 1993. Mutations in the PAX3 gene causing Waardenburg syndrome type 1 and type 2. Nat Genet 3:26–30.

137. Katoh, M. 2003. Identification and characterization of human SNAIL3 (SNAI3) gene in silico. Int J Mol Med 11:383–388.

138. Sefton, M., S. Sanchez, and M.A. Nieto. 1998. Conserved and divergent roles for members of the Snail family of transcription factors in the chick and mouse embryo. Development 125:3111–3121.

139. Sanchez-Martin, M., A. Rodriguez-Garcia, J. Perez-Losada, A. Sagrera, A.P. Read, and I. Sanchez-Garcia. 2002. SLUG (SNAI2) deletions in patients with Waardenburg disease. Hum Mol Genet 11:3231–3236.

140. LaBonne, C., and M. Bronner-Fraser. 1998. Neural crest induction in Xenopus: evidence for a two-signal model. Development 125:2403–2414.

141. Chazaud, C., M. Oulad-Abdelghani, P. Bouillet, D. Decimo, P. Chambon, and P. Dolle. 1996. AP-2.2, a novel gene related to AP-2, is expressed in the forebrain, limbs and face during mouse embryogenesis. Mech Dev 54:83–94.

142. Barrallo-Gimeno, A., J. Holzschuh, W. Driever, and E.W. Knapik. 2004. Neural crest survival and differentiation in zebrafish depends on mont blanc/tfap2a gene function. Development 131:1463–1477.

143. Knight, R.D., Y. Javidan, S. Nelson, T. Zhang, and T. Schilling. 2004. Skeletal and pigment cell defects in the lockjaw mutant reveal multiple roles for zebrafish tfap2a in neural crest development. Dev Dyn 229:87–98.

144. Brewer, S., W. Feng, J. Huang, S. Sullivan, and T. Williams. 2004. Wnt1-Cre-mediated deletion of AP-2alpha causes multiple neural crest-related defects. Dev Biol 267:135–152.

145. Huang, S., D. Jean, M. Luca, M.A. Tainsky, and M. Bar-Eli. 1998. Loss of AP-2 results in downregulation of c-KIT and enhancement of melanoma tumorigenicity and metastasis. Embo J 17:4358–4369.

146. Jean, D., J.E. Gershenwald, S. Huang, M. Luca, M.J. Hudson, M.A. Tainsky, and M. Bar-Eli. 1998. Loss of AP-2 results in up-regulation of MCAM/MUC18 and an increase in tumor growth and metastasis of human melanoma cells. J Biol Chem 273:16501–16508.

147. Goding, C.R. 2000. Mitf from neural crest to melanoma: signal transduction and transcription in the melanocyte lineage. Genes Dev 14:1712–1728.

148. Nakayama, A., M.T. Nguyen, C.C. Chen, K. Opdecamp, C.A. Hodgkinson, and H. Arnheiter. 1998. Mutations in microphthalmia, the mouse homolog of the human deafness gene MITF, affect neuroepithelial and neural crest-derived melanocytes differently. Mech Dev 70:155–166.

149. Tachibana, M., Y. Kobayashi, and Y. Matsushima. 2003. Mouse models for four types of Waardenburg syndrome. Pigment Cell Res 16:448–454.

150. Bear, J., Y. Hong, and M. Schartl. 2003. Mitf expression is sufficient to direct differentiation of medaka blastula derived stem cells to melanocytes. Development 130:6545–6553.

151. Tachibana, M., K. Takeda, Y. Nobukuni, K. Urabe, J.E. Long, K.A. Meyers, S.A. Aaronson, and T. Miki. 1996. Ectopic expression of MITF, a gene for Waardenburg syndrome type 2, converts fibroblasts to cells with melanocyte characteristics. Nat Genet 14:50–54.

152. Lister, J.A., C.P. Robertson, T. Lepage, S.L. Johnson, and D.W. Raible. 1999. nacre encodes a zebrafish microphthalmia-related protein that regulates neural-crest-derived pigment cell fate. Development 126:3757–3767.

153. Baxter, L.L., and W.J. Pavan. 2002. The oculocutaneous albinism type IV gene Matp is a new marker of pigment cell precursors during mouse embryonic development. Mech Dev 116:209–212.

154. Baxter, L.L., and W.J. Pavan. 2003. Pmel17 expression is Mitf-dependent and reveals cranial melanoblast migration during murine development. Gene Expr Patterns 3:703–707.

155. Du, J., A.J. Miller, H.R. Widlund, M.A. Horstmann, S. Ramaswamy, and D.E. Fisher. 2003. MLANA/MART1 and SILV/PMEL17/GP100 are transcriptionally regulated by MITF in melanocytes and melanoma. Am J Pathol 163:333–343.

156. Fang, D., Y. Tsuji, and V. Setaluri. 2002. Selective down-regulation of tyrosinase family gene TYRP1 by inhibition of the activity of melanocyte transcription factor, MITF. Nucleic Acids Res 30:3096–3106.

157. Miller, A.J., J. Du, S. Rowan, C.L. Hershey, H.R. Widlund, and D.E. Fisher. 2004. Transcriptional regulation of the melanoma prognostic marker melastatin (TRPM1) by MITF in melanocytes and melanoma. Cancer Res 64:509–516.

158. McGill, G.G., M. Horstmann, H.R. Widlund, J. Du, G. Motyckova, E.K. Nishimura, Y.L. Lin, S. Ramaswamy, W. Avery, H.F. Ding, S.A. Jordan, I.J. Jackson, S.J. Korsmeyer, T.R. Golub, and D.E. Fisher. 2002. Bcl2 regulation by the melanocyte master regulator Mitf modulates lineage survival and melanoma cell viability. Cell 109:707–718.

159. Yasumoto, K., K. Takeda, H. Saito, K. Watanabe, K. Takahashi, and S. Shibahara. 2002. Microphthalmia-associated transcription factor interacts with LEF-1, a mediator of Wnt signaling. Embo J 21:2703–2714.

160. Elworthy, S., J.A. Lister, T.J. Carney, D.W. Raible, and R.N. Kelsh. 2003. Transcriptional regulation of mitfa accounts for the sox10 requirement in zebrafish melanophore development. Development 130:2809–2818.

161. Saito, H., K. Yasumoto, K. Takeda, K. Takahashi, A. Fukuzaki, S. Orikasa, and S. Shibahara. 2002. Melanocyte-specific microphthalmia-associated transcription factor isoform activates its own gene promoter through physical interaction with lymphoid-enhancing factor 1. J Biol Chem 277:28787–28794.

162. Lalwani, A.K., A. Attaie, F.T. Randolph, D. Deshmukh, C. Wang, A. Mhatre, and E. Wilcox. 1998. Point mutation in the MITF gene causing Waardenburg syndrome type II in a three-generation Indian family. Am J Med Genet 80:406–409.

163. King, R., P.B. Googe, K.N. Weilbaecher, M.C. Mihm, Jr., and D.E. Fisher. 2001. Microphthalmia transcription factor expression in cutaneous benign, malignant melanocytic, and nonmelanocytic tumors. Am J Surg Pathol 25:51–57.

164. King, R., K.N. Weilbaecher, G. McGill, E. Cooley, M. Mihm, and D.E. Fisher. 1999. Microphthalmia transcription factor. A sensitive and specific melanocyte marker for MelanomaDiagnosis. Am J Pathol 155:731–738.

165. Clark, E.A., T.R. Golub, E.S. Lander, and R.O. Hynes. 2000. Genomic analysis of metastasis reveals an essential role for RhoC. Nature 406:532–535.

166. Dunn, K.J., Brady, M., Ochsenbauer-Jambor,C., Snyder, S., Incao, A., and W.J. Pavan. 2005. WNT1 and WNT3a promote expansion of melanocytes through distinct modes of action. Pigment Cell Res. 18:167–180.

167. Schaible, R. (1972). Comparative effects of piebald-spotting genes on clones of melanocytes in different vertebrate species. In Pigmentation: Its Genesis and Biologic Control (ed. V. Riley), pp. 343–357. New York: Appleton-Century-Crofts.

168. Hou L, Pavan WJ, Shin MK, Arnheiter H. 2004. Cell-autonomous and cell nonautonomous signaling through endothelin receptor B during melanocyte development. Development. 14:3239–3247.

169. Niemann S, Zhao C, Pascu F, Stahl U, Aulepp U, Niswander L, Weber JL, Muller U. 2004. Homozygous WNT3 mutation causes tetra-amelia in a large consanguineous family. Am J Hum Genet. 74:558–563.

170. Laurikkala J,Pispa J,Jung HS,Nieminen P,Mikkola M,Wang X, Saarialho-Kere U,Galceran J,Grosschedl R, Thesleff I. 2002. Regulation of hair follicle development by the TNF signal ectodysplasin and its receptor Edar. Development. 129:2541–2553.

171. Foster, J. W., Dominguez-Steglich, M. A., Guioli, S., Kwok, C., Weller, P. A., Stevanovic, M., Weissenbach, J., Mansour, S., Young, I. D., Goodfellow, P. N., Brook, J. D., Schafer, A. J. 1994 Campomelic dysplasia and autosomal sex reversal caused by mutations in an SRY-related gene. Nature 372: 525–530.

2

MITF

A Matter of Life and Death for Developing Melanocytes

*Heinz Arnheiter, Ling Hou,
Minh-Thanh T. Nguyen,
Keren Bismuth, Tamas Csermely,
Hideki Murakami, Susan Skuntz,
WenFang Liu, and Kapil Bharti*

CONTENTS

Summary

Since its discovery over a decade ago, the microphthalmia-associated transcription factor (MITF), has moved ever more to the center of pigment cell biology. Not only has MITF been found to regulate the expression of a number of genes involved in melanin biosynthesis, it is also essential in cell lineage determination, regulation of cell proliferation and cell survival, and replenishment of follicular melanocytes in the adult. To perform these multiple functions in a temporally and spatially appropriate manner, *Mitf* needs to be stringently regulated. Through the fruitful merging of genetics, biochemistry, and molecular and cell biology, it has become clear that *Mitf* is regulated both transcriptionally and posttranslationally in response to extracellular signaling and, hence, serves as a critical link between extracellular cues and gene expression. Intriguingly, many of the molecular pathways important for pigment cell development are also implicated in the formation of melanoma; therefore, the mechanisms controlling the development of pigment cells may provide invaluable insights into the cells' malignant transformation.

Key Words: Neural crest; melanoblast; retinal pigment epithelium; Kit; Kitl; transcription regulation; posttranslational regulation; serine phosphorylation; cell proliferation; cell differentiation.

From: *From Melanocytes to Melanoma: The Progression to Malignancy*
Edited by: V. J. Hearing and S. P. L. Leong © Humana Press Inc., Totowa, NJ

INTRODUCTION

Melanoma cells and developing melanocytes share many intriguing similarities. Both cells, for instance, engage in comparable complex behaviors that include the dissociation from an epithelial environment, invasion of the surrounding tissue, and migration to distant locations. Both cells respond to microenvironmental signals that regulate their growth, and both express common molecular markers, including microphthalmia-associated transcription factor (MITF), which links extracellular-signaling pathways with gene expression and seems crucial for the cells' survival. Hence, similar laws may govern melanocyte biology during development and malignant transformation, and understanding melanocyte development may help in understanding the formation and progression of melanoma.

Development of Mammalian Pigment Cells

Mammalian melanocytes are derived from multipotent precursors in the embryonic neural crest, which is formed from specific cells residing at the junction between the surface ectoderm and the neural plate (for a comprehensive review of the neural crest, *see* ref. *1*). Neural crest cells undergo an epithelial-to-mesenchymal transition, dissociate from each other, proliferate, and start to express distinct molecular markers. The expression of particular sets of markers is associated with biased cell fate choices that ultimately lead to the generation of a number of different cell types. These include, besides melanocytes, all cells of the peripheral nervous system, smooth muscle cells, and cartilage cells. The precursors to melanocytes are called "melanoblasts" and can be defined operationally as cells expressing the high mobility group transcription factor SOX10; MITF; the tyrosine kinase receptor, KIT; the G-coupled receptor, EDNRB; and the melanogenic enzyme, DCT (formerly called tyrosinase-related protein-2 or Tyrp-2); expression of these markers does not, however, preclude potential cell fate changes later in development. Melanoblasts migrate over considerable distances from the sites of their initial generation to their final destinations and start their journey approx 1 d later than other neural crest-derived cells. In areas where somites are present, melanoblasts migrate on a dorso-lateral path rather than the ventro-medial path along the side of the neural tube that is taken by other crest cells. Although the mechanisms responsible for these characteristic temporal and spatial migration patterns are not understood in detail, it appears that cadherins, integrins, and extracellular-signaling pathways operating through EDNRB are involved (reviewed in refs. *2* and *3*).

While traveling to their final destinations, melanoblasts sequentially express additional melanogenic genes, many of them regulated by MITF (for an overview, *see* ref. *4* and references therein). In the mouse, the sequence of expression of these genes culminates with the appearance of tyrosinase, the rate-limiting enzyme in melanin synthesis, approx 4–5 d after the first expression of MITF (for review, *see* refs. *4–6*). The emergence of tyrosinase marks the beginning of differentiation into mature, melanin-positive melanocytes that finally take up residence in skin and hair follicles, the oral mucosa, the choroid in the back of the eye, the iris, and several internal sites, such as the poorly understood periorbital Harderian gland, the leptomeninges (which form the connective tissue around the brain), and the inner ear (Fig. 1A). In the inner ear, melanocytes are located in a specialized part of the lateral wall of the cochlear duct, the stria vascularis, in which they participate by still unknown mechanisms in the regulation of the ionic homeostasis of the potassium-rich endolymph. In the absence of strial melano-cytes, regardless of the genetic cause, the electrical potential between endolymph and perilymph is close to 0 mV, instead of the normal 100 mV, and auditory hair cells no longer transduce mechano-sensory signals. In fact, in viable mice with *Kit* mutations, there often are asymmetries between left and right ears, and ears containing pigment cells in their stria display an endocochlear potential, whereas ears lacking strial pigmentation do not *(7,8)*. In addition, in human Waardenburg syndrome (of which there are several subtypes including one, Waardenburg IIa, linked to mutations in *MITF; see* ref. *9*), congenital deafness is associated with pigment disturbances in hair, skin, and iris that may serve as outward signs of melanocyte deficiencies in the inner ear. Importantly, however, it is melanocytes and not their melanin that is required for normal hearing; the lack of melanin *per se*, such as in albino organisms that retain unpigmented melanocytes in their stria, causes mild, if any, hearing problems *(10)*, although the sensitivity to ototoxic drugs may be increased *(11)*.

In the eye, neural crest-derived melanocytes populate the choroid and the anterior layer of the iris and act as light screens. In addition, as shown in Fig. 1B, the eye contains a specialized layer of pigment cells, the retinal pigment epithelium, or RPE, that is derived locally from the neuroepithelium of the optic vesicle. This neuroepithelium is developmentally bipotential and can give rise to either neuroretina or RPE, and dis-turbances in cell fate decisions between the future retina and the RPE can lead to devel-opmental abnormalities that ultimately result in coloboma, retinal malformations, and microphthalmia (for a recent review, *see* ref. *12*). Postnatally, disturbances in RPE cells can lead to retinal degeneration because of the critical functions that RPE cells play in photoreceptor cell physiology and maintenance.

Thus, it follows, that the biology of pigment cells reaches far beyond creating the variety and beauty of an animal's or person's pigmentation and touches on many other disciplines, including sensory organ physiology and oncology.

Melanocyte Development Is Controlled by a Genetic Network

Much of our knowledge about the network of the molecules controlling birth, prolif-eration, migration, differentiation, death, or malignant transformation of pigment cells comes from the successful integration of biochemistry, molecular biology, and genetics. Fig. 2 shows classical examples from mouse genetics depicting phenotypes associated with heterozygosity for certain mutant alleles of five distinct genes. They include *Sox10*, *Pax3, Kit ligand* (*Kitl*), *Kit*, and *Mitf*. Each of the mutant alleles produces similar white belly spots where neural crest-derived melanocytes are missing. Overlapping pheno-types often suggest that the products of the genes in question participate in common molecular pathways, and it is a gratifying finding that the five white spotting genes depicted in Fig. 2 indeed seem functionally linked in a common pathway. *Sox10* and *Pax3* encode transcription factors that, although more widely expressed than *Mitf*, acti-vate at least one of the many *Mitf* promoters in vitro *(13–15)*. *Kitl* and *Kit* encode a ligand/ receptor pair (for a recent review, *see* ref. *16*), whose activation leads to multiple post-translational modifications of MITF protein that affect MITF's transcriptional activities on target genes *(17–19)*. It thus appears that a network of extracellular and intracellular regulatory proteins all converge on the single transcription factor, MITF, which, in turn, serves as the nexus to a set of downstream target genes that execute the requisite program of melanogenesis (for a review, *see* ref. *20*). Here, we highlight these recent findings and

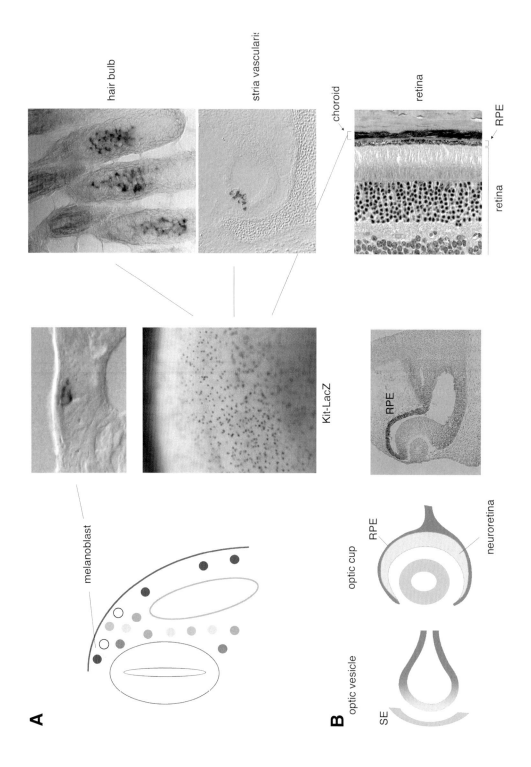

hair bulb

stria vascularis

choroid

retina

RPE

retina

melanoblast

Kit-LacZ

RPE

A

optic vesicle

optic cup

SE

RPE

neuroretina

B

30

focus in particular on mouse *Mitf*, because *Mitf* research started in mice, and mice provide a rich resource of *Mitf* mutations and will continue to yield important insights into the function of *Mitf*. For more comprehensive reviews on the transcriptional regulation of *Mitf* and its target genes, however, we refer the reader to Chapters 3 and 4 in this book, and to other recent reviews *(21,22)*.

MITF: EXPRESSION, ALLELES, AND DEVELOPMENTAL PHENOTYPES

The **Mitf** *Gene and Its Protein Products*

The *Mitf* gene was first isolated in 1993 from lines of mice with transgenic insertional mutations at the *microphthalmia* (*mi*) locus *(23,24)*. This locus was originally described more than 50 yrs earlier with a single mutant allele, *mi (25)*. Meanwhile, more than 30 additional alleles—many of them spontaneous, and some induced chemically, by irradiation or by targeted mutagenesis—have been isolated (refs. *26* and *27*, and unpublished results). Similar to mice with phenotypically severe *mi* alleles, mice homozygous for the transgenic insertion *Mitfvga-9*[1] lack neural crest-derived pigment cells in coat, eye, and inner ear; have an abnormal RPE; small, degenerating eyes; and are profoundly deaf *(23,28–30)*. In these transgenic mice, extraneous sequences are by chance inserted into the promoter region of a gene encoding a novel member of the basic helix-loop-helix–leucine zipper (bHLH-LZ) class of transcription factors *(23)* that we later termed *Mitf (31)* (Fig. 3). Such factors are known to participate in a variety of biological processes, including the regulation of cell fate specification, proliferation, and differentiation. The bHLH-LZ domain is the critical domain that allows these proteins to form obligatory homodimers and heterodimers and to bind specific DNA elements, Ephrussi (E)-boxes, 5'CANNTG3', in target gene promoters. Because all known *mi* alleles in mice turned out to have mutations in this gene, it is now firmly established that *Mitf* is indeed the single *mi* gene in this species *(32,33)*.

Fig. 1. (*opposite page*) Development of vertebrate pigment cells. (**A**) One source of pigment cells is the neural crest. In the trunk area of a wild-type mouse embryo, *Mitf*-positive melanoblasts (●) originate at the rooftop of the neural tube and then migrate underneath the surface ectoderm on a dorsolateral pathway. Other neural crest derivatives (gray circles) take the ventro-medial route. Some cells (○) may not yet express any cell type-specific marker and represent uncommitted stem cells. A Kit-LacZ transgene allows migrating *Kit*-positive melanoblasts to be labeled en face underneath the surface ectoderm. These melanoblasts migrate and differentiate and finally take up residence at various sites, such as in hair bulbs, the stria vascularis of the inner ear, or in the choroid behind the retina. (**B**) Another source of vertebrate pigment cells is the optic neuroepithelium which evaginates as an optic vesicle from the telencephalon. After invagination to form the optic cup, the part of the optic neuroepithelium exposed to growth factors emanating from the closely juxtaposed surface ectoderm (SE) finally gives rise to a domain that goes on to form the retina. The part closer to the brain will give rise to a domain that goes on to form the retinal pigment epithelium (RPE). Each part of the optic neuroepithelium is initially bipotential, that is, capable of giving rise to either retina or RPE, and addition or removal of growth factors or genetic manipulations can change the normal fate determinations *(119)*.

---

[1]"vga-9" was the ninth transgenic line made with a transgene comprised of a mouse vasopressin promoter, β-Gal reporter, and human vasopressin polyA signal.

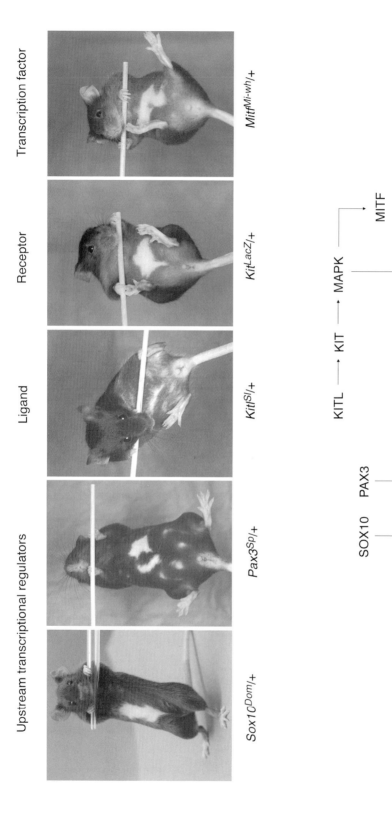

Fig. 2. Five genes controlling melanocyte development are linked in a common genetic pathway. Heterozygosity for particular alleles of these five genes causes similar belly spots in the mouse. They include the genes for the transcription factors SOX10 and PAX3, the ligand/receptor pair KITL/ KIT, and the transcription factor MITF. KIT signaling activates the mitogen-activated protein kinase (MAPK) pathway that can affect the transcription of the *Mitf* gene as well as modulate MITF activity through serine phosphorylation.

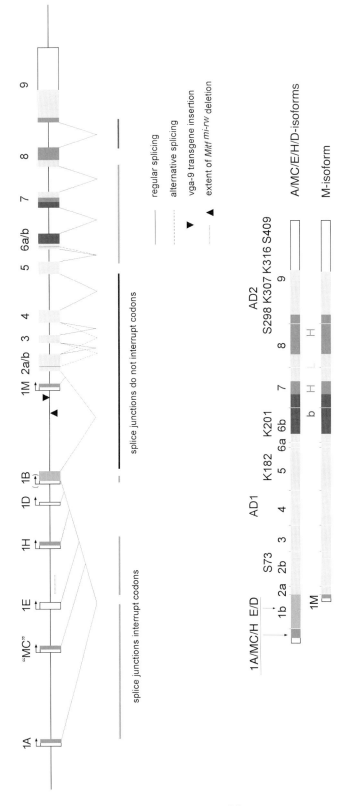

Fig. 3. *Mitf* gene structure and protein isoforms. The mouse *Mitf* gene on chromosome 6 spans approx 200 kbp and contains multiple exons. Most mRNA isoforms contain exons 2–9 and either the 1m exon, or exon 1b or part of exon 1b along with one of the upstream exons (1a, 1c, 1mc, 1ℎ). The site of the vga–9 transgene insertion and the 5′ and 3′ boundaries of the *Mitf mi–rw* deletion are indicated, as are standard and alternative splice forms. The basic (DNA-binding) domain is encoded by parts of exons 6 and 7, and the HLH-Zip domain by the remainder of exon 7, exon 8, and the beginning of exon 9. The encoded MITF proteins contain two activation domains (AD1 and AD2) and several residues that are subject to posttranslational modifications. They include the serines S73, S298, S307, and S409 as sites of phosphorylation, the lysines K182 and K316 as sites of sumoylation (*91,92*), and K201, reported as a site for ubiquitination (*19*).

33

Mitf is approx 100 megabasepairs (Mbp) from the centromere on mouse chromosome 6, and its human homolog, approx 70 Mbp from the telomere on chromosome 3p *(31)*. *Mitf* is most closely related to three other bHLH-LZ genes, *Tfeb*, *Tfe3*, and *Tfec*. The proteins encoded by these related genes and *MITF* can form stable dimeric combinations among each other but not with other bHLH-LZ or bHLH proteins *(34,35)*, and, together, constitute the MITF-TFE subfamily of bHLH-LZ proteins *(35)*. In both mouse and humans, *Mitf* transcription is initiated from at least nine distinct promoters, giving rise to mRNAs encoding proteins that differ at their amino-termini but usually share the sequences of eight exons (Fig. 3). Reverse transcription-polymerase chain reaction (RT-PCR) approaches, along with the analyses of *Mitf* mutations, have revealed a variety of alternatively spliced mRNAs lacking particular exons or parts of exons. Intriguingly, as shown in Fig. 3, the 3' splice junction of exon 1b; the 3' splice junction of exon 1m; all junctions of exons 2, 3, and 4; and the 5' junction of exon 5 correspond to in-frame codons. This means that exons 2, 3, and 4 can be spliced out safely without disrupting the remaining open reading frame, and their inclusion or exclusion could therefore be regulated depending on the developmental or proliferative state of a given cell. By contrast, selective elimination of the entire exons 5, 7, or 8, the latter two including sequences encoding the bHLH-LZ domain, would create mRNAs with premature stop codons, expected to be subject to nonsense-mediated degradation. Elimination of exon 6, however, does not lead to an interruption of the open reading frame, but, nevertheless, creates a nonfunctional protein, as seen in mice with the *Mitf mi–ew* mutation *(32)*. Also, the 3' splice junction of the exons 1a–1h interrupt the codons corresponding to the predicted amino-terminal reading frames, precluding the maintenance of open reading frames for a number of altenative potential splice arrangements such as splicing directly into exon 2. In fact, the elimination of exon 1b, as seen in *Mitf mi–rw* mice, in which the upstream exon A is spliced directly into exon 2, creates mRNAs with premature stop codons *(32,33)*.

Based on the observed gene structure, the single *Mitf* gene of mammals could theoretically give rise to at least 48 distinct, functional mRNAs and protein isoforms that retain the full bHLH-LZ domain. For some of these, such as splice forms lacking exon 6a, a genetic role has been established, but for many others, a specific role still needs to be explored by further mutational analyses. Intriguingly, the genes encoding the related proteins TFEB, TFE3, and TFEC are organized in a similarly complex manner *(36)*. Their capacity to dimerize with MITF when coexpressed may thus lead to a vast set of distinct dimers, each potentially with discrete stabilities and activities.

The Developmental Role of Mitf: *Expression Patterns and Genetics*

The cell-autonomous role of *Mitf* in melanocyte and RPE development is evident from its expression patterns and its genetics. Evolutionarily ancient—homologs are found in *Caenorhabditis elegans* and *Drosophila (37)*—*Mitf* is clearly expressed in developing pigment cells starting with urochordates, which have a notochord like vertebrates, but lack a neural crest *(38)*. Interestingly, tadpoles of the urochordate *Halocynthia roretzi* sport exactly two melanin-containing pigment cells, an anterior one called the otolith that serves as a balance organ akin to that in the inner ear of vertebrates, and a juxtaposed posterior one that is part of the ocellus, a primitive structure involved in light perception.

In vertebrates, *Mitf* is expressed in melanoblasts and melanin-containing melanocytes (called melanophores in fish, amphibia, and reptiles) and RPE cells *(30,39–41)*. This is not to say that *Mitf* is only found in pigment cells. For instance, in mammals, some isoforms are expressed in unrelated cell types such as osteoclasts *(42)*, NK cells *(43)*, macrophages *(44)*, B-cells *(45)*, and mast cells *(46)*, all of which are affected, if not by null alleles, at least by dominant-negative alleles of *Mitf*. *Mitf* is also expressed in heart *(23,30)*, in which its function has yet to be established. In fact, by RT-PCR techniques, *Mitf*, at least its exon 1b, is expressed widely, if not ubiquitously, as shown in the gene expression database GXD *(47)*. It would appear, then, that, evolutionarily, the *Mitf* gene must be under considerable constraints to maintain proper expression patterns and regulation to serve the needs of so many different cell types. It also implies that *Mitf* expression does not inevitably lead to the activation of the melanogenic program. Rather, it is the developmental history of cells, or the presence of specific Mitf isoforms, or a combination of history and isoforms, that is associated with the development of the respective lineages. Hence, despite the demonstration that *Mitf* or at least some isoforms are capable of recruiting cells other than melanocytes to become pigmented *(48)*, the broad term "melanocyte master regulator" should be applied with caution.

Whereas *C. elegans*, *D. melanogaster*, and *H. roretzi* each seem to have only one *Mitf* gene, teleost fish *(40,49)* and *Xenopus (50)* have two separate genes. One, *Mitf-a* (nomenclature according to ref. *40*), is expressed in the neural crest and the RPE, and the other, *Mitf-b*, in the RPE, epiphysis (zebrafish and frog), and olfactory bulb (zebrafish) but not, or less abundantly, in melanoblasts. In birds and mammals, there is no evidence for two separate genes, and tissue-specific roles may be fulfilled by the distinct isoforms. M-Mitf, the homolog of fish Mitf-a, for instance, is prominently expressed in the neural crest and not the RPE of mice, and A-Mitf (the homolog of fish Mitf-b) and D-Mitf are expressed in the RPE (ref. *51*, and unpublished results). Their respective roles can be assessed in organisms with distinct *Mitf* mutations, which are quite abundant in vertebrates.

Mutations in *Mitf-a* in the *nacre* zebrafish are associated with a selective loss of melanophores, while other types of pigment cells (xanthophores, iridophores, and RPE cells) are not affected *(39)*. Although no isolated mutation in zebrafish *Mitf-b* has yet been found, it is clear that *Mitf-b* retains the potential to generate melanophores, because it can rescue *Mitf-a* mutations, whereas the related zebrafish *Tfe3*, for instance, cannot *(40)*. *Mitf* mutations have also been found in quail *(52)*, hamster *(41)*, rat *(53,54)*, mice *(23,32,33)*, and humans *(9)*. In mice, even the mildest alleles affect neural crest-derived melanocytes, but only more severe mutations affect the RPE as well. The phenotypes associated with each of these alleles are far from being uniform or merely gradations in severity, however. Indeed, a trained eye can distinguish the 30 different mouse alleles and many of their heteroallelic combinations alone by visual inspection of their carriers.

A Variety of Alleles and Phenotypes: The Bane and Beauty of Mitf

One of the many reasons why distinct alleles cause such a variety of phenotypes lies in the fact that MITF is a protein with multiple, functionally distinct domains, some of which are subject to further posttranslational modifications. Mutations that eliminate or distort the protein's DNA binding basic domain, the dimerization domain, or one of its activation domains usually result in an early abrogation of the melanocyte lineage and a hyperproliferation of the RPE followed by subsequent derailment of eye development *(32,55)*. Hence, mice homozygous for such mutations are white, deaf, and microphthalmic, similar to mice lacking MITF protein altogether. Nevertheless, the complete lack of MITF protein is milder in its effects than the presence of an MITF protein that, although unable to bind DNA, still can dimerize or interact with other proteins and exert dominant-negative activities. Milder still are alleles that leave the bHLH-LZ domains intact but affect other protein domains. No doubt the mildest among all published alleles is *Mitfmi–sp* (*mi-spotted*), which, when homozygous, has no obvious pigmentation phenotype at all, although a reduction in tyrosinase levels in the skin has been observed. Only in combination with other *Mitf* alleles do carriers of *Mitfmi–sp* become conspicuous by the presence of white spots, and it is this fact that originally led to the discovery of *Mitfmi–sp* when it appeared *de novo* in a colony segregating *MitfMi–wh* (*Mi-white*) *(56)*. *Mitfmi–sp* is caused by the insertion of an extra base pair in exon 6a, leading to the exclusive expression of mRNAs lacking the exon 6a-associated six codons (encoding ACIFPT) normally present in at least half of the Mitf mRNAs *(32)*. Lack of these residues slightly lowers the protein's avidity for DNA *(35)* and its capacity to stimulate transcription. Another mild allele is *mi-vitiligo* (*Mitfmi–vit*), which leads to a combination of white spots and large pigmented areas that prematurely become gray as the animal goes through its molting cycles. Premature graying is likely caused by premature loss of melanocyte stem cells in the hair bulb niche *(57,58)*. A similar, though less extensive, premature graying is also seen with other alleles, but with certain alleles, such as *mi-red eyed-white* (*Mitfmi–rw*), pigmented spots do not seem to prematurely gray. Further, there are alleles such as *mi-brownish* (*Mitfmi-b*) or heteroallelic combinations between *MitfMi–wh* and several other alleles that lead to changes in the hue of pigmentation *(55,59)*. Such color changes show that *Mitf* does not only regulate melanoblast development but also the quality of melanin in the differentiated melanocyte, consistent with *Mitf*'s direct transcriptional stimulation of pigmentation genes or its effects on melanocyte dendricity or other aspects of melanocyte biology.

The different domains appended to the amino-termini of MITF may also contribute to allele-specific phenotypes. Available genetic evidence suggests, for instance, that selective deficiencies in M-MITF result in lack of pigmentation in the coat, choroid, and anterior layer of the iris, but not the RPE *(60)*, hinting at the possibility that selective deficiencies in other amino-terminal isoforms might likewise lead to cell type-specific phenotypes. It is not known, however, whether such cell type specificities are simply owing to differences in expression patterns or to functional differences between the different polypeptides. In other words, it is not known to what degree one isoform might substitute in vivo for another. Nevertheless, functional differences between isoforms have been suggested by a recent study showing that melanoma cells that lack M-Mitf expression (although expressing other isoforms), when reconstituted with an M-Mitf expression plasmid change their morphology and growth characteristics after in vivo transplantation *(61)*.

A further reason for allele-dependent phenotypic distinctions is heterodimerization of MITF with TFE proteins. The lack of either TFE3 or TFEC is without obvious phenotypic consequences in the mouse and the lack of TFEB is associated with disturbances in placental vascularization *(62)*. Combinations with *Mitf* mutations do not result in novel phenotypes except when both *Tfe3* and *Mitf* are missing. Mice lacking both TFE3 and MITF suffer from severe osteopetrosis that interferes with normal tooth eruption and is fatal at the time of weaning *(62)*. Indeed, mutations in *Mitf* alone, when homozygous, can lead to fatal osteopetrosis if the mutant MITF protein is still capable of heterodimerization with TFE3 but cannot bind DNA, thus mimicking the combined lack of TFE3 and MITF *(53,62)*. Importantly, however, the simple lack of MITF in osteoclasts does not result in osteopetrosis, and the lack of TFEB, TFE3, or TFEC does not seem to affect melanogenesis *(62)*. This suggests that although heterodimers between MITF and

TFE proteins are found in vivo, such as in osteoclasts *(53)*, they are not essential to the function of each protein. MITF-TFE proteins, therefore, do not seem to follow the rationale of regulation by heterodimerization that is seen with the MYC/MAD/MAX group of bHLH-LZ proteins or the myogenic MYOD group of bHLH proteins. This is surprising, because MITF, like these other proteins, also links cell proliferation with cell differentiation (*see* page 41).

From the genetic evidence it follows, then, that MITF must have multiple functions in melanogenesis: it recruits cells to the pigment lineage, regulates their proliferation and survival, induces their differentiation into mature melanocytes, regulates their differentiated state, and is responsible for their maintenance throughout adulthood.

REGULATION OF *Mitf*

Transcriptional Regulation

Not surprisingly, a factor as potent as MITF must be under stringent regulation to safeguard against two dangerous derailments: premature cell differentiation, potentially leading to deficiencies in cell numbers, or prolonged cell proliferation, potentially leading to an overproduction of immature cells. Ultimately, what needs to be regulated is *Mitf's* function in the broadest sense, which depends not only on Mitf mRNA and protein levels, but also on posttranslational modifications of MITF and the availability and activity of cofactors.

A first level of control is exerted, positively and negatively, by a combinatorial set of transcription factors that each binds specific motifs in the promoter elements of the *Mitf* gene and regulates Mitf mRNA expression. One of these, PAX3, is a paired homeodomain protein required for the proper generation of the neural crest and other lineages including, for instance, limb muscle precursors. For melanoblasts, PAX3 is limiting, because *Pax3* heterozygous mice have belly spots (Fig. 2), and *PAX3* heterozygous humans have the typical combination of pigment disturbances and deafness of Waardenburg I syndrome *(63)*. Another transcription factor is SOX10, associated with belly spots when mutated in mice (Fig. 2) and with Waardenburg-Shah syndrome when mutated in humans *(64)*. In fact, several groups have shown cooperativity of PAX3 and SOX10 on the M-Mitf promoter *(13,14)*. Additional positive regulators for M-Mitf include members of the LEF1/TCF family of proteins, which interact with β-catenin and link *Mitf* expression to Wnt-signaling *(65,66)*; this link provides the rationale for the observation that Wnt signaling increases the generation of melanocytes in zebrafish *(67)*, quail *(68)*, and mouse neural crest cell cultures *(69)*, and that Wnt1/Wnt3a double mutant mouse embryos have a substantial reduction in *Dct*-positive melanoblasts *(70)*. Intriguingly, LEF1 can interact with the bHLH-LZ domain of MITF and cooperate in the activation of the M-Mitf promoter, and this cooperation is even seen with a mutant MITF protein incapable of efficient DNA binding *(71,72)*. This observation is consistent with the facts that the M-Mitf promoter does not itself contain MITF binding sequences, and that *Mitf* mutations affecting DNA binding do not hamper early developmental *Mitf* expression. Consequently, by interacting with LEF1, MITF may potentially regulate its own expression.

There are a number of additional factors that have been implicated in the regulation of M-Mitf expression, mostly based on in vitro results. The bLZ protein cAMP responsive element binding protein (CREB), for instance, binds a cAMP-responsive element (CRE) in the M-Mitf promoter and links *Mitf* expression to cAMP responsiveness and, through CREB phosphorylation, to the mitogen-activated protein kinase (MAPK) pathway *(73;* for review *see* ref. *74).* Although CREB would come across as an all-purpose activator that is stimulated by many signal-transduction cascades and activates many target genes *(75),* the CRE of M-Mitf is quite tissue-specific, likely because its activation codepends on SOX10 *(76).* Additional factors involved in M-Mitf regulation include the transcription factor Onecut2, which belongs to a family of homeodomain proteins involved in lineage determination *(77),* and the POU domain protein BRN2, which has been proposed to serve as a negative regulator *(21).* Interestingly, *Brn2* expression is itself upregulated by Wnt signaling in vitro, as is M-Mitf expression, but *Brn2* is not seen in *Dct*-positive melanoblasts, only later in hair follicle melanocytes *(78).* Hence, *Brn-2* may not exert its potential negative activity on M-Mitf early in development. When prematurely activated in tyrosinase promoter/β-catenin transgenic mice, however, it interferes with normal melanogenesis *(78).*

Although the M-Mitf promoter has been studied in some detail, little is known about the regulation of the other promoters. A recent report shows that for RPE precursors, the paired domain proteins PAX2 and PAX6 act as critical, though redundant, positive regulators of *Mitf (79),* as do the homeodomain proteins OTX1/OTX2 *(80).* Furthermore, the paired-like homeodomain protein CHX10 represses MITF in the part of the neuroepithelium destined to become retina. In fact, the lack of MITF repression in the future neuroretina is part of the ocular phenotype in mice with *Chx10* mutations (refs. *81* and *82,* and *see* page 42).

Posttranslational Regulation

Besides regulation at the transcriptional level, MITF is also controlled post-translationally by several modifications, the best characterized of which is serine phosphorylation by MAPK signaling. As mentioned above, it is well established that MAPK signaling initiated by KITL-activated KIT is of critical importance to melanocyte development. In fact, potential links between KIT signaling and *mi* have been reported even before *Mitf* was cloned. For instance, a suggestion that the two genes might interact came from the observation that the extent of white spotting in mice heterozygous for both *Mitf/Mi–wh* and *KitW-36H* vastly exceeded that of their single heterozygous parents *(83),* a finding that we confirmed using the null allele *KitlacZ (4).* Importantly, however, combinations of *KitLacZ* with other *Mitf* alleles, including the null allele *Mitf^vga-9,* do not show such phenotypic enhancements, suggesting that *Kit* heterozygosity does not lead to further loss of melanocytes in combination with *Mitf* alleles unless acting through mutant MITF protein, in particular dominant-negative MITF (unpublished results; for further discussion of this point, *see* page 40). Another study showed that the tyrosine kinase receptor c-FMS, although capable of rescuing *Kit* mutant mast cells, was incapable of rescuing *mi* mutant mast cells *(84).* This suggested that either *Mitf* was downstream of the *Kit/c-fms* signal-transduction pathway or played entirely independent roles. In yet another study, however, *Kit* expression was found to be low in *mi* mutant mast cells, suggesting that *Mitf* was upstream of *Kit.* These latter two results are not necessarily conflicting, because they may simply reflect a feedback loop between *Kit* and *Mitf.* In fact, it was later shown that in primary melanoblast cultures, *Mitf* is required for upregulation and maintenance of *Kit* expression *(4,29),* and that in melanocyte or melanoma cell lines, KIT signaling regulates MITF protein through phosphorylation *(17–19).*

Following KIT signaling, phosphorylation occurs at two serine residues, serine-73 (S73), which is phosphorylated by the MAPK–stimulated extracellular signaling-regulated kinase ERK1/2 (17–19), and serine-409 (S409), which is phosphorylated by p90^{RSK}, itself activated by ERK1/2 and other kinases (18). Although S73-phosphorylated MITF can be conveniently detected because of its reduced electrophoretic mobility (17), S409 phosphorylation does not change the protein's electrophoretic mobility, which makes its detection less straightforward. Importantly, however, phosphorylation of neither one of these two serines is necessary for phosphorylation of the other, and either one can be phosphorylated regardless of the presence or absence of the genetically important exon 6a-encoded residues.

What is the biological consequence of MITF phosphorylation? It appears that unlike what is observed with other transcription factors, such as the SMAD proteins, phosphorylation does not regulate nuclear accumulation of MITF because both wild-type MITF, whether S73 phosphorylated or not, and MITF whose S73 and S409 have been substituted for nonphosphorylatable alanines, accumulate efficiently in the nucleus (unpublished results). Phosphorylation at S73 does, however, increase MITF's transcriptional activity on the tyrosinase promoter. This is inferred from the fact that a S73LA substitution yields a protein with a two- to threefold lower activity compared with wild type, as originally tested in the presence of constitutively active RAF and wild-type MEK (17), or later without these activators (18). The increased activity following S73 phosphorylation is thought to result from an increased association with the transcriptional cofactors CBP/p300 (85,86). CBP/p300 are histone acetyl transferases best known for their ability to modify chromatin architecture. It is not clear, however, whether the molecular target of these proteins is chromatin of Mitf target genes or MITF protein itself, which also has potential acetylation sites; acetylation has been demonstrated to modify the activity, for instance, of NF-κB (87). Alternatively, CBP/p300 might also act as bridging proteins between MITF and basal transcription factors, as scaffold proteins required for setting up the transcriptional machinery or as ubiquitin ligases.

Phosphorylation at S73 alone (19) or only in conjunction with phosphorylation at S409 (18) also renders MITF less stable. This loss of stability is thought to result from an increased polyubiquitination at lysine 201 (19) followed by proteasome-mediated degradation. For instance, 5 h after addition of KITL to human melanoma cells, there was a marked reduction of MITF, which could be prevented by addition of MAPK or proteasome inhibitors, or combined alanine substitutions at S73 and S409 (18). Despite an increase in stability, the double alanine substitutions rendered the protein transcriptionally inactive, yet still capable of binding DNA (18). In contrast to S73/409 unphosphorylated wild type or alanine-mono-substituted MITF, however, the doubly substituted MITF also displayed a surprising increase in electrophoretic mobility (ref. 18, unpublished results), suggesting either a change in conformation or in other modifications of MITF.

S409 phosphorylation has also been implicated in regulating the interaction of MITF with the zinc finger protein, PIAS3, which was found to repress the transcriptional activity of wild-type MITF but not of S409→D MITF, a substitution made to mimic the charge of phospho-S409 (88). Consistent with this finding, PIAS3 bound and inhibited wild-type MITF and S409→A mutated MITF but not S409→D mutated MITF. PIAS3, similar to other PIAS proteins, serves as E3 ligase for SUMO-1 (small ubiquitin-like modifier, a 101-residue-polypeptide), whose attachment to ε-amino groups of lysines embedded in an (I/L/V)KXE motif results in a branched polypeptide (for a recent review, *see* ref. *89*). Sumoylation has been shown to attenuate the activity of transcription factors, such as LEF1, by sequestering the sumoylated protein into nuclear bodies *(90)*. It would be intriguing if S409 phosphorylation modified MITF activity and/or stability by interfering with PIAS3-mediated sumoylation. It has recently been found that MITF is indeed sumoylated at two lysines, K182 and K316, and that sumoylation decreases MITF's transcriptional activity. This sumoylation depends on SUMO E1 activating enzyme (SAE I/SAE II) and E2 conjugating enzyme (Ubc9). Nevertheless, coexpression of PIAS members reduced the transcriptional activity of wild-type MITF and K182/K316→R mutated MITF to the same extent, suggesting that PIAS does not suppress MITF by modulating sumoylation *(91,92)*.

Besides phosphorylation at S73 and S409, phosphorylation at two additional serines has been implicated in the regulation of MITF. Signaling by the stress kinase p38 leads to phosphorylation at S307 and, concomitantly, to an increase in MITF's transcriptional activity *(93)*. This study was limited to osteoclasts, but because p38 is activated by UV (as are melanocytes), S307 phosphorylation might quite possibly play a role in melanocytes as well. It has also been proposed that S298 is phosphorylated by GSK-3β, which is inhibited in the canonical Wnt/β-catenin pathway but activated by cAMP, known to stimulate melanogenesis in an *Mitf*-dependent manner *(73,94,95)*. This serine is substituted for a proline in an individual with Waardenburg syndrome *(96)*. In vitro, substitutions for either proline or alanine impair MITF's activity *(96)*, but so do substitutions for aspartate or glutamate, despite the fact that these two residues mimic the charge of p-S298 *(94)*. In fact, to date, S298 fulfills only one of several criteria proposed for standard GSK-3β targets *(97)*, and until it is unequivocally proven that GSK-3β phosphorylates S298, one might explain the results also by assuming that substitutions at this residue might interfere with phosphorylation at other sites.

Regardless of the precise residue that becomes phosphorylated and the kinases that are involved, a consensus has emerged that phosphorylation increases MITF's transcriptional activity. Conversely, as seen, at least with S73 and S409 phosphorylation, it also decreases MITF stability. That stability can regulate the relative abundance of a transcription factor, and that relative abundance can determine the extent of target gene stimulation, has been amply demonstrated, for instance, for β-catenin or p53 *(98)*. At first sight, then, MITF's phosphorylation-dependent loss of stability and its gain of activity are two opposing principles, whereby one may win over the other, or they may cancel each other out, depending on when precisely and how efficiently phosphorylations and dephosphorylations occur during development (for a discussion of the importance of the kinetics of phosphorylation/dephosphorylation events in vitro, *see* ref. *99*). Interesting situations may arise with dominant-negative MITF proteins, whose stability can be regulated by phosphorylation but whose activity cannot be regulated because of their intrinsic inability to bind DNA. Such proteins should manifest their dominant-negativity more prominently if they are underphosphorylated. Intriguingly, as mentioned on page 38, white spotting is increased in *Kit* heterozygotes if they carry dominant-negative *Mitf* alleles but not if they carry *Mitf* null alleles (refs. *4* and *83*, and unpublished results). However, based on the tight coupling between instability and activity observed in a number of other transcription factors, including the bHLH-PAS factor AhR *(100)*, SMAD2 *(101)*, or STATs *(102)*, a different model of transcription regulation has emerged, in which ubiquitination and proteasome-mediated degradation of enhancer-bound factor are *prerequisite* for transcription initiation and elongation *(103)*. According to this model, a new molecule from the pool of unbound factor would have to be recruited to bind DNA for each round of transcription initiation, a mechanism that would allow for a stringent regulation of gene expression, provided the pool of unbound factor is limiting (which may again depend on the protein's stability). Future experiments will show whether MITF might operate along these lines or not. We find it to be of critical importance, however, that any in vitro results, however compelling, be confirmed in the intact organism, be it by testing targeted mutations or by rescue strategies using appropriate transgene constructs.

THE BUSINESS END OF *Mitf:* THE REGULATION OF CELL PROLIFERATION AND DIFFERENTIATION

In 1993, when *Mitf* was cloned, it was already known that the expression of melanocyte pigmentation genes, such as tyrosinase, depended on crucial *cis* elements called M-boxes *(104)*. In their core, M-boxes contain a CATGTG E-box, which, in a way, was puzzling because there is hardly anything melanocyte-specific about an E-box and no melanocyte-specific E-box-binding bHLH or bHLH-LZ proteins were known. The identification of *Mitf* as a bHLH-LZ gene was met with some relief because it went a long way toward explaining pigment gene regulation via E-boxes, not only in melanocytes but also in the RPE. However, although much has since been learned about target gene regulation and the multiple levels of the regulation of *Mitf* itself, many fundamental questions remain unanswered. For instance, E-boxes are found in many promoters, and even the refinement of the optimal MITF binding sequence *(105)* would not seem to provide the required element of specificity. Furthermore, *Mitf* is not specific to pigment cells, although during development it is most prominently expressed in the pigment lineage *(30)*. Hence, are pigment gene E-boxes characterized by a particularly high threshold of activation, and only MITF can meet this threshold because of its high level of expression in these cells? If so, which other factors, if experimentally expressed to similar levels, would substitute for *Mitf*? Or does *Mitf* cooperate with a distinct set of other factors to provide the necessary specificity? How does *Mitf* achieve the correct temporal sequence with which these target genes are expressed during development? What factors are responsible for the maintenance of target gene expression once *Mitf* is downregulated in differentiated cells, as is the case in the RPE? And finally, what precisely is the set of genes through which *Mitf* regulates the specification of precursor cells, the behavior of melanocyte stem cells, their survival, proliferation, migration, homing, and, ultimately, differentiation? Interestingly, an ever-growing list of genes including *Matp* (also known as *Aim-1*, underlying the *underwhite* mutation), *Mart1*, *Silver*, *OA1*, *Ink4a*, *Cdk2*, *Mif1*, and *Slug*, turn out to be targets of *Mitf (106–112)*, and their identification will undoubtedly shed light on some of these questions.

As pointed out on page 29, the lack of *Kit* or *Kitl*, similar to the lack of *Mitf*, leads to the demise of the melanocyte lineage. A lack of maintenance of KIT protein expression would therefore seem sufficient reason to explain the early loss of *Mitf* mutant melanoblasts *(29)*. However, things are rarely that simple. In fact, mutations in other genes, such as endothelin-3 (*Edn3*) and its receptor, Endothelin receptor B (*Ednrb*) may also lead to an early loss of melanoblasts *(113,114)*, but a direct link between *Mitf* and *Edn3/Ednrb* has not yet been established. We have recently found, however, that KITL generated by EDN3-responsive "nonmelanoblasts" can rescue *Ednrb*-deficient melanoblasts *(115)*, suggesting that there is perhaps an indirect link to nonmelanoblastic *Mitf* because of its response to KIT signaling. Furthermore, *Mitf* may regulate cell survival via yet another factor, the anti-apoptotic gene *Bcl2*. *Bcl2*-deficient mice are born pigmented but rapidly lose their pigmentation with the first hair cycle, earlier than *Mitfmi–vit/mi-vit* mice *(116)*. In vitro evidence suggests that *Bcl2* and *Mitf* might act in the same pathway. For instance, chromatin immunoprecipitation assays indicate that MITF associates with the Bcl2 promoter in melanoma cells, binds to an E-box in this promoter, and mutation of this E-box abolishes the stimulation of a reporter after MITF overexpression *(117)*. It has yet to be demonstrated, however, whether *Mitf* and *Bcl2* act in vivo in the same pathway. In fact, a recent study on hair graying suggests that they may not act in the same pathway *(58)*.

RPE cells react differently to *Mitf* mutations than melanocytes *(30)*. Rather than dying, RPE precursors survive and, in fact, hyperproliferate and transdifferentiate into a second neuroretina *(118,119)*. It is tempting to speculate, therefore, that if *Mitf* mutant melanoblasts could somehow be coerced to survive as well, they would hyperproliferate like RPE cells, suggesting that *Mitf* may serve as an inhibitor of cell proliferation. As listed in Table 1, although there is much indirect evidence suggesting that *Mitf* is antiproliferative, there are other studies arguing that it promotes proliferation.

To illustrate how *Mitf* might regulate cell proliferation negatively in vivo, let us turn away from pigment cells and consider retinal precursors. Early in mouse eye development (at the optic vesicle stage, *see* Fig. 1), *Mitf* is expressed in both the future retina and the future RPE. Experiments with explant cultures of such early eyes have shown that under the influence of the surface ectoderm, the juxtaposed presumptive neuroretina begins to express, or maintains expression of, the paired-like homeodomain transcription factor, CHX10 *(119)*. This factor is instrumental in the rapid downregulation of *Mitf* in the future neuroretina, because, in *Chx10* null mutant embryos, *Mitf* is no longer downregulated or is downregulated very slowly. This has the consequence that what should normally develop into a proliferating multilayered retina, now develops into a hypoplastic retina or, worse, a pigmented RPE-like monolayer in addition to the normal RPE *(81,82)*. If, however, a *Chx10*-mutant embryo also carries an *Mitf* mutation, the retina develops nearly normally, suggesting that an aberrant maintenance of wild-type *Mitf* expression slows down neuroretinal cell proliferation. Interestingly, like *Mitf* mutations, null mutations in p27Kip1 also correct the phenotype of a *Chx10* mutation *(114,115)*. p27Kip1, along with p21Cip1, belongs to a class of proteins that inhibit cdk2 and hence inhibit cyclinE/cdk2-mediated G1LS progression. One might postulate, therefore, that *Mitf* inhibits cell cycle progression in the *Chx10*-mutant retina by stimulating p27Kip1 expression. This is in line with the observation that p27Kip1 is normally expressed in the RPE during mid to late embryonic stages, when it might control the timing of cell cycle withdrawal *(122)*. A similar mechanism may operate in melanocytes, in which *Mitf* stimulates p21 expression *(123)*. Nevertheless, other studies show that *Mitf* activates the T box gene, *Tbx2*, which in turn represses the p21 promoter through a GTGGTA motif *(124)*. Moreover, Cdk2, whose product promotes G1→S progression, is stimulated by *Mitf* in some cell lines *(111,125)*. The decision on whether MTIF acts in a pro- or antiproliferative way may well depend on posttranslational modifications and on the relative abundance of each splice isoform. We recently found, for instance, that the isoform lacking exon 6a has little, if any, antiproliferative activity, in contrast to the isoform containing exon 6a *(126)*. It would therefore be of interest to analyze which isoforms are expressed in melanomas with *Mitf* gene amplifications *(127)*. In any event, it appears that there are multiple pathways with opposite activities, the perfect

Table 1
Evidence for a Role of *Mitf* in Regulating Cell Proliferation

Observation	Reference
1. Evidence consistent with inhibition of cell proliferation	
Hyperproliferation of RPE cells in *Mitf* mutants	*(30,118)*
Misexpression of *Mitf* in presumptive neuroretina reduces cell proliferation	*(81)*
Increased rate of melanoblast proliferation in the head region of *Mitfmi* heterozygous embryos	*(131)*
Activation of MITF by p38, itself associated with reduced cell proliferation	*(93)*
Mitogenic stimuli activate MAP kinase pathway and stimulate MITF degradation	*(18,19)*
Activated form of the E1A oncogene represses *Mitf*	*(132,133)*
Mitf stimulates p21 expression, an inhibitor of CyclinE/CDK2, which normally promotes G1→S progression	*(123)*
Mitf stimulates *Ink4a*, whose product promotes cell cycle exit	*(110)*
Overexpression of MITF inhibits DNA synthesis	*(123,126)*
2. Evidence consistent with promotion of cell proliferation	
In B16 melanoma cells, overexpression of wild-type β-catenin stimulates *Mitf* expression and increases the number of cells in S phase. This effect can be reversed by adding dominant-negative TCF or dominant-negative MITF.	*(130)*
Cdk2, which promotes G1→S progression, is positively regulated *Mitf (111)*. *Mtif* activates *Tbx2* which in turn suppresses p21, a negative regulator of cell cycle progression *(124)*.	

situation to allow fine-tuning of a system that is critical for achieving the appropriate balance between cell proliferation and differentiation.

All of this, of course, follows the assumption that MITF integrates the regulation of cell proliferation and differentiation solely in the capacity of what transcription factors are best known for, namely, binding enhancer motifs in target genes to stimulate or repress transcription. This, however, need not necessarily be so as MITF proteins with DNA binding mutations can retain their antiproliferative capacity upon transfection into heterologous cells *(126)*. That transcription factors can regulate cell proliferation without directly regulating transcription has been seen with other proteins as well. For instance, the homeodomain protein Six3, can promote cell proliferation by sequestering a negative regulator of cell cycle progression, geminin *(128)*. Another example is MYOD, which in proliferating, mitogen-stimulated myoblasts, is sequestered by the cyclin D1-responsive cyclin-dependent kinase, CDK4, and hence, prevented from activating muscle differentiation genes. This interaction goes both ways: MYOD also inhibits CDK4 activities, such as its inhibition of the retinoblastoma protein. Once mitogenic signals are reduced and cyclinD1 levels decrease, CDK4 is translocated to the cytoplasm, thereby allowing MYOD to form active complexes with E proteins and to activate muscle gene expression *(129)*. Taken together, the results suggest that cell proliferation and differentiation in this system are regulated by the relative levels of MYOD and CDK4:

overexpression of MYOD will override mitogenic stimulation, and overexpression of Cyclin D1 will override MYOD-mediated differentiation. If MITF regulation followed similar principles, conclusions based on cell lines in which MITF is expressed above its physiological levels would have to be taken with a grain of salt.

CONCLUSIONS AND PERSPECTIVES

Thus, it follows that similar pathways may regulate cell survival in melanoblasts and melanoma. In melanoma, the Wnt/β-catenin pathway is constitutively active, and when suppressed, for instance, by dominant-negative TCF, interferes with growth *(130)*. As mentioned, Wnt signaling is likewise critical for melanoblast development. Activating mutations in *BRAF*, which occur in a majority of melanoma, activate the MAPK-signaling pathway, and this pathway is likewise crucial for melanoblasts. For both signaling pathways, *Mitf* is a critical target. Moreover, *Brn2*, greatly overexpressed in melanoma, may suppress *Mitf* expression to some degree, and, hence, suppress an antiproliferative action of *Mitf*. *Brn2* is not expressed during early development, however, only later when melanoblasts are in the epidermis and in hair follicles, where it may function as a stimulator of cell proliferation.

These observations all suggest that a number of shared pathways operate during development, postnatal replenishment of melanocytes, and melanoma formation. No doubt, however, by homing in on a few pathways, often chosen because of the chance availability of striking genetic models or of convenient assays, we vastly simplify the intricate molecular complexities that characterize the generation of melanocytes and RPE cells and that are altered when these cells derail during malignant transformation. As time progresses, we expect that other pathways may gain favor and shine in the limelight of scientific interest, for shorter or longer periods. We hope that when all is said and done, a picture will emerge with each actor standing in his proper place on the common stage. This, we hope, will finally provide the required knowledge to design therapeutic strategies to lastingly control the growth and spread of melanoma.

ACKNOWLEDGMENTS

We express our thanks to Dr. S. Bertuzzi for providing the photomicrograph of the developing eye shown in Fig. 1B and to Dr. C. Goding for insightful suggestions and critical reading of the manuscript. In addition, we thank the National Institute of Neurological Disorders and Stroke Animal Health and Care Section for excellent animal care.

REFERENCES

1. Le Douarin NM, Kalcheim C. The Neural Crest. Cambridge University Press, Cambridge, UK: 1999.
2. Pla P, Moore R, Morali OG, Grille S, Martinozzi S, Delmas V, Larue L. Cadherins in neural crest cell development and transformation. J Cell Physiol 2001;189(2):121–132.
3. Pla P, Larue L. Involvement of endothelin receptors in normal and pathological development of neural crest cells. Int J Dev Biol 2003;47(5):315–325.
4. Hou L, Panthier JJ, Arnheiter H. Signaling and transcriptional regulation in the neural crest-derived melanocyte lineage: interactions between KIT and MITF. Development 2000;127(24):5379–5389.
5. Beermann F, Schmid E, Schutz G. Expression of the mouse tyrosinase gene during embryonic development: recapitulation of the temporal regulation in transgenic mice. Proc Natl Acad Sci USA 1992;89(7):2809–2813.
6. Ferguson CA, Kidson SH. The regulation of tyrosinase gene transcription. Pigment Cell Res 1997;10(3):127–138.
7. Cable J, Barkway C, Steel KP. Characteristics of stria vascularis melanocytes of viable dominant spotting (Wv/Wv) mouse mutants. Hear Res 1992;64(1):6–20.

8. Cable J, Huszar D, Jaenisch R, Steel KP. Effects of mutations at the W locus (c-kit) on inner ear pigmentation and function in the mouse. Pigment Cell Res 1994;7(1):17–32.

9. Tassabehji M, Newton VE, Read AP. Waardenburg syndrome type 2 caused by mutations in the human microphthalmia (MITF) gene. Nat Genet 1994;8(3):251–255.

10. Harrison RV, Palmer A, Aran JM. Some otological differences between pigmented and albino-type guinea pigs. Arch Otorhinolaryngol 1984;240(3):271–275.

11. Conlee JW, Bennett ML, Creel DJ. Differential effects of gentamicin on the distribution of cochlear function in albino and pigmented guinea pigs. Acta Otolaryngol 1995;115(3):367–374.

12. Ramon Martinez-Morales J, Rodrigo I, Bovolenta P. Eye development: a view from the retina pigmented epithelium. Bioessays 2004;26(7):766–777.

13. Bondurand N, Pingault V, Goerich DE, et al. Interaction among SOX10, PAX3 and MITF, three genes altered in Waardenburg syndrome. Hum Mol Genet 2000;9(13):1907–1917.

14. Potterf SB, Furumura M, Dunn KJ, Arnheiter H, Pavan WJ. Transcription factor hierarchy in Waardenburg Syndrome: regulation of MITF expression by SOX10 and PAX3. Hum Genet 2000;107(1):1–6.

15. Watanabe A, Takeda K, Ploplis B, Tachibana M. Epistatic relationship between Waardenburg syndrome genes MITF and PAX3. Nat Genet 1998;18(3):283–286.

16. Wehrle-Haller B. The role of Kit-ligand in melanocyte development and epidermal homeostasis. Pigment Cell Res 2003;16(3):287–296.

17. Hemesath TJ, Price ER, Takemoto C, Badalian T, Fisher DE. MAP kinase links the transcription factor Microphthalmia to c-Kit signalling in melanocytes. Nature 1998;391(6664):298–301.

18. Wu M, Hemesath TJ, Takemoto CM, et al. c-Kit triggers dual phosphorylations, which couple activation and degradation of the essential melanocyte factor Mi. Genes Dev 2000;14(3):301–312.

19. Xu W, Gong L, Haddad MM, et al. Regulation of microphthalmia-associated transcription factor MITF protein levels by association with the ubiquitin-conjugating enzyme hUBC9. Exp Cell Res 2000;255(2):135–143.

20. Goding C. Mitf from neural crest to melanoma: signal transduction and transcription in the melanocyte lineage. Genes Dev 2000;14:1712–1728.

21. Vance KW, Goding CR. The transcription network regulating melanocyte development and melanoma. Pigment Cell Res 2004;17:318–325.

22. Steingrimsson E, Copeland NG, Jenkins NA. Melanocytes and the Microphthalmia transcription factor network. Ann Rev Genet 2004;38:365–411.

23. Hodgkinson CA, Moore KJ, Nakayama A, et al. Mutations at the mouse microphthalmia locus are associated with defects in a gene encoding a novel basic-helix-loop-helix-zipper protein. Cell 1993;74(2):395–404.

24. Hughes MJ, Lingrel JB, Krakowsky JM, Anderson KP. A helix-loop-helix transcription factor-like gene is located at the mi locus. J Biol Chem 1993;268(28):20,687–20,690.

25. Hertwig P. Neue Mutationen und Kopplungsgruppen bei der Hausmaus. Z Indukt Abstammungs-u Vererbungsl 1942;80:220–246.

26. Blake JA, Richardson JE, Bult CJ, Kadin JA, Eppig JT. MGD: the Mouse Genome Database. Nucleic Acids Res 2003;31(1):193–195.

27. Hansdottir AG, Palsdottir K, Favor J, et al. The novel mouse microphthalmia mutations Mitfmi-enu5 and Mitfmi-bcc2 produce dominant negative Mitf proteins. Genomics 2004;83(5):932–935.

28. Tachibana M, Hara Y, Vyas D, et al. Cochlear disorder associated with melanocyte anomaly in mice with a transgenic insertional mutation. Mol Cell Neurosci 1992;3:433–445.

29. Opdecamp K, Nakayama A, Nguyen MT, Hodgkinson CA, Pavan WJ, Arnheiter H. Melanocyte development in vivo and in neural crest cell cultures: crucial dependence on the Mitf basic-helix-loop-helix-zipper transcription factor. Development 1997;124(12):2377–2386.

30. Nakayama A, Nguyen MT, Chen CC, Opdecamp K, Hodgkinson CA, Arnheiter H. Mutations in microphthalmia, the mouse homolog of the human deafness gene MITF, affect neuroepithelial and neural crest-derived melanocytes differently. Mech Dev 1998;70(1-2):155–166.

31. Tachibana M, Perez-Jurado LA, Nakayama A, et al. Cloning of MITF, the human homolog of the mouse microphthalmia gene and assignment to chromosome 3p14.1-p12.3. Hum Mol Genet 1994;3(4):553–557.

32. Steingrímsson E, Moore KJ, Lamoreux ML, et al. Molecular basis of mouse microphthalmia (mi) mutations helps explain their developmental and phenotypic consequences. Nat Genet 1994;8(3):256–263.

33. Hallsson JH, Favor J, Hodgkinson C, et al. Genomic, transcriptional and mutational analysis of the mouse microphthalmia locus. Genetics 2000;155(1):291–300.

34. Beckmann H, Kadesch T. The leucine zipper of TFE3 dictates helix-loop-helix dimerization specificity. Genes Dev 1991;5(6):1057–1066.
35. Hemesath TJ, Steingrimsson E, McGill G, et al. Microphthalmia, a critical factor in melanocyte development, defines a discrete transcription factor family. Genes Dev 1994;8(22):2770–2780.
36. Kuiper RP, Schepens M, Thijssen J, Schoenmakers EF, van Kessel AG. Regulation of the MiTF/TFE bHLH-LZ transcription factors through restricted spatial expression and alternative splicing of functional domains. Nucleic Acids Res 2004;32(8):2315–2322.
37. Hallsson JH, Haflidadottir BS, Stivers C, et al. The basic helix-loop-helix leucine zipper transcription factor Mitf is conserved in Drosophila and functions in eye development. Genetics 2004; 167(1):233–241.
38. Yajima I, Endo K, Sato S, et al. Cloning and functional analysis of ascidian Mitf in vivo: insights into the origin of vertebrate pigment cells. Mech Dev 2003;120(12):1489–1504.
39. Lister JA, Robertson CP, Lepage T, Johnson SL, Raible DW. Nacre encodes a zebrafish microphthalmia-related protein that regulates neural-crest-derived pigment cell fate. Development 1999;126(17):3757–3767.
40. Lister JA, Close J, Raible DW. Duplicate mitf genes in zebrafish: complementary expression and conservation of melanogenic potential. Dev Biol 2001;237(2):333–344.
41. Hodgkinson CA, Nakayama A, Li H, et al. Mutation at the anophthalmic white locus in Syrian hamsters: haploinsufficiency in the Mitf gene mimics human Waardenburg syndrome type 2. Hum Mol Genet 1998;7(4):703–708.
42. Weilbaecher KN, Motyckova G, Huber WE, et al. Linkage of M-CSF signaling to Mitf, TFE3, and the osteoclast defect in Mitf(mi/mi) mice. Mol Cell 2001;8(4):749–758.
43. Kataoka TR, Morii E, Oboki K, Kitamura Y. Strain-dependent inhibitory effect of mutant mi-MITF on cytotoxic activities of cultured mast cells and natural killer cells of mice. Lab Invest 2004;84(3):376–384.
44. Rohan PJ, Stechschulte DJ, Li Y, Dileepan KN. Macrophage function in mice with a mutation at the microphthalmia (mi) locus. Proc Soc Exp Biol Med 1997;215(3):269–724.
45. Lin L, Gerth AJ, Peng SL. Active inhibition of plasma cell development in resting B cells by microphthalmia-associated transcription factor. J Exp Med 2004;200(1):115–122.
46. Morii E, Oboki K, Ishihara K, Jippo T, Hirano T, Kitamura Y. Roles of MITF for development of mast cells in mice: effects on both precursors and tissue environments. Blood 2004;104(6):1656–1661.
47. Ringwald M, Eppig JT, Begley DA, et al. The mouse gene expression database (GXD). Nucleic Acids Res 2001;29(1):98–101.
48. Bear J, Hong Y, Schartl M. Mitf expression is sufficient to direct differentiation of medaka blastula derived stem cells to melanocytes. Development 2003;130(26):6545–6553.
49. Altschmied J, Delfgaauw J, Wilde B, et al. Subfunctionalization of duplicate mitf genes associated with differential degeneration of alternative exons in fish. Genetics 2002;161(1):259–267.
50. Kumasaka M, Sato H, Sato S, Yajima I, Yamamoto H. Isolation and developmental expression of Mitf in Xenopus laevis. Dev Dyn 2004;230(1):107–113.
51. Amae S, Fuse N, Yasumoto K, et al. Identification of a novel isoform of microphthalmia-associated transcription factor that is enriched in retinal pigment epithelium. Biochem Biophys Res Commun 1998;247(3):710–715.
52. Mochii M, Ono T, Matsubara Y, Eguchi G. Spontaneous transdifferentiation of quail pigmented epithelial cell is accompanied by a mutation in the Mitf gene. Dev Biol 1998;196(2):145–159.
53. Weilbaecher KN, Hershey CL, Takemoto CM, et al. Age-resolving osteopetrosis: a rat model implicating microphthalmia and the related transcription factor TFE3. J Exp Med 1998;187(5):775–785.
54. Opdecamp K, Vanvooren P, Riviere M, et al. The rat microphthalmia-associated transcription factor gene (Mitf) maps at 4q34-q41 and is mutated in the mib rats. Mamm Genome 1998;9(8):617–621.
55. Steingrimsson E, Arnheiter H, Hallsson JH, Lamoreux ML, Copeland NG, Jenkins NA. Interallelic complementation at the mouse Mitf locus. Genetics 2003;163(1):267–76.
56. Wolfe HG, Coleman DL. Mi-spotted: a mutation in the mouse. Genet Res Camb 1964;5:432–440.
57. Nishimura EK, Jordan SA, Oshima H, et al. Dominant role of the niche in melanocyte stem-cell fate determination. Nature 2002;416(6883):854–860.
58. Nishimura EK, Granter SR, Fisher DE. Mechanisms of hair graying: incomplete melanocyte stem cell maintenance in the niche. Science 2005;307(5710):720–724.
59. Steingrimsson E, Nii A, Fisher DE, et al. The semidominant Mi(b) mutation identifies a role for the HLH domain in DNA binding in addition to its role in protein dimerization. Embo J 1996;15(22): 6280–6289.

60. Yajima I, Sato S, Kimura T, et al. An L1 element intronic insertion in the black-eyed white (Mitf|mi-bw]) gene: the loss of a single Mitf isoform responsible for the pigmentary defect and inner ear deafness. Hum Mol Genet 1999;8(8):1431–1441.

61. Selzer E, Wacheck V, Lucas T, et al. The melanocyte-specific isoform of the microphthalmia tran-scription factor affects the phenotype of human melanoma. Cancer Res 2002;62(7):2098–2103.

62. Steingrimsson E, Tessarollo L, Pathak B, et al. Mitf and Tfe3, two members of the Mitf-Tfe family of bHLH-Zip transcription factors, have important but functionally redundant roles in osteoclast development. Proc Natl Acad Sci U S A 2002;99(7):4477–4482.

63. Tassabehji M, Read AP, Newton VE, et al. Mutations in the PAX3 gene causing Waardenburg syndrome type 1 and type 2. Nat Genet 1993;3(1):26–30.

64. Pingault V, Bondurand N, Kuhlbrodt K, et al. SOX10 mutations in patients with Waardenburg-Hirschsprung disease. Nat Genet 1998;18(2):171–173.

65. Dorsky RI, Raible DW, Moon RT. Direct regulation of nacre, a zebrafish MITF homolog required for pigment cell formation, by the Wnt pathway. Genes Dev 2000;14(2):158–162.

66. Takeda K, Yasumoto K, Takada R, et al. Induction of melanocyte-specific microphthalmia-associ-ated transcription factor by Wnt-3a. J Biol Chem 2000;275(19):14,013–14,016.

67. Dorsky RI, Moon RT, Raible DW. Control of neural crest cell fate by the Wnt signalling pathway. Nature 1998;396(6709):370–373.

68. Jin EJ, Erickson CA, Takada S, Burrus LW. Wnt and BMP signaling govern lineage segregation of melanocytes in the avian embryo. Dev Biol 2001;233(1):22–37.

69. Dunn KJ, Williams BO, Li Y, Pavan WJ. Neural crest-directed gene transfer demonstrates Wnt1 role in melanocyte expansion and differentiation during mouse development. Proc Natl Acad Sci USA 2000;97(18):10,050–10,055.

70. Ikeya M, Lee SM, Johnson JE, McMahon AP, Takada S. Wnt signalling required for expansion of neural crest and CNS progenitors. Nature 1997;389(6654):966–970.

71. Saito H, Yasumoto K, Takeda K, et al. Melanocyte-specific microphthalmia-associated transcription factor isoform activates its own gene promoter through physical interaction with lymphoid-enhanc-ing factor 1. J Biol Chem 2002;277(32):28,787–28,794.

72. Yasumoto K, Takeda K, Saito H, Watanabe K, Takahashi K, Shibahara S. Microphthalmia-associ-ated transcription factor interacts with LEF-1, a mediator of Wnt signaling. Embo J 2002;21(11): 2703–2714.

73. Bertolotto C, Abbe P, Hemesath TJ, et al. Microphthalmia gene product as a signal transducer in cAMP-induced differentiation of melanocytes. J Cell Biol 1998;142(3):827–835.

74. Busca R, Ballotti R. Cyclic AMP a key messenger in the regulation of skin pigmentation. Pigment Cell Res 2000;13(2):60–69.

75. Mayr B, Montminy M. Transcriptional regulation by the phosphorylation-dependent factor CREB. Nat Rev Mol Cell Biol 2001;2(8):599–609.

76. Huber WE, Price ER, Widlund HR, et al. A tissue-restricted cAMP transcriptional response: SOX10 modulates alpha-melanocyte-stimulating hormone-triggered expression of microphthalmia-associ-ated transcription factor in melanocytes. J Biol Chem 2003;278(46):45,224–45,230.

77. Jacquemin P, Lannoy VJ, O'Sullivan J, Read A, Lemaigre FP, Rousseau GG. The transcription factor onecut-2 controls the microphthalmia-associated transcription factor gene. Biochem Biophys Res Commun 2001;285(5):1200–1205.

78. Goodall J, Martinozzi S, Dexter TJ, et al. Brn-2 expression controls melanoma proliferation and is directly regulated by beta-catenin. Mol Cell Biol 2004;24(7):2915–2922.

79. Bäumer N, Marquardt T, Stoykova A, et al. Retinal pigmented epithelium determination requires the redundant activities of Pax2 and Pax6. Development 2003;130(13):2903–2915.

80. Martinez-Morales JR, Signore M, Acampora D, Simeone A, Bovolenta P. Otx genes are required for tissue specification in the developing eye. Development 2001;128(11):2019–2030.

81. Horsford DJ, Nguyen M-TT, Sellar GC, et al. Chx10 repression of Mitf is required for the mainte-nance of mammalian neuroretinal identity. Development 2005;132(1):177–187.

82. Rowan S, Chen C-MA, Young TL, Fisher DE, Cepko CL. Transdifferentiation of the retina into pigmented cells in ocular retardation mice defines a new function of the homeodomain gene Chx10. Development 2004;131(20):5139–5152.

83. Beechey CV, Harrison MA. A new spontaneous W allele, *W36H*. Mouse Genome 1994;92:502.

84. Dubreuil P, Forrester L, Rottapel R, Reedijk M, Fujita J, Bernstein A. The c-fms gene complements the mitogenic defect in mast cells derived from mutant W mice but not mi (microphthalmia) mice. Proc Natl Acad Sci U S A 1991;88(6):2341–2345.

85. Sato S, Roberts K, Gambino G, Cook A, Kouzarides T, Goding CR. CBP/p300 as a co-factor for the Microphthalmia transcription factor. Oncogene 1997;14(25):3083–3092.

86. Price ER, Ding HF, Badalian T, et al. Lineage-specific signaling in melanocytes. C-kit stimulation recruits p300/CBP to microphthalmia. J Biol Chem 1998;273(29):17,983–17,986.

87. Chen L, Fischle W, Verdin E, Greene WC. Duration of nuclear NF-kappaB action regulated by reversible acetylation. Science 2001;293(5535):1653–1657.

88. Levy C, Sonnenblick A, Razin E. Role played by microphthalmia transcription factor phosphorylation and its Zip domain in its transcriptional inhibition by PIAS3. Mol Cell Biol 2003;23(24):9073–9080.

89. Seeler JS, Dejean A. Nuclear and unclear functions of SUMO. Nat Rev Mol Cell Biol 2003;4(9):690–699.

90. Sachdev S, Bruhn L, Sieber H, et al. PIASy, a nuclear matrix-associated SUMO E3 ligase, represses LEF1 activity by sequestration into nuclear bodies. Genes Dev 2001;15(23):3088–3103.

91. Miller AJ, Levy C, Davis IJ, Razin E, Fisher DE. Sumoylation of MITF and its related family members TFE3 and TEFB. J Biol Chem 2005;280(1):146–155.

92. Murakami H, Arnheiter H. Sumoylation modulates transcriptional activity of MITF in a promoter-specific manner. Pigment Cell Res 2005;18:265–277.

93. Mansky KC, Sankar U, Han J, Ostrowski MC. Microphthalmia transcription factor is a target of the p38 MAPK pathway in response to receptor activator of NF-kappa B ligand signaling. J Biol Chem 2002;277(13):11,077–11,083.

94. Khaled M, Larribere L, Bille K, et al. Glycogen synthase kinase 3beta is activated by cAMP and plays an active role in the regulation of melanogenesis. J Biol Chem 2002;277(37):33,690–33,697.

95. Gaggioli C, Busca R, Abbe P, Ortonne JP, Ballotti R. Microphthalmia-associated transcription factor (MITF) is required but is not sufficient to induce the expression of melanogenic genes. Pigment Cell Res 2003;16(4):374–382.

96. Takeda K, Takemoto C, Kobayashi I, et al. Ser298 of MITF, a mutation site in Waardenburg syndrome type 2, is a phosphorylation site with functional significance. Hum Mol Genet 2000;9(1):125–132.

97. Frame S, Cohen P. GSK3 takes centre stage more than 20 years after its discovery. Biochem J 2001;359(Pt 1):1–16.

98. Haupt Y, Maya R, Kazaz A, Oren M. Mdm2 promotes the rapid degradation of p53. Nature 1997;387(6630):296–299.

99. Wellbrock C, Weisser C, Geissinger E, Troppmair J, Schartl M. Activation of p59(Fyn) leads to melanocyte dedifferentiation by influencing MKP-1-regulated mitogen-activated protein kinase signaling. J Biol Chem 2002;277(8):6443–6454.

100. Ma Q, Baldwin KT. 2,3,7,8-tetrachlorodibenzo-p-dioxin-induced degradation of aryl hydrocarbon receptor (AhR) by the ubiquitin-proteasome pathway. Role of the transcription activation and DNA binding of AhR. J Biol Chem 2000;275(12):8432–8438.

101. Lo RS, Massague J. Ubiquitin-dependent degradation of TGF-beta-activated smad2. Nat Cell Biol 1999;1(8):472–478.

102. Kim TK, Maniatis T. Regulation of interferon-gamma-activated STAT1 by the ubiquitin-proteasome pathway. Science 1996;273(5282):1717–1719.

103. Muratani M, Tansey WP. How the ubiquitin-proteasome system controls transcription. Nat Rev Mol Cell Biol 2003;4(3):192–201.

104. Lowings P, Yavuzer U, Goding CR. Positive and negative elements regulate a melanocyte-specific promoter. Mol Cell Biol 1992;12(8):3653–3662.

105. Aksan I, Goding CR. Targeting the microphthalmia basic helix-loop-helix-leucine zipper transcription factor to a subset of E-box elements in vitro and in vivo. Mol Cell Biol 1998;18(12):6930–6938.

106. Du J, Fisher DE. Identification of Aim-1 as the underwhite mouse mutant and its transcriptional regulation by MITF. J Biol Chem 2002;277(1):402 406.

107. Du J, Miller AJ, Widlund HR, Horstmann MA, Ramaswamy S, Fisher DE. MLANA/MART1 and SILV/PMEL17/GP100 are transcriptionally regulated by MITF in melanocytes and melanoma. Am J Pathol 2003;163(1):333–343.

108. Sanchez-Martin M, Perez-Losada J, Rodriguez-Garcia A, et al. Deletion of the SLUG (SNAI2) gene results in human piebaldism. Am J Med Genet 2003;122A(2):125–132.

109. Vetrini F, Auricchio A, Du J, et al. The microphthalmia transcription factor (Mitf) controls expression of the ocular albinism type 1 gene: link between melanin synthesis and melanosome biogenesis. Mol Cell Biol 2004;24(15):6550–6559.

110. Loercher AE, Tank EM, Delston RB, Harbour JW. MITF links differentiation with cell cycle arrest in melanocytes by transcriptional activation of INK4A. J Cell Biol 2005;168(1):35–40.

111. Du J, Widlund HR, Horstmann MA, et al. Critical role of CDK2 for melanoma growth linked to its melanocyte-specific transcriptional regulation by MITF. Cancer Cell 2004;6(6):565–576.

112. Busca R, Berra E, Gaggioli C, et al. Hypoxia-inducible factor 1α is a new target of microphthalmia-associated transcription factor (MITF) in melanoma cells. J Cell Biol 2005;170(1):49–59.

113. Baynash AG, Hosoda K, Giaid A, et al. Interaction of endothelin-3 with endothelin-B receptor is essential for development of epidermal melanocytes and enteric neurons. Cell 1994;79(7): 1277–1285.

114. Pavan WJ, Tilghman SM. Piebald lethal (sl) acts early to disrupt the development of neural crest-derived melanocytes. Proc Natl Acad Sci U S A 1994;91(15):7159–7163.

115. Hou L, Pavan WJ, Shin MK, Arnheiter H. Cell-autonomous and cell non-autonomous signaling through endothelin receptor B during melanocyte development. Development 2004;131(14): 3239–3247.

116. Veis DJ, Sentman CL, Bach EA, Korsmeyer SJ. Expression of the Bcl-2 protein in murine and human thymocytes and in peripheral T lymphocytes. J Immunol 1993;151(5):2546–2554.

117. McGill GG, Horstmann M, Widlund HR, et al. Bcl2 regulation by the melanocyte master regulator Mitf modulates lineage survival and melanoma cell viability. Cell 2002;109(6):707–718.

118. Müller G. Eine entwicklungsgeschichtliche Untersuchung über das erbliche Kolobom mit Mikrophthalmus bei der Hausmaus. Z Mikrosk Anat Forsch 1950;56:520–558.

119. Nguyen M, Arnheiter H. Signaling and transcriptional regulation in early mammalian eye development: a link between FGF and MITF. Development 2000;127(16):3581–3591.

120. Dyer MA. Regulation of proliferation, cell fate specification and differentiation by the homeodomain proteins Prox1, Six3, and Chx10 in the developing retina. Cell Cycle 2003;2(4):350–357.

121. Green ES, Stubbs JL, Levine EM. Genetic rescue of cell number in a mouse model of microphthalmia: interactions between Chx10 and G1-phase cell cycle regulators. Development 2003;130(3):539–552.

122. Defoe DM, Levine EM. Expression of the cyclin-dependent kinase inhibitor p27Kip1 by developing retinal pigment epithelium. Gene Expr Patterns 2003;3(5):615–619.

123. Carreira S, Goodall J, Aksan I, et al. Mitf cooperates with Rb1 and activates p21Cip1 expression to regulate cell cycle progression. Nature 2005;433(7027):764–769.

124. Prince S, Carreira S, Vance KW, Abrahams A, Goding CR. Tbx2 directly represses the expression of the p21(WAF1) cyclin-dependent kinase inhibitor. Cancer Res 2004;64(5):1669–1674.

125. Stennett LS, Riker AI, Kroll TM, et al. Expression of gp100 and CDK2 in melanoma cells is not co-regulated by a shared promotor region. Pigment Cell Res 2004;17(5):525–532.

126. Bismuth K, Mavic D, Arnheiter H. MITF and cell proliferation: The role of alternative splice forms. Pigment Cell Res 2005.

127. Garraway LA, Widlund HR, Rubin MA, et al. Integrative genomic analyses identify MITF as a lineage survival oncogene amplified in malignant meloma. Nature 2005;436(7047):117–122.

128. Del Bene F, Tessmar-Raible K, Wittbrodt J. Direct interaction of geminin and Six3 in eye development. Nature 2004;427(6976):745–749.

129. Wei Q, Paterson BM. Regulation of MyoD function in the dividing myoblast. FEBS Lett 2001;490(3):171–178.

130. Widlund HR, Horstmann MA, Price ER, et al. Beta-catenin–induced melanoma growth requires the downstream target Microphthalmia-associated transcription factor. J Cell Biol 2002;158(6): 1079–1087.

131. Hornyak TJ, Hayes DJ, Chiu LY, Ziff EB. Transcription factors in melanocyte development: distinct roles for Pax-3 and Mitf. Mech Dev 2001;101(1–2):47–59.

132. Yavuzer U, Keenan E, Lowings P, Vachtenheim J, Currie G, Goding CR. The Microphthalmia gene product interacts with the retinoblastoma protein in vitro and is a target for deregulation of melanocyte-specific transcription. Oncogene 1995;10(1):123–134.

133. Halaban R, Bohm M, Dotto P, Moellmann G, Cheng E, Zhang Y. Growth regulatory proteins that repress differentiation markers in melanocytes also downregulate the transcription factor microphthalmia. J Invest Dermatol 1996;106(6):1266–1272.

3

MITF

Critical Regulator of the Melanocyte Lineage

Erez Feige, Laura L. Poling, and David E. Fisher

Contents

Summary

The microphthalmia-associated transcription factor (MITF) is a basic helix-loop-helix–leucine zipper (bHLH-LZ) protein that acts as either a homo- or heterodimer with the related proteins TFEB, TFEC, and TFE3. Several isoforms of MITF have been identified, although only M-MITF is restricted to the melanocyte lineage. Although MITF is important in the development of multiple cell lineages, it plays a particularly important role in melanocyte differentiation and function. MITF mediates the pigmentation process through transcriptional regulation of melanogenic enzymes and processing factors. MITF is directly involved in regulation of multiple targets, some of which are established melanoma histopathological markers, as is MITF itself. As a point at which upstream signaling pathways converge, and as an activator of critical downstream cellular processes, MITF is a pivotal transcriptional regulator in the melanocyte lineage. This chapter will discuss the transcriptional and posttranslational control of MITF, will summarize the current knowledge of its target genes, and will portray our understanding of its roles in melanocytes and melanoma.

Key Words: Microphthalmia; melanocyte; melanoma; pigmentation; transcription.

INTRODUCTION

Microphthalmia-associated transcription factor (MITF) is a developmentally regulated and evolutionarily conserved transcription factor, with homologs identified from

From: *From Melanocytes to Melanoma: The Progression to Malignancy*
Edited by: V. J. Hearing and S. P. L. Leong © Humana Press Inc., Totowa, NJ

arthropods to mammals, including *Drosophila* (1), *Xenopus (2)*, zebrafish *(3)*, chicken *(4)*, mouse *(5)*, and human *(6)*. Mutations in the mouse *Mitf* locus have demonstrated that Mitf is implicated in regulation of several cell lineages. It is essential for neural crest-derived melanocytes *(5,7–9)*, as highlighted by the loss of melanocytes in mice (reviewed in ref. *10*) or melanophores in zebrafish null for *Mitf (3)*. In addition, Mitf is important for normal development of the retinal pigment epithelium (RPE), osteoclasts, and mast cells *(5,11,12)*, and some *Mitf* alleles result in small eyes, osteopetrosis, and mast cell loss. In humans, mutations in *MITF* are the cause of Waardenburg Syndrome type 2a (WS2a), characterized by hypopigmentation and sensorineural deafness resulting from loss of melanocytes in the skin, hair, and inner ear *(13)*.

Several isoforms of MITF have been identified, exhibiting diverse patterns of expression ranging from ubiquitous to cell type-specific, such as the restricted transcription of M-MITF in the melanocyte lineage. MITF expression, activity, and stability are tightly regulated through different promoters, alternative splicing, and posttranslational modifications. Data accumulating over the last decade have shed some light on the molecular mechanisms underlying MITF regulation and their roles in melanocytes. In addition, certain data suggest that MITF, or members of the *MITF/TFEB/TFEC/TFE3* (MiT) family of transcription factors, are implicated in human malignancy.

THE MiT FAMILY

MITF is a member of the MiT family of basic helix-loop-helix–leucine zipper (bHLH-LZ) transcription factors *(5)*. *MITF* maps to mouse chromosome 6 D3 *(11)* and chromosome 3p12.3-14.1 in humans *(6,13)*. Additional members of the MiT family are TFE3, TFEB, and TFEC, which have a similar genomic organization with conserved intron/exon boundaries *(14)*. The MiT members use the highly conserved basic and HLH-LZ regions to bind target DNA containing an E-box motif, CAC(G/A)TG *(15)*, and for homodimerization or heterodimerization *(15–17)*, respectively. The formation of heterodimers, such as MITF-TFE3 and MITF-TFEC, has been observed *(15,18–20)*; however, heterodimeric interactions may not be necessary for function, as suggested by redundant roles of MITF and TFE3 in osteoclast development *(21)*. Similar to MITF, the related family members TFEB and TFEC are found as alternative splice forms with differential first exon usage, indicating possible alternative promoters *(22)*. The relative expression levels of the MiT family members, combined with the alternative splice forms *(22)* and the formation of different homo/heterodimers, may contribute to tissue-specific distribution of MiT complexes.

MITF ISOFORMS

Several isoforms of MITF were identified (designated A, B, C, D, E, H, M, and Mc), which differ in their N-termini because of alternative promoters and first exons. However, all of the identified isoforms share downstream exons 2–9, which include the transactivation domain, basic region, HLH-LZ, and the known posttranslational modification target amino acids *(13,23–26)*. It is therefore unclear whether the various isoforms specify distinct functional activities for MITF or whether their different 5' ends only specify tissue expression patterns. Multiple cell types express MITF; A-, B-, C-, and H-MITF are ubiquitously expressed; and A-, C-, and H-MITF are enriched in the RPE *(5,12,25–30)*. D-MITF is also expressed in RPE cells, and can also be detected in macrophages and osteoclasts *(31)*. E- and Mc-MITF are expressed in mast cells *(18,32)*, and M-MITF is probably exclusive to melanocytes and melanoma *(29,33)*, although it has been suggested that M-MITF may be found in osteoclasts *(19)* and mast cells *(32)*.

In addition to the various MITF isoforms, two alternative splice forms have been discovered, which include or exclude six amino acids located near the basic region *(5,12)*. This isoform difference arises from an alternative splice acceptor choice, and the isoform that includes the six amino acids is absent, because of a splice-site mutation, in the mouse mutant *Mitf^{sp} (12)*. B-, H-, and M-MITF have been shown to be expressed containing or lacking the six amino acids, however the existence of these splice variants in other isoforms, and the functional significance of these six amino acids remains uncertain *(8,24,25)*. Because of the complexity of the *MITF* locus, this chapter will focus on the melanocyte-specific isoform, M-MITF.

MITF AND WAARDENBURG SYNDROME

Waardenburg Syndrome (WS) is a hereditary condition characterized by deficiency of melanocytes in the skin, hair, eyes, and inner ear, resulting in hypopigmentation and deafness. Clinically, WS is divided into four subtypes (WS1–4) according to clinical features beyond the core melanocyte-related abnormalities. The core syndrome is seen in the WS2 subtype *(34)*. Autosomal-dominant mutations of MITF result in WS2a and arise as a result of haploinsufficiency of the normal *MITF* allele *(13,35,36)*. Conversely, dominant-negative *MITF* alleles appear to produce the more severe, though highly related, albinism-deafness disorder, Tietz syndrome *(37,38)*.

Other subtypes of WS are characterized by abnormalities in addition to the features of WS2a. WS1 is associated with craniofacial deformities and WS3 (Waardenburg-Klein Syndrome) is associated with limb malformations. Both of these WS subtypes are caused by mutations in PAX3 *(39–41)*, a transcription factor that is important both in melanocytes and in other developmental lineages, such as muscle. In Waardenburg-Shah Syndrome 4 (WS4 or Waardenburg-Hirschsprung disease), additional neurological symptoms, including megacolon are observed, caused by defective enteric ganglia, derivatives of the embryonic neural crest *(42)*. WS4 is alternatively inherited in an autosomal recessive manner when associated with mutations of the endothelin-B receptor (EDNRB) *(43)* or its ligand, endothelin-3 (EDN3) *(44,45)*, or as an autosomal dominant trait when SOX10 is mutated *(42,46,47)*.

TRANSCRIPTIONAL REGULATION OF M-MITF

The regulation of *M-MITF* gene transcription appears to involve the interaction of multiple transcription factors that help confer the cell-type specific expression operating in the melanocyte lineage. The phenotypic convergence of WS2 with WS1, WS3, and WS4 has supported biochemical evidence that SOX10 and PAX3 are upstream regulators of MITF expression in melanocytes. Here, we will concentrate on the regulation of M-MITF by these, as well as by CREB and LEF-1/TCF transcription factors, shown to directly bind *cis*-acting consensus sequences and transactivate the *M-MITF* promoter/enhancer. Several transcription factors have been shown to bind and regulate the *M-MITF* promoter (*see* Fig. 1), and it is plausible that others will be discovered, because the *M-MITF* promoter/enhancer contains several evolutionarily conserved binding sites that have yet to be validated.

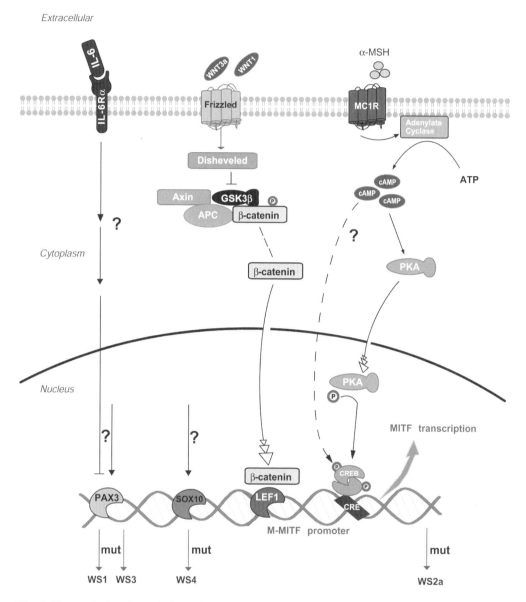

Fig. 1. Transcriptional regulation of the *M-MITF* promoter. The *M-MITF* promoter is regulated by the transcription factors CREB, LEF-1/TCF, SOX10, and PAX3. After binding of α-melanocyte stimulating hormone (α-MSH) to the melanocortin 1 receptor (MC1R), elevated cAMP levels produced by adenylate cyclase lead to phosphorylation of CREB, which binds cAMP-Responsive Element (CRE) to initiate M-MITF transcription. LEF-1/TCF-induced transcription depends on ligand (such as WNT1 or WNT3) binding to the Frizzled receptor, resulting in β-catenin release from its inhibiting complex, translocation to the nucleus, and activation of LEF-1/TCF. Although the signaling pathways affecting SOX10 and PAX3 are poorly understood, PAX3 can be affected by activated interleukin 6 receptor. Mutations in PAX3 and SOX10, as well as MITF, are associated with subtypes of the deafness-pigmentation disorder, Waardenburg Syndrome (WS), as indicated. (Graphical icons were adapted from www.biocarta.com.)

Regulation of M-MITF by CREB

M-MITF is a mediator of the pigmentation response in melanocytes, in which it is thought to bind and modulate the promoters of several major pigment enzymes via conserved E-box elements *(15,48,49)* in response to various stimuli, including the 12-amino acid peptide, α-melanocyte-stimulating hormone (α-MSH) *(50,51)*. α-MSH binds to the seven-transmembrane Melanocortin 1 receptor (MC1R), which signals to increase the intracellular cyclic adenosine monophosphate (cAMP) *(52)*. The elevated cAMP leads to phosphorylation and activation of the bZip factors CREB and ATF1 *(53)*. Activated CREB/ATF1 can bind to a consensus cAMP response element (CRE) in the promoter of its target genes.

A CRE site is located at –147, relative to the transcription start site, in the promoter of *M-MITF (8,50,54)*, and M-MITF expression can be induced via the α-MSH pathway and subsequently inhibited by an antagonist of MC1R *(50,51,55)*. This cAMP response of M-MITF through CREB/ATF1 likely explains the observed cAMP responsiveness of M-MITF target genes, such as *tyrosinase (Tyr)*. The cAMP response can also be activated with the application of various pharmaceuticals, such as forskolin, isobutyl-methylxanthine, and cholera toxin, circumventing the need for α-MSH stimulation *(56)*. With the addition of forskolin, MITF levels (RNA and protein) increase in a melanocyte-specific context *(51)*. However, because activation of CREB/ATF1 can be induced by various pathways in multiple cell lineages, an important question would be how expression of M-MITF is restricted to melanocytes. Recent data suggest that the specificity might be caused, at least in part, by cooperation between CREB/ATF1 and restricted SOX10 expression *(57)*.

Regulation by SOX10

SOX10 is a member of the *SRY box-containing* (SOX) high-mobility group (HMG) transcription factor family that is expressed in neural crest derivatives *(58)*. The study of the *Dom* (Dominant megacolon) mutant mouse which has *Sox10* mutations *(59)*, and the identification of WS4 patients with *SOX10* mutations *(42,60)*, helped identify SOX10 as a possible regulator of MITF. *In situ* hybridization using *Dom* mice, in which *Sox10* is ablated, has revealed disturbances of Mitf expression *(61)*. Although *Sox10* is not required for proper development or early migration of the neural crest, postmigratory neural crest cells in mice lacking *Sox10* undergo apoptosis before differentiation *(62)*.

SOX10 does play an important role in melanocyte differentiation as a direct regulator of M-MITF *(61,63–65)*. Several *SOX10* consensus binding elements are present in the *M-MITF* promoter *(61,63–65)*, and an additional two are present in the *M-MITF* distal enhancer *(66)*. Transactivation of the *M-MITF* promoter by SOX10 can be attenuated by constructs manifesting *SOX10* mutations identified in WS4 patients *(63–65)*. The transactivation can also be amplified by addition of PAX3, suggesting a possible synergy with SOX10 *(61,64,67)*. In addition, as stated in the previous paragraph, SOX10 has also been suggested to synergize with CREB/ATF1 to permit cAMP responsiveness of the *M-MITF* promoter in melanocytes *(57)*.

Regulation by PAX3

Mutations in *PAX3*, a paired homeodomain factor, have been associated with WS1 and WS3 *(40,41,67,68)*. WS1 patients have symptoms that overlap with WS2a patients, caused by mutation of *MITF*, consistent with a possible epistatic relationship of PAX-

3 to MITF *(69)*. The *M-MITF* promoter has been shown to be regulated by PAX3 in melanoblasts, melanocytes, and melanoma cell lines *(67,70)*. This transactivation failed when a melanoma cell line was transfected with constructs harboring *PAX3* mutations, as identified in WS1 patients *(67)*. The regulation of Mitf by Pax3 in mice seems to be further illustrated by the loss of melanocytes in the *splotch* mice, which harbor a *Pax3* mutation *(8,71)*. The role of Pax3 in the regulation of Mitf is further suggested by a study of B16/F10.9 melanoma cells, in which signaling via an interleukin-6 receptor/ interleukin-6 (IL6R/IL6) chimera led to a decrease in Pax3 mRNA and protein. This decrease was associated with downregulation of M-MITF mRNA and suppression of melanogenesis *(72)*.

Regulation by LEF-1/TCF

LEF-1/TCF, HMG-domain transcription factors, are nuclear proteins that mediate WNT signaling via an interaction with β-catenin *(73–75)*. The WNT proteins are secreted cysteine-rich glycoproteins that usually act in a paracrine fashion as the ligand for a seven-transmembrane Frizzled receptor. In the absence of WNT signals, β-catenin is complexed with the adenomatous polyposis coli tumor suppressor, axin, and glycogen synthase kinase-3β (GSK-3β). In this complex, GSK-3β phosphorylates β-catenin, thereby marking it for ubiquitination and subsequent degradation *(73)*. In the presence of WNT signals, the canonical pathway allows for the accumulation of β-catenin by inhibiting GSK-3β. The accumulated β-catenin migrates to the nucleus, where it functions as a coactivator for DNA binding factors of the LEF-1/TCF family and subsequently activates expression of target genes *(76–78)*.

The WNT-signaling pathway has been shown to play a role in the expansion *(79,80)* and differentiation of neural crest cells *(81–83)*. *M-MITF* is one of the targets of the WNT pathway as a downstream effector of WNT1 and WNT3a *(23,84–86)*. Wnt1 and Wnt3a appear to have redundant roles in melanocytes, as demonstrated by loss of melanocytes in *Wnt1⁻/⁻/Wnt3a⁻/⁻* mice *(80)*, whereas mutations in either one alone did not affect melanocytes *(87,88)*. The *M-MITF* promoter contains LEF-1/TCF consensus binding sites *(23,84)* and is directly regulated by WNT/β-catenin when complexed with LEF-1, thereby activating the *M-MITF* promoter in mammals as well as in zebrafish *(84,85,89)*.

The role of the WNT/MITF-signaling pathway in melanomagenesis is still being elucidated. Mutations in β-catenin that produce its stabilization have been found in melanoma cell lines *(90)*, but it is less clear whether these occur in primary melanoma. Nonetheless, some primary melanoma have been shown to have an accumulation of β-catenin in the nucleus, despite the lack of intrinsic mutations, suggesting that its stabilization has been dysregulated by an as yet poorly understood mechanism *(91)*. Importantly, M-MITF can rescue growth suppression of melanoma cell lines after disruption of the β-catenin/LEF-1/TCF complex *(89)*.

CRITICAL ROLES OF MITF IN THE MELANOCYTE LINEAGE

In light of the pigmentation defects in *Mitf^{mi/mi}* mutant mice and the melanocyte-specific expression of the M-MITF isoform, it was expected that MITF transcriptional targets would include genes affecting critical melanocyte functions, such as survival, proliferation, and differentiation. Indeed, data accumulating over the past decade have emphasized the importance of MITF in the melanocyte lineage, as a key regulator of various cellular processes.

Melanocyte Survival

Functional Mitf protein is required for melanocyte development and maintenance. Melanoblasts lacking Mitf die within 48 h of appearance *(30)*, demonstrating its necessity for their survival. However, Mitf presence is critical not only for melanoblasts, but also for the continued existence of differentiated cells of the melanocyte lineage. Postnatal melanocyte death and premature graying were found in hypomorphic alleles of the *microphthalmia* gene, such as in the *Mitf*$^{vit/vit}$ mice, which are born with slightly lighter than normal coat color that turns white prematurely *(12,92)*. A similar, although more accelerated, phenotype was observed with *Bcl2* knockout mice, which turn gray with the second hair follicle cycle *(93)*. This phenotype was reversed in 90% of *Bim*$^{-/-}$ *Bcl2*$^{-/-}$ double knockouts, but not in *Bim*$^{+/-}$ *Bcl2*$^{-/-}$ mice, emphasizing the delicate balance between proapoptotic and antiapoptotic proteins in melanocytes *(94)*. The identification of *BCL2* as an MITF direct target gene in melanocytes *(95)* underscored the importance of MITF in melanocyte survival, and hinted that it might contribute to the notorious resistance of melanoma to traditional chemotherapeutic treatments.

Pigment Production

Pigment production in the melanocyte lineage takes place only after cellular differentiation of unpigmented melanoblasts to melanocytes. Among the markers of melanocyte differentiation is the copper-binding protein tyrosinase (Tyr), is a melanosome membrane protein that catalyses the initial rate-limiting steps in the process of melanin biosynthesis, oxidizing tyrosine to dioxyphenylalanine (DOPA), and DOPA to DOPA quinone (reviewed in ref. *96*). Mutations in the *Tyr* locus result in various forms of hypopigmentation/albinism in mice (e.g., *albino, platinum/cp* mutations, refs. *97–99*), and are responsible for oculocutaneous albinism type I syndrome in humans, severely affecting pigmentation of the skin, hair, and eye (reviewed in ref. *100*). Expression of *Tyr* is restricted to melanocytes and RPE cells via a proximal promoter (reviewed in ref. *101*), and is probably amplified by an upstream distal enhancer *(49,102–104)*. The identification of *Tyrp1* and *dopachrome tautomerase (Dct)/Tyrp2*, *tyr*-related genes involved in later steps of melanin synthesis *(105–107)*, enabled analyses of promoter sequences, in a search for common elements that would account for the spatiotemporal expression of pigment-producing enzymes *(108–110)*. Detection of conserved DNA sequence elements in the promoters of all three genes, along with the finding that Mitf is capable of binding and transactivating this sequence element in vitro *(15)*, lead to the hypothesis that Mitf might regulate the expression of melanin biosynthesis enzymes. Indeed, reporter assays have demonstrated the ability of Mitf to transactivate the promoters of all three *Tyr* family enzymes, in an E-box-dependent manner *(15,48,49,111–114)*. In addition, inhibition of Mitf activity downregulated *Tyr* and *Tyrp1* transcription *(115,116)*, strengthening the upstream role of Mitf in regulation of pigmentation. Interestingly, overexpression of wild-type Mitf in either mouse B16 melanoma cells or human melanocytes did not upregulate Tyr levels, implying that Mitf alone is not sufficient to induce Tyr expression and might depend on cooperating protein(s) *(116)*. It is possible that a cooperative mechanism will also be implicated in the regulation of the *DCT* promoter. Although MITF can drive transactivation of a reporter gene from the *DCT* promoter *(111,114)*, a microarray screen for MITF target genes in melanocytes found that after stem cell factor (SCF) or 12-0-tetradecanoylphorbol-13-acetate (TPA) stimulation, *DCT* expression was cycloheximide-sensitive and MITF independent *(95)*. DCT is also expressed in the RPE cells of homozygous *MITF*^{vga-9} mice, although the *vga-9* mutation behaves like a null allele *(5,30)*. These data point to combinatorial regulation, and, indeed, recent studies reported synergism between MITF and LEF-1 *(117)* or SOX10 *(114)* in *DCT/TYRP2* reporter assays. Undoubtedly, MITF expression is crucial for pigment production, yet the exact mechanisms by which Mitf regulates pigmentation are still under investigation.

Additional MITF Target Genes

As a protein with restricted expression, MITF is a clinically important diagnostic marker for melanocytic neoplasms, including melanoma *(118–120)*. Recently, two other commonly used melanoma markers, SILV/Pmel17/GP100 and MLANA/MART1, were found to be regulated by MITF *(121)*. SILV is a melanosomal matrix protein, and although its function is still unknown, an insertion altering its C-terminus induces the *silver* coat color phenotype in mice *(122,123)*. MLANA/MART1 is a membrane protein whose expression is restricted to melanocytes and RPE cells, and has been suggested to play a role in early melanosome biosynthesis *(124,125)*. Expression levels of MITF, SILV, and MLANA/MART1 were found to be tightly correlated both in primary melanoma and melanoma cell lines, collectively representing the differentiation level of the tumor cells *(121)*.

Another melanocyte differentiation antigen regulated by MITF is MATP/AIM1 *(126)*, a potential sucrose transporter. Mutations in the mouse *Matp* gene are the cause of the *underwhite* phenotype, exhibiting fur and eye hypopigmentation, sometimes in an age-dependent fashion *(127)*. *MATP* is evolutionarily conserved, and a mutation in the medaka fish homolog, designated *b*, causes melanin loss and results in a goldfish-like phenotype caused by default nonmelanin pigments *(128)*. Interestingly, *MATP/AIM1* mutations were found in several oculocutaneous albinism type IV patients (*see* OMIM:606202), but their exact contribution to the phenotype is unknown.

Recently, MITF was found to be an important regulator of TRPM1/Melastatin1, a potential calcium channel protein *(129)*. Expression levels of TRPM1 inversely correlate with melanoma metastasis *(130)*, although the functional role and importance of TRPM1 are still enigmatic.

As the directory of MITF target genes is constantly growing, it is important to differentiate between immediate MITF-responsive promoters and secondarily affected genes. Several key transcription regulators were suggested to be either MITF targets or cyclo-heximide-resistant c-Kit/TPA and MITF-dependent targets in melanocytes, including the AP-1 subunits c-FOS and JUNB, ATF4, ELK1, and TBX2 *(95)*. It is plausible that the wide effect of MITF on the melanocyte lineage is at least partially mediated by regulation of such transcription factors. Although additional experiments are needed to verify the effect of MITF on the former ones, Tbx2 levels were shown to be regulated by Mitf in vitro, and Tbx2 is absent from Mitf-negative melanoblast precursor cells *(131)*. Acting as a transcriptional repressor, Tbx2 was found to negatively regulate the *Tyrp1* promoter *(132)*. However, because Tbx2 has been implicated in suppression of cell senescence through downregulation of Cdkn2a (p19^{ARF}) *(133)* and Cdkn1a (p21^{WAF1}) *(134)*, its effects in melanocytes might also be cell-cycle related.

An additional transcriptional repressor whose promoter was found to be regulated by MITF in vitro is *SNAI2/Slug (135)*. Like MITF, SNAI2 can bind E-box motifs, and mutations in *SNAI2* also result in melanocyte loss in human and mouse *(135,136)*. In this regard, the ability of SNAI2 to promote cell survival *(137)* and to downregulate E-cadherin expression in breast cancer *(138)* might suggest a role in melanoblast survival and/or migration, respectively, downstream of MITF. It is virtually certain that MITF is involved in regulation of additional target genes in melanocytes. Further identification of these targets may provide important clues to the key functional role for MITF in the melanocyte lineage.

POSTTRANSLATIONAL MODIFICATIONS OF MITF

As a key regulator of melanocyte processes, control of MITF expression and activity occurs at several levels, in addition to the transcriptional level described above. Although regulation of MITF RNA stability is poorly understood, posttranslational modifications control MITF transactivation capacity and stability *(see* Fig. 2). The phenotypic similarities between mutations in the *c-Kit* receptor tyrosine kinase, its ligand *Kitl/SCF,* and *Mitf* (described in *139),* suggested that the Mitf protein might be regulated by Kit-dependent phosphorylation. Biochemical analysis led to characterization of phosphorylation sites controlling the transactivation activity of MITF, and its half-life *(140).* On activation of the Kit/MAPK pathway, MITF is phosphorylated on Ser73 by MAPK1 (ERK2) *(140).* This modification allows it to recruit the transcriptional coactivator p300/CBP *(141).* MITF transactivation capacity may be further regulated by additional phosphorylation on Ser409 by the RPS6KA1 (RSK1) kinase (a direct target of ERK), which leads to ubiquitin-mediated proteolysis *(142).* Lysine 201 of MITF appears to be a potential ubiqitination site, because mutating it to alanine blocked proteasomal degradation of MITF *(143).* Activity of MITF seems to be dependent also on Ser298, positioned downstream of the bHLH-LZ domain. In vitro phosphorylation of Ser298 by GSK-3β was seen to enhance MITF transcriptional activity in reporter assays *(144).* The physiological importance of this residue is emphasized by characterization of a Ser298 mutation in individuals with WS2 *(39).* Although not reported in melanocytes, phosphorylation of MITF on Ser307 was found in osteoclasts after RANKL stimulation, in a p38-dependent manner *(145).* It is possible that the MITF protein is further modified on additional residues by various signaling pathways, yet to be found.

PROTEIN–PROTEIN INTERACTIONS OF MITF

In addition to its ability to form heterodimers with other MiT family members (TFE3, TFEB, and TFEC), MITF was found to interact with several other proteins, including transcription factors. As a suggested mechanism of self-amplification in melanocytes, MITF was reported to bind LEF-1, and to recruit it to its own promoter *(146).* In osteoclasts, MITF was reported to bind PU.1, an Ets family transcription factor expressed in hematopoietic cells *(147).* MITF acts downstream of PU.1 during osteoclast development, and mutations in PU.1 or MITF can cause osteopetrosis (reviewed in ref. *148).* An additional transcription factor that was shown to interact with MITF is Pax-6 *(149).* Because both *Mitf* mutations and *Pax-6* mutations cause eye abnormalities, this interaction might be important for normal RPE differentiation in vivo *(149).*

A yeast two-hybrid screen for MITF binding proteins identified UBC9, an E2 SUMO ligase, which was suggested to regulate MITF degradation through the ubiquitin-proteasome system *(143).* Interestingly, identification of an MITF interaction with PIAS3, an E3 SUMO ligase, suggests that an effect of UBC9 on MITF might be SUMO-

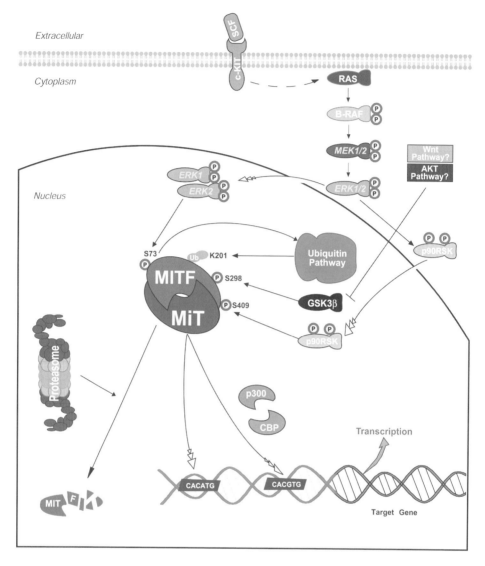

Fig. 2. Regulation of the MITF protein. After activation of the MAPK pathway, following c-KIT receptor binding by its ligand stem cell factor (SCF), MITF is phosphorylated at Ser73 by ERK2. p90RSK, acting downstream from activated ERK1/2, induces a second MITF phosphorylation, on Ser409. These modifications activate MITF, which, together with the coactivators p300/CBP, initiates transcription of target genes from E-Box elements. However, phosphorylation on Ser73 also sensitizes the protein to degradation by the proteasome via ubiquitination of Lys201. GSK-3β, acting downstream of the WNT/AKT pathways can phosphorylate MITF on Ser298. (Graphical icons were adapted from www.biocarta.com.)

mediated *(150,151)*. PIAS3 was found to downregulate the transcriptional activity of MITF, but MAPK/RSK1 phosphorylation on Ser409 of MITF disrupted PIAS3 binding and enhanced MITF transactivation capacity *(151)*. Another potential inhibitor of MITF is PKCI/HINT1, which is thought to regulate MITF in mast cells (reviewed in ref. *152*). Embryonic fibroblasts from *PKCI* null mice show cell-cycle irregularities and increased resistance to cytotoxicity by ionizing radiation, although the mice themselves have no noticeable phenotype *(153)*. Analogous to the MITF inhibition by PIAS3, MAPK-induced phosphorylation of MITF releases PKCI inhibition *(154)*.

MITF IN CANCER

A recurrent theme in cancer is the dysregulation of transcription factors. As effectors of multiple downstream genes, transcription factor levels and function are tightly regulated. However, when mutated or abnormally expressed, these proteins might lead to severe consequences, such as cancer. A well-known example is the MYC proto-oncogene, a bHLH-LZ protein that heterodimerizes with MAX to bind E-box sequences. Dysregulated expression of *c-MYC* is found in numerous cancer types, because of gene amplification or chromosomal translocation. Data emerging over the past few years have suggested that the MiT family of transcription factors might be involved in malignancy. Chromosomal translocations of *TFE3* were found in Papillary Renal Cell Carcinoma and in Alveolar Soft Part Sarcomas (reviewed in ref. *155*). In these instances, the bHLH-LZ domain of TFE3 was found fused downstream from a variety of different donor proteins, in each case forming a chimeric protein that retains the DNA-binding capacity of TFE3. Another mechanistically informative pathogenic event involves the recent identification of *TFEB* translocations in papillary renal cell carcinomas *(156–158)*. In these particular cases, a translocation was observed between chromosomes 6 and 11, and SILV/Pmel17/GP100 expression was observed in the tumor. The expression of this MITF target suggested the possibility that *TFEB* (located on chromosome 6) may be present at the translocation breakpoint. In this case, the translocation placed the entire open reading frame of TFEB downstream of the breakpoint, and the *alpha* gene into which TFEB was inserted contributed no open reading frame to the resulting transcript *(158)*. This translocation thus represents a pure example of promoter swapping and strongly suggests that the common mechanistic event in the MiT family translocations is dysregulated expression of a potentially normal MiT transcription factor *(157,158)*. Similar promoter substitution was shown to be the mechanism for *c-MYC*-induced Burkitt's lymphoma *(159,160)*. Considering the MiT family's capacity to regulate transcription via E-box elements similar to c-MYC, it is possible that a subset of c-MYC target genes may also be regulated by MiT proteins, and participate in cellular transformation, although this remains to be determined.

Although chromosomal abnormalities of the *MITF* gene have not been reported, MITF has emerged as a clinically useful histopathological marker for melanocytic lesions and has become incorporated as a common immunohistochemical target in melanoma diagnosis *(118,161–163)*. Interestingly, MITF levels often decrease during melanoma progression, although MITF signal has been detected in virtually all samples examined including amelanotic melanoma *(118,161–163)*. It is notable that expression of MITF targets such as TRPM1/melastatin1, HMB/pmel17/silver, and MLANA/Mart1 has also been seen to diminish in association with melanoma progression. The reason for this is unknown, but one may speculate that diminished MITF expression would be associated with a less differentiated phenotype (e.g., suppression of pigmentation), which may provide a growth advantage. Nonetheless, the observation that measurable MITF expression is usually retained may suggest that different target genes participate in the survival role of MITF as compared with differentiation/pigmentation, and that, mechanistically, these target genes might vary in the dose of MITF required for their regulation. Although the role of MITF in melanoma is certainly far from clear at this time, its ability to upregulate *BCL2 (95)*, an antiapoptotic gene, may be of particular importance. Moreover, a recent report showing cooperation between MITF and constitutively activated STAT3 in transformation of NIH-3T3 cells *(164)* points to a potential contribution of MITF in transformation, perhaps via upregulation of downstream targets, such as *c-Fos (95,164)*. The emerging picture from these data points to critical regulation of cellular survival and proliferation by MiT transcription factors.

CONCLUSIONS AND PERSPECTIVES

MITF is a remarkable factor in serving as a key master regulator of the entire neural crest-derived melanocyte lineage. Its loss of function produces dramatic phenotypes of melanocyte loss in numerous species, including humans. Furthermore, gain of function or dysregulated expression of its family members appear to be oncogenic in certain cell lineages. MITF plays a pivotal role in differentiation of melanocytes, largely through its ability to regulate pigment enzyme and processing gene expression. Yet, MITF clearly regulates other target genes, because pigmentation gene loss presumably cannot account for lack of melanocyte survival, as albino melanocytes are highly viable. The search for a more complete list of MITF transcriptional target genes, coupled to increased understanding of the signaling pathways and environmental cues that regulate MITF pretranslationally and posttranslationally, will stand to provide crucial information that may be of importance in both benign conditions (affecting pigmentation and deafness) as well as a variety of human malignancies, including melanoma and other MiT family-associated cancers.

ACKNOWLEDGMENTS

The authors acknowledge the outstanding contributions of numerous investigators to the work presented in this chapter. We also gratefully acknowledge the grant support of the National Institutes of Health, and the valuable advice and discussions from all members of the Fisher lab, past and present. D. E. F. is Jan and Charles Nirenberg Fellow in Pediatric Oncology at the Dana-Farber Cancer Institute.

REFERENCES

1. Hallsson JH, Haflidadottir BS, Stivers C, et al. The basic helix-loop-helix leucine zipper transcription factor mitf is conserved in Drosophila and functions in eye development. Genetics 2004; 167(1):233–241.
2. Kumasaka M, Sato H, Sato S, Yajima I, Yamamoto H. Isolation and developmental expression of Mitf in Xenopus laevis. Dev Dyn 2004;230(1):107–113.
3. Lister JA, Robertson CP, Lepage T, Johnson SL, Raible DW. Nacre encodes a zebrafish microphthalmia-related protein that regulates neural-crest–derived pigment cell fate. Development 1999;126(17):3757–3767.
4. Mochii M, Mazaki Y, Mizuno N, Hayashi H, Eguchi G. Role of Mitf in differentiation and transdifferentiation of chicken pigmented epithelial cell. Dev Biol 1998;193(1):47–62.
5. Hodgkinson CA, Moore KJ, Nakayama A, et al. Mutations at the mouse microphthalmia locus are associated with defects in a gene encoding a novel basic-helix-loop-helix-zipper protein. Cell 1993;74(2):395–404.
6. Tachibana M, Perez-Jurado LA, Nakayama A, et al. Cloning of MITF, the human homolog of the mouse microphthalmia gene and assignment to chromosome 3p14.1-p12.3. Hum Mol Genet 1994;3(4):553–557.

7. Opdecamp K, Nakayama A, Nguyen MT, Hodgkinson CA, Pavan WJ, Arnheiter H. Melanocyte development in vivo and in neural crest cell cultures: crucial dependence on the Mitf basic-helix-loop-helix-zipper transcription factor. Development 1997;124(12):2377–2386.

8. Goding CR. Mitf from neural crest to melanoma: signal transduction and transcription in the melanocyte lineage. Genes Dev 2000;14(14):1712–1728.

9. Hornyak TJ, Hayes DJ, Chiu LY, Ziff EB. Transcription factors in melanocyte development: distinct roles for Pax-3 and Mitf. Mech Dev 2001;101(1–2):47–59.

10. Moore KJ. Insight into the microphthalmia gene. Trends Genet 1995;11(11):442–448.

11. Hughes MJ, Lingrel JB, Krakowsky JM, Anderson KP. A helix-loop-helix transcription factor-like gene is located at the mi locus. J Biol Chem 1993;268(28):20,687–20,690.

12. Steingrimsson E, Moore KJ, Lamoreux ML, et al. Molecular basis of mouse microphthalmia (mi) mutations helps explain their developmental and phenotypic consequences. Nat Genet 1994; 8(3):256–263.

13. Tassabehji M, Newton VE, Read AP. Waardenburg syndrome type 2 caused by mutations in the human microphthalmia (MITF) gene. Nat Genet 1994;8(3):251–255.

14. Rehli M, Den Elzen N, Cassady AI, Ostrowski MC, Hume DA. Cloning and characterization of the murine genes for bHLH-ZIP transcription factors TFEC and TFEB reveal a common gene organization for all MiT subfamily members. Genomics 1999;56(1):111–120.

15. Hemesath TJ, Steingrimsson E, McGill G, et al. Microphthalmia, a critical factor in melanocyte development, defines a discrete transcription factor family. Genes Dev 1994;8(22):2770–2780.

16. Fisher DE, Carr CS, Parent LA, Sharp PA. TFEB has DNA-binding and oligomerization properties of a unique helix-loop-helix/leucine-zipper family. Genes Dev 1991;5(12A):2342–2352.

17. Zhao GQ, Zhao Q, Zhou X, Mattei MG, de Crombrugghe B. TFEC, a basic helix-loop-helix protein, forms heterodimers with TFE3 and inhibits TFE3-dependent transcription activation. Mol Cell Biol 1993;13(8):4505–4512.

18. Takemoto CM, Yoon YJ, Fisher DE. The identification and functional characterization of a novel mast cell isoform of the microphthalmia-associated transcription factor. J Biol Chem 2002;277(33): 30,244–30,252.

19. Mansky KC, Sulzbacher S, Purdom G, et al. The microphthalmia transcription factor and the related helix-loop-helix zipper factors TFE-3 and TFE-C collaborate to activate the tartrate-resistant acid phosphatase promoter. J Leukoc Biol 2002;71(2):304–310.

20. Weilbaecher KN, Hershey CL, Takemoto CM, et al. Age-resolving osteopetrosis: a rat model implicating microphthalmia and the related transcription factor TFE3. J Exp Med 1998;187(5):775–785.

21. Steingrimsson E, Tessarollo L, Pathak B, et al. Mitf and Tfe3, two members of the Mitf-Tfe family of bHLH-Zip transcription factors, have important but functionally redundant roles in osteoclast development. Proc Natl Acad Sci USA 2002;99(7):4477–4482.

22. Kuiper RP, Schepens M, Thijssen J, Schoenmakers EF, van Kessel AG. Regulation of the MiTF/TFE bHLH-LZ transcription factors through restricted spatial expression and alternative splicing of functional domains. Nucleic Acids Res 2004;32(8):2315–2322.

23. Saito H, Yasumoto K, Takeda K, Takahashi K, Yamamoto H, Shibahara S. Microphthalmia-associated transcription factor in the Wnt signaling pathway. Pigment Cell Res 2003;16(3):261–265.

24. Hallsson JH, Favor J, Hodgkinson C, et al. Genomic, transcriptional and mutational analysis of the mouse microphthalmia locus. Genetics 2000;155(1):291–300.

25. Udono T, Yasumoto K, Takeda K, et al. Structural organization of the human microphthalmia-associated transcription factor gene containing four alternative promoters. Biochim Biophys Acta 2000;1491(1-3):205–219.

26. Yasumoto K, Amae S, Udono T, Fuse N, Takeda K, Shibahara S. A big gene linked to small eyes encodes multiple Mitf isoforms: many promoters make light work. Pigment Cell Res 1998;11(6):329–336.

27. Shibahara S, Yasumoto K, Amae S, et al. Regulation of pigment cell-specific gene expression by MITF. Pigment Cell Res 2000;13(suppl 8):98–102.

28. Fuse N, Yasumoto K, Takeda K, et al. Molecular cloning of cDNA encoding a novel microphthalmia-associated transcription factor isoform with a distinct amino-terminus. J Biochem (Tokyo) 1999;126(6):1043–1051.

29. Amae S, Fuse N, Yasumoto K, et al. Identification of a novel isoform of microphthalmia-associated transcription factor that is enriched in retinal pigment epithelium. Biochem Biophys Res Commun 1998;247(3):710–715.

30. Nakayama A, Nguyen MT, Chen CC, Opdecamp K, Hodgkinson CA, Arnheiter H. Mutations in microphthalmia, the mouse homolog of the human deafness gene MITF, affect neuroepithelial and neural crest-derived melanocytes differently. Mech Dev 1998;70(1-2):155–166.

31. Takeda K, Yasumoto K, Kawaguchi N, et al. Mitf-D, a newly identified isoform, expressed in the retinal pigment epithelium and monocyte-lineage cells affected by Mitf mutations. Biochim Biophys Acta 2002;1574(1):15–23.

32. Oboki K, Morii E, Kataoka TR, Jippo T, Kitamura Y. Isoforms of mi transcription factor preferentially expressed in cultured mast cells of mice. Biochem Biophys Res Commun 2002;290(4): 1250–1254.

33. Fuse N, Yasumoto K, Suzuki H, Takahashi K, Shibahara S. Identification of a melanocyte-type promoter of the microphthalmia-associated transcription factor gene. Biochem Biophys Res Commun 1996;219(3):702–707.

34. Tachibana M, Kobayashi Y, Matsushima Y. Mouse models for four types of Waardenburg syndrome. Pigment Cell Res 2003;16(5):448–454.

35. Tachibana M. Evidence to suggest that expression of MITF induces melanocyte differentiation and haploinsufficiency of MITF causes Waardenburg syndrome type 2A. Pigment Cell Res 1997;10(1-2):25–33.

36. Nobukuni Y, Watanabe A, Takeda K, Skarka H, Tachibana M. Analyses of loss-of-function mutations of the MITF gene suggest that haploinsufficiency is a cause of Waardenburg syndrome type 2A. Am J Hum Genet 1996;59(1):76–83.

37. Smith SD, Kelley PM, Kenyon JB, Hoover D. Tietz syndrome (hypopigmentation/deafness) caused by mutation of MITF. J Med Genet 2000;37(6):446–448.

38. Amiel J, Watkin PM, Tassabehji M, Read AP, Winter RM. Mutation of the MITF gene in albinism-deafness syndrome (Tietz syndrome). Clin Dysmorphol 1998;7(1):17–20.

39. Tassabehji M, Newton VE, Liu XZ, et al. The mutational spectrum in Waardenburg syndrome. Hum Mol Genet 1995;4(11):2131–2137.

40. Tassabehji M, Read AP, Newton VE, et al. Waardenburg's syndrome patients have mutations in the human homologue of the Pax-3 paired box gene. Nature 1992;355(6361):635–636.

41. Baldwin CT, Hoth CF, Amos JA, da-Silva EO, Milunsky A. An exonic mutation in the HuP2 paired domain gene causes Waardenburg's syndrome. Nature 1992;355(6361):637–638.

42. Pingault V, Bondurand N, Kuhlbrodt K, et al. SOX10 mutations in patients with Waardenburg-Hirschsprung disease. Nat Genet 1998;18(2):171–173.

43. Puffenberger EG, Hosoda K, Washington SS, et al. A missense mutation of the endothelin-B receptor gene in multigenic Hirschsprung's disease. Cell 1994;79(7):1257–1266.

44. Edery P, Attie T, Amiel J, et al. Mutation of the endothelin-3 gene in the Waardenburg-Hirschsprung disease (Shah-Waardenburg syndrome). Nat Genet 1996;12(4):442–444.

45. Hofstra RM, Osinga J, Tan-Sindhunata G, et al. A homozygous mutation in the endothelin-3 gene associated with a combined Waardenburg type 2 and Hirschsprung phenotype (Shah-Waardenburg syndrome). Nat Genet 1996;12(4):445–447.

46. Touraine RL, Attie-Bitach T, Manceau E, et al. Neurological phenotype in Waardenburg syndrome type 4 correlates with novel SOX10 truncating mutations and expression in developing brain. Am J Hum Genet 2000;66(5):1496–1503.

47. Kuhlbrodt K, Schmidt C, Sock E, et al. Functional analysis of Sox10 mutations found in human Waardenburg-Hirschsprung patients. J Biol Chem 1998;273(36):23,033–23,038.

48. Bentley NJ, Eisen T, Goding CR. Melanocyte-specific expression of the human tyrosinase promoter: activation by the microphthalmia gene product and role of the initiator. Mol Cell Biol 1994;14(12): 7996–8006.

49. Yasumoto K, Yokoyama K, Shibata K, Tomita Y, Shibahara S. Microphthalmia-associated transcription factor as a regulator for melanocyte-specific transcription of the human tyrosinase gene. Mol Cell Biol 1994;14(12):8058–8070.

50. Bertolotto C, Abbe P, Hemesath TJ, et al. Microphthalmia gene product as a signal transducer in cAMP-induced differentiation of melanocytes. J Cell Biol 1998;142(3):827–835.

51. Price ER, Horstmann MA, Wells AG, et al. Alpha-Melanocyte-stimulating hormone signaling regulates expression of microphthalmia, a gene deficient in Waardenburg syndrome. J Biol Chem 1998;273(49):33,042–33,047.

52. Mountjoy KG, Robbins LS, Mortrud MT, Cone RD. The cloning of a family of genes that encode the melanocortin receptors. Science 1992;257(5074):1248–1251.

53. Roesler WJ, Park EA, McFie PJ. Characterization of CCAAT/enhancer-binding protein alpha as a cyclic AMP-responsive nuclear regulator. J Biol Chem 1998;273(24):14,950–14,957.

54. Bertolotto C, Bille K, Ortonne JP, Ballotti R. Regulation of tyrosinase gene expression by cAMP in B16 melanoma cells involves two CATGTG motifs surrounding the TATA box: implication of the microphthalmia gene product. J Cell Biol 1996;134(3):747–755.

55. Aberdam E, Bertolotto C, Sviderskaya EV, et al. Involvement of microphthalmia in the inhibition of melanocyte lineage differentiation and of melanogenesis by agouti signal protein. J Biol Chem 1998;273(31):19,560–19,565.

56. Busca R, Ballotti R. Cyclic AMP a key messenger in the regulation of skin pigmentation. Pigment Cell Res 2000;13(2):60–69.

57. Huber WE, Price ER, Widlund HR, et al. A tissue-restricted cAMP transcriptional response: SOX10 modulates alpha-melanocyte–stimulating hormone-triggered expression of microphthalmia-associated transcription factor in melanocytes. J Biol Chem 2003;278(46):45,224–45,230.

58. Bondurand N, Kobetz A, Pingault V, et al. Expression of the SOX10 gene during human development. FEBS Lett 1998;432(3):168–172.

59. Southard-Smith EM, Kos L, Pavan WJ. Sox10 mutation disrupts neural crest development in Dom Hirschsprung mouse model. Nat Genet 1998;18(1):60–64.

60. Herbarth B, Pingault V, Bondurand N, et al. Mutation of the Sry-related Sox10 gene in Dominant megacolon, a mouse model for human Hirschsprung disease. Proc Natl Acad Sci USA 1998; 95(9):5161–5165.

61. Bondurand N, Pingault V, Goerich DE, et al. Interaction among SOX10, PAX3 and MITF, three genes altered in Waardenburg syndrome. Hum Mol Genet 2000;9(13):1907–1917.

62. Mollaaghababa R, Pavan WJ. The importance of having your SOX on: role of SOX10 in the development of neural crest-derived melanocytes and glia. Oncogene 2003;22(20):3024–3034.

63. Lee M, Goodall J, Verastegui C, Ballotti R, Goding CR. Direct regulation of the Microphthalmia promoter by Sox10 links Waardenburg-Shah syndrome (WS4)-associated hypopigmentation and deafness to WS2. J Biol Chem 2000;275(48):37,978–37,983.

64. Potterf SB, Furumura M, Dunn KJ, Arnheiter H, Pavan WJ. Transcription factor hierarchy in Waardenburg syndrome: regulation of MITF expression by SOX10 and PAX3. Hum Genet 2000;107(1):1–6.

65. Verastegui C, Bille K, Ortonne JP, Ballotti R. Regulation of the microphthalmia-associated transcription factor gene by the Waardenburg syndrome type 4 gene, SOX10. J Biol Chem 2000;275(40): 30,757–30,760.

66. Watanabe K, Takeda K, Yasumoto K, et al. Identification of a distal enhancer for the melanocyte-specific promoter of the MITF gene. Pigment Cell Res 2002;15(3):201–211.

67. Watanabe A, Takeda K, Ploplis B, Tachibana M. Epistatic relationship between Waardenburg syndrome genes MITF and PAX3. Nat Genet 1998;18(3):283–286.

68. Baldwin CT, Lipsky NR, Hoth CF, Cohen T, Mamuya W, Milunsky A. Mutations in PAX3 associated with Waardenburg syndrome type I. Hum Mutat 1994;3(3):205–211.

69. Widlund HR, Fisher DE. Microphthalamia-associated transcription factor: a critical regulator of pigment cell development and survival. Oncogene 2003;22(20):3035–3041.

70. Galibert MD, Yavuzer U, Dexter TJ, Goding CR. Pax3 and regulation of the melanocyte-specific tyrosinase-related protein-1 promoter. J Biol Chem 1999;274(38):26,894–26,900.

71. Epstein DJ, Vekemans M, Gros P. Splotch (Sp2H), a mutation affecting development of the mouse neural tube, shows a deletion within the paired homeodomain of Pax-3. Cell 1991;67(4):767–774.

72. Kamaraju AK, Bertolotto C, Chebath J, Revel M. Pax3 down-regulation and shut-off of melanogenesis in melanoma B16/F10.9 by interleukin-6 receptor signaling. J Biol Chem 2002;277(17): 15,132–15,141.

73. Cadigan KM, Nusse R. Wnt signaling: a common theme in animal development. Genes Dev 1997;11(24):3286–3305.

74. Riese J, Yu X, Munnerlyn A, et al. LEF-1, a nuclear factor coordinating signaling inputs from wingless and decapentaplegic. Cell 1997;88(6):777–787.

75. Eastman Q, Grosschedl R. Regulation of LEF-1/TCF transcription factors by Wnt and other signals. Curr Opin Cell Biol 1999;11(2):233–240.

76. Behrens J, von Kries JP, Kuhl M, et al. Functional interaction of beta-catenin with the transcription factor LEF-1. Nature 1996;382(6592):638–642.

77. Huber O, Korn R, McLaughlin J, Ohsugi M, Herrmann BG, Kemler R. Nuclear localization of beta-catenin by interaction with transcription factor LEF-1. Mech Dev 1996;59(1):3–10.

78. Molenaar M, van de Wetering M, Oosterwegel M, et al. XTcf-3 transcription factor mediates beta-catenin–induced axis formation in Xenopus embryos. Cell 1996;86(3):391–399.

79. Saint-Jeannet JP, He X, Varmus HE, Dawid IB. Regulation of dorsal fate in the neuraxis by Wnt-1 and Wnt-3a. Proc Natl Acad Sci USA 1997;94(25):13,713–13,718.

80. Ikeya M, Lee SM, Johnson JE, McMahon AP, Takada S. Wnt signalling required for expansion of neural crest and CNS progenitors. Nature 1997;389(6654):966–970.

81. Dorsky RI, Moon RT, Raible DW. Control of neural crest cell fate by the Wnt signalling pathway. Nature 1998;396(6709):370–373.

82. Dunn KJ, Williams BO, Li Y, Pavan WJ. Neural crest-directed gene transfer demonstrates Wnt1 role in melanocyte expansion and differentiation during mouse development. Proc Natl Acad Sci USA 2000;97(18):10,050–10,055.

83. Jin EJ, Erickson CA, Takada S, Burrus LW. Wnt and BMP signaling govern lineage segregation of melanocytes in the avian embryo. Dev Biol 2001;233(1):22–37.

84. Dorsky RI, Raible DW, Moon RT. Direct regulation of nacre, a zebrafish MITF homolog required for pigment cell formation, by the Wnt pathway. Genes Dev 2000;14(2):158–162.

85. Takeda K, Yasumoto K, Takada R, et al. Induction of melanocyte-specific microphthalmia–associated transcription factor by Wnt-3a. J Biol Chem 2000;275(19):14,013–14,016.

86. Larue L, Kumasaka M, Goding CR. Beta-catenin in the melanocyte lineage. Pigment Cell Res 2003;16(3):312–317.

87. Thomas KR, Capecchi MR. Targeted disruption of the murine int-1 proto-oncogene resulting in severe abnormalities in midbrain and cerebellar development. Nature 1990;346(6287):847–850.

88. Takada S, Stark KL, Shea MJ, Vassileva G, McMahon JA, McMahon AP. Wnt-3a regulates somite and tailbud formation in the mouse embryo. Genes Dev 1994;8(2):174–189.

89. Widlund HR, Horstmann MA, Price ER, et al. Beta-catenin–induced melanoma growth requires the downstream target Microphthalmia-associated transcription factor. J Cell Biol 2002;158(6):1079–1087.

90. Rubinfeld B, Robbins P, El-Gamil M, Albert I, Porfiri E, Polakis P. Stabilization of beta-catenin by genetic defects in melanoma cell lines. Science 1997;275(5307):1790–1792.

91. Rimm DL, Caca K, Hu G, Harrison FB, Fearon ER. Frequent nuclear/cytoplasmic localization of beta-catenin without exon 3 mutations in malignant melanoma. Am J Pathol 1999;154(2):325–329.

92. Lerner AB, Shiohara T, Boissy RE, Jacobson KA, Lamoreux ML, Moellmann GE. A mouse model for vitiligo. J Invest Dermatol 1986;87(3):299–304.

93. Veis DJ, Sorenson CM, Shutter JR, Korsmeyer SJ. Bcl-2-deficient mice demonstrate fulminant lymphoid apoptosis, polycystic kidneys, and hypopigmented hair. Cell 1993;75(2):229–240.

94. Bouillet P, Cory S, Zhang LC, Strasser A, Adams JM. Degenerative disorders caused by Bcl-2 deficiency prevented by loss of its BH3-only antagonist Bim. Dev Cell 2001;1(5):645–653.

95. McGill GG, Horstmann M, Widlund HR, et al. Bcl2 regulation by the melanocyte master regulator Mitf modulates lineage survival and melanoma cell viability. Cell 2002;109(6):707–718.

96. Spritz RA. Molecular genetics of oculocutaneous albinism. Hum Mol Genet 1994;3 Spec No:1469–1475.

97. Halaban R, Moellmann G, Tamura A, et al. Tyrosinases of murine melanocytes with mutations at the albino locus. Proc Natl Acad Sci USA 1988;85(19):7241–7245.

98. Yokoyama T, Silversides DW, Waymire KG, Kwon BS, Takeuchi T, Overbeek PA. Conserved cysteine to serine mutation in tyrosinase is responsible for the classical albino mutation in laboratory mice. Nucleic Acids Res 1990;18(24):7293–7298.

99. Beermann F, Orlow SJ, Boissy RE, Schmidt A, Boissy YL, Lamoreux ML. Misrouting of tyrosinase with a truncated cytoplasmic tail as a result of the murine platinum (cp) mutation. Exp Eye Res 1995;61(5):599–607.

100. Oetting WS, Fryer JP, Shriram S, King RA. Oculocutaneous albinism type 1: the last 100 years. Pigment Cell Res 2003;16(3):307–311.

101. Ferguson CA, Kidson SH. The regulation of tyrosinase gene transcription. Pigment Cell Res 1997;10(3):127–138.

102. Ganss R, Montoliu L, Monaghan AP, Schutz G. A cell-specific enhancer far upstream of the mouse tyrosinase gene confers high level and copy number-related expression in transgenic mice. Embo J 1994;13(13):3083–3093.

103. Porter SD, Meyer CJ. A distal tyrosinase upstream element stimulates gene expression in neural-crest–derived melanocytes of transgenic mice: position-independent and mosaic expression. Development 1994;120(8):2103–2111.

104. Fryer JP, Oetting WS, King RA. Identification and characterization of a DNase hypersensitive region of the human tyrosinase gene. Pigment Cell Res 2003;16(6):679–684.

105. Jackson IJ. A cDNA encoding tyrosinase-related protein maps to the brown locus in mouse. Proc Natl Acad Sci USA 1988;85(12):4392–4396.

106. Jackson IJ, Chambers DM, Tsukamoto K, et al. A second tyrosinase-related protein, TRP-2, maps to and is mutated at the mouse slaty locus. Embo J 1992;11(2):527–535.

107. Tsukamoto K, Jackson IJ, Urabe K, Montague PM, Hearing VJ. A second tyrosinase-related protein, TRP-2, is a melanogenic enzyme termed DOPAchrome tautomerase. Embo J 1992;11(2):519–526.

108. Shibahara S, Taguchi H, Muller RM, et al. Structural organization of the pigment cell-specific gene located at the brown locus in mouse. Its promoter activity and alternatively spliced transcript. J Biol Chem 1991;266(24):15,895–15,901.

109. Lowings P, Yavuzer U, Goding CR. Positive and negative elements regulate a melanocyte-specific promoter. Mol Cell Biol 1992;12(8):3653–3662.

110. Yavuzer U, Goding CR. Melanocyte-specific gene expression: role of repression and identification of a melanocyte-specific factor, MSF. Mol Cell Biol 1994;14(5):3494–3503.

111. Bertolotto C, Busca R, Abbe P, et al. Different cis-acting elements are involved in the regulation of TRP1 and TRP2 promoter activities by cyclic AMP: pivotal role of M boxes (GTCATGTGCT) and of microphthalmia. Mol Cell Biol 1998;18(2):694–702.

112. Shibata K, Takeda K, Tomita Y, Tagami H, Shibahara S. Downstream region of the human tyrosinase-related protein gene enhances its promoter activity. Biochem Biophys Res Commun 1992;184(2):568–575.

113. Yasumoto K, Yokoyama K, Takahashi K, Tomita Y, Shibahara S. Functional analysis of microphthalmia-associated transcription factor in pigment cell-specific transcription of the human tyrosinase family genes. J Biol Chem 1997;272(1):503–509.

114. Ludwig A, Rehberg S, Wegner M. Melanocyte-specific expression of dopachrome tautomerase is dependent on synergistic gene activation by the Sox10 and Mitf transcription factors. FEBS Lett 2004;556(1-3):236–244.

115. Fang D, Tsuji Y, Setaluri V. Selective down-regulation of tyrosinase family gene TYRP1 by inhibition of the activity of melanocyte transcription factor, MITF. Nucleic Acids Res 2002;30(14):3096–3106.

116. Gaggioli C, Busca R, Abbe P, Ortonne JP, Ballotti R. Microphthalmia-associated transcription factor (MITF) is required but is not sufficient to induce the expression of melanogenic genes. Pigment Cell Res 2003;16(4):374–382.

117. Yasumoto K, Takeda K, Saito H, Watanabe K, Takahashi K, Shibahara S. Microphthalmia-associated transcription factor interacts with LEF-1, a mediator of Wnt signaling. EMBO J 2002;21(11):2703–2714.

118. King R, Weilbaecher KN, McGill G, Cooley E, Mihm M, Fisher DE. Microphthalmia transcription factor. A sensitive and specific melanocyte marker for melanoma diagnosis. Am J Pathol 1999;155(3):731–738.

119. O'Reilly FM, Brat DJ, McAlpine BE, Grossniklaus HE, Folpe AL, Arbiser JL. Microphthalmia transcription factor immunohistochemistry: a useful diagnostic marker in the diagnosis and detection of cutaneous melanoma, sentinel lymph node metastases, and extracutaneous melanocytic neoplasms. J Am Acad Dermatol 2001;45(3):414–419.

120. Dorvault CC, Weilbaecher KN, Yee H, et al. Microphthalmia transcription factor: a sensitive and specific marker for malignant melanoma in cytologic specimens. Cancer 2001;93(5):337–343.

121. Du J, Miller AJ, Widlund HR, Horstmann MA, Ramaswamy S, Fisher DE. MLANA/MART1 and SILV/PMEL17/GP100 are transcriptionally regulated by MITF in melanocytes and melanoma. Am J Pathol 2003;163(1):333–343.

122. Kwon BS, Chintamaneni C, Kozak CA, et al. A melanocyte-specific gene, Pmel 17, maps near the silver coat color locus on mouse chromosome 10 and is in a syntenic region on human chromosome 12. Proc Natl Acad Sci USA 1991;88(20):9228–9232.

123. Kwon BS, Kim KK, Halaban R, Pickard RT. Characterization of mouse Pmel 17 gene and silver locus. Pigment Cell Res 1994;7(6):394–397.

124. Rimoldi D, Muehlethaler K, Salvi S, et al. Subcellular localization of the melanoma-associated protein Melan-AMART-1 influences the processing of its HLA-A2–restricted epitope. J Biol Chem 2001;276(46):43,189–43,196.

125. De Maziere AM, Muehlethaler K, van Donselaar E, et al. The melanocytic protein Melan-A/MART-1 has a subcellular localization distinct from typical melanosomal proteins. Traffic 2002;3(9):678–693.

126. Du J, Fisher DE. Identification of Aim-1 as the underwhite mouse mutant and its transcriptional regulation by MITF. J Biol Chem 2002;277(1):402–406.

127. Sweet HO, Brilliant MH, Cook SA, Johnson KR, Davisson MT. A new allelic series for the underwhite gene on mouse chromosome 15. J Hered 1998;89(6):546–551.

128. Fukamachi S, Shimada A, Shima A. Mutations in the gene encoding B, a novel transporter protein, reduce melanin content in medaka. Nat Genet 2001;28(4):381–385.

129. Miller AJ, Du J, Rowan S, Hershey CL, Widlund HR, Fisher DE. Transcriptional regulation of the melanoma prognostic marker melastatin (TRPM1) by MITF in melanocytes and melanoma. Cancer Res 2004;64(2):509–516.

130. Duncan LM, Deeds J, Hunter J, et al. Down-regulation of the novel gene melastatin correlates with potential for melanoma metastasis. Cancer Res 1998;58(7):1515–1520.

131. Carreira S, Liu B, Goding CR. The gene encoding the T-box factor Tbx2 is a target for the microphthalmia-associated transcription factor in melanocytes. J Biol Chem 2000;275(29):21,920–21,927.

132. Carreira S, Dexter TJ, Yavuzer U, Easty DJ, Goding CR. Brachyury-related transcription factor Tbx2 and repression of the melanocyte-specific TRP-1 promoter. Mol Cell Biol 1998;18(9):5099–5108.

133. Jacobs JJ, Keblusek P, Robanus-Maandag E, et al. Senescence bypass screen identifies TBX2, which represses Cdkn2a (p19(ARF)) and is amplified in a subset of human breast cancers. Nat Genet 2000;26(3):291–299.

134. Prince S, Carreira S, Vance KW, Abrahams A, Goding CR. Tbx2 directly represses the expression of the p21(WAF1) cyclin-dependent kinase inhibitor. Cancer Res 2004;64(5):1669–1674.

135. Sanchez-Martin M, Rodriguez-Garcia A, Perez-Losada J, Sagrera A, Read AP, Sanchez-Garcia I. SLUG (SNAI2) deletions in patients with Waardenburg disease. Hum Mol Genet 2002;11(25):3231–3236.

136. Sanchez-Martin M, Perez-Losada J, Rodriguez-Garcia A, et al. Deletion of the SLUG (SNAI2) gene results in human piebaldism. Am J Med Genet 2003;122A(2):125–132.

137. Inukai T, Inoue A, Kurosawa H, et al. SLUG, a ces-1-related zinc finger transcription factor gene with antiapoptotic activity, is a downstream target of the E2A-HLF oncoprotein. Mol Cell 1999;4(3):343–352.

138. Hajra KM, Chen DY, Fearon ER. The SLUG zinc-finger protein represses E-cadherin in breast cancer. Cancer Res 2002;62(6):1613–1618.

139. Silvers WK. The Coat Color of Mice: A Model for Mammalian Gene Action and Interaction. Springer-Verlag, New York, NY: 1979.

140. Hemesath TJ, Price ER, Takemoto C, Badalian T, Fisher DE. MAP kinase links the transcription factor Microphthalmia to c-Kit signalling in melanocytes. Nature 1998;391(6664):298–301.

141. Price ER, Ding HF, Badalian T, et al. Lineage-specific signaling in melanocytes. C-kit stimulation recruits p300/CBP to microphthalmia. J Biol Chem 1998;273(29):17,983–17,986.

142. Wu M, Hemesath TJ, Takemoto CM, et al. c-Kit triggers dual phosphorylations, which couple activation and degradation of the essential melanocyte factor Mi. Genes Dev 2000;14(3):301–312.

143. Xu W, Gong L, Haddad MM, et al. Regulation of microphthalmia-associated transcription factor MITF protein levels by association with the ubiquitin-conjugating enzyme hUBC9. Exp Cell Res 2000;255(2):135–143.

144. Takeda K, Takemoto C, Kobayashi I, et al. Ser298 of MITF, a mutation site in Waardenburg syndrome type 2, is a phosphorylation site with functional significance. Hum Mol Genet 2000;9(1):125–132.

145. Mansky KC, Sankar U, Han J, Ostrowski MC. Microphthalmia transcription factor is a target of the p38 MAPK pathway in response to receptor activator of NF-kappa B ligand signaling. J Biol Chem 2002;277(13):11,077–11,083.

146. Saito H, Yasumoto K, Takeda K, et al. Melanocyte-specific microphthalmia-associated transcription factor isoform activates its own gene promoter through physical interaction with lymphoid-enhancing factor 1. J Biol Chem 2002;277(32):28,787–28,794.

147. Luchin A, Suchting S, Merson T, et al. Genetic and physical interactions between Microphthalmia transcription factor and PU.1 are necessary for osteoclast gene expression and differentiation. J Biol Chem 2001;276(39):36,703–36,710.

148. Hershey CL, Fisher DE. Mitf and Tfe3: members of a b-HLH-ZIP transcription factor family essential for osteoclast development and function. Bone 2004;34(4):689–696.

149. Planque N, Leconte L, Coquelle FM, Martin P, Saule S. Specific Pax-6/microphthalmia transcription factor interactions involve their DNA-binding domains and inhibit transcriptional properties of both proteins. J Biol Chem 2001;276(31):29,330–29,337.

150. Levy C, Nechushtan H, Razin E. A new role for the STAT3 inhibitor, PIAS3: a repressor of microphthalmia transcription factor. J Biol Chem 2002;277(3):1962–1966.

151. Levy C, Sonnenblick A, Razin E. Role played by microphthalmia transcription factor phosphorylation and its Zip domain in its transcriptional inhibition by PIAS3. Mol Cell Biol 2003;23(24): 9073–9080.

152. Nechushtan H, Razin E. The function of MITF and associated proteins in mast cells. Mol Immunol 2002;38(16-18):1177–1180.

153. Su T, Suzui M, Wang L, Lin CS, Xing WQ, Weinstein IB. Deletion of histidine triad nucleotide-binding protein 1/PKC-interacting protein in mice enhances cell growth and carcinogenesis. Proc Natl Acad Sci USA 2003;100(13):7824–7829.

154. Razin E, Zhang ZC, Nechushtan H, et al. Suppression of microphthalmia transcriptional activity by its association with protein kinase C-interacting protein 1 in mast cells. J Biol Chem 1999;274(48): 34,272–34,276.

155. Argani P, Ladanyi M. Recent advances in pediatric renal neoplasia. Adv Anat Pathol 2003; 10(5):243–260.

156. Argani P, Hawkins A, Griffin CA, et al. A distinctive pediatric renal neoplasm characterized by epithelioid morphology, basement membrane production, focal HMB45 immunoreactivity, and t(6;11)(p21.1;q12) chromosome translocation. Am J Pathol 2001;158(6):2089–2096.

157. Davis IJ, Hsi BL, Arroyo JD, et al. Cloning of an Alpha-TFEB fusion in renal tumors harboring the t(6;11)(p21;q13) chromosome translocation. Proc Natl Acad Sci USA 2003;100(10):6051–6056.

158. Kuiper RP, Schepens M, Thijssen J, et al. Upregulation of the transcription factor TFEB in t(6;11)(p21;q13)-positive renal cell carcinomas due to promoter substitution. Hum Mol Genet 2003;12(14):1661–1669.

159. Taub R, Kirsch I, Morton C, et al. Translocation of the c-myc gene into the immunoglobulin heavy chain locus in human Burkitt lymphoma and murine plasmacytoma cells. Proc Natl Acad Sci USA 1982;79(24):7837–7841.

160. Dalla-Favera R, Bregni M, Erikson J, Patterson D, Gallo RC, Croce CM. Human c-myc onc gene is located on the region of chromosome 8 that is translocated in Burkitt lymphoma cells. Proc Natl Acad Sci USA 1982;79(24):7824–7827.

161. Salti GI, Manougian T, Farolan M, Shilkaitis A, Majumdar D, Das Gupta TK. Micropthalmia transcription factor: a new prognostic marker in intermediate-thickness cutaneous malignant melanoma. Cancer Res 2000;60(18):5012–5016.

162. Miettinen M, Fernandez M, Franssila K, Gatalica Z, Lasota J, Sarlomo-Rikala M. Microphthalmia transcription factor in the immunohistochemical diagnosis of metastatic melanoma: comparison with four other melanoma markers. Am J Surg Pathol 2001;25(2):205–211.

163. Granter SR, Weilbaecher KN, Quigley C, Fisher DE. Role for microphthalmia transcription factor in the diagnosis of metastatic malignant melanoma. Appl Immunohistochem Mol Morphol 2002;10(1):47–51.

164. Joo A, Aburatani H, Morii E, Iba H, Yoshimura A. STAT3 and MITF cooperatively induce cellular transformation through upregulation of c-fos expression. Oncogene 2004;23(3):726–734.

4 Melanocytes and the Transcription Factor Sox10

Michael Wegner

Contents

Summary

The high-mobility group (HMG) domain transcription factor Sox10 influences melanocyte development on at least two levels. Sox10 is required for survival, proliferation, and the maintenance of pluripotent neural crest stem cells, thereby controlling the size of the stem cell pool and indirectly influencing the number of generated melanocytes. Sox10 also directly affects melanocyte specification. Expression of Mitf, the key regulator of melanocyte development, is controlled by Sox10, which binds to and activates the M promoter of the Mitf gene in close cooperation with other signaling pathways. Although its epistatic relationship to Mitf is sufficient to explain the role of Sox10 in melanocyte specification, analyses of expression and target genes suggest that Sox10 has additional functions in melanocytes apart from and following Mitf activation. Additionally, Sox10 is highly expressed in melanoma. It may influence melanoma properties and could therefore be of diagnostic and therapeutic value.

Key Words: Sry-box; HMG; neural crest; Mitf; synergy; Pax3; Waardenburg disease; dopachrome tautomerase; tyrosinase-related protein 2; β-catenin.

INTRODUCTION

Transcription factors play vital roles in the development of most cell types, tissues, and organs. Sox proteins are one such group of transcription factors. They are characterized by possession of a common DNA-binding domain, the Sry-box *(1,2)* that was first identified in Sry, a protein encoded on the mammalian Y chromosome and responsible for male sex determination *(3,4)*. This Sry-box is a variant of the HMG domain that occurs in several sequence-specific and many nonsequence-specific DNA binding proteins *(5)*. In Sox proteins, it allows minor groove DNA binding in a sequence-specific manner. Because binding concomitantly introduces a strong bend into the DNA *(6)*, Sox

From: *From Melanocytes to Melanoma: The Progression to Malignancy*
Edited by: V. J. Hearing and S. P. L. Leong © Humana Press Inc., Totowa, NJ

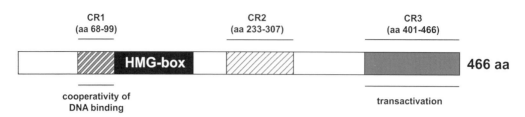

Fig. 1. Topology of conserved and functional domains in the transcription factor Sox10. Positions of conserved regions 1–3 (CR1–CR3) relative to the high-mobility group domain (HMG) of Sox10 are shown. Where known, functions of conserved domains are listed.

proteins are believed to fulfill architectural functions in chromatin in addition to their role as transcription factors *(7)*.

Sox proteins appear limited in their occurrence in animals, and have been detected in many different invertebrate and vertebrate species *(2,8)*. In mammals, such as mouse and humans, 20 different Sox proteins are present. According to amino acid similarities, both within and outside their HMG domain, these 20 Sox proteins can be further subdivided into eight groups, A–H *(2,8)*. Group E consists of Sox8, Sox9, and Sox10. In addition to the HMG domain, these proteins share three additional regions of high amino acid homology *(9)*. One of these regions is an amino-terminal extension of the HMG domain (CR1 in Fig.1), which alters the DNA binding characteristics of group E Sox proteins, because it allows them to cooperatively bind on DNA to adjacent recognition elements *(10,11)*. The second domain is located in the carboxy-terminal region of the protein and coincides with the transcriptional activation domain of Sox9 and Sox10 *(9,12,13)*. Whereas clear biochemical functions were ascribed to these regions, none has yet been attributed to the third region of homology in the central part of the protein (CR2 in Fig.1).

Sox10 has been identified and studied in many model organisms including human *(14)*, mouse *(15,16)*, rat *(9)*, chicken *(17,18)*, *Xenopus laevis (19,20)*, zebrafish *(21)*, and the puffer fish *Fugu rubripes (22)*. Sox10 proteins are highly homologous between even distantly related species. Thus, amino acid identity of *Xenopus* Sox10 and mammalian Sox10 is 71% *(20)*; and rodent and human Sox10 are 97% identical *(9)*. In all analyzed species, Sox10 has a similar expression pattern in the developing embryo, with strong expression in the early neural crest and many of its derivatives, followed by a later phase of expression in glial cells of the central nervous system. In *Xenopus*, early neural crest expression appears to be furthermore dependent on Wnt and Fgf signaling and is genetically downstream of snail *(19,20)*. However, subtle differences in Sox10 expression may exist between different species. In *Xenopus*, for instance, *Sox10* seems to be turned on sooner in cells of the premigratory neural crest than in mice *(15,19,20)*.

Although originally expressed in all neural crest cells, Sox10 is not essential for those cranial neural crest cells that form bones and mesenchyme of the face and skull. In contrast, many other neural crest cells are affected on inactivation of Sox10. The glial cells of the peripheral nervous system *(23)*, the precursor cells for the enteric nervous system, and pigment cells *(15,16,24)* are completely missing in the absence of Sox10.

Defects are similar in all species in which inactivations of the *Sox10* gene have been observed, including humans, mice, and zebrafish. These overall phenotypic similarities notwithstanding, slight differences exist between various species. Whereas heterozygous loss of Sox10 is already sufficient in mice and men to cause partial defects of pigmentation and enteric nervous system formation *(14,15)*, no such haploinsufficiency has been observed in the zebrafish *(21)*.

In zebrafish, *Sox10* is inactivated in several allelic variants of the *colorless* mutant *(21)*. In mice, a spontaneous, truncating mutation (Dominant megacolon, Dom, $Sox10^{dom}$) *(15,16)* and a targeted mutation that removes the complete open reading frame of *Sox10* ($Sox10^{lacZ}$) *(23)* have both been reported. Additionally, *SOX10* mutations were found in human patients suffering from combined Waardenburg-Hirschsprung disease *(14)*, sometimes associated with additional central or peripheral neuropathies *(25–28)*. Waardenburg disease is characterized by partial pigmentation defects of skin and hair combined with sensorineural deafness, whereas Hirschsprung disease results from aganglionosis of the distal colon. Sensorineural deafness in Waardenburg disease is generally believed to result from a melanocyte loss in the stria vascularis of the inner ear. However, the strong Sox10 expression in the olfactory placode and later in the olfactory epithelium is also compatible with a direct effect on inner ear epithelial cells in the case of *Sox10* mutations *(29)*.

Sox10 performs multiple functions at its various sites of expression. Thus, Sox10 has been implicated in maintaining the pluripotency of neural crest stem cells *(30)*; in promoting their survival and proliferation *(31)*; in influencing fate decisions *(23,32)*; and, at a later stage, in terminal differentiation of already specified precursor cells *(33)*.

Because Sox10 influences specification of several neural crest-derived cell lineages, it cannot exert its function alone but must cooperate with other cell-restricted signaling pathways and transcription factors that are differentially present or active in the various neural crest lineages. Thus, Sox10 is necessary for specification of peripheral glia and melanocytes, but clearly not sufficient.

SOX10 AND MELANOCYTES

The role of Sox10 in melanocyte development has been studied both through loss-of-function and gain-of-function analyses. Deletion of Sox10 in the mouse leads to a near complete absence of melanocytes from very early stages *(15,23,24)*, independent of the marker that was used for melanocyte detection. Injection of Sox10 RNA into one blastomere of a two-cell *Xenopus* embryo not only led to a strong expansion of neural crest cells, but also caused these neural crest cells to preferably turn into melanocytes *(19)*. This increase in the melanocyte pool size was only observed when ectopic Sox10 expression took place before gastrulation, arguing that its effect on the melanocyte lineage is an early one *(19)*. It has also been reported that Sox10 expression is rapidly downregulated from pigment cell precursors in zebrafish *(34)*, again arguing that Sox10 functions early in the melanocyte lineage, either during melanocyte specification or immediately afterwards. Because Sox10 expression at this early stage is largely confined to neural crest cells and their derivatives, a cell-intrinsic function is very likely. Formal proof was obtained by phenotypic rescue of melanocytes after selective expression of ectopic Sox10 in neural crest cells from Sox10-deficient mice *(35)*.

In mammals, Sox10 expression in the melanocyte lineage appears to last longer than in zebrafish, because Sox10 can be readily detected in most melanocyte precursors migrating along the lateral pathway in mammals but not in zebrafish *(15,21,23)*. This argues for a species-specific difference of Sox10 expression in the melanocyte lineage. Whether Sox10 expression in mammals is maintained in fully differentiated melanocytes in vivo has not been stringently tested. However, Sox10 is strongly expressed in cultures of primary and transformed melanocytes *(36–38)*. If its expression in mammalian melanocytes lasts into later stages of lineage development, Sox10 is likely to have additional effects on melanocytes apart from the specification event. These effects are, however, difficult to analyze with the currently available loss-of-function mutants. Their study requires a system that allows a temporally and spatially controlled ablation of Sox10.

SOX10 AND MITF EXPRESSION

How can the early function of Sox10 during melanocyte specification be explained on a mechanistic level? From specification onwards, many aspects of melanocyte development rely on the M-specific isoform of the bHLH protein, Mitf, which, through its target genes, influences proliferation, survival, and expression of differentiation markers in this cell lineage *(see* Chapters 2 and 3). Evidence for a genetic interaction between both genes in vivo came from crosses of heterozygous Mitf[+/mi] and Sox10[+/Dom] mice *(39)*. The resulting double heterozygous mice exhibited a dramatically increased hypopigmentation relative to the single heterozygous mice. Although this observation leaves the question of the epistatic relationship between both proteins unanswered, analysis of Sox10-deficient mice and zebrafish showed that M-Mitf (and its zebrafish homolog mitfa) is not expressed in the absence of Sox10 *(34,40)*, suggesting that expression of M-Mitf is directly controlled by Sox10.

In mammals, expression of the M-Mitf isoform is under control of the melanocyte-specific M promoter. Transcription from the human and murine M promoter is strongly activated by Sox10 *(37,39–41)*. Several putative binding sites for Sox10 were identified by sequence inspection (Fig. 2). Binding studies revealed that among these putative Sox10 binding sites, one had, by far, the highest affinity for Sox10. This site is conserved between the mouse and human promoters and is localized in the human promoter at –268 to –262, relative to the transcription start site *(37,39,40)*. Mutation of this site had the most dramatic effect on Sox10-dependent activation of the M promoter. However, Sox10 responsiveness was not completely abolished after mutation of this site and could be reduced further by additional mutation of some of the other sites. These results imply that Sox10 exerts its effect on the M promoter via multiple binding sites, of which one, however, is functionally predominant *(37,39–41)*. Whether binding of Sox10 to the M promoter is sufficient for Mitf activation under normal conditions in vivo has not been addressed so far. The identification of a 298-bp enhancer element in the human *MITF* gene located approx 14.5 kb upstream from the transcriptional start site, with additional Sox10 binding sites and Sox10 responsiveness, might at least point to participation of additional regulatory elements within the *Mitf* gene *(29)*.

Similar studies on the Mitf promoter have also been performed in zebrafish and essentially led to the same results *(34)*. The proximal Mitf promoter from zebrafish proved responsive to Sox10 and contained many Sox10-binding sites, of which one at –157 had the strongest effect, with other sites playing accessory roles. Despite this obvious similarity to the mammalian system, it is noteworthy that the sequences of the most important site in the mammalian and zebrafish promoters are not conserved *(34,40)* and represent fairly different versions of the Sox binding consensus element 5'-$^A/_T$$^A/_T$ CAA$^T/_A$G-3' *(2)*. In contrast to the studies on the human MITF promoter, analysis of the zebrafish promoter was not only performed in tissue culture, but also in embryos *(34)*, thus confirming the in vivo relevance of this regulatory pathway.

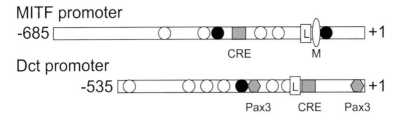

Fig. 2. Topology of mapped binding sites in the promoters of the *MITF* and *Dct* genes. The proximal promoter regions of the *MITF* gene (positions –685 to +1) and the *Dct* gene (positions –535 to +1) contain binding sites for CREB (gray rectangle, CRE); β-catenin/LEF1 (unfilled rectangle, L); Mitf (ellipse, M); Pax3 (gray hexagon); and Sox10 (circles). Functionally dominant Sox10 binding sites are shown as black circles.

Sox10 is not the only transcription factor known to influence the activity of the M promoter (Fig. 2). This promoter had previously been shown in mammals to be responsive to the canonical Wnt pathway via LEF1-binding, and to α-melanocyte-stimulating hormone (α-MSH) via binding of the cAMP-response element binding protein (CREB) *(42–45)*. The paired-domain protein Pax3, which is strongly expressed in early neural crest cells, had similarly been shown to influence M-Mitf expression by direct binding to the M promoter *(46)*.

Thus, cross talk between Sox10 and any of these activation pathways may exist. The existence of such cross talk is easily conceivable for Pax3 and Sox10, which are both expressed in neural crest cells before specification to the melanocyte lineage and the corresponding onset of Mitf expression. Indeed, Pax3 was found to synergistically activate Sox10-dependent activation of the M promoter *(39,40)*. Efficient synergistic activation of the M promoter required both Pax3 and Sox10 to bind to DNA. Interestingly, the functionally most important Sox10 binding site is located immediately adjacent to one of two Pax3 binding sites in the proximal M promoter (Fig. 2). It is currently unknown, however, whether synergy is primarily mediated by this composite element of adjacent Pax3 and Sox10 binding sites in the M promoter.

Interestingly, a residual synergistic effect between Sox10 and Pax3 was still observed after mutation of all of the Sox10 binding sites *(40)*. The most parsimonious explanation for this finding is that, under these circumstances, Sox10 is recruited indirectly to the M promoter by binding to Pax3. This synergy appears to depend on a region of Sox10 that corresponds approximately to the CR2 region of homology in the central part of group E Sox proteins (Fig. 1). Whether this region is directly involved in physical interactions with Pax3 is unclear at present, because one other study found interaction with Pax3 to be mediated by the HMG domain of Sox10 *(47)*. It also needs to be mentioned that some studies on the M promoter failed to detect synergy between Sox10 and Pax3 *(37,41)*. Given the fact that different cell lines were used in the various studies and that the experimental setup varied, it is difficult to comment on these differences. Nevertheless, synergy between Pax3 and Sox10 would effectively restrict Mitf expression in vivo to cells in which both transcription factors are coexpressed (i.e., neural crest cells), and from cells in which either Pax3 or Sox10 are expressed alone (i.e., myoblasts and oligodendrocytes).

An interesting cross talk has also been identified between α-MSH-dependent stimulation of the Mitf promoter and Sox10 *(48)*. The α-MSH pathway is primarily needed to activate pigmentation genes in melanocytes through Mitf. Although α-MSH functions via a classical cAMP response element (CRE) in the M promoter, to which CREB binds *(43,44)*, it does so in a strictly tissue-restricted manner that cannot easily be explained by the CRE element or by CREB. Interestingly, Sox10 appears to be responsible for the tissue-restricted function of the CRE based on two findings *(48)*. First, the M promoter loses most of its responsiveness toward α-MSH after mutation of the major Sox10 binding site. Second, tissue restriction of the α-MSH effect is overcome after ectopic expression of Sox10 in nonmelanocyte cell lines. CRE and Sox10 binding sites are separated by approx 100 basepairs (Fig. 2), thus making direct protein–protein contact between both proteins unlikely, unless the existence of a complex three-dimensional enhanceosome on the M promoter is invoked. Again, the combinatorial use of two transactivation pathways allows the establishment of tissue-specificity, which would not be possible through either signal alone.

No data exist so far regarding the relationship between Wnt signaling through the β-catenin/LEF1 complex and Sox10-dependent activation of the Mitf promoter. What is intriguing, however, is the fact that both LEF1 and Sox10 contain a sequence-specific HMG domain as a DNA binding domain. Although both proteins have quite similar DNA binding characteristics, the β-catenin/LEF1 complex and Sox10 are reported to function through different binding elements in the M promoter of the *Mitf* gene *(39,40,42,45)*. Several Sox proteins have also been reported to interact with β-catenin, thereby interfering with Wnt signaling *(49)*, arguing that β-catenin/LEF1 and Sox10 should influence each other during Mitf activation.

MOLECULAR SOX10 FUNCITON

Loss of melanocytes in Sox10-deficient animal models can be easily explained as a consequence of lost Mitf expression. At least in zebrafish, there is good evidence for the paramount importance of the epistatic relationship between Sox10 and Mitf. Thus, ectopic neural crest-specific expression of Mitf in Sox10-deficient zebrafish embryos was as efficient in rescuing melanophore development as was the analogous ectopic Sox10 expression *(34)*, clearly indicating that Mitf, under these circumstances, can compensate for Sox10 during melanocyte development.

This, of course, does not rule out that in other species or even during normal development in zebrafish, Mitf cannot fully compensate for the loss of Sox10. There is evidence that at least one other gene in addition to *Mitf* is regulated by Sox10 in melanocytes, although this gene is not essential for melanocyte development *(23,38,50)*. This gene is the *dopachrome tautomerase/tyrosinase-related protein-2 (Dct)*. The number of Dct-expressing cells in Sox10[+/Dom] or Sox10[+/lacZ] mouse embryos was reduced more than the number of melanoblasts detected with other markers, indicating that some melanoblasts fail to express Dct *(23,50)*. This inhibition of Dct expression was transient and most pronounced between 10.5 dpc and 12.5 dpc *(50)*. Importantly, no such selective reduction of Dct expression was observed in mice carrying heterozygous *Mitf* mutations, excluding the possibility that reduced Dct expression is secondary to Sox10 dosage effects on Mitf expression.

Analysis of the Dct upstream regulatory region over a length that had previously shown to be sufficient for melanocyte specific expression, revealed many similarities to regulation of the Mitf promoter by Sox10 *(38)*. As was the case for the Mitf promoter, the Dct upstream region contained several putative Sox10 binding sites (Fig. 2). These sites exhibited different affinities for Sox10, and bound Sox10 either as monomers or as dimers. The two sites with the highest affinities were again those with biggest contribution to Sox10-dependent activation of the Dct promoter, whereas other sites contributed to overall activation to a lesser extent. Interestingly, Sox10-dependent activation of the Dct promoter could be synergistically increased by Mitf *(38)*, which independently binds to the Dct promoter *(51)*. Thus, synergy could be severely reduced by mutation of a composite element within the Dct promoter that consisted of adjacent Sox10 and Mitf binding sites (Fig. 2), or by combinatorial mutation of all major Sox10 binding sites *(38)*. The mechanism of synergy is not clear yet. Again, synergistic activation might be essential to ensure the correct spatiotemporal Dct expression. As Sox10 expression precedes Mitf expression, Sox10-dependent Dct activation might be particularly important during the onset of Dct expression, when Mitf expression is still relatively low. Finally, it deserves to be mentioned that the Dct promoter also contains binding sites for CREB and the β-catenin/LEF1 complex (Fig. 2) *(51,52)*. Future studies will have to address whether there is also a functional interaction between Sox10 and these regulators.

SOX10 AND MELANOMA

Recently, tumor-infiltrating cytotoxic T-lymphocytes from a patient with dramatic clinical response to melanoma immunotherapy have been found to be reactive against Sox10 *(36)*. This argues that Sox10 is expressed in melanoma, a fact that could be verified by direct expression studies. Recognition by tumor-infiltrating cytotoxic T-lymphocytes correlates with a fairly high level of Sox10 expression. A second study reported that Sox10 is differentially expressed in different sublineages of K-1735 murine melanoma *(53)*. This differential expression correlated with the metastatic potential of the respective sublineages, being high in those with high metastatic potential. Upregulation of Sox10 in highly metastatic melanoma sublineages might indicate that Sox10, in addition to its many other functions, is also involved in positively regulating cell migration, a function hypothesized for Sox10 in the peripheral nervous system of zebrafish, but so far unproven *(54)*. If increased Sox10 expression is needed for increased cell mobility, interfering with Sox10 upregulation in melanoma might offer an opportunity to counteract metastasis.

Whether levels of Sox10 expression differ between melanocytes and melanoma has, however, not stringently been analyzed. The fact that Sox10 has also been identified as an antigen in cases of autoimmune-based vitiligo *(55)* argues for a strong expression already in the nontransformed state of normal melanocytes. Even if high expression is not specific for melanoma, Sox10 might still be useful as a source for peptides used in vaccination of melanoma patients who have to undergo immunotherapy. However, it needs to be pointed out that the occurrence of Sox10 in other cells apart from melanocytes might be problematic in such a strategy, because it might also direct the immune system of patients against myelinating glia of the peripheral and the central nervous system and thus cause demyelinating neuropathies.

CONCLUSIONS AND PERSPECTIVES

Sox10 is firmly established as an essential regulator of melanocyte development. However, its functions after melanocyte specification still need to be defined. Valuable insights will be derived from conditional mouse mutants that allow a temporally fine-tuned interference with Sox10 expression at later stages of melanocyte development. Equally important is a more complete characterization of Sox10 target genes in melanocytes through expression profiling or comparable approaches. By studying these target genes, common regulatory principles will be identified as well as transcription factors, with which Sox10 cooperates as part of the transcriptional network that imparts and maintains melanocyte identity. It will allow us to understand why Sox10 activates genes in melanocytes that are not turned on in other Sox10-expressing cells, and how Sox10 might be able to activate different sets of target genes at different phases of melanocyte development. Finally, it will help to clarify potential functions of Sox10 in melanoma.

ACKNOWLEDGMENTS

Work in the author's lab on Sox10 has been funded by grants from the Deutsche Forschungsgemeinschaft, the Thyssen-Stiftung, and the Volkswagen-Stiftung.

REFERENCES

1. Bowles J, Schepers G, Koopman P. Phylogeny of the SOX family of developmental transcription factors based on sequence and structural indicators. Dev Biol 2000;227:239–255.
2. Wegner M. From head to toes: the multiple facets of Sox proteins. Nucleic Acids Res 1999;27: 1409–1420.
3. Gubbay J, Collignon J, Koopman P, et al. A gene mapping to the sex-determining region of the mouse Y chromosome is a member of a novel family of embryonically expressed genes. Nature 1990;346:245–250.
4. Sinclair AH, Berta P, Palmer MS, et al. A gene from the human sex-determining region encodes a protein with homology to a conserved DNA-binding motif. Nature 1990;346:240–244.
5. Laudet V, Stehelin D, Clevers H. Ancestry and diversity of the HMG box superfamily. Nucleic Acids Res 1993;21:2493–2501.
6. Werner MH, Huth JR, Gronenborn AM, Clore GM. Molecular basis of human 46X,Y sex reversal revealed from the three-dimensional solution structure of the human SRY-DNA complex. Cell 1995;81:705–714.
7. Werner MH, Burley SK. Architectural transcription factors: proteins that remodel DNA. Cell 1997;88:733–736.
8. Schepers GE, Taesdale RD, Koopman P. Twenty pairs of Sox: extent, homology, and nomenclature of the mouse and human Sox transcription factor families. Dev Cell 2002;3:167–170.
9. Kuhlbrodt K, Herbarth B, Sock E, Hermans-Borgmeyer I, Wegner M. Sox10, a novel transcriptional modulator in glial cells. J Neurosci 1998;18:237–250.
10. Peirano RI, Wegner M. The glial transcription factor Sox10 binds to DNA both as monomer and dimer with different functional consequences. Nucleic Acids Res 2000;28:3047–3055.
11. Peirano RI, Goerich DE, Riethmacher D, Wegner M. Protein zero expression is regulated by the glial transcription factor Sox10. Mol Cell Biol 2000;20:3198–3209.
12. Südbeck P, Schmitz ML, Baeuerle PA, Scherer G. Sex reversal by loss of the C-terminal transactivation domain of human SOX9. Nature Genet 1996;13:230–232.
13. Pusch C, Hustert E, Pfeifer D, et al. The SOX10/Sox10 gene from human and mouse: sequence, expression, and transactivation by the encoded HMG domain transcription factor. Hum Genet 1998;103:115–123.
14. Pingault V, Bondurand N, Kuhlbrodt K, et al. Sox10 mutations in patients with Waardenburg-Hirschsprung disease. Nature Genet 1998;18:171–173.
15. Southard-Smith EM, Kos L, Pavan WJ. Sox10 mutation disrupts neural crest development in *Dom* Hirschsprung mouse model. Nature Genet 1998;18:60–64.
16. Herbarth B, Pingault V, Bondurand N, et al. Mutation of the Sry-related Sox10 gene in *Dominant megacolon*, a mouse model for human Hirschsprung disease. Proc Natl Acad Sci USA 1998;95: 5161–5165.
17. Bell KM, Western PS, Sinclair AH. Sox8 expression during chick embryogenesis. Mech Dev 2000;94:257–260.

18. Schneider C, Wicht H, Enderich J, Wegner M, Rohrer H. Bone morphogenetic proteins are required in vivo for the generation of sympathetic neurons. Neuron 1999;24:861–870.

19. Aoki Y, Saint-Germain N, Gyda M, et al. Sox10 regulates the development of neural crest-derived melanocytes in Xenopus. Dev Biol 2003;259:19–33.

20. Honore SM, Aybar MJ, Mayor R. Sox10 is required for the early development of the prospective neural crest in Xenopus embryos. Dev Biol 2003;260:79–96.

21. Dutton KA, Pauliny A, Lopes SS, et al. Zebrafish colourless encodes sox10 and specifies non-ectomesenchymal neural crest fates. Development 2001;128:4113–4125.

22. Koopman P, Schepers G, Brenner S, Venkatesh B. Origin and diversity of the Sox transcription factor gene family: genome-wide analysis in Fugu rubripes. Gene 2004;328:177–186.

23. Britsch S, Goerich DE, Riethmacher D, et al. The transcription factor Sox10 is a key regulator of peripheral glial development. Genes Dev 2001;15:66–78.

24. Kapur RP. Early death of neural crest cells is responsible for total enteric aganglionosis in Sox10(Dom)/Sox10(Dom) mouse embryos. Pediatr Dev Pathol 1999;2:559–569.

25. Inoue K, Shilo K, Boerkoel CF, et al. Congenital hypomyelinating neuropathy, central dysmyelination, and Waardenburg-Hirschsprung disease: phenotypes linked by SOX10 mutation. Ann Neurol 2002;52:836–842.

26. Pingault V, Bondurand N, Le Caignec C, et al. The SOX10 transcription factor: evaluation as a candidate gene for central and peripheral hereditary myelin disorders. The Clinical E.N.B.D.D. Clinical European Network on Brain Dysmyelinating Disease. J Neurol 2001;248:496–499.

27. Southard-Smith EM, Angrist M, Ellison JS, et al. The Sox10(Dom) mouse: modeling the genetic variation of Waardenburg- Shah (WS4) syndrome. Genome Res 1999;9:215–225.

28. Touraine RL, Attie-Bitach T, Manceau E, et al. Neurological phenotype in Waardenburg syndrome type 4 correlates with novel SOX10 truncating mutations and expression in developing brain. Am J Hum Genet 2000;66:1496–1503.

29. Watanabe K-I, Takeda K, Yasumoto K-I, et al. Identification of a distal enhancer for the melanocyte-specific promoter of the MITF gene. Pigment Cell Res 2002;15:201–211.

30. Kim J, Lo L, Dormand E, Anderson DJ. SOX10 maintains multipotency and inhibits neuronal differentiation of neural crest stem cells. Neuron 2003;38:17–31.

31. Sonnenberg-Riethmacher E, Miehe M, Stolt CC, Goerich DE, Wegner M, Riethmacher D. Development and degeneration of dorsal root ganglia in the absence of the HMG-domain transcription factor Sox10. Mech Dev 2001;109:253–265.

32. Paratore C, Goerich DE, Suter U, Wegner M, Sommer L. Survival and glial fate acquisition of neural crest cells are regulated by an interplay between the transcription factor Sox10 and extrinsic combinatorial signaling. Development 2001;128:3949–3961.

33. Stolt CC, Rehberg S, Ader M, et al. Terminal differentiation of myelin-forming oligodendrocytes depends on the transcription factor Sox10. Genes Dev 2002;16:165–170.

34. Elworthy S, Lister JA, Carney TJ, Raible DW, Kelsh RN. Transcriptional regulation of mitfa accounts for the sox10 requirement in zebrafish melanophore development. Development 2003;130:2809–2818.

35. Hou L, Loftus SK, Incao A, Chen A, Pavan WJ. Complementation of melanocyte development in Sox10 mutant neural crest using lineage-directed gene transfer. Dev Dyn 2004;229:54–62.

36. Khong HT, Rosenberg SA. The Waardenburg syndrome type 4 gene, SOX10, is a novel tumor-associated antigen identified in a patient with a dramatic response to immunotherapy. Cancer Res 2002;62:3020–3023.

37. Verastegui C, Bille K, Ortonne J-P, Ballotti R. Regulation of the microphthalmia-associated transcription factor gene by the Waardenburg syndrome type 4 gene, SOX10. J Biol Chem 2000;275: 30,757–30,760.

38. Ludwig A, Rehberg S, Wegner M. Melanocyte-specific expression of dopachrome tautomerase is dependent on synergistic gene activation by the Sox10 and Mitf transcription factors. FEBS Lett 2004;556:236–244.

39. Potterf BS, Furumura M, Dunn KJ, Arnheiter H, Pavan WJ. Transcription factor hierarchy in Waardenburg syndrome: regulation of MITF expression by SOX10 and PAX3. Hum Genet 2000;107:1–6.

40. Bondurand N, Pingault V, Goerich DE, et al. Interaction between SOX10, PAX3 and MITF, three genes implicated in Waardenburg syndrome. Hum Mol Genet 2000;9:1907–1917.

41. Lee M, Goodall J, Verastegui C, Ballotti R, Goding CR. Direct regulation of the microphthalmia promoter by Sox10 links Waardenburg-Shah syndrome (WS4)-associated hypopigmentation and deafness to WS2. J Biol Chem 2000;275:37,978–37,983.

42. Takeda K, Yasumoto K, Takada R, et al. Induction of melanocyte-specific microphthalmia-associated transcription factor by Wnt-3a. J Biol Chem 2000;275:14,013–14,016.

43. Price ER, Horstmann MA, Wells AG, et al. Alpha-Melanocyte–stimulating hormone signaling regulates expression of microphthalmia, a gene deficient in Waardenburg syndrome. J Biol Chem. 1998;273:33,042–33,047.

44. Fuse N, Yasumoto K, Suzuki H, Takahashi K, Shibahara S. Identification of a melanocyte-type promoter of the microphthalmia-associated transcription factor gene. Biochem Biophys Res Comm 1996;219:702–707.

45. Dorsky RI, Raible DW, Moon RT. Direct regulation of nacre, a zebrafish MITF homolog required for pigment cell formation, by the Wnt pathway. Genes Dev 2000;14:158–162.

46. Watanabe A, Takeda K, Ploplis B, Tachibana M. Epistatic relationship between Waardenburg syndrome genes MITF and PAX3. Nature Genetics 1998;18:283–286.

47. Lang D, Epstein JA. Sox10 and Pax3 physically interact to mediate activation of a conserved c-RET enhancer. Hum Mol Genet 2003;12:937–945.

48. Huber WE, Price R, Widlund HR, et al. A tissue restricted cAMP transcriptional response: SOX10 modulates MSH-triggered expression of MITF in melanocytes. J Biol Chem 2003;278:45,224–45,230.

49. Zorn AM, Barish GD, Williams BO, Lavender P, Klymkowsky MW, Varmus HE. Regulation of Wnt signaling by Sox proteins: XSox17 alpha/beta and XSox3 physically interact with beta-catenin. Mol Cell 1999;4:487–498.

50. Potterf SB, Mollaaghababa R, Hou L, et al. Analysis of SOX10 function in neural crest-derived melanocyte development: SOX10-dependent transcriptional control of dopachrome tautomerase. Dev Biol 2001;237:245–257.

51. Bertolotto C, Busca R, Abbe P, et al. Different cis-acting elements are involved in the regulation of TRP1 and TRP2 promoter activities by cyclic AMP: pivotal role of M boxes (GTCATGTGCT) and of microphthalmia. Mol Cell Biol 1998;18:694–702.

52. Yasumoto KI, Takeda K, Saito H, Watanabe K-I, Takahashi K, Shibahara S. Microphthalmia-associated transcription factor interacts with LEF-1, a mediator of Wnt signaling. EMBO J 2002;21:2703–2714.

53. Tani M, Shindo-Okada N, Hashimoto Y, et al. Isolation of a novel Sry-related gene that is expressed in high-metastatic K-1735 murine melanoma cells. Genomics 1997;39:30–37.

54. Gilmour ST, Maischein H-M, Nüsslein-Volhard C. Migration and function of a glial subtype in the vertebrate peripheral nervous system. Neuron 2002;34:577–588.

55. Hedstrand H, Ekwall O, Olsson MJ, et al. The transcription factors SOX9 and SOX10 are vitiligo autoantigens in autoimmune polyendocrine syndrome type I. J Biol Chem 2001;276:35,390–35,395.

5

Human Cutaneous Pigmentation

A Collaborative Act in the Skin,
Directed by Paracrine, Autocrine,
and Endocrine Factors and the Environment

Zalfa A. Abdel-Malek and Ana Luisa Kadekaro

CONTENTS

Summary

Cutaneous pigmentation is the outcome of exquisite interactions among various cell types in the skin, the best described of which are the interactions between epidermal melanocytes and keratinocytes, and between melanocytes and dermal fibroblasts. Melanocytes are the site of melanin synthesis, and keratinocytes are the recipients of melanosomes, melanin-containing organelles. The wide variation in constitutive pigmentation among humans is caused by enormous differences in the rate of synthesis of the two forms of melanin, eumelanin and pheomelanin, and the rate of transfer of melanosomes to keratinocytes. Cutaneous pigmentation is regulated by a wide array of factors, some of which are endocrine, and many are paracrine and/or autocrine. Many of those factors regulate constitutive pigmentation and also participate in the ultraviolet radiation (UVR)- or inflammation-induced hyperpigmentation. There is convincing evidence that the tanning response to UVR exposure is mediated by a spectrum of locally produced cytokines and growth factors, such as α-melanocyte-stimulating hormone (α-MSH) and adrenocorticotropic hormone (ACTH), and endothelin-1 (ET-1). Currently, more is known about the regulation of melanin synthesis than about the control of melanosome transfer. Only in the past few years

From: *From Melanocytes to Melanoma: The Progression to Malignancy*
Edited by: V. J. Hearing and S. P. L. Leong © Humana Press Inc., Totowa, NJ

was significant progress made in defining some of the molecular aspects and genes involved in the latter process. The significance of cutaneous pigmentation lies in its principal role in photoprotection against the carcinogenic effects of UVR. Numerous epidemiological and clinical studies have concluded that the incidence of UVR-induced skin cancer correlates inversely with constitutive pigmentation and the ability to tan. An important role of some of the paracrine/autocrine factors, such as nerve growth factor (NGF), stem cell factor (SCF), ET-1, α-MSH, or ACTH, is to protect melanocytes from stress-induced apoptosis, e.g., that induced by exposure to UVR. This survival effect is of tremendous importance given the significance of the melanocyte in photoprotection and its limited capacity to proliferate and self-renew. It is plausible that at least some of those factors might link the survival pathways to the DNA repair pathways in melanocytes. If this is the case, then the ability of melanocytes to respond to those survival factors might be a determinant of skin cancer, particularly melanoma, susceptibility.

Key Words: Human melanocytes; endocrine factors; paracrine factors; autoimmune factors; facultative pigmentation; constitutive pigmentation; photoprotection.

SKIN PIGMENTATION: THE OUTCOME OF MELANIN SYNTHESIS AND DISTRIBUTION IN THE EPIDERMIS

Melanocytes are cells that are specialized in the synthesis of melanin(s), the pigment that provides the skin and hair with their distinctive coloration. In humans, the vast majority of melanocytes reside in the epidermis and within the hair follicles, and some are present in other anatomical sites, mainly the eyes and inner ear. To date, most of the current knowledge about the regulation of human pigmentation is either based on studies of human epidermal melanocytes, or extrapolated from studies on follicular melanocytes in other mammals, mainly mice. In general, epidermal and follicular melanocytes are considered to be similar in the manner they are regulated. However, these two melanocyte populations differ in several aspects, including their life span, interaction with the surrounding epithelial and mesenchymal cells, and responses to environmental factors, particularly ultraviolet radiation (UVR).

In humans, skin pigmentation is the outcome of the synthesis of melanin by epidermal melanocytes and the distribution of melanin to surrounding keratinocytes (1). In the human epidermis, melanocytes comprise less than 10% of the entire epidermal cell population, whereas keratinocytes are the major structural cells. Melanocytes interact physically via their dendrites with the neighboring keratinocytes. Melanin-containing melanosomes are transferred along the dendrites of melanocytes to keratinocytes, and this donation of melanosomes is critical for normal skin pigmentation. The physical interaction of melanocytes with keratinocytes has led to the concept of the epidermal melanin unit, which underscores the importance of communication between these two cell types for normal pigmentation (2). Keratinocytes have a high self-renewal capacity and undergo a well-defined differentiation program that culminates in apoptotic-like cell death (3). In contrast, melanocytes in the epidermis are generally highly differentiated and slowly proliferating, and have a poor ability to regenerate. The significance of the melanocytes lies in their role in photoprotection against the damaging effects of UVR, the worst of which is skin cancer; hence, it is crucial to maintain their survival in the epidermis (4,5).

The wide diversity of skin color in humans is caused by the extensive variation in constitutive pigmentation, which, in turn, is determined by three main factors: the rate of synthesis of melanin by melanocytes, the relative amounts of eumelanin (the brown-black pigment) and pheomelanin (the red-yellow pigment) synthesized by melanocytes, and the number and size of melanosomes and the rate of their transfer to keratinocytes (1,6,7). In dark skin, melanosomes are larger and more numerous than in light skin, and are transferred as single entities from melanocytes to keratinocytes, whereas, in light skin, melanosomes are transferred as clusters *(1,8)*. Moreover, the relative eumelanin to pheomelanin contents in dark skin are always higher than those in light skin *(6)*. Melanin content in different pigmentary phenotypes is directly proportional to the activity of tyrosinase, the rate-limiting enzyme in the melanin synthetic pathway, and to the levels of tyrosinase, and tyrosinase-related proteins (TYRP), TYRP-1 and TYRP-2 *(9–12)*.

Keratinocytes also interact with melanocytes via the synthesis of biochemical mediators that regulate the survival, function, and proliferation of melanocytes *(13–18)*. In turn, the melanocytes, via donation of melanin to the keratinocytes, confer protection for the entire epidermis from damage caused by intrinsic or extrinsic environmental insults, such as inflammation or solar UVR, respectively *(19–21)*. Increased melanin synthesis by melanocytes is suggested to be part of the stress response, and to be induced by DNA damage *(22)*. Melanin, particularly eumelanin, is thought to be efficient in scavenging reactive oxygen species produced during inflammation or exposure to UVR *(23,24)*. Melanin, mainly eumelanin, also acts as a physical barrier that shields the skin from impinging UVR and limits its penetration through the epidermal layers *(25,26)*. These properties of melanin account for its photoprotective role against UVR-induced DNA damage and carcinogenesis. This important function of melanin is supported by many epidemiological studies demonstrating an inverse relationship between pigmentation and the risk for skin cancer, including melanoma *(27–29)*.

REGULATION OF PIGMENTATION BY ENDOCRINE FACTORS

Cutaneous pigmentation is the outcome of a complex process that is regulated by an array of factors that are either locally synthesized in the skin, or produced by distant organs or tissues and transported to the skin by the circulation. The importance of endocrine factors is demonstrated by the pigmentary changes observed under certain physiological and pathological conditions that involve endocrine alterations, such as pregnancy *(30)* or Addison's disease *(31,32)*, respectively. Hyperpigmentation observed in women during pregnancy is thought to be a result of changes in the levels of female reproductive hormones, such as estrogen *(33,34)*, and possibly increased melanocortins. The increased darkening of the genitalia in men and women relative to other organs is attributed to the effects of male and female reproductive hormones, respectively *(35,36)*. Melasma, which is often associated with pregnancy and augmented by sun exposure, is thought to be caused by high levels of estrogens, and melanocortins that are synthesized at a higher level in the epidermis in response to UVR *(33,34)*. In addition, increased pigmentation observed in patients with Addison's disease that results from increased adrenocorticotropic hormone (ACTH) levels is now recognized to be a result of the stimulatory effect of ACTH on human melanocytes via activation of the melanocortin 1 receptor (MC1R). Some of these clinical observations deserve to be rigorously investigated to identify the exact nature of the causative melanogenic factors and the mechanisms by which they affect skin pigmentation.

REGULATION OF PIGMENTATION BY PARACRINE
AND AUTOCRINE FACTORS

Cutaneous pigmentation is not solely regulated by endocrine factors. The traditional concept that human pigmentation is entirely subject to regulation by endocrine factors has led to some erroneous conclusions, e.g., about the significance of melanocortins in human pigmentation. In the past, it was assumed that melanocortins are only synthesized by distal organs, mainly the pituitary gland, and, because physiologically relevant levels of melanocortins could not be detected in human serum, their physiological role in human pigmentation was undermined and even discounted (37–39). A role for paracrine and autocrine factors in the regulation of skin pigmentation was first supported by the clinical observation of postinflammatory hyperpigmentation. It was proposed that inflammatory mediators, such as immune-inflammatory cytokines and eicosanoids are involved in this process (21,40). This notion was supported by the findings that the production of certain cytokines, such as interleukin (IL)-1, IL-6, and tumor necrosis factor-α (TNF-α) (41,42) and eicosanoids, such as prostaglandin (PG) E$_2$, leukotriene (LT) B$_4$, LTC$_4$, and LTD$_4$ (43,44), and histamine (45,46), all of which affect human melanocytes, is increased in the skin during inflammation.

It is established that human melanocytes (hMC) are a target for many cytokines produced by immune cells. In this review, the contributions of epidermal keratinocytes and dermal fibroblasts, the two major cell types in the skin, to the regulation of melanocytes, as well as the effects of known autocrine factors will be addressed. A list of paracrine and autocrine factors for melanocytes is included in Table 1.

The first experimental evidence for the role of paracrine factors in the regulation of hMC was provided by the observation that medium conditioned by cultured human keratinocytes increased melanogenesis and dendricity of cultured hMC (47). Although many factors affect the melanocytes directly, some factors have indirect effects on melanocytes. For example, calcitonin gene-related peptide (CGRP) that is synthesized by human keratinocytes has no direct effects on melanocytes, but conditioned media derived from human keratinocytes treated with CGRP increase hMC proliferation and melanogenesis (48). These findings suggest that CGRP stimulates keratinocytes to synthesize paracrine factors that are mitogenic and melanogenic for hMC.

Similarly, fibroblasts secrete factors that modulate hMC proliferation. Conditioned medium from cultured human fibroblasts had mitogenic effects on cultured hMC (49). Basic fibroblast growth factor (bFGF; FGF-2) is one paracrine factor that is synthesized by keratinocytes as well as fibroblasts (13,49). Other factors that are synthesized by both keratinocytes and fibroblasts include stem cell factor (SCF), also known as steel factor or kit ligand, and hepatocyte growth factor (HGF)/scatter factor, both of which are mitogenic for hMC; and nerve growth factor (NGF), which promotes melanocyte survival (49–56). Fibroblasts also express the gene for neurotrophin-3 (NT-3), which, like NGF, increases the survival of melanocytes (57). Recently, it was reported that the drastic reduction in melanocytes in palmoplantar human skin (i.e., on palms and soles) is caused, at least in part, by increased expression of dickkopf 1 (DDK1) in palmoplantar fibroblasts, which inhibits the proliferation and melanogenesis of hMC (58).

The feasibility of culturing hMC has allowed for rapid advances in understanding the regulation of human pigmentation and provided an optimal in vitro model to test the effects of various factors, including UVR. Cultured hMC were shown to respond to the immune inflammatory cytokines IL-1α, IL-1β, IL-6, and TNF-α with dose-dependent inhibition of proliferation and melanogenesis (59). Another inhibitory cytokine for hMC is transforming growth factor β (TGFβ), known to be an important autocrine regulator of epithelial cell proliferation and differentiation (60,61). Treatment of cultured hMC with TGFβ-1 inhibited their proliferation, suggesting a paracrine role for this cytokine (61). In addition, cultured hMC synthesize the primary cytokines IL-1α and

Table 1
List of the Major Paracrine and Autocrine Factors
That Affect Human Melanocyte Proliferation, Melanogenesis, and/or Survival

Cytokine/growth factor	Cell source	Effect on melanocyte		
		Proliferation	Survival	Melanogenesis
IL-1α	KC/MC	–	ND	–
IL-1β	KC/MC	–	ND	–
IL-6	KC	–	ND	–
TNF-α	KC	–	ND	–
ACTH	KC/MC	+	+	+
α-MSH	KC/MC	+	+	+
β-Endorphin	KC/MC	+	ND	+
ET-1	KC	+	+	+
ASP	KC	–	–	–
NGF	KC/FB	ND	ND	ND
NT-3	KC	ND	+	ND
B-FGF	KC/FB	+	+	+
HGF/scatter factor	KC/FB	+	ND	ND
SCF	KC/FB	+	+	ND
CGRP	KC	+	ND	+
PGE2	KC	+	ND	+
PGF2α	MC	+	ND	+
LTB4	MC	+	ND	–
LTC4	KC	+	ND	+
LTD4	KC	+	ND	+
PGF 2α	KC/MC	ND	ND	ND
12-HETE	MC	ND	ND	ND
TGFβ	KC/FB	–	ND	–
DDK1	FB	–	ND	–

IL, interleukin; TNF-α, tumor necrosis factor-α; ACTH, adrenocorticotropic hormone; α-MSH, α-melanocyte-stimulating hormone; ET-1, endothelin-1; ASP, agouti signaling protein; NGF, nerve growth factor; NT-3, neurotrophin-3; B-FGF, basic fibroblast growth factor; HGF, hepatocyte growth factor; SCF, stem cell factor; CGRP, calcitonin gene-related peptide; PG, prostaglandin; LT, leukotriene; 12-HETE, 12-hydroxyeicosatetranoic acid; TGFβ, transforming growth factor β; DDK1, dickkopf 1.

IL-1β, suggesting that these factors act as autocrine regulators *(62)*. Interestingly, the primary cytokine IL-1α has been shown to upregulate the synthesis and release of endothelin-1 (ET-1) by human keratinocytes and α-melanocyte stimulating hormone (α-MSH) by human keratinocytes and melanocytes; both factors are known to stimulate hMC proliferation and melanogenesis *(15,16,18,63–65)*. These observations point to the exquisite ability of the skin to balance the production of inhibitory and stimulatory factors to regulate melanocyte function.

Response of hMC to Eicosanoids

Eicosanoids represent two main families of arachidonic acid-derived metabolites: prostaglandins and thromboxanes that are generated from the cyclooxygenase pathway, and leukotrienes and hydroxyeicosatetraenoic acids (HETEs) that are the products of the lipoxygenase pathway. Eicosanoids have long been known for their participation in the inflammatory response and for their inhibitory effects on melanoma cells *(66–68)*. Mouse Cloudman S91 melanoma cells were found to respond to PGE_1 and PGE_2 with dose-dependent inhibition of proliferation and increase in tyrosinase activity, and to PGA_1 and PGD_2 with reduction in proliferation and tyrosinase activity *(69)*. Normal hMC were shown to respond to LTC_4 and LTD_4 with a pronounced increase in proliferation *(70)*. Comparison of the responses of hMC to PGE_2, thromboxane B_2, LTC_4, and LTD_4, revealed that all four eicosanoids increased the amount of TYRP-1 as well as the cell perimeter, cell area, and number of dendrites; with LTC_4 being the most effective *(71)*. Both LTD_4 and LTC_4 increased tyrosinase activity. In comparison, PGD_2, LTB_4, LTE_4, and 12-HETE increased the amount of TYRP-1 protein and melanocyte perimeter, but not cell area or dendricity. Additionally, hMC were found to respond to LTB_4 with increased proliferation and inhibition of tyrosinase activity (Abdel-Malek et al., unpublished results), suggesting that hMC express peroxisome proliferator-activated receptors (PPAR)-α, which are activated by their natural ligand LTB_4 *(72)*. Human melanocytes also responded to PGJ2, which binds to PPARγ, by increasing tyrosinase activity (Abdel-Malek et al., unpublished results). Recently, it was reported that hMC express EP1 and EP3 receptors, the receptors for PGE_2, as well as FP receptors, the receptors for $PGF_{2\alpha}$ *(73)*. Activation of these receptors by their ligands or agonists resulted in increased dendrite arborization by hMC, an effect that is expected to enhance melanosome transfer from melanocytes to keratinocytes. It was shown that activation of protease-activated receptor 2 (PAR 2), which is expressed on human keratinocytes and increases phagocytosis of melanosomes, enhanced the release of PGE_2 and $PGF_{2\alpha}$ *(73)*. Not only keratinocytes, but also hMC have the capacity to metabolize arachidonic acid into specific products of the cyclooxygenase and lipoxygenase pathways. Human melanocytes synthesize $PGF_{2\alpha}$, 12-HETE, and LTB_4, suggesting that these arachidonic acid metabolites might function as autocrine factors *(74)*.

Paracrine Factors That Activate Tyrosine Kinase Receptors

The discovery that bFGF, which is synthesized by keratinocytes and dermal fibroblasts, is a mitogen for hMC further substantiated the role of paracrine factors in regulating skin pigmentation *(13,49)*. The mitogenic effect of bFGF has been exploited for improving the proliferation of cultured hMC. It is recognized that hMC express specific bFGF receptors, namely FGF receptor-1, and that bFGF activates signaling pathways, namely its own tyrosine kinase receptor and protein kinase C, that are critical for hMC proliferation and survival *(75)*. Unlike most other paracrine factors, bFGF is not secreted by keratinocytes *(13)*, which raises the question of how it interacts with melanocytes. One possibility is that keratinocytes secrete bFGF together with extracellular matrix components. This possibility is supported by the observation that extracellular matrix produced by cells in response to bFGF mimics all the effects of bFGF on these cells *(76)*. Another growth factor that is synthesized by human keratinocytes and fibroblasts and is mitogenic for hMC is hepatocyte growth factor (HGF) *(49,52,77–79)*. Similar to bFGF, HGF regulates hMC directly by binding to its specific tyrosine kinase receptor, c-Met *(80)*.

The effects of SCF are mediated by activation of its specific tyrosine kinase receptor, c-kit *(81)*. SCF is synthesized by various skin cells, including epidermal keratinocytes and dermal fibroblasts *(49,82)*. Stem cell factor is a critical survival factor for various cell types, including melanocytes, hemopoietic cells, and germline cells (50,83,84). It has been known for a long time that mutations that disrupt either the gene for SCF or its tyrosine kinase receptor, c-KIT, result in white spotting in mice, resulting from failure of melanoblasts to migrate to the skin from the neural crest during embryonic development (85). In humans, piebaldism that is characterized by congenital loss of melanocytes from patches of skin and hair results from a mutation in the Kit gene (86). Stem cell factor is a mitogen for hMC in culture (87). When adult human skin grafted onto nude mice was injected with recombinant human SCF, an increase in melanocyte number and expression of TRP-1 and pmel 17 (silver protein) was noted (88). Conversely, injection of these xenografts with the KIT-inhibitory antibody resulted in melanocyte loss. These results demonstrate that SCF and c-KIT not only play a critical role during embryonic development and melanoblast migration to the skin, but also insure melanocyte survival in adult skin. Treatment of hMC with SCF modulated the expression of various integrins, and had differential effects on attachment and migration depending on extracellular matrix ligands (89). Moreover, SCF had profound effects on the organization of the cytoskeleton, exemplified by increasing actin stress fiber formation, and the phosphorylation of the focal contact protein, paxillin (90). These effects provide an explanation for why mutations in the SCF gene affect melanoblast migration. In addition to bFGF receptors, c-Met, and c-Kit, hMC express the tyrosine kinase receptor, trk, which is activated by the neurotrophic factors NGF and NT-3, and trk-c, which is activated by NT-3 (57). Both NGF and NT-3 are synthesized in the skin and promote the survival of hMC (56,57,91).

ROLE OF ENDOTHELIN-1 IN REGULATING hMC

Endothelin-1 is a 21-amino-acid peptide that is synthesized by keratinocytes and is mitogenic and melanogenic for hMC (15,63,65,92). The effects of ET-1 are mediated primarily by binding to the endothelin-B receptor (ETBR), which is predominantly expressed on hMC (65). The ETBR is a G_q protein-coupled receptor with seven transmembrane domains (93). Binding of this receptor by its ligand activates a complex signaling pathway that includes increased intracellular calcium mobilization, activation of PKC and nonreceptor tyrosine kinases (93–98). During embryonic development, ET-3, which binds to ETBR with the same affinity as ET-1, is essential for the migration of neural crest-derived melanoblasts to the epidermis (65,99). Mutations that disrupt the expression of the gene for ET-3 or ETBR result in Hirschsprung's disease, characterized by spotting, caused by loss of melanocytes from certain skin areas, and megacolon (100). The pigmentary phenotype that arises from either mutation underscores the importance of endothelins and ETBR in the survival and migration of melanoblasts from the neural crest during embryonic development. Moreover, the synthesis of ET-1 by human keratinocytes suggests its importance as a paracrine regulator of melanocytes.

Neuroendocrine Factors That Affect hMC

Nerve Growth Factor and Neurotrophin-3

There is substantial evidence that several known neuroendocrine factors are synthesized in human skin. The neurotrophins NGF and NT-3 are synthesized by keratinocytes, and NGF is synthesized by fibroblasts and possibly by melanocytes as well (57,91,101,102). Both neurotrophins serve as survival factors for human melanocytes (56,57). The synthesis of NGF by human keratinocytes is induced by substance P and neurokinin A, both of which are released by cutaneous sensory nerves (103).

The Melanocortins and MC1R

Proopiomelanocortin (POMC) is synthesized and processed into its bioactive peptides, α-MSH and ACTH, as well as β-endorphin in the skin *(16,17,104,105)*. Corticotropin-releasing hormone, which stimulates the expression of POMC in the pituitary, is also expressed in human skin *(106)*. Thus, it is conceivable that in the skin, as in the pituitary, the production of POMC is regulated by corticotropin-releasing hormone. The melanocortins, ACTH, α-MSH, β-MSH, and γ-MSH, are a family of structurally related peptides that are derived from one precursor protein, POMC *(107)*. Posttranslational modification of POMC by the enzymes proconvertase 1 and 2 yields the 39-amino-acid peptide ACTH, and results in the subsequent cleavage of ACTH into the 13-amino-acid peptide, α-MSH, respectively *(108)*. All four melanocortins share a common tetrapeptide sequence, His-Phe-Arg-Trp, which is thought to be essential for their pigmentary effects. Important functions of melanocortins include regulation of steroidogenesis by ACTH, melanogenesis by ACTH, α-MSH, and β-MSH, and food intake by α-MSH and possibly γ-MSH *(109)*.

Classically, α-MSH has been known as the physiological regulator of integumental pigmentation of many vertebrate species *(110–113)*. α-MSH regulates rapid color change by inducing melanosome dispersion in fish, amphibians, and reptiles. In mammals, α-MSH increases eumelanin synthesis, as best demonstrated in mouse follicular melanocytes decades ago *(114)*. The role of melanocortins in regulating human pigmentation was enigmatic until the early 1990s, when it was confirmed by the cloning of MC1R from hMC and the demonstration that this receptor can be activated by ACTH and α-MSH, resulting in stimulation of proliferation and melanogenesis, specifically eumelanogenesis, of cultured hMC *(18,115–118)*. Subsequently, it was shown that the human MC1R recognizes ACTH and α-MSH with similar affinity, has a lower affinity for β-MSH, and the least affinity for γ-MSH *(64)*. These findings, together with the evidence for the presence of ACTH and α-MSH in the human epidermis, suggested that among the melanocortins, these two peptides are the most relevant for the regulation of human pigmentation, whereas γ-MSH is the least effective *(16,17)*.

Of interest are the findings that ACTH and α-MSH increase the expression of the MC1R mRNA levels, suggesting that these ligands upregulate the expression of their receptor, thus sustain, or even augment, the response of hMC to melanocortins *(64,119)*. An increase in MC1R mRNA was also observed after treatment of hMC with ET-1 *(65,119)*. Thus ET-1 interacts with melanocortins not only at the level of cross talk among their mutual signaling pathways, but also by enhancing the response of hMC to melanocortins. The MC1R mRNA levels are also increased after treatment of hMC with β-estradiol *(119)*. This effect might contribute to increased skin pigmentation, such as that seen during pregnancy and in melasma.

In mouse follicular melanocytes, the MC1R is a key to the switch between eumelanin and pheomelanin synthesis *(120–122)*. Activation of the MC1R by binding of α-MSH induces the synthesis of eumelanin by follicular melanocytes, and temporal expression of agouti-signaling protein (ASP), the physiological antagonist of α-MSH, blocks α-MSH binding and results in pheomelanin synthesis *(123)*. The regulation of ASP expression and blockade of the MC1R by ASP binding results in the agouti phenotype that is characterized by a eumelanotic band, followed by a pheomelanotic band, then a eumelanotic band caused by cessation of ASP expression and resumption of eumelanin synthesis. The human agouti gene was cloned and its product, the human ASP, purified

(124). Expression of the human *agouti* gene in transgenic mice resulted in a yellow coat color, providing evidence that this gene is homologous to its mouse counterpart in that it regulates pheomelanin synthesis *(125)*. The human ASP blocks the melanogenic and mitogenic effects of α-MSH on cultured hMC *(126)*. These effects of ASP are mediated by competing with α-MSH for binding to the MC1R. These results unequivocally demonstrate that hMC respond to ASP, suggesting a role for ASP in regulating human pigmentation. Unlike the *MC1R* gene, which is highly polymorphic, the *agouti* gene is not. So far, only two allelic variants of the human *agouti* gene have been identified, and found to be caused by alterations in the noncoding region of the gene *(127,128)*. These results undermine the role of *agouti* gene in the diversity of human pigmentation.

Genetic studies carried out in various Northern European populations and Australia revealed that the human *MC1R* gene is highly polymorphic, suggesting the significance of this gene in determining constitutive pigmentation in humans. So far, more than 35 allelic variants of the *MC1R* gene have been identified, most of which are point mutations that result in a single amino acid substitution. Interestingly, the wild-type *MC1R* gene is predominant in African populations *(129)*. Some of the allelic variants of the *MC1R* gene, namely Arg142His, Arg151Cys, Arg160Trp, and Asp294His substitutions, are loss-of-function mutations that are strongly associated with red hair phenotype, poor tanning ability, and, importantly, with increased risk for melanoma and possibly nonmelanoma skin cancer *(130–135)*. A number of alleles, such as Val60Leu, Val92Met, and Arg163Gln substitutions, are thought to have lower penetrance for red hair phenotype, yet still seem to contribute to the risk for melanoma and skin cancer in general *(135)*. The associations with hair color, ability to tan, and skin cancer susceptibility indicate that the *MC1R* gene is an important regulator of constitutive, as well as facultative pigmentation. Moreover, these associations implicate the *MC1R* gene as a melanoma, and possibly a nonmelanoma, skin cancer susceptibility gene.

β-Endorphin

Another POMC-derived peptide that has recently been implicated in the regulation of hMC is the opioid peptide β-endorphin. It was demonstrated that β-endorphin is present in human skin, particularly epidermal melanocytes and keratinocytes, and that its μ-opiate receptor is expressed by these cells *(104)*. More recently, the expression of β-endorphin and μ-opiate receptor was shown in human follicular melanocytes *in situ* and in vitro *(136)*. Human epidermal, as well as follicular, melanocytes responded to β-endorphin with increased proliferation, dendricity, and melanin content, suggesting a paracrine/autocrine role for β-endorphin in regulating pigmentation of human skin and hair.

FURTHER ROLE OF KERATINOCYTES, FIBROBLASTS, AND MELANOCYTES IN THE DIVERSITY OF HUMAN PIGMENTATION

Because keratinocyte and fibroblasts regulate the function of melanocytes, it is plausible that they contribute directly to the diversity of skin color in humans. It has been shown that expression and activation of PAR2 in keratinocytes correlate with skin pigmentation, because dark skin has a higher expression and broader distribution of PAR2 than light skin *(137)*. Moreover, it is plausible that keratinocytes or fibroblasts in dark skin synthesize higher basal levels of melanogenic factors or lower levels of melanogenic inhibitors than keratinocytes or fibroblasts in light skin. It is also conceivable that hMC in different color skin differ in their ability to synthesize autocrine factors. Melanocytes in different individuals may differ in the expression of receptors for certain stimulatory or inhibitory factors. None of these possibilities is mutually exclusive, and investigating them in normal skin with different constitutive melanin content will undoubtedly lead to a better understanding of the basis for the wide diversity of constitutive pigmentation in humans.

ROLE OF PHYSIOLOGICAL REGULATORS IN THE RESPONSE OF MELANOCYTES TO UVR

The major environmental agent that affects human pigmentation is solar UVR. A hallmark of sun exposure is increased skin pigmentation, known as the tanning response *(1,4)*. Exposure to the sun results in immediate skin darkening, caused by the photooxidation of pre-existing melanin, and reorganization of intermediate filaments in melanocytes and keratinocytes to facilitate melanosome transfer. Immediate skin darkening occurs within minutes after sun exposure and is thought to be primarily caused by long wavelength UVA rays. Prolonged sun exposure results in delayed tanning response, which becomes evident within 2–3 d, and is induced by UVA and UVB rays. This response involves increased melanin synthesis as well as transfer of newly formed melanin to keratinocytes. In general, facultative pigmentation induced by UVR is dependent on constitutive pigmentation, and an individual's tanning ability correlates directly with constitutive melanin content in the skin.

The ability to tan has been used as a criterion to classify humans into six different phototypes: skin types 1–6 *(1)*. Skin type 1 and 2 phototypes are characterized by their inability to tan, susceptibility to burn readily, and having fair skin and blue eyes. Skin type 3 individuals tan efficiently and rarely burn, and skin types 4–6 tan well, do not burn, and have dark skin color. These skin phototypes have also been used to determine the risk for skin cancer, with skin phototypes 1 and 2 having the highest risk for melanoma and nonmelanoma skin cancer. This concept has been supported by many epidemiological studies and clinical observations *(27,28,138)*. However, the skin phototype classification is arbitrary, and there are ongoing attempts to develop better quantitative assessment of pigmentary phenotypes based on more accurate criteria *(139,140)*. One criterion that is considered is the minimal erythemal dose that correlates in normal skin directly with constitutive pigmentation and inversely with the ability to tan.

The ability of the skin to tan is a critical photoprotective mechanism and an important determinant of the risk for skin cancer. Experimental evidence for this comes from the observations that the extent of UVR-induced DNA damage is substantially higher in light-colored skin than in dark-colored skin. This was demonstrated by the generation of more cyclobutane pyrimidine dimers and 6,4-photoproducts in light skin compared with dark skin, and in cultured hMC derived from light skin compared with their counterparts from dark skin in response to the same dose of UVR *(20,140,141)*. Moreover, hMC with a high melanin content respond *in situ*, as well as in vitro, more readily to UVR with increased melanin synthesis and melanosome transfer, compared with melanocytes with a low melanin content *(140,141)*. The importance of UVR-induced DNA damage in photocarcinogenesis is best illustrated in patients with xeroderma pigmentosum, who are deficient in nucleotide excision repair, and have a high incidence and early onset of skin cancer. In addition, UVR-signature mutations, e.g., in the *p53* gene, are common in nonmelanoma skin cancer, and similar signature mutations in the *CDKN2A* gene are present in sporadic melanoma tumors *(142–145)*.

As stated in "Skin Pigmentation: The Outcome of Melanin Synthesis and Distribution in the Epidermis," it is common knowledge that melanin reduces the penetration of UVR through the epidermal layers (26) and scavenges reactive oxygen species that are generated in the skin on sun exposure (24). Eumelanin is thought to have a greater ability to filter and scatter UVR and quench reactive oxygen species than pheomelanin (23,26,146). Experimentally, it has been shown that modulation of eumelanin and pheomelanin contents of cultured hMC affects the induction of DNA photoproducts (147). As expected, increasing eumelanin content reduced the generation of cyclobutane pyrimidine dimers in hMC.

The pigmentary response to UVR is mediated by an array of paracrine and autocrine factors whose synthesis is stimulated by UVR (Fig. 1). Among those factors are bFGF; ET-1, the melanocortins α-MSH and ACTH, SCF, NGF, as well as PGE_2 and PGF_{2a} (15,16,55,148–150). Exposure to UVR also increases the synthesis of the cytokines IL-1 and TNF-α (14,151). Interleukin-1, in turn, stimulates the synthesis of ET-1 by keratinocytes, and of α-MSH and ACTH by both melanocytes and keratinocytes (15,16). ET-1 and the melanocortins α-MSH and ACTH play a pivotal role in UVR-induced melanin synthesis by hMC (65,152,153). Blocking ET-1 by a specific antibody inhibited the UVR-induced melanogenesis by hMC (152). Human melanocytes expressing loss of function mutations in the MC1R gene have a poor melanogenic response to UVR (130,131). The cAMP pathway, the main signaling pathway induced by α-MSH, is required for the melanogenic response to UVR, because cultured hMC show increased melanogenesis after UVR irradiation only in the presence of a cAMP inducer in their culture medium (153). As mentioned in "the Melanocortins and MC1R," treatment of cultured hMC with ET-1 or either α-MSH or ACTH increases the levels of MC1R mRNA, which is expected to increase the ability of hMC to respond to melanocortins (64,119). Therefore, UVR increases the MC1R mRNA levels indirectly by stimulating the synthesis of ET-1 and melanocortins.

REGULATION OF MELANOSOME MOVEMENT AND TRANSFER FROM MELANOCYTES TO KERATINOCYTES

Most of the studies on the regulation of human skin pigmentation focused on the control of melanin synthesis by melanocytes. Serious investigation of the molecular mechanisms that govern melanosome movement and transfer began only few years ago. It is acknowledged that the transfer of melanosomes from melanocytes to keratinocytes is pivotal for normal pigmentation, and defects in this process result in hypopigmentation, as seen in Griscelli's syndrome (154). The following is a brief summary highlighting the major advances in this area of research. An important discovery was the expression of PAR2 by human keratinocytes and its role in melanosome transfer and regulation of pigmentation (155). The significance of PAR2 was further substantiated by the findings that modulation of its activity affected skin pigmentation via altering melanosome transfer (156). Activation of PAR2 resulted in skin darkening and inhibition of PAR2 reduced pigmentation. Subsequent studies demonstrated that irradiation of the skin of human subjects with UVR upregulated PAR2 expression, thus providing evidence for the association of PAR2 with the upregulation of human skin pigmentation by UVR in vivo (157).

For melanosomes to be transferred from melanocytes to keratinocytes, they need to be transported within the melanocyte from the perikaryon to the tips of the dendrites.

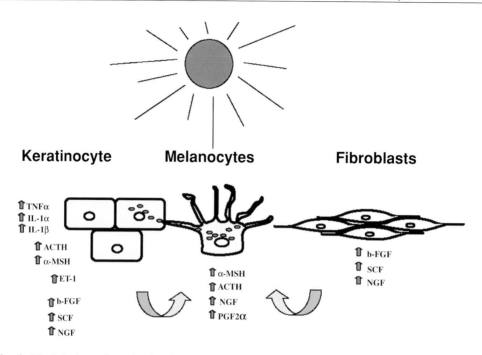

Fig. 1. Modulation of synthesis of various paracrine and autocrine regulators of melanocytes by ultraviolet radiation (UVR). Exposure of the skin or cultured skin cells to UVR increased the synthesis of the cytokines interleukin-1 (IL-1), tumor necrosis factor-α (TNF-α), and endothelin-1 (ET-1) by keratinocytes; the melanocortins adrenocorticotropic hormone (ACTH) and α-melanocyte stimulating hormone (α-MSH) by keratinocytes and melanocytes; the production of nerve growth factor (NGF) by keratinocytes, melanocytes, and fibroblasts; and basic fibroblast growth factor (bFGF) and stem cell factor (SCF) by keratinocytes and fibroblasts.

Melanocytic dendrites are dynamic microtubule-containing structures, and their extension and arborization is regulated by a plethora of growth factors, including α-MSH, ET-1, and NGF, as well as by UVR *(158)*. In general, the extent of dendricity of hMC correlates directly with their melanogenic activity. In hMC, dendrite extension is modulated by the small GTP-binding proteins Rac and rho *(158)*. Dendricity of melanocytes is promoted by Rac and inhibited by rho. Melanosome movement along the dendrites requires the cooperation of cytoskeleton-associated motor proteins *(154)*. These include myosin Va and Rab 27a. Within melanocytes, melanosomes associate with myosin Va to move short distances along actin filaments and long distances along microtubules. However, motor proteins that associate with actin seem to interact directly with motor proteins that associate with microtubules, adding to the complexity of the regulation of melanosome movement.

MAINTENANCE OF MELANOCYTE SURVIVAL AND GENOMIC STABILITY

Given the significance of the melanocyte in photoprotection against sun-induced skin cancer, it is important to insure its survival in the epidermis. In normal skin, melanocytes are maintained for many years of the life of an individual. One known reason for this longevity is the resistance of melanocytes to apoptosis, particularly resulting from high constitutive expression of the antiapoptotic Bcl2 *(159,160)*. Unlike keratinocytes that have a high self-renewal and proliferation capacity, the vast majority of epidermal melanocytes are highly differentiated and have a low proliferation and self-renewal capacity. Some of the paracrine and autocrine factors that regulate melanocyte function and proliferation also function as survival factors that rescue hMC from apoptosis caused by environmental insults, such as exposure to UVR or chemical toxins. NGF was shown to increase the survival of UVR-irradiated hMC by maintaining a high level of Bcl2 *(56)*. Similarly, NT3 also had survival effects on cultured hMC *(57)*. Recently, it was demonstrated that ET-1, as well as α-MSH and ACTH, reduce the UVR-induced apoptosis of hMC by activating specific survival pathways, which in turn increase the level of Bcl2 and, thus, prevent its reduction by UVR *(161)*. Similarly, SCF was found to have an antiapoptotic effect on hMC *(162)*.

It is now evident that the inositol-3,4,5-triphosphate (IP3) kinase pathway plays an important role in melanocyte survival. Growth factors, such as α-MSH and ET-1, as well as SCF and HGF, activate IP3 kinase, as determined by phosphorylation and activation of its substrate Akt *(162–164)*. In turn, Akt inhibits the proapoptotic Bad, allowing for the dimerization of Bcl2 or Bcl_{xl} with Bax, thus preventing apoptosis *(165)*. Activated Akt also phosphorylates the transcription factor cyclin AMP response element binding protein (CREB) *(166)*, which activates the melanocyte-specific microphthalmia-associated transcription factor (Mitf) *(167)*. In turn, Mitf upregulates the expression of Bcl2 and promotes melanocyte survival *(168)*. It is important to note that melanocyte survival is only beneficial if accompanied by genomic stability, otherwise melanocytes would become prone to malignant transformation. An attractive speculation is that, in hMC, activation of Mitf is somehow linked to DNA repair. One gene whose expression is upregulated by Mitf is breast cancer susceptibility gene 2 (*BRCA2*), known to be involved in the DNA damage response *(168,169)*. *BRCA2* binds to RAD51 to insure the efficient repair of DNA double strand breaks *(170,171)*. Mutations in the *BRCA2* gene are associated not only with breast cancer, but with several other types of cancer, mainly prostate and pancreatic cancer, and possibly melanoma *(169)*. In hMC, α-MSH that activates Mitf not only promotes survival, but also reduces the extent of UVR-induced DNA photoproducts, thus promoting genomic stability. The exact mechanism for this novel and important effect of α-MSH is not yet known. Unraveling the mechanisms that regulate hMC survival will have enormous implications on vitiligo, a disease thought to be caused by melanocyte apoptosis, on one hand, and melanoma, which resists apoptosis, on the other.

REFERENCES

1. Pathak MA, Jimbow K, Fitzpatrick T. Photobiology of pigment cell. In: Seiji M, ed. Phenotypic Expression in Pigment Cells. University of Tokyo Press, Tokyo, Japan, 1980, pp. 655–670.
2. Fitzpatrick TB, Szabo G, Seiji M, Quevedo WC. Biology of the melanin pigmentary system. In: Fitzpatrick TB, Eisen AZ, Wolff K, Freeberg IM, Austen KF, eds. Dermatology in General Medicine. McGraw-Hill, New York, NY, 1979, pp. 131–163.
3. Fuchs E. Epidermal differentiation: the bare essentials. J Cell Biol 1990;111:2807–2814.
4. Dillman AM. Photobiology of skin pigmentation. In: Levine N, ed. Pigmentation and Pigmentary Disorders. CRC, Boca Raton, FL, 1993, pp. 61–94.
5. Gilchrest BA, Zhai S, Eller MS, Yarosh DB, Yaar M. Treatment of human melanocytes and S91 melanoma cells with the DNA repair enzyme T4 endonuclease V enhances melanogenesis after ultraviolet irradiation. J Invest Dermatol 1993;101:666–672.
6. Kadekaro AL, Kavanagh RJ, Wakamatsu K, Ito S, Pipitone MA, Abdel-Malek ZA. Cutaneous photobiology. The melanocyte vs. the sun: who will win the final round? Pigment Cell Res 2003;16:434–47.

7. Hunt G, Kyne S, Ito S, Wakamatsu K, Todd C, Thody AJ. Eumelanin and pheomelanin contents of human epidermis and cultured melanocytes. Pigment Cell Res 1995;8:202–208.

8. Szabo G. Racial differences in the fate of melanosomes in human epidermis. Nature 1969;222:1081.

9. Halaban R, Pomerantz SH, Marshall S, Lambert DT, Lerner AB. Regulation of tyrosinase in human melanocytes grown in culture. J Cell Biol 1983;97:480–488.

10. Abdel-Malek Z, Swope V, Collins C, Boissy R, Zhao H, Nordlund J. Contribution of melanogenic proteins to the heterogeneous pigmentation of human melanocytes. J Cell Sci 1993;106:1323–1331.

11. Abdel-Malek ZA, Swope VB, Nordlund JJ, Medrano EE. Proliferation and propagation of human melanocytes in vitro are affected by donor age and anatomical site. Pigment Cell Res 1994;7:116–122.

12. Iwata M, Corn T, Iwata S, Everett MA, Fuller BB. The relationship between tyrosinase activity and skin color in human foreskins. J Invest Dermatol 1990;95:9–15.

13. Halaban R, Langdon R, Birchall N, et al. Basic fibroblast growth factor from human keratinocytes is a natural mitogen for melanocytes. J Cell Biol 1988;107:1611–1619.

14. Kock A, Schwarz T, Kirnbauer R, et al. Human keratinocytes are a source for tumor necrosis factor α: evidence for synthesis and release upon stimulation with endotoxin or ultraviolet light. J Exp Med 1990;172:1609–1614.

15. Imokawa G, Yada Y, Miyagishi M. Endothelins secreted from human keratinocytes are intrinsic mitogens for human melanocytes. J Biol Chem 1992;267:24,675–24,680.

16. Chakraborty AK, Funasaka Y, Slominski A, et al. Production and release of proopiomelanocortin (POMC) derived peptides by human melanocytes and keratinocytes in culture: regulation by ultraviolet B. Biochim Biophys Acta 1996;1313:130–138.

17. Wakamatsu K, Graham A, Cook D, Thody AJ. Characterization of ACTH peptides in human skin and their activation of the melanocortin-1 receptor. Pigment Cell Res 1997;10:288–297.

18. Abdel-Malek Z, Swope VB, Suzuki I, et al. Mitogenic and melanogenic stimulation of normal human melanocytes by melanotropic peptides. Proc Natl Acad Sci U S A 1995;92:1789–1793.

19. Pathak MA, Hori Y, Szabo G, Fitzpatrick TB. The photobiology of melanin pigmentation in human skin. In: Kawamura T, Fitzpatrick TB, Seiji M, eds. Biology of Normal and Abnormal Melanocytes. University Park Press, Baltimore, MD, 1971, pp. 149–169.

20. Kobayashi N, Nakagawa A, Muramatsu T, et al. Supranuclear melanin caps reduce ultraviolet induced DNA photoproducts in human epidermis. J Invest Dermatol 1998;110:806–810.

21. Nordlund JJ, Abdel-Malek ZA. Mechanisms for post-inflammatory hyperpigmentation and hypopigmentation. In: Bagnara J, ed. Advances in Pigment Cell Research Proceedings of the XIII International Pigment Cell Society. Alan R. Liss, New York, NY, 1988, pp. 219–236.

22. Gilchrest BA, Eller MS. DNA photodamage stimulates melanogenesis and other photoprotective responses. J Investig Dermatol Symp Proc 1999;4:35–40.

23. Menon IA, Persad S, Ranadive NS, Haberman HF. Photobiological effects of eumelanin and pheomelanin. In: Bagnara JT, Klaus SN, Paul E, Schartl M, eds. Biological, Molecular and Clinical Aspects of Pigmentation. University of Tokyo Press, Tokyo, Japan, 1985, pp. 77–86.

24. Bustamante J, Bredeston L, Malanga G, Mordoh J. Role of melanin as a scavenger of active oxygen species. Pigment Cell Res 1993;6:348–353.

25. Pathak MA, Fitzpatrick TB. The role of natural photoprotective agents in human skin. In: Fitzpatrick TB, Pathak MA, Haber LC, Seiji M, Kukita A, eds. Sunlight and Man. University of Tokyo Press, Tokyo, Japan, 1974, pp. 725–750.

26. Kaidbey KH, Poh Agin P, Sayre RM, Kligman AM. Photoprotection by melanin—a comparison of black and Caucasian skin. J Am Acad Dermatol 1979;1:249–260.

27. Sober AJ, Lew RA, Koh HK, Barnhill RL. Epidemiology of cutaneous melanoma. An update. Dermatol Clin 1991;9:617–629.

28. Pathak MA. Ultraviolet radiation and the development of non-melanoma and melanoma skin cancer: clinical and experimental evidence. Skin Pharmacol 1991;4(suppl 1):85–94.

29. Gilchrest BA, Eller MS, Geller AC, Yaar M. The pathogenesis of melanoma induced by ultraviolet radiation. N Engl J Med 1999;340:1341–1348.

30. Levine N, Hori Y, Kubota Y. Acquired hypermelanotic disorders. In: Levine N, ed. Pigmentation and Pigmentary Disorders. CRC, Bota Raton, FL, 1993, pp. 211–238.

31. Dunlop D. Eighty-six cases of Addison's disease. Br Med J 1963;5362:887–891.

32. Nerup J. Addison's disease—clinical studies. A report of 108 cases. Acta Endocrinol (Copenh) 1974;76:127–41.

33. Smith AG, Shuster S, Thody AJ, Peberky M. Chloasma, oral contraceptives, and plasma immunoreactive β-melanocyte-stimulating hormone. J Invest Dermatol 1977;68:169–170.

34. Stulberg DL, Clark N, Tovey D. Common hyperpigmentation disorders in adults: Part II. Melanoma, seborrheic keratoses, acanthosis nigricans, melasma, diabetic dermopathy, tinea versicolor, and postinflammatory hyperpigmentation. Am Fam Physician 2003;68:1963–1968.
35. Snell RS. The pigmentary changes occurring in the breast skin during pregnancy and following estrogen treatment. J Invest Dermatol 1964;43:181–186.
36. Wilson MJ, Spaziani E. The melanogenic response to testosterone in scrotal epidermis; the effects on tyrosinase activity and protein synthesis. Acta Endocrin 1976;81:435–448.
37. Friedmann PS, Wren F, Buffey J, MacNeil S. α-MSH causes a small rise in cAMP but has no effect on basal or ultraviolet-stimulated melanogenesis in human melanocytes. Br J Dermatol 1990; 123:145–151.
38. Halaban R, Tyrrell L, Longley J, Yarden Y, Rubin J. Pigmentation and proliferation of human melanocytes and the effects of melanocyte-stimulating hormone and ultraviolet B light. Ann N Y Acad Sci 1993;680:290–301.
39. Fuller BB, Rungta D, Iozumi K, et al. Hormonal regulation of melanogenesis in mouse melanoma and in human melanocytes. Ann N Y Acad Sci 1993;680:302–319.
40. Tomita Y, Maeda K, Tagami H. Mechanisms for hyperpigmentation in postinflammatory pigmentation, urticaria pigmentosa and sunburn. Dermatologica 1989;179(suppl 1):49–53.
41. Thestrup-Pedersen K, Larsen CS, Kristensen M, Zachariae C. Interleukin-1 release from peripheral blood monocytes and soluble interleukin-2 and cd8 receptors in serum from patients with atopic dermatitis. Acta Derm Venereol 1990;70:395–399.
42. Ferreri NR, Millet I, Paliwal V, et al. Induction of macrophage TNF alpha, IL-1, IL-6, and PGE2 production by DTH-initiating factors. Cell Immunol 1991;137:389–405.
43. Ford-Hutchinson AW, Rackman A. Leukotrienes as mediators of skin inflammation. Br J Dermatol 1983;109(suppl 25):26–29.
44. Fogh K, Herlin T, Kragballe K. Eicosanoids in skin of patients with atopic dermatitis: prostaglandin E_2 and leukotriene B_4 are present in biologically active concentrations. J Allergy Clin Immunol 1989;83:450–455.
45. Tomita Y, Maeda K, Tagami H. Histamine stimulates normal human melanocytes in vitro: one of the possible inducers of hyperpigmentation in urticaria pigmentosa. J Dermatol Sci 1993;6:146–154.
46. Yoshida M, Takahashi Y, Inoue S. Histamine induces melanogenesis and morphologic changes by protein kinase A activation via H2 receptors in human normal melanocytes. J Invest Dermatol 2000;114:334–342.
47. Gordon PR, Mansur CP, Gilchrest BA. Regulation of human melanocyte growth, dendricity, and melanization by keratinocyte derived factors. J Invest Dermatol 1989;92:565–572.
48. Toyoda M, Luo Y, Makino T, Matsui C, Morohashi M. Calcitonin gene-related peptide upregulates melanogenesis and enhances melanocyte dendricity via induction of keratinocyte-derived melanotrophic factors. J Investig Dermatol Symp Proc 1999;4:116–125.
49. Imokawa G, Yada Y, Morisaki N, Kimura M. Biological characterization of human fibroblast-derived mitogenic factors for human melanocytes. Biochem J 1998;330:1235–1239.
50. Matsui Y, Zsebo KM, Hogan BL. Embryonic expression of a haematopoietic growth factor encoded by the Sl locus and the ligand for c-kit. Nature 1990;347:667–669.
51. Longley BJ Jr, Morganroth GS, Tyrrell L, et al. Altered metabolism of mast-cell growth factor (c-kit ligand) in cutaneous mastocytosis. N Engl J Med 1993;328:1302–1307.
52. Matsumoto K, Tajima H, Nakamura T. Hepatocyte growth factor is a potent stimulator of human melanocyte DNA synthesis and growth. Biochem Biophys Res Commun 1991;176:45–51.
53. Yaar M, Grossman K, Eller M, Gilchrest BA. Evidence for nerve growth factor-mediated paracrine effects in human epidermis. J Cell Biol 1991;115:821–828.
54. Di-Marco E, Marchisio PC, Bondanza S, Franzi AT, Cancedda R, De Luca M. Growth regulated synthesis and secretion of biologically active nerve growth factor by human keratinocytes. J Biol Chem 1991;266:21,718–21,722.
55. Tron VA, Coughlin MD, Jang DE, Stanisz J, Sauder DN. Expression and modulation of nerve growth factor in murine keratinocytes (PAM 212). J Clin Invest 1990;85:1085–1089.
56. Zhai S, Yaar M, Gilchrest BA. Nerve growth factor rescues pigment cells from ultraviolet induced apoptosis by upregulating BCL-2 levels. Exp Cell Res 1996;224:335–343.
57. Yaar M, Eller MS, DiBenedetto P, et al. The trk family of receptors mediates nerve growth factor and neurotrophin-3 effects in melanocytes. J Clin Invest 1994;94:1550–1562.
58. Yamaguchi Y, Itami S, Watabe H, et al. Mesenchymal-epithelial interactions in the skin: increased expression of dickkopf1 by palmoplantar fibroblasts inhibits melanocyte growth and differentiation. J Cell Biol 2004;165:275–285.

59. Swope VB, Abdel-Malek ZA, Kassem L, Nordlund JJ. Interleukins 1α and 6 and tumor necrosis factor-α are paracrine inhibitors of human melanocyte proliferation and melanogenesis. J Invest Dermatol 1991;96:180–185.

60. Blobe GC, Schiemann WP, Lodish HF. Role of transforming growth factor β in human disease. N Engl J Med 2000;342:1350–1358.

61. Krasagakis K, Garbe C, Schrier PI, Orfanos CE. Paracrine and autocrine regulation of human melanocyte and melanoma cell growth by transforming growth factor beta in vitro. Anticancer Res 1994;14:2565–2571.

62. Swope VB, Sauder DN, McKenzie RC, et al. Synthesis of interleukin-1α and β by normal human melanocytes. J Invest Dermatol 1994;102:749–753.

63. Swope VB, Medrano EE, Smalara D, Abdel-Malek Z. Long-term proliferation of human melanocytes is supported by the physiologic mitogens α-melanotropin, endothelin-1, and basic fibroblast growth factor. Exp Cell Res 1995;217:453–459.

64. Suzuki I, Cone R, Im S, Nordlund J, Abdel-Malek Z. Binding capacity and activation of the MC1 receptors by melanotropic hormones correlate directly with their mitogenic and melanogenic effects on human melanocytes. Endocrinology 1996;137:1627–1633.

65. Tada A, Suzuki I, Im S, et al. Endothelin-1 is a paracrine growth factor that modulates melanogenesis of human melanocytes and participates in their responses to ultraviolet radiation. Cell Growth Differ 1998;9:575–584.

66. Bach MK. Mediators of anaphylaxis and inflammation. Ann Rev in Microbiol 1982;36:371–413.

67. Bregman MD, Peters E, Sander D, Meyskens FL Jr. Dexamethasone, prostaglandin A, and retinoic acid modulation of murine and human melanoma cells grown in soft agar. J Natl Cancer Inst 1983;71:927–932.

68. Bregman MD, Funk C, Fukushima M. Inhibition of human melanoma growth by prostaglandin A, D and J analogues. Cancer Res 1986;46:2740–2744.

69. Abdel-Malek Z, Swope VB, Amornsiripanitch N, Nordlund JJ. In vitro modulation of proliferation and melanization of S91 melanoma cells by prostaglandins. Cancer Res 1987;47:3141–3146.

70. Morelli JG, Yohn JJ, Lyons MB, Murphy RC, Norris DA. Leukotrienes C_4 and D_4 as potent mitogens for cultured human melanocytes. J Invest Dermatol 1989;93:719–722.

71. Tomita Y, Maeda K, Tagami H. Melanocyte-stimulating properties of arachidonic acid metabolites: possible role in postinflammatory pigmentation. Pigment Cell Res 1992;5:357–361.

72. Krey G, Braissant O, L'Horset F, et al. Fatty acids, eicosanoids, and hypolipidemic agents identified as ligands of peroxisome proliferator-activated receptors by coactivator-dependent receptor ligand assay. Mol Endocrinol 1997;11:779–791.

73. Scott G, Leopardi S, Printup S, Malhi N, Seiberg M, Lapoint R. Proteinase-activated receptor-2 stimulates prostaglandin production in keratinocytes: analysis of prostaglandin receptors on human melanocytes and effects of PGE_2 and PGF_{2a} on melanocyte dendricity. J Invest Dermatol 2004;122:1214–1224.

74. Leikauf GD, Abdel-Malek ZA, Swope VB, Doupnik CA, Nordlund JJ. Constitutive biosynthesis of 12-hydroxy-5,8,10,14-eicosatetraenoic acid and 6-keto prostaglandin F_{1a} by human melanocytes and Cloudman S91 melanoma cells. In: Hammerstrom S, Marnett LW, eds. Prostaglandins, Leukotrienes and Cancer. Boston, MA: Kluwer Academic Press; 1994.

75. Pittelkow MR, Shipley GD. Serum-free culture of normal human melanocytes: growth kinetics and growth factor requirements. J Cell Physiol 1989;140:565–576.

76. Gospodarowicz D, Cohen DC, Fujii DK. Regulation of cell growth by the basal lamina and plasma factors: relevance to embryonic control of cell proliferation. In: Sato G, Pardee A, Sirbasku D, eds. Cold Spring Harbor Conferences on Cell Proliferation 9: Growth of Cells in Hormonally Deficient Media. Vol. 9. Cold Spring Harbor Laboratory, Cold Spring Harbor, NY, 1982, pp. 95–124.

77. Cooper CS, Park M, Blair DG, et al. Molecular cloning of a new transforming gene from a chemically transformed human cell line. Nature 1984;311:29–33.

78. Park M, Dean M, Cooper CS, et al. Mechanism of met oncogene activation. Cell 1986;45:895–904.

79. Bladt F, Riethmacher D, Isenmann S, Aguzzi A, Birchmeier C. Essential role for the c-met receptor in the migration of myogenic precursor cells into the limb bud. Nature 1995;376:768–771.

80. Halaban R, Rubin JS, Funasaka Y, et al. Met and hepatocyte growth factor/scatter factor signal transduction in normal melanocytes and melanoma cells. Oncogene 1992;7:2195–2206.

81. Zsebo KM, Williams DA, Geissler EN, et al. Stem cell factor is encoded at the Sl locus of the mouse and is the ligand for the *c-kit* receptor. Cell 1990;63:213–214.

82. Grabbe J, Welker P, Dippel E, Czarnetzki BM. Stem cell factor, a novel cutaneous growth factor for mast cells and melanocytes [Review]. Arch Dermatol Res 1994;287:78–84.

83. Manova K, Bacharova RF. Expression of c-kit encoded at the W locus of mice in developing embryonic germ cells and presumptive melanoblasts. Dev Biol 1991;146:312–324.

84. Keshet E, Lyman SD, Williams DE, et al. Embryonic RNA expression patterns of the c-kit receptor and its cognate ligand suggest multiple functional roles in mouse development. EMBO J 1991;10:2425–2435.

85. Besmer P, Manova K, Duttlinger R, et al. The {Ikit} ligand (steel factor) and its receptor {Ic-kit/W}: pleiotropic roles in gametogenesis and melanogenesis. Development 1993;(suppl):125–137.

86. Giebel LB, Spritz RA. Mutation of the *KIT* (mast/stem cell growth factor receptor) proto-oncogene in human piebaldism. Proc Natl Acad Sci U S A 1991;88:8696–8699.

87. Funasaka Y, Boulton T, Cobb M, et al. c-Kit–Kinase induces a cascade of protein tyrosine phosphorylation in normal human melanocytes in response to mast cell growth factor and stimulates mitogen-activated protein kinase but is down-regulated in melanomas. Mol Biol Cell 1992;3:197–209.

88. Grichnik JM, Burch JA, Burchette J, Shea CR. The SCF/KIT pathway plays a critical role in the control of normal human melanocyte homeostasis. J Invest Dermatol 1998;111:233–238.

89. Scott G, Ewing J, Ryan D, Abboud C. Stem cell factor regulates human melanocyte-matrix interaction. Pigment Cell Res 1994;7:44–51.

90. Scott G, Liang H, Luthra D. Stem cell factor regulates the melanocyte cytoskeleton. Pigment Cell Res 1996;9:134–141.

91. Pincelli C, Yaar M. Nerve growth factor: its significance in cutaneous biology. J Investig Dermatol Symp Proc 1997;2:31–36.

92. Yohn JJ, Morelli JG, Walchak SJ, Rundell KB, Norris DA, Zamora MR. Cultured human keratinocytes synthesize and secrete endothelin-1. J Invest Dermatol 1993;100:23–26.

93. Rubanyi GM, Polokoff MA. Endothelins: molecular biology, biochemistry, pharmacology, physiology, and pathophysiology. Pharmacol Rev 1994;46:325–415.

94. Baynash AG, Hosoda K, Giaid A, et al. Interaction of endothelin-3 with endothelin-B receptor is essential for development of epidermal melanocytes and enteric neurons. Cell 1994;79:1277–1285.

95. Imokawa G, Yada Y, Kimura M. Signalling mechanisms of endothelin-induced mitogenesis and melanogenesis in human melanocytes. Biochem J 1996;314:305–312.

96. McCallion AS, Chakravarti A. EDNRB/EDN3 and Hirschsprung disease type II. Pigment Cell Res 2001;14:161–169.

97. Tada A, Pereira E, Beitner Johnson D, Kavanagh R, Abdel-Malek ZA. Mitogen and ultraviolet-B–induced signaling pathways in normal human melanocytes. J Invest Dermatol 2002;118:316–322.

98. Lee HO, Levorse JM, Shin MK. The endothelin receptor-B is required for the migration of neural crest-derived melanocyte and enteric neuron precursors. Dev Biol 2003;259:162–175.

99. Inoue A, Yanagisawa M, Kimura S, et al. The human endothelin family: three structurally and pharmacologically distinct isopeptides predicted by three separate genes. Proc Natl Acad Sci USA 1989;86:2863–2867.

100. Puffenberger EG, Hosoda K, Washington SS, et al. A missense mutation of the endothelin-B receptor gene in multigenic Hirschsprung's disease. Cell 1994;79:1257–1266.

101. Murase K, Murakami Y, Takayanagi K, Furukawa Y, Hayashi K. Human fibroblast cells synthesize and secrete nerve growth factor in culture. Biochem Biophys Res Commun 1992;184:373–379.

102. Stefanato CM, Yaar M, Bhawan J, et al. Modulations of nerve growth factor and Bcl-2 in ultraviolet-irradiated human epidermis. J Cutan Pathol 2003;30:351–357.

103. Burbach GJ, Kim KH, Zivony AS, et al. The neurosensory tachykinins substance P and neurokinin A directly induce keratinocyte nerve growth factor. J Invest Dermatol 2001;117:1075–1082.

104. Kauser S, Schallreuter KU, Thody AJ, Gummer C, Tobin DJ. Regulation of human epidermal melanocyte biology by beta-endorphin. J Invest Dermatol 2003;120:1073–1080.

105. Suzuki I, Kato T, Motokawa T, Tomita Y, Nakamura E, Katagiri T. Increase of pro-opiomelanocortin mRNA prior to tyrosinase, tyrosinase-related protein 1, dopachrome tautomerase, Pmel-17/gp100, and P-protein mRNA in human skin after ultraviolet B irradiation. J Invest Dermatol 2002;118:73–78.

106. Slominski A, Ermak G, Mazurkiewicz JE, Baker J, Wortsman J. Characterization of corticotropin-releasing hormone (CRH) in human skin. J Clin Endocrinol Metab 1998;83:1020–1024.

107. Eberle AN. Proopiomelanocortin and the melanocortin peptides. In: Cone RD, ed. The Melanocortin Receptors. Humana, Totowa, NJ, 2000, pp. 3–67.

108. Seidah NG, Day R, Marcinkiewicz M, Chretien M. Mammalian paired basic amino acid convertases of prohormones and proproteins. Ann N Y Acad Sci 1993;680:135–146.

109. Abdel-Malek ZA. Melanocortin receptors: their functions and regulation by physiological agonists and antagonists. Cell Mol Life Sci 2001;58:434–441.

110. Sawyer TK, Hruby VJ, Hadley ME, Engel MH. α-Melanocyte stimulating hormone: chemical nature and mechanism of action. Am Zool 1983;23:529–540.

111. Castrucci AM, Hadley ME, Hruby VJ. Melanotropin bioassays: in vitro and in vivo comparisons. Gen Comp Endocrinol 1984;55:104–111.

112. Castrucci AML, Hadley ME, Sawyer TK, et al. α-Melanotropin: the minimal active sequence in the lizard skin bioassay. Gen Comp Endocrinol 1989;73:157–163.

113. Visconti MA, Ramanzini GC, Camargo CR, Castrucci AM. Elasmobranch color change: a short review and novel data on hormone regulation. J Exp Zool 1999;284:485–491.

114. Geschwind II, Huseby RA, Nishioka R. The effect of melanocyte-stimulating hormone on coat color in the mouse. Rec Prog Hormone Res 1972;28:91–130.

115. Mountjoy KG, Robbins LS, Mortrud MT, Cone RD. The cloning of a family of genes that encode the melanocortin receptors. Science 1992;257:1248–1251.

116. Chhajlani V, Wikberg JES. Molecular cloning and expression of the human melanocyte stimulating hormone receptor cDNA. FEBS Lett 1992;309:417–420.

117. Hunt G, Kyne S, Wakamatsu K, Ito S, Thody AJ. Nle^{4}DPhe^7 α-melanocyte–stimulating hormone increases the eumelanin:phaeomelanin ratio in cultured human melanocytes. J Invest Dermatol 1995;104:83–85.

118. Hunt G, Donatien PD, Lunec J, Todd C, Kyne S, Thody AJ. Cultured human melanocytes respond to MSH peptides and ACTH. Pigment Cell Res 1994;7:217–221.

119. Scott MC, Suzuki I, Abdel-Malek ZA. Regulation of the human melanocortin 1 receptor expression in epidermal melanocytes by paracrine and endocrine factors, and by UV radiation. Pigment Cell Res 2002;15:433–439.

120. Tamate HB, Takeuchi T. Action of the *e* locus of mice in the response of phaeomelanic hair follicles to α-melanocyte–stimulating hormone in vitro. Science 1984;224:1241–1242.

121. Robbins LS, Nadeau JH, Johnson KR, et al. Pigmentation phenotypes of variant extension locus alleles result from point mutations that alter MSH receptor function. Cell 1993;72:827–834.

122. Abdel-Malek ZA, Scott MC, Furumura M, et al. The melanocortin 1 receptor is the principal mediator of the effects of agouti signaling protein on mammalian melanocytes. J Cell Sci 2001;114:1019–1024.

123. Siracusa LD. The *agouti* gene: turned on to yellow. Trends Genet 1994;10:423–428.

124. Kwon HY, Bultman SJ, Loffler C, et al. Molecular structure and chromosomal mapping of the human homolog of the agouti gene. Proc Natl Acad Sci U S A 1994;91:9760–9764.

125. Wilson BD, Ollmann MM, Kang L, Stoffel M, Bell GI, Barsh GS. Structure and function of *ASP*, the human homolog of the mouse *agouti* gene. Hum Mol Genet 1995;4:223–230.

126. Suzuki I, Tada A, Ollmann MM, et al. Agouti signaling protein inhibits melanogenesis and the response of human melanocytes to α-melanotropin. J Invest Dermatol 1997;108:838–842.

127. Voisey J, Box NF, van Daal A. A polymorphism study of the human Agouti gene and its association with MC1R. Pigment Cell Res 2001;14:264–267.

128. Kanetsky PA, Swoyer J, Panossian S, Holmes R, Guerry D, Rebbeck TR. A polymorphism in the agouti signaling protein gene is associated with human pigmentation. Am J Hum Genet 2002;70:770–775.

129. Harding RM, Healy E, Ray AJ, et al. Evidence for variable selective pressures at MC1R. Am J Hum Genet 2000;66:1351–1361.

130. Box NF, Wyeth JR, O'Gorman LE, Martin NG, Sturm RA. Characterization of melanocyte stimulating hormone receptor variant alleles in twins with red hair. Hum Mol Genet 1997;6:1891–1897.

131. Smith R, Healy E, Siddiqui S, et al. Melanocortin 1 receptor variants in Irish population. J Invest Dermatol 1998;111:119–122.

132. Palmer JS, Duffy DL, Box NF, et al. Melanocortin-1 receptor polymorphisms and risk of melanoma: is the association explained solely by pigmentation phenotype? Am J Hum Genet 2000;66:176–186.

133. Bastiaens MT, ter Huurne JAC, Kielich C, et al. Melanocortin-1 receptor gene variants determine the risk of non-melanoma skin cancer independent of fair skin type and red hair. Am J Hum Genet 2001;68:884–894.

134. Scott MC, Wakamatsu K, Ito S, et al. Human *melanocortin 1 receptor* variants, receptor function and melanocyte response to ultraviolet radiation. J Cell Sci 2002;115:2349–2355.

135. Duffy DL, Box NF, Chen W, et al. Interactive effects of MC1R and OCA2 on melanoma risk phenotypes. Hum Mol Genet 2004;13:447–461.

136. Kauser S, Thody AJ, Schallreuter KU, Gummer CL, Tobin DJ. beta-Endorphin as a regulator of human hair follicle melanocyte biology. J Invest Dermatol 2004;123:184–195.

137. Babiarz-Magee L, Chen N, Seiberg M, Lin CB. The expression and activation of protease-activated receptor-2 correlate with skin color. Pigment Cell Res 2004;17:241–251.

138. Epstein JH. Photocarcinogenesis, skin cancer and aging. J Am Acad Dermatol 1983;9:487–502.

139. Rees JL. Genetics of hair and skin color. Annu Rev Genet 2003;37:67–90.

140. Tadokoro T, Kobayashi N, Zmudzka BZ, et al. UV-induced DNA damage and melanin content in human skin differing in racial/ethnic origin. FASEB J 2003 [online]. April 8, 2003;express article 10.1096/fj.02-0865fje.

141. Barker D, Dixon K, Medrano EE, et al. Comparison of the responses of human melanocytes with different melanin contents to ultraviolet B irradiation. Cancer Res 1995;55:4041–4046.

142. Brash DE, Rudolph JA, Simon JA, et al. A role for sunlight in skin cancer: UV-induced p53 mutations in squamous cell carcinoma. Proc Natl Acad Sci U S A 1991;88:10,124–10,128.

143. Ziegler A, Jonason AS, Leffell DJ, et al. Sunburn and p53 in the onset of skin cancer. Nature 1994;372:773–776.

144. Pollock PM, Yu F, Qiu L, Parsons PG, Hayward NK. Evidence for u.v. induction of *CDKN2* mutations in melanoma cell lines. Oncogene 1995;11:663–668.

145. Flores JF, Walker GJ, Glendening JM, et al. Loss of the p16INK4a and p15INK4b genes, as well as neighboring 9p21 markers, in sporadic melanoma. Cancer Res 1996;56:5023–5032.

146. Chedekel MR, Smith SK, Post PW, Pokora A, Vessell DL. Photodestruction of pheomelanin: role of oxygen. Proc Natl Acad Sci U S A 1978;75:5395–5399.

147. Smit NPM, Vink AA, Kolb RM, et al. Melanin offers protection against induction of cyclobutane pyrimidine dimers and 6-4 photoproducts by UVB in cultured human melanocytes. Photochem Photobiol 2001;74:424–430.

148. Hachiya A, Kobayashi A, Ohuchi A, Takema Y, Imokawa G. The paracrine role of stem cell factor/c-kit signaling in the activation of human melanocytes in ultraviolet-B–induced pigmentation. J Invest Dermatol 2001;116:578–586.

149. Imokawa G. Autocrine and paracrine regulation of melanocytes in human skin and in pigmentary disorders. Pigment Cell Res 2004;17:96–110.

150. Black AK, Greaves MW, Hensby CN, Plummer NA. Increased prostaglandins E2 and F_{2a} in human skin at 6 and 24 h after ultraviolet B irradiation (290–320 nm). Br J Clin Pharmacol 1978;5:431–436.

151. Kupper TS, Chua AO, Flood P, McGuire J, Gubler U. Interleukin 1 gene expression in cultured human keratinocytes is augmented by ultraviolet irradiation. J Clin Invest 1987;80:430–436.

152. Imokawa G, Miyagishi M, Yada Y. Endothelin-1 as a new melanogen: coordinated expression of its gene and the tyrosinase gene in UVB-exposed human epidermis. J Invest Dermatol 1995;105:32–37.

153. Im S, Moro O, Peng F, et al. Activation of the cAMP pathway by α-melanotropin mediates the response of human melanocytes to UVB light. Cancer Res 1998;58:47–54.

154. Westbroek W, Lambert J, Naeyaert JM. The dilute locus and Griscelli syndrome: gateways towards a better understanding of melanosome transport. Pigment Cell Res 2001;14:320–327.

155. Seiberg M, Paine C, Sharlow E, et al. The protease-activated receptor-2 regulates pigmentation via keratinocyte-melanocyte interactions. Exp Cell Res 2000;254:25–32.

156. Seiberg M, Paine C, Sharlow E, et al. Inhibition of melanosome transfer results in skin lightening. J Invest Dermatol 2000;115:162–167.

157. Scott G, Deng A, Rodriguez-Burford C, et al. Protease-activated receptor 2, a receptor involved in melanosome transfer, is upregulated in human skin by ultraviolet irradiation. J Invest Dermatol 2001;117:1412–1420.

158. Scott G. Rac and rho: the story behind melanocyte dendrite formation. Pigment Cell Res 2002;15:322–330.

159. Klein-Parker HA, Warshawski L, Tron VA. Melanocytes in human skin express bcl-2 protein. J Cutan Pathol 1994;21:297–301.

160. Plettenberg A, Ballaun C, Pammer J, et al. Human melanocytes and melanoma cells constitutively express the bcl-2 proto-oncogene in situ and in cell culture. Am J Pathol 1995;146:651–659.

161. Kadekaro AL, Kanto H, Kavanagh RJ, Schwemberger S, Babcock G, Abdel-Malek ZA. A novel role for the paracrine factors endothelin-1 and alpha-melanocortin as survival factors for human melanocytes. Pigment Cell Res 2003;16:416(Abstract).

162. Larribere L, Khaled M, Tartare-Deckert S, et al. PI3K mediates protection against TRAIL-induced apoptosis in primary human melanocytes. Cell Death Differ 2004.

163. Kadekaro AL, Kavanagh R, Kanto H, et al. α-Melanocortin and endothelin-1 activate antiapoptotic pathways and reduce DNA damage in human melanocytes. Cancer Res 2005;65:4292–4299.

164. Rouzaud F, Kadekaro AL, Abdel-Malek ZA, Hearing VJ. MC1R and the response of melanocytes to ultraviolet radiation. Mutat Res 2005;571:133–152.
165. Datta SR, Dudek H, Tao X, et al. Akt phosphorylation of BAD couples survival signals to the cell-intrinsic death machinery. Cell 1997;91:231–241.
166. Pugazhenthi S, Nesterova A, Sable C, et al. Akt/protein kinase B up-regulates Bcl-2 expression through cAMP-response element-binding protein. J Biol Chem 2000;275:10,761–10,766.
167. Price ER, Horstmann MA, Wells AG, et al. α-Melanocyte-stimulating hormone signaling regulates expression of *microphthalmia*, a gene deficient in Waardenburg syndrome. J Biol Chem 1998;273: 33,042–33,047.
168. McGill GG, Horstmann M, Widlund HR, et al. Bcl2 regulation by the melanocyte master regulator Mitf modulates lineage survival and melanoma cell viability. Cell 2002;109:707–718.
169. Liede A, Karlan BY, Narod SA. Cancer risks for male carriers of germline mutations in BRCA1 or BRCA2: a review of the literature. J Clin Oncol 2004;22:735–742.
170. Wong AK, Pero R, Ormonde PA, Tavtigian SV, Bartel PL. RAD51 interacts with the evolutionarily conserved BRC motifs in the human breast cancer susceptibility gene *brca2*. J Biol Chem 1997;272:31,941–31,944.
171. Chen PL, Chen CF, Chen Y, Xiao J, Sharp ZD, Lee WH. The BRC repeats in BRCA2 are critical for RAD51 binding and resistance to methyl methanesulfonate treatment. Proc Natl Acad Sci USA 1998;95:5287–5292.

6

Melanocyte Distribution and Function in Human Skin

Effects of Ultraviolet Radiation

Yuji Yamaguchi and Vincent J. Hearing

CONTENTS

Summary

Catalytic entities involved in melanin synthesis (including tyrosinase [TYR], tyrosinase-related protein 1 [TYRP1], and dopachrome tautomerase [DCT]) and structural proteins important to the integrity of melanosomes (including GP100/Pmel17) play active roles in the maintenance of the function and structure of those organelles produced by melanocytes. Constitutive skin pigmentation is regulated by a number of distinct factors (including melanocyte dendricity, transport of melanosomes to dendrites, and transfer of melanosomes to keratinocytes and their subsequent distribution) and can be affected by paracrine factors (from neighboring keratinocytes and fibroblasts) and the environment, including ultraviolet (UV) radiation, that regulate melanocyte proliferation and function. Because UV is inherently associated with photocarcinogenesis in the skin, including melanoma, we discuss melanocyte density and function, melanin content and distribution, DNA damage (measured by 6,4-phytoproducts [64PP] and cyclobutane pyrimidine dimers [CPD]) and apoptosis (measured by terminal deoxynucleotidyl transferase-mediated dUTP-biotin nick end labeling [TUNEL] staining) in response to UV in three different types of skin. In sum, UV-induced DNA damage in the lower epidermis is not effectively prevented in light/fair skin and UV-induced apoptosis is not seen in light skin after low doses of UV. These observations suggest that the combination of decreased DNA damage and more efficient removal of UV-damaged cells plays an important role in the decreased photocarcinogenesis seen in darker skin.

Key Words: Melanocyte; skin; photoprotection; pigmentation.

From: *From Melanocytes to Melanoma: The Progression to Malignancy*
Edited by: V. J. Hearing and S. P. L. Leong © Humana Press Inc., Totowa, NJ

INTRODUCTION

Visible pigmentation of the skin, hair, and eyes depends on the function of melanocytes in those tissues and can be influenced by a wide variety of factors that work at different levels. Melanocytes in the skin are found in two distinct populations, those residing at the dermal–epidermal junction, which give rise to skin color, and those residing in hair follicles, which give rise to hair color. A complex process of critical steps in development, proliferation, and differentiation of melanocyte precursors (termed melanoblasts) must occur with high fidelity to achieve uniform and appropriate pigmentation, including factors that affect melanoblast development and migration in the developing embryo; melanocyte survival and proliferation once in place *in situ*; melanocyte function in response to environmental stimuli; and melanin granule distribution and subsequent processing by neighboring keratinocytes. Numerous genes affect those processes either directly or indirectly, and more than 120 such genes have been identified in mammals to date *(1)*; no doubt that number will increase in the future.

The pigment (termed melanin) is produced within specific membrane-bound organelles known as melanosomes, which are produced only by melanocytes. Several of the known pigment-related genes encode proteins that are localized in melanosomes, and play active roles in the structure and function of that organelle, either as catalytic entities involved in melanin synthesis (TYR, TYRP1, DCT) or as structural proteins important to the integrity of melanosomes (GP100). During their biogenesis and the synthesis and deposition of melanin, the melanosomes are transported toward the periphery of melanocytes and are transferred to neighboring keratinocytes by a process that is poorly understood at this point. In dark skin and hair, relatively copious quantities of melanins are produced and are distributed uniformly in those tissues, leading to maximum absorption of light (and darkest color), whereas in lighter color skin and hair, decreased amounts of melanins are produced that are typically organized in clusters, which reduces their absorption of light (and hence minimizes visible color). Thus, the color of skin and hair is regulated at many points, and environmental cues, such as ultraviolet (UV) radiation, can dramatically affect visible pigmentation. This chapter summarizes what we know about how constitutive skin pigmentation is regulated and mechanisms involved in responses to the environment, including parameters that increase the risk of photocarcinogenesis in the skin.

MELANOSOMAL COMPONENTS REQUIRED
FOR MELANIN SYNTHESIS

The critical requirement for tyrosinase in the production of melanin from the amino acid tyrosine has been known for some time. Tyrosinase was initially characterized in mushrooms *(2,3)* and, several decades later, was shown to also function in melanin synthesis in mammals *(4–7)*. The initial reaction involving the hydroxylation of tyrosine to 3,4-dihydroxyphenylalanine (DOPA) is the critical one and proceeds at negligible rates in the absence of functional tyrosinase. Once synthesized, DOPA can give rise to the biopolymer melanin via an extensive series of reactions, generally known as the Raper-Mason scheme *(8–10)*. The process involves a complex series of oxidations and rearrangements that result in the formation of indole-quinone ring structures that readily polymerize to high molecular weight pigmented biopolymers *(11,12)*. It has been subsequently shown that different types of melanins can be formed depending on other posttyrosinase enzymes and also on the availability of sulfhydryl groups, the different types of melanins having distinct properties with respect to visible color and other biochemical and photoprotective properties *(13–15)*. Other regulatory points in the melanogenic cascade have been described, including: inhibitors (that modulate tyrosinase activity), posttyrosinase enzymes (that regulate the nature of the melanins produced), intracellular pH, proteasome activity, and intracellular trafficking that modulates the processing and sorting of melanogenic enzymes.

It is important to note that the early concept of direct tyrosinase regulation of melanin formation remains essentially correct because it is certainly true that in the absence of active tyrosinase there will be no melanin formation, e.g., as occurs in oculocutaneous albinism type 1. However, we now know that there are many ways in which tyrosinase activity is regulated in the melanocyte and that it is not solely at the level of transcription of a functional tyrosinase gene; there are many instances in which active tyrosinase is present yet little or no melanin is produced (e.g., oculocutaneous albinism types 2, 3, and 4). We also now know that there are many other switchpoints in the melanin biosynthetic pathway that modulate what type of melanin is produced and how much of it is produced. It should be noted from the outset that we are only now starting to unravel the highly complex series of interactions that are involved in the biogenesis and function of melanin granules, as underscored by the complexity of their proteomic analyses *(16,17)*.

MELANOCYTE PROPERTIES REQUIRED FOR PIGMENTATION

In addition to the requirement for the catalytic machinery to synthesize melanins, other properties of melanocytes and their interactions with keratinocytes are equally relevant to the control of visible skin pigmentation. For example, factors that affect the distribution, proliferation, and survival of melanocytes in various tissues are of critical importance (reviewed in refs. *18–20*) and a number of hypopigmentary and hyperpigmentary disorders have been described that result from lesions at this level, including piebaldism and vitiligo. If environmental cues, such as UV radiation or melanocyte-stimulating hormone (MSH), are functional *in situ* but responsive melanocytes are absent, there will be no pigmentation in that tissue. Similarly, important regulatory effects occur at the cellular level, both within and without melanocytes. Some factors functional at that level include melanocyte structure (e.g., dendrite formation), interactions with keratinocytes (both as a source of regulatory factors and as a repository of donated melanosomes), and other such cellular processes that affect the ultimate distribution and processing of melanosomes in tissues.

Melanocytes are highly responsive cells that interact closely with their environment, and such responses are often elicited by specific receptors that respond to hormones, growth factors, differentiation factors, and so on *(21–26)*. Some of those factors are produced within melanocytes in an autocrine fashion, although the vast majority of them derive from the environment or from neighboring keratinocytes and fibroblasts (e.g., UV radiation, MSH, endothelins, basic fibroblast growth factor, and dickkopf 1). Palmoplantar human skin (i.e., skin on the palms and the soles) is generally hypopigmented, partly because fibroblasts are heterogeneous (topographically different) in terms of the maintenance of expression patterns of *HOX (27)* and *dickkopf* genes *(26)*. *HOX* genes play important roles in regulating the patterning in the primary and secondary axes of the developing embryo and may regulate topographic differentiation and positional memory in adult tissue. Palmoplantar fibroblasts secrete high levels of dickkopf 1 (an inhibitor of the canonical Wnt-signaling pathway), which decreases melanocyte growth and differentiation through β-catenin-mediated regulation of microphthalmia transcription factor (MITF). Additionally, the pigmented nonpalmoplantar epidermis becomes hypopigmented when it is grafted onto palmoplantar wounds, suggesting that the topographic regulation of melanocyte differentiation and/or proliferation is differentially regulated via mesenchymal–epithelial interactions by fibroblasts derived from palmoplantar or nonpalmoplantar skin *(28–30)*.

Melanocyte Dendricity

The efficiency of melanosome transfer to keratinocytes is markedly affected by the dendricity of melanocytes and their cell–cell communications with those cells. In fact, melanocytes are stimulated to proliferate and to become more dendritic by factors secreted by keratinocytes *(31–33)*. The formation of dendrites requires the function of actin and Rac1/RhoA have been shown to be important effectors in this regard *(34,35)*, regulating both the extension of dendrites and their retraction. That dendricity is actively regulated by physiological factors, such as MSH and UV radiation.

Transport of Melanosomes to Dendrites

The transport of melanosomes within melanocytes to the cellular peripheries has recently become well characterized by virtue of mouse models wherein that process is compromised. At least three genes (all pigment-related loci) interact to regulate such transport, and each of those genes has been implicated in human pigmentary disorders, such as Griscelli syndrome. In brief, the melanosome uses a tether composed of two distinct proteins to link itself to myosin motors that move those organelles through the cytoplasm *(36–40)*. Mutations in any of those proteins (Rab27a, melanophilin, or myosin Va) will interrupt the distribution of melanosomes and thus have dramatic effects on the efficiency of pigment transfer in the skin. However, movement through the cytoplasm is only half of the story, and once at the periphery of the dendrites, the melanosomes need to be captured by actin filaments to remain there and eventually transfer out of the cell. Dynactin–kinesin complexes are involved in retaining melanosomes at the ends of the dendrites *(38,40–44)* and may even play roles in their eventual transfer to keratinocytes.

Transfer of Melanosomes to Keratinocytes and Subsequent Distribution

Despite intensive effort, little is known about the mechanism of melanosome transfer to keratinocytes, although it is quite apparent that it is actively regulated by melanocytes and by keratinocytes, and can be affected by the environment, e.g., MSH and UV *(45–51)*. It is clear that melanosome transfer is involved in several hypopigmentary conditions *(52,53)*, and recently protease activated receptor 2 (PAR2), which is expressed by keratinocytes, has been shown to be involved in this process *(53,54)*.

RESPONSES TO THE ENVIRONMENT

As noted above, constitutive skin pigmentation is regulated by a number of distinct factors, and can be dramatically affected by autocrine and/or paracrine factors that regulate melanocyte proliferation and/or function. MSH working through the melanocortin-1 receptor (MC1R) receptor is an excellent example of one such ligand–receptor complex that affects skin and hair pigmentation. The function of that receptor has been shown to be closely linked to skin type and hair color, also to susceptibility to various forms of skin cancer *(55–60)*. However, responses to UV (commonly called the tanning reaction) are perhaps the most well known, and because UV is inherently associated with photocarcinogenesis (including melanoma) it will be the special focus of this section.

Melanocyte Density and Distribution in the Skin

Although differences in melanocytes in different sites of the body in Asians have been reported (the density of melanocytes in palmoplantar skin is 2.5 ± 0.3 melanocytes/mm and in nonpalmoplantar skin is 13.3 ± 1.7 melanocytes/mm) *(26)*, similarities or differences in melanocytes in different types of skin have not been critically examined until recently. We recently initiated a study examining the effects of UV on human skin of various racial/ethnic backgrounds *(61)*. Examination of those skin specimens when stained for melanocyte-specific markers (TYR, TYRP1, DCT, MART1, MITF, and gp100) allowed melanocyte density and distribution to be quantitated in the different types of skin (Fig. 1). The densities of melanocytes in unirradiated skin of Asian, Black, and White subjects were virtually identical, ranging from 12.2 to 12.8 melanocytes/mm *(51)*, which agreed closely with an earlier study *(62)* reporting the density of melanocytes in White skin (17.1 ± 8.8 melanocytes/mm). The similar densities of melanocytes in the skin of Asian, Black, and White subjects was particularly interesting because, based on appearance, one might expect significant differences in melanocyte density in the various types of skin. At 1 or 7 d after 1 minimal erythema dose (MED) UV exposure, the densities of melanocytes were not significantly altered in any of the three racial groups, although chronic exposure of human skin to UV does increase the melanocyte density in human skin *(63)*, and presumably this takes longer than 1 wk.

Melanocyte Function in Response to UV

UV stimulates pigmentation in human skin, commonly called the tanning reaction. Such changes in skin color are readily visible, but few studies have examined the molecular consequences of UV on human skin of various racial groups and phototypes, or have detailed the specific mechanism(s) involved in the tanning phenomenon. Two types of tanning response are known: immediate pigment darkening, which can occur within minutes after UV exposure, and delayed tanning, which takes several days or longer to become apparent. It was unknown whether delayed tanning results from increased synthesis of melanins, changes in the distribution of existing melanin, increases in enzyme function, and so on. We have used the skin biopsies before and after UV exposure to measure the expression of melanocyte markers in response to UV, as well as melanin content and its distribution *(51)*.

MITF is considered the master regulator of melanocyte function because it regulates the expression, at least in part, of genes encoding the melanosome proteins TYR, TYRP1, DCT, gp100, and MART1 *(64–67)*. Expression of those genes has been shown to be regulated in a paracrine manner by MSH, which functions through MC1R, and by ASP, an antagonist of that receptor *(68,69)*, and it is only recently that their responses to UV have been reported in skin from different races *(51)*. The expression of those genes was examined by immunohistochemistry and their abundance before and after UV exposure was measured. In sum, constitutive levels of MITF expression in unirradiated skin were

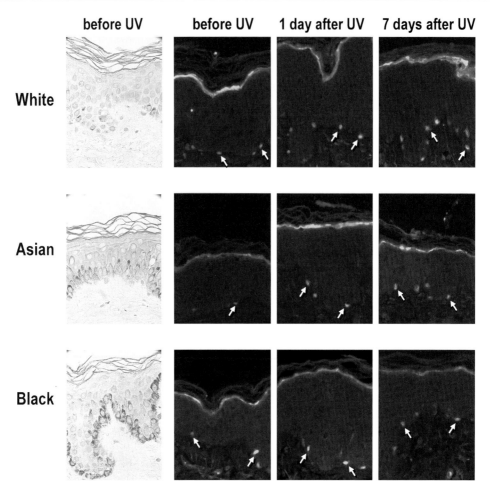

Fig. 1. Melanin and melanocyte distribution in different types of human skin. Panels in the left column are representative images of skin specimens (before UV exposure) stained with Fontana-Masson silver stain to emphasize melanin. Panels in the three columns to the right are representative immunohistochemical images to identify melanocytes by nuclear staining of MITF (some positive cells are marked by arrows) before, or 1 d or 7 d after 1 MED UV exposure.

a bit higher in Black subjects, as might be anticipated by the higher levels of melanocyte function in the darker skin, but MITF levels in Asian and in White skin were surprisingly high and were greater than 50% of those found in Black skin. All three types of skin responded to UV with similar increases in the expression of MITF, and those responses occurred within 1 d after UV. The increases in MITF were still present 7 d after this single moderate UV dose (Fig. 1). Levels of tyrosinase and the other melanosomal proteins (TYRP1, DCT, MART1, and GP100) were similarly increased between 1 and 7 d after this single 1 MED UV exposure.

Melanin Content and Distribution in Response to UV

Melanin content before and after exposure to UV has been determined by a highly specific HPLC analysis system and by quantitative measurement of Fontana-Masson staining *(61)*. The total amount of melanin in unirradiated skin from Asian and from White subjects is very similar, whereas the amount in Black skin is about fourfold higher. Interestingly, despite the appearance of a significant visible tan within 7 d, the total amount of melanin was essentially unchanged in all three types of skin 1 d after UV exposure, and had increased only slightly (6–14%) 7 d later.

Melanin distribution in various layers of the epidermis reveals why there can be significant increases in visible skin pigmentation within 1 wk in the absence of dramatic increases in melanin content. Before UV exposure, the percent of total melanin in the lower layer of the epidermis ranged from 54 to 68%, the content of melanin in the middle layer ranged from 25 to 30%, whereas only 7 to 16% of the melanin is was found in the upper layer *(51)*. However, 1 wk after UV exposure, the percent of melanin was decreased in the basal layer in all three skin types (from 8 to 13%), whereas it was increased in the middle layer of the skin (from 4 to 14%). The redistribution of melanin in the epidermis after UV exposure was initially noticed more than 80 yr ago *(70–73)*. It is known that the amount and composition of chromophores, such as melanin, in the skin are of primary importance in skin color *(74)*, but the distribution of melanin and melanosomes as well as the shape of melanosomes also have a great influence *(75,76)*. Our results show clearly that the redistribution of existing melanin toward the surface of the skin plays a major role in early tanning responses after UV exposure.

UV INDUCTION OF DNA DAMAGE
TO MELANOCYTES: EARLY STEPS TO MALIGNANCY

UV exposure can have a wide range of acute and delayed adverse effects in the skin *(77,78)* and can result in photocarcinogenesis, particularly in fair/light skin. The rates of basal/squamous cell carcinomas and malignant melanoma in the United States are 50 and 13 times higher in Whites than in Blacks or African Americans, respectively *(79–82)*. As discussed above, pigmentation of the skin is determined by the types and amounts of melanin that melanocytes produce and their distribution in keratinocytes, and can vary greatly among individuals of various ethnic/racial origins *(13,83)*. Characterization of melanocyte and keratinocyte responses to UV in various types of skin showed an inverse relationship between melanin content and DNA damage induced by UV exposure *in situ* *(61)*. Analysis of skin from the back biopsied before, or 7 min, 1 d, or 1 wk after a single 1 MED UV exposure, showed great variation among individuals in the amounts of DNA damage incurred and the rates of its removal. The skin of subjects from all groups suffered significant DNA damage, measured as cyclobutane pyrimidine dimers (CPD) and as (6-4)-photoproducts (64PP), and increasing contents of constitutive melanin correlated inversely with amounts of DNA damage.

Supranuclear melanin caps often cover the nuclei of keratinocytes exposed to UV *(84)* and the capacity of melanin to prevent DNA damage in underlying tissues can be quite dramatic. The distribution of melanin in the upper layers of the skin no doubt plays a significant role in determining its photoprotective value to underlying cells. UV-induced DNA damage to the lower epidermal layer of the skin may be more crucial to photocarcinogenesis than is damage to the upper layer because the lower epidermis contains not only melanocytes, but also keratinocyte stem cells and transient amplifying cells that are highly proliferative, are not lost via desquamation, and thus could eventually give rise to various types of skin cancers.

DNA Damage in Different Types of Skin

Comparison of DNA damage in the lower epidermis with that in the upper epidermis showed that overall levels of 64PP were similar in the upper half of the epidermis in all races but were significantly lower in dark skin immediately after UV exposure compared with fair skin *(85)*. However, there were no significant differences in 64PP levels at 1 and 7 d after UV exposure among the racial/ethnic groups, demonstrating that the repair of 64PP is quick and is similar among those various types of skin (Fig. 2). Similar but more dramatic results were seen for CPD in UV-exposed skin from subjects with fair, intermediate, or dark skin. CPD damage in the lower epidermis and upper epidermis were similar in fair skin immediately after UV radiation, or at 1 d or 7 d later. However, in intermediate skin and more dramatically in dark skin, CPD damage in the lower epidermis was significantly less than in the upper epidermis at all times (7 min, 1 d, and 7 d) after UV radiation.

Taken together, these results show that UV penetrates deeper in less pigmented skin to generate CPD and that the repair of CPD is impaired in fair skin compared with dark skin after the 1 MED UV exposure. This suggests that skin containing more melanin incurs less DNA damage in the lower epidermis and that DNA damage in the upper epidermis is similar among racial/ethnic groups immediately after UV. The sum of these results demonstrate that:

1. Skin containing more melanin suffers significantly less DNA damage not only in the upper epidermis but also in the lower epidermis.
2. The initial DNA damage the subjects suffered correlates inversely with its repair.
3. Recovery from CPD damage in the epidermis takes significantly longer than seen for 64PP.

DNA Damage in Melanocytes After UV Irradiation

Because DNA damage detected as CPD immediately after 1 MED UV was significant, even deep in the epidermis, we characterized DNA damage in melanocytes in various types of skin measured by double staining for CPD and for tyrosinase *(26)*. The number of melanocytes with detectable levels of CPD was significantly higher in fair skin than in intermediate and in dark skin, and the constitutive melanin content of the skin correlated inversely with the percent of melanocytes with DNA damage immediately after UV *(85)*.

Melanin Facilitates the Induction of Apoptosis by UV

Cells that are damaged in the epidermis after UV exposure often undergo apoptosis *(86)*, presumably to prevent cells with significantly damaged DNA (and potentially risky mutations) from proliferating. We used the TUNEL assay to measure apoptotic cells in the skin of different racial/ethnic groups after exposure to 1 MED or to a constant dose of $180–200 \text{ J/m}^2$ UV *(85)*. Surprisingly, sevenfold more apoptotic cells were observed in dark skin than in fair skin after 1 MED UV (Fig. 3), although the DNA damage in dark skin was significantly less than in fair or in intermediate skin, as noted above. A similar study using an approximately identical dose ($180–200 \text{ J/m}^2$ UV) revealed that TUNEL-positive apoptotic cells were observed at more than threefold higher levels in dark skin 1 d after UV than in fair skin.

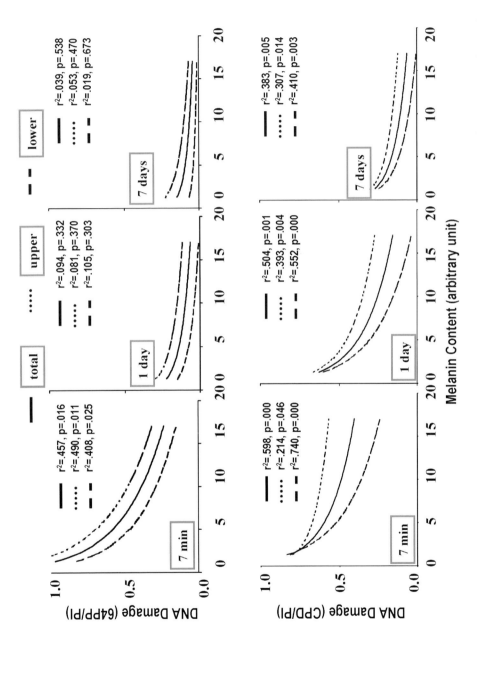

Fig. 2. Comparison of DNA damage in various types of human skin. The graphs compare DNA damage ([6-4]-photoproducts, 64PP, in the upper panels; cyclobutane pyrimidine dimers, CPD, in the lower panels) in the upper epidermis with that in the lower epidermis, sorted by constitutive melanin content. Each graph shows curves of DNA damage in the total epidermis (solid lines), the upper epidermis (dotted lines), and the lower epidermis (dashed lines). Data are sorted by constitutive melanin pigmentation (measured by Fontana-Masson silver staining) at 7 min, at 1 d or at 7 d after 1 MED UV exposure. r^2, correlation coefficient. Details are as discussed in ref. 85.

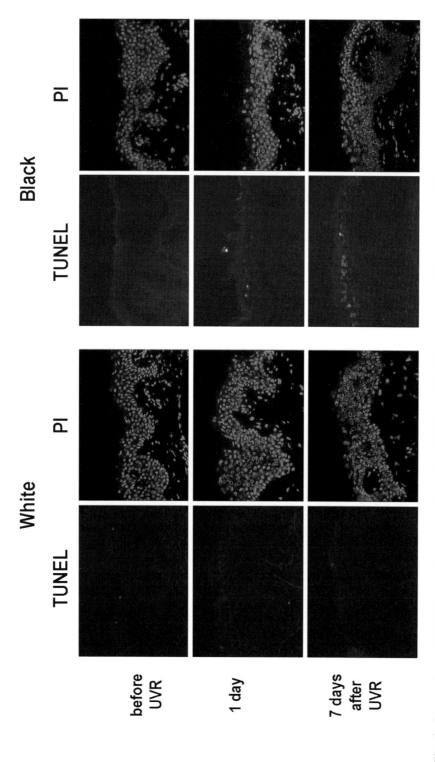

Fig. 3. Comparison of TUNEL-positive apoptotic cells in White and in Black skin after UV exposure. TUNEL-positive cells are shown as white (originally green fluorescence) in the left panels of each group, nuclei are stained by PI (right panels in each group). Sevenfold more apoptotic cells are observed in Black (dark skin) than in White (light/fair skin) 2 d after 1 MED UV.

A reasonable explanation for those effects would be that the melanin within keratinocytes is involved in the increased apoptosis after UV exposure because the only appreciable difference among skin in various racial/ethnic groups is the amount and distribution of melanin pigment in those cells. Characterization of reconstructed three-dimensional human skin equivalents (termed MelanoDerm) containing melanocytes derived from Black, Asian, or White donors (each using keratinocytes from the same Latino donor) showed similar results (85). The differences in melanin distribution are significant among these composites and they represent typical skin morphologies (including pigmentation) of those types of skin (87). MelanoDerm cultures unirradiated or UVB-irradiated at 25 or 50 J/m^2 were harvested 2 d later and characterized by TUNEL assay. Significantly more apoptotic cells were found in Black skin equivalents than in Asian or White skin equivalents at both UVB doses.

The position of the TUNEL-positive cells in the middle to upper layers of the skin after UV exposure suggests that they are keratinocytes rather than melanocytes. The mechanism(s) underlying this effect are, of course, of great interest but are currently unknown. One possible mechanism is that the UV energy absorbed by melanin in the upper epidermis may cause selective damage to pigmented structures, and a 351 nm pulse laser causes highly selective injury to melanocytes containing melanosomes (88). In other words, low doses of UV may cause melanin-specific photothermolysis, which could be considered another form of photoprotection, because it would enhance the removal of cells, many of which would have significant DNA damage. In this context, it was recently shown that eumelanin or pheomelanin was equally able to elicit apoptotic cells in the skin of mice exposed to UV (89,90).

CONCLUSIONS AND PERSPECTIVES

Melanocyte and keratinocyte responses to UV are critical for the immediate increase in skin pigmentation that occurs after a single UV exposure. The amount and the distribution of melanin in keratinocytes, particularly in the upper layers of the skin are quite important. UV increases the secretion of melanosomes by melanocytes, and concurrently increases the ingestion of melanosomes by keratinocytes (49). The mechanisms that regulate pigment transfer and the subcellular machinery involved in that process within melanocytes and keratinocytes are slowly being unraveled. Microarray or proteomic analysis of human skin before and after UV radiation might be a useful approach to further define genes and/or proteins that are critical to that process. The redistribution of melanin to upper layers of the skin following a single, relatively mild dose of UV is critical to the increased pigmentation and increased photoprotection of the skin.

In summary, two distinct mechanisms seem to underlie the dramatic differences in photocarcinogenesis of light and dark skin. First, UV-induced DNA damage in the lower epidermis (including keratinocyte stem cells and melanocytes) is not effectively prevented in White skin, whereas DNA damage in the upper epidermis is quite similar among all types of skin, which demonstrates that pigmented epidermis is an efficient UV filter. Prolonged DNA repair required by the initial severe level of UV damage may result in inherited mutations in critical genes involved in photocarcinogenesis. Second, UV-induced apoptosis is not apparent in White skin after low doses of UV, whereas it is significant in Black or African American skin, which suggests that UV-damaged cells are more efficiently removed in darker skin. The combination of decreased DNA damage and more efficient removal of UV-damaged cells no doubt plays an important role in the decreased photocarcinogenesis seen in darker skin. The fact that melanocytes in light skin show dramatically more DNA damage after UV exposure than darker skin no doubt explains, at least in part, why the incidence of melanoma is 13-fold higher in light skin than in dark skin.

REFERENCES

1. Bennett DC, Lamoreux ML. The color loci of mice—a genetic century. Pigment Cell Res 2003; 16:333–344.
2. Bourquelot E, Bertrand A. Le bleuissement et le noircissement des champignons. Comp Rend Soc Biol 1895;2:582–584.
3. Bertrand G. Sur une novelle oxydase, ou ferment soluble oxydant, d'origine vegetale. Comp Rend Acad Sci Paris 1896;122:1215–1217.
4. Bloch B. Chemische untersuchungen uber das specifische pigmentbildende ferment der haut, die dopaoxydase. Zeits Physiol Chem 1916;98:227–254.
5. Bloch B, Schaaf F. Pigment studien. Biochem Zeits 1925;162:181–206.
6. Lerner AB, Fitzpatrick TB, Calkins E, Summerson WH. Mammalian tyrosinase: preparation and properties. J Biol Chem 1949;178:185–195.
7. Lerner AB, Fitzpatrick TB. Biochemistry of melanin formation. Physiol Rev 1950;30:91–126.
8. Raper HS. XIV. The tyrosinase-tyrosine reaction. VI. Production from tyrosine of 5,6-dihydroxyindole and 5,6-dihydroxyindole-2-carboxylic acid—the precursors of melanin. Biochem J 1927;21:89–96.
9. Mason HS. Structure of melanins. In: Gordon M, ed. Pigment Cell Biology. Academic, New York, NY: 1959, pp. 563–582.
10. Mason HS. The structure of melanin. In: Montagna W, Hu F, eds. Advances in Biology of the Skin. Vol VIII, The Pigmentary System. Pergamon, Oxford, UK, 1967: pp. 293–312.
11. Riley PA. The evolution of melanogenesis. In: Zeise L, Chedekel MR, Fitzpatrick TB, eds. Melanin: Its Role in Human Photoprotection. Valdenmar, Overland Park, Kansas, 1995: pp. 1–10.
12. Land EJ, Riley PA. Spontaneous redox reactions of dopaquinone and the balance between the eumelanic and phaeomelanic pathways. Pigment Cell Res 2000;13:273–277.
13. Kaidbey KH, Agin PP, Sayre RM, Kligman AM. Photoprotection by melanin—a comparison of black and Caucasian skin. J Amer Acad Dermatol 1979;1:249–260.
14. Chedekel MR. Photophysics and photochemistry of melanin. In: Zeise L, Chedekel MR, Fitzpatrick TB, eds. Melanin: Its Role in Human Photoprotection. Valdenmar, Overland Park, Kansas, 1995: pp. 11–22.
15. Jimbow K, Reszka K, Schmitz S, Salopek T, Thomas P. Distribution of eu- and pheomelanins in human skin and melanocytic tumors, and their photoprotective vs. phototoxic properties. In: Zeise L, Chedekel MR, Fitzpatrick TB, eds. Melanin: Its Role in Human Photoprotection. Valdenmar, Overland Park, Kansas, 1995: pp. 155–176.
16. Kushimoto T, Basrur V, Matsunaga J, et al. A new model for melanosome biogenesis based on the purification and mapping of early melanosomes. Proc Natl Acad Sci USA 2001;98:10,698–10,703.
17. Basrur V, Yang F, Kushimoto T, et al. Proteomic analysis of early melanosomes: identification of novel melanosomal proteins. J Prot Res 2003;2:69–79.
18. Hearing VJ, King RA. Determinants of skin color: melanocytes and melanization. In: Levine N, ed. Pigmentation and Pigmentary Abnormalities. CRC, New York, NY, 1993: pp. 3–32.
19. Spritz RA, Hearing VJ. Genetic disorders of pigmentation. In: Hirschhorn K, Harris H, eds. Advances in Human Genetics. Plenum, New York, NY, 1994: pp. 1–45.
20. King RA, Hearing VJ, Oetting WS. Abnormalities of pigmentation. In: Rimoin DL, Connor JM, Pyeritz RE, eds. Emery and Rimoin's Principles and Practice of Medical Genetics. 3rd ed. Churchill Livingstone, New York, NY, 1997: pp. 1171–1203.
21. Halaban R. The regulation of normal melanocyte proliferation. Pigment Cell Res 2000;13:4–14.
22. Abdel-Malek ZA, Scott MC, Suzuki I, et al. The melanocortin-1 receptor is a key regulator of human cutaneous pigmentation. Pigment Cell Res 2000;13(suppl 8):156–162.
23. Tada A, Pereira E, Beitner-Johnson D, Kavanagh R, Abdel-Malek ZA. Mitogen- and ultraviolet-B–induced signaling pathways in normal human melanocytes. J Invest Dermatol 2002;118:316–322.
24. Imokawa G, Yada Y, Morisaki N, Kimura M. Biological characterization of human fibroblast-derived mitogenic factors for human melanocytes. Biochem J 1998;330:1235–1239.

25. Imokawa G. Autocrine and paracrine regulation of melanocytes in human skin and in pigmentary disorders. Pigment Cell Res 2004;17:96–110.
26. Yamaguchi Y, Itami S, Watabe H, et al. Mesenchymal-epithelial interactions in the skin: increased expression of dickkopf1 by palmoplantar fibroblasts inhibits melanocyte growth and differentiation. J Cell Biol 2004;165:275–285.
27. Chang HY, Chi JT, Dudoit S, et al. Diversity, topographic differentiation, and positional memory in human fibroblasts. Proc Natl Acad Sci USA 2002;99:12,877–12,882.
28. Yamaguchi Y, Itami S, Tarutani M, Hosokawa K, Miura H, Yoshikawa K. Regulation of keratin 9 in nonpalmoplantar keratinocytes by palmoplantar fibroblasts through epithelial-mesenchymal interactions. J Invest Dermatol 1999;112:483–488.
29. Yamaguchi Y, Kubo T, Tarutani M, et al. Epithelial-mesenchymal interactions in wounds: treatment of palmoplantar wounds by nonpalmoplantar pure epidermal sheet grafts. Arch Dermatol 2001; 137:621–628.
30. Yamaguchi Y, Yoshikawa K. Cutaneous wound healing; an update. J Dermatol 2001;28:521–534.
31. Kippenberger S, Bernd A, Bereiter-Hahn J, Ramirez-Bosca A, Kaufmann R. The mechanism of melanocyte dendrite formation: the impact of differentiating keratinocytes. Pigment Cell Res 1998;11:34–37.
32. Yoon TJ, Hearing VJ. Co-culture of mouse epidermal cells for studies of pigmentation. Pigment Cell Res 2003;16:159–163.
33. Lei TC, Virador V, Vieira WD, Hearing VJ. A melanocyte-keratinocyte co-culture model to assess regulators of pigmentation in vitro. Anal Biochem 2002;305:260–268.
34. Scott G, Cassidy L. Rac1 mediates dendrite formation in response to melanocyte stimulating hormone and ultraviolet light in a murine melanoma model. J Invest Dermatol 1998;111:243–250.
35. Scott G. Rac and Rho: the story behind melanocyte dendrite formation. Pigment Cell Res 2002;15:322–330.
36. Wu X, Hammer JA III. Making sense of melanosome dynamics in mouse melanocytes. Pigment Cell Res 2000;13:241–247.
37. Wu X, Wang F, Rao K, Sellers JR, Hammer JA. Rab27a is an essential component of melanosome receptor for myosin Va. Mol Biol Cell 2002;13:1735–1749.
38. Rogers SL, Gelfand VI. Membrane trafficking, organelle transport, and the cytoskeleton. Curr Opin Cell Biol 2000;12:57–62.
39. Deacon SW, Gelfand VI. Of yeast, mice, and men: Rab proteins and organelle transport. J Cell Biol 2001;152:F21–F23.
40. Deacon SW, Serpinskaya AS, Vaughan PS, et al. Dynactin is required for bidirectional organelle transport. J Cell Biol 2003;160:297–301.
41. Gross SP, Tuma MC, Deacon SW, Serpinskaya AS, Reilein AR, Gelfand VI. Interactions and regulation of molecular motors in Xenopus melanophores. J Cell Biol 2002;156:855–865.
42. Goldstein LS, Yang Z. Microtubule-based transport systems in neurons: the roles of kinesins and dyneins. Ann Rev Neurosci 2000;23:39–71.
43. Vancoillie G, Lambert J, Haeghen YV, et al. Colocalization of dynactin subunits P150Glued and P50 with melanosomes in normal human melanocytes. Pigment Cell Res 2000;13:449–457.
44. Aspengren S, Wallin M. A role for spectrin in dynactin-dependent melanosome transport in Xenopus laevis melanophores. Pigment Cell Res 2004;17:295–301.
45. Yamamoto O, Bhawan J. Three modes of melanosome transfers in Caucasian facial skin: hypothesis based on an ultrastructural study. Pigment Cell Res 1994;7:158–169.
46. Seiberg M, Paine C, Sharlow E, et al. Inhibition of melanosome transfer results in skin lightening. J Invest Dermatol 2000;115:162–167.
47. Seiberg M. Keratinocyte–melanocyte interactions during melanosome transfer. Pigment Cell Res 2001;14:236–242.
48. Scott G, Leopardi S, Printup S, Madden BC. Filopodia are conduits for melanosome transfer to keratinocytes. J Cell Sci 2002;115:1441–1451.
49. Virador V, Muller J, Wu X, et al. Influence of α-melanocyte stimulating hormone and ultraviolet radiation on the transfer of melanosomes to keratinocytes. FASEB J 2002;16:105–107.
50. Tadokoro T, Kobayashi N, Beer JZ, et al. The biochemistry of melanogenesis and its regulation by ultraviolet radiation. In: Ortonne JP, Ballotti R, eds. Mechanisms of Suntanning. Martin Dunitz Publishing, London, UK, 2002: pp. 67–78.
51. Tadokoro T, Yamaguchi Y, Zmudzka BZ, Beer JZ, Hearing VJ. Physiological regulation of melanocyte proliferation and differentiation in human skin of different racial/ethnic groups in response to ultraviolet radiation. J Invest Dermatol 2005;124:1326–1332.

52. Hakozaki T, Minwalla L, Zhuang J, et al. The effect of niacinamide on reducing cutaneous pigmentation and suppression of melanosome transfer. Brit J Dermatol 2002;147:20–31.
53. Sakuraba K, Hayashi N, Kawashima M, Imokawa G. Down-regulated PAR-2 is associated in part with interrupted melanosome transfer in pigmented basal cell epithelioma. Pigment Cell Res 2004;17:371–378.
54. Babiarz-Magee L, Chen N, Seiberg M, Lin CB. The expression and activation of protease-activated receptor-2 correlate with skin color. Pigment Cell Res 2004;17:241–251.
55. Ichii-Jones F, Lear JT, Heagerty AHM, et al. Susceptibility to melanoma: influence of skin type and polymorphism in the melanocyte stimulating hormone receptor gene. J Invest Dermatol 1998;111 :218–221.
56. Funasaka Y, Chakraborty AK, Hayashi Y, et al. Modulation of melanocyte-stimulating hormone receptor expression on normal human melanocytes: evidence for a regulatory role of ultraviolet B, interleukin-1α, interleukin-1β, endothelin-1 and tumour necrosis factor–α. Brit J Dermatol 1998;139:216–224.
57. Lu D, Haskell-Luevano C, Vage DI, Cone RD. Functional variants of the MSH receptor (MC1-R), *agouti*, and their effects on mammalian pigmentation. In: Spiegel AM, ed. Contemporary Endocrinology: G Proteins, Receptors and Disease. Humana, Totawa, NJ, 1999: pp. 231–259.
58. Rees JL. The melanocortin 1 receptor (MC1R): more than just red hair. Pigment Cell Res 2000; 13:135–140.
59. Flanagan N, Healy E, Ray A, et al. Pleiotropic effects of the melanocortin 1 receptor (*MC1R*) gene on human pigmentation. Hum Mol Gen 2000;9:2531–2537.
60. Sturm RA. Skin colour and skin cancer—*MC1R*, the genetic link. Melanoma Res 2002;12:405–416.
61. Tadokoro T, Kobayashi N, Zmudzka BZ, et al. UV-induced DNA damage and melanin content in human skin differing in racial/ethnic origin and photosensitivity. FASEB J 2003;17:1177–1179.
62. Whiteman DC, Parsons PG, Green AC. Determinants of melanocyte density in adult human skin. Arch Dermatol Res 1999;291:511–516.
63. Stierner U, Rosdahl IK, Augustsson A, Kågedal B. UVB irradiation induces melanocyte increase in both exposed and shielded human skin. J Invest Dermatol 1989;92:561–564.
64. Tachibana M. MITF: a stream flowing for pigment cells. Pigment Cell Res 2000;13:230–240.
65. Shibahara S, Takeda K, Yasumoto K, et al. Microphthalmia-associated transcription factor (MITF): multiplicity in structure, function and regulation. J Invest Dermatol 2001;(suppl 6):99–104.
66. Yasumoto K, Takeda K, Saito H, Watanabe K, Takahashi K, Shibahara S. Microphthalmia-associated transcription factor interacts with LEF-1, a mediator of Wnt signaling. EMBO J 2002;21:2703–2714.
67. Du J, Miller AJ, Widlund HR, Horstmann MA, Ramaswamy S, Fisher DE. MLANA/MART1 and SILV/PMEL17/GP100 are transcriptionally regulated by MITF in melanocytes and melanoma. Amer J Path 2003;163:333–343.
68. Sakai C, Ollmann M, Kobayashi T, et al. Modulation of murine melanocyte function in vitro by agouti signal protein. EMBO J 1997;16:3544–3552.
69. Abdel-Malek ZA, Scott MC, Furumura M, et al. The melanocortin 1 receptor is the principal mediator of the effects of agouti signaling protein on mammalian melanocytes. J Cell Sci 2001;114:1019–1024.
70. Hausser KW, Vahle W. Die Abhaengigkeit des Lichterythems und der Pigmentbildung von der Schwingungszahl (Wellenlaenge) der erregenden Strahlung. Strahlentherapie 1922;13:41–71.
71. Miescher G. Untersuchungen ueber die Bedeutung des Pigments fuer den UV. Lichtschutz der Haut. Strahlentherapie 1932;435:201–216.
72. Hausser KW. Ueber die spezifische Wirkung des langwelligen ultravioletten Lichts auf die menschliche Haut. Strahlentherapie 1938;62:315–322.
73. Hamperl H, Henschke U, Schulze R. Vergleich de Hautreaktion beim Bestrahlungserythem und bei der direkten Pigmenticrung. Virchows Arch [Pathol Anat] 1939;304:19–33.
74. Quevedo WCJ, Holstein TJ. General biology of mammalian pigmentation. In: Nordlund JJ, Boissy RE, Hearing VJ, King RA, Oetting WS, eds. The Pigmentary System: Physiology and Pathophysiology. 1st ed. Oxford Univ Press, New York, NY, 1998: pp. 43–58.
75. Alaluf S, Atkins D, Barrett K, Blount M, Carter N, Heath A. The impact of epidermal melanin on objective measurements of human skin colour. Pigment Cell Res 2002;15:119–126.
76. Thong H-Y, Jee S-H, Sun C-C, Boissy RE. The patterns of melanosome distribution in keratinocytes of human skin as one determining factor of skin colour. Brit J Dermatol 2003;149:498–505.
77. Matsumura Y, Ananthaswamy HN. Molecular mechanisms of photocarcinogenesis. Front Biosci 2002;7:765–783.

78. Wei Q, Lee JE, Gershenwald JE, et al. Repair of UV light-induced DNA damage and risk of cutaneous malignant melanoma. J Natl Cancer Inst 2003;95:308–315.

79. Preston DS, Stern RS. Nonmelanoma cancers of the skin. New Eng J Med 1992;327:1649–1662.

80. Halder RM, Bridgeman-Shah S. Skin cancer in African Americans. Cancer 1995;75:667–673.

81. English DR, Armstrong BK, Kricker A, Fleming C. Sunlight and cancer. Cancer Causes Control 1997;8:271–283.

82. Gilchrest BA, Eller MS, Geller AC, Yaar M. The pathogenesis of melanoma induced by ultraviolet radiation. New Eng J Med 1999;340:1341–1348.

83. Szabo G, Gerald AB, Pathak MA, Fitzpatrick TB. Racial differences in the fate of melanosomes in human epidermis. Nature 1969;222:1081.

84. Kobayashi N, Nakagawa A, Muramatsu T, et al. Supranuclear melanin caps reduce ultraviolet induced DNA photoproducts in human epidermis. J Invest Dermatol 1998;110:806–810.

85. Yamaguchi Y, Takahashi K, Zmudzka BZ, et al. Response of human skin to ultraviolet radiation: melanin-containing cells in the upper epidermis protect against DNA damage in the lower epidermis and increase the rate of apoptosis. Submitted.

86. Wikonkal NM, Brash DE. Ultraviolet radiation signature mutations in photocarcinogenesis. J Invest Dermatol 1999;4:6–10.

87. Yoon TJ, Lei TC, Yamaguchi Y, Batzer J, Wolber R, Hearing VJ. Reconstituted 3-dimensional human skin as a novel in vitro model for studies of pigmentation. Anal Biochem 2003;318:260–269.

88. Anderson RR, Parrish JA. Selective photothermolysis: precise microsurgery by selective absorption of pulsed radiation. Science 1983;220:524–527.

89. Song S, Lambert PF. Different responses of epidermal and hair follicular cells to radiation correlate with distinct patterns of p53 and p21 induction. Amer J Path 1999;155:1121–1127.

90. Takeuchi S, Zhang W, Wakamatsu K, et al. Melanin acts as a potent UVB photosensitizer to cause a novel mode of cell death in murine skin. Proc Natl Acad Sci USA 2004;101:15,076–15,081.

II MELANOCYTE TRANSFORMATION AND PROGRESSION TO MELANOMA

7
Altered Signal Transduction in Melanoma

Pablo López Bergami, Anindita Bhoumik, and Ze'ev Ronai

CONTENTS

Summary

Our understanding of signal transduction pathways involved in the regulation of melanoma development and resistance to treatment has advanced significantly in recent years. Here we focus on the current understanding of major cascades—from the receptors (including HGF, TNFR-associated factors, and Wnt), to kinases (including phosphatidylinositol phosphate 3'-phosphate and mitogen-activated protein kinase), to the affected corresponding transcription factors (including activating transcription factor 2 [ATF2], nuclear factor-κB, β-catenin, and Stat)—that contribute to the course of melanoma development.

Key Words: Stress kinases; JNK; p38; TRAF; apoptosis; Wnt; NF-κB; ATF2; Stat; PI3K; MET.

WNT PATHWAY

Wnt1

The *Wnt* genes code for secreted cysteine-rich growth factors that mediate cell-to-cell signaling via a paracrine mechanism during development and ontogeny. Secreted Wnts associate with cell surfaces and the extracellular matrix, and many have been shown to

From: *From Melanocytes to Melanoma: The Progression to Malignancy*
Edited by: V. J. Hearing and S. P. L. Leong © Humana Press Inc., Totowa, NJ

associate closely with the Frizzled family of receptors *(1)*. Wnt pathways are involved in the control of gene expression, cell behavior, cell adhesion, and cell polarity, mainly by inhibiting the degradation of β-catenin (Fig. 1).

The β-catenin protein is a central component of the Wnt (wingless) signal-transduction pathway, which plays an important role in development and tumorigenesis *(2–4)*. Intracellular levels of β-catenin are tightly regulated by a multiprotein complex composed of the APC tumor-suppressor protein, axin, and glycogen synthetase kinase (GSK)-3 *(2–4)*. In the absence of a Wnt signal, this complex promotes the phosphorylation of serine and threonine residues in the amino-terminal region of β-catenin by GSK-3. Phosphorylated β-catenin can be bound by the F-box and WD40 domain-containing protein, β-Trcp *(5)*, and is thereby targeted for degradation via the ubiquitin–proteasome pathway *(6–9)*.

Activation of Frizzled receptors inhibits GSK-3 via the Disheveled (Dsh) protein *(10)*. Inhibition of GSK-3-dependent phosphorylation of β-catenin allows β-catenin to accumulate in the cytoplasm and then translocate into the nucleus *(11)*. Once there, β-catenin promotes transcription by binding to members of the T-cell factor (TCF)/lymphoid enhancer factor (LEF)-1 family of transcription factors *(3,4)*. Activation of TCF/LEF-1 by binding to β-catenin induces the transcription of various target genes, including proto-oncogenes, such as *MYC* and *CCND1*, whose products promote cell growth and proliferation *(12,13)*. Within the cell nucleus, activity of the β-catenin–TCF/LEF-1 complex can be inhibited by the protein ICAT (inhibitor of β-catenin and TCF), which blocks the interaction between β-catenin and TCF and thereby interferes with Wnt signaling *(14)*.

Cytogenetic and molecular genetic studies have implicated a number of chromosomal and genetic changes in melanoma pathogenesis. The genes known to be aberrant in variable subsets of malignant melanomas include tumor-suppressor genes, such as *CDKN2A* and *PTEN,* as well as proto-oncogenes, such as *CDK4*, *NRAS*, and *MYC (15–17)*. Mutations of genes encoding members of the Wnt-signaling cascade, in particular *CTNNB1* and *APC,* are frequent in various types of human cancer, including, among others, colorectal carcinoma, hepatocellular carcinoma, and hepatoblastoma, as well as primitive neuroectodermal tumors *(2–4,18,19)*. Because activation of β-catenin appeared to be frequent in melanoma *(20)*, during recent years several groups studied the occurrence of genetic modifications and changes in expression of *CTNNB1* and *APC. APC* mutations were found in sporadic cases of primary melanoma *(20–22)*. Hypermethylation of APC promoter 1A was present in 13% of cell lines and in 17% of melanoma biopsies. However, cell lines with APC promoter 1A hypermethylation did not show increased Wnt signaling, probably because of residual APC activity expressed from promoter 1B *(22)*.

Oncogenic activation of β-catenin by amino acid substitutions or deletions has been demonstrated in a significant percentage (23%) of melanoma cell lines *(21)*. Conversely, β-catenin mutations are rare in primary melanoma *(20,23)*. Nonetheless, almost one-third of primary human melanoma specimens display aberrant nuclear accumulation of β-catenin, although generally without evidence of direct mutations within the β-catenin or *APC* gene *(20,23,24)*. Metastatic melanomas were found to contain nuclear and cytoplasmic accumulation of β-catenin and increased TCF/LEF-dependent transcription *(25)*. These observations are consistent with the hypothesis that the Wnt pathway contributes to the behavior of melanoma cells and might be inappropriately deregulated in the genesis of this disease. Moreover, evaluation of activated β-catenin using phospho-

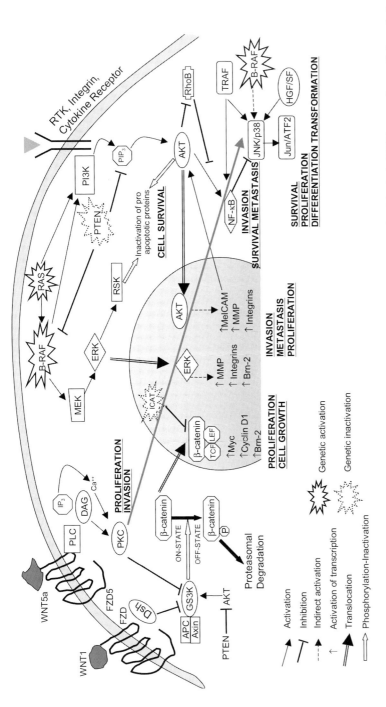

Fig. 1. Altered signal transduction pathways in melanoma. From left to right: Wnt1 signals via Frizzled (FZD) to activate disheveled protein (Dsh), resulting in inhibition of glycogen synthetase kinase-3 and stabilization of β-catenin (on-state). β-catenin translocates to nucleus and promotes transcription by binding to T-cell factor (TCF)/lymphoid enhancer factor (LEF) transcription factors. Genetic or epigenetic modifications in several genes (i.e., *APC*, *β-catenin*, *ICAT*) contribute to the activation of β-catenin seen in melanoma. Wnt5a expression has been shown to increase in melanoma, leading to protein kinase C (PKC) activation. PKC also increases β-catenin translocation. Activating mutations in Ras and B-RAF leads to constitutive activation of the MEK–ERK pathway in melanoma. PTEN inactivation has been observed in 40–50% of melanomas, resulting in activation of Akt signaling. PTEN inactivation potentiates both B-RAF–MEK–ERK and β-catenin signaling, whereas Ras and B-RAF mutations contribute to activation of the ERK–PI3K–AKT pathway. Activated Akt, as well as dysregulated TRAFs, contribute to nuclear factor (NF)-κB activation. B-RAF, hepatocyte growth factor (HGF)/scatter factor (SF), and tumor necrosis factor receptor-associated factors (TRAF) activate the mitogen-activated protein kinase (MAPK) pathway. The consequences of the activation of each pathway on melanoma biology are underlined.

antibodies revealed that nuclear phospho-β-catenin was more common in metastatic lesions and that high levels of nuclear phospho-β-catenin are associated with significantly worse overall survival *(26)*.

The finding that more melanomas have nuclear and/or cytoplasmic β-catenin accumulation than carry detectable mutations in *CTNNB1* or *APC* suggests that the pathway may be activated in such tumors through aberrations in other genes.

Recently, *ICAT* was identified as a gene that regulates the Wnt-signaling pathway. ICAT dysregulation may lead to activation of this pathway and tumorigenesis *(24)*. The *ICAT* gene has been mapped to 1p36.2 and shown to encode a negative regulator of the pathway *(14)*. ICAT protein inhibits the association of β-catenin with TCF-4 in the cell nucleus and represses transactivation of β-catenin–TCF-4 target genes in a dose-dependent manner *(14)*. Therefore, ICAT may function as a tumor suppressor and its inactivation may lead to tumorigenesis *(14)*. Messenger RNA expression analyses revealed ICAT transcript levels reduced to 20% or less relative to normal skin and benign nevi in more than two-thirds of melanomas, including most of the cases in which loss of heterozygosity was detected on 1p36. This suggests that loss of ICAT expression may contribute to melanoma progression and metastasis by virtue of altered β-catenin–TCF-4 regulation in the cell nucleus *(24)*. The mechanism underlying the markedly reduced *ICAT* mRNA levels in melanomas is unclear at present.

Regardless of the underlying mechanism, constitutive activation of the Wnt/β-catenin signaling pathway is a notable feature of malignant melanoma. The identification of target genes downstream from this pathway is therefore crucial to our understanding of the disease. The POU domain transcription factor, Brn-2, has been found to be directly controlled by the Wnt/β-catenin signaling pathway in melanoma cell lines and in transgenic mice *(27)*. Strikingly, expression of Brn-2 is not only upregulated by β-catenin but is also elevated in response to mitogen-activated protein kinase (MAPK) signaling downstream from receptor tyrosine kinases (RTKs) and, in particular, downstream from B-RAF *(28)*, which is known to be activated by mutation in about 70% of melanomas and nevi *(15,29)*. Consistent with upregulation of these two pathways, Brn-2 expression is strongly upregulated in melanoma. Overexpression of this gene has been associated with increased proliferation and tumorigenicity in melanoma *(27,30)*.

A key role of Wnt signaling in melanocyte development is the activation of the promoter for the gene encoding the microphthalmia-associated transcription factor (MITF; *31,32*). MITF *(33,34)* is essential for development of the melanocyte lineage and has key functions in control of cell proliferation and survival and in differentiation *(35)*.

Recently, it was demonstrated that β-catenin's contribution to growth of melanoma cells depends on its downstream target, MITF. Moreover, suppression of melanoma clonogenic growth by disruption of the β-catenin–TCF/LEF complex is rescued by constitutive MITF. Thus, β-catenin regulation of MITF expression represents a tissue-restricted pathway that significantly influences the growth and survival behavior of this notoriously treatment-resistant neoplasm *(36)*.

Wnt5a

Wnt signaling has been shown to be important not only in development but also in tumorigenesis. Wnt5a is upregulated in cancers of the lung, breast, and prostate and is downregulated in pancreatic cancer *(37–39)*.

Expression profiling studies aimed at identifying molecular subclasses of tumors found a series of genes whose expression differed in cutaneous melanomas with differing invasive phenotypes *(40,41)*. Among genes that created the distinct classes were those important in cell motility and invasive ability. *WNT5a* was identified as a particularly robust marker of highly aggressive behavior *(40)*. The study by Bittner et al. confirmed early studies of Wnt5a RNA expression in tumors and indicated that overall, many tumors showed increased Wnt5a expression relative to their normal tissue of origin, and accordingly, that melanomas showed increased Wnt5a expression relative to skin *(38)*. Furthermore, Wnt5a protein expression in human melanoma biopsies directly correlates with increasing tumor grade, cell motility, and invasion of metastatic melanoma *(42)*, and inversely correlates with patient survival *(40)*. Importance of the Wnt5a–Frizzled pathway in melanoma was confirmed by analysis of SAGE libraries from melanoma tissues. This study allowed identification of several genes from the Wnt5a–Frizzled family (among others) that are preferentially expressed in melanoma *(43)*.

Unlike that of other Wnt family members (e.g., Wnt1 and Wnt8), Wnt5a expression does not profoundly affect β-catenin stabilization. Instead, Wnt5a activity activates protein kinase C (PKC) *(44)*. In vitro analysis of melanoma cell lines differing in Wnt5a expression levels revealed that increased expression corrolated with PKC activation and increased motility and invasiveness of melanoma cells *(42)*. As additional support for the idea that this pathway contributes to the invasive phenotype of the melanoma cells, the authors demonstrated that inhibition of this pathway by desensitization of the Wnt5a receptor, *Frizzled5*, by an antibody that interfered with activation by Wnt5a resulted in decreased activation of the PKC pathway and inhibition of in vitro motility and invasion phenotype of the melanoma cells *(42)*. Increased expression of Wnt5a in melanoma tumors is localized, occurring in cells at the site of active invasion and in cells showing morphological features associated with aggressive tumor behavior. In connection with Wnt5a, it is noteworthy that PKC has been identified as a contributing factor in skin tumorigenesis. In models of melanoma, PKC-α activation is typically associated with increased tumor cell proliferation and invasiveness, and decreased differentiation *(45)*. PKC has long been known to be more abundantly expressed in melanoma cells than in melanocytes *(46)*. However, there is no consensus regarding whether this difference arises as part of the normal process of melanocyte differentiation or as a result of malignant transformation. Further, the upstream events involved in PKC activation in melanoma are not clear. Along these lines, the study by Weeraratna suggests involvement of the Wnt5a pathway in PKC activation in melanoma *(42)*. It has also been shown that increase or inhibition of PKC activity results in corresponding changes in Wnt5a expression *(47)*. These observations suggest the possibility that the activities of Wnt5a and PKC drive a positive feedback loop, perhaps a Wnt5a autocrine loop, and that increase in the activity of either may result in increased melanoma motility (Fig. 1).

PHOSPHATIDYLINOSITOL-3 KINASE–AKT PATHWAY

The presence of a tumor suppressor gene or genes on chromosome 10q had long been suspected, because loss of heterozygosity on regions of chromosome 10q was observed frequently in various cancers *(48–52)*. In melanoma, loss of chromosome 10 was first reported by Parmiter et al. *(53)* and studied extensively since then *(50,51)*. In 1997, using homozygous deletion mapping in gliomas and breast tumors, *PTEN* was identified as a candidate tumor suppressor gene on chromosome 10q. Subsequently, *PTEN* mutations were reported in malignant melanoma, squamous cell carcinoma, endometrial cancer, and thyroid tumors, in addition to glioma, prostate, and breast tumors.

The *PTEN* gene encodes a phosphatase whose primary function is to degrade the products of phosphatidylinositol-3 kinase (PI3K) by dephosphorylating phosphatidylinositol 3,4,5-trisphosphate and phosphatidylinositol 3,4-bisphosphate at the 3 position *(58)*. Loss of functional PTEN from tumor cells causes accumulation of these critical second messenger lipids, which, in turn, increase Akt phosphorylation and activity, leading to decreased apoptosis and/or increased mitogen signaling *(59–64)*. Reintroduction of PTEN into cells lacking it has been shown to lower Akt activity and induce cell cycle arrest, apoptosis, or both; however, it is unknown whether PTEN functions similarly in melanoma cells *(65)*.

A *PTEN* mutation rate of 30–50% in melanoma cell lines has been reported by several groups. Among cell lines with a *PTEN* mutation, 57–70% showed homozygous deletion of the *PTEN* gene *(55,66,67)*. However *PTEN* mutations in uncultured melanoma samples are rare (5–20%). Importantly, mostly metastatic melanomas contain *PTEN* mutations *(66–70,71,72)*. These findings suggest either that PTEN loss occurs late in melanoma tumorigenesis or that alteration of PTEN takes place in early melanomas, which is difficult to detect (e.g., because of relative change in the level of expression, epigenetic downregulation of expression, or homozygous deletion), as occurs in the instance of homozygous deletion of chromosome 9p21 (at CDKN2A) *(73)*. If this is the case, chromosome 10q24 *PTEN* deletions in melanomas may have been underdetected. Zhou et al., who supported this view, found no PTEN protein expression in 15% (5/34) and low expression in 50% (17/34) of melanoma samples (4 primary and 30 metastatic) *(74)*. Surprisingly, among the five melanomas with no PTEN protein expression, four showed no deletion or mutation of the *PTEN* gene, indicating the action of an epigenetic mechanism of biallelic functional inactivation of PTEN *(74)*. These observations have led to speculation that besides *PTEN* mutation, other mechanisms, such as epigenetic silencing *(54,75,76)* or altered subcellular localization, *(77)* are important in PTEN inactivation, and that the sum of these events could account for PTEN dysfunction in as many as 40–50% of sporadic melanomas *(74)*.

Functional mapping of melanoma suppressor genes on chromosome 10 has also identified PTEN as a potentially important factor in the disease. Robertson et al. used an approach that involved transfer of a normal copy of chromosome 10 into melanoma cells lacking PTEN protein. Over time, this resulted in spontaneous breakage and deletions of the wild-type copy of PTEN introduced into a culture *(78,79)*. Ectopic expression of PTEN was demonstrated to suppress melanoma cell growth *(79)* and melanoma tumorigenicity and metastasis *(80)*. Collectively, the molecular and functional mapping reports could be interpreted as indicating that PTEN plays an important role in melanoma tumorigenesis.

Because PTEN functions as an antagonist of PI3K-mediated signaling, a consequence of PTEN loss is the increase in Akt activity (Fig. 1). Akt/protein kinase B (PKB), a serine/threonine kinase, is a core component of the PI3K-signaling pathway activated through phosphorylation of Ser-473/474 and Thr-308/309 *(81)*. Several studies have shown that Akt/PKB activates the transcription of a wide range of genes, especially those involved in immune activation, cell proliferation, apoptosis, and cell survival (Fig. 2; *82*). Mecha-

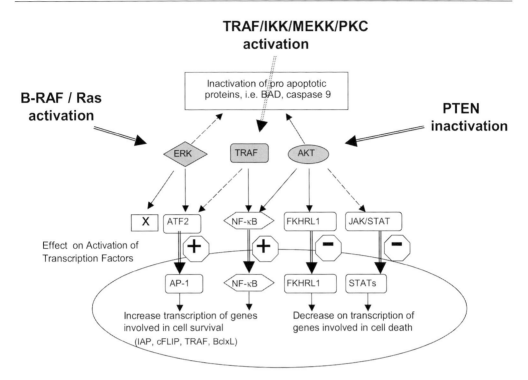

Fig. 2. Altered pathways in melanoma: effects on apoptosis. Constitutive activation of ERK and AKT and upregulation of tumor necrosis factor receptor-associated factors (TRAF) members in melanoma inhibit apoptosis by inactivating proapoptotic components or by altering the degree of activation of transcription factors that control expression of genes involved in cell death and cell survival. Akt activity induces FKHRL1 cytoplasmic retention, IKK activation, and reduces tyrosine phosphorylation of signal transducers and activators of transcription (STATs). AP-1 transcription factors are activated by ERK phosphorylation and, indirectly, by TRAF upregulation (through mitogen-activated protein kinases [MAPKs]). Balance between the signaling pathways is altered during the course of melanoma development and progression, thereby providing one of the underlying mechanisms for acquired resistance of melanoma to undergo apoptosis following treatment.

nisms associated with the ability of Akt to suppress apoptosis include phosphorylation and inactivation of many proapoptosis proteins, such as Bad *(64)*, and caspase-9 *(83)*. Downstream effects of Akt activation are also mediated by inactivation of the forkhead family of transcription factors *(84)*, and activation of NF-κB *(85)*.

Akt overexpression or activation has been documented in various human tumors, and the role of the PI3K–Akt pathway in several tumors has been identified *(86,87)*. However, little is known regarding possible Akt alterations or its role in human melanoma. Screening of the pleckstrin homology domain *(88)* and codons 308 and 473 *(89)* of Akt yielded no mutations. Considering the frequency of PTEN loss or, more importantly, its low expression in melanoma, dysregulation of Akt activity is expected. Accordingly, two recent studies addressed this issue using an antibody specific for phospho-Akt Ser-473.

Dhawan et al. found that two of five melanoma cell lines, Hs294T and WM115, were highly phosphorylated at Ser-473, as compared with normal controls. MAPK assays confirmed higher Akt activity in those cell lines. Akt activation was also assessed in 29 paraffin-embedded melanocyte lesions, including junctional, compound and dermal nevi (benign), dysplastic nevi (precancerous), lentigo maligna, and metastatic melanoma. Normal and slightly dysplastic nevi exhibited no significant Akt expression, in marked contrast to the dramatic Akt immunoreactivity seen in severely dysplastic nevi and melanomas (66.3% positive) *(90)*. Interestingly, phosphorylated Akt was located in the tumor cell membrane, the cytoplasm, and the nucleus *(90)*, which is indicative of Akt activation *(91)*. The second study showed no Ser473 phosphorylation in melanocytes (FOM73), whereas various levels of activation were observed in a set of melanoma cell lines of varying progression stage. Increase in Akt protein levels was also noted in two of three metastatic cell lines (WM164 and 1205Lu), because constitutive activation of Akt occurred in melanocyte lesions at different stages *(92)*.

As described for other cell types *(93)*, the PI3K–Akt pathway plays a critical role in survival of melanocyte cells (Fig. 2; *94–98*). The mechanisms of AKT-mediated protection from cell death appear to be multifactorial *(93)*. Accordingly, inhibition of RhoB *(94)* and Janus kinase (JAK)–signal transducers and activators of transcription (Stat) *(96)*; and activation of MelCAM *(92)*, matrix metalloproteinases (MMPs) *(99)*, and NF-κB *(90)* were identified among the downstream effectors that mediated the PI3K–Akt effect on melanoma progression and cell survival.

Although relatively small in number, the studies reviewed here provide clear evidence that the PI3K–Akt pathway is activated in melanoma cells and suggest that it contributes to melanoma development.

The cell adhesion protein MelCAM plays a critical role in cell-cell interactions during melanoma development, and increased expression is strongly associated with acquisition of malignancy by human melanoma *(100)*. Active Akt is responsible for upregulation of MelCAM in melanoma cell lines. Moreover, a reciprocal regulation loop between Akt and MelCAM has been demonstrated. Along these lines, activation of the MelCAM/ Akt–signaling axis was shown to increase survival, most likely by inhibition of the proapoptosis protein, Bad *(92)*.

Unlike other guanosine triphosphatase (GTPase) family members, such as RhoA, Ras, Rac1, and Cdc42, RhoB has been shown to inhibit invasiveness and metastasis *(101)*. A recent study by Jian et al. showed that RhoB antagonizes Ras–PI3K–Akt malignancy. Therefore, suppression of RhoB expression is one of the mechanisms by which the Ras–PI3K–Akt pathway induces tumor survival, transformation, invasion, and metastasis *(94)*.

PI3K and Akt have recently been shown to induce expression of MMP-2 and MMP-9 by a mechanism involving Akt activation of NF-κB binding to the MMP promoter *(102,103)*. Thus, a possible mechanism by which RhoB inhibits tumor migration and invasion is blocking the ability of the Ras–PI3K–Akt pathway to activate NF-κB. Consistent with this is the demonstration by Fritz et al. that ectopic expression of RhoB inhibits NF-κB-dependent transcriptional activation *(104)*. Finally, the PI3K–Akt-induced resistance of nonadherent cells to apoptosis (anoikis) is antagonized by RhoB, giving further support to the notion that the prosurvival Ras–PI3K–Akt pathway must suppress RhoB expression for nonadherent cancer cells to migrate and invade. This pathway has also been implicated in positive regulation of MMP-2 and MMP-1, but, in this case, by favoring cooperative interactions with laminin that lead to remodeling of the tumor cell microenvironment *(99)*.

MAPK–B-RAF

The Ras proteins regulate cell proliferation, survival, and differentiation by activating a number of effector proteins (Fig. 1), including the RalGDS exchange factors, the PI3Ks, and the three RAF protein kinases (A-RAF, B-RAF, and C-RAF). For many years, Ras signaling has been implicated in initiation and progression of melanoma. Approximately 15–20% of human melanomas have mutations in Ras genes *(67,105)*. Most such mutations are at codon-61 of N-Ras, with K-Ras and H-Ras mutations being relatively rare *(105,106)*, but Ras activation in melanocytes is not sufficient to induce melanoma in mouse models unless the cell cycle progression inhibitor p16INK4A is also deleted *(101)*.

Although Ras clearly plays a role in human melanoma, its importance has recently been shadowed by the discovery that the Ras effector B-RAF is mutated in up to 82% of cutaneous melanocyte nevi *(107)*, 66% of primary melanomas *(29)*, and 40–68% of metastatic melanomas *(108,109)*. The correlation of mutational status and clinical course revealed that the presence of B-RAF/N-Ras mutations in primary tumors did not negatively affect tumor progression or overall patient survival. In contrast, in metastatic lesions, the presence of B-RAF/N-Ras mutations was associated with a significantly poorer prognosis, i.e., decreased survival *(110)*. Because B-RAF and N-Ras mutations appear to be mutually exclusive *(23,29,111)*, alterations in MAPK signaling appears to play a major role in the pathogenesis of most melanomas.

More than 80% of the oncogenic B-RAF alleles described to date consist of the missense exchange from valine to glutamic acid in residue 599 (V599E). The mutation engenders constitutive and maximal activation of B-RAF kinase activity, likely by mimicking phosphorylation of S598/T601 in native B-RAF *(29)*. Interestingly, mutations V599R and V599K, which represent almost 15% of mutations at this position, also displayed increased kinase and transforming activity *(110)*. The remaining oncogenic B-RAF mutations cluster near the V599 site or in the G loop ATP-binding region at residues 463–468. In vitro studies demonstrated a 10- to 12-fold increase in kinase activity at V599E B-RAF that led to enhanced activation of the MEK–ERK pathway in COS cells *(29)*. When transfected into NIH 3T3 cells, the V599E B-RAF kinase mutant was 70–138 times more potent in mediating transformation compared with wild-type B-RAF *(29)*. Accordingly, ERK was found to be constitutively active in almost all melanoma cell lines and in tumor tissues tested, in contrast to normal melanocytes and several early-stage radial growth phase (RGP) melanoma cell lines *(112)*. Furthermore, elevated ERK signaling appears to be required for melanocyte proliferation in culture *(113–115)*.

As demonstrated for Ras *(116,117)*, mutated B-RAF also transforms cultured mouse and human melanocytes, suggesting a role in melanoma initiation *(118)*. B-RAF depletion blocked MEK-ERK signaling and cell cycle progression in human melanoma cells harboring oncogenic B-RAF, but not in melanoma cells harboring oncogenic Ras or in Ras-transformed melanocytes. Thus, although mutated B-RAF can act as a potent oncogene in the early stages of melanoma by signaling through MEK and ERK, it is not required for such signaling in Ras-transformed melanocytes because of innate redundancy within the pathway *(118)*.

The finding that the V599E B-RAF allele could be detected in as many as 80% of benign nevi pointed to a possible role of oncogenic B-RAF in nevus formation and melanoma initiation *(107)*. However, to date, no evidence indicates that benign nevi harboring V599E B-RAF actually progress to malignancy. In fact, most may represent nonprogressing terminally differentiated lesions that are analogous to nondysplastic colorectal aberrant crypt foci *(119,120)*. A more recent study found B-RAF lesions in only 10% of earliest stage or RGP melanomas. These findings imply that B-RAF mutations cannot be involved in the initiation of the great majority of melanomas but instead reflect a progression event with important prognostic implications in the transition from the RGP to the vertical growth phase (VGP) and/or metastatic melanoma *(121)*.

Several lines of evidence suggest that B-RAF mutation may not be essential in all forms of melanocyte neoplasia and that distinct pathways of melanoma formation exist *(122–124)*. Along this line, B-RAF mutation was not detected in mucosal melanomas, vulvar melanomas, and more than 90% of sinonasal and uveal melanomas *(125–128)*. These data suggest that despite sharing a common progenitor cell, the neural crest-derived melanocyte, the melanoma subtypes appear to follow different genetic pathways of tumorigenesis *(123,124)*. These distinct genetic alterations may underlie well-recognized differences in risk factors and behavioral patterns among the various melanoma subtypes *(122,129,130)*. The very low incidence of B-RAF mutations in melanomas arising in non-sun-exposed sites suggests that ultraviolet (UV) exposure plays a role in the genesis of B-RAF mutations in cutaneous melanoma, despite the absence of the characteristic C>T or CC>TT mutation signature associated with UV exposure, and points to the possibility that mechanisms other than pyrimidine dimer formation are important in UV-induced mutagenesis *(127,130)*.

However, like Ras, oncogenic B-RAF is not sufficient to induce melanoma because B-RAF mutations are also found in 80% of nevi classed as benign melanocyte lesions *(107,121)*. Therefore, other genetic events appear necessary for melanoma genesis. Along these lines, two recent studies identified association of mutated V599E B-RAF with p16/ARF loss and TP53 and PTEN mutations *(131,132)*. Thus, it has been proposed that a possible cooperation between B-RAF activation and loss of either P16/ARF or PTEN contributes to melanoma development *(132)*.

How does activation of B-RAF affect the oncogenic behavior of such tumors? How signaling events downstream from B-RAF affect the underlying program of gene expression is not completely understood. Several lines of evidence indicate that ERK activation is strongly associated with melanoma development (Fig. 1). ERK is constitutively activated in melanoma cell lines and in tumor tissues *(112)*, and elevated ERK signaling appears to be required for melanocyte proliferation in culture *(113–115)*. These findings suggest that activating mutations in Ras and B-RAF are important, but are not the only contributors to ERK activation. In line with this, constitutive ERK activation can occur in the absence of B-RAF mutations, as demonstrated by Weber in uveal malignant melanomas *(133)*. In addition, despite their low combined B-RAF and N-Ras mutation frequency, Spitz nevi showed strong MAPK pathway activation as measured by cytoplasmic expression of dually phosphorylated ERK1/2. Moreover, ERK activation can be partially inhibited using inhibitors of fibroblast growth factor (FGF) and hepatocyte growth factor (HGF) but not interleukin-8 signaling pathways. These data suggest that melanoma growth, invasion, and metastasis are attributable to constitutively activated ERK, apparently mediated by excessive growth factors through autocrine mechanisms and B-RAF kinase activation *(112)*.

Constitutive activation of ERK has been shown to contribute to melanoma tumorigenesis by increasing cell proliferation, tumor invasion, and metastasis, and by inhibiting apoptosis (Fig. 2). Activated ERK plays a pivotal role in cell proliferation by controlling the G1-phase to S-phase transition. Constitutively active ERK contributes to the growth of melanoma cells by negative regulation of the p27/Kip1 inhibitor *(134,135)* and upregulation of c-Myc activity *(135)*. Inhibition of ERK activity is associated with less proliferation *(135)* and G1-phase cell cycle arrest, mediated by upregulation of the cyclin-dependent kinase (Cdk) inhibitor, p27/Kip1, and hypophosphorylation of retinoblastoma protein. The downregulation of Cdk2 kinase activity seen after inhibition of ERK is likely caused by an augmented level of p27/Kip1 associated with cyclin E-Cdk2 complexes *(134)*.

Another target of ERK is the Brn-2 POU domain transcription factor, which is highly expressed in melanoma cell lines but not in melanocytes or melanoblasts. Expression of Brn-2 is positively regulated by B-RAF and MAPK signaling. Overexpression of Brn-2 in melanocytes results in increased proliferation, and depletion of Brn-2 in melanoma cells expressing activated B-RAF leads to decreased proliferation *(28)*.

ERK is believed to play a role in increasing proliferation by inhibiting differentiation. During differentiation of melanocytes, increase in intracellular cyclic adenosine monophosphate (cAMP) leads to stimulation of the Ras–MEK–ERK pathway and expression of MITF. MITF induces expression of the melanogenic enzyme tyrosinase, among other targets. Conversely, constitutive activity ERK limits differentiation in melanoma by targeting MITF for degradation *(35,136,137)*.

The constitutively hyperactivated ERK pathway mediates melanoma-specific survival signaling by differentially regulating RSK-mediated phosphorylation and inactivation of the proapoptotic protein Bad *(138)*. ERK-mediated inhibition of JAK–Stat *(96)* is another pathway of the MAPK effect on melanoma cell survival (Fig. 2).

ERK contributes to tumor invasion and metastasis by regulating expression of proteins, such as MMPs and integrins. A critical step in the process of metastasis is degradation of the extracellular matrix to allow cellular migration. Two families of proteases are secreted by the invading cells, the urokinase plasminogen activation (uPA) and MMPs, which are involved in matrix remodeling. The expression and activity of MMPs and urokinase are tightly controlled by MAPKs *(139–141)*. The Ras–Raf–MEK–ERK pathway is constitutively active in melanoma and is the dominant pathway driving the production of collagenase-1 (MMP-1) *(142–144)*. Furthermore, blocking MEK–ERK activity inhibits melanoma cell proliferation and abrogates collagen degradation, decreasing their metastatic potential *(145)*. Thus, constitutive activation of this MAPK pathway not only promotes increased proliferation of melanoma cells but also is important in the acquisition of an invasive phenotype *(145)*.

Integrins are heterodimeric proteins that regulate adhesion and interaction between cells and the extracellular matrix. It has been demonstrated that sustained, and not transient, activation of the Raf–MEK–ERK signaling pathway specifically controls the expression of individual integrin subunits and may participate in changes in cell adhesion and migration that accompany the process of oncogenic transformation *(146)*.

HGF–MET–PAX3

Among early observations made in the context of changes that take place in melanomas are altered expression and activity of receptors with tyrosine kinase activity that are required both for proliferation of normal melanocytes and for uncontrolled growth of melanomas *(147)*. Normal human melanocytes depend on exogenous growth factors, such as basic FGF (bFGF), HGF/scatter factor (SF), or mast cell growth factor (MGF), all of which stimulate receptors with tyrosine kinase activity. In contrast, human melanoma cells of advanced stages (i.e., in VGP) grow autonomously, in part, as a result of constant production and secretion of bFGF and activation of the bFGF receptor kinase *(148,149)*. Upregulation of FGF expression is attributed at least in part to the c-MYB proto-oncogene *(150)*. bFGF upregulation efficiently induces growth *(151)*, resulting in a transformed phenotype in normal human melanocytes, pointing to its important role in melanoma progression *(152,153)*. Conversely, expression of dominant negative FGF receptor inhibits proliferation and reduces survival of melanoma cells *(154)*. bFGF has been implicated in regulation of cyclin-dependent kinases, including CDK4, which phosphorylates retinoblastoma (Rb) protein and dissociates Rb-E2F1 inhibitory complexes, allowing progression through the cell cycle. Constitutive CDK4 activity in melanomas may result from inactivation of the negative regulator p16INK4 *(148)*.

Expression of Met, the tyrosine kinase receptor for HGF/SF, is significantly upregulated in Ras-transformed cells (Fig. 1). Inhibition of Met signaling by a dominant negative construct efficiently attenuated metastasis of melanoma tumors, suggesting that Met plays a prominent role during Ras-mediated tumor growth and metastasis *(155)*. Expression of c-Met is higher in both cytoplasmic and membrane fractions in VGP tumors, as well as in melanomas with high mitotic index or with lymphatic vascular invasion and nodal, as well as visceral, metastases. High expression in both membrane and cytoplasm was proved a significant prognostic factor in overall survival in a univariate analysis *(156)*. HFG/SF has also been implicated in the regulation of the uveal melanoma interconverted phenotype *(157)*. Animal model studies revealed the role of c-Met in the development of malignant melanoma and in the acquisition of the metastatic phenotype *(158,159)*. Regulation of HGF expression and the cause of its upregulation are not yet clear, although a recent study pointed to the role of Stat3 in the regulation of HGF transcription *(160)*. Activated HGF/SF promotes the proliferation of melanoma cells through p38-MAPK, ATF2, and cyclin D1 *(161)*. Significantly, transgenic mice overexpressing HGF subjected to UV irradiation at a few days of age form melanomas that histologically resemble the human counterpart *(162)*.

Pax3 is a member of a Pax family of developmentally regulated transcription factors critical in physiological embryonic development. Pax3 is expressed in human melanomas and contributes to tumor cell survival *(163,164)*. Pax proteins are defined by the presence of a 128-amino acid DNA-binding domain termed the paired domain, and some Pax proteins, such as Pax3, also contain a second DNA-binding domain, the paired-type homeodomain. The carboxyl-termini of these proteins act as transcriptional activation domains *(165)*. Pax3 plays an essential role in the establishment of melanogenic and myogenic cell lineages, as suggested by the severe phenotypes in mice and in humans with reduced functional Pax3 protein *(166)*. The *Pax3* gene causes Waardenburg syndrome, characterized by pigmentation abnormalities and hearing impairment attributable to the absence of melanocytes *(167)*. Interestingly, in humans, a t(2;13) chromosomal translocation juxtaposing the amino-terminal DNA binding domains of Pax3 with the transcriptional activation domain of FKHR (a Forkhead family member) results in a fusion protein that is a more potent transcriptional activator than Pax3 itself; it causes a tumor of muscle and pediatric alveolar rhabdomyosarcoma *(168)*.

Pax3 binds to the tyrosinase-related protein-1 promoter and increases its activity *(164)*. A naturally occurring Pax3 loss-of-function mutation in mice (*Splotch Sp*) leads to severe pigmentation defects and failure to establish hypaxial skeletal muscle cells *(169)*.

Although the Pax3-dependent survival pathway is not fully understood, the best-studied Pax3 target gene is the proto-oncogene c-*met*, which encodes the tyrosine kinase receptor for HGF/SF *(170)*. Stimulation of c-met expression by Pax3 is likely to represent an important pathway in melanoma development. Additional Pax3 target genes that may play a role in cell survival include another member of the tyrosine kinase receptor family, IGF-1R *(171)*, as well as the antiapoptosis survival guide gene bcl-$_{XL}$ *(172)*. In most melanomas, expression of Pax3, through its effect on cell survival, is likely to contribute to development and/or maintenance. Pax3 might therefore represent a possible novel target for therapeutic intervention in melanomas.

JAK–STAT

The Stat proteins are a family of transcription factors involved in activation of target genes in response to cytokines and growth factors *(173,174)*. The binding of these ligands to their cognate receptors leads to tyrosine kinase activation and phosphorylation of latent Stat monomers in the cytoplasm *(175)*. Tyrosine-phosphorylated Stats undergo homodimerization or heterodimerization via reciprocal SH2-phosphotyrosine interactions, followed by translocation to the nucleus and transcription of various genes *(174)*. Some of the genes regulated by Stats encode the Bcl-x, cyclin D1, p21WAF, and c-Myc proteins involved in apoptosis and cell cycle control.

The duration of individual Stat proteins' activity under normal physiological conditions usually lasts from a few minutes to several hours. However, numerous studies have demonstrated constitutive activation of Stats (in particular, Stat1, Stat3, and Stat5) in a large number of human tumor cell lines *(176–179)* and in a wide variety of tumors, including blood malignancies (leukemia, lymphomas, and multiple myeloma), as well as solid tissues (such as head and neck, breast, and prostate cancers) *(178,180,181)*. Constitutive expression of Stat3 suppresses tumor expression of proinflammatory cytokines and chemokines that activate innate immunity and dendritic cells, thereby blocking the production and sensing of inflammatory signals by multiple components of the immune system *(182)*.

Although Stat1 activation is elevated in some tumors and cell lines, the function of this molecule has been associated with growth suppression rather than malignant transformation and it thus can be considered a potential tumor suppressor *(183)*. Along these lines, malignant melanoma associates with deficient IFN-induced Stat1 phosphorylation *(184)*, as well as with Stat2 and p48-ISGF3g *(185)*. Aberrant signaling of Stat3 and Stat5 participates in the development and progression of human cancers either by preventing apoptosis (Fig. 2), inducing cell proliferation (Fig. 1), or both *(179)*. Stat3's contribution to melanoma resistance to treatment is mediated, in part, through its cooperation with c-Jun, resulting in downregulation of Fas receptor expression *(186)*. Stat3 is constitutively activated by c-Src tyrosine kinase, as demonstrated in melanoma cell lines, in which it is important for cell growth and survival *(187)*. Significantly, melanoma cells undergo apoptosis when either Src kinase activity or Stat3 signaling is inhibited, which is accompanied by downregulation of expression of the antiapoptosis genes *Bcl-$_{x(L)}$* and *Mcl-1*. Stat activity in melanoma cells was also shown to be affected by PI3K signaling in concert with ERK *(188,189)*. These observations generate substantial interest in the possible use of Stat3 as a target for cancer drug discovery and therapeutic intervention *(190)*.

TRAF, P38, ATF2, JNK, c-Jun, and NF-κB

TRAF–TNFR

Members of the tumor necrosis factor receptor (TNFR) superfamily play important roles in regulating the cellular response to cytokines, stress, and DNA damage *(191)*. Stimulation of a TNFR results in receptor trimerization and the recruitment of TNFR-associated factors (TRAFs) and/or TNFR-associated death domain protein (TRADD) to the cytoplasmic regions of the receptors *(191)*. TRAF2 is a prototypical member of the TRAF family of proteins that is recruited to TNFR1 through its interaction with the adaptor protein, TRADD *(192)*, or its oligomerization *(193)*. TRAF2 can also interact directly with other members of the TNFR superfamily, including CD40, CD30, CD27, 4-1BB, and RANK, which are primarily implicated in immune functions *(191,194,195)*. TRAF2 also interacts with RIP, GCK, ASK1, and NIK and plays a critical role in the regulation of most stress kinases, including ASK1, MEKK1, and IKK *(196–198)* and their corresponding transcription factors, including p53, c-Jun, and NF-κB *(199–201)*. TRAF2 can negatively regulate apoptosis signals from TNFR1 through interaction with IAPs or Stat1, which also affects activation of NF-κB *(202,203)*.

These functions position TRAF2 as an important mediator of antiapoptosis signals. TRAF2 activity has been shown to be regulated by multiple mechanisms, such as its oligomerization or binding to other TRAF family members, as shown for TRAF6 *(191)*, its targeting for degradation *(204)*, and its ubiquitination-dependent translocation to the insoluble membrane domains, which is required for activation of JNK but not IKK or p38. TRAF2, as well as other members of the TRAF family, is upregulated in various tumors, including melanomas *(205)*. Failure to degrade TRAF2 following irradiation is associated with resistance of melanoma cells to apoptosis *(205)*. Indeed, expression of a RING finger-deleted TRAF2, which serves as a dominant negative, resulted in sensitization of metastatic melanoma to apoptosis (Fig. 2), and coincided with upregulation of p38 and TNF-α and downregulation of NF-κB activities *(206)*. Because TRAF2 serves as a gatekeeper of stress signaling, and because it is upregulated in human tumors, including melanomas, its downstream targets are likely to be equally affected and to alter melanoma development and resistance to treatment.

All three major TRAF2-regulated-signaling pathways have been implicated in melanoma pathophysiology. Activation of JNK was shown to be critical in hypoxia-induced apoptosis of human melanoma cells *(207)*. Conversely, p38 can protect melanoma cells from apoptosis through its effect on NF-κB *(203)*. The ratio between p38 and ERK was shown to be an important determinant of tumor dormancy in several tumor types but not melanoma *(208)*, an observation that highlights the role of the interplay between diverse signaling cascades and their implications for pathophysiological alterations in melanoma.

TRAF–NF-κB

A target of TRAF2, as well as TRAF6 activities is IKK, which is responsible for the phosphorylation and subsequent degradation of IkB, resulting in release of IkB from the cytoplasm into the nuclei. Degradation of IkB by βTRCP and the SCF ubiquitin ligase complex is among the primary mechanisms underlying the activation of NF-κB, through its release into the nucleus, where it mediates its transcriptional activities *(209,210)*. Indeed, inhibition of βTRCP activity in human melanoma cells reduces NF-κB activity and renders the cells more sensitive to treatment *(209)*. NF-κB belongs to the Rel family, which contains five mammalian Rel/NF-κB proteins: RelA (p65), c-Rel, RelB, NF-κB1 (p50/p105), and NF-κB2 (p52/100) *(211,212)*.

NF-κB has been implicated in the regulation of proapoptosis and antiapoptosis gene expression, thereby controlling the balance between cell survival and apoptosis (Fig. 2). NF-κB is constitutively activated in metastatic melanoma cells in culture *(213–216)*. Constitutive activation of Akt/PKB in melanoma was reported to result in upregulation of NF-κB, which has been associated with tumor progression and invasiveness *(217,218)*. NF-κB also plays a role in the interaction between melanoma cells and tumor vasculature. The p65 subunit of NF-κB has been implicated in melanoma metastasis via its effects on melanoma cell invasiveness *(219)*.

TRAF–AP-1

Through its effect on MEKK1–MKK4/7–JNK, TRAF proteins tightly regulate the activities of AP-1 components. Upregulation of TRAF2 in melanoma is likely to cause the constitutive activity of TRAF2 targets, including AP-1. Members of the AP-1 transcriptional complex include c-Jun, JunB, JunD, c-Fos, FosB, Fra-1, and Fra-2, all of which contain a leucine zipper and form either homodimers or heterodimers through this domain. The different dimer combinations recognize different sequence elements in the promoters and enhancers of target genes *(220,221)*. Components of the AP-1 complex are induced by the tumor promoter 12-*O*-tetra-decanoylphorbol-13-acetate (TPA), growth factors, cytokines, and oncoproteins, which are implicated in the proliferation, survival, differentiation, and transformation of cells *(222)*. The complex of AP-1 proteins binds to the TRE sequence, which is ubiquitously positioned on a wide range of genes implicated in the stress response as in growth and development. Overexpression of AP-1 complex proteins has often been reported in human tumors. These transcription factors react to changes in growth and environmental conditions to adjust the gene expression profile in a way that allows the cell to adapt to the new environment *(223)*. AP-1 target genes are differentially regulated by distinct AP-1 dimers. The dynamic changes in Jun and Fos composition after stress-stimuli balance discrete signals that play a key role in determining whether cells undergo apoptosis, survival, or senescence *(224)*. *c-Jun*, *jun-B*, and *c-fos* genes have been shown to play a role in the transformation of melanocytes into malignant melanoma *(225)*, suggesting a potential role of *AP-1* genes in cell transformation. Further changes in the composition of AP-1 components studied during progression of melanoma were revealed in mouse melanoma B16 tumor models *(226)*. Additionally, it has been demonstrated that the AP-1 binding site is a key regulatory element necessary for full stimulation of *mda-7* gene transcription; expression of this gene is reduced expression as melanocytes progress to metastatic melanomas *(227)*. Expression of mda-7 inversely correlates with melanoma progression and culminates in cancer-specific apoptosis *(228)*.

TRAF–ATF2

The ability of TRAF2 to activate ASK1–MKK3/6–p38 causes the efficient phosphorylation-dependent activation of ATF2. ATF2 is a member of the bZIP family of transcription factors, which elicits its transcriptional activities after heterodimerization with c-Jun, as with Rb, CREB, and p65/NF-κB *(229–231)* following its phosphorylation by the stress kinases, JNK or p38-MAPK *(232,233)*. ATF2 has been implicated in the regulation of tumor necrosis factor-α (TNF-α), transforming growth factor-β (TGF-β), interleukin 6, cyclin A, and E-selectin *(234–236)*. ATF2 activities have also been associated with tumor development and progression *(237)*. Activation of ATF2 by HGF/SF through p38-MAPK and SAPK/JNK mediates proliferation signals in melanoma cells *(161)*. ATF2 has been implicated as one of the primary transcription factors that heterodimerize with c-Jun *(230,238)* and bind to Jun2-like elements in human melanoma cells *(239)*. ATF2 plays an important role in the acquisition of resistance to chemotherapy and radiation therapy in human melanoma *(240,241)*. ATF2 alters melanoma's susceptibility to apoptosis (Fig. 2), in part, as a result of its ability to alter the balance between tumor necrosis factor and Fas signaling *(205)*.

As a transcription factor, ATF2 is active within the nuclear compartment, where it elicits its transcriptional activities. Of particular interest is the finding that nuclear ATF2 expression is more frequently found in metastatic sites (lymph nodes, bone metastases, or visceral metastases) than in primary cutaneous specimens, and that it correlates with poor prognosis *(242)*. Strong nuclear staining in a melanoma tumor specimen *(242)* suggests that ATF2 is constitutively active.

Inhibition of ATF2 activities, either by expression of its dominant negative forms or via short peptides that out-compete the endogenous protein, has been found to be an efficient mechanism for sensitizing human and mouse melanoma cells to radiation-induced apoptosis *(240,243,244)*. These studies suggest a critical role for ATF2 in melanoma progression and resistance to therapy. The notorious resistance of melanoma cells to drug treatment can be overcome by inhibition of ATF2 activities using a 50-amino-acid peptide derived from ATF2 (ATF2$^{50-100}$). ATF2$^{50-100}$ induces apoptosis by sequestering ATF2 to the cytoplasm, inhibiting its transcriptional activities. ATF2$^{50-100}$ binds to JNK, resulting in increased JNK activity with concomitant activation of Jun and JunD. Inhibition of ATF2 in concert with increased JNK/Jun and JunD activities appears to reflect the mechanism by which this peptide is capable of sensitizing melanoma cells to apoptosis and inhibits their tumorigenicity *(239)*. Significantly, expression of the ATF2 peptide in mouse melanoma models prone to metastasize (B16F10 and SW1) resulted in inhibition of melanoma growth in the corresponding syngeneic mouse model. Such inhibition was observed when the peptide was constitutively expressed, induced in the developed tumor (via inducible promoter) or delivered by an adenovirus construct *(243)*. Further, in a syngeneic mouse system, injection of HIV-TAT fused to the 50-amino-acid peptide (which is produced in bacteria and purified in vitro) into tumors causes their efficient regression *(239)*, whereas the 50-amino-acid peptide induces both spontaneous and inducible apoptosis (i.e., apoptosis after drug treatment). A shorter, 10-amino-acid version of this peptide efficiently induces spontaneous apoptosis, which suffices to inhibit growth of mouse melanoma tumors *(239)*. These observations point to the ability to sensitize melanoma to treatment and inhibit its growth in vivo by inducing apoptosis. Experiments performed with human melanoma cultures in nude mouse models also revealed inhibition of human tumor growth after expression of the ATF2 peptide, which was enhanced after administration of either p38 inhibitor or a chemotherapeutic drug *(229)*.

Our current understanding of ATF2 in human melanoma suggests that it may serve as a clinical marker for monitoring melanoma development and as a target for therapy of this tumor type.

TGF-β

The TGF-β family includes multiple factors that elicit diverse functions in development and growth control *(245–248)*. TGF-β binds to membrane receptors that have a cytoplasmic serine/threonine kinase domain. Binding of the ligand causes the assembly of a receptor complex that phosphorylates proteins of the SMAD family that bind DNA and recruit transcriptional coactivators *(245)*. Phosphorylation causes SMAD translocation into the nucleus, where they assemble complexes that directly control gene expression.

TGF-β suppresses the growth of normal human melanocytes, but this response is lost in approximately two-thirds of ocular melanoma cells *(249)*. TGF-β1 expression in human melanoma cells stimulates the neighboring stroma cells through increased production and deposition of extracellular matrix proteins. The activation of stroma leads to a tumor cell survival advantage and increased metastasis *(250)*.

INTERACTIONS AMONG THE MAJOR PATHWAYS

The connection between the PI3K–Akt and the Raf–MEK–Erk pathway is well documented. Ras can activate Akt and both Ras and B-RAF binds and activates PI3K. Conversely, PI3K and Akt can directly alter B-RAF kinase activity and PTEN downregulates not only Akt but also MAPK *(251)*. The functional consequence of these multiple contacts is that PI3K–Akt and B-RAF–MEK–ERK strengthen one another's activities to promote tumorigenesis—essentially by positively regulating cell survival, cell cycle progression, tumor angiogenesis, and tumor invasion.

Remarkably, in melanoma, these two pathways not only cooperate with one another but also are both constitutively active as a result of mutations in B-RAF and inactivation of PTEN.

In contrast to the tight relationship between the PI3K–Akt and B-RAF–MEK–ERK pathways, the Wnt pathways are independent from the B-RAF–MEK–ERK pathways (Fig. 1). On the contrary, PTEN and Akt are involved in preventing nuclear translocation of β-catenin and TCF-mediated transcriptional activation *(252)*. This regulation is mediated by inhibition of GSK-3 after being phosphorylated by Akt *(253,254)*.

Cross-signaling is also expected at the level of stress kinases and MAPK. Constitutively active B-RAF is expected to affect ATF2 activities, based on its ability to induce Ral GDS-dependent phosphorylation of ATF2. Upregulation of HGF/SF also contributes to increase ATF2 activity via p38 activation. The increase in TRAF family members observed in various tumors, including melanomas, can enhance the activity of NF-κB and MAPK pathways. Further, the effects of NF-κB on JNK signaling and on apoptosis provide an alternative pathway for activation of stress-signaling cascades (Fig. 2).

TARGETING CONSTITUTIVELY ACTIVATED PATHWAYS IN MELANOMA TREATMENT

The important role that B-RAF plays in melanoma prompted development of anticancer agents that target key components of the MAPK pathway. Indeed, drugs targeting Raf proteins have already entered clinical trials *(255,256)*. Recently, oral administration of a MEK inhibitor prevented formation of pulmonary metastases and caused rapid regression of established pulmonary metastases in mice injected with a human melanoma cell line with the V599E B-RAF mutation *(257)*. Using a RAF inhibitor, Karasarides et al. were able to block B-RAF signaling in vivo and induce a substantial growth delay in melanoma tumor xenografts *(258)*. Because, in melanoma, constitutive activation of the PI3K–Akt pathway seems to occur simultaneously with B-RAF–ERK pathway activation, and because primary cutaneous melanomas are suitable for nonsystemic treatments, Bedogni et al. tried to block these two pathways with topical treatment with PI3K and MEK inhibitors. This treatment inhibited the growth of TPRas transgenic melanomas in severe combined immunodeficient mice, blocked invasive behavior, and reduced angiogenesis. The reduction of tumor angiogenesis was achieved through inhibition of vascular endothelial growth factor production by tumor cells *(259)*.

RNA interference is also being considered as a way to deplete mutated B-RAF *(258)*. RNAi inhibited the growth of most melanoma cell lines in vitro as well as in vivo, effects accompanied by decrease of both B-RAF protein and ERK phosphorylation. Furthermore, B-RAF RNAi inhibited matrigel invasion of melanoma cells accompanied by a decrease of matrix metalloproteinase activity and β1-integrin expression. Interestingly, the mutated V599E B-RAF-specific small interfering RNA inhibited the growth and MAPK activity only of melanoma cell lines with this mutation *(260)*. These results make it clear that the mutated V599E B-RAF is essentially involved in the malignant phenotype of melanoma cells through MAPK activation and is an attractive molecular target for melanoma treatment.

Recently, microarray gene expression profiling was used to identify highly specific gene expression changes driven by B-RAF activation compared with wild-type cells *(261)*. In that study, as few as 83 genes were able to discriminate between the B-RAF mutant and B-RAF wild-type cells. The identification of this expression signature in B-RAF mutant cells requires further analysis of the individual genes to better understand the molecular events controlling melanoma development. Because half of the discriminating genes encode proteins with unknown function, unveiling their roles may provide new therapeutic targets to treat melanomas carrying B-RAF mutations *(261)*.

Stat has also been efficiently targeted by small peptides to result in tumor regression, an aspect that is yet to be explored in melanoma. Finally, inhibitors of TRAF2, NF-κB, and ATF2 have been used in the context of melanoma and have offered promising results in preclinical studies.

CONCLUSIONS AND PERSPECTIVES

In this chapter, we have highlighted some of the major changes in signal transduction-related regulatory events that dictate melanoma phenotypes in the course of development and progression. Much of the information summarized in this chapter was reported over the past few years, which is the best testimony for the important advances in our understanding of mechanisms underlying melanoma biology. Clearly, the kinases and their receptors, as well as their substrates, are likely to serve as good targets for drug design, and as elucidated in different sections of this chapter, active research toward potential clinical trials is going on. Thus, it is our hope that the important progress will continue at the same pace and that corresponding translational studies will be able to introduce new therapeutic measures for melanoma.

REFERENCES

1. Yang-Snyder J, Miller JR, Brown JD, Lai CJ, Moon RT. A frizzled homolog functions in a vertebrate Wnt signaling pathway. Curr Biol 1996;6:1302–1306.
2. Barker N, Clevers H. Catenins, Wnt signaling and cancer. Bioessays 2000;22:961–965.
3. Bienz M, Clevers H. Linking colorectal cancer to Wnt signaling. Cell 2000;103:311–320.
4. Seidensticker MJ, Behrens J. Biochemical interactions in the Wnt pathway. Biochim Biophys Acta 2000;1495:168–182.
5. Margottin F, Bour SP, Durand H, et al. A novel human WD protein, hbeta TrCp, that interacts with HIV-1 Vpu connects CD4 to the ER degradation pathway through an F-box motif. Mol Cell 1998;1:565–574.
6. Hart M, Concordet JP, Lassot I, et al. The F-box protein beta-TrCP associates with phosphorylated beta-catenin and regulates its activity in the cell. Curr Biol 1999;9:207–210.
7. Latres E, Chiaur DS, Pagano M. The human F box protein beta-Trcp associates with the Cul1/Skp1 complex and regulates the stability of beta-catenin. Oncogene 1999;18:849–854.
8. Polakis P. More than one way to skin a catenin. Cell 2001;105:563–566.
9. Fuchs SY, Spiegelman VS, Kumar KG. The many faces of beta-TrCP E3 ubiquitin ligases: reflections in the magic mirror of cancer. Oncogene 2004;23:2028–2036.
10. Cook D, Fry MJ, Hughes K, Sumathipala R, Woodgett JR, Dale TC. Wingless inactivates glycogen synthase kinase-3 via an intracellular signalling pathway which involves a protein kinase C. EMBO J 1996;15:4526–4536.
11. Funayama N, Fagotto F, McCrea P, Gumbiner BM. Embryonic axis induction by the armadillo repeat domain of beta-catenin: evidence for intracellular signaling. J Cell Biol 1995;128:959–968.
12. He TC, Sparks AB, Rago C, et al. Identification of c-MYC as a target of the APC pathway. Science 1998;281:1509–1512.
13. Lin SY, Xia W, Wang JC, et al. Beta-catenin, a novel prognostic marker for breast cancer: its roles in cyclin D1 expression and cancer progression. Proc Natl Acad Sci U S A 2000;97:4262–4266.
14. Tago K, Nakamura T, Nishita M, et al. Inhibition of Wnt signaling by ICAT, a novel beta-catenin-interacting protein. Genes Dev 2000;14:1741–1749.
15. Pollock PM, Trent JM. The genetics of cutaneous melanoma. Clin Lab Med 2000;20:667–690.
16. Saida T. Recent advances in melanoma research. J Dermatol Sci 2001;26:1–13.
17. Castellano M, Parmiani G. Genes involved in melanoma: an overview of INK4a and other loci. Melanoma Res 1999;9:421–432.
18. Koch A, Denkhaus D, Albrecht S, Leuschner I, von Schweinitz D, Pietsch T. Childhood hepatoblastomas frequently carry a mutated degradation targeting box of the beta-catenin gene. Cancer Res 1999;59:269–273.
19. Koch A, Waha A, Tonn JC, et al. Somatic mutations of WNT/wingless signaling pathway components in primitive neuroectodermal tumors. Int J Cancer 2001;93:445–449.
20. Rimm DL, Caca K, Hu G, Harrison FB, Fearon ER. Frequent nuclear/cytoplasmic localization of beta-catenin without exon 3 mutations in malignant melanoma. Am J Pathol 1999;154:325–329.
21. Rubinfeld B, Robbins P, El-Gamil M, Albert I, Porfiri E, Polakis P. Stabilization of beta-catenin by genetic defects in melanoma cell lines. Science 1997;275:1790–1792.
22. Worm J, Christensen C, Gronbaek K, Tulchinsky E, Guldberg P. Genetic and epigenetic alterations of the APC gene in malignant melanoma. Oncogene 2004;23:5215–5226.
23. Omholt K, Platz A, Ringborg U, Hansson J. Cytoplasmic and nuclear accumulation of beta-catenin is rarely caused by CTNNB1 exon 3 mutations in cutaneous malignant melanoma. Int J Cancer 2001;92:839–842.
24. Reifenberger J, Knobbe CB, Wolter M, et al. Molecular genetic analysis of malignant melanomas for aberrations of the WNT signaling pathway genes CTNNB1, APC, ICAT and BTRC. Int J Cancer. 2002;100:549–556.
25. Murakami T, Toda S, Fujimoto M, et al. Constitutive activation of Wnt/beta-catenin signaling pathway in migration-active melanoma cells: role of LEF-1 in melanoma with increased metastatic potential. Biochem Biophys Res Commun 2001;288:8–15.
26. Kielhorn E, Provost E, Olsen D, et al. Tissue microarray-based analysis shows phospho–beta-catenin expression in malignant melanoma is associated with poor outcome. Int J Cancer 2003;103:652–656.
27. Goodall J, Martinozzi S, Dexter TJ, et al. Brn-2 expression controls melanoma proliferation and is directly regulated by beta-catenin. Mol Cell Biol 2004;27:2915–2922.

28. Goodall J, Wellbrock C, Dexter TJ, Roberts K, Marais R, Goding CR. The Brn-2 transcription factor activated BRAF to melanoma proliferation. Mol Cell Biol 2004;24:2924–2932.

29. Davies H, Bignell GR, Cox C, et al. Mutations of the BRAF gene in human cancer. Nature 2002;417:949–954.

30. Thomson JA, Murphy K, Baker E, Sutherland GR, Parsons PG, Sturm RA. The brn-2 gene regulates the melanocytic phenotype and tumorigenic potential of human melanoma cells. Oncogene 1995;11:690–700.

31. Dorsky RI, Raible DW, Moon RT. Direct regulation of nacre, a zebrafish MITF homolog required for pigment cell formation, by the Wnt pathway. Genes Dev 2000;14:158–162.

32. Takeda K, Yasumoto K, Takada R, et al. Induction of melanocyte-specific microphthalmia-associated transcription factor by Wnt-3a. J Biol Chem 2000;275:14,013–14,016.

33. Hodgkinson CA, Moore KJ, Nakayama A, et al. Mutations at the mouse microphthalmia locus are associated with defects in a gene encoding a novel basic-helix-loop-helix-zipper protein. Cell 1993;74:395–404.

34. Hughes MJ, Lingrel JB, Krakowsky JM, Anderson KP. A helix-loop-helix transcription factor-like gene is located at the mi locus. J Biol Chem 1993;268:20,687–20,690.

35. Goding CR. Mitf from neural crest to melanoma: signal transduction and transcription in the melanocyte lineage. Genes Dev 2000;14:1712–1728.

36. Widlund HR, Horstmann MA, Price ER, et al. Beta-catenin–induced melanoma growth requires the downstream target Microphthalmia-associated transcription factor. J Cell Biol 2002;158:1079–1087.

37. Crnogorac-Jurcevic T, Efthimiou E, Capelli P, et al. Gene expression profiles of pancreatic cancer and stromal desmoplasia. Oncogene 2001;20:7437–7446.

38. Iozzo RV, Eichstetter I, Danielson KG. Aberrant expression of the growth factor Wnt-5A in human malignancy. Cancer Res. 1995;55:3495–3499.

39. Lejeune S, Huguet EL, Hamby A, Poulsom R, Harris AL. Wnt5a cloning, expression, and up-regulation in human primary breast cancers. Clin Cancer Res 1995;1:215–222.

40. Bittner M, Meltzer P, Chen Y, et al. Molecular classification of cutaneous malignant melanoma by gene expression profiling. Nature 2000;406:536–540.

41. Carr KM, Bittner M, Trent JM. Gene-expression profiling in human cutaneous melanoma. Oncogene 2003;22:3076–3080.

42. Weeraratna AT, Jiang Y, Hostetter G, et al. Wnt5a signaling directly affects cell motility and invasion of metastatic melanoma. Cancer Cell 2002;1:279–288.

43. Weeraratna AT, Becker D, Carr KM, et al. Generation and analysis of melanoma SAGE libraries: SAGE advice on the melanoma transcriptome. Oncogene 2004;23:2264–2274.

44. Kuhl M, Sheldahl LC, Park M, Miller JR, Moon RT. The Wnt/Ca2+ pathway: a new vertebrate Wnt signaling pathway takes shape. Trends Genet 2000;16:279–283.

45. Lahn MM, Sundell KL. The role of protein kinase C-alpha (PKC-alpha) in melanoma. Melanoma Res. 2004;14:85–89.

46. Powell MB, Rosenberg RK, Graham MJ, et al. Protein kinase C beta expression correlates with biological responses to 12-0-tetradecanoylphorbol 13-acetate. J Cancer Res Clin Oncol 1993; 119:199–206.

47. Jonsson M, Smith K, Harris AL. Regulation of Wnt5a expression in human mammary cells by protein kinase C activity and the cytoskeleton. Br J Cancer 1998;78:430–438.

48. Fults D, Pedone C. Deletion mapping of the long arm of chromosome 10 in glioblastoma multiforme. Genes Chromosomes Cancer 1993;7:173–177.

49. Isshiki K, Elder DE, Guerry D, Linnenbach AJ. Chromosome 10 allelic loss in malignant melanoma. Genes Chromosomes Cancer 1993;8:178–184.

50. Herbst RA, Weiss J, Ehnis A, Cavenee WK, Arden KC. Loss of heterozygosity for 10q22-10qter in malignant melanoma progression. Cancer Res 1994;54:3111–3114.

51. Healy E, Rehman I, Angus B, Rees JL. Loss of heterozygosity in sporadic primary cutaneous melanoma. Genes Chromosomes Cancer 1995;12:152–156.

52. Ittmann M. Allelic loss on chromosome 10 in prostate adenocarcinoma. Cancer Res 1996;56: 2143–2147.

53. Parmiter AH, Balaban G, Clark WH Jr, Nowell PC. Possible involvement of the chromosome region 10q24–q26 in early stages of melanocytic neoplasia. Cancer Genet Cytogenet 1988;30:313–317.

54. Dahia PL, Marsh DJ, Zheng Z, et al. Somatic deletions and mutations in the Cowden disease gene, PTEN, in sporadic thyroid tumors. Cancer Res 1997;57:4710–4713.

55. Guldberg P, Thor Straten P, Birck A, Ahrenkiel V, Kirkin AF, Zeuthen J. Disruption of the MMAC1/ PTEN gene by deletion or mutation is a frequent event in malignant melanoma. Cancer Res 1997;57:3660–3663.
56. Tashiro H, Blazes MS, Wu R, et al. Mutations in PTEN are frequent in endometrial carcinoma but rare in other common gynecological malignancies. Cancer Res 1997;57:3935–3940.
57. Poetsch M, Lorenz G, Kleist B. Detection of new PTEN/MMAC1 mutations in head and neck squamous cell carcinomas with loss of chromosome 10. Cancer Genet Cytogenet 2002;132:20–24.
58. Simpson L, Parsons R. PTEN: life as a tumor suppressor. Exp Cell Res 2001;264:29–41.
59. Dudek H, Datta SR, Franke TF, et al. Regulation of neuronal survival by the serine-threonine protein kinase Akt. Science 1997;275:661–665.
60. Kauffmann-Zeh A, Rodriguez-Viciana P, Ulrich E, et al. Suppression of c-Myc–induced apoptosis by Ras signalling through PI(3)K and PKB. Nature 1997;385:544–548.
61. Kennedy SG, Wagner AJ, Conzen SD, et al. The PI 3-kinase/Akt signaling pathway delivers an anti-apoptotic signal. Genes Dev 1997;11:701–713.
62. Kulik G, Klippel A, Weber MJ. Antiapoptotic signalling by the insulin-like growth factor I receptor, phosphatidylinositol 3-kinase, and Akt. Mol Cell Biol 1997;17:1595–1606.
63. Songyang Z, Baltimore D, Cantley LC, Kaplan DR, Franke TF. Interleukin 3-dependent survival by the Akt protein kinase. Proc Natl Acad Sci U S A 1997;94:11,345–11,350.
64. Datta SR, Dudek H, Tao X, et al. Akt phosphorylation of BAD couples survival signals to the cell-intrinsic death machinery. Cell 1997;91:231–241.
65. Cheney IW, Johnson DE, Vaillancourt MT, et al. Suppression of tumorigenicity of glioblastoma cells by adenovirus-mediated MMAC1/PTEN gene transfer. Cancer Res 1998;58:2331–2334.
66. Teng DH, Hu R, Lin H, et al. MMAC1/PTEN mutations in primary tumor specimens and tumor cell lines. Cancer Res 1997;57:5221–5225.
67. Tsao H, Zhang X, Benoit E, Haluska FG. Identification of PTEN/MMAC1 alterations in uncultured melanomas and melanoma cell lines. Oncogene 1998;16:3397–3402.
68. Birck A, Ahrenkiel V, Zeuthen J, Hou-Jensen K, Guldberg P. Mutation and allelic loss of the PTEN/ MMAC1 gene in primary and metastatic melanoma biopsies. J Invest Dermatol 2000;114:277–280.
69. Reifenberger J, Wolter M, Boström J, Schulte K, Ruzicka T, Reifenberger G. Allelic losses on chromosome arm 10q and mutation of the PTEN (MMAC1) tumour suppressor gene in primary and metastatic malignant melanomas. Virchows Arch 2000;436:487–493.
70. Celebi JT, Shendrik I, Silvers DN, Peacocke MJ. Identification of PTEN mutations in metastatic melanoma specimens. J Med Genet 2000;37:653–657.
71. Boni R, Vortmeyer AO, Burg G, Hofbauer G, Zhuang Z. The PTEN tumour suppressor gene and malignant melanoma. Melanoma Res 1998;8:300–302.
72. Poetsch M, Dittberner T, Woenckhaus C. PTEN/MMAC1 in malignant melanoma and its importance for tumor progression. Cancer Genet Cytogenet 2001;125:21–26.
73. Cairns P, Polascik TJ, Eby Y, et al. Frequency of homozygous deletion at p16/CDKN2 in primary human tumours. Nat Genet 1995;11:210–212.
74. Zhou XP, Gimm O, Hampel H, Niemann T, Walker MJ, Eng C. Epigenetic PTEN silencing in malignant melanomas without PTEN mutation. Am J Pathol 2000;157:1123–1128.
75. Whang YE, Wu X, Suzuki H, et al. Inactivation of the tumor suppressor PTEN/MMAC1 in advanced human prostate cancer through loss of expression. Proc Natl Acad Sci USA 1998;95:5246–5250.
76. Salvesen HB, MacDonald N, Ryan A, et al. PTEN methylation is associated with advanced stage and microsatellite instability in endometrial carcinoma. Int J Cancer 2001;91:22–26.
77. Whiteman DC, Zhou XP, Cummings MC, Pavey S, Hayward NK, Eng C. Nuclear PTEN expression and clinicopathologic features in a population-based series of primary cutaneous melanoma. Int J Cancer 2002;99:63–67.
78. Robertson GP, Herbst RA, Nagane M, Huang HJ, Cavenee WK. The chromosome 10 monosomy common in human melanomas results from loss of two separate tumor suppressor loci. Cancer Res 1999;59:3596–3601.
79. Robertson GP, Furnari FB, Miele ME, et al. In vitro loss of heterozygosity targets the PTEN/MMAC1 gene in melanoma. Proc Natl Acad Sci USA 1998;95:9418–9423.
80. Hwang PH, Yi HK, Kim DS, Nam SY, Kim JS, Lee DY. Suppression of tumorigenicity and metastasis in B16F10 cells by PTEN/MMAC1/TEP1 gene. Cancer Lett 2001;172:83–91.
81. Harlan JE, Yoon HS, Hajduk PJ, Fesik SW. Structural characterization of the interaction between a pleckstrin homology domain and phosphatidylinositol 4,5-bisphosphate. Biochemistry 1995;34: 9859–9864.

82. Karin M, Lin A. NF-B at the crossroads of life and death. Nat Immunol 2002;3:221–227.
83. Cardone MH, Roy N, Stennicke HR, et al. Regulation of cell death protease caspase-9 by phospho-rylation. Science 1998;282:1318–1321.
84. Brunet A, Bonni A, Zigmond MJ, et al. Akt promotes cell survival by phosphorylating and inhibiting a Forkhead transcription factor. Cell 1999;96:857–868.
85. Romashkova JA, Makarov SS. NF-B is a target of AKT in anti-apoptotic PDGF signalling. Nature 1999;401:86–90.
86. Aoki M, Batista O, Bellacosa A, Tsichlis P, Vogt PK. The akt kinase: molecular determinants of oncogenicity. Proc Natl Acad Sci USA 1998;95:14,950–14,955.
87. Nicholson KM, Anderson NG. The protein kinase B/Akt signalling pathway in human malignancy. Cell Signal 2002;14:381–395.
88. Waldmann V, Wacker J, Deichmann M. Absence of mutations in the pleckstrin homology (PH) domain of protein kinase B (PKB/Akt) in malignant melanoma. Melanoma Res 2002;12:45–50.
89. Waldmann V, Wacker J, Deichmann M. Mutations of the activation-associated phosphorylation sites at codons 308 and 473 of protein kinase B are absent in human melanoma. Arch Dermatol Res 2001;293:368–372.
90. Dhawan P, Singh AB, Ellis DL, Richmond A. Constitutive activation of Akt/protein kinase B in melanoma leads to up-regulation of nuclear factor-kappaB and tumor progression. Cancer Res 2002;62:7335–7342.
91. Andjelkovic M, Alessi DR, Meier R, et al. Role of translocation in the activation and function of protein kinase B. J Biol Chem 1997;272:31,515–31,524.
92. Li G, Kalabis J, Xu X, et al. Reciprocal regulation of MelCAM and AKT in human melanoma. Oncogene 2003;22:6891–6899.
93. Vivanco I, Sawyers CL. The phosphatidylinositol 3-kinase AKT pathway in human cancer. Nat Rev Cancer 2002;2:489–501.
94. Jiang K, Sun J, Cheng J, Djeu JY, Wei S, Sebti S. Akt mediates Ras downregulation of RhoB, a suppressor of transformation, invasion, and metastasis. Cancer Res 2003;63:2881–2890.
95. Stewart AL, Mhashilkar AM, Yang XH, et al. PI3 kinase blockade by Ad-PTEN inhibits invasion and induces apoptosis in RGP and metastatic melanoma cells. Mol Med 2002;8:451–461.
96. Krasilnikov M, Ivanov VN, Dong J, Ronai Z. ERK and PI3K negatively regulate STAT-transcrip-tional activities in human melanoma cells: implications towards sensitization to apoptosis. Oncogene 2003;22:4092–4101.
97. Stahl JM, Cheung M, Sharma A, Trivedi NR, Shanmugam S, Robertson GP. Loss of PTEN promotes tumor development in malignant melanoma. Cancer Res 2003;63:2881–2890.
98. Larribere L, Khaled M, Tartare-Deckert S. PI3K mediates protection against TRAIL-induced apoptosis in primary human melanocytes. Cell Death Differ 2004;1038:4401–4475.
99. Hess AR, Seftor EA, Seftor RE, Hendrix MJ. Phosphoinositide 3-kinase regulates membrane Type 1-matrix metalloproteinase (MMP) and MMP-2 activity during melanoma cell vasculogenic mim-icry. Cancer Res 2003;63:4757–4762.
100. Johnson JP. Cell adhesion molecules in the development and progression of malignant melanoma. Cancer Metastasis Rev 1999;18:345–357.
101. Chen Z, Sun J, Pradines A, Favre G, Adnane J, Sebti SM. Both farnesylated and geranylgeranylated RhoB inhibit malignant transformation and suppress human tumor growth in nude mice. J Biol Chem 2000;275:17,974–17,978.
102. Kim D, Kim S, Koh H, et al. Akt/PKB promotes cancer cell invasion via increased motility and metalloproteinase production. FASEB J 2001;15:1953–1962.
103. Park BK, Zeng X, Glazer RI. Akt1 induces extracellular matrix invasion and matrix metalloproteinase-2 activity in mouse mammary epithelial cells. Cancer Res 2001;61:7647–7653.
104. Fritz G, Kaina B. Ras-related GTPase Rhob represses NF-kappaB signaling. J Biol Chem 2001;276:3115–3122.
105. van Elsas A, Zerp S, van der Flier S, et al. Analysis of N-Ras mutations in human cutaneous mela-noma: tumour heterogeneity detected by polymerase chain reaction/single-stranded conformation polymerism analysis. Rec Results Cancer Res 1995;139:57–67.
106. Carr J, MacKie RM. Point mutations in the N-Ras oncogene in malignant melanoma and congenital naevi. Br J Dermatol 1994;131:72–77.
107. Pollock PM, Harper UL, Hansen KS, et al. High frequency of BRAF mutations in nevi. Nat Genet 2003;33:19–20.

108. Gorden A, Osman I, Gai W, et al. Analysis of BRAF and N-Ras mutations in metastatic melanoma tissues. Cancer Res. 2003;63:3955–3957.

109. Kumar R, Angelini S, Czene K, et al. BRAF mutations in metastatic melanoma: a possible association with clinical outcome. Clin Cancer Res 2003;9:3362–3368.

110. Houben R, Becker JC, Kappel A, et al. Constitutive activation of the Ras-Raf signaling pathway in metastatic melanoma is associated with poor prognosis. J Carcinog 2004;3:6.

111. Ball NJ, Yohn JJ, Morelli JG, Norris DA, Golitz LE, Hoeffler JP. Ras mutations in human melanoma: a marker of malignant progression. J Investig Dermatol 1994;102:285–290.

112. Satyamoorthy K, Li G, Gerrero MR, et al. Constitutive mitogen-activated protein kinase activation in melanoma is mediated by both BRAF mutations and autocrine growth factor stimulation. Cancer Res. 2003;63:756–759.

113. Bohm M, Moellmann G, Cheng E, et al. Identification of p90RSK as the probable CREB-Ser133 kinase in human melanocytes. Cell Growth Differ 1995;6:291–302.

114. Imokawa G, Kobayasi T, Miyagishi M. Intracellular signaling mechanisms leading to synergistic effects of endothelin-1 and stem cell factor on proliferation of cultured human melanocytes. Cross-talk via trans-activation of the tyrosine kinase c-kit receptor. J Biol Chem 2000;275:33,321–33,328.

115. Wellbrock C, Weisser C, Geissinger E, Troppmair J, Schartl M. Activation of p59(Fyn) leads to melanocyte dedifferentiation by influencing MKP-1–regulated mitogen-activated protein kinase signaling. J Biol Chem 2002;277:6443–6454.

116. Wilson RE, Dooley TP, Hart IR. Induction of tumorigenicity and lack of in vitro growth requirement for 12-O-tetradecanoylphorbol-13-acetate by transfection of murine melanocytes with v-Ha-Ras. Cancer Res 1989;49:711–716.

117. Albino AP, Sozzi G, Nanus DM, Jhanwar SC, Houghton AN. Malignant transformation of human melanocytes: induction of a complete melanoma phenotype and genotype. Oncogene 1992;7:2315–2321.

118. Wellbrock C, Ogilvie L, Hedley D, et al. V599EB-RAF is an oncogene in melanocytes. Cancer Res 2004;64:2338–2342.

119. Takayama T, Ohi M, Hayashi T, et al. Analysis of K-Ras, APC, and beta-catenin in aberrant crypt foci in sporadic adenoma, cancer, and familial adenomatous polyposis. Gastroenterology 2001;121:599–611.

120. Yamashita N, Minamoto T, Ochiai A, Onda M, Esumi H. Frequent and characteristic K-Ras activation and absence of p53 protein accumulation in aberrant crypt foci of the colon. Gastroenterology 1995;108:434–440.

121. Dong J, Phelps RG, Qiao R, et al. BRAF oncogenic mutations correlate with progression rather than initiation of human melanoma. Cancer Res 2003;63:3883–3885.

122. Saldanha G, Purnell D, Fletcher A, Potter L, Gillies A, Pringle JH. High BRAF mutation frequency does not characterize all melanocytic tumor types. Int J Cancer 2004;111:705–710.

123. Rivers JK. Is there more than one road to melanoma? Lancet 2004;363:728–730.

124. Tomicic J, Wanebo HJ. Mucosal melanomas. Surg Clin N Am 2003;83:237–252.

125. Cohen Y, Goldenberg-Cohen N, Parrella P, et al. Lack of BRAF mutation in primary uveal melanoma. Invest Ophthalmol Vis Sci 2003;44:2876–2878.

126. Edmunds SC, Cree IA, Di Nicolantonio F, Hungerford JL, Hurren JS, Kelsell DP. Absence of BRAF gene mutations in uveal melanomas in contrast to cutaneous melanomas. Br J Cancer 2003;88:1403–1405.

127. Edwards RH, Ward MR, Wu H, et al. Absence of BRAF mutations in UV-protected mucosal melanomas. J Med Genet 2004;41:270–272.

128. Klc E, Bruggenwirth HT, Verbiest MM, et al. The Ras-BRAF kinase pathway is not involved in uveal melanoma. Melanoma Res 2004;14:203–205.

129. Maldonado JL, Fridlyand J, Patel H, et al. Determinants of BRAF mutations in primary melanomas. J Natl Cancer Inst 2003;95:1878–1890.

130. Cohen Y, Rosenbaum E, Begum S, et al. Clin exon 15 BRAF mutations are uncommon in melanomas arising in nonsun-exposed sites. Cancer Res 2004;10:3444–3447.

131. Daniotti M, Oggionni M, Ranzani T, et al. BRAF alterations are associated with complex mutational profiles in malignant melanoma. Oncogene 2004;23:5968–5977.

132. Tsao H, Zhang X, Fowlkes K, Haluska FG. Relative reciprocity of NRas and PTEN/MMAC1 alterations in cutaneous melanoma cell lines. Cancer Res 2000;60:1800–1804.

133. Weber A, Hengge UR, Urbanik D, et al. Absence of mutations of the BRAF gene and constitutive activation of extracellular-regulated kinase in malignant melanomas of the uvea. Lab Invest 2003;83:1771–1776.

134. Kortylewski M, Heinrich PC, Kauffmann ME, Bohm M, MacKiewicz A, Behrmann I. Mitogen-activated protein kinases control p27/Kip1 expression and growth of human melanoma cells. Biochem J 2001;357:297–303.

135. Lefebre G, Calipel A, Mouriaux F, Hecquet C, Malecaze F, Mascarelli F. Opposite long-term regulation of c-Myc and p27Kip1 through overactivation of Raf-1 and the MEK/ERK module in proliferating human choroidal melanoma cells. Oncogene 2003;22:8813–8822.

136. Wu M, Hemesath TJ, Takemoto CM, et al. c-Kit triggers dual phosphorylations, which couple activation and degradation of the essential melanocyte factor Mi. Genes Dev 2000;14:301–312.

137. Kim DS, Hwang ES, Lee JE, Kim SY, Kwon SB, Park KC. Sphingosine-1–phosphate decreases melanin synthesis via sustained ERK activation and subsequent MITF degradation. J Cell Sci 2003;116:1699–706.

138. Eisenmann KM, VanBrocklin MW, Staffend NA, Kitchen SM, Koo HM. Mitogen-activated protein kinase pathway-dependent tumor-specific survival signaling in melanoma cells through inactivation of the proapoptotic protein bad. Cancer Res. 2003;63:8330–8337.

139. Aguirre Ghiso JA, Kovalski K, Ossowski L. Tumor dormancy induced by downregulation of urokinase receptor in human carcinoma involves integrin and MAPK signaling. J Cell Biol 1999; 147:89–104.

140. Santibanez JF, Iglesias M, Frontelo P, Martinez J, Quintanilla M. Involvement of the Ras/MAPK signaling pathway in the modulation of urokinase production and cellular invasiveness by transforming growth factor-beta (1) in transformed keratinocytes. Biochem Biophys Res Commun 2000;273:521–527.

141. Genersch E, Hayess K, Neuenfeld Y, Haller H. Sustained ERK phosphorylation is necessary but not sufficient for MMP-9 regulation in endothelial cells: involvement of Ras-dependent and -independent pathways. J Cell Sci 2000;113:4319–4330.

142. Tower GB, Coon CC, Benbow U, Vincenti MP, Brinckerhoff CE. Erk 1/2 differentially regulates the expression from the 1G/2G single nucleotide polymorphism in the MMP-1 promoter in melanoma cells. Biochim Biophys Acta 2002;1586:265–274.

143. Ishii Y, Ogura T, Tatemichi M, Fujisawa H, Otsuka F, Esumi H. Induction of matrix metalloproteinase gene transcription by nitric oxide and mechanisms of MMP-1 gene induction in human melanoma cell lines. Int J Cancer 2003;103:161–168.

144. Ramos MC, Steinbrenner H, Stuhlmann D, Sies H, Brenneisen P. Induction of MMP-10 and MMP-1 in a squamous cell carcinoma cell line by ultraviolet radiation. Biol Chem 2004;385:75–86.

145. Huntington JT, Shields JM, Der CJ, et al. Overexpression of collagenase 1 (MMP-1) is mediated by the ERK pathway in invasive melanoma cells: role of BRAF mutation and FGF signaling. J Biol Chem 2004;279:33,168–33,176.

146. Woods D, Cherwinski H, Venetsanakos E, et al. Induction of beta3-integrin gene expression by sustained activation of the Ras-regulated Raf-MEK-extracellular signal-regulated kinase signaling pathway. Mol Cell Biol 2001;21:3192–3205.

147. Halaban R. Growth factors and tyrosine protein kinases in normal and malignant melanocytes. Cancer Metastasis Rev 1991;10:129–140.

148. Halaban R. Growth factors and melanomas. Semin Oncol 1996;23:673–681.

149. Easty DJ, Bennett DC. Protein tyrosine kinases in malignant melanoma. Melanoma Res 2000; 10:401–411.

150. Miglarese MR, Halaban R, Gibson NW. Regulation of fibroblast growth factor 2 expression in melanoma cells by the c-MYB proto-oncoprotein. Cell Growth Differ 1997;8:1199–1210.

151. Richmond A, Lawson DH, Nixon DW, Stevens JS, Chawla RK. In vitro growth promotion in human malignant melanoma cells by fibroblast growth factor. Cancer Res 1982;42:3175–3180.

152. Nesbit M, Nesbit HK, Bennett J, et al. Basic fibroblast growth factor induces a transformed phenotype in normal human melanocytes. Oncogene 1999;18:6469–6476.

153. Meier F, Caroli U, Satyamoorthy K, et al. Fibroblast growth factor-2 but not Mel-CAM and/or beta3 integrin promotes progression of melanocytes to melanoma. Exp Dermatol 2003;12:296–306.

154. Ozen M, Medrano EE, Ittmann M. Inhibition of proliferation and survival of melanoma cells by adenoviral-mediated expression of dominant negative fibroblast growth factor receptor. Melanoma Res 2004;14:13–21.

155. Furge KA, Kiewlich D, Le P, et al. Suppression of Ras-mediated tumorigenicity and metastasis through inhibition of the Met receptor tyrosine kinase. Proc Natl Acad Sci USA 2001;98:10,722–10,727.

156. Cruz J, Reis-Filho JS, Silva P, Lopes JM. Expression of c-met tyrosine kinase receptor is biologically and prognostically relevant for primary cutaneous malignant melanomas. Oncology 2003;65:72–82.

157. Hendrix MJ, Seftor EA, Seftor RE, et al. Regulation of uveal melanoma interconverted phenotype by hepatocyte growth factor/scatter factor (HGF/SF). AM J Pathol 1998;152:855–863.

158. Otsuka T, Takayama H, Sharp R, et al. c-Met autocrine activation induces development of malignant melanoma and acquisition of the metastatic phenotype. Cancer Res 1998;58:5157–5167.

159. Elia G, Ren Y, Lorenzoni P, et al. Mechanisms regulating c-met overexpression in liver-metastatic B16-LS9 melanoma cells. J Cell Biochem 2001;81:477–487.

160. Tomida M, Satio T. The human hepatocyte growth factor (HGF) gene is transcriptionally activated by leukemia inhibitory factor through the Stat binding element. Oncogene 2004;23:679–686.

161. Recio JA, Merlino G. Hepatocyte growth factor/scatter factor activates proliferation in melanoma cells through p38 MAPK, ATF-2 and cyclin D1. Oncogene 2002;21:1000–1008.

162. Noonan FP, Recio JA, Takayama H, et al. Neonatal sunburn and melanoma in mice. Nature 2001;413:271–272.

163. Scholl FA, Kamarashev J, Murmann OV, Geertsen R, Dummer R, Schafer BW. PAX3 is expressed in human melanomas and contributes to tumor cell survival. Cancer Res 2001;61:823–826.

164. Galibert MD, Yavuzer U, Dexter TJ, Goding CR. Pax3 and regulation of the melanocyte-specific tyrosinase-related protein-1 promoter. J Biol Chem 1999;274:26,894–26,900.

165. Dahl E, Koseki H, Balling R. Pax genes and organogenesis. BioEssays 1997;19:755–765.

166. Bober E, Franz T, Arnold HH, Gruss P, Tremblay P. PAX3 is required for the development of limb muscles: a possible role for the migration of dermomyotomal muscle progenitor cells. Development 1994;120:603–612.

167. Tassabehji M, Read AP, Newton VE, et al. Mutations in the PAX3 gene causing Waardenburg syndrome type 1 and type 2. Nat Genet 1993;3:26–30.

168. Barr FG, Galili N, Holick J, Biegel JA, Rovera G, Emanuel BS. Rearrangement of the PAX3 paired box gene in the paediatric solid tumour alveolar rhabdomyosarcoma. Nat Genet 1993;3:113–117.

169. Epstein DJ, Vekemans M, Gros P. Splotch (Sp2H), a mutation affecting development of the mouse neural tube, shows a deletion within the paired homeodomain of Pax-3. Cell 1991;67:767–774.

170. Epstein JA, Shapiro DN, Cheng J, Lam PY, Maas RL. Pax3 modulates expression of the c-Met receptor during limb muscle development. Proc Natl Acad Sci USA 1996;93:4213–4218.

171. Wang W, Kumar P, Wang W, et al. Insulin-like growth factor II and PAX3-FKHR cooperate in the oncogenesis of rhabdomyosarcoma. Cancer Res 1998;58:4426–4433.

172. Margue CM, Bernasconi M, Barr FG, Schafer BW. Transcriptional modulation of the anti-apoptotic protein BCL-XL by the paired box transcription factors PAX3 and PAX3/FKHR. Oncogene 2000;19:2921–2929.

173. Ihle JN, Kerr IM. Jaks and stats in signaling by the cytokine receptor superfamily. Trends Genet 1995;11:69–74.

174. Darnell JE Jr. STATs and gene regulation. Science 1997;277:1630–1635.

175. Darnell JE Jr, Kerr IM, Stark GR. Jak-STAT pathways and transcriptional activation in response to IFNs and other extracellular signaling proteins. Science 1994;264:1415–1421.

176. Turkson J, Jove R. STAT proteins: novel molecular targets for cancer drug discovery. Oncogene 2000;19:6613–6626.

177. Garcia R, Jove R. Activation of STAT transcription factors in oncogenic tyrosine kinase signaling. J Biomed Sci 1998;5:79–85.

178. Catlett-Falcone R, Dalton WS, Jove R. STAT proteins as novel targets for cancer therapy. Signal transducer and activator of transcription. Curr Opin Oncol 1999;11:490–496.

179. Bowman T, Garcia R, Turkson J, Jove R. STATs in oncogenesis. Oncogene 2000;19:2474–2488.

180. Song JI, Grandis JR. STAT signaling in head and neck cancer. Oncogene 2000;19:2489–2495.

181. Coffer PJ, Koenderman L, de Groot RP. The role of STATs in myeloid differentiation and leukemia. Oncogene 2000;19:2511–2522.

182. Wang T, Niu G, Kortylewski M, et al. Regulation of the innate and adaptive immune responses by Stat-3 signaling in tumor cells. Nat Med 2004;10:48–54.

183. Bromberg JF, Horvath CM, Wen Z, Schreiber RD, Darnell JE Jr. Transcriptionally active Stat1 is required for the antiproliferative effects of both interferon γ and interferon γ. Proc Natl Acad Sci USA 1996;93:7673–7678.

184. Kovarik J, Boudny V, Kocak I, Lauerova L, Fait V, Vagundova M. Malignant melanoma associates with deficient IFN-induced STAT1 phosphorylation. Int J Mol Med 2003;12:335–340.

185. Wong LH, Krauer KG, Hatzinisiriou I, et al. Interferon-resistant human melanoma cells are deficient in ISGF3 components, STAT1, STAT2, and p48-ISGF3gamma. J Biol Chem 1997;272: 28,779–28,785.

186. Ivanov VN, Bhoumik A, Krasilnikov M, et al. Cooperation between STAT3 and c-jun suppresses Fas transcription. Mol Cell 2001;7:517–528.

187. Niu G, Bowman T, Huang M, et al. Roles of activated Src and Stat3 signaling in melanoma tumor cell growth. Oncogene 2002;21:7001–7010.

188. Ivanov VN, Krasilnikov M, Ronai Z. Regulation of Fas expression by STAT3 and c-Jun is mediated by phosphatidylinositol 3-kinase-AKT signaling. J Biol Chem 2002;277:4932–4944.

189. Krasilnikov M, Ivanov VN, Dong J, Ronai Z. ERK and PI3K negatively regulate STAT-transcriptional activities in human melanoma cells: implications towards sensitization to apoptosis. Oncogene 203;22:4092–4101.

190. Turkson J, Jove R. STAT proteins: novel molecular targets for cancer drug discovery. Oncogene 2000;19:6613–6626.

191. Arch RH, Gedrich RW, Thompson CB. Translocation of TRAF proteins regulates apoptotic threshold of cells. Biochem Biophys Res Commun 2000;272:936–945.

192. Hsu H, Shu HB, Pan MG, Goeddel DV. TRADD-TRAF2 and TRADD-FADD interactions define two distinct TNF receptor 1 signal transduction pathways. Cell 1996;84:299–308.

193. Baud V, Liu ZG, Bennett B, Suzuki N, Xia Y, Karin M. Signaling by proinflammatory cytokines: oligomerization of TRAF2 and TRAF6 is sufficient for JNK and IKK activation and target gene induction via an amino-terminal effector domain. Genes Dev 1999;13:1297–1308.

194. Duckett CS, Thompson CB. CD30-dependent degradation of TRAF2: implications for negative regulation of TRAF signaling and the control of cell survival. Genes Dev 1997;11:2810–2821.

195. Galibert L, Tometsko ME, Anderson DM, Cosman D, Dougall WC. The involvement of multiple tumor necrosis factor receptor (TNFR)-associated factors in the signaling mechanisms of receptor activator of NF-kappaB, a member of the TNFR superfamily. J Biol Chem 1998;273:34,120–34,127.

196. Rothe M, Pan MG, Henzel WJ, Ayres TM, Goeddel DV. The TNFR2-TRAF signaling complex contains two novel proteins related to baculoviral inhibitors of apoptosis proteins. Cell 1995;83: 1243–1252.

197. Liu H, Su YC, Becker E, Treisman J, Skolnik EY. A Drosophila TNF-receptor–associated factor (TRAF) binds the ste20 kinases Misshapen and activates Jun kinase. Curr Biol 1999;9:101–104.

198. Natoli G, Costanzo A, Ianni A, et al. Activation of SAPK/JNK by TNF receptor 1 through a noncytotoxic TRAF2-dependent pathway. Science 1997;275:200–203.

199. Shi CS, Kehrl JH. Activation of stress-activated protein kinase/c-Jun N-terminal kinase, but not NF-kappaB, by the tumor necrosis factor (TNF) receptor 1 through a TNF receptor-associated factor 2- and germinal center kinase related-dependent pathway. J Biol Chem 1997;272:32,102–32,107.

200. Nishitoh H, Saitoh M, Mochida Y, et al. ASK1 is essential for JNK/SAPK activation by TRAF2. Mol Cell 1998;2:389–395.

201. Devin A, Lin Y, Yamaoka S, Li Z, Karin M, Liu ZG. The alpha and beta subunits of IkappaB kinase (IKK) mediate TRAF2-dependent IKK recruitment to tumor necrosis factor (TNF) receptor 1 in response to TNF. Mol Cell Biol 2001;21:3986–3994.

202. Shu HB, Takeuchi M, Goeddel DV. The tumor necrosis factor receptor 2 signal transducers TRAF2 and c-IAP1 are components of the tumor necrosis factor receptor 1 signaling complex. Proc Natl Acad Sci USA 1996;93:13,973–13,978.

203. Wang Y, Wu TR, Cai S, Welte T, Chin YE. Stat1 as a component of tumor necrosis factor alpha receptor 1-TRADD signaling complex to inhibit NF-kappaB activation. Mol Cell Biol 2000;20: 4505–4512.

204. Habelhah H, Frew IJ, Laine A, et al. Stress-induced decrease in TRAF2 stability is mediated by Siah2. EMBO J 2002;21:5756–5765.

205. Ivanov VN, Kehrl JH, Ronai Z. Role of TRAF2/GCK in melanoma sensitivity to UV-induced apoptosis. Oncogene 2000;19:933–942.

206. Ivanov VN, Fodstad O, Ronai Z. Expression of ring finger-deleted TRAF2 sensitizes metastatic melanoma cells to apoptosis via up-regulation of p38, TNFalpha and suppression of NF-kappaB activities. Oncogene 2001;20:2243–2253.

207. Kunz M, Ibrahim S, Koczan D, et al. Activation of c-Jun NH2-terminal kinase/stress-activated protein kinase (JNK/SAPK) is critical for hypoxia-induced apoptosis of human malignant melanoma. Cell Growth Differ 2001;12:137–145.

208. Aguirre-Ghiso JA, Estrada Y, Liu D, Ossowski L. ERK (MAPK) activity as a determinant of tumor growth and dormancy; regulation by p38(SAPK). Cancer Res 2003;63:1684–1695.

209. Fuchs SY, Chen A, Xiong Y, Pan ZQ, Ronai Z. HOS, a human homolog of Slimb, forms an SCF complex with Skp1 and Cullin1 and targets the phosphorylation-dependent degradation of IkappaB and beta-catenin. Oncogene 1999;18:2039–2046.

210. Yaron A, Hatzubai A, Davis M, et al. Identification of the receptor component of the IkappaBalpha-ubiquitin ligase. Nature 1998;396:590–594.

211. Ghosh S, Karin M. Missing pieces in the NF-kappaB puzzle. Cell 2002;109:S81–S96.

212. Baldwin AS Jr. The NF-kappa B and I kappa B proteins: new discoveries and insights. Annu Rev Immunol 1996;14:649–683.

213. McNulty SE, Tohidian NB, Meyskens FL. RelA, p50 and inhibitor of kappa B alpha are elevated in human metastatic melanoma cells and respond aberrantly to ultraviolet light B. Pigment Cell Res 2001;14:456–465.

214. Meyskens FL Jr, Buckmeier JA, McNulty SE, Tohidian NB. Activation of nuclear factor-kappa B in human metastatic melanoma cells and the effect of oxidative stress. Clin Cancer Res 1999;5:1197–1202.

215. Devalaraja MN, Wang DZ, Ballard DW, Richmond A. Elevated constitutive IkappaB kinase activity and IkappaB-alpha phosphorylation in Hs294T melanoma cells lead to increased basal MGSA/GRO-alpha transcription. Cancer Res 1999;59:1372–1377.

216. Yang J, Richmond A. Constitutive IkappaB kinase activity correlates with nuclear factor-kappaB activation in human melanoma cells. Cancer Res 2001;61:4901–4909.

217. Dhawan P, Singh AB, Ellis DL, Richmond A. Constitutive activation of Akt/Protein Kinase B in melanoma leads to up-regulation of nuclear factor-kappaB and tumor progression. Cancer Research 2002;62:7335–7342.

218. Kashani-Sabet M, Shaikh L, Miller JR 3rd, et al. NF-kappa B in the vascular progression of melanoma. J Clin Oncol 2004;22:617–623.

219. Kashani-Sabet M, Liu Y, Fong S. Identification of gene function and functional pathways by systemic plasmid-based ribozyme targeting in adult mice. Proc Natl Acad Sci USA 2002;99:3878–3883.

220. Chinenov Y, Kerppola TK. Close encounters of many kinds: Fos-Jun interactions that mediate transcription regulatory specificity. Oncogene 2001;20:2438–2452.

221. Vogt PK. Fortuitous convergences: the beginnings of JUN. Nature Rev Cancer 2002;2:465–469.

222. Angel P, Karin M. The role of Jun, Fos and the AP-1 complex in cell-proliferation and transformation. Biochim Biophys Acta 1991;1072:129–157.

223. Shaulian E, Karin M. AP-1 as a regulator of cell life and death. Nat Cell Biol 2002;4:131–136.

224. Angel P, Szabowski A, Schorpp-Kistner M. Function and regulation of AP-1 subunits in skin physiology and pathology. Oncogene 2001;20:2413–2423.

225. Yamanishi DT, Buckmeier JA, Meyskens FL Jr. Expression of c-Jun, JunB, and c-Fos proto-oncogenes in human primary melanocytes and metastatic melanomas. J Invest Dermatol 1991;97:349–353.

226. Rutberg SE, Goldstein IM, Yang YM, Stackpole CW, Ronai Z. Expression and transcriptional activity of AP-1, CRE, and URE binding proteins in B16 mouse melanoma subclones. Mol Carcinog 1994;10:82–87.

227. Madireddi MT, Dent P, Fisher PB. AP-1 and C/EBP transcription factors contribute to mda-7 gene promoter activity during human melanoma differentiation. J Cell Physiol 2000;185:36–46.

228. Fisher PB, Gopalkrishnan RV, Chada S, et al. mda-7/IL-24, a novel cancer selective apoptosis inducing cytokine gene: from the laboratory into the clinic. Cancer Biol Ther 2003;2:S23–S37.

229. Bhoumik A, Gangi L, Ronai Z. Inhibition of melanoma growth and metastasis by ATF2-derived peptides. Cancer Res 2004;64:8222–8230.

230. van Dam H, Castellazzi M. Distinct roles of Jun: Fos and Jun: ATF dimers in oncogenesis. Oncogene 2001;20:2453–2464.

231. Kaszubska W, Hooft van Huijsduijnen R, Ghersa P, et al. Cyclic AMP-independent ATF family members interact with NF-kappa B and function in the activation of the E-selectin promoter in response to cytokines. Mol Cell Biol 1993;13:7180–7190.

232. Kim SJ, Wagner S, Liu F, O'Reilly MA, Robbins PD, Green MR. Retinoblastoma gene product activities expression of the human TGF-beta 2 gene through transcription factor ATF-2. Nature 1992;358:331–334.

233. Gupta S, Campbell D, Derijard B, Davis RJ. Transcription factor ATF2 regulation by the JNK signal transduction pathway. Science 1995;267:389–393.

234. Tsai EY, Jain J, Pesavento PA, Rao A, Goldfeld AE. Tumor necrosis factor alpha gene regulation in activated T cells involves ATF-2/Jun and NFATp. Mol Cell Biol 1996;16:459–467.

235. Shimizu M, Nomura Y, Suzuki H, et al. Activation of the rat cyclin A promoter by ATF2 and Jun family members and its suppression by ATF4. Exp Cell Res 1998;239:93–103.

236. van Dam H, Duyndam M, Rottier R, et al. Heterodimer formation of cJun and ATF-2 is responsible for induction of c-Jun by the 243 amino acid adenovirus E1A protein. EMBO 1993;12:479–487.

237. Huguier S, Baguet J, Perez S, van Dam H, Castellazzi M. Transcription factor ATF2 cooperates with v-Jun to promote growth factor-independent proliferation in vitro and tumor formation in vivo. Mol Cell Biol 1998;18:7020–7029.

238. van Dam H, Huguier S, Kooistra K, et al. Autocrine growth and anchorage independence: two complementing Jun-controlled genetic programs of cellular transformation. Genes Dev 1998;12:1227–1239.

239. Bhoumik A, Jones N, Ronai Z. Transcriptional switch by activating transcription factor 2-derived peptide sensitizes melanoma cells to apoptosis and inhibits their tumorigenicity. Proc Natl Acad Sci USA 2004;101:4222–4227.

240. Ronai Z, Yang YM, Fuchs SY, Adler V, Sardana M, Herlyn M. ATF2 confers radiation resistance to human melanoma cells. Oncogene 1998;16:523–531.

241. Ivanov VN, Bhoumik A, Ronai Z. Death receptors and melanoma resistance to apoptosis. Oncogene 2003;22:3152–3161.

242. Berger A, Harriet K, Ning L, et al. Subcellular localization of activating transcription factor 2 in melanoma specimens predicts patient survival. Cancer Res 2003;63:8103–8107.

243. Bhoumik A, Ivanov V, Ronai Z. Activating transcription factor 2-derived peptides alter resistance of human tumor cell lines to ultraviolet irradiation and chemical treatment. Clin Cancer Res 2001;7:331–342.

244. Bhoumik A, Huang TG, Ivanov V, et al. An ATF2-derived peptide sensitizes melanomas to apoptosis and inhibits their growth and metastasis. J Clin Investig 2002;110:643–650.

245. Massagué J. TGFβ signal transduction. Annu Rev Biochem 1998;67:753–791.

246. Schier AF, Shen MM. Nodal signalling in vertebrate development. Nature 2000;403:385–389.

247. Whitman M. SMADs and early developmental signaling by the TGFβ superfamily. Genes Dev 1998;12:2445–2462.

248. Massagué J, Blain SW, Lo RS. TGF-β signaling in growth control, cancer and heritable disorders. Cell 2000;103:295–309.

249. Myatt N, Aristodemou P, Neale MH. Abnormalities of the transforming growth factor-beta pathway in ocular melanoma. J Pathol 2000;192:511–518.

250. Berking C, Takemoto R, Schaider H, et al. Transforming growth factor-beta1 increases survival of human melanoma through stroma remodeling. Cancer Res 2001;61:8306–8316.

251. Wu H, Goel V, Haluska FG. PTEN signaling pathways in melanoma. Oncogene 2003;22:3113–3122.

252. Persad S, Troussard AA, McPhee TR, Mulholland DJ, Dedhar S. Tumor suppressor PTEN inhibits nuclear accumulation of beta-catenin and T cell/lymphoid enhancer factor 1-mediated transcriptional activation. J Cell Biol 2001;153:1161–1174.

253. Hajduch E, Alessi DR, Hemmings BA, Hundal HS. Constitutive activation of protein kinase B by membrane targeting promotes glucose and system A amino acid transport, protein synthesis, and inactivation of glycogen synthase kinase 3 in L6 muscle cells. Diabetes1998;47:1006–1013.

254. van Weeren PC, de Bruyn KM, de Vries-Smits AM, van Lint J, Burgering BM. Essential role for protein kinase B (PKB) in insulin-induced glycogen synthase kinase 3 inactivation: characterization of dominant-negative mutant of PKB. J Biol Chem 1998;273:13,150–13,156.

255. Rudin CM, Holmlund J, Fleming GF, et al. Phase I trial of ISIS 5132, an antisense oligonucleotide inhibitor of c-raf-1, administered by 24-hour weekly infusion to patients with advanced cancer. Clin Cancer Res 2001;7:1214–1220.

256. Mercer KE, Pritchard CA. Raf proteins and cancer: B-Raf is identified as a mutational target. Biochim Biophys Acta 2003;165:25–40.

257. Collisson EA, De A, Suzuki H, Gambhir SS, Kolodney MS. Treatment of metastatic melanoma with an orally available inhibitor of the Ras-Raf-MAPK cascade. Cancer Res 2003;63:5669–5673.

258. Karasarides M, Chiloeches A, Hayward R, et al. B-RAF is a therapeutic target in melanoma. Oncogene 2004;23:6292–6298.
259. Bedogni B, O'Neill MS, Welford SM, et al. Topical treatment with inhibitors of the phosphatidyli-nositol 3'-kinase/Akt and Raf/mitogen-activated protein kinase kinase/extracellular signal-regulated kinase pathways reduces melanoma development in severe combined immunodeficient mice. Cancer Res 2004;64:2552–2560.
260. Sumimoto H, Miyagishi M, Miyoshi H, et al. Inhibition of growth and invasive ability of melanoma by inactivation of mutated BRAF with lentivirus-mediated RNA interference. Oncogene 2004;23:6031–6039.
261. Pavey S, Johansson P, Packer L, et al. Microarray expression profiling in melanoma reveals a BRAF mutation signature. Oncogene 2000;23:4060–4067.

8

BRN2 in Melanocytic Cell Development, Differentiation, and Transformation

Anthony L. Cook, Glen M. Boyle, J. Helen Leonard, Peter G. Parsons, and Richard A. Sturm

CONTENTS

Summary

POU domain transcription factors are critical regulators of many developmental processes, and can also be reactivated during malignancy. The *BRN2* gene encoding the N-Oct-3 DNA binding activity is one such factor that is expressed in melanocytic cells. Cultured unpigmented epidermal human melanoblasts express high levels of BRN2 protein and DNA binding activity similar to metastatic melanoma cell lines, but this decreases after differentiation to a pigmented melanocyte phenotype. BRN2 expression can be increased by several melanocytic growth factors, some of which signal through the BRAF pathway, which is frequently mutated in melanoma. Ablation of BRN2 in melanoma cell lines produces a loss of melanocytic markers, decreased proliferation, and loss of tumorigenicity. Microarray analysis of these cell lines suggests that BRN2 resides upstream of other melanocytic transcription factors, such as SOX10, MITF, and SLUG, but below or in a separate hierarchy to PAX3. Because of the sensitivity of cells to POU protein expression levels in determination of cell fate, downregulation of BRN2 may act as a molecular switch in melanocytic cells to coordinate the onset of melanogenesis with differentiation, but which can be aberrantly reactivated in melanoma.

Key Words: POU; melanoblast; melanoma; microarray; antisense RNA.

THE BRN2 POU DOMAIN TRANSCRIPTION FACTOR

POU domain transcription factors constitute a conserved family of developmental and tissue-specific regulators of many diverse cell types (*1*). The POU domain was first described in 1988 based on the sequence similarity of the DNA binding domains of four

From: *From Melanocytes to Melanoma: The Progression to Malignancy*
Edited by: V. J. Hearing and S. P. L. Leong © Humana Press Inc., Totowa, NJ

transcription factors: the mammalian factors Pit-1, Oct-1 and Oct-2, and the nematode factor, Unc-86 *(2,3)*. To date, a total of six mammalian POU protein subclasses have been described and grouped according to the extent of amino acid identity. All cell types express the ubiquitous Oct-1 factor *(4)*, whereas other family members show expression that is more restricted. For example, the Pit-1 factor is expressed in the neural tube and pituitary during embryogenesis, but is restricted to the pituitary in adult tissues *(5)*. The Class III POU domain transcription factor BRN2 (POU3F2; also known as N-Oct-3 when complexed with DNA) has been implicated in the development of neural and glial cell lineages *(6–8)*, and is also expressed in several malignant tissues, such as glioblastoma and neuroblastoma *(9)*, small cell lung carcinoma *(10)*, Merkel cell carcinoma *(11)*, and melanoma *(9, 12–14)*.

Several groups independently identified, cloned, and characterized the *BRN2* gene and cDNA. The gene was initially identified in a redundant RT-PCR-based screen of rat brain tissue (hence its designated name) and shown to be expressed in nervous tissue *(15)*. Subsequently, the murine *BRN2* gene was cloned, and, like other Class III POU factors, was found to be encoded by a single exon *(16)*. N-Oct-3 DNA binding activity was identified as the product of the *BRN2* gene after in vitro transcribed and translated protein from a cDNA clone was shown to migrate with the same mobility as the N-Oct-3 complex of a human brain extract *(17)*. The octamer binding profile of mammalian cells transfected with a *BRN2* expression construct produced up to three complexes, namely N-Oct-3, N-Oct-5a, and N-Oct-5b *(17)*. The two N-Oct-5 complexes were initially considered to result from alternative translation initiation, however, later studies showed that these activities were caused by proteolytic clipping of the BRN2 protein during extract preparation *(18,19)*.

DNA Binding

The POU domain is a bipartite DNA binding structure, consisting of an N-terminal POU-specific (POU$_S$) domain and a C-terminal POU homeodomain (POU$_H$) joined by a flexible amino acid linker of varying length *(3)*. POU domain-containing proteins bind monomerically to the 5'-ATGCAAAT-3' octamer sequence *(20)*. The 5' ATGC motif and the 3' AAAT sequence can be considered as half sites *(21)*, because the crystal structure of the Oct-1 POU domain bound to this sequence demonstrated that each subdomain binds to separate halves of the octamer motif on opposite faces of the DNA helix *(22)*. This crystal structure also revealed that the POU$_S$ and POU$_H$ domains form helix-turn-helix motifs, using the second and third helix of the subdomain.

Because of the flexibility of the linker region, POU domain proteins are able to adopt different arrangements of the POU subdomains on the DNA molecule *(23)*. This allows for:

1. Differences in orientation of the recognition sequence (and hence orientation of the POU$_S$ and POU$_{H}$ domains) caused by changes in octamer half site orientation.
2. Introduction of extra bases into the recognition motif, which separate the half sites, both of which lead to the third difference.
3. Differences in the positioning of the subdomains relative to each other when bound to DNA.

Accordingly, BRN2 is able to bind to both consensus octamer motifs as well as divergent sequences that are bound with higher affinity *(24)*.

Redox sensitivity of BRN2 DNA binding activity in vitro has also been documented *(19)*. Formation of the N-Oct-3 complex in DNA binding experiments revealed the presence of metal ions, such as iron (III) and nickel in the binding buffer caused a reduction in BRN2 activity. These ions had an oxidizing effect on the BRN2 molecule, because the inclusion of the reducing agent dithiothreitol in the reaction mix prevented the effects on N-Oct-3 complex formation *(19)*. Similarly, the inclusion of hydrogen peroxide or diamide resulted in a loss of N-Oct-3 activity, which was also abrogated by the presence of dithiothreitol in the assay. Notably, the DNA binding activity of the Oct-2 factor is also inhibited by oxidation of the protein *(25)*.

In addition to monomeric interactions with DNA recognition sequences, POU domain proteins of the neural system, such as BRN2, have also been shown to have the capacity to bind DNA homodimerically in a highly cooperative manner on appropriate DNA motifs, which consist of four tandem half sites *(24)*, and, subsequently, BRN2 co-dimers on this site were documented using melanoma cell line nuclear extracts *(26)*. More recently, a BRN2 dimerization motif in the promoter of the aromatic L-amino acid decarboxylase gene has been characterized and shown to be transactivated by BRN2 in co-transfection assays *(27)*. Notably, this motif differs from the consensus BRN2 dimerization site because of the insertion of two bases between the central half sites of the motif and a single base substitution *(24,27)*. Characterization of POU domain dimerization has shown that the sequence of DNA elements permissive for dimeric binding can vary the spatial arrangement of the POU_S and POU_H subdomains of each protein, which, in turn, alters POU–POU protein interactions and recruitment of other transcriptional co-regulators, which increases the complexity of possible tertiary interactions *(23,28,29)*.

Expression of Octamer Binding Proteins in Melanoma

The *POU3F2* genomic locus encoding BRN2 has been mapped to 6q16 *(30,31)*, outside the region most common for deletion in cutaneous melanoma at 6q22-27 *(32)*, a result consistent with BRN2 expression being detected in most melanoma cell lines examined *(12,14)*. BRN2 appears to be important for development of malignant melanoma because its expression in human melanoma cell lines is much higher than in primary melanocytes *(12,14,33)*, and human melanoma cell lines expressing antisense *BRN2* lose the ability to form tumors in immunodeficient mice *(31)*.

BRN1/N-Oct-2 DNA binding activity has also been found in nuclear extracts of melanoma biopsies and cell lines, but all samples also contained the BRN2/N-Oct-3 complex *(14)*. In both adult and embryonic rat nervous system *BRN1*, and *BRN2* exhibit similar expression patterns, including coexpression in the neural tube *(15)*. Intriguingly, Nakai et al *(34)* reported that in $BRN2^{-/-}$ mice, the DNA binding activity of BRN1 (N-Oct-2 complex) was increased, implying a compensatory mechanism. However, the lack of N-Oct-2 activity in BRN2-ablated melanoma cells *(31)* may suggest this is not obviously the case for melanocytic cells. Notably, BRN1 and BRN2 are both Class III POU proteins and these factors display partial functional redundancy in oligodendrocytes *(35)* and cortical neurons *(36,37)*.

BRN2 AND MELANOCYTIC DIFFERENTIATION

Conditions for the in vitro propagation of unpigmented human melanoblasts from neonatal foreskin tissue have been developed and we have recently reported the differentiation of these cells to melanocytes in response to culture medium changes *(38)*. The ability of these differentiated melanoblasts to synthesize melanin was supported by visual examination of harvested cell pellets, as well as experimental evidence, such as

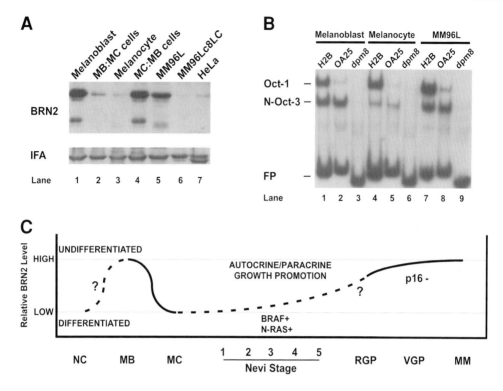

Fig. 1. (A) BRN2 expression in melanocytic cells. Immunoblot analysis of BRN2 expression in melanoblasts, MB:MC cells, melanocytes, MC:MB cells, MM96L melanoma cells, BRN2-ablated MM96Lc8LC cells, and nonmelanocytic HeLa cells (lanes 1–7, respectively). IFA expression was used as a loading control. **(B)** EMSA analysis of N-Oct-3 (BRN2) DNA-binding activity in melanoblasts (lanes 1–3), melanocytes (lanes 4–6), and MM96L melanoma cells (lanes 7–9). H2B, OA25, and dpm8 are wild-type, divergent, and mutant octamer probes, respectively. The positions of the ubiquitously expressed Oct-1 and N-Oct-3 activities are shown to the left of the figure. FP, free probe. **(C)** Schematic representation of BRN2 expression levels during melanocytic differentiation and malignancy in vivo. Timing of common causal mutations in melanoma associated genes are indicated. NC, neural crest; MB, melanoblast; MC, melanocyte; RGP, radial growth phase; VGP, vertical growth phase; MM, metastatic melanoma.

DOPA reactivity and analysis of melanosome maturation visualized by transmission electron microscopy *(38)*.

Using this system, the expression profile and DNA-binding activity of BRN2 during in vitro melanocytic differentiation were examined (Fig. 1). Immunoblot analysis showed that melanoblasts expressed higher amounts of BRN2 than melanocytes, at a level more comparable to the MM96L metastatic melanoma cell line (Fig. 1A, compare lanes 1, 3, and 5). After induction of differentiation (Fig. 1A, lane 2), the level of BRN2 decreased to resemble that of melanocyte cultures. Additionally, culture of differentiated melanocytes in melanoblast growth medium caused an induction of BRN2 protein levels (Fig. 1A, lane 4), which was accompanied by a decrease in cell pellet pigmentation and DOPA reactivity *(38)*.

Examination of BRN2 DNA binding during in vitro melanoblast differentiation was also conducted using wild-type (H2B), divergent (OA25), and mutant (dpm8) octamer sequences (ref. *38* and Fig. 1B). Consistent with the higher BRN2 protein levels, melanoblasts (Fig. 1B, lanes 1–3) had more N-Oct-3 (BRN2) DNA-binding activity than melanocytes (Fig. 1B, lanes 4–6), and again these levels more closely resembled those of the MM96L melanoma cell line (Fig. 1B, lanes 7–9). These changes in the expression levels and DNA-binding activity of BRN2 were also confirmed using immunohistochemical methods *(38)*. Interestingly, expression of BRN2 can be modulated in human melanoma cell lines, with differentiating agents, such as butyric acid and dimethyl sulfoxide, decreasing expression *(13)*, implying a role for BRN2 in maintaining the undifferentiated melanocytic phenotype.

POU domain factors are typically developmental regulators and a role for BRN2 during melanocytic development is highly likely. This is supported by the finding that cell lines derived from murine neural crest explant cultures express varying amounts of BRN2 *(38)*. However, recent data has suggested that *BRN2* is not expressed in early neural crest-derived migrating melanoblasts, identified by *LacZ* reporter gene expression placed under the control of a *DCT* promoter in transgenic mice at embryonic day 11.5 *(39)*. This discrepancy may in part be explained by the period during which the neural crest cell lines were cloned after neural tube harvest *(40)*. Thus, it may be that *BRN2* is expressed at stages of melanocytic development later than embryonic day 11.5.

This possibility is supported by other findings. First, the melanoblast cultures were established from neonatal foreskin epidermis *(38)*, and are therefore representative of an epidermal melanoblast population, as has been described to reside in the murine hair follicle *(41)*. Second, despite not detecting *BRN2* in migrating melanoblasts, *BRN2* expression was found in epidermal melanocytic cells *(39)*, and third, the effects of homozygous *BRN2* deletion are first observed at embryonic day 12.5, before death by postnatal day 10 *(34,42)*. Whatever the reason for these experimental differences, BRN2 is undoubtedly expressed in melanocytic cells and does contribute to the melanocytic phenotype. One possible function may be that BRN2 expression allows acquisition of a phenotype permissive for melanoblast migration into the hair follicle and/or crossing of the basal layer and into the epidermis.

From the summation of these studies, it appears that there is a reciprocal relationship between BRN2 and the differentiated status of melanocytic cells, such that undifferentiated (melanoblasts) or de-differentiated (malignant melanoma) cells express more BRN2 (Fig. 1C). The relative expression level of a single transcription factor can have a dramatic effect on a cell. This is particularly evident for the role of the POU domain factor Oct-3/4 (POU5F1) in controlling cell fate decisions of murine ES cells *(43)*. Thus, a threshold level of Oct-3/4 is required to maintain the pluripotency of the ES cells, with increased or decreased expression inducing differentiation or de-differentiation, respectively. Notably, less than a twofold change in Oct-3/4 was required to induce differentiation, suggesting exquisite sensitivity to levels of POU protein expression. Downregulation of BRN2 after differentiation is not specific to the melanocytic lineage. During Schwann cell differentiation in vitro, expression of BRN2 is also decreased *(44)*, and, interestingly, this cell type shares expression of several transcription factors with melanocytic cells in addition to BRN2, such as SOX10 and PAX3 *(44,45)*. Additionally, another Class III POU domain protein, Oct-6, is also repressed during Schwann cell, oligodendrocyte, and ES cell differentiation *(46–48)*.

BRN2 AND MELANOMA

Dysregulation of transcription factor expression is likely to have severe consequences for the cell. This is well evidenced by the ability of several POU domain factors to produce a malignant phenotype in several experimental models. For example, exogenous expression of the Oct-1 and Oct-2 POU domains in T-cells of transgenic mice induced lymphoma formation *(49)*, and Oct-3/4 overexpression has been shown to confer malignancy on both ES cells and fibroblasts *(50)*. In neuroblastoma cell lines, the expression level of BRN3b (POU4F2) is important for regulation of cell behavior, because overexpression increased proliferation in culture and in xenograft models, in addition to promoting invasiveness in vitro, whereas antisense RNA-mediated ablation produced the opposite effects compared with control cell lines *(51)*. Given the expression level and DNA-binding activity differences of BRN2 between cultured melanocytes and melanoma cell lines, it seems likely that BRN2 has a positive effect on melanomagenesis.

Any pair of the melanocytic mitogens fibroblast growth factor-2, (FGF2), stem cell factor (SCF), and endothelin-3 (EDN3) can act synergistically to increase expression and DNA binding activity of BRN2 in cultured human melanocytes *(38)*. Several studies have also shown that combinations of SCF, EDN1, EDN3, and FGF2 act synergistically on cultured human melanocytes to activate MAPK *(52–54)*. More recently, the simultaneous adenoviral delivery of FGF2, SCF, and EDN3, and subsequent ultraviolet B (UVB)-exposure of xenografted human neonatal foreskin tissue was shown to induce histopathologically recognizable melanoma *(55)*. It would be of interest to determine whether a recently described adenoviral vector encoding BRN2 *(56)* recapitulated these results when used in similar experiments. Additionally, these growth factor and UV radiation-induced lesions expressed activated MAPK, and *BRAF* mutations were present in a minority of cells in some cases *(55)*. Most human melanomas have an activated MAPK pathway, mediated via both *BRAF* mutations and autocrine growth factor mechanisms, whereas normal melanocytes and nevus cells in vivo do not constitutively express phosphorylated MAPK *(57)*. Inhibition of either the FGF2 or scatter factor (SF) autocrine loops (using either FGF2-specific antisense RNA or SF-neutralizing antibodies, respectively) in a metastatic melanoma cell line carrying a *BRAF* mutation caused a loss of MAPK activation, clearly indicating signaling additional to constitutively active BRAF is required for MAPK activation in melanoma *(57)*.

Recent work has linked melanocyte proliferation from activated BRAF to BRN2 *(58)*. Overexpression of BRN2 led to increased proliferation of melanocytes, whereas downregulation of BRN2 in a melanoma cell line using siRNA led to a decrease in proliferation. BRN2 expression was found to be strongly upregulated by MAP-kinase-dependent signaling mediated via an EGFR-fusion construct and, further, BRN2 expression was reduced after downregulation of BRAF using siRNA. These results are consistent with the high frequency of *BRAF* mutation and increased BRN2 expression in many melanoma cell lines, with the similar cell morphology seen for both BRAF- and BRN2-ablated melanoma cell lines, and with the subsequent lack of tumorigenicity of these transfected cell lines. Furthermore, BRAF signaling or constitutive activation in melanoma links high levels of BRN2 expression to increased proliferation.

BRN2 was also found to be a direct target for β-catenin/Lef1 through binding of this complex to its promoter region *(39)*. In the same study, siRNA-mediated downregulation of BRN2 in melanoma cells overexpressing β-catenin resulted in decreased proliferation of these cells, and ectopic β-catenin has been shown to induce *BRN2* expression in murine melanocytes in vivo and in melanoma cell lines. Importantly, frequent nuclear accumulation of β-catenin, which promotes cellular proliferation *(59,60)*, has been seen in primary melanoma specimens. One class of extracellular ligand that signals via β-catenin is WNT proteins, which act to stabilize β-catenin, thereby allowing nuclear translocation

(61). Notably, several groups have shown that WNT proteins, such as WNT1 and WNT3A, promote murine melanocytic commitment *(62–64)*. However, not all WNT proteins use this signaling pathway. Thus, although WNT5A has been associated with invasive melanoma in other microarray screening studies *(65)*, and subsequent functional data supports this finding *(66)*, it was also found that ectopic WNT5A had no effect on β-catenin expression or its nuclear translocation.

Thus, BRN2 appears to be the focus for convergence of the BRAF and β-catenin signaling pathways *(39,58)*, two key melanoma-associated transduction mechanisms that are linked to cellular proliferation. This underlines the importance of BRN2 dysregulation in melanocytic cells for the progression of melanoma cells toward metastasis.

EXPRESSION PROFILING OF BRN2-ABLATED MELANOMA CELLS

In an attempt to elucidate novel transcriptional targets of BRN2, and to find a molecular explanation for the reduction in melanocytic tumorigenicity after BRN2 ablation, expression profiling analysis using microarrays was performed with melanoma cell lines expressing (MM96Lc8D) or ablated for BRN2 (MM96Lc8LC) *(31)*. These two cell lines have previously been shown to differ morphologically (Fig. 2A) as well as to differentially express several pigmentation-associated genes *(31)*. Note that the BRN2-ablated cells are similar in morphology to melanoma cell lines, in which BRAF expression is silenced using RNAi techniques *(58,67)*. Other research groups have also been successful in ablating BRN2 expression in melanoma cell lines, using either antisense RNA or RNAi methods *(39,68)*, but, as yet, these cells have not been examined using microarray technology.

The results presented here (Table 1 and Fig. 2B) will focus on the reduction or loss of gene expression after ablation of BRN2. Importantly, all experiments gave consistent results for the genes previously shown to be differentially expressed between the MM96Lc8D and MM96Lc8LC cell lines *(31)*. Many genes were verified to be expressed differentially using an alternate method of analysis, either semiquantitative reverse transcriptase polymerase chain reaction (RT-PCR) or immunoblot (Fig. 2B and C, respectively).

Pigmentation

Initial characterization of the BRN2-ablated melanoma cell lines revealed a loss of several pigmentation markers, including the tyrosinase-related protein (TYRP) family members *TYR*, *TYRP1*, and *DCT (TYRP2)*, attributed to the concomitant loss of *MITF* in these cells *(31)*. Thus, these genes were able to serve as internal controls during hybridization signal analysis and, consistent with previous studies, were also found to have differential expression as judged by microarray screening. Immunoblot analysis for TYR and TYRP1 expression confirmed this result at the protein level. Other genes involved in melanogenesis, such as *SILV*, and *MART1* showed decreased expression in MM96Lc8LC cells; it is notable that the promoters of these two genes have recently been shown to also be regulated by MITF *(69)*.

Genes involved in the intracellular trafficking of both melanogenic enzymes and melanosomes themselves, as well as melanosome biogenesis, also displayed decreased expression levels as a consequence of BRN2 ablation. For example, Rab38 is involved in the transport of TYRP1 to mature melanosomes, because mutation of *Rab38* in mice produces a phenocopy of oculocutaneous albinism consistent with *Tyrp1* mutation *(70)*.

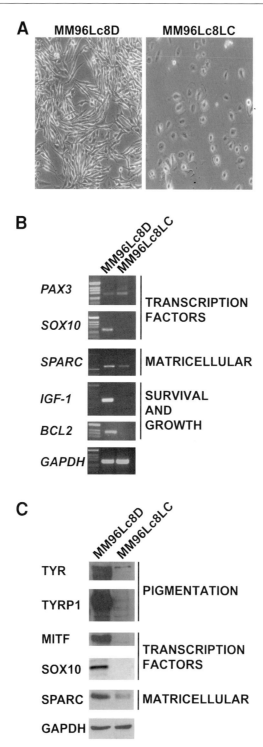

Fig. 2. (A) Expression profiling of BRN2-ablated melanoma cell lines. Phase-contrast photomicrographs of MM96Lc8D (left) and BRN2-ablated MM96Lc8LC (right) melanoma cell lines. **(B)** RT-PCR and/or **(C)** immunoblot confirmation of differential gene expression levels between MM96Lc8D and MM96Lc8LC melanoma cell lines identified by microarray hybridization.

Table 1
Selected Downregulated Genes Following BRN2 Ablation[a]

GenBank Acc. No.	Mean ratio	Common name	Description	Function	Confirmed
W79081	49.54	SILV	Silver homolog (mouse)	Melanogenesis	—
H86270	46.84	TYRP1	Tyrosinase-related protein 1	Melanogenesis	IB
N66177	26.12	MITF	Microphthalmia-associated transcription factor	Transcription factor	IB
N72893	22.52	DCT	Dopachrome tautomerase	Melanogenesis	IB
R93847	20.75	IGF1	Insulin-like growth factor 1	Growth/proliferation	RT
N35680	18.29	MART1	Melanoma antigen recognized by T cells 1	Melanogenesis	—
N42770	17.92	TYR	Tyrosinase (oculocutaneous albinism IA)	Melanogenesis	IB
H17696	12.32	MBP	Myelin basic protein	Melanogenesis	—
R72919	9.17	SOX10	Sex-determining region Y (SRY)-box 10	Transcription factor	RT,IB
R97323	8.23	TIMP3	Tissue inhibitor of metalloproteinase 3		—
W35163	8.13	NAV2	Neuron navigator 2		—
BM911128	6.50	SPARC	Secreted protein, acidic, cysteine-rich (osteonectin)	Matricellular Interactions	RT,IB
N28287	5.43	SLUG	Snail homolog 2 (Drosophila)	Transcription factor	—
N42447	4.38	RAB38	RAB38, member RAS oncogene family	Transport	—
BI761161	4.20	CD63	CD63 antigen (melanoma 1 antigen)	Melanosome biogenesis?	—
R21466	4.19	GPM6B	Glycoprotein M6B		—
H16558	2.87	MYO5A	Myosin VA (heavy polypeptide 12, myoxin)	Melanosome transport	—
BM910117	2.81	RAB25	RAB25, member RAS oncogene family		—
W24394	2.75	A2M	α-2 macroglobulin		RT
H73130	2.63	BCL2	B-cell CLL/lymphoma 2	Survival	RT
W40490	2.62	RAB5B	RAB5B, member RAS oncogene family		—
N29275	2.39	EDNRB	Endothelin receptor type B	Growth/proliferation	RT
H98469	2.17	RAB27A	RAB27A, member RAS oncogene family	Melanosome transport	—

[a]MM96Lc8D and MM96Lc8LC cells were grown to 70% confluence and RNA harvested on two separate occasions. Microarray expression profiling was performed in a reciprocal "dye swap", and common reference experimental design, using three separate platforms. Selected differentially expressed genes are shown. Average ratio differences were determined following background subtraction and normalization using the LOWESS algorithm in GeneSpring 6.0 (Silicon Genetics, Redwood, CA). IB, immunoblot; RT, semiquantitative RT-PCR.

Both RAB27A and MYO5A *(71)*, are involved in melanosome transport, with RAB27A indirectly interacting with MYO5A. CD63 is a membrane protein associated with endosomes and lysosomes *(72)*, which are organelles considered to be the precursors of melanosomes *(73)*. Furthermore, immunofluorescent studies have shown that CD63 and TYRP1 are partially colocalized in a lightly pigmented melanoma cell line *(74)*. All four of these genes were repressed in the MM96Lc8LC cell line, consistent with results obtained for TYRP family genes, and which are further suggestive of a role for BRN2 in maintaining the melanocytic phenotype.

Transcription Factors

Several transcription factors have been implicated in murine and human melanocytic development and differentiation *(75)*, including the MITF, SOX10, PAX3, and SLUG proteins. Mutations within each of these genes can cause Waardenburg syndrome, an inherited disorder resulting in pigmentary disturbances of the skin, hair, and eyes, among other clinical features. Previous work has shown that expression of MITF is absent in BRN2-ablated cells *(31)*, and, in turn, that expression of MITF is thought to be controlled by SOX10 and PAX3 *(76–79)*. The microarray analysis presented here shows that expression of *SOX10* is also decreased after BRN2 ablation, whereas no change in *PAX3* expression was detected. Further, these results were confirmed by semiquantitative RT-PCR, and lack of SOX10 protein was confirmed by immunoblot.

Recently, the promoter of the *SLUG* (SNAI2) gene was shown to be regulated by MITF in co-transfection experiments *(80)*. Hence, because BRN2 ablation causes a loss of MITF, it is not surprising that SLUG expression is decreased in the MM96Lc8LC cell line. SLUG belongs to the SNAIL family of zinc-finger domain transcription factors that bind to E-box motifs *(81)*. The E-box motif is also bound by the MITF transcription factor *(82)*, and it has been postulated that SNAIL family factors compete with basic helix-loop-helix factors for DNA binding at the promoters of target genes *(81)*. Interestingly, the SNAIL protein acts as a repressor of E-cadherin in melanocytic cells *(83)*, whereas SLUG acts in a similar manner in breast cancer cells *(84)*. The SLUG and SNAIL factors act in a coordinated fashion during epithelial–mesenchymal transitions *(85,86)*, a process involved in cancer progression. SNAIL initially represses E-cadherin to allow acquisition of a migratory phenotype and then SLUG maintains the migratory/ mesodermal phenotype. Li et al. have demonstrated that the melanocytic mitogen SF contributes to an autocrine loop to repress E-cadherin and Desmoglein-1 in both melanoma cells and primary melanocytes *(87)*. Thus, it is tempting to suggest that SF-mediated repression of E-cadherin involves upregulation of SNAIL and/or SLUG factors. In support of this, the ability of either EDN1 or EDN3 to increase both SNAIL and N-cadherin expression and concomitantly repress that of E-cadherin in melanoma cell lines has recently been demonstrated *(88)*.

Tumor Survival and Growth

Recently, the antiapoptotic gene *BCL2* has been shown to be under the control of the transcription factor MITF *(89)* in the melanocytic lineage. Consistent with these findings, ablation of BRN2 and the resulting decrease in levels of MITF led to a decreased expression of *BCL2*. This difference was found using the cDNA microarrays and confirmed by RT-PCR (Fig. 2B).

Upregulation of SPARC/osteonectin has been shown following ectopic expression of β_3-integrin in RGP melanoma cells *(90)*. Further, ablation of SPARC expression by antisense RNA has been shown to abrogate tumorigenicity in a nude mouse model *(91)*. cDNA microarray analysis of the nontumorigenic MM96Lc8LC cells revealed a decreased expression compared with BRN2-expressing melanoma cells, a result consistent with the lack of tumorigenicity of both SPARC and BRN2-ablated cell lines. RT-PCR and immunoblot analysis of the two cell lines confirmed the microarray hybridization result. TIMP3 was also more lowly expressed after BRN2 ablation. TIMP3 has been reported to be induced during melanoma progression *(92)*, thus, a loss of TIMP3 expression is consistent with the nontumorigenic phenotype of these cells.

Metastatic and late vertical growth phase melanoma cell lines are unresponsive to IGF1, unlike melanocytes and melanoma cell lines derived from radial or early vertical growth phase tumors *(93)*. Furthermore, IGF1 signaling can be mediated by IL-8 *(94)*. Intriguingly, these two growth factors displayed opposing regulation after BRN2 ablation, with *IGF1* expression being lost and *IL-8* being upregulated, suggestive of a possible compensatory mechanism. Several other interleukins, such as *IL-1β*, *IL-6*, and *IL-24* similarly showed increased expression in MM96Lc8LC cells after microarray analysis and RT-PCR confirmation (data not shown).

Microarray screening also demonstrated that *EDNRB* expression was decreased after BRN2 ablation; this was confirmed by RT-PCR. Intriguingly, in mice heterozygous for a mutant *SOX10* allele, expression of *EDNRB* was developmentally delayed *(95)*, suggesting that the lack of *EDNRB* in MM96Lc8LC cells may in part be caused by the loss of SOX10. However, the BRN2 protein may also have a direct role in regulation of the EDNRB expression because of the presence of octamer motifs in the promoter that can be bound by BRN2 *(96)*.

The data presented here focuses on genes whose expression is lost after BRN2 ablation. A more pertinent question is to determine which promoters are either reactivated or repressed as a consequence of a higher BRN2 expression level during melanocytic transformation. In vitro systems for induction of BRN2 in melanocytic cells have been reported *(38,39,58)*, and, thus, analysis of gene expression profiles of these cells compared with cultured melanocytes and melanoma cell lines may provide some answers to this question.

POSITIONING BRN2 IN THE MELANOCYTIC GENE REGULATORY HIERARCHY

To date, the precise function of the BRN2 protein in melanocytic cells remains to be fully clarified. It is known that BRN2-ablated melanoma cells (MM96Lc8LC cell line, Fig. 1A) revert to a less mature cell type, lacking tumorigenicity as well as many markers of differentiated melanocytes, such as TYRP family members, MC1R, and MITF (ref. *31*, Fig. 2 and Table 1), implicating BRN2 in sustaining the melanocytic phenotype. Of particular note is the absence of expression of several transcription factors that constitute a transcriptional hierarchy operational in melanocytic cells (Fig. 3A), and which are causal genes for Waardenburg syndrome *(75)*. Thus, given that MM96Lc8LC cells lack both MITF and SOX10, and that SOX10 regulates MITF expression *(78,79,97)*, it seems plausible that the paucity of MITF expression caused by BRN2 ablation is in part caused by a lack of SOX10. In a similar manner, the absence of *SLUG* transcripts may in part be a reflection that these cells lack MITF.

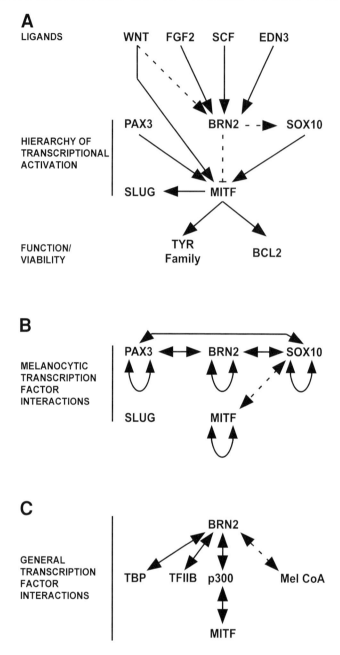

Fig. 3. Melanocytic gene regulatory hierarchies and interactions. Several transcription factors expressed in melanocytic cells constitute a network of interactions that not only have a transcriptional relationship (**A**, indicated by arrows), but also have a direct interaction relationship with both melanocytic (**B**, double headed arrows) and general transcriptional cofactors (**C**). Dashed arrows indicate an implied relationship or interaction that has not been experimentally verified.

Another layer of complexity is added to this hierarchy by the ability of several of these proteins to physically interact with both themselves and each other (Fig. 3B). For example, the ability of SOX10 and PAX3 to mediate synergistic transcriptional activation is well characterized, not only in melanocytic cells *(76,78)*, but also in other lineages *(45,98)*. Additionally, synergism between MITF and SOX10 for *DCT* promoter transactivation has recently been reported, although no physical interaction between these proteins was able to be demonstrated *(99)*. The BRN2 protein interacts with both SOX10 and PAX3, tested in mammalian two-hybrid systems and in GST-fusion protein pull-down experiments *(26)*, however, no melanocytic gene promoter or co-binding site for BRN2 with either SOX10 or PAX3 has been characterized to date.

It is thought that both the POU and SOX families of transcription factors coevolved, allowing acquisition of specific developmental codes during metazoan evolution *(100)*. Consistent with this, a number of studies have provided direct evidence for a specific combinatorial POU-SOX code, which permits specific members of each family to inter-act and produce a functional regulator able to promote or repress transcription *(101)*. The crystal structure of the of Oct-1 POU domain–Sox2 HMG domain–DNA ternary complex has been described, and showed that the HMG domain C-terminal interacted with the N-terminal of the POU$_S$ subdomain via regions highly conserved in both protein families *(1,102)*. Interestingly, this same surface of the SOX protein is also responsible for mediating interactions with PAX proteins *(102)*. Hence, the implications of competition between POU–SOX–PAX family transcription factors for co-dimer formation in melanocytic cells is likely to be complex, owing to the coexpression of SOX10, PAX3, and BRN2, and the ability of these proteins to interact with each other *(26)*.

BRN2 not only interacts with cell-type-specific transcription factors, but also with the general transcriptional machinery cofactors p300, TBP, and TFIIB in GST-fusion protein pull-down experiments *(26)*. Notably, co-immunoprecipitation studies have shown that the MITF factor also interacts with p300 in both cultured melanocytes and melanoma cell lines *(103)*. Other POU proteins have also been reported to interact with basal transcriptional regulators. For example, TBP interacts with Oct-1 and Oct-2 *(104,105)*, and, additionally, Oct-1 also interacts with TFIIB *(106)*. Furthermore, the POU domain is sufficient to induce transcription from a downstream promoter when bound to an enhancer by recruitment of TBP to otherwise inactive promoter elements *(105)*.

The BRN2 protein also contains a 25-residue sequence (amino acids 125–149), which consists of entirely glutamine residues, with the only exception a histidine in position 4 of the sequence *(17)*. Using the 122–154 region of the BRN2 protein as bait, several proteins that interact with this motif in a yeast two-hybrid system were identified in a screen of a human embryonic cDNA library *(107,108)*. For one of these proteins, PQBP-1, this interaction was further characterized and found to occur via polar amino acid-rich regions and co-transfection reporter assays revealed that PQBP-1 has a negative effect on BRN2-mediated transactivation *(107)*.

Identification of BRN2 target promoters is of importance in understanding the role of this protein in melanocytic cells. Although microarray analysis of BRN2-ablated cell lines provides multiple candidate genes, elucidation of transcriptional targets is complicated by the fact that loss of BRN2 affects other transcription factors, such as SOX10 and MITF. Thus, merely showing a loss of expression after BRN2 ablation does not immediately suggest direct regulation by the BRN2 protein. Notwithstanding this caveat, several genes are candidates for regulation by BRN2. BRN2 ablation in a melanoma cell line causes a complete loss of TYRP family gene expression, most likely as a result of the concomitant loss of *MITF* expression in these cells *(31)*. Other studies have suggested that, in melanocytic cells, BRN2 is a repressor of the *MITF* promoter *(109)* and the *TYR* promoter *(33)*. Microarray analysis suggests that BRN2 ablation in a melanoma cell line resulted in a loss of SOX10 expression (Fig. 2B and Table 1), suggesting that one role of BRN2 may be to regulate the *SOX10* promoter. Others have shown a role for BRN2 in regulation of *gadd45* expression in response to UVB radiation, because ablation of BRN2 using antisense RNA techniques abrogated this response *(68)*.

Obviously, the consequences of self dimerization and/or co-dimerization by BRN2 and its transcriptional cofactors on appropriate DNA sequences is pivotal to understanding the differences in transcription factor expression levels that direct gene regulation in melanocytes. This is exemplified by the B-cell-specific coactivator for Oct-1 and Oct-2, OBF1, which is precluded from interacting with Oct-1 dimers on certain promoter elements because of shielding of the Oct-1 surface by the POU_S–POU_H dimer interface *(28,29)*, but when able to bind, acts to stabilize the Oct-1 dimer on DNA *(110)*. Because BRN2 is expressed in several cell types, there may be a melanocyte-specific equivalent of OBF1, which interacts with BRN2 to mediate specific transcriptional regulation (Mel CoA in Fig. 3C). Hence, knowledge of the physical interactions between POU proteins and their transcriptional co-regulators, as well as the DNA sequence of their target promoters is required to understand fully the capacity of these molecules to function as a molecular switch in maintaining the differentiated phenotype or promoting cell growth leading to malignancy.

CONCLUSIONS AND PERSPECTIVES

Understanding of the role BRN2 has in melanoma has progressed significantly since its initial description as a melanocytic octamer binding protein *(12,13)*, in which, broadly speaking, BRN2 functions in tumorigenicity and cellular proliferation *(31,39,58)*. It appears that BRN2 upregulation is a critical step in melanoma progression. If expression levels seen in vitro are relevant to clinical melanomagenesis, then they should be observable in human skin lesions, in which they may act as useful prognostic indicators of early stage melanoma. Several studies have identified pathways capable of augmenting BRN2 expression in melanocytes *(38,39,58)*, and which, when combined with UV radiation, experimentally induce melanoma. Thus, examination of BRN2 expression levels in these specimens may identify the stage at which homeostatic regulation of BRN2 is lost by melanocytes (Fig. 1C). Subsequent comparison of BRN2 expression levels by melanocytes in normal skin with those at the sites of melanocytic nevi and in melanoma would address the clinical significance of this conclusion.

ACKNOWLEDGMENTS

The authors thank Dr. Colin Goding (Marie Curie Research Institute, UK) for communication of manuscripts before publication and Dr. Sandra Pavey, Dr. Graeme Walker, and Dr. Nick Hayward (QIMR) for communicating unpublished data. A.L.C. was supported by a University of Queensland Postgraduate Scholarship. R.A.S. is a Senior Research Fellow of the Australian NHMRC. The work was funded in part by a grant from the Royal Brisbane Hospital Research Foundation and by NHMRC Program Grant 199600. The Institute for Molecular Bioscience is a Special Research Center of the Australian Research Council.

REFERENCES

1. Ryan AK, Rosenfeld MG. POU domain family values: flexibility, partnerships, and developmental codes. Genes Dev 1997;11:1207–1225.
2. Herr W, Sturm RA, Clerc RG, et al. The POU domain: a large conserved region in the mammalian pit-1, oct-1, oct-2, and Caenorhabditis elegans unc-86 gene products. Genes Dev 1988;2:1513–1516.
3. Sturm RA, Herr W. The POU domain is a bipartite DNA-binding structure. Nature 1988;336:601–604.
4. Sturm RA, Das G, Herr W. The ubiquitous octamer-binding protein Oct-1 contains a POU domain with a homeo box subdomain. Genes Dev 1988;2:1582–1599.
5. Wegner M, Drolet DW, Rosenfeld MG. POU-domain proteins: structure and function of developmental regulators. Curr Opin Cell Biol 1993;5:488–498.
6. Fujii H, Hamada H. A CNS-specific POU transcription factor, Brn-2, is required for establishing mammalian neural cell lineages. Neuron 1993;11:1197–1206.
7. Schreiber E, Merchant RE, Wiestler OD, Fontana A. Primary brain tumors differ in their expression of octamer deoxyribonucleic acid-binding transcription factors from long-term cultured glioma cell lines. Neurosurgery 1994;34:129–135.
8. Hagino-Yamagishi K, Saijoh Y, Ikeda M, Ichikawa M, Minamikawa-Tachino R, Hamada H. Predominant expression of Brn-2 in the postmitotic neurons of the developing mouse neocortex. Brain Res 1997;752:261–268.
9. Schreiber E, Harshman K, Kemler I, Malipiero U, Schaffner W, Fontana A. Astrocytes and glioblastoma cells express novel octamer-DNA binding proteins distinct from the ubiquitous Oct-1 and B cell type Oct-2 proteins. Nucleic Acids Res 1990;18:5495–5503.
10. Schreiber E, Himmelmann A, Malipiero U, Tobler A, Stahel R, Fontana A. Human small cell lung cancer expresses the octamer DNA-binding and nervous system-specific transcription factor N-Oct 3 (brain-2). Cancer Res 1992;52:6121–6124.
11. Thomson JAF, Leonard JH, McGregor K, Sturm RA, Parsons PG. A nonconsensus octamer-recognition sequence (TAATGARAT-motif) identifies a novel DNA binding protein in human Merkel cell carcinoma cell lines. Int J Cancer 1994;58:285–290.
12. Cox PM, Temperley SM, Kumar H, Goding CR. A distinct octamer-binding protein present in malignant melanoma cells. Nucleic Acids Res 1988;16:11,047–11,056.
13. Sturm RA, Bisshop F, Takahashi H, Parsons PG. A melanoma octamer binding protein is responsive to differentiating agents. Cell Growth Differ 1991;2:519–524.
14. Thomson JAF, Parsons PG, Sturm RA. In vivo and in vitro expression of octamer binding proteins in human melanoma metastases, brain tissue, and fibroblasts. Pigment Cell Res 1993;6:13–22.
15. He X, Treacy MN, Simmons DM, Ingraham HA, Swanson LW, Rosenfeld MG. Expression of a large family of POU-domain regulatory genes in mammalian brain development. Nature 1989;340:35–41.
16. Hara Y, Rovescalli AC, Kim Y, Nirenberg M. Structure and evolution of four POU domain genes expressed in mouse brain. Proc Natl Acad Sci U S A 1992;89:3280–3284.
17. Schreiber E, Tobler A, Malipiero U, Schaffner W, Fontana A. cDNA cloning of human N-Oct3, a nervous-system specific POU domain transcription factor binding to the octamer DNA motif. Nucleic Acids Res 1993;21:253–258.
18. Atanasoski S, Schreiber E, Fontana A, Herr W. N-Oct 5 is generated by in vitro proteolysis of the neural POU-domain protein N-Oct 3. Oncogene 1997;14:1287–1294.
19. Smith AG, Brightwell G, Smit SE, Parsons PG, Sturm RA. Redox regulation of Brn-2/N-Oct-3 POU domain DNA binding activity and proteolytic formation of N-Oct-5 during melanoma cell nuclear extraction. Melanoma Res 1998;8:2–10.
20. Scholer HR. Octamania: the POU factors in murine development. Trends in Genetics 1991;7:323–329.
21. Klemm JD, Pabo CO. Oct-1 POU domain-DNA interactions: cooperative binding of isolated subdomains and effects of covalent linkage. Genes Dev 1996;10:27–36.
22. Klemm JD, Rould MA, Aurora R, Herr W, Pabo CO. Crystal structure of the Oct-1 POU domain bound to an octamer site: DNA recognition with tethered DNA-binding modules. Cell 1994;77:21–32.
23. Herr W, Cleary MA. The POU domain: versatility in transcriptional regulation by a flexible two-in-one DNA-binding domain. Genes Dev 1995;9:1679–1693.
24. Rhee JM, Gruber CA, Brodie TB, Trieu M, Turner EE. Highly cooperative homodimerization is a conserved property of neural POU proteins. J Biol Chem 1998;273:34,196–34,205.
25. Rigoni P, Xu L, Harshman K, Schaffner W, Arnosti DN. Conserved cysteine residues of Oct-2 POU domain confer sensitivity to oxidation but are dispensable for sequence-specific DNA binding. Biochim Biophys Acta 1993;1173:141–146.

26. Smit DJ, Smith AG, Parsons PG, Muscat GE, Sturm RA. Domains of Brn-2 that mediate homodimerization and interaction with general and melanocytic transcription factors. Eur J Biochem 2000;267:6413–6422.

27. Dugast-Darzacq C, Egloff S, Weber MJ. Cooperative dimerization of the POU domain protein Brn-2 on a new motif activates the neuronal promoter of the human aromatic L-amino acid decarboxylase gene. Brain Res Mol Brain Res 2004;120:151–163.

28. Tomilin A, Remenyi A, Lins K, et al. Synergism with the coactivator OBF-1 (OCA-B, BOB-1) is mediated by a specific POU dimer configuration. Cell 2000;103:853–864.

29. Remenyi A, Tomilin A, Pohl E, et al. Differential dimer activities of the transcription factor Oct-1 by DNA-induced interface swapping. Mol Cell 2001;8:569–580.

30. Atanasoski S, Toldo SS, Malipiero U, Schreiber E, Fries R, Fontana A. Isolation of the human genomic brain-2/N-Oct 3 gene (POUF3) and assignment to chromosome 6q16. Genomics 1995;26:272–280.

31. Thomson JAF, Murphy K, Baker E, Sutherland GR, Parsons PG, Sturm RA. The brn-2 gene regulates the melanocytic phenotype and tumorigenic potential of human melanoma cells. Oncogene 1995;11:691–700.

32. Chin L, Merlino G, DePinho RA. Malignant melanoma: modern black plague and genetic black box. Genes Dev 1998;12:3467–3481.

33. Eisen T, Easty DJ, Bennett DC, Goding CR. The POU domain transcription factor Brn-2: elevated expression in malignant melanoma and regulation of melanocyte-specific gene expression. Oncogene 1995;11:2157–2164.

34. Nakai S, Kawano H, Yudate T, et al. The POU domain transcription factor Brn-2 is required for the determination of specific neuronal lineages in the hypothalamus of the mouse. Genes Dev 1995;9:3109–3121.

35. Schreiber J, Enderich J, Sock E, Schmidt C, Richter-Landsberg C, Wegner M. Redundancy of class III POU proteins in the oligodendrocyte lineage. J Biol Chem 1997;272:32,286–32,293.

36. Sugitani Y, Nakai S, Minowa O, et al. Brn-1 and Brn-2 share crucial roles in the production and positioning of mouse neocortical neurons. Genes Dev 2002;16:1760–1765.

37. McEvilly RJ, de Diaz MO, Schonemann MD, Hooshmand F, Rosenfeld MG. Transcriptional regulation of cortical neuron migration by POU domain factors. Science 2002;295:1528–1532.

38. Cook AL, Donatien PD, Smith AG, et al. Human melanoblasts in culture: expression of BRN2 and synergistic regulation by fibroblast growth factor-2, stem cell factor, and endothelin-3. J Invest Dermatol 2003;121:1150–1159.

39. Goodall J, Martinozzi S, Dexter TJ, et al. Brn-2 expression controls melanoma proliferation and is directly regulated by beta-catenin. Mol Cell Biol 2004;24:2915–2922.

40. Murphy M, Bernard O, Reid K, Bartlett PF. Cell lines derived from mouse neural crest are representative of cells at various stages of differentiation. J Neurobiol 1991;22:522–535.

41. Nishimura EK, Jordan SA, Oshima H, et al. Dominant role of the niche in melanocyte stem-cell fate determination. Nature 2002;416:854–860.

42. Schonemann MD, Ryan AK, McEvilly RJ, et al. Development and survival of the endocrine hypothalamus and posterior pituitary gland requires the neuronal POU domain factor Brn-2. Genes Dev 1995;9:3122–3135.

43. Niwa H, Miyazaki J, Smith AG. Quantitative expression of Oct-3/4 defines differentiation, dedifferentiation or self-renewal of ES cells. Nat Genet 2000;24:372–376.

44. Jaegle M, Ghazvini M, Mandemakers W, et al. The POU proteins Brn-2 and Oct-6 share important functions in Schwann cell development. Genes Dev 2003;17:1380–1391.

45. Kuhlbrodt K, Herbarth B, Sock E, Hermans-Borgmeyer I, Wegner M. Sox10, a novel transcriptional modulator in glial cells. J Neurosci 1998;18:237–250.

46. Suzuki N, Rohdewohld H, Neuman T, Gruss P, Scholer HR. Oct-6: a POU transcription factor expressed in embryonal stem cells and in the developing brain. EMBO J 1990;9:3723–3732.

47. Collarini EJ, Kuhn R, Marshall CJ, Monuki ES, Lemke G, Richardson WD. Down-regulation of the POU transcription factor SCIP is an early event in oligodendrocyte differentiation in vitro. Development 1992;116:193–200.

48. Jaegle M, Mandemakers W, Broos L, et al. The POU factor Oct-6 and Schwann cell differentiation. Science 1996;273:507–510.

49. Qin XF, Luo Y, Suh H, et al. Transformation by homeobox genes can be mediated by selective transcriptional repression. EMBO J 1994;13:5967–5976.

50. Gidekel S, Pizov G, Bergman Y, Pikarsky E. Oct-3/4 is a dose-dependent oncogenic fate determinant. Cancer Cell 2003;4:361–370.

51. Irshad S, Pedley RB, Anderson J, Latchman DS, Budhram-Mahadeo VS. The Brn-3b transcription factor regulates the growth, behaviour and invasiveness of human neuroblastoma cells in vitro and in-vivo. J Biol Chem 2004;279:21,617–21,627.

52. Bohm M, Moellmann G, Cheng E, et al. Identification of p90RSK as the probable CREB-Ser133 kinase in human melanocytes. Cell Growth Differ 1995;6:291–302.

53. Tada A, Suzuki I, Im S, et al. Endothelin-1 is a paracrine growth factor that modulates melanogenesis of human melanocytes and participates in their responses to ultraviolet radiation. Cell Growth Differ 1998;9:575–584.

54. Imokawa G, Kobayasi T, Miyagishi M. Intracellular signaling mechanisms leading to synergistic effects of endothelin-1 and stem cell factor on proliferation of cultured human melanocytes. Cross-talk via trans-activation of the tyrosine kinase c-kit receptor. J Biol Chem 2000;275:33,321–33,328.

55. Berking C, Takemoto R, Satyamoorthy K, et al. Induction of melanoma phenotypes in human skin by growth factors and ultraviolet B. Cancer Res 2004;64:807–811.

56. Wong LF, Murphy D. Adenoviral-mediated over-expression of Brn2 in the rat paraventricular nucleus: no effect on vasopressin or corticotrophin releasing factor RNA levels. Mol Cell Endocrinol 2003;200:165–175.

57. Satyamoorthy K, Li G, Gerrero MR, et al. Constitutive mitogen-activated protein kinase activation in melanoma is mediated by both BRAF mutations and autocrine growth factor stimulation. Cancer Res 2003;63:756–759.

58. Goodall J, Wellbrock C, Dexter TJ, Roberts K, Marais R, Goding CR. The Brn-2 transcription factor links activated BRAF in melanoma to melanocyte proliferation. Mol Cell Biol 2004;24:2923–2931.

59. Rimm DL, Caca K, Hu G, Harrison FB, Fearon ER. Frequent nuclear/cytoplasmic localization of beta-catenin without exon 3 mutations in malignant melanoma. Am J Pathol 1999;154:325–329.

60. Widlund HR, Horstmann MA, Price ER, et al. Beta-catenin–induced melanoma growth requires the downstream target Microphthalmia-associated transcription factor. J Cell Biol 2002;158:1079–1087.

61. Huelsken J, Behrens J. The Wnt signalling pathway. J Cell Sci 2002;115:3977–3978.

62. Dorsky RI, Moon RT, Raible DW. Control of neural crest cell fate by the Wnt signalling pathway. Nature 1998;396:370–373.

63. Dunn KJ, Williams BO, Li Y, Pavan WJ. Neural crest-directed gene transfer demonstrates Wnt1 role in melanocyte expansion and differentiation during mouse development. Proc Natl Acad Sci USA 2000;97:10,050–10,055.

64. Ikeya M, Lee SM, Johnson JE, McMahon AP, Takada S. Wnt signalling required for expansion of neural crest and CNS progenitors. Nature 1997;389:966–970.

65. Bittner M, Meltzer P, Chen Y, et al. Molecular classification of cutaneous malignant melanoma by gene expression profiling. Nature 2000;406:536–540.

66. Weeraratna AT, Jiang Y, Hostetter G, et al. Wnt5a signaling directly affects cell motility and invasion of metastatic melanoma. Cancer Cell 2002;1:279–288.

67. Hingorani SR, Jacobetz MA, Robertson GP, Herlyn M, Tuveson DA. Suppression of BRAF(V599E) in human melanoma abrogates transformation. Cancer Res 2003;63:5198–5202.

68. Lefort K, Rouault JP, Tondereau L, Magaud JP, Dore JF. The specific activation of gadd45 following UVB radiation requires the POU family gene product N-oct3 in human melanoma cells. Oncogene 2001;20:7375–7385.

69. Du J, Miller AJ, Widlund HR, Horstmann MA, Ramaswamy S, Fisher DE. MLANA/MART1 and SILV/PMEL17/GP100 are transcriptionally regulated by mitf in melanocytes and melanoma. Am J Pathol 2003;163:333–343.

70. Loftus SK, Larson DM, Baxter LL, et al. Mutation of melanosome protein RAB38 in chocolate mice. Proc Natl Acad Sci USA 2002;99:4471–4476.

71. Wu X, Wang F, Rao K, Sellers JR, Hammer JA 3rd. Rab27a is an essential component of melanosome receptor for Myosin va. Mol Biol Cell 2002;13:1735–1749.

72. Metzelaar MJ, Wijngaard PL, Peters PJ, Sixma JJ, Nieuwenhuis HK, Clevers HC. CD63 antigen. A novel lysosomal membrane glycoprotein, cloned by a screening procedure for intracellular antigens in eukaryotic cells. J Biol Chem 1991;266:3239–3245.

73. Marks MS, Seabra MC. The melanosome: membrane dynamics in black and white. Nat Rev Mol Cell Biol 2001;2:738–748.

74. Chen H, Salopek TG, Jimbow K. The role of phosphoinositide 3-kinase in the sorting and transport of newly synthesized tyrosinase-related protein-1 (TRP-1). J Investig Dermatol Symp Proc 2001;6:105–114.

75. Bennett DC, Lamoreux ML. The color loci of mice—a genetic century. Pigment Cell Res 2003;16:333–344.

76. Bondurand N, Pingault V, Goerich DE, et al. Interaction among SOX10, PAX3 and MITF, three genes altered in Waardenburg syndrome. Hum Mol Genet 2000;9:1907–1917.
77. Watanabe A, Takeda K, Ploplis B, Tachibana M. Epistatic relationship between Waardenburg syndrome genes MITF and PAX3. Nat Genet 1998;18:283–286.
78. Potterf SB, Furumura M, Dunn KJ, Arnheiter H, Pavan WJ. Transcription factor hierarchy in Waardenburg syndrome: regulation of MITF expression by SOX10 and PAX3. Hum Genet 2000;107:1–6.
79. Lee M, Goodall J, Verastegui C, Ballotti R, Goding CR. Direct regulation of the Microphthalmia promoter by Sox10 links Waardenburg-Shah syndrome (WS4)-associated hypopigmentation and deafness to WS2. J Biol Chem 2000;275:37,978–37,983.
80. Sanchez-Martin M, Rodriguez-Garcia A, Perez-Losada J, Sagrera A, Read AP, Sanchez-Garcia I. SLUG (SNAI2) deletions in patients with Waardenburg disease. Hum Mol Genet 2002;11: 3231–3236.
81. Hemavathy K, Ashraf SI, Ip YT. Snail/slug family of repressors: slowly going into the fast lane of development and cancer. Gene 2000;257:1–12.
82. Goding CR. Mitf from neural crest to melanoma: signal transduction and transcription in the melanocyte lineage. Genes Dev 2000;14:1712–1728.
83. Poser I, Dominguez D, de Herreros AG, Varnai A, Buettner R, Bosserhoff AK. Loss of E-cadherin expression in melanoma cells involves up-regulation of the transcriptional repressor Snail. J Biol Chem 2001;276:24,661–24,666.
84. Hajra KM, Chen DY, Fearon ER. The SLUG zinc-finger protein represses E-cadherin in breast cancer. Cancer Res 2002;62:1613–1618.
85. Cano A, Perez-Moreno MA, Rodrigo I, et al. The transcription factor snail controls epithelial-mesenchymal transitions by repressing E-cadherin expression. Nat Cell Biol 2000;2:76–83.
86. Bolos V, Peinado H, Perez-Moreno MA, Fraga MF, Esteller M, Cano A. The transcription factor Slug represses E-cadherin expression and induces epithelial to mesenchymal transitions: a comparison with Snail and E47 repressors. J Cell Sci 2003;116:499–511.
87. Li G, Schaider H, Satyamoorthy K, Hanakawa Y, Hashimoto K, Herlyn M. Downregulation of E-cadherin and Desmoglein 1 by autocrine hepatocyte growth factor during melanoma development. Oncogene 2001;20:8125–8135.
88. Bagnato A, Rosano L, Spinella F, Di Castro V, Tecce R, Natali PG. Endothelin B receptor blockade inhibits dynamics of cell interactions and communications in melanoma cell progression. Cancer Res 2004;64:1436–1443.
89. McGill GG, Horstmann M, Widlund HR, et al. Bcl2 regulation by the melanocyte master regulator Mitf modulates lineage survival and melanoma cell viability. Cell 2002;109:707–718.
90. Sturm RA, Satyamoorthy K, Meier F, et al. Osteonectin/SPARC induction by ectopic beta(3) integrin in human radial growth phase primary melanoma cells. Cancer Res 2002;62:226–232.
91. Ledda MF, Adris S, Bravo AI, et al. Suppression of SPARC expression by antisense RNA abrogates the tumorigenicity of human melanoma cells. Nat Med 1997;3:171–176.
92. Airola K, Karonen T, Vaalamo M, et al. Expression of collagenases-1 and -3 and their inhibitors TIMP-1 and -3 correlates with the level of invasion in malignant melanomas. Br J Cancer 1999;80:733–743.
93. Satyamoorthy K, Li G, Vaidya B, Patel D, Herlyn M. Insulin-like growth factor-1 induces survival and growth of biologically early melanoma cells through both the mitogen-activated protein kinase and beta-catenin pathways. Cancer Res 2001;61:7318–7324.
94. Satyamoorthy K, Li G, Vaidya B, Kalabis J, Herlyn M. Insulin-like growth factor-I–induced migration of melanoma cells is mediated by interleukin-8 induction. Cell Growth Differ 2002;13:87–93.
95. Southard-Smith EM, Kos L, Pavan WJ. Sox10 mutation disrupts neural crest development in Dom Hirschsprung mouse model. Nat Genet 1998;18:60–64.
96. Smith AG. The regulation of melanocytic gene expression by the Brn-2 transcription factor [PhD Thesis]. The University of Queensland, Brisbane, Australia, 1999.
97. Verastegui C, Bille K, Ortonne JP, Ballotti R. Regulation of the microphthalmia-associated transcription factor gene by the Waardenburg syndrome type 4 gene, SOX10. J Biol Chem 2000;275: 30,757–30,760.
98. Lang D, Epstein JA. Sox10 and Pax3 physically interact to mediate activation of a conserved c-RET enhancer. Hum Mol Genet 2003;12:937–945.
99. Ludwig A, Rehberg S, Wegner M. Melanocyte-specific expression of dopachrome tautomerase is dependent on synergistic gene activation by the Sox10 and Mitf transcription factors. FEBS Lett 2004;556:236–244.

100. Dailey L, Basilico C. Coevolution of HMG domains and homeodomains and the generation of transcriptional regulation by Sox/POU complexes. J Cell Physiol 2001;186:315–328.

101. Kuhlbrodt K, Herbarth B, Sock E, Enderich J, Hermans-Borgmeyer I, Wegner M. Cooperative function of POU proteins and SOX proteins in glial cells. J Biol Chem 1998;273:16,050–16,057.

102. Remenyi A, Lins K, Nissen LJ, Reinbold R, Scholer HR, Wilmanns M. Crystal structure of a POU/HMG/DNA ternary complex suggests differential assembly of Oct4 and Sox2 on two enhancers. Genes Dev 2003;17:2048–2059.

103. Sato S, Roberts K, Gambino G, Cook A, Kouzarides T, Goding CR. CBP/p300 as a co-factor for the Microphthalmia transcription factor. Oncogene 1997;14:3083–3092.

104. Zwilling S, Annweiler A, Wirth T. The POU domains of the Oct1 and Oct2 transcription factors mediate specific interaction with TBP. Nucleic Acids Res 1994;22:1655–1662.

105. Bertolino E, Singh H. POU/TBP cooperativity: a mechanism for enhancer action from a distance. Mol Cell 2002;10:397–407.

106. Nakshatri H, Nakshatri P, Currie RA. Interaction of Oct-1 with TFIIB. Implications for a novel response elicited through the proximal octamer site of the lipoprotein lipase promoter. J Biol Chem 1995;270:19,613–19,623.

107. Waragai M, Lammers CH, Takeuchi S, et al. PQBP-1, a novel polyglutamine tract-binding protein, inhibits transcription activation by Brn-2 and affects cell survival. Hum Mol Genet 1999;8:977–987.

108. Imafuku I, Waragai M, Takeuchi S, et al. Polar amino acid-rich sequences bind to polyglutamine tracts. Biochem Biophys Res Commun 1998;253:16–20.

109. Goding CR. Beta-catenin activation of Brn-2 expression leads to repression of Mitf and increased melanocyte proliferation. Pigment Cell Res 2002;15:56(Abstract).

110. Lins K, Remenyi A, Tomilin A, et al. OBF1 enhances transcriptional potential of Oct1. EMBO J 2003;22:2188–2198.

9

The Dynamic Roles of Cell-Surface Receptors in Melanoma Development

Dong Fang and Meenhard Herlyn

Contents

Summary

Cell-surface receptors on melanocytic cells change dramatically during transformation. These molecules facilitate adhesive functions and modulate growth, survival, and invasion. In this review, we focus on cadherins for cell–cell adhesion and frizzled (Fzd) receptors for growth control. Both receptors activate the β-catenin pathway, which is critical for melanocyte differentiation and melanoma progression. Cadherins are physically associated with receptor tyrosine kinases that mediate growth signals. The switch from epithelial cadherin in melanocytes to neural cadherin in melanoma cells appears to profoundly change cell-signaling partners for each cell type.

Key Words: Melanoma; transformation; cadherin; Wnt-signaling pathway; tyrosine kinase receptor.

INTRODUCTION

Pigment-producing melanocytes are localized in the basal layer of the skin. Each melanocyte is coordinately associated with 5 to 10 basal keratinocytes, forming the "epidermal-melanin unit" of up to 35 cells *(1)*. Within this unit, each melanocyte transports melanin-containing melanosomes into neighboring keratinocytes. Pigmentation deposited in the skin protects us from the deleterious effects of ultraviolet radiation. The functions and biological properties of melanocytes are finely controlled by their symbiotic keratinocytes. The regulation of melanocytes by keratinocytes is facilitated through cell surface receptors that either establish adhesive contacts or mediate ligands from the other cells. Disturbances in normal melanocyte–keratinocyte contacts may lead to a transformed phenotype of melanocytes. For example, epithelial (E)-cadherin, which is

From: *From Melanocytes to Melanoma: The Progression to Malignancy*
Edited by: V. J. Hearing and S. P. L. Leong © Humana Press Inc., Totowa, NJ

the major adhesion molecule mediating melanocyte–keratinocyte adhesion, is downregulated in melanoma cells before their invasion into the adjacent dermal compartment and is accompanied by an increase in neural (N)-cadherin expression *(2)*. This chapter will focus on the alterations in cell surface receptors of melanocytic cells and their cellular signaling pathways during transformation of melanocytes. We will predominantly discuss cadherin and Wnt-signaling pathways.

CADHERIN MOLECULES IN CELL–CELL ADHESION AND SIGNAL TRANSDUCTION

Adhesion molecules have important roles in cell–cell communication. Cadherins are a family of functionally related glycoproteins involved in calcium-dependent cell–cell adhesion and signaling. They are transmembrane proteins comprised of an extracellular domain, a membrane-spanning domain, and a highly conserved cytoplasmic domain. Cadherins contribute to epithelial cell–cell adhesion, cell shape, differentiation, epithelial to mesenchymal transition, and invasion. Cadherins are expressed in a cell- and tissue-specific manner. The expression patterns of major cadherins in skin cells are summarized in Table 1. E-cadherin serves as the major adhesion molecule in the adherence junction of keratinocytes in the skin, whereas N-cadherin is expressed by both endothelial cells and fibroblasts. E-cadherins bind to unphosphorylated β-catenin, γ-catenin (plakoglobin), and p120-catenin, forming an E-cadherin–catenin unit at the cell membrane to functionally maintain cell–cell contact. The link to the actin cytoskeleton is established through α-catenin (Fig. 1). E-cadherin mediates cellular signaling by dissociating β-catenin from the complex, which then accumulates in the cytoplasm, enters the nucleus to bind the transcription factor lymphoid enhancer factor/T-cell factor (LEF/TCF), and then transactivates downstream target genes.

Melanocytes also express E-cadherin, allowing them to bind to keratinocytes *(3)*. Expression of E-cadherin by melanocytes is regulated by growth factors produced by either keratinocytes or fibroblasts. Keratinocyte-derived endothelin-1 (ET-1) downregulates E-cadherin on melanocytes *(4)*. Fibroblast-derived hepatocyte growth factor/scatter factor can also downregulate the expression of E-cadherin *(5)*. Similarly, platelet-derived growth factor (PDGF) can downregulate E-cadherin expressed by melanocytes *(6)*. This downregulation will allow the melanocytes to decouple from keratinocytes before cell division or migration over the basement membrane. Keratinocytes and melanocytes also express desmoglein 1 *(5)*, likely also desmocollin. Desmoglein 1 is regulated by growth factors similar to E-cadherin. The distribution pattern for P-cadherin in the epidermis is less clear, in large part because of difficulties with antibodies. Keratinocytes express P-cadherin and likely also melanocytes. VE-cadherin is specific for endothelial cells but is expressed by melanoma cells *(7)*.

Cadherins contribute to embryonic development of various tissues (Table 2). Gene knockout experiments in mice show that, for example, E-cadherin is involved in the development of trophectodermal epithelium *(8)*; N-cadherin is required for embryonic morphogenesis of the neural tube, heart, and somites *(9)*; and P-cadherin expression is associated with mammary gland development *(10)*. Changes in expression of E-cadherin correlate with malignant transformation in a variety of tumor systems *(11)*. In the skin, E-cadherin is negatively associated with melanoma development and progression and it is absent in nevus or melanoma cells *(12,13)*. Loss of E-cadherin on melanocytes appears

Table 1
Regulation and Function of Cadherins on Normal and Malignant Skin Cells

Cadherin	Chromosome	Keratinocyte		Melanocytes	Langerhans cells	Fibroblasts	Endothelial cells	Melanoma cells	Squamous carcinoma cells
		Basal layer	Super layer						
Type I:									
E-cadherin (cdh1)	16q22.1	+	+	+	+	–	–	–	
N-cadherin (cdh2)	18q11.2	–	–	–		+	+	+	+
P-cadherin (cdh3)	16q22.1	+	–	+		–		±	
Type II:									
VE-cadherin (cdh5)	16q22.1	–	–	–			+	+	–
Others:									
Desmoglein 1, 2, 3, 4 (DSG1, DSG2, DSG3, DSG4)	18q12.1-q12.2	+	+	+					
Desmocollin 1, 2, 3 (DSC1, DSC2, DSC3)	18q12.1	+	+						

+, positive expression; ±, variable expression; – not expressed; empty space, no information available.

171

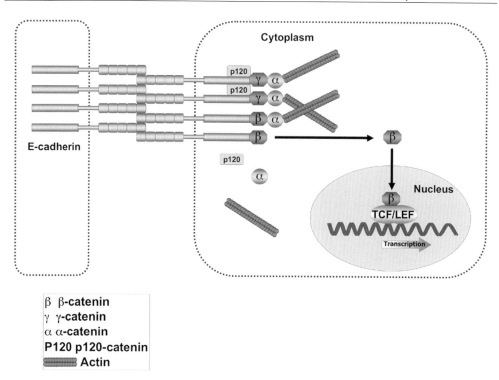

Fig. 1. Signaling pathway mediated by cadherin. Epithelial (E)-cadherin molecules interact with neighboring cells in a zipper-like fashion. This homophilic interaction is mediated by the most amino-terminal cadherin domain on each E-cadherin molecule containing the histidine–alanine–valine motif. α-catenin, β-catenin, γ-catenin (plakoglobin), and p120-catenin form a cytoplasmic complex that links E-cadherin homodimers to the actin cytoskeleton. The cadherin–catenin complex is regulated by various pathways. In this case, β-catenin molecules are dissociated from the complex and released into the cytoplasm. Enhanced cytoplasmic β-catenin translocates into the nuclei to transactivate its target genes.

to be one of the first critical steps during melanoma progression *(2)*. Restoring E-cadherin expression in melanoma cells inhibits invasion of melanoma cells into dermis through downregulation of melanoma cell adhesion molecule-CAM (Mel-CAM) and β3 integrin *(13)*, suggesting that loss of adhesive capacity allows the melanocytes to escape from control by neighboring keratinocytes.

Expression of N-cadherin in melanoma cells is associated with increased invasive potential during tumor progression *(2)*. Altered *N*-glycans of N-cadherin were found in metastatic but not in primary melanoma cells, suggesting different carbohydrate profiles for N-cadherin in melanoma cells for different stages of progression *(14)*. N-cadherin enhances migration of melanoma cells over dermal fibroblasts *(15)*. It also acts as a survival factor for the malignant cells by upregulation of the antiapoptosis molecule, Bad *(15)*. N-cadherin mediates gap junctional communications between malignant cells, between melanoma cells and fibroblasts, and between melanoma cells and endothelial cells *(16)*. Mel-CAM can act as a co-receptor for N-cadherin-mediated gap junctional communication *(17)*.

Table 2
Functional Consequences of Ablation of Genes in the Cadherin and Wnt Pathway

Gene	Functional consequences of gene knockout	Reference
E-cadherin (cdh1)	Defects in embryonic development of trophectodermal epithelium	8
N-cadherin (cdh2)	Defects in embryonic morphogenesis, including the neural tube, early heart, somites, and so on.	9
P-cadherin (cdh3)	Defects in mammary gland development	10
β-catenin	Defects in development of ectodermal cell layer and anterior–posterior axis formation	72,73
Wnt-1	Defects in embryonic development of midbrain patterning, T-cell maturation	18–20
Wnt-3	Defect in axis formation	74
Wnt-3a	Homozygous null mutants die at embryonic day 10.5–12.5 with failed development of caudal somites, notochord, and structures rostral to hindlimbs	21 and http://www.inform-atics.jax.org
Wnt-1/Wnt-3a (compound mutants)	Defects in expansion of neural crest and central nervous system progenitors, including melanocytes	22
Wnt-4	Defects in T-cell maturation	75
Wnt-1/Wnt-4[a] (compound mutants)	Defects in T-cell maturation and dysregu-lation of immature thymocyte precursors	75

[a]Wnt-4 was shown to be primarily mediated by the calcium pathway instead of the β-catenin pathway.

ROLES OF FRIZZLED RECEPTORS

Wnt signals are indispensable for embryonic development (Table 2). Wnt proteins may be differentially involved in the development of a variety of cells and tissues. For example, Wnt-1 is required for midbrain patterning, central nervous system development, and T-cell maturation (18–20); whereas Wnt3a is essential for somite and tailbud formation (21). Double knockouts of Wnt1 and Wnt3a cause deficiencies in neural crest derivatives, including lack of melanocytes (22). In avian and fish embryos, Wnt proteins act as the differentiation inducer of the neural crest (23,24), and Wnt3a induces melanocytic differentiation of neural crest cells in vitro (25,26). Wnt3a transactivates one of the melanocyte-associated transcription factors, the nacre/MITF gene (27,28).

Wnts are secreted glycoproteins that bind to frizzled (Fzd) seven-transmembrane span receptors and are thus involved in cell–cell signaling. Fzd receptors have been identified in both vertebrates and invertebrates. There are 10 known members in humans and mice, 4 in flies, and 3 in worms (29). Intracellular signaling of the Wnt pathway diversifies into at least three other pathways:

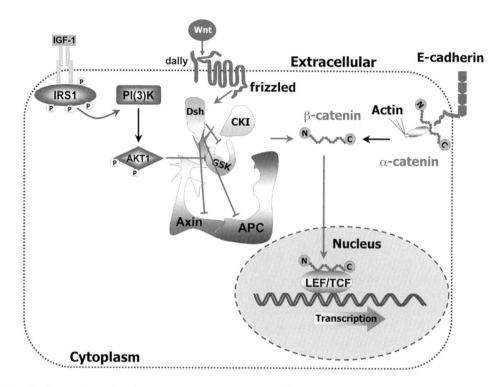

Fig. 2. β-catenin activation through outside signals. β-catenin plays a central role in various signaling pathways mediated by Wnt, insulin-like growth factor (IGF)-1, and epithelial (E)-cadherin. Wnt binds to frizzled (Fzd) seven-transmembrane span receptors. The proteoglycan dally acts as a co-receptor for Wnts. Interactions of Wnt/Fzd lead to stabilization of cytosolic β-catenin. In the absence of Wnts, β-catenin is phosphorylated by casein kinase Iα (CKIα) and/or CKIε at Ser45. Initial phosphorylation at Ser45, in turn, causes glycogen synthase kinase (GSK)-3β to phosphorylate serine/threonine residues 41, 37, and 33. Phosphorylation of these residues prompts ubiquitylation of β-catenin and degradation in proteasomes. Phosphorylation of β-catenin occurs in a multiprotein complex containing the scaffold protein, axin, which can form a homodimer or a heterodimer with the related protein, conductin/axin2, the tumor suppressor gene product APC. In the presence of Wnts, disheveled (Dsh) blocks β-catenin degradation. Stabilized β-catenin enters the nucleus and associates with LEF/TCF transcription factors, which leads to the transcription of Wnt target genes. Binding of the growth factor IGF-1 to the IGF-1 receptor tyrosine kinase induces a conformational change in the IGF-1 receptor tyrosinase kinase and its trans-phosphorylation, which, in turn, leads to phosphorylation of insulin receptor substrate (IRS-1). This activates PI(3)K. Activation of PI(3)K results in the production of phosphatidylinositol-3,4,5-trisphosphate, which provides a membrane-binding site for the serine/threonine kinase Akt/PKB. Akt is phosphorylated after translocation to the membrane by the kinase Pdk-1. Once activated, Akt blocks β-catenin degradation through phosphorylation of GSK-3β. β-catenin also mediates the signaling pathway of cadherin, as described above.

1. The β-catenin pathway (canonical Wnt pathway; stimulated by Wnt1, Wnt2, Wnt3, Wnt3a, and Wnt8), which activates target genes in the nucleus.
2. The planar cell polarity pathway, which involves Jun N-terminal kinase (JNK) and cytoskeletal rearrangements.
3. The Wnt/calcium pathway (noncanonical Wnt pathway), which is stimulated by Wnt4, Wnt5a, Wnt5b, Wnt7, and Wnt11.

The relatively well-studied canonical and calcium pathways are outlined in Fig. 2. In humans, 19 distinct Wnt proteins have been identified *(29)*. Distinct sets of Wnt and Fzd

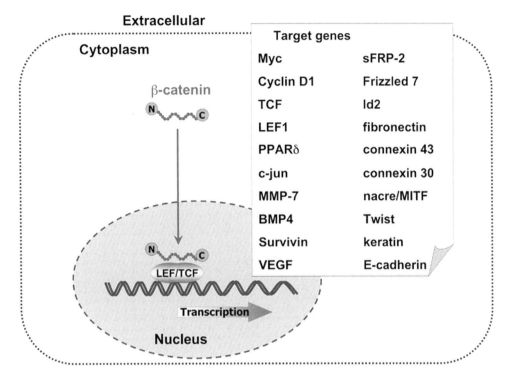

Fig. 3. Nuclear targets for β-catenin signaling. The following genes are upregulated by β-catenin signaling: *c-myc, Cyclin D, TCF, LEF1, PPAR-δ, c-jun, MMP-7, BMP4, Survivin, VEGF, sFRP-2, Frizzled 7, Id2, fibronectin, connexin 43, connexin 30, nacre/MITF, Twist, Keratin.* The following genes are downregulated by β-catenin signaling: *osteocalcin, E-cadherin.*

ligand-receptor pairs can activate each of these pathways and result in unique cellular responses. Because of their diversity, it is unclear how the Fzd members differ in function and ligand specificity.

The β-catenin pathway is critically involved in development (Table 2). Defects in knockouts are observed primarily in ectodermal cell layers and anterior–posterior axis formation. A large number of target genes of β-catenin have been identified (Fig. 3), including c-myc *(30)*, cyclin D *(31,32)*, TCF *(33)*, LEF1 *(34)*, PPARδ *(35)*, c-Jun *(36)*, MMP-7 *(37)*, BMP4 *(38)*, survivin *(39)*, VEGF *(40)*, sFRP-2 *(41)*, Frizzled 7 *(42)*, Id2 *(43)*, fibronectin *(43)*, connexin 43 *(44)*, connexin 30 *(45)*, twist *(46)*, and keratin *(47)*. Few genes are downregulated by β-catenin signaling, including osteocalcin *(48)* and E-cadherin *(49)*.

The Wnt/β-catenin signaling plays a critical role in self-renewal of stem cells and acts as their growth factor *(50,51)*. Wnt signaling is endogenously activated in undifferentiated stem cells and appears to be indispensable for self-renewal and proliferation of stem and progenitor cells. After differentiation, Wnt expression is downregulated *(52)*. Our own preliminary studies suggest that Wnt signaling, mediated by Wnt3a, plays an important role in melanocytic differentiation of human embryonic stem cells. This differentiation process depends on continuous presence of the ligand.

In addition to the critical roles for Wnt–Fzd signaling during development, the pathway is also involved in tumorigenesis, including melanoma development *(53)*. Gene

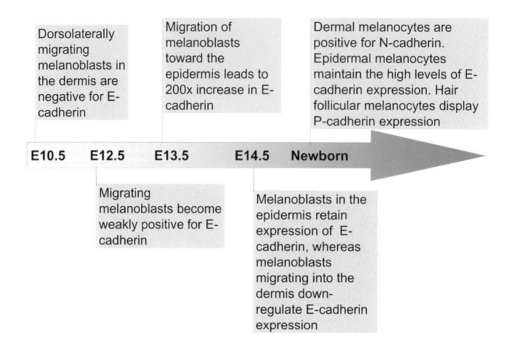

Fig. 4. Cadherin shift during embryonic development determines melanocyte locations. Melanocyte progenitors migrate along the dorsolateral pathway to the dermis during embryonic development. Types and levels of cadherin expression correlate to the locations of the progenitor cells.

expression profiling found that Wnt5a expression correlates with increasing tumor progression stage *(54)*. Immunohistology revealed changes in Wnt and Fzd expression patterns with progression of melanoma cells *(55)*. Reduced activity or absence of soluble Fzd receptor protein 1 permits the transduction of noncanonical Wnt signals, at least in colorectal tumorigenesis *(56)*. Much less is known in melanoma, but Wnt–Fzd signals are most likely involved in development of this disease as in other tumors *(53,57,58)*.

β-catenin plays a central role in transducing multiple signals. Besides being activated by Wnt and E-cadherin signaling, β-catenin also mediates insulin-like growth factor (IGF)-1 signals (Fig. 2). IGF-1 induces survival and growth of biological early melanoma cells through β-catenin stabilization, as indicated by nuclear and cytoplasmic localization *(59,60)*. Potentially, this could occur through activating mutations in the *β-catenin* gene *(61)*, but mutations are relatively rare.

CADHERIN SHIFT BY MELANOCYTES AND THEIR PRECURSORS DURING MURINE DEVELOPMENT

Epidermal melanocytes are derived from neural crest cells, which are a transient population of cells arising from the dorsal neural tube. Melanocyte precursors migrate along the dorsolateral pathway, and cross the basement membrane into the epidermis, where they differentiate to melanocytes *(62)*. During migration and differentiation of murine melanoblasts, there is a significant shift in expression of cadherins (Fig. 4). Dorsolaterally migrating melanoblasts in the dermis lack E-cadherin at 10.5 d *post coitum*. Within 2 d, they become weakly positive. At 13.5 d, melanoblast migration into the epidermis is accompanied by an approx 200-fold increase in E-cadherin expression

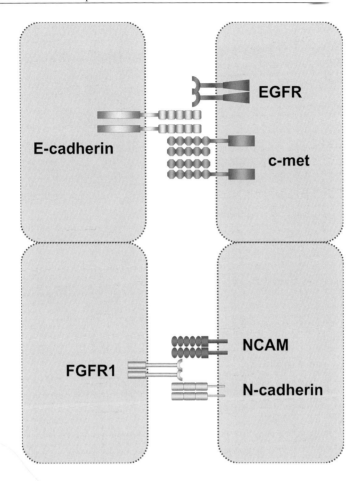

Fig. 5. Association of epithelial (E)-cadherin and neutral (N)-cadherin with receptor tyrosine kinase. E-cadherin can initiate signal transduction pathways through the involvement of tyrosine kinase receptors for epidermal growth factor (EGFR) and/or c-met. N-cadherin-mediated signaling pathways can be associated with fibroblast growth factor receptor (FGFR) and neural cell adhesion molecule (NCAM).

(63). One or two days later, most melanocytes downregulate E-cadherin, leave the epidermis, and migrate into hair follicles, where they express P-cadherin. Few remaining epidermal melanocytes continue to express E-cadherin, whereas dermal melanocytes express N-cadherin. After birth, epidermal melanocytes maintain high levels of E-cadherin expression, whereas dermal melanocytes continue to express N-cadherin and hair follicular melanocytes express P-cadherin *(63,64)*. Pigmented murine melanocytes are first detected at E16.5 and increase dramatically after birth *(65,66)*.

ASSOCIATION OF CADHERIN WITH TYROSINE KINASE RECEPTORS

In addition to homophilic and heterophilic binding, cadherins can interact with growth factor receptors. Hepatocyte growth factor receptor, c-met, forms a complex with E-cadherin in tumor cells, including melanoma cells (Fig. 5) *(5,67,68)*. In immortalized nontumorigenic keratinocytes, E-cadherin also stimulates the MAPK pathway through ligand-independent activation of epidermal growth factor receptor (EGFR) *(67,68)*.

E-cadherin could negatively regulate ligand-dependent activation of divergent classes of receptor tyrosine kinases by inhibiting their ligand-dependent activation in association with decreases in receptor mobility and in ligand-binding affinity. EGFR regulation by E-cadherin was associated with complex formation between EGFR and E-cadherin, which is dependent on the extracellular domain of E-cadherin but was independent of β-catenin binding or p120-catenin binding *(69)*. These results suggest that dysregulation of E-cadherin signaling or downregulation of expression may have profound effects on receptor tyrosine kinase signaling. Similar to E-cadherin, N-cadherin also appears to closely interact with a tyrosine kinase. N-cadherin promotes neuronal cell survival by activating fibroblast growth factor receptor *(70,71)*. However, little is known about the underlying mechanisms.

REFERENCES

1. Fitzpatrick TB, Szabo G, Seiji M, Quevedo WC Jr. Biology of the melanin pigmentary system. In: Fitzpatrick TB, Eise AZ, Wolf K, Freedberg IM, Ansten KF, eds. Dermatology in General Medicine, 2nd ed. McGraw-Hill, New York, NY: 1979, p. 131.
2. Hsu MY, Wheelock MJ, Johnson KR, Herlyn M. Shifts in cadherin profiles between human normal melanocytes and melanomas. J Investig Dermatol Symp Proc 1996;1:188–194.
3. Tang A, Eller MS, Hara M, Yaar M, Hirohashi S, Gilchrest BA. E-cadherin is the major mediator of human melanocyte adhesion to keratinocytes in vitro. J Cell Sci 1994;107(Pt 4):983–992.
4. Jamal S. Endothelin-1 down-regulates E-cadherin in melanocytic cells by apoptosis-independent activation of caspase-8. J Am Acad Dermatol 2000;43:703–704.
5. Li G, Schaider H, Satyamoorthy K, Hanakawa Y, Hashimoto K, Herlyn M. Downregulation of E-cadherin and Desmoglein 1 by autocrine hepatocyte growth factor during melanoma development. Oncogene 2001;20:8125–8135.
6. Schaider H, et al. Unpublished.
7. Hendrix MJ, Seftor EA, Meltzer PS, et al. Expression and functional significance of VE-cadherin in aggressive human melanoma cells: role in vasculogenic mimicry. Proc Natl Acad Sci USA 2001;98:8018–8023.
8. Larue L, Ohsugi M, Hirchenhain J, Kemler R. E-cadherin null mutant embryos fail to form a trophectoderm epithelium. Proc Natl Acad Sci USA 1994;91:8263–8267.
9. Radice GL, Rayburn H, Matsunami H, Knudsen KA, Takeichi M, Hynes RO. Developmental defects in mouse embryos lacking N-cadherin. Dev Biol 1997;181:64–78.
10. Radice GL, Ferreira-Cornwell MC, Robinson SD, et al. Precocious mammary gland development in P-cadherin-deficient mice. J Cell Biol 1997;139:1025–1032.
11. Christofori G, Semb H. The role of the cell-adhesion molecule E-cadherin as a tumour-suppressor gene. Trends Biochem Sci 1999;24:73–76.
12. Danen EH, de Vries TJ, Morandini R, Ghanem GG, Ruiter DJ, van Muijen GN. E-cadherin expression in human melanoma. Melanoma Res 1996;6:127–131.
13. Hsu MY, Meier FE, Nesbit M, et al. E-cadherin expression in melanoma cells restores keratinocyte-mediated growth control and down-regulates expression of invasion-related adhesion receptors. Am J Pathol 2000;156:1515–1525.
14. Ciolczyk-Wierzbicka D, Gil D, Hoja-Lukowicz D, Litynska A, Laidler P. Carbohydrate moieties of N-cadherin from human melanoma cell lines. Acta Biochim Pol 2002;49:991–998.
15. Li G, Satyamoorthy K, Herlyn M. N-cadherin-mediated intercellular interactions promote survival and migration of melanoma cells. Cancer Res 2001;61:3819–3825.
16. Hsu M, Andl T, Li G, Meinkoth JL, Herlyn M. Cadherin repertoire determines partner-specific gap junctional communication during melanoma progression. J Cell Sci 2000;113(Pt 9):1535–1542.
17. Satyamoorthy K, Muyrers J, Meier F, Patel D, Herlyn M. Mel-CAM-specific genetic suppressor elements inhibit melanoma growth and invasion through loss of gap junctional communication. Oncogene 2001;20:4676–4684.
18. McMahon AP, Bradley A. The Wnt-1 (int-1) proto-oncogene is required for development of a large region of the mouse brain. Cell 1990;62:1073–1085.

19. Thomas KR, Capecchi MR. Targeted disruption of the murine int-1 proto-oncogene resulting in severe abnormalities in midbrain and cerebellar development. Nature 1990;346:847–850.

20. Mulroy T, McMahon JA, Burakoff SJ, McMahon AP, Sen J. Wnt-1 and Wnt-4 regulate thymic cellularity. Eur J Immunol 2002;32:967–971.

21. Takada S, Stark KL, Shea MJ, Vassileva G, McMahon JA, McMahon AP. Wnt-3a regulates somite and tailbud formation in the mouse embryo. Genes Dev 1994;8:174–189.

22. Ikeya M, Lee SM, Johnson JE, McMahon AP, Takada S. Wnt signalling required for expansion of neural crest and CNS progenitors. Nature 1997;389:966–970.

23. Wilson SI, Rydstrom A, Trimborn T, et al. The status of Wnt signalling regulates neural and epidermal fates in the chick embryo. Nature 2001;411:325–330.

24. Garcia-Castro MI, Marcelle C, Bronner-Fraser M. Ectodermal Wnt function as a neural crest inducer. Science 2002;297:848–851.

25. Dorsky RI, Moon RT, Raible DW. Control of neural crest cell fate by the Wnt signalling pathway. Nature 1998;396:370–373.

26. Jin EJ, Erickson CA, Takada S, Burrus LW. Wnt and BMP signaling govern lineage segregation of melanocytes in the avian embryo. Dev Biol 2001;233:22–37.

27. Dorsky RI, Raible DW, Moon RT. Direct regulation of nacre, a zebrafish MITF homolog required for pigment cell formation, by the Wnt pathway. Genes Dev 2000;14:158–162.

28. Takeda K, Yasumoto K, Takada R, et al. Induction of melanocyte-specific microphthalmia-associated transcription factor by Wnt-3a. J Biol Chem 2000;275:14,013–14,016.

29. Miller JR. The Wnts. Genome Biol 2002;3(Reviews):3001.

30. He TC, Sparks AB, Rago C, et al. Identification of c-MYC as a target of the APC pathway. Science 1998;281:1509–1512.

31. Shtutman M, Zhurinsky J, Simcha I, et al. The cyclin D1 gene is a target of the beta-catenin/LEF-1 pathway. Proc Natl Acad Sci USA 1999;96:5522–5527.

32. Tetsu O, McCormick F. Beta-catenin regulates expression of cyclin D1 in colon carcinoma cells. Nature 1999;398:422–426.

33. Roose J, Huls G, van Beest M, et al. Synergy between tumor suppressor APC and the beta-catenin-Tcf4 target Tcf1. Science 1999;285:1923–1926.

34. Hovanes K, Li TW, Munguia JE, et al. Beta-catenin-sensitive isoforms of lymphoid enhancer factor-1 are selectively expressed in colon cancer. Nat Genet 2001;28:53–57.

35. He TC, Chan TA, Vogelstein B, Kinzler KW. PPARdelta is an APC-regulated target of nonsteroidal anti-inflammatory drugs. Cell 1999;99:335–345.

36. Mann B, Gelos M, Siedow A, et al. Target genes of beta-catenin-T cell-factor/lymphoid-enhancer-factor signaling in human colorectal carcinomas. Proc Natl Acad Sci USA 1999;96:1603–1608.

37. Brabletz T, Jung A, Dag S, Hlubek F, Kirchner T. Beta-catenin regulates the expression of the matrix metalloproteinase-7 in human colorectal cancer. Am J Pathol 1999;155:1033–1038.

38. Kim JS, Crooks H, Dracheva T, et al. Oncogenic beta-catenin is required for bone morphogenetic protein 4 expression in human cancer cells. Cancer Res 2002;62:2744–2748.

39. Zhang T, Otevrel T, Gao Z, Ehrlich SM, Fields JZ, Boman BM. Evidence that APC regulates survivin expression: a possible mechanism contributing to the stem cell origin of colon cancer. Cancer Res 2001;61:8664–8667.

40. Zhang X, Gaspard JP, Chung DC. Regulation of vascular endothelial growth factor by the Wnt and K-ras pathways in colonic neoplasia. Cancer Res 2001;61:6050–6054.

41. Lescher B, Haenig B, Kispert A. sFRP-2 is a target of the Wnt-4 signaling pathway in the developing metanephric kidney. Dev Dyn 1998;213:440–451.

42. Willert J, Epping M, Pollack JR, Brown PO, Nusse R. A transcriptional response to Wnt protein in human embryonic carcinoma cells. BMC Dev Biol 2002;2:8.

43. Gradl D, Kuhl M, Wedlich D. The Wnt/Wg signal transducer beta-catenin controls fibronectin expression. Mol Cell Biol 1999;19:5576–5587.

44. van der Heyden MA, Rook MB, Hermans MM, et al. Identification of connexin43 as a functional target for Wnt signalling. J Cell Sci 1998;111(Pt 12):1741–1749.

45. McGrew LL, Takemaru K, Bates R, Moon RT. Direct regulation of the Xenopus engrailed-2 promoter by the Wnt signaling pathway, and a molecular screen for Wnt-responsive genes, confirm a role for Wnt signaling during neural patterning in Xenopus. Mech Dev 1999;87:21–32.

46. Howe LR, Watanabe O, Leonard J, Brown AM. Twist is up-regulated in response to Wnt1 and inhibits mouse mammary cell differentiation. Cancer Res 2003;63:1906–1913.

47. DasGupta R, Fuchs E. Multiple roles for activated LEF/TCF transcription complexes during hair follicle development and differentiation. Development 1999;126:4557–4568.
48. Kahler RA, Westendorf JJ. Lymphoid enhancer factor-1 and beta-catenin inhibit Runx2-dependent transcriptional activation of the osteocalcin promoter. J Biol Chem 2003;278:11,937–11,944.
49. Jamora C, DasGupta R, Kocieniewski P, Fuchs E. Links between signal transduction, transcription and adhesion in epithelial bud development. Nature 2003;422:317–322.
50. Reya T, Duncan AW, Ailles L, et al. A role for Wnt signalling in self-renewal of haematopoietic stem cells. Nature 2003;423:409–414.
51. Willert K, Brown JD, Danenberg E, et al. Wnt proteins are lipid-modified and can act as stem cell growth factors. Nature 2003;423:448–452.
52. Sato N, Meijer L, Skaltsounis L, Greengard P, Brivanlou AH. Maintenance of pluripotency in human and mouse embryonic stem cells through activation of Wnt signaling by a pharmacological GSK-3–specific inhibitor. Nat Med 2004;10:55–63.
53. Polakis P. Wnt signaling and cancer. Genes Dev 2000;14:1837–1851.
54. Weeraratna AT, Jiang Y, Hostetter G, et al. Wnt5a signaling directly affects cell motility and invasion of metastatic melanoma. Cancer Cell 2002;1:279–288.
55. Pham K, Milovanovic T, Barr RJ, Truong T, Holcombe RF. Wnt ligand expression in malignant melanoma: pilot study indicating correlation with histopathological features. Mol Pathol 2003;56:280–285.
56. Caldwell GM, Jones C, Gensberg K, et al. The Wnt antagonist sFRP1 in colorectal tumorigenesis. Cancer Res 2004;64:883–888.
57. Barker N, Clevers H. Catenins, Wnt signaling and cancer. Bioessays 2000;22:961–965.
58. Taipale J, Beachy PA. The Hedgehog and Wnt signalling pathways in cancer. Nature 2001;411:349–354.
59. Rimm DL, Caca K, Hu G, Harrison FB, Fearon ER. Frequent nuclear/cytoplasmic localization of beta-catenin without exon 3 mutations in malignant melanoma. Am J Pathol 1999;154:325–329.
60. Satyamoorthy K, Li G, Vaidya B, Patel D, Herlyn M. Insulin-like growth factor-1 induces survival and growth of biologically early melanoma cells through both the mitogen-activated protein kinase and beta-catenin pathways. Cancer Res 2001;61:7318–7324.
61. Rubinfeld B, Robbins P, El-Gamil M, Albert I, Porfiri E, Polakis P. Stabilization of beta-catenin by genetic defects in melanoma cell lines. Science 1997;275:1790–1792.
62. Mayer TC. The migratory pathway of neural crest cells into the skin of mouse embryos. Dev Biol 1973;34:39–46.
63. Nishimura EK, Yoshida H, Kunisada T, Nishikawa SI. Regulation of E- and P-cadherin expression correlated with melanocyte migration and diversification. Dev Biol 1999;215:155–166.
64. Jouneau A, Yu YQ, Pasdar M, Larue L. Plasticity of cadherin-catenin expression in the melanocyte lineage. Pigment Cell Res 2000;13:260–272.
65. Hirobe T, Takeuchi T. Induction of melanogenesis in the epidermal melanoblasts of newborn mouse skin by MSH. J Embryol Exp Morphol 1977;37:79–90.
66. Hirobe T. Histochemical survey of the distribution of the epidermal melanoblasts and melanocytes in the mouse during fetal and postnatal periods. Anat Rec 1984;208:589–594.
67. Hiscox S, Jiang WG. Association of the HGF/SF receptor, c-met, with the cell-surface adhesion molecule, E-cadherin, and catenins in human tumor cells. Biochem Biophys Res Commun 1999;261:406–411.
68. Pece S, Gutkind JS. Signaling from E-cadherins to the MAPK pathway by the recruitment and activation of epidermal growth factor receptors upon cell-cell contact formation. J Biol Chem 2000;275:41,227–41,233.
69. Qian X, Karpova T, Sheppard AM, McNally J, Lowy DR. E-cadherin-mediated adhesion inhibits ligand-dependent activation of diverse receptor tyrosine kinases. Embo J 2004;23:1739–1784.
70. Cavallaro U, Niedermeyer J, Fuxa M, Christofori G. N-CAM modulates tumour-cell adhesion to matrix by inducing FGF-receptor signalling. Nat Cell Biol 2001;3:650–657.
71. Skaper SD, Facci L, Williams G, Williams EJ, Walsh FS, Doherty P. A dimeric version of the short N-cadherin binding motif HAVDI promotes neuronal cell survival by activating an N-cadherin/fibroblast growth factor receptor signalling cascade. Mol Cell Neurosci 2004;26:17–23.
72. Haegel H, Larue L, Ohsugi M, Fedorov L, Herrenknecht K, Kemler R. Lack of beta-catenin affects mouse development at gastrulation. Development 1995;121:3529–3537.
73. Huelsken J, Vogel R, Brinkmann V, Erdmann B, Birchmeier C, Birchmeier W. Requirement for beta-catenin in anterior-posterior axis formation in mice. J Cell Biol 2000;148:567–578.

74. Liu P, Wakamiya M, Shea MJ, Albrecht U, Behringer RR, Bradley A. Requirement for Wnt3 in vertebrate axis formation. Nat Genet 1999;22:361–365.
75. Mulroy T, McMahon JA, Burakoff SJ, McMahon AP, Sen J. Wnt-1 and Wnt-4 regulate thymic cellularity. Eur J Immunol 2002;32:967–971.

10

Familial Melanoma Genes, Melanocyte Immortalization, and Melanoma Initiation

Dorothy C. Bennett

Contents

Summary

The most common types of pigmented lesions have been classified by Clark and colleagues into a series of increasingly malignant types. We have proposed a general model for the genetic events underlying this series of lesions and progression from one lesion type to another. The current form of this model, the evidence that gave rise to it, and the areas of uncertainty that remain are presented here. In particular, evidence for the following is discussed:

1. Involvement of the process of cell senescence in the proliferative arrest seen in nevi.
2. A role for apoptosis and keratinocyte-dependence in the flat growth pattern of radial growth-phase melanomas.
3. The genetic suppression of both senescence and apoptosis in more advanced melanomas.

The protein p16, encoded by the familial melanoma locus cyclin-dependent kinase inhibitor 2A (*CDKN2A*), appears to play a central role in the senescence of nevi and probably also in the keratinocyte-dependence of thin melanomas, in interaction with two other key tumor suppressors, retinoblastoma (RB)-1 and p53.

Key Words: Melanoma; nevus; cell senescence; p16; CDKN2A; RB1; telomere; immortalization; apoptosis.

From: *From Melanocytes to Melanoma: The Progression to Malignancy*
Edited by: V. J. Hearing and S. P. L. Leong © Humana Press Inc., Totowa, NJ

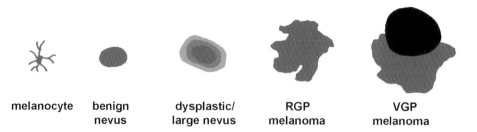

| melanocyte | benign nevus | dysplastic/ large nevus | RGP melanoma | VGP melanoma |

Fig. 1. Clark et al.'s classification of pigmented lesions. The melanocyte is not to scale. RGP, radial growth phase; VGP, vertical growth phase. A VGP melanoma may not necessarily have a visible RGP area. *See* pages 184–185 for further details.

INTRODUCTION

There is, as yet, no type of solid cancer for which the minimal genetic events required to produce that lesion are definitely known and proven. Genetic models have been produced for some tumor types, such as the widely cited model of Vogelstein and colleagues for colorectal cancer and its variants *(1)*, but so far without a conclusive demonstration that the proposed events are necessary or sufficient to produce the cancer. It is possible that cutaneous melanoma may be among the first solid cancers to be genetically "solved" in this way, because an early epidemiological analysis suggested that melanoma might be genetically relatively simple, compared with other solid cancers, in terms of the number of cellular events needed to produce it. This was based on age–incidence curves; the number of independent causal events (interpreted as genetic changes) required to produce each type of cancer could be estimated from a best fit between theoretical and observed curves. Among the cancer types analyzed, melanoma was estimated to require the fewest events for its development *(2)*. The estimated number of events was only one, although it now seems likely that at least three genetic changes are needed to produce even an early melanoma, as discussed from page 189. The fact that $n = 1$ gives the best mathematical fit suggests that one of the necessary events is substantially more rare than the others, thus being rate-limiting. This chapter will review our current knowledge of the genetic basis of human melanoma and the common benign pigmented lesions. A relatively simple genetic model for sporadic melanoma will be discussed, which brings these data together and relates them to the widely-used clinical classification of pigmented lesions by Clark et al. *(3–5)*, supporting the idea that few genetic events are required to produce a metastatic melanoma. I will begin with some sections of background information needed to understand the biological and genetic events to be discussed.

THE CLARK MODEL FOR PRIMARY MELANOMA DEVELOPMENT

Figure 1 shows a version of the series of primary pigmented lesions described by Clark et al. *(3–5)*. These are sometimes taken to represent a linear progression, in which each lesion is the direct precursor of the next, but it seems best simply to regard them as clinically distinct types of lesion, each of which may apparently develop directly from normal skin as well as from one of the more benign types. Various evidence, including clinical and molecular (as will be discussed), indicates that the pathways by which different cases of advanced melanoma develop may vary.

The first lesion type (Fig. 1) is the benign nevus or mole, small and well-delineated, of which, most of us have a good many on our skin. The clinical definition of the dysplastic nevus is somewhat disputed, but this is broadly agreed to mean a nevus that has one or more features more typical of a melanoma, such as being unusually large, having an irregular or indistinct border and/or uneven pigmentation. Atypical mole has also been suggested as a better clinical term for such lesions, which does not imply a particular histopathological pattern (dysplasia). Next is the radial growth-phase (RGP) melanoma. This lesion grows progressively, but only "radially," forming a flat plaque within the epidermis or with small dermal nests close to the epidermis. Lastly, a vertical growth-phase (VGP) melanoma forms large nodule(s) in the dermis; this key feature is predictive of the potential to metastasize *(4)*. Interestingly, melanoma differs from most other solid cancers in that acquiring the ability to metastasize does not appear to be a separate step from becoming able to invade neighboring tissues *(4)*.

CELL SENESCENCE: TYPES AND MOLECULAR MECHANISMS

I will now introduce the main concepts of cellular senescence and immortalization, as needed to understand the apparent connection with melanoma progression. These concepts have been reviewed more fully by a number of authors, both generally *(6–8)* and as applied specifically to melanocytes *(9,10)*. Normal somatic mammalian cells (as studied in cell culture) can undergo only a limited number of cell divisions, called their proliferative life-span, although this number varies between animal species, between cell types, and with culture conditions *(9)*. When cells reach the end of this life-span, they irreversibly stop growing, and this arrest is called cellular senescence, as first described by Hayflick *(11)*. We now know that cellular senescence can be affected by more than one molecular pathway *(6,7,12)*. For example, the mechanisms are radically different between mouse cells and human cells; telomere shortening (*see* next paragraph) is important in the senescence of most normal human cells, but not that of normal mouse cells, which have extremely long telomeres *(7)*. This review will concentrate on human cell senescence, in relation to human melanoma.

Even among human cells of different types, different kinds of senescence can be distinguished (Fig. 2). M1 senescence, typical of human fibroblasts, is the best understood. The key initiating signal for M1 senescence appears to be critical shortening of telomeres (the multiple DNA hexamer repeats at the ends of the chromosomes), which become shorter with each division in somatic cells. In germline cells and a few others, together with most cancer cells, telomere length is maintained by the reverse transcriptase, telomerase *(13)*. However, most human somatic cells lack the catalytic subunit, human telomerase reverse transcriptase (hTERT). If these cells undergo numerous divisions, the telomeres shorten, as does a single-stranded loop at the very end *(14)*, resulting in unfolding of the loop, recognition of the single-stranded DNA, and activation of DNA damage-signaling mechanisms, which activate p53 through a pathway involving checkpoint kinase 2 (CHK2) *(15)*. Cellular growth arrest (M1 senescence) results partly from this active p53, which transcriptionally upregulates the growth-inhibitor protein, p21, and partly from the parallel upregulation of another important growth inhibitor, p16^{INK4A} or p16, by a less-understood pathway. p16 will be discussed further on page 187, as the product of a melanoma susceptibility gene. At present, we will just note that p16 activates the tumor suppressor and growth inhibitor, RB1 (retinoblastoma), and the two other members of the RB protein family, RBL1/p107 (retinoblas-

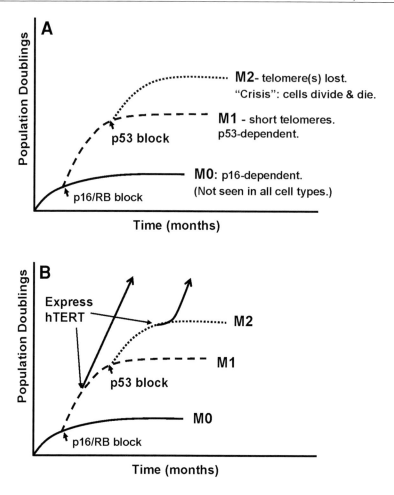

Fig. 2. Types of cellular senescence. *See* pages 185–187 for explanation.

toma-like 1) and RBL2/p130. p16 does this by inhibiting cyclin-dependent kinase 4 (CDK4), which can inhibit RB activity through phosphorylation. Either the RB proteins (activated by p16) or activated p53 are independently capable of arresting human cell growth during M1 senescence; in other words, cell senescence will still occur through RB if p53 signaling is disrupted, and vice versa *(6,12,16)*. p16 is not present in most normal cells *(17)*, but its synthesis is activated at cellular senescence *(8,18)*. It is not clear how this synthesis occurs in response to extended cell proliferation *(8)*, except that, in senescence of human fibroblasts, an increase and a decrease, respectively, in the amounts of transcription factors ETS1 and ID1 have been implicated in the upregulation of p16 *(19)*. There seems to be no information, however, on how these changes in ETS1 and ID1 levels would result from extended cell proliferation.

The second form of cell senescence in Fig. 2, M0 senescence, is precipitated by p16 alone, without involvement of p53. This type of senescence has been reported in various human epithelial cells under stressful culture conditions *(20,21)*, in human fibroblasts also under stressful conditions *(21)*, and in human melanocytes under the most favorable culture conditions known (including growth with "feeder cells") *(10,22,23)*. Again, we know little of how p16 expression becomes induced in M0 senescence or "stress," although there is some evidence for roles for transcription factors ETS2, ID1 *(19)*, and BMI1 *(24)*. At any rate, the outcome is activation of RB proteins and proliferative arrest. As Fig. 2B shows, expression of exogenous hTERT allows cells to overcome or circumvent M1 senescence, after which they can divide apparently without limit (immortalization). However, this is not true of cells in M0 senescence. These require inactivation of the p16/RB pathway as well as expression of hTERT before they can be immortalized *(20,23,25)*.

THE *CDKN2A* LOCUS, ITS TWO GENE PRODUCTS, AND MELANOMA

Approximately 10% of cutaneous melanoma cases worldwide occur in a loosely familial context, that is, one or more relatives also have melanoma, suggesting inheritance of a susceptibility gene *(26,27)*. There are several detailed recent reviews on melanoma genetics *(26–28)*. To date, mutations of four different genes at three different loci are known to confer susceptibility to melanoma. These are the *INK4A* (p16) and *ARF* sequences at the *CDKN2A* locus (chromosome 9p21); *CDK4* (chromosome 12q14), encoding the principal kinase that p16 inhibits; and the recently identified and uncloned locus, *CMM4* (cutaneous malignant melanoma 4; chromosome 1p22) *(29)*. Melanoma-associated mutations of *INK4A* and *CDK4* seem to be functionally equivalent, because both block the association of p16 with CDK4, and hence p16's ability to activate the RB family *(30,31)*. Accordingly, these mutations could interfere with cellular senescence, especially M0 senescence, as observed in melanocytes (*see* pages 186–187). It is interesting that both *INK4A* and *CDK4* mutations are associated relatively specifically with melanoma; the only other cancer that clearly occurs at a higher than normal rate in families carrying *INK4A* mutations appears to be pancreatic cancer *(32,33)*.

The *CDKN2A* locus is highly unusual, possibly unique in vertebrates, in that the same DNA sequence is used to encode two different, unrelated proteins in different reading frames, although the two gene products do have separate sequences as their first exons *(34,35)*. One of the products is p16, the other (as mentioned above) is called ARF (alternative reading frame), also known as p14[ARF] in humans and p19[Arf] in the mouse (reflecting the different protein sizes in the two species). ARF also appears to have a role in human melanoma. Nearly all tested melanoma-associated mutations in *CDKN2A* functionally affect p16 protein, whereas many of them do not affect ARF function *(34,36)*. Nonetheless, a few of these mutations apparently have no effect on p16 and do disrupt ARF function. Such mutations have been reported both in melanoma families and in sporadic melanomas *(37–39)*. *ARF* is thus included here among the melanoma susceptibility genes.

Like p16, ARF is a powerful inhibitor of cell proliferation. Its best-known function is stabilization of p53, through inhibition of the ubiquitin ligase MDM2 (mouse double minute 2 homolog, also sometimes—less correctly—called HDM2 in the human). MDM2 can ubiquitinylate p53, leading to its degradation *(40,41)*. In the mouse, Arf is an essential player in cellular senescence; fibroblasts from mice with normal p16 but deleted Arf fail to senesce, and the mice are susceptible to a variety of tumor types, although melanoma is not observed *(42)*. However, there is good evidence that human ARF, surprisingly, plays no part in senescence of normal fibroblasts *(43)*. This may be connected with the role of telomere shortening in activating p53 in human but not mouse cells. In the mouse, a pathway involving Arf may substitute for the short telomere/CHK2 pathway in activating p53 after a certain amount of cell division. Returning to humans, ARF does appear to have some tumor suppressor function, because individuals heterozygous for a germline ARF mutation appear susceptible to melanoma and probably some types of neural tumors *(26,38)*. It is not, however, clear how ARF acts as a tumor suppressor in humans. One possibility is through RB proteins, because MDM2 can interact in an inhibitory fashion with RB1 *(44)*, thus, ARF may also be able to prevent this. Another possibility is that ARF may be involved in a kind of premature M1-like senescence induced by activation of single mitogenic oncogenes, such as *HRAS* or *MYC*, because ARF expression and upregulation of p53 as well as p16 are reported in human fibroblasts under these conditions *(45–47)*.

EFFECTS OF *CDKN2A* DEFICIENCIES IN CULTURED MOUSE AND HUMAN MELANOCYTES

Cell culture studies have yielded some interesting and unexpected information on the biology of *CDKN2A* deficiency in melanocytes, which will be reviewed here for comparison with the biology of early melanoma. Mouse melanocytes with a *Cdkn2a* deletion, which abolishes the synthesis of both p16 and Arf, have been cultured and compared with wild-type melanocytes from the same inbred mouse strain. The wild-type melanocytes senesced within 5–6 wk. However, like fibroblasts from these p16 and Arf-null mice *(48)*, the melanocytes grew very well in culture and showed almost no cell senescence, showing that p16, Arf, or both are required for mouse melanocyte senescence *(49)*. Fibroblasts with a single copy of the deletion were reported to senesce similarly to wild-type mouse fibroblasts *(48)*, but melanocyte cultures with only a single copy showed only partial senescence followed by immortalization of all cultures *(49)*, indicating that two intact copies of this locus are needed for normal cell senescence in melanocytes (but not fibroblasts). This suggests that particularly high protein levels of p16, Arf, or both are needed for normal mouse melanocyte senescence, which may be relevant to the melanoma susceptibility of humans who carry a single copy of a mutation in p16.

Melanocyte cultures were also prepared from two human familial melanoma patients, both of whom (very unusually) had mutations in both copies of the p16 coding sequence but normal ARF function. The patients are described by Gruis et al. *(50)* and Huot et al. *(51)*, and the melanocytes by Sviderskaya et al. *(23)*. These cultures, unexpectedly, showed very little net growth in a medium in which normal human melanocytes grow well, although mitotic cells could be observed. The explanation proved to be a high rate of apoptosis in these cells. Further experimentation revealed that the excessive apoptosis was suppressed by coculture with keratinocytes, or with two peptides produced by keratinocytes, stem cell factor, and endothelin 1 *(23)*. Under these conditions, the p16-deficient melanocytes divided for far longer than normal adult human melanocytes. They did eventually senesce, with upregulation of p53 and p21 *(23)*. This is reminiscent of the epithelial cell types that undergo M0 senescence under some conditions; if RB function is blocked, then these cells bypass M0, proliferate extensively, and then enter a new senescent phase that is M1-like, because it involves p53 and p21. This second senescent phase can be circumvented by expression of hTERT, leading to cell immortalization *(20)*. The p16-deficient melanocytes could likewise be immortalized using hTERT alone *(23)*.

Recent unpublished work indicates similar biology between these human p16-deficient melanocytes and melanocytes from mice that are likewise deficient for p16 but

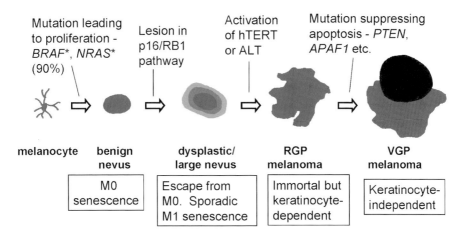

Fig. 3. Genetic model for melanoma progression, correlated with the clinical model of Clark et al. Adapted and updated from Bennett *(10)*. Note that not all the stages shown may necessarily be observed in a given case; for example, the genetic changes may happen in a different order.

have normal Arf *(52)*. These mouse melanocytes grow normally in the beginning, then slow down at the expected time of senescence, with apparent cell death. However, the slowing-down can be reversed by either keratinocyte feeder cells or stem cell factor with endothelin 1, in the presence of which, the cells grow well and do not senesce *(53,* abstract only). This finding preliminarily implicates Arf in the excessive cell death and keratinocyte-dependence of p16-deficient melanocytes, at least in the mouse, because mouse melanocytes null for both p16 and Arf did not show this cell death *(49)*.

POSSIBLE GENETIC BASIS FOR THE CLARK MODEL AND SUPPORTING EVIDENCE

These observations of excessive apoptosis (suppressed by keratinocytes) and deficient cell senescence in p16-deficient melanocytes, combined with emerging evidence on genetic alterations and abnormal gene expression in pigmented lesions, led to a hypothesis for the genetic basis for the Clark series of lesions *(10)*. The current version of this model is presented in Fig. 3, and the evidence for each proposed step is now discussed. It has also been reviewed in detail elsewhere *(28)*.

Proliferative Mutation in the Nevus

First, it is suggested that a benign nevus is a clone of melanocytes that has undergone a single mutation that overcomes the mechanism that normally limits the local population density of normal epidermal melanocytes, allowing the clone to proliferate into a colony of densely packed melanocytes. The most likely causal mutations are activating mutations of *BRAF* and *NRAS*, because approx 90% of benign nevi are reported to carry one or other of these two mutations, usually *BRAF* (approx 80% of nevi, whether benign, congenital, or dysplastic), and, in general, the two are mutually exclusive *(54–56)*. As inferred from other cell types, these mutations are functionally very similar and would activate the MAPK intracellular signaling pathway, promoting cell proliferation and inhibiting apoptosis; moreover, expression of an activated *BRAF* sequence has been shown to be both mitogenic and oncogenic in mouse melanocytes *(57)*.

M0 Senescence in the Benign Nevus

It is proposed that the reason that benign nevi stop growing and can remain static for many years is that their cells undergo cell senescence. This idea has already been proposed by several groups *(9,58,59)*. There was circumstantial support for the idea, in that nevi grow initially and then stop growing, showing virtual absence of the proliferation marker Ki67 *(60)*; moreover, nevus cells appear to show poor ability to divide when put into cell culture, compared with normal melanocytes, and the nevus cultures are reported to include giant, highly dendritic cells that are sometimes multinucleate, all properties observed in senescent cells, including melanocytes (reviewed in ref. 9). Descriptions of nevus cell cultures and their proliferation are somewhat variable, which may be attributable to varying proportions of normal melanocytes present in the cultures; nonetheless, they are generally reported to have low proliferative potential *(9)*. The idea that nevi are senescent was recently tested further by examination of additional cellular properties in nevi and other pigmented lesions *(25)*. It was found that benign nevi nearly all expressed substantial levels of p16, and all showed acidic β-galactosidase, a marker with some specificity for senescent cells *(61)*, neither of which was present in normal melanocytes in adjacent skin *(25)*. p16 has been reported in nevi before, but it does not seem to have been realized that this is abnormal as compared with normal melanocytes *(62,63)*. Gray-Schopfer et al. also reported that benign nevi rarely expressed detectable p53 or p21, indicating that their type of senescence was M0, just as seen in cultured melanocytes *(25)*. This provides an attractive explanation for the observation that families with p16 mutations and susceptibility to melanoma often show dysplastic nevus syndrome, a tendency to have large numbers of nevi, many of which may be unusually large and/or classifiable as dysplastic *(27)*. If the growth arrest of nevi is p16-dependent cell senescence, then it makes sense for a germline defect in p16 to be associated with larger nevi through deficient (delayed) cell senescence. This theory does not explain why only some individuals with p16 mutations have dysplastic nevus syndrome *(27)*.

Escape From M0 Senescence in Dysplastic Nevi

The model in Fig. 3 proposes that dysplastic nevi contain or consist of cells that have bypassed M0 senescence, which would necessarily involve a defect in the p16/RB pathway. Alterations and deletions of p16 are reported in some dysplastic nevi, although not in benign nevi *(64,65)* (it remains unclear how p16 loss may happen in pigmented lesions; Gray-Schopfer et al. reported a tendency for reduced or more patchy expression of p16 in dysplastic nevi *(25)*, consistent with the previous studies). It was predicted that dysplastic nevi might reach a state of p53-dependent senescence, as seen with p16-deficient human melanocytes in culture, but immunohistochemical data did not support the presence of p21 in most of these lesions *(25)*. It is therefore possible, instead, that cells in dysplastic nevi are generally not senescent but still proliferating.

Cell Immortalization and Telomere Maintenance in Melanoma; Apoptosis in RGP

It has been reported in general that more than 90% of human cancers express hTERT, and that the rest can extend their telomeres by an abnormal mechanism called ALT (alternative lengthening of telomeres), which appears to involve recombination *(66)*. Melanomas appear to conform to the generality concerning telomere maintenance; whereas benign and dysplastic nevi have little or no telomerase, the majority of melanomas are reported to have substantial levels of telomerase activity *(67–69)*. Lower telomerase activity in thinner melanomas was provisionally concluded to be an artefact caused by contamination by normal cells, when all melanomas but not host cells were found to express the telomerase template RNA subunit hTR by *in situ* hybridization *(67)*. However, further evidence is needed on the question of telomerase activity in RGP melanomas, because there does not appear to be clear evidence regarding whether these lesions also express hTERT, also needed for activity of telomerase. Although this gap in the data should be noted, our model (Fig. 3) proposes that the critical difference between melanomas and nevi is cellular immortalization. We postulate that RGP melanomas will often have the minimal genetic changes that would achieve both growth and immortalization, namely:

1. A mutation leading to cell proliferation.
2. A deficit in the p16/RB pathway.
3. The activation of telomerase (or possibly sometimes ALT).

A mutation leading to cell proliferation would usually be attributable to the *BRAF* and *NRAS* mutations already mentioned, which are also found in approx 70% of melanomas *(55,56,70)*, and the activation of telomerase (or possibly sometimes ALT) has just been discussed. Actual mutations of p16 are not very common in sporadic melanoma *(34)*, but expression of p16 appears to be very commonly reduced in RGP as well as in advanced melanomas *(25,63,71,72)*, and other RB pathway lesions are also reported in melanoma *(73;* reviewed in ref. *28)*. Accordingly, RGP melanoma cells are expected to resemble p16-deficient melanocytes, including the high rate of apoptosis in the absence of keratinocytes or keratinocyte-derived growth factors *(23)*. This fits with the growth pattern of RGP melanomas, namely, growth only in or near the epidermis *(4)*— it would be expected that the RGP cells would undergo apoptosis if they move beyond the diffusion range of keratinocyte-derived growth factors. Incidentally, benign nevus cells, which are not p16-deficient, would not be expected to be so keratinocyte-dependent, which accords with their ability to grow in the dermis.

SUPPRESSION OF APOPTOSIS IN VGP MELANOMA

If RGP melanoma cells grow near the epidermis because they are keratinocyte-dependent, one would expect VGP cells, which grow deeper in the dermis, not to be keratinocyte-dependent. This fits with the known ability of advanced primary and metastatic melanoma cells to grow well in cell culture without any other cells, and indeed with very few growth factors *(74,75)*. There are thousands of cell lines derived from such melanomas. We therefore postulate that VGP melanoma cells possess all the same genetic changes as listed for RGP, but in addition have one or more alterations that inhibit apoptosis. This fits well with our knowledge of common genetic alterations in VGP and metastatic melanoma cells. As shown (Fig. 3), many of these common alterations do reduce apoptosis, as follows. Oncogenic activation of p53 is reported in approx 10% of advanced melanomas *(76,77)*. Loss or silencing (by methylation) of apoptotic protease activating factor 1 (APAF1), an effector of apoptosis that is transcriptionally activated by p53, is also common in melanoma *(78,79)*. A variety of protein tyrosine kinases become overexpressed in melanoma cells, at least as measured in cultured melanoma lines (reviewed in ref. *80)*; signaling from these kinases would be expected to suppress apoptosis through phosphoinositide signaling, activating the antiapoptotic protein kinase, AKT *(81)*. Likewise, approx 15% of uncultured melanomas have inactivating mutations in phosphatase and tensin homolog (PTEN) *(82,83)*. PTEN is a phosphatase that degrades the phosphoinositide and AKT activator, PIP3, thus, PTEN inactivation is another route to excessive AKT activity and reduced apoptosis.

Other modulators of apoptosis are members of the B-cell lymphoma 2 (BCL2) protein family, found in mitochondrial membranes, and incidentally, modulated in activity by AKT. Normal melanocytes already have high levels of the suppressor of apoptosis, BCL2 *(84,85)*, and apparently require this for survival when synthesizing pigment *(85)*. Bush and Li *(86)* recently reviewed alterations in the BCL2 protein family, which include both proapoptotic and antiapoptotic factors. They concluded that, although most family members show no consistent trend in their expression related to melanoma progression, there are consistent reports of overexpression of antiapoptotic factor BCL2L1 (BCL-X_L) in melanomas. A last major antiapoptotic pathway to be mentioned is that of β-catenin activation. Activating mutations of β-catenin itself can be found in melanoma but are rare *(87)*. It is more common to find defects or transcriptional silencing of adenomatous polyposis coli protein, which normally facilitates destruction of β-catenin *(88)*. Also fairly common is overexpression of the transcription factor and proto-oncoprotein, SKI, which can also activate β-catenin *(89)*. In summary, there are many genetic and epigenetic routes by which apoptosis becomes inhibited in melanoma, and the collation given here is probably far from exhaustive. Many of the same pathways also promote cell proliferation, thus, they would confer a double advantage for tumor growth.

CONCLUSIONS AND PERSPECTIVES

The model presented here seems consistent with our knowledge to date about the biology and genetics of melanoma progression. It can explain some puzzling aspects of the biology of pigmented lesions, such as why nevus cells should be able to grow relatively deep in the dermis, whereas the apparently more malignant RGP melanoma cells do not. At present, however, various aspects of the model are unproven and speculative, and some details may well change as more information emerges. What does seem very likely, in a nutshell, is that cell senescence is important in nevi and escape from senescence is important in melanoma.

A number of interesting questions are raised by these considerations. One key remaining question is that of how p16 is activated during M0 senescence. We now know in some detail how shortening of telomeres can activate p53, but we seem to have little idea of which other mechanism for counting cell divisions might result in the increasing expression of p16. It does not appear to be connected with telomere shortening, because telomere maintenance by the forced expression of hTERT does not prevent this type of senescence. Transcription factors ETS1 and ETS2 were reported to be involved in this activation of p16, respectively, in M1 senescence and in the type of accelerated senescence that follows oncogene activation, together with falling expression of ID1 *(19)* and BMI1 *(24)*. These findings were in human fibroblasts. If they are applicable to other cell types, then the question becomes rephrased as: what determines this changing expression of these transcription factors in dividing normal cells?

Another obvious question is whether cell senescence does indeed act as a barrier to other types of cancer, proposed as probable by those who study it. If so, then, in organs in which cancers can develop, there should commonly be benign, static lesions composed of senescent cells following a mitogenic mutation. This can be tested in future by looking for the expression of senescence markers in the known types of static lesions, such as epithelial cysts and polyps.

A related question is that of why *INK4A* should be a susceptibility gene only for melanoma and, less commonly, pancreatic cancer. This seems to suggest that escape from M0/p16-mediated senescence may not be rate limiting for the initiation of most cancer types, other than melanoma and, presumably, pancreatic cancer. If not, then what is more usually rate-limiting? It is tempting to suggest M1/p53-mediated senescence. Mutations of the p53 coding sequence *TP53* are notoriously common in cancer; germline *TP53* mutations predispose to a wide variety of cancers, as do mutations in *CHK2*, which activates p53 during senescence *(90)*. This is the set of cancers in which we might predict expression of normal p53 and p21, and probably p16 also, in the commonest types of static benign lesions.

Lastly, returning to melanoma, it is of special interest to determine whether cell senescence markers may have any value for diagnosis or prognosis. Initial studies indicate a connection with progression, but it remains to be seen whether, using any of these markers, exact criteria may be developed that have better prognostic value than (for example) those offered by Clark et al. over a decade ago. It may at least be hoped that further clarification of our biological understanding of the processes that restrict the growth of benign pigmented lesions may be one route to the identification of therapeutic targets for better treatment of metastatic melanoma.

ACKNOWLEDGMENTS

Work in the author's laboratory reviewed here was supported by European Commission Contract QLK4-1999-01084 and by Wellcome Trust Grants 046038 and 064583. I am grateful to many colleagues for stimulating discussions about this topic.

REFERENCES

1. Arends JW. Molecular interactions in the Vogelstein model of colorectal carcinoma. J Pathol 2000;190:412–416.
2. Cook PJ, Doll R, Fellingham SA. A mathematical model for the age distribution of cancer in man. Int J Cancer 1969;4:93–112.
3. Clark WH, Elder DE, Guerry D, Epstein MN, Greeve MH, Van Horn M. A study of tumor progression: the precursor lesions of superficial spreading and nodular melanoma. Hum Pathol 1984;15: 1147–1165.
4. Clark WH, Elder DE, Guerry D, et al. Model predicting survival in stage I melanoma based on tumor progression. J Natl Cancer Inst 1989;81:1893–1904.
5. Crotty K, McCarthy S, Mihm MC. The histological diagnosis and classification of melanoma. In: Thompson JF, Morton DL, Kroon BBR, eds. Textbook of melanoma. Martin Dunitz, New York, NY: 2004, pp. 115–121.
6. Wynford-Thomas D. Cellular senescence and cancer. J Pathol 1999;187:100–111.
7. Newbold RF. The significance of telomerase activation and cellular immortalization in human cancer. Mutagenesis 2002;17:539–550.
8. Sharpless NE, DePinho RA. Telomeres, stem cells, senescence, and cancer. J Clin Invest 2004;113:160–168.
9. Bennett DC, Medrano EE. Molecular regulation of melanocyte senescence. Pigment Cell Res 2002;15:242–250.
10. Bennett DC. Human melanocyte senescence and melanoma susceptibility genes. Oncogene 2003;22:3063–3069.
11. Hayflick L. The limited in vitro lifetime of human diploid cell strains. Exp Cell Res 1965;37:614–636.

12. Bond JA, Haughton MF, Rowson JM, et al. Control of replicative life span in human cells: barriers to clonal expansion intermediate between M1 senescence and M2 crisis. Mol Cell Biol 1999;19: 3103–3114.

13. Blackburn EH. Telomere states and cell fates. Nature 2000;408:53–56.

14. Stewart SA, Ben Porath I, Carey VJ, O'Connor BF, Hahn WC, Weinberg RA. Erosion of the telomeric single-strand overhang at replicative senescence. Nat Genet 2003;33:492–496.

15. d'Adda di Fagagna F, Reaper PM, Clay-Farrace L, et al. A DNA damage checkpoint response in telomere-initiated senescence. Nature 2003;426:194–198.

16. Ramirez RD, Herbert BS, Vaughan MB, et al. Bypass of telomere-dependent replicative senescence (M1). upon overexpression of Cdk4 in normal human epithelial cells. Oncogene 2003;22:433–444.

17. Zindy F, Quelle DE, Roussel MF, Sherr CJ. Expression of the p16[INK4a] tumor suppressor versus other INK4 family members during mouse development and aging. Oncogene 1997;15:203–211.

18. Hara E, Smith R, Parry D, Tahara H, Stone S, Peters G. Regulation of p16CDKN2 expression and its implications for cell immortalization and senescence. Mol Cell Biol 1996;16:859–867.

19. Ohtani N, Zebedee Z, Huot TJG, et al. Opposing effects of Ets and Id proteins on p16[INK4a] expression during cellular senescence. Nature 2001;409:1067–1070.

20. Kiyono T, Foster SA, Koop JI, McDougall JK, Galloway DA, Klingelhutz AJ. Both RB/p16[INK4a] inactivation and telomerase activity are required to immortalize human epithelial cells. Nature 1998;396:84–88.

21. Ramirez RD, Morales CP, Herbert BS, et al. Putative telomere-independent mechanisms of replicative aging reflect inadequate growth conditions. Genes Dev 2001;15:398–403.

22. Bandyopadhyay D, Medrano EE. Melanin accumulation accelerates melanocyte senescence by a mechanism involving p16{+INK4a}/CDK4/pRB and E2F1. Ann N Y Acad Sci 2000;908:71–84.

23. Sviderskaya EV, Gray-Schopfer VC, Hill SP, et al. p16/cyclin-dependent kinase inhibitor 2A deficiency in human melanocyte senescence, apoptosis, and immortalization: possible implications for melanoma progression. J Natl Cancer Inst 2003;95:723–732.

24. Itahana K, Zou Y, Itahana Y, et al. Control of the replicative life span of human fibroblasts by p16 and the polycomb protein Bmi-1. Mol Cell Biol 2003;23:389–401.

25. Gray-Schopfer VC, Cheong SC, Chow J, et al. Cellular senescence in melanocytic nevi: a mechanism for melanoma suppression by p16. 2005, submitted.

26. Hayward NK. Genetics of melanoma predisposition. Oncogene 2003;22:3053–3062.

27. Kefford RF, Mann GJ, Newton Bishop J. Genetic predisposition to melanoma. In: Thompson JF, Morton DL, Kroon BBR, eds. Textbook of Melanoma. Martin Dunitz, New York, NY: 2004, pp. 56–64.

28. Gray-Schopfer VC, Bennett DC. The genetics of melanoma. In: Nordlund JJ, Boissy RE, Hearing VJ, King RA, Oetting WS, Ortonne JP, eds. The Pigmentary System. Physiology and Pathophysiology. Oxford University Press, New York, NY: 2005, in press.

29. Gillanders E, Juo SH, Holland EA, et al. Localization of a novel melanoma susceptibility locus to 1p22. Am J Hum Genet 2003;73:301–313.

30. Zuo L, Weger J, Yang Q, et al. Germline mutations in the p16[INK4a] binding domain of CDK4 in familial melanoma. Nat Genet 1996;12:97–99.

31. Soufir N, Avril MF, Chompret A, et al. Prevalence of p16 and CDK4 germline mutations in 48 melanoma-prone families in France. The French Familial Melanoma Study Group. Hum Mol Genet 1998;7:209–216.

32. Hayward N. New developments in melanoma genetics. Curr Oncol Rep 2000;2:300–306.

33. Tucker MA, Goldstein AM. Melanoma etiology: where are we? Oncogene 2003;22:3042–3052.

34. Ruas M, Peters G. The p16INK4a/CDKN2A tumor suppressor and its relatives. Biochim Biophys Acta 1998;1378:F115–F177.

35. Sherr CJ. The INK4a/ARF network in tumour suppression. Nature Rev Mol Cell Biol 2001;2:731–737.

36. Sharpless NE, DePinho RA. The INK4A/ARF locus and its two gene products. Curr Opinion Genet Dev 1999;9:22–30.

37. Rizos H, Puig S, Badenas C, et al. A melanoma-associated germline mutation in exon 1beta inactivates p14ARF. Oncogene 2001;20:5543–5547.

38. Randerson-Moor JA, Harland M, Williams S, et al. A germline deletion of p14(ARF) but not CDKN2A in a melanoma-neural system tumour syndrome family. Hum Mol Genet 2001;10:55–62.

39. Hewitt C, Lee WC, Evans G, et al. Germline mutation of ARF in a melanoma kindred. Hum Mol Genet 2002;11(11):1273–1279.

40. Pomerantz J, Schreiber-Agus N, Liegeois NJ, et al. The INK4a tumor suppressor gene product, p19[ARF], interacts with MDM2 and neutralizes MDM2's inhibition of p53. Cell 1998;92:713–723.

41. Momand J, Wu HH, Dasgupta G. MDM2—master regulator of the p53 tumor suppressor protein. Gene 2000;242:15–29.

42. Kamijo T, Zindy F, Roussel MF, et al. Tumor suppression at the mouse *INK4a* locus mediated by the alternative reading frame product p19*ARF*. Cell 1997;91:649–659.

43. Wei W, Hemmer RM, Sedivy JM. Role of p14[ARF] in replicative and induced senescence of human fibroblasts. Mol Cell Biol 2001;21:6748–6757.

44. Hsieh JK, Chan FSG, O'Connor DJ, Mittnacht S, Zhong S, Lu X. RB regulates the stability and the apoptotic function of p53 via MDM2. Mol Cell 1999;3:181–193.

45. Serrano M, Lin AW, McCurrach ME, Beach D, Lowe SW. Oncogenic *ras* provokes premature cell senescence associated with accumulation of p53 and p16[INK4a]. Cell 1997;88:593–602.

46. Lin AW, Barradas M, Stone JC, van Aelst L, Serrano M, Lowe SW. Premature senescence involving p53 and p16 is activated in response to constitutive MEK/MAPK mitogenic signaling. Genes Dev 1998;12:3008–3019.

47. Drayton S, Rowe J, Jones R, et al. Tumor suppressor p16INK4a determines sensitivity of human cells to transformation by cooperating cellular oncogenes. Cancer Cell 2003;4:301–310.

48. Serrano M, Lee HW, Chin L, Cordon-Cardo C, Beach D, DePinho RA. Role of the *INK4a* locus in tumor suppression and cell mortality. Cell 1996;85:27–37.

49. Sviderskaya EV, Hill SP, Evans-Whipp TJ, et al. p16[Ink4a] in melanocyte senescence and differentiation. J Natl Cancer Inst 2002;94:446–454.

50. Gruis NA, van der Velden PA, Sandkuijl LA, et al. Homozygotes for *CDKN2* (p1) germline mutation in Dutch familial melanoma kindreds. Nat Genet 1995;10:351–353.

51. Huot TJ, Rowe J, Harland M, et al. Biallelic mutations in p16[INK4a] confer resistance to Ras- and Ets-induced senescence in human diploid fibroblasts. Mol Cell Biol 2002;22:8135–8143.

52. Krimpenfort P, Quon KC, Mooi WJ, Loonstra A, Berns A. Loss of p16[Ink4a] confers susceptibility to metastatic melanoma in mice. Nature 2001;413:83–86.

53. Sviderskaya EV, Hill SP, Krimpenfort P, Bennett DC. p16[Ink4a] in mouse melanocyte senescence. Pigment Cell Res 2004;17:568.

54. Pollock PM, Harper UL, Hansen KS, et al. High frequency of *BRAF* mutations in nevi. Nat Genet 2003;33:19–20.

55. Omholt K, Platz A, Kanter L, Ringborg U, Hansson J. NRAS and BRAF mutations arise early during melanoma pathogenesis and are preserved throughout tumor progression. Clin Cancer Res 2003;9:6483–6488.

56. Yazdi AS, Palmedo G, Flaig MJ, et al. Mutations of the BRAF gene in benign and malignant melanocytic lesions. J Invest Dermatol 2003;121:1160–1162.

57. Wellbrock C, Ogilvie L, Hedley D, et al. V599EB-RAF is an oncogene in melanocytes. Cancer Res 2004;64(7):2338–2342.

58. Mooi WJ, Peeper DS. Pathogenesis of melanocytic naevi: growth arrest linked with cellular senescence? Histopathol 2002;41:120–146.

59. Bastian BC. The longer your telomeres, the larger your nevus? Am J Dermatopathol 2003;25:83–84.

60. Healy E, Belgaid C, Takata M, et al. Prognostic significance of allelic losses in primary melanoma. Oncogene 1998;16:2213–2218.

61. Dimri GP, Lee X, Basile G, et al. A biomarker that identifies senescent human cells in culture and in aging skin in vivo. Proc Natl Acad Sci USA 1995;92:9363–9367.

62. Talve L, Sauroja I, Collan Y, Punnonen K, Ekfors T. Loss of expression of the *p16INK4/CDKN2* gene in cutaneous malignant melanoma correlates with tumor cell proliferation and invasive stage. Int J Cancer 1997;74:255–259.

63. Keller-Melchior R, Schmidt R, Piepkorn M. Expression of the tumor suppressor gene product p16[INK4] in benign and malignant melanocytic lesions. J Invest Dermatol 1998;110:932–938.

64. Park WS, Vortmeyer AO, Pack S, et al. Allelic deletion at chromosome 9p21(p16) and 17p13(p53) in microdissected sporadic dysplastic nevus. Hum Pathol 1998;29(2):127–130.

65. Papp T, Pemsel H, Rollwitz I, et al. Mutational analysis of N-ras, p53, CDKN2A (p16(INK4a)), p14(ARF), CDK4, and MC1R genes in human dysplastic melanocytic naevi. J Med Genet 2003;40:E14.

66. Londono-Vallejo JA, Der-Sarkissian H, Cazes L, Bacchetti S, Reddel RR. Alternative lengthening of telomeres is characterized by high rates of telomeric exchange. Cancer Res 2004;64:2324–2327.

67. Ramirez RD, D'Atri S, Pagani E, et al. Progressive increase in telomerase activity from benign melanocytic conditions to malignant melanoma. Neoplasia 1999;1:42–49.

68. Glaessl A, Bosserhoff AK, Buettner R, Hohenleutner U, Landthaler M, Stolz W. Increase in telomerase activity during progression of melanocytic cells from melanocytic naevi to malignant melanomas. Arch Dermatol Res 1999;291:81–87.

69. Rudolph P, Schubert C, Tamm S, et al. Telomerase activity in melanocytic lesions: a potential marker of tumor biology. Am J Pathol 2000;156:1425–1432.

70. Davies H, Bignell GR, Cox C, et al. Mutations of the *BRAF* gene in human cancer. Nature 2002;417:949–954.

71. Straume O, Sviland L, Akslen LA. Loss of nuclear p16 protein expression correlates with increased tumor cell proliferation (Ki-67) and poor prognosis in patients with vertical growth phase melanoma. Clin Cancer Res 2000;6:1845–1853.

72. Pavey SJ, Cummings MC, Whiteman DC, et al. Loss of p16 expression is associated with histological features of melanoma invasion. Melanoma Res 2002;12:539–547.

73. Bartkova J, Lukas J, Guldberg P, et al. The p16-cyclin D/Cdk4-pRb pathway as a functional unit frequently altered in melanoma pathogenesis. Cancer Res 1996;56:5475–5483.

74. Herlyn M, Thurin J, Balaban G, et al. Characteristics of cultured human melanocytes isolated from different stages of tumor progression. Cancer Res 1985;45:5670–5676.

75. Herlyn M, Balaban G, Bennicelli J, et al. Primary melanoma cells of the vertical growth phase: similarities to metastatic cells. J Natl Cancer Inst 1985;74:283–289.

76. Albino AP, Vidal MJ, McNutt NS, et al. Mutation and expression of the p53 gene in human malignant melanoma. Melanoma Res 1994;4:35–45.

77. Castellano M, Parmiani G. Genes involved in melanoma: an overview of *INK4a* and other loci. Melanoma Res 1999;9:421–432.

78. Soengas MS, Capodieci P, Polsky D, et al. Inactivation of the apoptosis effector Apaf-1 in malignant melanoma. Nature 2001;409:207–211.

79. Baldi A, Santini D, Russo P, et al. Analysis of APAF-1 expression in human cutaneous melanoma progression. Exp Dermatol 2004;13:93–97.

80. Easty DJ, Bennett DC. Protein tyrosine kinases in malignant melanoma. Melanoma Res 2000; 10:401–411.

81. Blume-Jensen P, Hunter T. Oncogenic kinase signalling. Nature 2001;411:355–365.

82. Guldberg P, Thor SP, Birck A, Ahrenkiel V, Kirkin AF, Zeuthen J. Disruption of the MMAC1/PTEN gene by deletion or mutation is a frequent event in malignant melanoma. Cancer Res 1997;57: 3660–3663.

83. Pollock PM, Walker GJ, Glendening JM, et al. PTEN inactivation is rare in melanoma tumours but occurs frequently in melanoma cell lines. Melanoma Res 2002;12:565–575.

84. Plettenberg A, Ballaun C, Pammer J, et al. Human melanocytes and melanoma cells constitutively express the Bcl-2 proto-oncogene in situ and in cell culture. Am J Pathol 1995;146:651–659.

85. Yamamura K, Kamada S, Ito S, Nakagawa K, Ichihashi M, Tsujimoto Y. Accelerated disappearance of melanocytes in bcl-2–deficient mice. Cancer Res 1996;56:3546–3550.

86. Bush JA, Li G. The role of Bcl-2 family members in the progression of cutaneous melanoma. Clin Exp Metastasis 2003;20:531–539.

87. Omholt K, Platz A, Ringborg U, Hansson J. Cytoplasmic and nuclear accumulation of beta-catenin is rarely caused by CTNNB1 exon 3 mutations in cutaneous malignant melanoma. Int J Cancer 2001;92:839–842.

88. Worm J, Christensen C, Gronbaek K, Tulchinsky E, Guldberg P. Genetic and epigenetic alterations of the APC gene in malignant melanoma. Oncogene 2004;23:5215–5226.

89. Chen D, Xu W, Bales E, et al. SKI activates Wnt/beta-catenin signaling in human melanoma. Cancer Res 2003;63:6626–6634.

90. Bell DW, Varley JM, Szydlo TE, et al. Heterozygous germ line hCHK2 mutations in Li-Fraumeni syndrome. Science 1999;286:2528–2531.

11 Genetic Progression From Melanocyte to Malignant Melanoma

Boris C. Bastian

Summary

Melanocytes can give rise to a variety of benign and malignant neoplasms that differ in their appearance and, more importantly, in their biological behavior. Melanocytic nevi are self-limited proliferations of melanocytes, whereas melanocytes in melanoma continue to proliferate and therefore constitute a severe threat to the host. There is emerging evidence that the initiating events, such as mutations in oncogenes, such as *BRAF* and *RAS*, may be similar in nevi and melanoma. However, the exact nature of the mechanism that restricts proliferation in nevi that presumably fails in melanoma is currently unclear. Among melanomas, clinical and histopathological presentation can vary significantly. Several factors, such as anatomic location, sun-exposure patterns, and patient age have been associated with different histopathological and clinical patterns of melanoma *(1,2)*. In this chapter, I review genetic changes in different types of nevi and melanomas and discuss potential biological consequences and possible impacts on classification and therapy.

Key Words: Melanoma; melanocytic nevus; genetics; minimal residual disease; chromosomal aberrations; BRAF; RAS; cyclin D1.

MELANOCYTIC NEVI

Nevi can vary dramatically in size, clinical, and microscopic appearance. One way that melanocytic nevi are classified is a division into congenital and acquired types. Applied strictly, this would put all nevi that are present at birth in the congenital category, and all others in the acquired category. However, the exact history is commonly not available in patients that present after birth. Instead, clinical or histopathological criteria are frequently used for classifying nevi into congenital or acquired. In general, congenital nevi tend to be larger than acquired nevi. As a rule, giant congenital nevi, i.e., nevi larger than 20 cm in size, which can sometimes cover significant portions of the body,

From: *From Melanocytes to Melanoma: The Progression to Malignancy*
Edited by: V. J. Hearing and S. P. L. Leong © Humana Press Inc., Totowa, NJ

are always already present at birth. In addition to the larger size of congenital nevi, they also tend to show increased numbers of terminal hairs growing out of the lesion. Pathologists frequently use histomorphological criteria, such as melanocytes present around dermal adnexae or splayed between collagen bundles of the deep reticular dermis to diagnose congenital nevi. However, there are studies showing no correlation of histomorphology with presence or absence of the lesion at birth (3,4). Birth as a time point is not directly linked to a defined state of development. Babies can be born too early, too late, or just on time. Although there are obvious limits to this variation, these differences could well matter given the pace of development *in utero*. For these reasons, the boundary between congenital and acquired nevi is blurry and perhaps ill chosen.

Other types of nevi are categorized according to their clinical appearance. For instance, blue nevi are intradermal proliferations of melanocytes that appear as bluish skin lesions because of their pigment distribution. Dysplastic (also termed atypical) nevi have been described as histopathological entities that are both precursor and marker for melanoma risk (5). Although subsequent studies have confirmed that dysplastic nevi represent an inherited feature (6) that is associated with an increased risk for melanoma (7), no studies have been able to establish the histopathological features originally described as diagnostic of dysplastic nevi as an independent risk factor. Therefore, dysplastic nevi seem to represent a quantitative trait that indicates increased melanoma risk rather than a clinico-pathological entity (8,9).

Spitz nevi are benign melanocytic neoplasms that can resemble melanoma on histopathological examination. They were first described as "juvenile melanoma" by Sophie Spitz in 1948, and were initially regarded as a subset of childhood melanoma that follows a benign course (10). Spitz nevi account for approx 1% of surgically removed melanocytic nevi (11). Both Spitz nevi and melanoma can be composed of melanocytes with abundant cytoplasm and large nuclei. These nuclei can be pleomorphic and contain macronucleoli. Mitotic figures, sometimes numerous, occur in both neoplasms. Misdiagnosis of Spitz nevus as melanoma and vice versa has been repeatedly reported (12–14). A retrospective study of 102 melanocytic tumors occurring in patients under age 17 yr that were originally diagnosed as melanoma found that only 60 cases were classified as melanoma after re-examination by a panel of experts (15). Forty-two lesions were reclassified as nevi, 22 of those as Spitz nevi.

Problems with correct histopathological assessment are not restricted to Spitz nevi and can occur with all types of melanocytic nevi (15–17). Together with lymphoma, misdiagnosis of melanocytic lesions head the list of malpractice cases (18,19). The hazard of mistaking a nevus for melanoma is that the patient may be subjected to needless surgery and adjunctive therapy, become unable to plan for the future, be psychologically traumatized, and have difficulties in obtaining health insurance. For obvious reasons, the misdiagnosis of a melanoma as nevus can have sequelae that are even more dramatic. A better understanding on the mechanistic differences between nevi and melanoma could potentially lead to improved, more objective methods of classification, with higher diagnostic accuracy.

Recent studies have shown that, similar to melanoma (20,21), melanocytic nevi frequently show oncogenic mutations in members of the MAP-kinase pathway, such as *BRAF* and *RAS* (22–24). These findings indicate that the initiating oncogenic lesions may be similar in nevi and in melanoma and may be of little help for diagnostic purposes. It is of interest, however, that the types of oncogenic lesions appear to differ between different types of nevi. Whereas Spitz nevi have been shown to have recurrent mutations in *HRAS*, mutations in *BRAF* appear to be absent in Spitz nevi *(25)*. In addition, *BRAF* mutations have been found to be infrequent in blue nevi *(25)*. Future studies are necessary to identify the common oncogenic events in these and other types of nevi.

We have performed comparative genomic hybridization (CGH) and found significant differences between nevi and melanomas. As shown in Fig. 1, whereas most melanomas (more than 95% in our hands) show chromosomal aberrations, the majority of nevi had either no aberrations or a very restricted set that showed very little overlap with melanoma *(26–28)*.

We found that approx 20% of Spitz nevi show increased copy number of chromosome 11p *(23,27)*. Studies that are more recent revealed that this gain is caused by an isochromosome 11p, an aberration that we did not find in a series of 170 melanomas (to be published). The frequent gain of chromosome 11p helped us to identify *HRAS* as at least one of the critical genes driving this aberration, because 80% of Spitz nevi with the 11p copy number increase carry a mutated *HRAS* on that chromosome *(23)*. *HRAS* is a potent oncogene and we were surprised to find it to be mutated in a substantial portion of Spitz nevi *(23)*. Follow-up of these patients for up to 7 yr did not show any signs of recurrences or relapses, indicating that these lesions were indeed benign. As pointed out earlier, Spitz nevi can share several features with melanoma. Considering the hallmarks of cancer as defined by Hanahan and Weinberg *(29)*, Spitz nevus cells show several— but not all — essential features of cancer. The presence of *HRAS* mutations makes them independent from at least some external growth stimuli. They appear to be resistant to apoptotic stimuli, possibly resulting from the constitutive activation of the MAP-kinase pathway, because apoptosis has been reported to be low *(30)*. Spitz nevi can show significant vascularity, showing that they are also able to induce their own blood supply. The major difference between Spitz nevi and melanoma lies in the fact that melanoma cells are able to proliferate indefinitely. This pivotal difference probably applies to all nevi.

To address potential mechanisms that could prevent benign nevi with oncogenic mutations, such as *RAS* mutations, from progression to melanoma, we recently performed a study looking at cell-cycle inhibitor expression in nevi with and without oncogenic mutations. Specifically, we analyzed MAP-kinase activation using immunohistochemistry for phospho-ERK, cyclin D1, and MITF expression in 17 Spitz nevi with and 18 Spitz nevi without 11p copy number increase. Because our previous studies showed that *HRAS* mutations were frequently accompanied by increased copy numbers of the mutated allele *(23)*, a sustained and marked activation of the MAP-kinase-signaling cascade can be assumed to be present in these Spitz nevi. We found relatively high levels of phospho-ERK and cyclin D1 expression, suggesting MAP-kinase pathway activation in both groups of Spitz nevi, independent of the mutation or copy number status of *HRAS (31)*. This may indicate that mutations other than *HRAS* activate the MAP-kinase pathway in the Spitz nevi without *HRAS* mutations. Interestingly, Spitz nevi with 11p copy number increases showed significantly higher levels of cyclin D1 expression and lower levels of MITF expression, suggesting stronger MAP-kinase pathway activation in this group. Contrasting this apparent activation, the proliferation rate, as assessed by Mib1 expression, was low in both groups. An analysis of cell-cycle inhibitory proteins, including p16, p21, and p27, showed that the majority of Spitz nevus cells expressed high levels of p16, with cells of the cases that had increased copy number of 11p expressing significantly higher levels than those of Spitz nevi with normal copy number of 11p. The

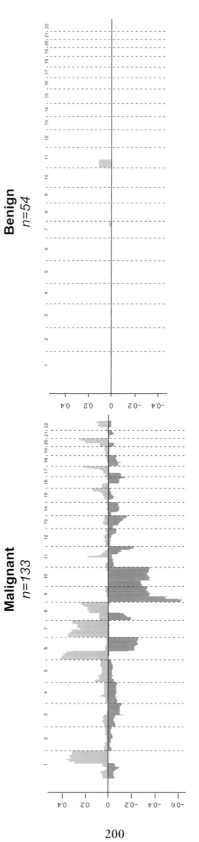

Fig. 1. Copy number differences in melanoma (**A**) and melanocytic nevi (**B**). The *y*-axes shows the proportion of copy number increases (gray) and decreases lost (black) by chromosomal bin (28).

association between MAP-kinase activation and induction of p16 parallels in vitro experiments with various cell types. In vitro, constitutive activation of the MAP-kinase pathway through activated oncogenes in normal cells leads to a p16-mediated permanent growth arrest (32). This condition has been termed premature senescence or oncogene-induced senescence (33). P16 has been shown to be essential for melanocyte senescence as well (34,35), and found to be expressed in other types of melanocytic nevi (36).

It is therefore tempting to speculate that Spitz nevi, and possibly melanocytic nevi in general, represent an example of oncogene-induced senescence in vivo. In the presence of an intact p16 tumor suppressor pathway, melanocytes could withstand full transformation by activated oncogenes. The observation that Spitz nevi with increased copy number of chromosome 11p expressed significantly higher levels of p16 also suggests a direct link between MAP-kinase pathway activation and p16 expression levels in melanocytes. Future studies are necessary to establish the nature of this link and to examine potential candidate mediators, such as the ETS transcription factors (37).

Independent of the type, all nevi represent a finite proliferation of melanocytes that eventually cease to grow. The previously described association between age at which nevi occur and the final nevus size may provide insight into possible additional mechanism(s) that can prevent uncontrolled proliferation. Bona fide congenital nevi, i.e., nevi present at birth, may be caused by mutations of melanocyte precursors that occur before the migrating melanoblasts have reached their target, the skin. This may explain why, in large congenital nevi, melanocytes can be encountered in large numbers in extracutaneous sites, such as the meninges. The larger size of these lesions may thus be related to the increased replicative potential of the affected cells, possibly linking telomere length to nevus size (38). Future studies are necessary to elucidate which mechanism(s) lead to induction of cell cycle arrest through p16 or other factors in different types of nevi.

In summary, these observations suggest that nevi are oncogene-induced finite proliferations of melanocytes, in which intact checkpoints prevent an unchecked proliferation resulting in telomere erosion, chromosomal breaks, and instability.

DIFFERENCES BETWEEN TYPES OF MELANOMA

In addition to problems in classifying melanocytic lesions as benign or malignant, there is controversy about whether melanoma is one disease or consists of biologically and histologically distinct subtypes. It has long been noted that the presentation of melanoma can vary significantly, and a classification was proposed to separate melanoma into superficial spreading melanoma (SSM), lentigo maligna melanoma (LMM), nodular melanoma (NM), and acral lentiginous melanoma (ALM) (39,40). The criteria proposed for this classification are based on the growth pattern of the radial growth phase of a melanoma: a so-called pagetoid pattern with solitary and nested melanocytes scattered throughout the epidermis in SSM, as opposed to a lentiginous pattern with single melanocytes arrayed along the dermo–epidermal junction in LMM and ALM. NM was defined as an invasive melanoma without any notable radial growth. These histological patterns show some correlation with anatomic location (SSM and NM on trunk and extremities; LMM on the face; and ALM on the palms, soles, and subungual sites), sun-exposure patterns (acute–intermittent in SSM and NM, chronic in LMM, and no association in ALM), and patient age (SSM and NM more frequent in patient under 60 yr, LMM and ALM more frequent in patients over 60 yr). However, these associations overlap significantly and it is currently unclear whether there truly are biologically distinct types of cutaneous melanomas, and, if so, what defines them. This overlap is illustrated by the fact that the histological patterns of SSM and NM can also occur in melanomas evolving on palms and soles *(41)*, and the histological pattern of ALM has been reported for melanomas on acral skin outside of the palms and soles, such as the dorsa of hands and feet *(42)*.

Genetic approaches have been of significant help to classify hematopoietic neoplasias *(43)* and, as illustrated by recent advances in the treatment of chronic myeloid leukemia, the identification of distinct aberrations followed by the identification of the precise genetic defect has paved the way to specific treatments *(44)*. With the advent of targeted therapy for cancer, it therefore becomes critically important to understand the genetic denominators of the disease.

Ocular melanoma shows a stereotypic pattern of metastasis to the liver and frequent aberrations of chromosome 3, separating it from cutaneous melanoma *(45–51)*. Using CGH, we found evidence that among cutaneous melanomas, those that are located on acral skin (palms, soles, and subungual sites) differ from other types by a uniquely high frequency of focused amplifications *(52)*.

Over the last years, we have analyzed several hundred melanomas using conventional, chromosome-based CGH, and array CGH to compare the patterns of chromosomal aberrations between different types of melanoma. We found confirmation of our earlier studies that melanomas on the soles, palms, and subungual skin invariably show gene amplifications independent of the microscopic growth pattern, and that such amplifications occur only in a minority of melanomas on the remainder of the skin; suggesting that anatomic location, i.e., location on glabrous (non-hair-bearing) skin, not histological pattern, defines a distinct melanoma type *(26,28,52)*. Therefore, we suggest using the term acral melanoma (AM) instead of acral lentiginous melanoma. AMs also showed certain aberrations that occurred with significantly different frequency when compared with melanomas on nonglabrous skin. For example, AMs showed significantly more frequent amplifications involving chromosome 11q13, a region that harbors the cyclin D1 gene. We demonstrated that cyclin D1 amplification is always accompanied by overexpression of the protein *(53)*. The biological relevance of cyclin D1 amplification/overexpression was demonstrated by antisense treatment in cell lines. When treated with an antisense-expressing adenovirus, the melanoma cell lines overexpressing cyclin D1 underwent massive apoptosis, whereas normal melanocytes remained unaffected. In a mouse xenograft model, antisense treatment lead to marked shrinkage of tumors through massive apoptosis. Cell lines or tumors treated with a control virus remained largely unaffected *(53)*. Interestingly, cyclin D1 was also found to be overexpressed in a subset of melanomas without amplifications, indicating that mechanisms other than amplification can lead to overexpression in melanoma *(53,54)*.

Another region found frequently amplified in AM is chromosome 5p15. This region contains the gene for the catalytic component of telomerase (hTERT). FISH studies confirmed that hTERT was amplified in cases with 5p15 amplification. Amplifications of hTERT have been reported in other cancers as well *(55)*. Chromosome 12q14 was another region that was preferentially gained in AMs. The area contains several cancer related genes, including cyclin-dependent kinase 4, a gene mutated in some melanomas *(56)*.

We also found differences between melanomas arising on chronically sun-damaged skin (CSD) and not chronically sun-damaged skin (no CSD). The majority of our CSD cases were LMMs, and the majority of our no CSD cases were SSMs. CSDs showed much more frequent deletions involving distal chromosome 13q than any of the other types *(28)*.

Using a cohort of 115 primary invasive melanomas, we recently showed that the frequency of BRAF varies strongly depending on the type of melanoma *(57)*. We found mutations to be significantly ($p < 0.00005$) more common in melanomas occurring on skin subject to intermittent sun exposure (23/43), than in those on chronically sun-damaged skin (1/12) or on skin relatively or completely unexposed, such as the palms, soles, and subungual sites (6/39), and mucosal membranes (2/21). The rare mutations in mucosal melanoma have been confirmed by others *(58,59)*.

More recent data using array CGH measurements confirm the differences in the patterns of DNA copy number changes among different melanoma types and refine the boundaries of the regions differentially involved among different types of melanoma *(59a)*. We measured DNA copy number aberrations in 35 melanomas from AM, such as the palms, soles, and subungual sites; 25 SSM from cutaneous but not acral sites; and 21 melanomas from mucosal sites (MM). AM tumors came from sites with limited sun exposure, whereas MM sites are totally unexposed. The fraction of genome that was at aberrant copy number was significantly higher in MMs than in AMs and SSMs (29.2% [range, 10.8–44.6%] vs 22.51% [range, 9.1–59.1%] and 19.6% [range, 7.5–44%], respectively; $p < 0.05$). Identification of aberrations that occurred with a significant difference in frequency among the three groups was accomplished using a permutation-based threshold to compensate for the multiple comparisons that are required in the analysis. This approach is a conservative way to address multiple comparison problems in large data sets. The conservatism is demonstrated by the comparison of the copy number differences between men and women in the overall group. Only clones that mapped to the X-chromosome were found to be significantly different between the two groups, so that the correction resulted in no false-positive calls. When this method was used to compare melanomas on skin with CSD, without CSD, AM, and mucosal melanoma, we found that classification algorithms using the k-nearest neighbor method could correctly classify melanomas into one of the four classes in 80% of the cases.

The differences in the mutation frequencies in BRAF and in the patterns of chromosomal aberrations strongly supports the notion of the existence of distinct melanoma types. With the development of targeted therapeutic strategies for melanoma, these differences will become clinically relevant.

GENETIC PROGRESSION FROM MELANOCYTES TO MELANOMA

During our studies on AM, we found that the amplifications arose very early during the progression and allowed us to study of the early evolution of the disease. We used FISH with probes targeted to the sites of amplifications to topographically map the aberrations on tissue sections of the melanomas. In AM, melanocytes with amplifications were present in the invasive and the *in situ* portions of the tumor. To our surprise, we found that, in several cases, the amplifications could also be detected in histologically normal-appearing melanocytes in a stretch of adjacent epidermis of up to 5 mm (Fig. 2). These cells were equidistantly spaced and showed no marked atypicality, appeared histologically to be normal melanocytes, and were termed field cells *(52)*. The finding of amplifications in the *in situ* portion and in field cells suggested that the amplifications were present before the tumors became invasive and even before they became recognizable as *in situ*. This was confirmed by several additional observations: first, amplifica-

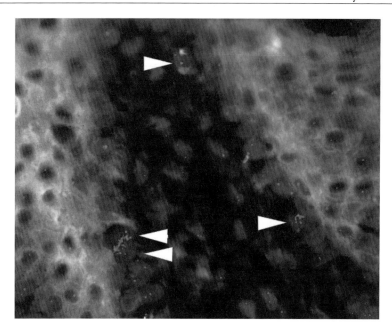

Fig. 2. Field cells in acral melanoma detected by fluorescence *in situ* hybridization. Single basal melanocytes with amplifications of cyclin D1 highlighted by the arrowheads. Please *see* color insert following p. 430.

tions were also encountered in tumors that were solely *in situ*; second, in some tumors, the amplification levels were higher in the invasive component than in the *in situ* or field-cell component, suggesting that clonal evolution selected for higher copy number; third, in some tumors, additional amplifications of other genomic regions were found in the invasive component that were absent the *in situ* or field-cell component. All these observations indicate that amplifications arise very early in AM, even before the cancer becomes detectable microscopically, and that one of the cells with an amplification acquired additional abnormalities and then became invasive.

The existence of field cells has potential implications for the recommendation of safety margins. The National Comprehensive Cancer Network recommends that cutaneous melanoma be excised with a margin of clinically normal-appearing skin of 0.5–2 cm, depending on the thickness of the melanoma. Four randomized trials, with a total of 2406 participants, showed that safety margins decrease the rate of persistent melanoma but do not impact overall survival in melanoma *(60)*. The width of these margins is entirely empirically based, and the nature of minimal residual melanoma addressed by this procedure is unknown.

Clinical and histological data suggests that there are at least two different types of local recurrences once a melanoma has been excised with histologically clear margins: one form that manifests itself as predominantly intradermal nodular proliferations of melanocytes appearing around or within the scar; and a second form in which the melanoma reappears with a clear intraepidermal component. The second form occurs often with a considerable latency of several years. The latency and histological pattern of this type of persistence suggest that it is caused by intraepidermal melanoma cells left behind after surgery.

Several arguments suggest that field cells are the source of clinically relevant minimal residual disease in melanoma that arises through the second mechanism. Clinical data indicates that margins predominantly prevent local recurrence of and do not increase survival. Thus, the residual cells are likely to be noninvasive or they represent metastatic deposits indicative of systemic dissemination of the disease. In our series, we observed one melanoma that recurred three times at the excision site. All excision specimens were read as 'margins free of neoplasm' by conventional pathology, but FISH detected field cells at the margin in every excision. This strongly suggests that field cells are responsible for local recurrences.

Field cells in AMs were easily detectable by FISH because of the presence of high-level amplifications. We also attempted to detect field cells in the few SSMs and LMMs that had gene amplifications. However, in these melanoma types, FISH showed that the amplifications were confined to the invasive portion and could not be demonstrated in the radial growth phase or *in situ* portions. This indicated that the amplifications occur late in progression in SSMs and LMMs, rather than early, as in AM, and cannot be used to detect field cells in these melanoma types. However, other aberrations, such as a loss of chromosome 9p or gain of chromosome 17, were detectable in the *in situ* portion of these melanoma types using FISH. More recent work, using a combination of FISH and immunohistochemistry, allowed us to individually karyotype single basal melanocytes in histologically uninvolved skin adjacent to melanoma samples. Using this method, we could demonstrate chromosomal aberrations in the basal melanocytes in the histologically uninvolved epidermis adjacent to LMMs. Future studies are necessary to elucidate whether field cells are restricted to certain types of melanoma, such as melanoma with a lentiginous growth pattern, or are present in all melanomas. The findings so far indicate that, at least in AM and probably in LMM, there is a stage of melanoma progression that precedes melanoma *in situ*, which is currently considered the earliest presentation of melanoma. More detailed studies of field cells hold the promise of identifying genomic alterations that occur early in melanoma progression.

The observation of significant genomic aberrations in very early lesions of melanoma, such as gene amplifications, suggests that genomic instability may occur early on in the evolution in melanoma. Clinically, AM *in situ* and LMM undergo a very slow progression, sometimes taking several decades to form an invasive growth. This suggests that the cells of these early lesions either do not proliferate very rapidly or that proliferation is paralleled by significant cell death, keeping the net increase in cell number relatively small.

When one considers the frequent chromosomal aberrations in melanomas, as described, and the relative absence thereof in nevi, one can hypothesize what may happen during this phase of melanoma evolution. The field cell and melanoma *in situ* phases of progression may be a period analogous to what has been described as crisis in cell culture models *(61)*. Crisis is a term used for the massive cell death occurring when mammalian cells in culture pass their replicative lifespan. Most human differentiated cells have a finite replicative lifespan and stop dividing after a certain number of divisions. For example, human diploid fibroblasts can undergo 60–80 population doublings in culture until they cease dividing and enter a senescent state, at which point they stay metabolically active and can be maintained in culture for several years. The molecular mechanisms that determine the intrinsic replicative lifespan of human cells seem to be controlled by a single process—telomere shortening *(33)*. Telomeres are the repetitive DNA sequences bound by a complex of proteins at the end of chromosomes. Telomeres shorten slightly with each cell division until they reach a critical length, at which time a signal requiring p53 and RB is triggered, leading to permanent cell-cycle arrest. This replicative senescence limits the number of cell divisions and is regarded as a major tumor suppressive mechanism *(33)*. Cells in which the damage signal is disabled (e.g., by mutations in the p53 or RB pathways, including p16) continue to proliferate beyond their replication limit. After several additional rounds of cell division, the telomere attrition becomes critical, leading to open DNA ends and end-to-end fusion of chromatids. During this state (termed "crisis") cells carry on dividing but show high rates of apoptosis, which is triggered by gross chromosomal abnormalities. Crisis can be seen as a *transient* period of random genomic restructuring and selection, which ultimately gives rise to new clones that have an altered but stabilized genome. Crisis is thus characterized as a period in which the apoptotic rate is higher than the proliferation rate, leading to a (temporal) decrease of cell number. During crisis, the cancer is "spinning its wheels" and may be even slipping backwards in terms of net cell proliferation.

Given the fact that chromosomal aberrations can already be detected at the *in situ* stage of melanoma and the observation that it often takes many years for a melanoma *in situ* to become an invasive cancer, one can speculate that the early progression stages of melanoma may represent a stage of genomic rearrangement in which an increased melanocyte proliferation rate is paralleled by an increased apoptotic rate. The rate of cell death may even outpace proliferation, transiently leading to partial regression of the lesion. Regression of melanoma that we now attribute solely to effectors of the immune system could, thus, also be at least partially a reflection of crisis *(62)*. The genomic restructuring during crisis represents a period of evolution ultimately leading to a more aggressive phenotype. To maintain any favorable genetic constellation that emerges and to weather crisis, cancer cells ultimately have to restabilize their telomeres. Most human tumors, including melanomas *(63)*, stabilize their telomeres through activation of telomerase; the remainder stabilize their telomeres by a different mechanism, termed alternative lengthening of telomeres. After this step, cells have become immortal. If cells lack telomerase, crisis is prolonged and genomic instability is more pronounced *(64)*. Conversely, if cells are transduced with oncogenes and telomerase, chromosomal aberrations do not seem to occur, even after many passages *(65)*.

Therefore, gross chromosomal abnormalities can be seen as evidence that a cancer went through crisis. Our studies on 133 melanomas showed that more than 95% have chromosomal aberrations, mostly involving gains or losses of partial chromosomes, whereas the majority of nevi do not *(28)*. The marked chromosomal aberrations in melanomas and the absence thereof in melanocytic nevi, therefore, may indicate that the melanomas went through crisis, whereas the nevi did not. An intact G1/S checkpoint function, possibly mediated through p16, may be an essential feature preventing unchecked proliferation and entry into crisis.

Whether caused by crisis or not, the marked differences in the pattern of chromosomal aberrations between melanoma and benign nevi are likely to be of diagnostic help in cases that are now ambiguous.

REFERENCES

1. Clark WH Jr, Elder DE, Van Horn M. The biologic forms of malignant melanoma. Hum Pathol 1986;17:443–450.
2. Clark WH, From L, Bernadino EA, Mihm MC. The histogenesis and biological behaviour of pimary human malignant melanoma. Am J Pathol 1969;55:39–52.

3. Clemmensen OJ, Kroon S. The histology of "congenital features" in early acquired melanocytic nevi. J Am Acad Dermatol 1988;19:742–746.

4. Everett MA. Histopathology of congenital pigmented nevi. Am J Dermatopathol 1989;11:11–12.

5. Elder DE, Goldman LI, Goldman SC, Greene MH, Clark WH Jr. Dysplastic nevus syndrome: a phenotypic association of sporadic cutaneous melanoma. Cancer 1980;46:1787–1794.

6. Goldgar DE, Cannon-Albright LA, Meyer LJ, Piepkorn MW, Zone JJ, Skolnick MH. Inheritance of nevus number and size in melanoma and dysplastic nevus syndrome kindreds. J Natl Cancer Inst 1991;83:1726–1733.

7. Tucker MA, Halpern A, Holly EA, et al. Clinically recognized dysplastic nevi. A central risk factor for cutaneous melanoma [see comments]. JAMA 1997;277:1439–1444.

8. Piepkorn M, Meyer LJ, Goldgar D, et al. The dysplastic melanocytic nevus: a prevalent lesion that correlates poorly with clinical phenotype. J Am Acad Dermatol 1989;20:407–415.

9. Meyer LJ, Piepkorn M, Goldgar DE, et al. Interobserver concordance in discriminating clinical atypia of melanocytic nevi, and correlations with histologic atypia. J Am Acad Dermatol 1996;34:618–625.

10. Spitz S. Melanoma of childhood. Am J Pathol 1948;24:591–609.

11. Casso EM, Grin-Jorgensen CM, Grant-Kels JM. Spitz nevi. J Am Acad Dermatol 1992;27:901–913.

12. Peters MS, Goellner JR. Spitz nevi and malignant melanomas of childhood and adolescence. Histopathology 1986;10:1289–1302.

13. Okun MR. Melanoma resembling spindle and epithelioid nevus. Arch Dermatol 1979;115:1416–1420.

14. Goldes J, Holmes S, Satz M, Cich J, Dehner L. Melanoma masquerading as Spitz nevus following acute lymphoblastic leukemia. Pediatr Dermatol 1984;1:295–298.

15. Spatz A, Ruiter D, Hardmeier T, et al. Melanoma in childhood: an EORTC-MCG multicenter study on the clinico-pathological aspects. Int J Cancer 1996;68:317–324.

16. Farmer ER, Gonin R, Hanna MP. Discordance in the histopathologic diagnosis of melanoma and melanocytic nevi between expert pathologists. Hum Pathol 1996;27:528–531.

17. Veenhuizen KC, De Wit PE, Mooi WJ, Scheffer E, Verbeek AL, Ruiter DJ. Quality assessment by expert opinion in melanoma pathology: experience of the pathology panel of the Dutch Melanoma Working Party [see comments]. J Pathol 1997;182:266–272.

18. Troxel DB, Sabella JD. Problem areas in pathology practice. Uncovered by a review of malpractice claims [see comments]. Am J Surg Pathol 1994;18:821–831.

19. Jackson R. Malignant melanoma: a review of 75 malpractice cases. Int J Dermatol 1997;36:497–498.

20. Albino AP, Nanus DM, Mentle IR, et al. Analysis of ras oncogenes in malignant melanoma and precursor lesions: correlation of point mutations with differentiation phenotype. Oncogene 1989;4:1363–1374.

21. Davies H, Bignell GR, Cox C, et al. Mutations of the BRAF gene in human cancer. Nature 2002;417:949–954.

22. Carr J, Mackie RM. Point mutations in the N-ras oncogene in malignant melanoma and congenital naevi. Br J Dermatol 1994;131:72–77.

23. Bastian BC, LeBoit PE, Pinkel D. Mutations and copy number increases of *HRAS* in Spitz nevi with distinctive histopathologic features. Am J Pathol 2000;157:967–972.

24. Pollock PM, Harper UL, Hansen KS, et al. High frequency of BRAF mutations in nevi. Nat Genet 2002;25:25.

25. Yazdi AS, Palmedo G, Flaig MJ, et al. Mutations of the BRAF gene in benign and malignant melanocytic lesions. J Invest Dermatol 2003;121:1160–1162.

26. Bastian BC, LeBoit PE, Hamm H, Bröcker EB, Pinkel D. Chromosomal gains and losses in primary cutaneous melanomas detected by comparative genomic hybridization. Cancer Res 1998;58:2170–2175.

27. Bastian BC, Wesselmann U, Pinkel D, LeBoit PE. Molecular cytogenetic analysis of Spitz nevi show clear differences to melanoma. J Invest Dermatol 1999;113:1065–1069.

28. Bastian BC, Olshen A, LeBoit PE, Pinkel D. Classification of melanocytic tumors by DNA copy number changes. Am J Pathol 2003;163:1765–1770.

29. Hanahan D, Weinberg RA. The hallmarks of cancer. Cell 2000;100:57–70.

30. Wesselmann U, Becker LR, Brocker EB, LeBoit PE, Bastian BC. Eosinophilic globules in spitz nevi: no evidence for apoptosis. Am J Dermatopathol 1998;20:551–554.

31. Maldonado JL, Fridlyand J, Timmerman L, Bastian BC. Mechanisms of cell cycle arrest in Spitz nevi with constitutive activation of the MAP-kinase pathway. Am J Pathol 2004;164:1783–1787.

32. Serrano M, Lin AW, McCurrach ME, Beach D, Lowe SW. Oncogenic ras provokes premature cell senescence associated with accumulation of p53 and p16INK4a. Cell 1997;88:593–602.

33. Mathon NF, Lloyd AC. Cell senescence and cancer. Nat Rev Cancer 2001;1:203–213.
34. Bandyopadhyay D, Medrano EE. Melanin accumulation accelerates melanocyte senescence by a mechanism involving p16INK4a/CDK4/pRB and E2F1. Ann N Y Acad Sci 2000;908:71–84.
35. Sviderskaya EV, Hill SP, Evans-Whipp TJ, et al. p16(Ink4a) in melanocyte senescence and differentiation. J Natl Cancer Inst 2002;94:446–454.
36. Funk JO, Schiller PI, Barrett MT, Wong DJ, Kind P, Sander CA. p16INK4a expression is frequently decreased and associated with 9p21 loss of heterozygosity in sporadic melanoma. J Cutan Pathol 1998;25:291–296.
37. Ohtani N, Zebedee Z, Huot TJ, et al. Opposing effects of Ets and Id proteins on p16INK4a expression during cellular senescence. Nature 2001;409:1067–1070.
38. Bastian BC. The longer your telomeres, the larger your nevus? Am J Dermatopathol 2003;25:83–84.
39. Clark WH Jr, From L, Bernardino EA, Mihm MC. The histogenesis and biologic behavior of primary human malignant melanomas of the skin. Cancer Res 1969;29:705–727.
40. Reed RJ. Acral lentiginous melanoma. In: Hartmann W, Kay S, Reed RJ, eds. New Concepts in Surgical Pathology of the Skin. New York, NY:John Wiley and Sons; 1976:89–90.
41. Feibleman CE, Stoll H, Maize JC. Melanomas of the palm, sole, and nailbed: a clinicopathologic study. Cancer 1980;46:2492–2504.
42. Kuchelmeister C, Schaumburg-Lever G, Garbe C. Acral cutaneous melanoma in Caucasians: clinical features, histopathology and prognosis in 112 patients. Br J Dermatol 2000;143:275–280.
43. Harris NL, Jaffe ES, Stein H, et al. A revised European-American classification of lymphoid neoplasms: a proposal from the International Lymphoma Study Group. Blood 1994;84:1361–1392.
44. Mauro MJ, Druker BJ. STI571: targeting BCR-ABL as therapy for CML. Oncologist 2001;6:233–238.
45. Gordon KB, Thompson CT, Char DH, et al. Comparative genomic hybridization in the detection of DNA copy number abnormalities in uveal melanoma. Cancer Res 1994;54:4764–4768.
46. White VA, McNeil BK, Thiberville L, Horsman DE. Acquired homozygosity (isodisomy) of chromosome 3 during clonal evolution of a uveal melanoma: association with morphologic heterogeneity. Genes Chromosomes Cancer 1996;15:138–143.
47. Elavathil LJ, LeRiche J, Rootman J, Gallagher RP, Phillips D. Prognostic value of DNA ploidy as assessed with flow cytometry in uveal melanoma. Can J Ophthalmol 1995;30:360–365.
48. Ghazvini S, Char DH, Kroll S, Waldman FM, Pinkel D. Comparative genomic hybridization analysis of archival formalin-fixed paraffin-embedded uveal melanomas. Cancer Genet Cytogenet 1996;90:95–101.
49. Prescher G, Bornfeld N, Friedrichs W, Seeber S, Becher R. Cytogenetics of twelve cases of uveal melanoma and patterns of nonrandom anomalies and isochromosome formation. Cancer Genet Cytogenet 1995;80:40–46.
50. Coleman K, Baak JP, van Diest PJ, et al. DNA ploidy status in 84 ocular melanomas: a study of DNA quantitation in ocular melanomas by flow cytometry and automatic and interactive static image analysis. Hum Pathol 1995;26:99–105.
51. Speicher MR, Prescher G, du Manoir S, et al. Chromosomal gains and losses in uveal melanomas detected by comparative genomic hybridization. Cancer Res 1994;54:3817–3823.
52. Bastian BC, Kashani-Sabet M, Hamm H, et al. Gene amplifications characterize acral melanoma and permit the detection of occult cells in the surrounding skin. Cancer Res 2000;60:1968–1973.
53. Sauter ER, Yeo UC, Von Stemm A, et al. Cyclin D1 is a candidate oncogene in cutaneous melanoma. Cancer Res 2002;62:3200–3206.
54. Florenes VA, Faye RS, Maelandsmo GM, Nesland JM, Holm R. Levels of cyclin D1 and D3 in malignant melanoma: deregulated cyclin D3 expression is associated with poor clinical outcome in superficial melanoma. Clin Cancer Res 2000;6:3614–3620.
55. Zhang A, Zheng C, Lindvall C, et al. Frequent amplification of the telomerase reverse transcriptase gene in human tumors. Cancer Res 2000;60:6230–6235.
56. Wolfel T, Hauer M, Schneider J, et al. A p16INK4a-insensitive CDK4 mutant targeted by cytolytic T lymphocytes in a human melanoma. Science 1995;269:1281–1284.
57. Maldonado JL, Fridlyand J, Patel H, et al. Determinants of BRAF mutations in primary melanoma. J Natl Cancer Inst 2003;95:1878–1890.
58. Cohen Y, Rosenbaum E, Begum S, et al. Exon 15 BRAF mutations are uncommon in melanomas arising in nonsun-exposed sites. Clin Cancer Res 2004;10(10):3444–3447.
59. Edwards RH, Ward MR, Wu H, et al. Absence of BRAF mutations in UV-protected mucosal melanomas. J Med Genet 2004;41:270–272.

59a. Curtin JA, Fridlyand J, Kageshita T, et al. Distinct sets of genetic alterations in melanoma. N Engl J Med 2005, in press.

60. Lens MB, Dawes M, Goodacre T, Bishop JA. Excision margins in the treatment of primary cutaneous melanoma: a systematic review of randomized controlled trials comparing narrow vs wide excision. Arch Surg 2002;137:1101–1105.

61. Sherr CJ, DePinho RA. Cellular senescence: mitotic clock or culture shock? Cell 2000;102:407–410.

62. Bastian BC. Hypothesis: a role for telomere crisis in spontaneous regression of melanoma. Arch Dermatol 2003;139:667–668.

63. Ramirez RD, D'Atri S, Pagani E, et al. Progressive increase in telomerase activity from benign melanocytic conditions to malignant melanoma. Neoplasia 1999;1:42–49.

64. Greenberg RA, Chin L, Femino A, et al. Short dysfunctional telomeres impair tumorigenesis in the INK4a(delta2/3) cancer-prone mouse. Cell 1999;97:515–525.

65. Zimonjic D, Brooks MW, Popescu N, Weinberg RA, Hahn WC. Derivation of human tumor cells in vitro without widespread genomic instability. Cancer Res 2001;61:8838–8844.

12

The Multiple Roles of the Oncogenic Protein SKI in Human Malignant Melanoma

Dahu Chen, Qiushi Lin, I. Saira Mian, Jon Reed, and Estela E. Medrano

Summary

Cellular localization, association with different protein partners, and posttranslational modifications can dramatically change protein function. SKI and the highly homologous protein snoN are potent repressors of transforming growth factor-β signaling through their association with the Smad proteins. In fact, SKI can act as molecular switch converting the Smad proteins from an activating to a repressing entity on chromatin. SKI also plays additional roles in melanomas: in association with the LIM protein FHL2 activates β-catenin signaling, a pathway associated with cancer progression. This chapter reviews the transcriptional co-repressor and co-activator activities of SKI and discusses their biological significance for melanoma tumor progression.

Key Words: SnoN; Smad2; Smad3; FHL2; β-catenin; MITF.

INTRODUCTION

The protein products of the proto-oncogene *SKI* and the *SKI*-related novel gene (*sno*) are implicated in processes as diverse as differentiation and transformation *(1–4)*. Overexpression of SKI correlates with progression of melanoma *(5)* and esophageal squamous cell carcinoma *(6)*. Although SKI was believed to be a nuclear protein, melanomas display aberrant cellular trafficking of this protein *(5)*. In preinvasive melanomas *in situ*, SKI is observed predominantly in the nucleus of intraepidermal melanoma cells (Fig. 1A). However, primary invasive melanomas display both nuclear and cytoplasmic

From: *From Melanocytes to Melanoma: The Progression to Malignancy*
Edited by: V. J. Hearing and S. P. L. Leong © Humana Press Inc., Totowa, NJ

localization of SKI. In melanoma metastasis, SKI localizes to both the nuclear and cytoplasmic compartments, or predominantly to the cytoplasmic compartment (Fig. 1B,C). Interestingly, cytoplasmic SnoN is associated with poor prognosis in breast cancer (7). It remains to be established whether cytoplasmic SKI in preinvasive melanomas also has prognostic value.

Here, we review the oncogenic activities associated with overexpression of SKI and discuss possible novel activities of this protein that could lead to silencing and inactivation of tumor suppressors and repression of apoptosis.

DECONSTRUCTING SKI

Ski was originally identified as the transforming protein of Sloan Kettering Viruses (8). The ski protein family includes chicken c-ski; mouse Ski; human SKI; sno, two paralogs (skiA and skiB) in zebra fish (9), and the recently identified *Caenorhabditis elegans* homolog, Daf-5 (10). The Ski proteins were initially considered transcription factors; however, it was later demonstrated that they do not directly bind to DNA (11,12). The identification of proteins associated with SKI has been critical for unraveling its activities, which include repression of transforming growth factor-β (TGF-β) and activation of Wnt-signaling pathways (discussed in detail in "The Repressor and Activator Functions of SKI").

Structural domains located in the human SKI and mouse Ski proteins include, from the amino-terminus, a proline rich area (amino acids 61–89), helix-loop-helix motifs, a cysteine/histidine rich area, a region of basic amino acids, and a leucine zipper-like domain (Fig. 2A). The Dach domain, common to the SKI/Sno/Dachshund family of proteins, contains a putative domain of 100 amino acids that contains a conserved CLPQ motif. SKI and snoN also share a region of homology at the carboxy-terminus (13–17). Computational analysis using MARCOIL suggests that the C-terminus positions 532–710 adopt a coiled-coil conformation. However, it appears that it is not a single contiguous coiled-coil, but two to three coils separated by one to two hinge regions (Fig. 2A).

The amino-terminal residues 75–304 are sufficient for the transforming activity of c-Ski (17). Homodimerization of Ski, mediated by a bipartite C-terminal domain consisting of five tandem repeats and a leucine zipper (Fig. 2A), correlates with efficient DNA binding and cellular transformation (18). However, coexpression of c-ski and c-SnoN results in the preferential formation of heterodimers. Tethered c-ski:Sno heterodimers that lack tandem repeat/leucine zipper domains are more active in cellular transformation than either of their monomeric counterparts, tethered ski:ski homodimers or full-length SnoN and c-ski (2).

Ski transcripts are detected in the mouse embryo at 8.5 to 9.5 d *post-coitum*, during migration of neural crest cells, including melanocytes and dorsal root ganglia (19). SKI and SnoN share a large region of homology in the amino-terminus, and the biological activities of these related oncogenes appear to be similar (20). However, Ski and snoN play different roles during development. Whereas *Ski* null mice die shortly after birth, displaying defects in neurulation, craniofacial patterning, and skeletal development (21,22), mice lacking *sno* die at an early stage of embryogenesis, indicating that *sno* is required for blastocyst formation (23). Ski activities appear to be required for the expansion of a subset of precursors in the neuroepithelial and skeletal muscle lineages, because no major defects were detected in other neural crest-derived cells, including melanocytes.

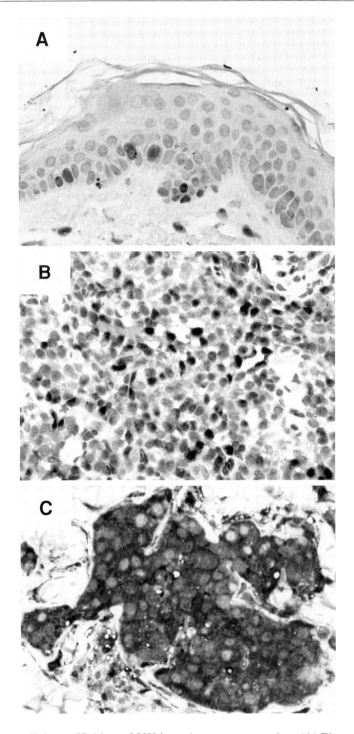

Fig. 1. Aberrant cellular trafficking of SKI in melanoma progression. **(A)** Elevated expression of SKI with predominant nuclear localization in a melanoma *in situ* (intra-epidermal malignant melanoma). **(B)** Increased levels of predominantly nuclear SKI in many (but not all) of the melanoma cells in this metastatic lesion. **(C)** Elevated, predominantly cytoplasmic, expression of SKI in a different metastatic lesion. All panels immunolabeled for SKI as described previously *(5)*; original magnification ×250.

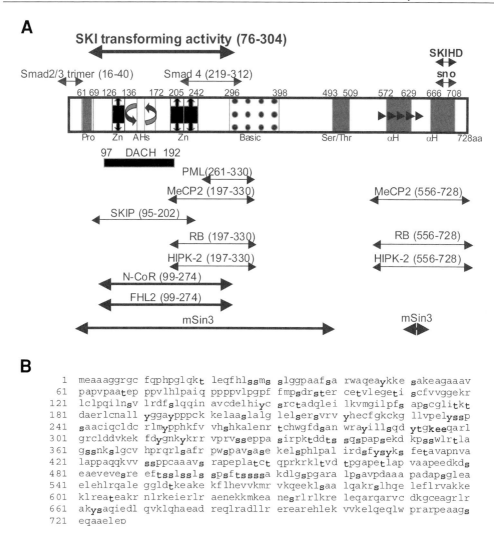

Fig. 2. The human SKI protein. **(A)** Cartoon depicting motifs and domains required for different protein–protein association. Pro, a proline rich domain; Zn, a leucine zipper-like domain; AHs, helix-loop-helix motifs; Basic, a region of basic amino acids; αH, a unique tandem repeats of α-helical domains that is involved in the dimerization of the SKI family through coiled-coil interactions. Arrowheads indicate 3 tandem repeats of 25 amino acids located at residues 572–645. SKI-HD, SKI homodimerization domain. SKI domains required for association with multiple proteins are indicated by a double arrow line. **(B)** Amino acid sequence. Serine, threonine, and tyrosine residues are indicated in bold.

ski⁻ᐟ⁻ melanocytes isolated from the skin of pups delivered by cesarian section at embryonic day 18.5 can be readily established in culture *(24)*; indicating that Ski is not essential for melanoblast migration, proliferation, or differentiation. The *ski* and *snoN* heterozygous mice are an example of as yet unexplained paradoxes regarding function of the Ski and sno proteins. When challenged with carcinogens, heterozygous *sno⁺ᐟ⁻* mice show increased number of lymphomas compared with wild-type mice *(25)*; a phenotype shared by *ski⁺ᐟ⁻* animals *(26)*. These activities apparently contradict previous data showing that Ski is a transforming protein *(18,27)*. However, Ski protein levels may be critical determinants of its function. For example, Ski is required for the transcriptional repression mediated by the retinoblastoma protein RB *(28)*; in contrast, a high level of SKI suppresses RB function. Thus, SKI could function either as a tumor suppressor or as an oncogene/tumor promoter.

Little is known regarding posttranslational modifications of the SKI protein. The chicken c-ski protein is phosphorylated on serine residues; the carboxy-terminal region is either the site of phosphorylation or is required for phosphorylation *(15)*. The human SKI protein contains multiple serines, threonines, and tyrosine residues (Fig. 1B). Computational analysis of the human SKI protein suggests that it is also a phosphoprotein, because it contains 39 serine, 7 threonine, and 2 tyrosine potential phosphorylation sites.

The human *SKI* maps to chromosome 1p36 *(29)*, a common region of alterations in human cancers, including melanomas *(30)*. Because an early study did not find alterations in *SKI* restriction enzyme patterns or increases in gene dosage in human melanoma cell lines *(31)*, its overexpression in human melanoma tissues *(5,32)* likely results from yet to be defined transcriptional and/or posttranscriptional events.

THE REPRESSOR FUNCTIONS OF SKI

The nuclear receptor co-repressor (N-CoR) protein contains a conserved bipartite nuclear receptor interaction domain (NRID) and three independent repressor domains that can actively repress a heterologous DNA-binding domain (reviewed in ref. *33*). N-CoR can interact with the Sin3 co-repressor, which, in turn, binds to the histone deacetylase (HDAC), HDAC1 *(34)*. Different HDAC proteins, including HDAC1, HDAC2, and HDAC3, are found in N-CoR complexes. HDACs deacetylate the ε-amino group of lysyl residues in histones, resulting in nonpermissive, compact heterochromatin structures.

High Levels of SKI Repress TGF-β Signaling:
A Major Pathway Involved in Tumor Progression

N-CoR plays a critical role in the transcriptional repression of some but not all SKI complexes. For example, SKI/N-CoR association is required for repression of Mad, the thyroid hormone receptor *(35)*, vitamin D receptor, and bone morphogenetic protein signaling, but not for Smad signaling *(36)*. High levels of SKI repress TGF-β signaling; a major pathway involved in tumor progression. Binding of TGF-β to its receptors initiates a signaling cascade transduced by the Smad family of transcriptional coactivators (reviewed in refs. *37–39*). Ligand-mediated receptor activation results in carboxy-terminal phosphorylation of Smad2 and Smad3, formation of heterotrimeric complexes with the common partner Smad4, nuclear translocation, and transcriptional activation of TGF-β target genes.

The GTCTAGAC sequence, which is bound by c-ski-containing proteins *(39a)*, was also identified as a Smad binding element (SBE). The Smad proteins cooperate with a diverse number of transcription factors in response to TGF-β. SBEs contain the four basepairs (5'AGAC-3' or its reverse complement 5'AGAC-3') that are directly bound by Smad3 and Smad4 proteins *(40)*. Several groups including ours demonstrated, through a variety of approaches that included affinity chromatography, GST pull-downs, and yeast two-hybrid screening *(41–43)*, that mouse Ski and human SKI associate with a multi-Smad complex that specifically bind the SBE. Nuclear SKI binds the MH2 domains of Smad2 and Smad3, forming repressor complexes that curtail TGF-β signaling in melanomas and other cell types *(32)*.

Increased levels of $p21^{Waf-1}$ appear to be essential for TGF-β-mediated inhibition of the cyclin-dependent kinase CDK2 and growth inhibition (reviewed in ref. *44*). High levels of SKI prevent $p21^{Waf-1}$ induction through a Smad-dependent mechanism that involves transcriptional repression *(5)*. Thus, elevated expression of SKI facilitates cell cycle progression by targeting the RB pathway in at least two ways: high levels can directly repress retinoblastoma protein (RB) activity, and, indirectly, increase CDK2 activity by repressing TGF-β-mediated induction of $p21^{Waf-1}$.

In turn, cytoplasmic SKI associates with Smad3 and prevents its nuclear translocation in response to TGF-β*(5)*. SKI retains Smads in the cytoplasm by the formation of Smads inactive complexes though the suppression of Smad2 phosphorylation *(45)* and association with the protein C184M *(46)*. Thus, the biological consequence of SKI/Smad interaction in the cytoplasm appears to be similar to NLS mutations in Smad3, because this mutant remains in the cytoplasm and functions as dominant-negative inhibitor of TGF-β signaling *(47)*.

High Levels of SKI Repress RB Function: A Lesion Reciprocal to $p16^{INK4a}$ Loss

RB functions as a potent repressor of genes required in the S phase of the cell cycle. The RB protein family associate via the pocket domain with mSin3-HDAC complexes containing exclusively class I HDACs. These proteins do not interact directly with RB family proteins; they use the protein RBP1 to target the pocket *(48)*. c-Ski directly interacts with RB, forming complexes containing mSin3 and HDAC. Overexpression of SKI can partially represses RB activity *(28)*. However, SKI in association with the Ski-interacting protein 1 (Skip1) can completely overcome the G1 arrest and flat cell phenotype induced by RB *(49)*. Thus, SKI can cause lesions in the RB pathway similar to deletions or mutations of the cyclin-dependent kinase inhibitor $p16^{INK4a}$, an event associated with mouse and human melanoma formation and progression (reviewed in refs. *50–52*).

The SKI Protein Is Required
for Methyl CpG-Mediated Transcriptional Repression

MeCP2, a member of the family of methyl-CpG-binding proteins, directly binds to the co-repressor mSin3, which also interacts with class I histone deacetylase, recruiting them to methyl-CpG regions to suppress transcription. c-Ski and SnoN are required for MeCP2-mediated transcriptional repression *(29)*. Recent data demonstrated that MeCP2 associates with and facilitates histone methylation at Lys9 of histone H3, a key epigenetic modification involved in gene silencing *(53)*. Increased cellular proliferation associated with high levels of SKI may be the result of enhanced methyl CpG gene silencing of growth inhibitory genes *(29)*. It has been proposed that association of MeCP2 with DNA could serve to identify novel targets of epigenetic inactivation in human cancer *(54)*. Determining whether SKI participates in such activity could help to identify global patterns of gene expression required for immortality and cellular transformation of melanoma and other tumors overexpressing SKI or snoN.

Promyelocytic Leukemia Protein Complexes

Promyelocytic leukemia protein (PML) is a critical component of the senescence response *(55)*. Overexpression of PML results in senescence of human diploid fibroblasts, which is characterized by a modest increase in p53 levels and activity, accumulation of hypophosphorylated RB and a reduced expression of E2F-dependent genes *(56)*. PML interaction with the co-repressors c-Ski, N-CoR, mSin3A, and HDAC1 is required for transcriptional repression mediated by RB. However, high levels of SKI could alter the stoichiometry of the complexes because it interacts with PML and RB through the same amino acid sequence (Fig. 2A). Altered complex composition could, in turn, lead to altered PML function. If this hypothesis were confirmed, high levels of SKI could result in lesions similar to loss of PML protein expression, which is associated with tumor grade and progression in a variety of human tumors *(57)*, and with decreased apoptosis *(58)*. Because *pml*$^{-/-}$ mice and cells are protected from apoptosis triggered by a number of stimuli, including ionizing radiation, interferon, ceramide, Fas, and TNF, repression of PML function by SKI could lead to the well-known resistance of melanoma tumors to apoptosis signals *(57)*.

THE ACTIVATOR FUNCTIONS OF SKI
IN THE WNT-SIGNALING PATHWAY

The Wnt-signaling pathway controls cell fate determination in neural crest cells, which give rise to melanocytes *(59)*. Activation of Wnt signaling involves the inhibition of β-catenin degradation by the proteasome, which results in its nuclear accumulation and transcriptional activation of LEF/TCF target genes (reviewed in refs. *60* and *61*).

Aberrant activation of β-catenin signaling by either mutations in β-catenin *(62)* or by the elevation in wild-type β-catenin nuclear content *(63)* has been linked to melanoma progression. We have recently demonstrated that SKI interacts with FHL2 *(64)*, a LIM-only protein that functions as a co-repressor or coactivator of β-catenin, depending on the promoter or cellular context *(65,66)* . LIM domains are characterized by the cysteine-rich consensus $CX2CX_{16-23}HX_2CX_2CX_2CX_{16-21}CX_{2-3}(C/H/D)$ *(67)*, and function as adapters and modifiers in protein interactions *(68)*. The FHL2-interacting domain resides within amino acids 99–274 of the SKI molecule. This same domain is required for its association with N-CoR and the transcriptional repression activities of SKI *(35)*. This suggests that distinct SKI complexes, having repressive or activating activities, may coexist in the cell, and, by targeting different promoters, diversify the functions of SKI.

SKI Is an Activator of the MITF and Nr-CAM Genes

It was recently demonstrated that β-catenin is a potent mediator of melanoma growth by mechanisms involving MITF *(68)*. MITF can target the expression of *Bcl2*, and disruption of MITF in melanoma cells induces massive apoptosis *(69)*. Thus, activation of the β-catenin pathway and MITF expression appears to be essential for growth and survival of melanoma cells. In addition, SKI and FHL2 are potent activators of Nr-CAM, a protein involved in melanoma proliferation, motility, and tumorigenicity *(70)*. Overexpression of SKI appears to be sufficient for increasing both MITF and Nr-CAM

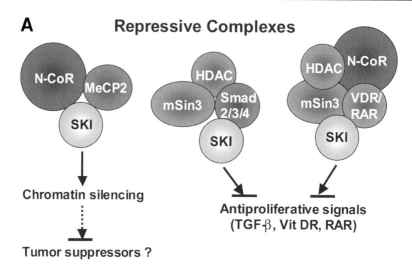

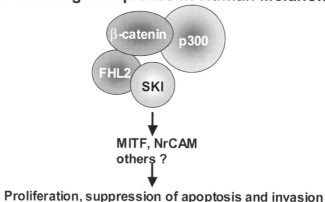

Fig. 3. The multiple functions of SKI in human melanoma. (**A**) SKI repressive complexes. SKI in association with Smad2 and Smad3 is a potent repressor of TGF-β signaling in human melanoma. (**B**) SKI in association with FHL2 is a potent activator of β-catenin.

mRNA over the basal levels. Cutaneous melanomas display nuclear expression of β-catenin *(63)*. However, in contrast with other human cancers, localization of β-catenin in melanomas does not correlate with mutations. We suggest that the nuclear accumulation of β-catenin may result from its interaction with active SKI/FHL2 complexes.

CONCLUSIONS AND PERSPECTIVES

Is SKI a Likely Target for Melanoma Therapy?

SKI is associated with a cascade of events known to increase cell cycle alterations and growth potential, invasion, and cell survival (Fig. 3). The extent of TGF-β resistance often correlates with metastatic progression *(71)*. However, TGF-β-mediated growth inhibition in melanomas can be restored by downregulation of SKI protein levels *(5)*. But will that help in vivo? Current evidence suggests that that might be the case. Melanoma tumors are known to secrete large amounts of TGF-β to the microenvironment *(72)*. In the absence of SKI, TGF-β could limit tumor growth by an autocrine mechanism, because no measurable defects at its receptors have been found in melanomas *(73)*. In addition, low levels of SKI could curtail the oncogenic activities of β-catenin by restricting its nuclear localization. In conclusion, SKI may be a valuable target in the treatment of human malignant melanoma, because it regulates two major pathways involved in cancer progression: the Wnt/β-catenin- and the TGF-β-signaling pathways.

ACKNOWLEDGMENT

Work mentioned in this review that was performed in the E.E.M. laboratory was supported by an RO-1 grant from the National Cancer Institute.

REFERENCES

1. Colmenares C, Stavnezer E. The ski oncogene induces muscle differentiation in quail embryo cells. Cell 1989;59:293–303.
2. Cohen SB, Zheng G, Heyman HC, Stavnezer E. Heterodimers of the SnoN and Ski oncoproteins form preferentially over homodimers and are more potent transforming agents. Nucleic Acids Res 1999;27:1006–1014.
3. Charge SB, Brack AS, Hughes SM. Aging-related satellite cell differentiation defect occurs prematurely after Ski-induced muscle hypertrophy. Am J Physiol Cell Physiol 2002;283:C1228–C1241.
4. He J, Tegen SB, Krawitz AR, Martin GS, Luo K. The transforming activity of Ski and SnoN is dependent on their ability to repress the activity of Smad proteins. J Biol Chem 2003;278:30,540–30,547.
5. Reed JA, Bales E, Xu W, Okan NA, Bandyopadhyay D, Medrano EE. Cytoplasmic localization of the oncogenic protein ski in human cutaneous melanomas in vivo: functional implications for transforming growth factor Beta signaling. Cancer Res 2001;61:8074–8078.
6. Fukuchi M, Nakajima M, Fukai Y, et al. Increased expression of c-Ski as a co-repressor in transforming growth factor-beta signaling correlates with progression of esophageal squamous cell carcinoma. Int J Cancer 2004;108:818–824.
7. Zhang F, Lundin M, Ristimaki A, et al. Ski-related novel protein N (SnoN), a negative controller of transforming growth factor-beta signaling, is a prognostic marker in estrogen receptor-positive breast carcinomas. Cancer Res 2003;63:5005–5010.
8. Stavnezer E, Gerhard DS, Binari RC, Balazs I. Generation of transforming viruses in cultures of chicken fibroblasts infected with an avian leukosis virus. J Virol 1981;39:920–934.
9. Kaufman CD, Martinez-Rodriguez G, Hackett PB Jr. Ectopic expression of c-ski disrupts gastrulation and neural patterning in zebrafish. Mech Dev 2000;95:147–162.
10. da Graca LS, Zimmerman KK, Mitchell MC, et al. DAF-5 is a Ski oncoprotein homolog that functions in a neuronal TGF beta pathway to regulate C. elegans dauer development. Development 2004;131:435–446.
11. Tarapore P, Richmond C, Zheng G, et al. DNA binding and transcriptional activation by the Ski oncoprotein mediated by interaction with NFI. Nucleic Acids Res 1997;25:3895–3903.
12. Nagase T, Mizuguchi G, Nomura N, Ishizaki R, Ueno Y, Ishii S. Requirement of protein co-factor for the DNA-binding function of the human ski proto-oncogene product. Nucleic Acids Res 1990;18:337–343.
13. Nagase T, Nomura N, Ishii S. Complex formation between proteins encoded by the ski gene family. J Biol Chem 1993;268:13,710–13,716.
14. Heyman HC, Stavnezer E. A carboxyl-terminal region of the ski oncoprotein mediates homodimerization as well as heterodimerization with the related protein SnoN. J Biol Chem 1994;269:26,996–27,003.
15. Sutrave P, Copeland TD, Showalter SD, Hughes SH. Characterization of chicken c-ski oncogene products expressed by retrovirus vectors. Mol Cell Biol 1990;10:3137–3144.
16. Zheng G, Blumenthal KM, Ji Y, Shardy DL, Cohen SB, Stavnezer E. High affinity dimerization by Ski involves parallel pairing of a novel bipartite alpha-helical domain. J Biol Chem 1997;272:31,855–31,864.

17. Zheng G, Teumer J, Colmenares C, Richmond C, Stavnezer E. Identification of a core functional and structural domain of the v-Ski oncoprotein responsible for both transformation and myogenesis. Oncogene 1997;15:459–471.

18. Colmenares C, Sutrave P, Hughes SH, Stavnezer E. Activation of the c-ski oncogene by overexpression. J Virol 1991;65:4929–4935.

19. Lyons GE, Micales BK, Herr MJ, et al. Protooncogene c-ski is expressed in both proliferating and postmitotic neuronal populations. Dev Dyn 1994;201:354–365.

20. Pearson-White S, Crittenden R. Proto-oncogene Sno expression, alternative isoforms and immediate early serum response. Nucleic Acids Res 1997;25:2930–2937.

21. Berk M, Desai SY, Heyman HC, Colmenares C. Mice lacking the ski proto-oncogene have defects in neurulation, craniofacial, patterning, and skeletal muscle development. Genes Dev 1997;11:2029–2039.

22. Colmenares C, Heilstedt HA, Shaffer LG, et al. Loss of the SKI proto-oncogene in individuals affected with 1p36 deletion syndrome is predicted by strain-dependent defects in Ski$^{-/-}$ mice. Nat Genet 2001;30:106–109.

23. Shinagawa T, Dong HD, Xu M, Maekawa T, Ishii S. The sno gene, which encodes a component of the histone deacetylase complex, acts as a tumor suppressor in mice. EMBO J 2000;19:2280–2291.

24. Chen D, Xu W, Bales E, et al. SKI activates Wnt/beta-catenin signaling in human melanoma. Cancer Res 2003;63:6626–6634.

25. Shinagawa T, Dong HD, Xu M, Maekawa T, Ishii S. The sno gene, which encodes a component of the histone deacetylase complex, acts as a tumor suppressor in mice. EMBO J 2000;19:2280–2291.

26. Shinagawa T, Nomura T, Colmenares C, Ohira M, Nakagawara A, Ishii S. Increased susceptibility to tumorigenesis of ski-deficient heterozygous mice. Oncogene 2001;20:8100–8108.

27. Dahl R, Kieslinger M, Beug H, Hayman MJ. Transformation of hematopoietic cells by the Ski oncoprotein involves repression of retinoic acid receptor signaling. Proc Natl Acad Sci USA 1998;95:11,187–11,192.

28. Tokitou F, Nomura T, Khan MM, et al. Viral ski inhibits retinoblastoma protein (Rb)-mediated transcriptional repression in a dominant negative fashion. J Biol Chem 1999;274:4485–4488.

29. Kokura K, Kaul SC, Wadhwa R, et al. The Ski protein family is required for MeCP2-mediated transcriptional repression. J Biol Chem 2001;276:34,115–34,121.

30. Kaghad M, Bonnet H, Yang A, et al. Monoallelically expressed gene related to p53 at 1p36, a region frequently deleted in neuroblastoma and other human cancers. Cell 1997;90:809–819.

31. Fumagalli S, Doneda L, Nomura N, Larizza L. Expression of the c-ski proto-oncogene in human melanoma cell lines. Melanoma Res 1993;3:23–27.

32. Xu W, Angelis K, Danielpour D, et al. Ski acts as a co-repressor with Smad2 and Smad3 to regulate the response to type beta transforming growth factor. Proc Natl Acad Sci USA 2000;97:5924–5929.

33. Jepsen K, Rosenfeld MG. Biological roles and mechanistic actions of co-repressor complexes. J Cell Sci 2002;115:689–698.

34. Alland L, Muhle R, Hou H Jr, et al. Role for N-CoR and histone deacetylase in Sin3-mediated transcriptional repression. Nature 1997;387:49–55.

35. Nomura T, Khan MM, Kaul SC, et al. Ski is a component of the histone deacetylase complex required for transcriptional repression by Mad and thyroid hormone receptor. Genes Dev 1999;13:412–423.

36. Ueki N, Hayman MJ. Direct interaction of Ski with either Smad3 or Smad4 is necessary and sufficient for Ski-mediated repression of transforming growth factor-beta signaling. J Biol Chem 2003;278:32,489–32,492.

37. Massague J, Chen YG. Controlling TGF-beta signaling. Genes Dev 2000;14:627–644.

38. Piek E, Heldin CH, ten Dijke P. Specificity, diversity, and regulation in TGF-beta superfamily signaling. FASEB J 1999;13:2105–2124.

39. Derynck R, Akhurst RJ, Balmain A. TGF-beta signaling in tumor suppression and cancer progression. Nat Genet 2001;29:117–129.

39a. Nicol R, Stavaezer E. Transcriptional repression by v-Ski and c-Ski mediated by a specific DNA-binding site. J Biol Chem 1998;273:3588–3597.

40. Zawel L, Dai JL, Buckhaults P, et al. Human Smad3 and Smad4 are sequence-specific transcription activators. Mol Cell 1998;1:611–617.

41. Luo K, Stroschein SL, Wang W, et al. The Ski oncoprotein interacts with the Smad proteins to repress TGFbeta signaling. Genes Dev 1999;13:2196–2206.

42. Sun Y, Liu X, Eaton EN, Lane WS, Lodish HF, Weinberg RA. Interaction of the Ski oncoprotein with Smad3 regulates TGF-beta signaling. Mol Cell 1999;4:499–509.

43. Akiyoshi S, Inoue H, Hanai J, et al. c-Ski acts as a transcriptional co-repressor in transforming growth factor-beta signaling through interaction with smads. J Biol Chem 1999;274:35,269–35,277.

44. Moustakas A, Pardali K, Gaal A, Heldin CH. Mechanisms of TGF-beta signaling in regulation of cell growth and differentiation. Immunol Lett 2002;82:85–91.

45. Prunier C, Pessah M, Ferrand N, Seo SR, Howe P, Atfi A. The oncoprotein Ski acts as an antagonist of transforming growth factor-beta signaling by suppressing Smad2 phosphorylation. J Biol Chem 2003;278:26,249–26,257.

46. Kokura K, Kim H, Shinagawa T, Khan MM, Nomura T, Ishii S. The Ski-binding protein C184M negatively regulates tumor growth factor-beta signaling by sequestering the Smad proteins in the cytoplasm. J Biol Chem 2003;278:20,133–20,139.

47. Xiao Z, Liu X, Lodish HF. Importin beta mediates nuclear translocation of Smad 3. J Biol Chem 2000;275:23,425–23,428.

48. Lai A, Kennedy BK, Barbie DA, et al. RBP1 recruits the mSIN3-histone deacetylase complex to the pocket of retinoblastoma tumor suppressor family proteins found in limited discrete regions of the nucleus at growth arrest. Mol Cell Biol 2001;21:2918–2932.

49. Prathapam T, Kuhne C, Banks L. Skip interacts with the retinoblastoma tumor suppressor and inhibits its transcriptional repression activity. Nucleic Acids Res 2002;30:5261–5268.

50. Yang FC, Merlino G, Chin L. Genetic dissection of melanoma pathways in the mouse. Semin Cancer Biol 2001;11:261–268.

51. Bardeesy N, Bastian BC, Hezel A, Pinkel D, DePinho RA, Chin L. Dual inactivation of RB and p53 pathways in RAS-induced melanomas. Mol Cell Biol 2001;21:2144–2153.

52. Tietze MK, Chin L. Murine models of malignant melanoma. Mol Med Today 2000;6:408–410.

53. Fuks F, Hurd PJ, Wolf D, Nan X, Bird AP, Kouzarides T. The methyl-CpG-binding protein MeCP2 links DNA methylation to histone methylation. J Biol Chem 2003;278:4035–4040.

54. Ballestar E, Paz MF, Valle L, et al. Methyl-CpG binding proteins identify novel sites of epigenetic inactivation in human cancer. EMBO J 2003;22:6335–6345.

55. Ferbeyre G, de Stanchina E, Querido E, Baptiste N, Prives C, Lowe SW. PML is induced by oncogenic ras and promotes premature senescence. Genes Dev 2000;14:2015–2027.

56. Mallette FA, Goumard S, Gaumont-Leclerc MF, Moiseeva O, Ferbeyre G. Human fibroblasts require the Rb family of tumor suppressors, but not p53, for PML-induced senescence. Oncogene 2004;23:91–99.

57. Gurrieri C, Capodieci P, Bernardi R, et al. Loss of the tumor suppressor PML in human cancers of multiple histologic origins. J Natl Cancer Inst 2004;96:269–279.

58. Bernardi R, Pandolfi PP. Role of PML and the PML-nuclear body in the control of programmed cell death. Oncogene 2003;22:9048–9057.

59. Dorsky RI, Moon RT, Raible DW. Control of neural crest cell fate by the Wnt signalling pathway. Nature 1998;396:370–373.

60. Conacci-Sorrell M, Zhurinsky J, Ben Ze'ev A. The cadherin-catenin adhesion system in signaling and cancer. J Clin Invest 2002;109:987–991.

61. Willert K, Nusse R. Beta-catenin: a key mediator of Wnt signaling. Curr Opin Genet Dev 1998; 8:95–102.

62. Rubinfeld B, Robbins P, El Gamil M, Albert I, Porfiri E, Polakis P. Stabilization of beta-catenin by genetic defects in melanoma cell lines. Science 1997;275:1790–1792.

63. Demunter A, Libbrecht L, Degreef H, Wolf-Peeters C, van den Oord JJ. Loss of membranous expression of beta-catenin is associated with tumor progression in cutaneous melanoma and rarely caused by exon 3 mutations. Mod Pathol 2002;15:454–461.

64. Chen D, Xu W, Bales E, et al. SKI activates Wnt/beta-catenin signaling in human melanoma. Cancer Res 2003;63:6626–6634.

65. Martin B, Schneider R, Janetzky S, et al. The LIM-only protein FHL2 interacts with {beta}-catenin and promotes differentiation of mouse myoblasts. J Cell Biol 2002;159:113–122.

66. Wei Y, Renard CA, Labalette C, et al. Identification of the LIM protein FHL2 as a coactivator of beta-catenin. J Biol Chem 2003;278:5188–5194.

67. Schmeichel KL, Beckerle MC. Molecular dissection of a LIM domain. Mol Biol Cell 1997;8:219–230.

68. Dawid IB, Breen JJ, Toyama R. LIM domains: multiple roles as adapters and functional modifiers in protein interactions. Trends Genet 1998;14:156–162.

69. McGill GG, Horstmann M, Widlund HR, et al. Bcl2 regulation by the melanocyte master regulator Mitf modulates lineage survival and melanoma cell viability. Cell 2002;109:707–718.

70. Conacci-Sorrell ME, Ben Yedidia T, Shtutman M, Feinstein E, Einat P, Ben Ze'ev A. Nr-CAM is a target gene of the beta-catenin/LEF-1 pathway in melanoma and colon cancer and its expression enhances motility and confers tumorigenesis. Genes Dev 2002;16:2058–2072.

71. Stone JG, Spirling LI, Richardson MK. The neural crest population responding to endothelin-3 in vitro includes multipotent cells. J Cell Sci 1997;110:1673–1682.

72. Shih IM, Herlyn M. Autocrine and paracrine roles for growth factors in melanoma. In Vivo 1994;8:113–123.

73. Holbrook NJ, Fornace AJ. Response to adversity: molecular control of gene activation following genotoxic stress. New Biol 1991;3:825–833.

13 RB/E2F Regulation and Dual Activity in the Melanocytic System

Ruth Halaban

CONTENTS

Summary

Retinoblastoma (RB) is a tumor suppressor that represses the expression of E2F-regulated genes required for cell cycle progression. It is inactivated in melanomas and other cancer cells by phosphorylation catalyzed by persistent cyclin-dependent kinase (CDK) activity. CDK activity is sustained in melanoma cells mostly by the elimination of the CDK inhibitor, $p16^{INK4A}$, and by high levels of cyclins, whose expression is maintained by stimuli emanating from activated cell-surface receptors and/or by mutated intracellular intermediates, such as N-Ras and B-Raf. However, RB also suppresses the expression of apoptosis genes, and its presence protects normal melanocytes from cell death. Its high expression in human melanoma cells and tumors suggests a similar positive effect on the viability of the malignant cells as well. The release and suppression of E2F transcriptional activity is likely to depend on promoter-specific RB/E2F interaction. Phosphorylated RB is displaced from cell cycle genes but not from others. In addition, RB gene repression is dependent on the nature of RB/E2F interaction and the composition of RB-bound proteins possessing specific chromatin modification activities recruited to the promoter. Deciphering the differences in RB/E2F complex formation in normal and malignant melanocytes is likely to shed light on the mechanism by which RB can exert tumor suppressing and promoting activities in this cellular system. The RB/E2F pathway provides opportunities for efficient therapy at multiple levels. Novel drugs can reactivate RB potential to suppress growth cycle-promoting genes. In addition, the high E2F transcriptional activity in melanoma cells can be exploited to deliver cytotoxic molecules specifically to tumors, sparing the normal tissues.

Key Words: Melanoma; CDK; apoptosis; chromatin modification; HDAC; DNMT; cell cycle; signal transduction.

From: *From Melanocytes to Melanoma: The Progression to Malignancy*
Edited by: V. J. Hearing and S. P. L. Leong © Humana Press Inc., Totowa, NJ

INTRODUCTION

Retinoblastoma (RB) is one of the best-characterized tumor suppressors. Its existence was postulated over three decades ago by Knudson, whose insightful observations on hereditary predisposition to RB led him to formulate the "two-hit" model for cancer development (ref. *1*, for a recent review see ref. *2*). In this model, susceptible individuals carry a germline with an inactivating RB mutation and develop cancer when subsequent mutations at one or more loci accumulate in the target somatic cell. The localization of *RB* to chromosomal band 13q14 *(3,4)*, and cloning of the gene by two independent groups *(5,6)*, launched intense investigations on the genetics, regulation, and function of this tumor suppressor. RB is now recognized to participate in the regulation of the cell cycle, senescence, developmental processes, tissue homeostasis, and responses to chemotherapy (reviewed in *7*). Its inactivation in almost every cancer has been widely documented and its intricate mode of operation and its regulation have been summarized by excellent reviews (refs. *7–13* and others cited in the text).

RB belongs to a family of proteins known as "pocket proteins," which include RB, p107, and p130 *(14,15)*. Although the three proteins have some overlapping functions, and all are inactivated in various cancer cells including melanoma (*see* for example, refs. *16,17*), RB emerged as the most relevant tumor suppressor. In this review, I will summarize briefly the prevailing concepts regarding RB function and regulation, with a focus on implications pertinent to normal melanocytes and melanoma.

TRANSCRIPTIONAL REGULATION BY RB/E2F

RB functions as a transcriptional repressor by association with other transcription factors, in particular those belonging to the E2F family *(8,18)*. Although numerous other DNA-binding proteins interact with RB (reviewed in ref. *19*), the E2F family members (E2F1–4), particularly E2F1, are the main players in mediating the RB regulatory responses *(18,20)*.

RB exerts its effect on E2F-regulated gene transcription by two independent mechanisms. It inhibits E2F transcription by physically interacting with and masking the E2F's transactivation domain (Fig. 1A,B) (reviewed in refs. *8,21,22*). In addition, it represses transcription by recruiting "chromatin remodeling factors" that suppress gene expression (Fig. 1C). RB attracts histone deacetylase (HDAC) and its repressive machinery to promoter sites *(23,24)*. Acetylation of histone 3 lysine 9 (acetH3-K9) is associated with open chromatin and transcribed genes, and deacetylation of this residue induces transcriptional repression (Fig. 1D) *(25,28)*. In addition, RB recruits histone H3 methyltransferase and members of the ATP-dependent chromatin-remodeling complex, SWI/SNF (refs. *25,28–31*; reviewed in ref. *32*). Methylation of lysine 9 (meH3-K9) is associated with inactive chromatin, whereas methylation of lysine 4 (meH3-K4) is associated with active chromatin *(33–36)*. The meH3-K9 provides a binding site for heterochromatin protein 1, an essential component of gene silencing at heterochromatin sites *(31,37)*. The *dihydrofolate reductase (DHFR)* promoter is an example of an E2F1-regulated gene that undergoes transition from an inactive hypermethylated meH3-K9 form while in the growth arrest (G0) phase of the cell cycle to an active hyperacetylated state, acetH3-K9, at the initiation of DNA synthesis (G1/S). These temporal changes are mediated by E2F associated with RB in complex with the histone methyl transferase, SUV39H1 or HDAC1, respectively *(28,29)*.

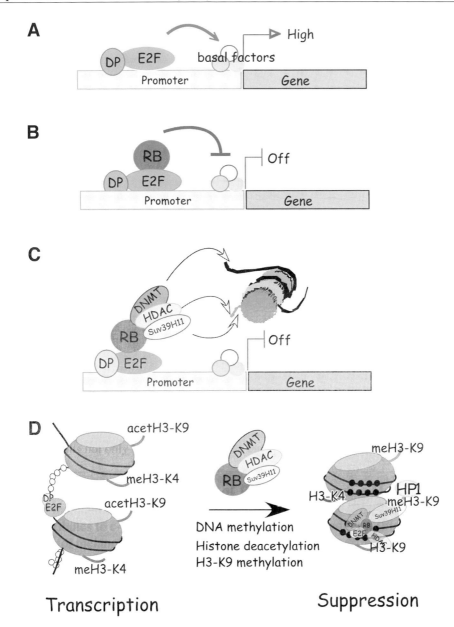

Fig. 1. Control of RB/E2F gene expression. (**A**) E2F family members in complex with dimerization partner (DP) bind consensus E2F sites in promoters of genes and promote gene expression in cooperation with the basal transcription initiation machinery (basal factors). (**B**) RB-binding blocks activation by inhibiting the interaction between the E2F activation domain and basal transcription initiation factors. (**C**) RB directly or indirectly recruits chromatin modification enzymes, such as DNA methyltransferase (DNMT), histone deacetylase (HDAC), Suv39H1, and heterochromatin protein 1, to the E2F sites, which enhances a suppressive configuration, preventing access to the basal transcription initiation machinery or other transcription factors. (**D**) Open nucleosome structure conducive for transcription is promoted by demethylation of CpG-rich sites (indicated as open circles on DNA), histone acetylation, and H3-K4 methylation. In contrast, DNA methylation (full circles on DNA), histone deacetylation, and H3-K9 methylation favors a close nucleosome structure that silences gene expression *(22,30,32,77,78)*.

RB may also mediate long-term silencing of specific genes by association with DNA methyltransferase 1 (DNMT1), enforcing a repressive chromatin state (Fig. 1D). DNMTs catalyze *de novo* methylation of DNA at the C-5 position of cytosine (5-methyl cytosine). This modification occurs almost exclusively in clusters of CpG dinucleotides surrounding the 5' ends of genes known as CpG-rich islands *(38,39)*. The presence of methylated cytosines alters the chromatin structure, and, in most cases, represses the embedded promoter by recruitment of methyl-CpG-binding domain proteins, such as MeCP1 and MeCP2 *(38)*. MeCP, in turn, silences transcription by attracting the HDAC repressive machinery *(40)*. MeCP also associates with histone methyltransferase in vivo, which methylates Lys 9 of histone H3, which further induces an inactive chromatin state (refs. *38,41*; reviewed in ref. *42*). RB association with DNMT1 represses the E2F1-responsive *p16INK4A/ARF* promoter in in vivo studies *(24,43)*. This observation, and the fact that *CDKNA/B*, the locus for *p16INK4A/ARF*, can be permanently silenced by DNA methylation in uveal *(44)* and in sporadic melanomas *(45)*, may imply the involvement of RB in this process. Furthermore, other tumor suppressor genes, genes whose protein products confer growth disadvantage, metastatic potential, or protection from DNA damage are also silenced in melanoma tumors by DNA methylation *(46,48)*. Therefore, more studies are needed to resolve the question of whether RB participates in the long-term silencing of critical genes that contribute to melanoma genesis.

REGULATION OF RB ACTIVITY

RB suppressive activity is modulated by external stimuli that trigger intracellular cascades of events that influence RB interaction with E2F transcription factors. Growth stimuli lead to release of RB from E2F by phosphorylation at specific serine and threonine sites (refs. *49,50*; reviewd in ref. *51*) (Fig. 2). On the other hand, apoptotic signals induce the dissociation of the RB/E2F complex by targeting RB to proteolytic degradation (reviewed in ref. *11*). Although much is known about RB-phosphorylation-mediated regulation, the degradation mode of control is an emerging theme (*see* page 233–234).

Hypophosphorylated RB binds to E2F and suppresses E2F-dependent gene transcription. Phosphorylation releases RB from E2F-bound promoters during the G1 (resting) phase of the cell cycle, leading to the accumulation of transcriptionally active E2F and activation of genes required for progression into the S phase *(51–53)*. A panel of serine/threonine kinases, collectively known as cyclin-dependent kinases (CDKs), coordinates the phosphorylation of RB (reviewed in refs. *12,49,54*) (Fig. 2A). Dephosphorylation is accomplished by the serine/threonine protein phosphatases PP1 and PP2A (refs. *55,56* and references within). The CDKs, mainly CDK3, CDK4, CDK6, and CDK2 are sequentially activated by their respective cyclins to allow quiescent cells to progress from the arrested/resting stages G0/G1 into DNA synthesis (S phase) (Fig. 2B).

The levels of cyclins fluctuate in response to external stimuli (Fig. 2B). CDK3 is activated by the C-type cyclin to rescue cells from growth arrest (G0); CDK4 and CDK6 are activated by the D-type cyclins (cyclins D1, D2, and D3) in early G1 phase; and CDK2 is activated by the E-type cyclins (cyclin E1 and E2) in late G1 and G1/S transition, and then by the A-type cyclins (cyclin A1 and A2) during S phase *(12,57–59)* (Fig. 2B). The latest concept is that the cyclin D/CDK4 or cyclin D/CDK6 hypophosphorylated RB binds to E2F and prevents transcription of E2F-responsive genes. Phosphorylation by

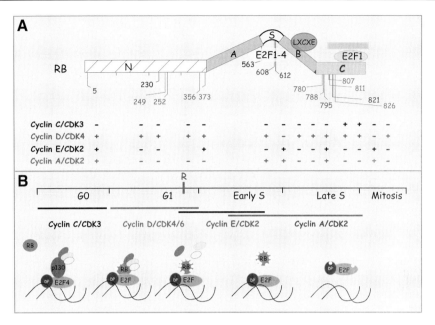

Fig. 2. RB structural/functional domains, cyclin dependent kinase (CDK) phosphorylation sites, and the cell cycle phase at which CDKs are activated. **(A)** The figure shows the N- and C-termini, the pocket A and B, and the spacer (S) domains of RB. The minimum growth-suppressive region of RB is comprised of the pocket and the C-terminus. Several amino acids in A and B constitute the high affinity-binding domain to E2F family members (E2F1–4) *(182,183)*. The additional low-affinity site specific for E2F1 is present in the C-domain *(167)*. The LXCXE domain in pocket B contains conserved Y709, K713, Y756, and R757, involved in contacting LXCXE-containing proteins, such as viral oncogenes (large T antigen, E1A, and E7), histone deacetylase, histone methyl transferase, SWI/SNF, and RF-Cp145 (reviewed in ref. *19*). The C-domain also possesses binding sites for MDM2 and C-Abl (reviewed in ref. *19*). The 16 potential serine/threonine (S/T) cyclin/CDK phosphorylation sites are located throughout the length of the protein but outside of the A/B domains. Although certain phosphorylation sites are unique for cyclin D1/CDK4 (S249/T252, T356, S790, S788, S807, and S811) and for cyclin A/CDK2 and/or cyclin E/CDK2 (S612 and T821), others are shared by several enzyme complexes *(53)*. The phosphorylation status of S230 and S563 is not yet clear. **(B)** A diagram showing the temporary activation of CDK, RB phosphorylation, and E2F association during progression from the resting state into G1, the restriction point (R) and into DNA synthesis. Only fully phosphorylated RB (RB with multiple circles) is released from E2F, allowing cells to pass R, the critical point of no return into late G1 and DNA synthesis. Cyclin A/CDK2 also phosphorylates the E2F/DP complex, freeing it from promoter sites. Notice that unphosphorylated RB is not bound to E2F in G0-arrested cells, and suppressive complexes are composed of p130 and E2F4 *(53)*. The emerging notion is that E2F4 and E2F5 are the family members that function as repressors when bound to pocket proteins, while E2F1, 2, and 3 in the unbound form act as activators of transcription *(184)*. This is an idealized diagram, because it is now recognized that phosphorylated RB may remain bound to some E2F promoters, as discussed in the text.

cyclin E/CDK2 at additional sites inactivates RB, releasing its grip on E2F, allowing transcriptional activation of cell cycle genes, such as those involved in cell cycle progression (*cyclin D1, cyclin E, cyclin A, cdc2, p107,* and *p21^{WAF1}*), DNA synthesis (*DHFR* and *DNA polymerase α*), and transcription factors (*c-MYC, c-MYB, B-MYB,* as well as *E2F1, 2, 4,* and *5*) *(21,60–64)*. Cyclin A/CDK2 complexes bind to E2F and phosphorylate both E2F and DP during the late S phase, neutralizing the DNA-binding capacity of the heterodimer, a step required for proper further cell cycle progression and to restrain the expression of tumor suppressors, such as p53, preventing the onset of apoptotic cell death *(65,66)*. Although cyclin D/CDK4 or cyclin D/CDK6 are not sufficient to inactivate RB, they are linked to cell growth by promoting directly or indirectly the activation of metabolic genes in early G1 and protecting the cells from entering G0 *(53)*. In G0-arrested cells, the unphosphorylated RB is not bound to E2F, and the major repressive complex at this phase is p130/E2F4 *(53,67)*.

CDK activity is also governed by association with the CDK kinase inhibitors (CKI) and by phosphorylation/dephosphorylation events *(68–70)*. The CKI are divided into the INK4 or WAF/KIP family based on activity and sequence homology. The INK4 family members of CKI bind to CDK4 and CDK6, preventing their association with D-type cyclins. Inactivation of INK4A is common in cancer in general and melanoma genesis in particular (*see* page 229). The CKI from the WAF/KIP family (p21^{WAF1}, p27^{KIP1}, and p57^{KIP2}) form heterotrimeric complexes with cyclin D/CDK4, cyclin D/CDK6, and cyclin E/CDK2. Although p21^{WAF1} and p27^{KIP1} inhibit all CDK4, CDK6, and CDK2 activity at high concentration, further analysis revealed that at physiological concentrations, cyclin E/CDK2 activity is inhibited, whereas complex formation between CDK4 or CDK6 and cyclin D is augmented by p27^{KIP1} and p21^{WAF1}, enhancing their kinase activity *(71–73)*. In agreement with these observations, inactivating mutations in *p16INK4A* facilitates immortalization of human melanocytes in culture but does not alter growth factor requirement *(74)*. Likewise, mouse melanocytes with targeted disruption in the *p16INK4A*, p21^{WAF1}, or *p27KIP1* became immortalized as their wild-type counterparts and did not lose their dependency on external growth factor. However, the disruption in *p21WAF1* or *p27KIP1*, but not *p16INK4A* accelerated melanocyte death in growth factor-deprived medium, suggesting that their presence protects the cells from apoptosis.

RB/E2F AND NORMAL MELANOCYTE PROLIFERATION

In vitro studies with genetically modified mouse melanocytes documented the need for E2F1 for proper proliferation. Melanocytes cultured from an E2F1-knockout mouse display repressed growth rate relative to wild-type melanocytes (Fig. 3). The population doubling time of E2F1-null melanocytes was 6–8 d, compared with approx 3 and 1.6 d for E2F1$^{+/-}$ and wild-type cells, respectively (Fig. 3). Furthermore, transgenic melanocytes expressing dominant-positive mutant E2F1 (a mutant protein that binds RB but not to E2F promoter sites), escaped the need for external growth factor (Fig. 3) *(75)*. This release from external constraints is caused by RB sequestration by the mutant protein and the accumulation of free endogenous E2F transcriptional activity *(75)*.

Probing of normal human melanocytes grown in culture revealed a role for additional RB and E2F family members in cell cycle progression (Fig. 4) *(76)*. As expected, melanocyte mitogens tightly control the phosphorylated state of RB, p107, and p130 and their interaction with E2F transcription factors. Gel shift DNA analyses demonstrated that E2F2 and E2F4 were the major unbound E2F-binding activity in proliferating early passage normal melanocytes, whereas E2F1 was hardly detected (Fig. 4). Growth arrest in response to deprivation from external growth factors was associated with decreased total E2F DNA-binding activity and the formation of mostly E2F4/p130 and some RB/

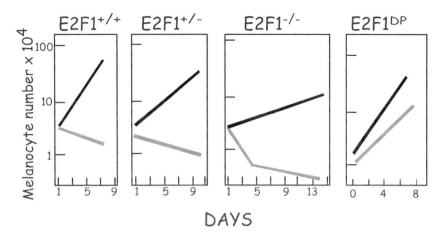

Fig. 3. Melanocyte growth properties are modulated by E2F1. The curves show the growth kinetics of melanocytes from wild-type (E2F$^{+/+}$), knockout mice heterozygous (E2F$^{+/-}$) or homozygous (E2F$^{-/-}$) for the E2F1-disrupted allele, and wild-type melanocytes expressing a dominant-positive mutant E2F1$_{E132}$ (E2F1^{DP}). Melanocytes were grown in the presence (black line) or absence (gray) of the growth stimulator 12-*O*-tetradecanoyl phorbol-13-acetate *(75)*.

E2F2 and/or RB/E2F4 suppressive complexes *(76)*. In contrast, late-passage melanocytes exposed to the growth factors displayed a "growth-arrest" pattern of E2F/DNA-binding activity, i.e., a drastic reduction in free, unbound E2F and a prominent shift toward inhibitory E2F4/p130 complex (Fig. 4) *(76)*. These data are in agreement with the general notion that E2F4/p130 are the major growth-suppressive complexes in growth-arrested cells (reviewed in ref. *77,184*). Furthermore, senescence-associated changes in heterochromatin organization of specific promoters directed by RB were recently reported in human fibroblasts *(78)*. In this case, stable p130 and RB complexes accumulated on silenced cyclin A and PCNA E2F-responsive promoters that were embedded in heterochromatin containing meH3-K9 and heterochromatin protein 1 proteins *(78)*. The persistent and stable association of inhibitory pocket protein/E2F complexes on genes required for cell proliferation can explain the unresponsiveness of senescing cells, including melanocytes, to external mitogens *(79)*.

RB/E2F AND MELANOMA

In human melanoma cells, all three RB pocket proteins are hyperphosphorylated, and several E2F family members (E2F1, E2F2, E2F3, and E2F4) are highly expressed in unbound, transcriptionally active forms even in the absence of melanocyte mitogens *(16,76,80)*. Constitutive phosphorylation by unrestrained CDK4, CDK6, and CDK2 activities is the major reason for the inactivation of pocket proteins in melanoma. Although melanoma is the most common type of second primary tumor diagnosed among retinoblastoma survivors and their families *(81–83)*, inactivation of RB by mutations is rare in sporadic tumors and melanoma-prone families *(80,84)*. The other mode of RB inactivation, through association with tumor viruses capable of inducing mouse melanoma, such as SV40 and E1a, *(85,86)*, has not been shown to be operative in human melanomas.

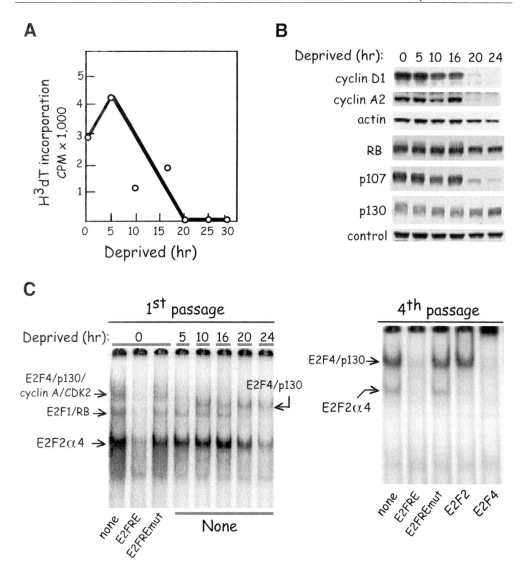

Fig. 4. Activation of RB family members in normal human melanocytes by growth factor deprivation. The figures show that starvation of first passage melanocytes induces a rapid growth arrest (**A**), and depletion of cyclin D1, cyclin A2, and p107, accompanied by the accumulation of faster migrating, underphosphorylated forms of RB and p130 (**B**). Downregulation of cyclins and p107 is likely to be in response to growth suppressive E2F4/p130, apparent within 10 h of starvation, as determined by gel-shift analysis employing double-stranded DNA encoding the E2F-responsive element in the *dihydrofolate reductase* promoter (E2FRE) (**C**, 1st passage). In contrast, E2F4/p130 suppressive complexes are present in senescing melanocytes even in the presence of growth factor (**C**, 4th passage). Notice that proliferating melanocytes display not only free E2F activity (E2F2α4), but also large protein DNA complexes composed of RB/E2F1 and E2F4/p130/cyclin A/CDK2, as determined by the addition of the respective antibodies to the gel-shift assays *(76)*. The specificity of the E2F/DNA complex formation is indicated by displacement of the radioactive probe with excess cold E2FRE but not with mutant E2FRE (E2FREmut). In the case of fourth passage cells, the assay was performed also in the presence of antibodies to E2F2 or E2F4, demonstrating suppression of free E2F2 and E2F4 DNA complexes, respectively, and a shift in the E2F4/p130 large molecular-weight aggregates. (For more details, *see* ref. *76*.)

Two complementary events lead to constitutive CDK activation in melanoma: suppression of CKI and upregulation of cyclins. Chromosome analyses followed by the identification of inherent mutations provided the initial evidence that loss of p16^{INK4A} function can contribute to melanoma initiation and/or predisposition. In melanoma tumors, the *CDKN2*A locus, encoding p16$^{INK4A/p14ARF}$ on chromosome band 9p21, is frequently deleted *(87–90)* or silenced by promoter hypermethylation *(44,45)*. Furthermore, families carrying inactivation mutations in *CDKN2A* are predisposed to develop melanoma *(83,91,92)*. The mutations in p16^{INK4A} release restraints on CDK4 or CDK6 activity because they reduce the ability of the protein to bind to and inhibit CDK4 or CDK6 *(93)*. A mirror-image germline point mutation in *CDK4* (a substitution of arginine at position 24 to cysteine, R24C) that abolishes the ability of the protein to bind p16^{INK4A} and leads to increased CDK4 kinase activity was also found, but, thus far, only in 3 melanoma families *(83,94,95)*. Interestingly, in many other types of human neoplasms, the R24C CDK4 mutation could not be detected *(96,97)*, and, thus far, no kinase-activating mutations have been identified in *CDK2 (98,99)*.

The loss or inactivation of the other two tumor suppressors on the 9p21 chromosomal region that abrogate cell cycle control, *p14AR*^{F} (an alternative splice form of p16^{INK4A}) and *INK4B* (*p15INK4A*), were also reported in melanomas. p14^{ARF} interacts with HDM2 to prevent p53 degradation. Its loss unleashes the HDM2 ubiquitination of p53, subsequent degradation of the protein by the proteasome, and loss of apoptotic signals mediated by this tumor suppressor. More than 40% of the mutations in melanoma kindred that diminish p16^{INK4A} function also impair p14^{ARF}, affecting the two independent pathways that enhance deregulated growth (*see*, for example, ref. *100*; reviewed in ref. *101*).

Knockout mice with deleted *p16^{INK4A}*, and knock-in mice expressing the CDK4 R24C allele, validate the importance of restraining CDK4 activity in melanoma genesis. These mice are susceptible to melanoma development and other cancers, particularly after carcinogenic treatments (*101–106*; reviewed in ref. *107*).

Downregulation of p27^{KIP1} also contributes to unrestricted CDK activity in melanomas. Immunohistochemistry of melanoma specimens revealed that loss of p27^{KIP1} protein expression correlated with tumor progression and was associated with worse prognosis *(108,109)*. In contrast, p21^{WAF1} is overexpressed in metastatic melanomas compared with common acquired nevi, and its upregulation was apparent already in advanced primary melanoma tumors compared with thin ones *(110,111)*. It has been suggested that p21^{WAF1} provides protection from p53-induced apoptosis thereby enhancing tumor cell survival *(112)*.

Constitutive expression of cyclins is one of the major culprits for melanoma-cell dysregulated proliferation, because loss of p16^{INK4A}, by itself, is not sufficient to alter the cell dependency on growth factors *(75)* or to induce melanomas in humans *(113)*. Cyclin D1, cyclin E, and cyclin A are maintained at high levels in cultured melanoma cells and tumors *(76,114–117)*. In some melanomas, cyclin D1 overexpression is caused by gene amplification *(118–120)*. On average, approx 10% of melanoma tumors harbor amplification of *CD1* (the locus of cyclin D1 on chromosome 11q13, previously known as *PRAD1*) *(118,120)*. However, there are significant differences in the frequency of *CD1* amplification among different melanoma subtypes. The locus is most frequently amplified in acral melanoma, a subclass that occurs on the palms and soles, as well as under the nails, areas normally protected from UV irradiation (44% of cases) *(121)*. On the other hand, 17 and 7% of lentigo maligna and superficial-spreading melanoma cases

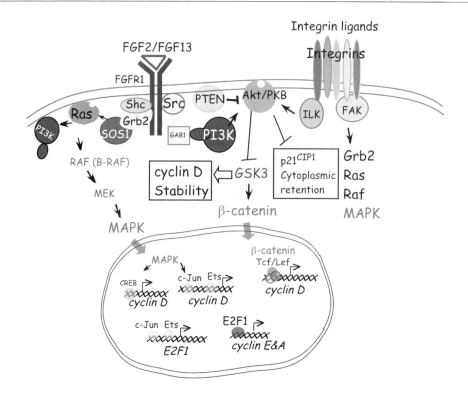

Fig. 5. A simplified diagram showing the constitutive receptor mediated signaling in melanoma cells that is likely to lead to persistent cyclin dependent kinase (CDK) activity. The figure shows the activation of fibroblast growth factor receptor 1 (FGFR1) receptor tyrosine kinase by autocrine stimulation with FGF2 and FGF13 and the activation of integrins by changes in the expression of several components as described in the text (p231). Activation of cell surface receptor lead to activation of the Ras/MAPK (mitogen-activated protein kinase), phosphatidylinositol 3-kinase (PI3K) and protein kinase B/Akt (PKB/Akt), the latter resulting in inactivation of glycogen synthase kinase 3 (GSK3) and activation of β-catenin. Consequently, the activated MAPK and β-catenin translocate to the nucleus and in turn activate transcription factors that upregulated *cyclin D* and *E2F1* gene expression (cyclic AMP responsive element binding factor known as CREB, Tcf, c-Jun, Ets and Tcf/Lef). *E2F1* in turn, activates other genes including *cyclin E*, and *cyclin A*, required for CDK activation. Inhibition of GSK3 kinase activity also leads to stabilization of cyclin D, and activation of Akt leads to cytoplasmic retention of p21[WAF1].

demonstrated *CD1* amplification, respectively, whereas no *CD1* amplification was found in nodular melanoma *(121)* or in other sporadic metastatic melanomas *(122)*. Thus far, no gene amplifications were reported in any of the other cyclins, and among the CDK, only CDK2 was reported to be overexpressed *(116,117)*.

   The wide spread overexpression of cyclin D1 and other cyclins, in the face of infrequent amplification, suggests the involvement of other mechanisms. Under normal conditions, the levels of cyclins fluctuate during the cell cycle in response to ligand-activated cell-surface receptors *(58,123)*. The major signaling pathways triggered by the receptors, the mitogen-activated protein kinase (MAPK; also known as extracellular signal-regulated kinase, or ERK) pathway (reviewed in refs. *124* and *125*), and the phosphatidylinositol 3-kinase (PI3K) pathway (reviewed in refs. *124* and *125*) (Fig. 5), are constitutively active in melanoma cells. The continuous activation of receptor tyrosine kinases, such as fibroblast growth factor receptor 1 (FGFR1) or insulin-like growth factor-1 receptor (IGF-1R), in melanomas has been well established (reviewed in refs. *16* and *114*). FGFR1 is activated by aberrant production of the protooncogene fibroblast growth factor-2 (FGF2; also known as basic FGF, bFGF) and possibly by FGF13 *(126)*. The IGF-1R, on the other hand, is self-activated by receptor overexpression *(17,127)*. The biological significance of constitutive receptor kinase activity has been validated by targeted inhibition that, in each case, led to melanoma cell growth arrest in vitro and in vivo (*17*; reviewed in refs. *16, 114,* and *128–131*). Inhibition of FGFR1 caused downregulation of cyclin D1 and cyclin D2 expression, inhibition of cyclin D/ CDK4 activity and, as a consequence, reduction of RB phosphorylation in human breast cancers *(132)*, and is likely to have a similar effect on melanoma cells.

MAPK and PI3K can be activated in melanomas also via the integrin pathway, because several components of the integrin pathway are overexpressed in a synergistic manner. These include integrins (ITGA7, ITGA4, ITGA6, ITGB3, ITGB1, and ITGA5), integrin ligands (Cyr61, TNC1, FN1, and CTGF), and integrin-linked kinase (ILK) *(126,133–137)*. ILK is a mediator of integrin signal transduction (*see*, for example, *138*), and its constitutive activity is further enhanced in melanomas by downregulation of the serine/threonine phosphatase, ILKAP *(126)*, which selectively suppresses ILK1 activity. Activation of the MAPK and PI3K increase cyclin D1 levels through protein stabilization and upregulation of gene expression, as delineated in Fig. 5.

Finally, mutational activation of signaling intermediates in the receptor-mediated cascade can serve as the driving force for increased cyclin expression. Among the intermediates activated by mutations in melanomas are N-Ras and B-RAF *(139,140*; reviewed in refs. *141–143*). The transforming ability of persistent MAPK activation was validated by its experimental manipulation. The introduction of activated Ras *(86)*, or constitutively active MAPK kinase (MEK) into immortalized melanocytes facilitated the growth of the transduced cells as tumors in nude mice *(144)*. In addition, genetically modified mice that overexpress a constitutively active receptor tyrosine kinase (Ret) *(145)*, a potent ligand for receptor kinase (HGF/SF), or activated Ras, developed melanoma tumors (*146–148*; reviewed in refs. *149* and *150*). Similarly, inhibiting MAPK signaling in melanoma cells directly or via downregulation of activated B-Raf caused growth arrest and promoted apoptosis *(151,152)*.

DUAL ROLE FOR RB

Paradoxically, active RB suppresses cell proliferation but its presence is required to maintain cell viability. This latter role of RB was first apparent in RB$^{-/-}$ mouse embryo phenotype (reviewed in refs. *11* and *64*). RB-null mice die *in utero* because of massive apoptosis in the nervous system, lens, and skeletal muscles in response to E2F1 deregulation *(153–156)*. Elegant studies by Dowdy and collaborators demonstrated a similar effect on melanocytes *(157)*. To overcome the embryonic lethality associated with RB deficiency, these investigators devised conditional ablation of RB in somatic cells by employing RB^{LoxP} mice and TAT-Cre protein delivery system. Subcutaneous injection of TAT-Cre protein into cycling hair follicles induced excision of RB exon 19 (the LoxP recombination site), followed by suppression of RB protein levels, loss of melanocytes, and depigmentation (Fig. 6A,B). Likewise, direct elimination of endogenous RB in

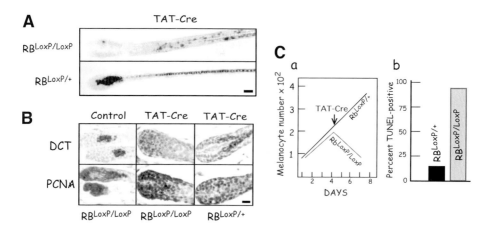

Fig. 6. RB is required to suppress apoptosis in normal melanocytes. (**A**) Nonpigmented hair shaft of TAT-Cre-treated RB[LoxP/LoxP] hair follicles compared with pigmented RB[LoxP/+] hair shaft. (**B**) Loss of melanocytes in TAT-Cre-treated RB[LoxP/LoxP] hair shaft compared with normal and RB[LoxP/+] controls, as evaluated by immunoreactivity with antibodies directed to the melanocyte-specific enzyme, dopachrome tautomerase (DCT, formerly known as TRP2). In contrast, all TAT-Cre-treated hair follicles were positive for PCNA, indicating normal follicular development. (**C**) RB acts in a melanocyte-autonomous fashion. Proliferation of cultured RB[LoxP/+] (black line) and RB[LoxP/LoxP] (gray line) primary murine melanocytes before and after treatment with a single TAT-Cre protein, arrow (**a**). Histogram showing high levels of apoptosis in RB[LoxP/LoxP] (gray column) relative to RB[LoxP/+] melanocytes in response to TAT-Cre protein, as indicated by DNA fragmentation detected by TUNEL assay (**b**). (Figures reprinted with permission from ref. *157*). Please *see* color insert following p. 430.

cultured RB[LoxP] melanocytes by TAT-Cre protein induced growth arrest and apoptotic cell death (Fig. 6C). These experiments demonstrated that RB is required for normal mouse melanocyte proliferation, and that other family members (p107 and p130) cannot substitute for RB.

A positive effect of RB on viability may be operative also in malignant cells. In contrast to what is expected from a tumor suppressor, normal, nonmutated RB is highly expressed in most cancers, including melanomas, relative to normal cells *(76,84,114,158)* (Fig. 7A). Furthermore, antisense-mediated reduction in RB levels in adenocarcinoma and myeloid leukemia cells induced growth arrest and apoptosis *(159)*. These results imply that RB can act also as a tumor promoter.

RB is present in melanoma cells in its hypophosphorylated and hyperphosphorylated forms at higher levels compared with normal melanocytes (Fig. 7A), and RB/E2F complexes are also more abundant in exponentially growing melanoma cells relative to normal melanocytes, indicating that the association between the two proteins is not compromised *(76)*. Immunofluorescent analysis with antibodies that detect the total protein (IF8) or its S608-phosphorylated form confirmed nuclear localization, the expected site of RB action (Fig. 7B). This phenotype was not restricted to melanoma cells in cultures but was also observed in melanoma tumors (Fig. 7C). Immunohistochemistry of a melanoma tissue microarray composed of approx 550 specimens showed that all patients had strong RB nuclear immunoreactivity in a large percentage of their melanoma cells (at least 50%; R. Halaban, unpublished results). Further analysis revealed

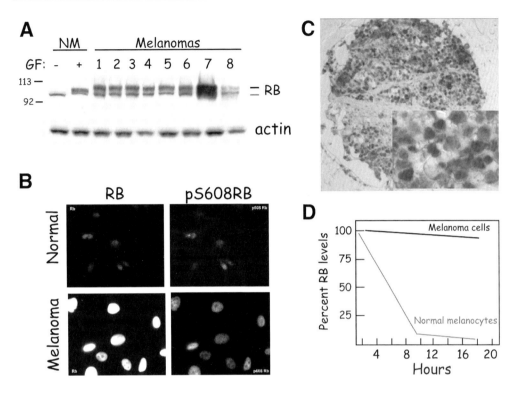

Fig. 7. RB is highly abundant in melanoma cells relative to normal melanocytes. (**A**) Western blot showing expression of RB in normal melanocytes (NM) vs melanoma cell strains from different tumors (1–8). The normal human melanocytes derived from newborn foreskins were cultured in the presence of growth factors and then shifted to growth factor-free medium for 24 h (–), or grown continuously in the presence of agents required for proliferation (+). The melanoma cells from individual donors from advanced primary (1) or metastatic lesions (7, 8) were grown without melanocyte growth factors. The cell extracts were subjected to Western blotting with anti-pRB monoclonal antibodies (IF8), and then with anti-actin rabbit polyclonal antibodies to assess protein loading in each well. Gray and black lines on the right-hand side point at the fast- and slow-migrating RB immunoreactive bands, and indicate the hypophosphorylated and hyper-phosphorylated forms, respectively. (**B**) RB nuclear localization as seen by immunofluorescence analysis of normal human melanocytes (Normal) and melanoma cells, employing RB mAb IF8, which recognizes all RB forms (RB) and phospho-specific polyclonal antibodies that recognize only the S608RB phosphorylated form (pS608RB). Courtesy of Sergio Trombetta, Cell Biology, Yale University School of Medicine. (**C**) A histospot from melanoma TMA showing RB immu-noreactivity with the monoclonal antibody, IF8. Original magnification: ×10 and ×40 (inset). Courtesy of Drs. Harriet Kluger, Mr. Aaron Berger, and Dr. David Rimm, Department of Pathol-ogy, Yale University School of Medicine. (**D**) RB stability in melanoma cells (black line) vs normal melanocytes (gray line) (curves are based on radioactive pulse-chase experiments de-scribed in ref. *76*). Please *see* color insert following p. 430.

that RB is highly stable in melanoma cells, whereas it is rapidly degraded in normal melanocytes (with a half-life of over 18 h compared with approx 4 h, respectively; Fig. 7D). The reason for RB stabilization in melanoma cells has not yet been fully investigated, but preliminary results suggest that it is mediated by persistent receptor kinase activity. Inhibition of the IGF-1R by the tyrphostin, AG1024, induced rapid proteasomal degradation of RB in melanoma cells *(17)*. These observations raise the question of whether the growth-suppressive function of RB in melanoma is compromised by the absence of cofactors, or whether active RB exerts a positive effect, as demonstrated for normal melanocytes *(157)*.

The positive effect of RB on cell viability can be mediated by transcriptional repression of a subclass of E2F-responsive genes. Studies with knockout mice demonstrated that E2F1 is required to induce apoptosis in RB-null mice, a process that was mediated by *p53* and apoptosis protease-activating factor 1 *(Apaf) (156,160,161)*. E2F1 induces the accumulation of p53 directly and indirectly, by activating *p53* and *p19AR*[F] transcription (human p14ARF), respectively. Consequently, p53 protein levels are increased in response to synthesis and stability, because of p19[ARF] inhibition of MDM2-mediated degradation. p53 is further instrumental in its own stabilization, because it also activates *p19ARF*. In addition, RB suppresses other E2F1-responsive genes whose products are involved in apoptosis, such as p21[WAF1] *(162)*; several caspase proenzymes *(163)*; and the p53-related gene, *p73 (164)*.

How can active RB enhance two opposing processes, suppression of proliferation and promotion of viability? At least three independent mechanisms have been proposed, all invoking promoter-specific regulation by active repression. In the model proposed by Chau and Wang, differential sensitivity to the phosphorylated state of RB distinguishes promoters of cell cycle genes from apoptosis genes *(11)*. CDK phosphorylation releases the repressive association of RB from E2F bound to promoters of genes during G1 to S transition, but not from promoters of apoptosis genes. Instead, degradation of RB is required to disrupt the repressive complexes at the promoters of pro-apoptosis genes, a process mediated by caspases *(11)*, or by ubiquitination and proteasomal degradation, as seen in melanoma *(17)*. Results from unbiased analysis of CpG-rich promoter occupancy experiments provide evidence that RB/E2F complexes associate with specific promoter sites in a cell cycle-regulated and -unregulated manner *(20)*. Employing RB and E2F chromatin immunoprecipitation assays combined with microarray analysis, Farnham and collaborators showed that RB occupies some promoter sites only during G0/G1 phase, some only during S phase, and others were bound constitutively by RB *(20)*. Furthermore, the use of phospho-specific RB antibodies directed at four different residues known to be substrates for CDKs (S780, S795, or S807 and S811; Fig. 2) demonstrated that phosphorylation abolished binding to some but not all target sequences. For example, phospho-RB remained bound to the β-lactamase and Myc promoters *(20)*.

In another model suggested by Fotedar et al. *(165)*, active repression of cell cycle-promoting genes and apoptotic genes is mediated by different classes of RB/LXCXE-associated proteins *(165)*. Whereas some genes, such as *cyclin E* and *DHFR*, are generally repressed by recruitment of RB/E2F1/HDAC complexes and deacetylation of histone termini *(23)*, other genes, such as *p73* (which is required for p53-independent, E2F1-induced cell death) are repressed by RB/E2F1 in association with RF-Cp145, the large subunit of replication factor C. RF-Cp145 is an ATPase, and this enzymatic activity is required to elicit RB-mediated active repression. Therefore, it is envisioned that RF-Cp145 in complex with RB/E2F induces a repressive chromatin configuration by an ATP-dependent remodeling process shown for SWI/SNF ATPase complexes *(165,166)*. This model is supported by observations that implicate HDAC repression of E2F-regulated promoters in G1 of the cell cycle and SWI/SNF in the absence of HDAC at the latter S transition (reviewed in refs. *18* and *23*). For example, RB/HDAC/SWI/SNF repressed the *cyclin E* gene, whereas RB/SWI/SNF, in the absence of HDAC, maintained repression of *cyclin A* and *CDC2 (23)*.

Finally, Dick and Dyson suggested that RB suppression of E2F1-induced apoptosis is mediated by a novel E2F1 RB C-terminus-binding domain (as indicated in Fig. 2) *(167)*. The low affinity novel domain in amino acids 792–928 of RB exclusively binds E2F1 (termed specific, or S) and not other E2F family members, and, thus, is different from the general A/B pocket site, which binds all four E2F members (E2F1–4) at high affinity (termed general, or G) *(167)* (Fig. 2). RBΔE2F-G mutant RB compromised in the A/B pocket region is a more potent suppressor of E2F1/DP1-induced cell death in response to DNA damage than wild-type RB. How RBΔE2F-G suppresses E2F1-mediated apoptosis has not yet been resolved, but one suggestion is that it does so by blocking E2F1-induced transcription of some promoters but not others *(167)*.

It is clear that cells evolved a complex mechanism to maintain a proper balance between proliferation and apoptosis, and the full details by which RB/E2F participates in this process remain to be elucidated. One has to take in account not only the nature of the RB association with E2F, but also the differences in the ability of various E2F family members to activate or repress transcription *(18,184)*. It is tempting to consider the possibility that two major imbalances exist between normal and malignant melanocytes. On one hand, there is upregulation of free E2F transcriptional activity that maintains persistent uncontrolled expression of cell cycle genes in melanoma cells. In addition, the highly expressed RB in melanoma cells relative to normal melanocytes may serve to suppress the expression of E2F-regulated apoptosis genes in a promoter-specific manner by a mechanism that remains to be determined. In support of this view, is the observation that adenovirus-mediated E2F1 gene transfer to melanoma cells induced growth inhibition, rapid loss of cell viability, and widespread apoptosis *(168,169)*.

THE RB/E2F PATHWAY AND CLINICAL IMPLICATIONS

The multiple levels by which the RB/E2F pathway is deregulated in melanoma and other cancers provide several potential targets for cancer therapy. One of the original approaches capitalizing on this pathway was to reactivate RB suppressive potential by inhibiting CDK activity. A series of potent CDK inhibitors that act by competing with ATP for binding at the CDK catalytic site have been recently identified *(170,171)*. Among this group is flavopiridol, an inhibitor of CDK1, 2, 4, and 7 that blocks cell cycle progression and induces apoptosis in several cancer cell types, including melanoma *(76 and references within)*. This agent induced progressive loss of phosphorylated forms of all three pocket proteins, RB, p107, and p130, as well as reduction in RB and p107 protein levels, and a sharp decrease in free E2F-binding activity *(76)*. However, thus far, administration of flavopiridol did not improve the clinical status of melanoma patients *(172)*.

Other approaches include targeting the aberrant signal transduction pathway that maintains RB phosphorylation and stability (*see*, for example, ref. *173*). Targeting receptor kinases can be an effective way, as demonstrated by the use of the tyrphostin, AG1024, *(17)* and the FGFR1 inhibitors mentioned on page 231. Recently, targeting Raf kinases by molecular manipulation or with a low-molecular weight inhibitor (BAY-43-9006) have shown promising results with potential for clinical application (reviewed in refs. *142* and *174*). Currently, BAY-43-9006 is under phase I/II clinical trials in combination with standard chemotherapeutics (reviewed in ref. *175*). It remains to be seen whether it will be effective in the treatment of melanomas, as was shown for another ATP analog, Gleevec (STI-571), the inhibitor of PDGF, c-Abl, c-Kit and vascular endothelial growth factor (VEGF), in the treatment of chronic myelogenous leukemia and gastrointestinal stromal tumors (reviewed in ref. *176*).

The "free" E2F can also be directly targeted with novel therapeutic approaches involving application of DNA technology. Double-stranded DNA with high affinity for E2F can serve as a decoy to bind endogenous E2F, sequester it from host promoter sites, and block the activation of genes mediating cell cycle progression (reviewed in ref. *177*). On the other hand, the abundant E2F transcriptional activity can be exploited to express cytotoxic molecules at high levels specifically in tumor cells using a gene under the E2F-responsive promoter. For example, the high E2F promoter activity in C6 glioma cells was used to express the herpes thymidine kinase gene at extremely high levels specifically in the cancer cells *(178)*. More recently, several groups constructed human adenoviruses that replicated in an E2F-dependent manner and were selectively cytotoxic to human tumor cells but not to normal cells in vitro and in vivo *(179–181)*. In these oncolytic adenoviruses, the expression of E1A, the early viral gene essential for replication, is under the control of the E2F-responsive promoter, therefore, viral particles replicate only in E2F-rich tumor cells but not in normal cells. These approaches should be evaluated in clinical trials for melanoma patients.

CONCLUSIONS AND PERSPECTIVES

RB and its 2 homologues, p107 and p130, regulate a myriad of E2F-responsive genes whose relative expression determine the course of several cellular processes, such as proliferation, differentiation, and apoptosis. All three family members are aberrantly inactivated in melanomas by phosphorylation catalyzed by persistent CDK activity. CDK activity is sustained in melanoma cells mostly by the elimination of the CDK inhibitor, p16^{INK4A}, and by high levels of cyclins, whose expression is maintained by stimuli emanating from activated cell-surface receptors and/or by mutated intracellular intermediates, such as N-Ras and B-Raf. Phosphorylation releases RB repressive activity from some, but not all, E2F-bound promoters. In melanoma cells, transcription of E2F-mediated growth-promoting genes is turned on, whereas apoptosis genes are silenced. The intricate mechanism by which RB exerts differential promoter activity is a challenge for future studies. Thus far, evidence exists that it depends on RB-specific interaction with E2F family members and association with chromatin-modifying enzymes. The high expression of RB in melanoma cells suggests that the protein performs a positive function, such as suppression of growth-arrest genes. Because RB is not permanently disabled by mutations, novel drugs can be devised to reactivate its tumor suppressive activity in melanoma. Alternatively, the high E2F transcriptional activity in melanoma cells can be exploited to deliver cytotoxic molecules specifically to tumors, sparing the normal tissues.

REFERENCES

1. Knudson AG. Mutation and cancer: statistical study of retinoblastoma. Proc Natl Acad Sci USA 1971;68:820–823.
2. Knudson AG. Hereditary cancer: two hits revisited [Review]. J Cancer Res Clin Oncol 1996;122:135–140.
3. Francke U, Kung F. Sporadic bilateral retinoblastoma and 13q- chromosomal deletion. Med Pediatr Oncol 1976;2:379–385.

4. Knudson AG Jr, Meadows AT, Nichols WW, Hill R. Chromosomal deletion and retinoblastoma. N Engl J Med 1976;295:1120–1123.

5. Friend SH, Bernards R, Rogelj S, et al. A human DNA segment with properties of the gene that predisposes to retinoblastoma and osteosarcoma. Nature 1986;323:643–646.

6. Lee WH, Bookstein R, Hong F, Young LJ, Shew JY, Lee EY. Human retinoblastoma susceptibility gene: cloning, identification, and sequence. Science 1987;235:1394–1399.

7. Liu H, Dibling B, Spike B, Dirlam A, Macleod K. New roles for the RB tumor suppressor protein. Curr Opin Genet Dev 2004;14:55–64.

8. Nevins JR. The RB/E2F pathway and cancer. Hum Mol Genet 2001;10:699–703.

9. Ben-Porath I, Weinberg RA. When cells get stressed: an integrative view of cellular senescence. J Clin Invest 2004;113:8–13.

10. Fan G, Steer CJ. The role of retinoblastoma protein in apoptosis. Apoptosis 1999;4:21–29.

11. Chau BN, Wang JY. Coordinated regulation of life and death by RB. Nat Rev Cancer 2003;3:130–138.

12. Malumbres M, Hunt SL, Sotillo R, et al. Driving the cell cycle to cancer. Adv Exp Med Biol 2003;532:1–11.

13. Sherr CJ. Principles of tumor suppression. Cell 2004;116:235–246.

14. Tonini T, Hillson C, Claudio PP. Interview with the retinoblastoma family members: do they help each other? J Cell Physiol 2002;192:138–150.

15. Classon M, Harlow E. The retinoblastoma tumour suppressor in development and cancer. Nat Rev Cancer 2002;2:910–917.

16. Halaban R, Miglarese MR, Smicun Y, Puig S. Melanomas, from the cell cycle point of view (Review). Int J Mol Med 1998;1:419–425.

17. von Willebrand M, Zacksenhaus E, Cheng E, Glazer P, Halaban R. The tyrphostin AG1024 accelerates the degradation of phosphorylated forms of retinoblastoma protein (pRB) and restores pRB tumor suppressive function in melanoma cells. Cancer Res 2003;63:1420–1429.

18. Frolov MV, Dyson NJ. Molecular mechanisms of E2F-dependent activation and pRB-mediated repression. J Cell Sci 2004;117:2173–2181.

19. Morris EJ, Dyson NJ. Retinoblastoma protein partners. Adv Cancer Res 2001;82:1–54.

20. Wells J, Yan PS, Cechvala M, Huang T, Farnham PJ. Identification of novel pRB binding sites using CpG microarrays suggests that E2F recruits pRB to specific genomic sites during S phase. Oncogene 2003;22:1445–1460.

21. Nevins JR. Toward an understanding of the functional complexity of the E2F and retinoblastoma families. Cell Growth Diff 1998;9:585–593.

22. Kaelin WG Jr. Functions of the retinoblastoma protein. Bioessays 1999;21:950–958.

23. Zhang HS, Gavin M, Dahiya A, et al. Exit from G1 and S phase of the cell cycle is regulated by repressor complexes containing HDAC-RB-hSWI/SNF and RB-hSWI/SNF. Cell 2000;101:79–89.

24. Robertson KD, Ait-Si-Ali S, Yokochi T, Wade PA, Jones PL, Wolffe AP. DNMT1 forms a complex with RB, E2F1 and HDAC1 and represses transcription from E2F-responsive promoters. Nat Genet 2000;25:338–342.

25. Brehm A, Miska EA, McCance DJ, Reid JL, Bannister AJ, Kouzarides T. Retinoblastoma protein recruits histone deacetylase to repress transcription. Nature 1998;391:597–601.

26. Magnaghi-Jaulin L, Groisman R, Naguibneva I, et al. Retinoblastoma protein represses transcription by recruiting a histone deacetylase. Nature 1998;391:601–605.

27. Luo RX, Postigo AA, Dean DC. RB interacts with histone deacetylase to repress transcription. Cell 1998;92:463–473.

28. Nicolas E, Roumillac C, Trouche D. Balance between acetylation and methylation of histone H3 Lysine 9 on the E2F-responsive dihydrofolate reductase promoter. Mol Cell Biol 2003;23:1614–1622.

29. Vaute O, Nicolas E, Vandel L, Trouche D. Functional and physical interaction between the histone methyl transferase Suv39H1 and histone deacetylases. Nucleic Acids Res 2002;30:475–481.

30. Vandel L, Nicolas E, Vaute O, Ferreira R, Ait-Si-Ali S, Trouche D. Transcriptional repression by the retinoblastoma protein through the recruitment of a histone methyltransferase. Mol Cell Biol 2001;21:6484–6494.

31. Nielsen SJ, Schneider R, Bauer UM, et al. RB targets histone H3 methylation and HP1 to promoters. Nature 2001;412:561–565.

32. Ferreira R, Naguibneva I, Pritchard LL, Ait-Si-Ali S, Harel-Bellan A. The RB/chromatin connection and epigenetic control: opinion. Oncogene 2001;20:3128–3133.

33. Bernstein BE, Humphrey EL, Erlich RL, et al. Methylation of histone H3 Lys 4 in coding regions of active genes. Proc Natl Acad Sci U S A 2002;99:8695–8700.

34. Varga-Weisz PD, Dalgaard JZ. A mark in the core: silence no more! Mol Cell 2002;9:1154–1156.
35. Lachner M, Jenuwein T. The many faces of histone lysine methylation. Curr Opin Cell Biol 2002;14:286–298.
36. Heard E, Rougeulle C, Arnaud D, Avner P, Allis CD, Spector DL. Methylation of histone H3 at Lys-9 is an early mark on the X chromosome during X inactivation. Cell 2001;107:727–738.
37. Yamamoto K, Sonoda M. Self-interaction of heterochromatin protein 1 is required for direct binding to histone methyltransferase, SUV39H1. Biochem Biophys Res Commun 2003;301:287–292.
38. Bird A. DNA methylation patterns and epigenetic memory. Genes Dev 2002;16:6–21.
39. Costello JF, Plass C. Methylation matters. J Med Genet 2001;38:285–303.
40. Nan X, Ng HH, Johnson CA, et al. Transcriptional repression by the methyl-CpG-binding protein MeCP2 involves a histone deacetylase complex. Nature 1998;393:386–389.
41. Fuks F, Hurd PJ, Wolf D, Nan X, Bird AP, Kouzarides T. The methyl-CpG-binding protein MeCP2 links DNA methylation to histone methylation. J Biol Chem 2003;278:4035–4040.
42. Jones PA, Baylin SB. The fundamental role of epigenetic events in cancer. Nat Rev Genet 2002; 3:415–428.
43. Pradhan S, Kim GD. The retinoblastoma gene product interacts with maintenance human DNA (cytosine-5) methyltransferase and modulates its activity. EMBO J 2002;21:779–788.
44. van der Velden PA, Metzelaar-Blok JA, Bergman W, et al. Promoter hypermethylation: a common cause of reduced p16^{INK4a} expression in uveal melanoma. Cancer Res 2001;61:5303–5306.
45. Gonzalgo ML, Bender CM, You EH, et al. Low frequency of p16/CDKN2A methylation in sporadic melanoma: comparative approaches for methylation analysis of primary tumors. Cancer Res 1997;57:5336–5347.
46. Hoon DS, Spugnardi M, Kuo C, Huang SK, Morton DL, Taback B. Profiling epigenetic inactivation of tumor suppressor genes in tumors and plasma from cutaneous melanoma patients. Oncogene 2004;23:4014–4022.
47. Worm J, Bartkova J, Kirkin AF, et al. Aberrant p27Kip1 promoter methylation in malignant melanoma. Oncogene 2000;19:5111–5115.
48. Zhang H, Schneider J, Rosdahl I. Expression of p16, p27, p53, p73 and Nup88 proteins in matched primary and metastatic melanoma cells. Int J Oncol 2002;21:43–48.
49. Lundberg AS, Weinberg RA. Functional inactivation of the retinoblastoma protein requires sequential modification by at least two distinct cyclin-cdk complexes. Mol Cell Biol 1998;18:753–761.
50. Brown VD, Phillips RA, Gallie BL. Cumulative effect of phosphorylation of pRB on regulation of E2F activity. Mol Cell Biol 1999;19:3246–3256.
51. Mittnacht S. Control of pRB phosphorylation. Curr Opin Genet Dev 1998;8:21–27.
52. Adams PD. Regulation of the retinoblastoma tumor suppressor protein by cyclin/cdks. Biochim Biophys Acta 2001;1471:M123–133.
53. Ezhevsky SA, Ho A, Becker-Hapak M, Davis PK, Dowdy SF. Differential regulation of retinoblastoma tumor suppressor protein by G$_1$ cyclin-dependent kinase complexes in vivo. Mol Cell Biol 2001;21:4773–4784.
54. Connell-Crowley L, Harper JW, Goodrich DW. Cyclin D1/Cdk4 regulates retinoblastoma protein-mediated cell cycle arrest by site-specific phosphorylation. Mol Biol Cell 1997;8:287–301.
55. Tamrakar S, Rubin E, Ludlow JW. Role of pRB dephosphorylation in cell cycle regulation. Front Biosci 2000;1:D121–137.
56. Rubin E, Mittnacht S, Villa-Moruzzi E, Ludlow JW. Site-specific and temporally-regulated retinoblastoma protein dephosphorylation by protein phosphatase type 1. Oncogene 2001;20:3776–3785.
57. Sherr CJ. D-type cyclins. Trends Biochem Sci 1995;20:187–190.
58. Sherr CJ. Cancer cell cycles. Science 1996;274:1672–1677.
59. Malumbres M, Barbacid M. To cycle or not to cycle: a critical decision in cancer. Nat Rev Cancer 2001;1:222–231.
60. Jacks T, Weinberg RA. Cell-cycle control and its watchman. Nature 1996;381:643–644.
61. Grana X, Garriga J, Mayol X. Role of the retinoblastoma protein family, pRB, p107 and p130 in the negative control of cell growth. Oncogene 1998;17:3365–3383.
62. Johnson DG, Schneider-Broussard R. Role of E2F in cell cycle control and cancer. Front Biosci 1998;27:d447–448.
63. Hiyama H, Iavarone A, Reeves SA. Regulation of the CDK inhibitor p21 gene during cell cycle progression is under the control of the transcription factor E2F. Oncogene 1998;16:1513–1523.
64. Lipinski MM, Jacks T. The retinoblastoma gene family in differentiation and development. Oncogene 1999;18:7873–7882.

65. Krek W, Xu G, Livingston DM. Cyclin A-kinase regulation of E2F-1 DNA binding function underlies suppression of an S phase checkpoint. Cell 1995;83:1149–1158.
66. Xu M, Sheppard KA, Peng CY, Yee AS, Piwnica-Worms H. Cyclin A/CDK2 binds directly to E2F-1 and inhibits the DNA-binding activity of E2F-1/DP-1 by phosphorylation. Mol Cell Biol 1994;14:8420–8431.
67. Trimarchi JM, Lees JA. Sibling rivalry in the E2F family. Nat Rev Mol Cell Biol 2002;3:11–20.
68. Sherr CJ, Roberts JM. CDK inhibitors: positive and negative regulators of G1-phase progression. Genes Dev 1999;13:1501–1512.
69. Murray AW. Recycling the cell cycle: cyclins revisited. Cell 2004;116:221–234.
70. Lee MH, Yang HY. Negative regulators of cyclin-dependent kinases and their roles in cancers. Cell Mol Life Sci 2001;58:1907–1922.
71. Blain SW, Montalvo E, Massagué J. Differential interaction of the cyclin-dependent kinase (Cdk) inhibitor p27^{Kip1} with cyclin A-Cdk2 and cyclin D2-Cdk4. J Biol Chem 1997;272:25,863–25,872.
72. LaBaer J, Garrett MD, Stevenson LF, et al. New functional activities for the p21 family of CDK inhibitors. Genes Dev 1997;11:847–862.
73. Cheng M, Olivier P, Diehl JA, et al. The p21^{Cip1} and p27^{Kip1} CDK 'inhibitors' are essential activators of cyclin D-dependent kinases in murine fibroblasts. EMBO J 1999;18:1571–1583.
74. Sviderskaya EV, Hill SP, Evans-Whipp TJ, et al. p16^{Ink4a} in melanocyte senescence and differentiation. J Natl Cancer Inst 2002;94:446–454.
75. Halaban R, Cheng E, Zhang Y, Mandigo CE, Miglarese MR. Release of cell cycle constraints in mouse melanocytes by overexpressed mutant E2F1$_{E132}$, but not by deletion of p16^{INK4A} or p21$^{WAF1/CIP1}$. Oncogene 1998;16:2489–2501.
76. Halaban R, Cheng E, Smicun Y, Germino J. Deregulated E2F transcriptional activity in autonomously growing melanoma cells. J Exp Med 2000;191:1005–1015.
77. Cam H, Dynlacht BD. Emerging roles for E2F: Beyond the G1/S transition and DNA replication. Cancer Cell 2003;3:311–316.
78. Narita M, Nunez S, Heard E, et al. RB-mediated heterochromatin formation and silencing of E2F target genes during cellular senescence. Cell 2003;113:703–716.
79. Bennett DC, Medrano EE. Molecular regulation of melanocyte senescence. Pigm Cell Res 2002;15:242–250.
80. Bartkova J, Lukas J, Guldberg P, et al. The p16-cyclin D/Cdk4-pRB pathway as a functional unit frequently altered in melanoma pathogenesis. Cancer Res 1996;56:5475–5483.
81. Bataille V, Hiles R, Bishop JA. Retinoblastoma, melanoma and the atypical mole syndrome. Br J Dermatol 1995;132:134–138.
82. Moll AC, Imhof SM, Bouter LM, Tan KE. Second primary tumors in patients with retinoblastoma. A review of the literature. Ophthalmic Genet 1997;18:27–34.
83. Kefford RF, Newton Bishop JA, Bergman W, Tucker MA. Counseling and DNA testing for individuals perceived to be genetically predisposed to melanoma: a consensus statement of the Melanoma Genetics Consortium. J Clin Oncol 1999;17:3245–3251.
84. Horowitz JM, Park S-H, Bogenman E, et al. Frequent inactivation of the retinoblastoma anti-oncogene is restricted to a subset of human tumor cells. Proc Natl Acad Sci USA 1990;87:2775–2779.
85. Mintz B, Silvers WK. Transgenic mouse model of malignant skin melanoma. Proc Natl Acad Sci USA 1993;90:8817–8821.
86. Dotto GP, Moellmann G, Ghosh S, Edwards M, Halaban R. Transformation of murine melanocytes by basic fibroblast growth factor cDNA and oncogenes and selective suppression of the transformed phenotype in a reconstituted cutaneous environment. J Cell Biol 1989;109:3115–3128.
87. Cowan JM, Halaban R, Francke U. Cytogenetic analysis of melanocytes from premalignant nevi and melanomas. J Natl Cancer Inst 1988;80:1159–1164.
88. Kamb A, Gruis NA, Weaver-Feldhaus J, et al. A cell cycle regulator potentially involved in genesis of many tumor types. Science 1994;264:436–440.
89. Kamb A, Shattuck-Eidens D, Eeles R, et al. Analysis of the p16 gene (CDKN2) as a candidate for the chromosome 9p melanoma susceptibility locus. Nat Genet 1994;8:23–26.
90. Dracopoli NC, Fountain JW. CDKN2 mutations in melanoma. Cancer Surv 1996;26:115–132.
91. Chaudru V, Chompret A, Bressac-de Paillerets B, Spatz A, Avril MF, Demenais F. Influence of genes, nevi, and sun sensitivity on melanoma risk in a family sample unselected by family history and in melanoma-prone families. J Natl Cancer Inst 2004;96:785–795.
92. Tucker MA, Goldstein AM. Melanoma etiology: where are we? Oncogene 2003;22:3042–3052.
93. Russo AA, Tong L, Lee JO, Jeffrey PD, Pavletich NP. Structural basis for inhibition of the cyclin-dependent kinase Cdk6 by the tumour suppressor p16INK4a. Nature 1998;395:237–243.

94. Wolfel T, Hauer M, Schneider J, et al. A p16[INK4a]-insensitive CDK4 mutant targeted by cytolytic T lymphocytes in a human melanoma. Science 1995;269:1281–1284.

95. Zuo L, Weger J, Yang Q, et al. Germline mutations in the p16[INK4a] binding domain of CDK4 in familial melanoma. Nat Genet 1996;12:97–99.

96. Vax VV, Bibi R, Diaz-Cano S, et al. Activating point mutations in cyclin-dependent kinase 4 are not seen in sporadic pituitary adenomas, insulinomas or Leydig cell tumours. J Endocrinol 2003;178:301–310.

97. Mori N, Yang R, Kawamata N, Miller CW, Mizoguchi H, Koeffler HP. Absence of R24C mutation of the CDK4 gene in leukemias and solid tumors. Int J Hematol 2003;77:259–262.

98. Flores JS, Pollock PM, Walker GJ, et al. Analysis of the CDKN2A, CDKN2B and CDK4 genes in 48 Australian melanoma kindreds. Oncogene 1997;15:2999–3005.

99. Walker G, Hayward N. No evidence of a role for activating CDK2 mutations in melanoma. Melanoma Res 2001;11:343–348.

100. Rizos H, Darmanian AP, Holland EA, Mann GJ, Kefford RF. Mutations in the INK4a/ARF melanoma susceptibility locus functionally impair p14[ARF]. J Biol Chem 2001;276: 41,424–41,434.

101. Sharpless E, Chin L. The INK4a/ARF locus and melanoma. Oncogene 2003;22:3092–3098.

102. Sotillo R, Garcia JF, Ortega S, et al. Invasive melanoma in Cdk4-targeted mice. Proc Natl Acad Sci USA 2001;98:13,312–13,317.

103. Sharpless NE, Bardeesy N, Lee KH, et al. Loss of p16[Ink4a] with retention of p19[Arf] predisposes mice to tumorigenesis. Nature 2001;413:86–91.

104. Krimpenfort P, Quon KC, Mooi WJ, Loonstra A, Berns A. Loss of p16Ink4a confers susceptibility to metastatic melanoma in mice. Nature 2001;413:83–86.

105. Rane SG, Cosenza SC, Mettus RV, Reddy EP. Germ line transmission of the Cdk4(R24C) mutation facilitates tumorigenesis and escape from cellular senescence. Mol Cell Biol 2002;22:644–656.

106. Sotillo R, Dubus P, Martin J, et al. Wide spectrum of tumors in knock-in mice carrying a Cdk4 protein insensitive to INK4 inhibitors. EMBO J 2001;20:6637–6647.

107. Ortega S, Malumbres M, Barbacid M. Cyclin D-dependent kinases, INK4 inhibitors and cancer. Biochim Biophys Acta 2002;1602:73–87.

108. Woenckhaus C, Fenic I, Giebel J, et al. Loss of heterozygosity at 12p13 and loss of p27KIP1 protein expression contribute to melanoma progression. Virchows Arch 2004;445: 491–497.

109. Florenes VA, Maelandsmo GM, Kerbel RS, Slingerland JM, Nesland JM, Holm R. Protein expression of the cell-cycle inhibitor p27Kip1 in malignant melanoma: inverse correlation with disease-free survival. Am J Pathol 1998;153:305–312.

110. Maelandsmo GM, Holm R, Fodstad O, Kerbel RS, Florenes VA. Cyclin kinase inhibitor p21[WAF1/CIP1] in malignant melanoma: reduced expression in metastatic lesions. Am J Pathol 1996;149:1813–1822.

111. Trotter MJ, Tang L, Tron VA. Overexpression of the cyclin-dependent kinase inhibitor p21[WAF1/CIP1] in human cutaneous malignant melanoma. J Cutan Pathol 1997;24:265–271.

112. Gorospe M, Cirielli C, Wang X, Seth P, Capogrossi MC, Holbrook NJ. p21[Waf1/Cip1] protects against p53-mediated apoptosis of human melanoma cells. Oncogene 1997;14:929–935.

113. Kamb A. Cyclin-dependent kinase inhibitors and human cancer. Cur Top Microbiol Immunol 1998;227:139–148.

114. Halaban R. Melanoma cell autonomous growth: the RB/E2F pathway. Cancer Metastasis Rev 1999;8:333–343.

115. Bales ES, Dietrich C, Bandyopadhyay D, et al. High levels of expression of p27KIP1 and cyclin E in invasive primary malignant melanomas. J Invest Dermatol 1999;113:1039–1046.

116. Tang L, Li G, Tron VA, Trotter MJ, Ho VC. Expression of cell cycle regulators in human cutaneous malignant melanoma. Melanoma Res 1999;9:148–154.

117. Georgicva J, Sinha P, Schadendorf D. Expression of cyclins and cyclin dependent kinases in human benign and malignant melanocytic lesions. J Clin Pathol 2001;54:229–235.

118. Halaban R, Funasaka Y, Lee P, Rubin J, Ron D, Birnbaum D. Fibroblast growth factors in normal and malignant melanocytes. Ann NY Acad Sci 1991;638:232–243.

119. Bastian BC, LeBoit PE, Hamm H, Brocker EB, Pinkel D. Chromosomal gains and losses in primary cutaneous melanomas detected by comparative genomic hybridization. Cancer Res 1998;58: 2170–2175.

120. Gaudray P, Szepetowski P, Escot C, Birnbaum D, Theillet C. DNA amplification at 11q13 in human cancer: from complexity to perplexity. Mutat Res 1992;276:317–328.

121. Sauter ER, Yeo UC, von Stemm A, et al. Cyclin D1 is a candidate oncogene in cutaneous melanoma. Cancer Res 2002;62:3200–3206.

122. Maelandsmo GM, Florenes VA, Hovig E, et al. Involvement of the pRB/p16/cdk4/cyclin D1 pathway in the tumorigenesis of sporadic malignant melanomas. Br J Cancer 1996;73:909–916.

123. Sherr CJ, Weber JD. The ARF/p53 pathway. Curr Opin Genet Dev 2000;10:94–99.

124. Pearson G, Robinson F, Beers Gibson T, et al. Mitogen-activated protein (MAP) kinase pathways: regulation and physiological functions. Endocr Rev 2001;22:153–183.

125. Raman M, Cobb MH. MAP kinase modules: many roads home. Curr Biol 2003;13:R886–888.

126. Hoek K, Rimm DL, Williams KR, et al. Expression profiling reveals novel pathways in the transformation of melanocytes to melanomas. Cancer Res 2004;64:5270–5282.

127. Quong RY, Bickford ST, Ing YL, Terman B, Herlyn M, Lassam NJ. Protein kinases in normal and transformed melanocytes. Melanoma Res 1994;4:313–319.

128. Becker D, Lee PL, Rodeck U, Herlyn M. Inhibition of the fibroblast growth factor receptor 1 (FGFR-1) gene in human melanocytes and malignant melanomas leads to inhibition of proliferation and signs indicative of differentiation. Oncogene 1992;7:2303–2313.

129. Wang Y, Becker D. Antisense targeting of basic fibroblast growth factor and fibroblast growth factor receptor-1 in human melanomas blocks intratumoral angiogenesis and tumor growth. Nature Med 1997;3:887–893.

130. Ozen M, Medrano EE, Ittmann M. Inhibition of proliferation and survival of melanoma cells by adenoviral-mediated expression of dominant negative fibroblast growth factor receptor. Melanoma Res 2004;14:13–21.

131. Yayon A, Ma YS, Safran M, Klagsbrun M, Halaban R. Suppression of autocrine cell proliferation and tumorigenesis of human melanoma cells and fibroblast growth factor transformed fibroblasts by a kinase-deficient FGF receptor 1: evidence for the involvement of Src- family kinases. Oncogene 1997;14:2999–3009.

132. Koziczak M, Holbro T, Hynes NE. Blocking of FGFR signaling inhibits breast cancer cell proliferation through downregulation of D-type cyclins. Oncogene 2004;23:3501–3508.

133. Leung-Hagesteijn C, Mahendra A, Naruszewicz I, Hannigan GE. Modulation of integrin signal transduction by ILKAP, a protein phosphatase 2C associating with the integrin-linked kinase, ILK1. EMBO J 2001;20:2160–2170.

134. Trikha M, Timar J, Lundy SK, et al. The high affinity alphaIIb beta3 integrin is involved in invasion of human melanoma cells. Cancer Res 1997;57:2522–2528.

135. Dai DL, Makretsov N, Campos EI, et al. Increased expression of integrin-linked kinase is correlated with melanoma progression and poor patient survival. Clin Cancer Res 2003;9:4409–4414.

136. Seftor RE, Seftor EA, Hendrix MJ. Molecular role(s) for integrins in human melanoma invasion. Cancer Metastasis Rev 1999;18:359–375.

137. Van Belle PA, Elenitsas R, Satyamoorthy K, et al. Progression-related expression of beta3 integrin in melanomas and nevi. Hum Pathol 1999;30:562–567.

138. Tan C, Cruet-Hennequart S, Troussard A, et al. Regulation of tumor angiogenesis by integrin-linked kinase (ILK). Cancer Cell 2004;5:79–90.

139. Alsina J, Gorsk DH, Germino FJ, et al. Detection of mutations in the mitogen-activated protein kinase pathway in human melanoma. Clin Cancer Res 2003;9:6419–6425.

140. Calipel A, Lefevre G, Pouponnot C, Mouriaux F, Eychene A, Mascarelli F. Mutation of B-Raf in human choroidal melanoma cells mediates cell proliferation and transformation through the MEK/ERK pathway. J Biol Chem 2003;278:42,409–42,418.

141. Mercer KE, Pritchard CA. Raf proteins and cancer: B-Raf is identified as a mutational target. Biochim Biophys Acta 2003;1653:25–40.

142. Tuveson DA, Weber BL, Herlyn M. BRAF as a potential therapeutic target in melanoma and other malignancies. Cancer Cell 2003;4:95–98.

143. Wan PT, Garnett MJ, Roe SM, et al. Mechanism of activation of the RAF-ERK signaling pathway by oncogenic mutations of B-RAF. Cell 2004;116:855–867.

144. Govindarajan B, Bai X, Cohen C, et al. Malignant transformation of melanocytes to melanoma by constitutive activation of mitogen-activated protein kinase kinase (MAPKK) signaling. J Biol Chem 2003;278:9790–9795.

145. Kato M, Liu W, Akhand AA, et al. Linkage between melanocytic tumor development and early burst of Ret protein expression for tolerance induction in metallothionein-I/ret transgenic mouse lines. Oncogene 1999;18:837–842.

146. Noonan FP, Recio JA, Takayama H, et al. Neonatal sunburn and melanoma in mice. Nature 2001;413:271–272.

147. Bardeesy N, Bastian BC, Hezel A, Pinkel D, DePinho RA, Chin L. Dual inactivation of RB and p53 pathways in RAS-induced melanomas. Mol Cell Biol 2001;21:2144–2153.

148. Kannan K, Sharpless NE, Xu J, O'Hagan RC, Bosenberg M, Chin L. Components of the RB pathway are critical targets of UV mutagenesis in a murine melanoma model. Proc Natl Acad Sci USA 2003;100:1221–1225.

149. Chin L. The genetics of malignant melanoma: lessons from mouse and man. Nat Rev Cancer 2003;3:559–570.

150. Yang FC, Merlino G, Chin L. Genetic dissection of melanoma pathways in the mouse. Semin Cancer Biol 2001;11:261–268.

151. Hingorani SR, Jacobetz MA, Robertson GP, Herlyn M, Tuveson DA. Suppression of BRAF(V599E) in human melanoma abrogates transformation. Cancer Res 2003;63:5198–5202.

152. Eisenmann KM, VanBrocklin MW, Staffend NA, Kitchen SM, Koo HM. Mitogen-activated protein kinase pathway-dependent tumor-specific survival signaling in melanoma cells through inactivation of the proapoptotic protein bad. Cancer Res 2003;63:8330–8337.

153. Jacks T, Fazeli A, Schmitt EM, Bronson RT, Goodell MA, Weinberg RA. Effects of an RB mutation in the mouse [see comments]. Nature 1992;359:295–300.

154. Lee EY, Chang CY, Hu N, et al. Mice deficient for RB are nonviable and show defects in neurogenesis and haematopoiesis. Nature 1992;359:288–294.

155. Tsai KY, Hu Y, Macleod KF, Crowley D, Yamasaki L, Jacks T. Mutation of E2f-1 suppresses apoptosis and inappropriate S phase entry and extends survival of RB-deficient mouse embryos. Mol Cell 1998;2:293–304.

156. Pan H, Yin C, Dyson NJ, Harlow E, Yamasaki L, Van Dyke T. Key roles for E2F1 in signaling p53-dependent apoptosis and in cell division within developing tumors. Mol Cell 1998;2:283–292.

157. Yu BD, Becker-Hapak M, Snyder EL, Vooijs M, Denicourt C, Dowdy SF. Distinct and nonoverlapping roles for pRB and cyclin D:cyclin-dependent kinases 4/6 activity in melanocyte survival. Proc Natl Acad Sci USA 2003;100:14,881–14,886.

158. Yamamoto H, Soh JW, Monden T, et al. Paradoxical increase in retinoblastoma protein in colorectal carcinomas may protect cells from apoptosis. Clin Cancer Res 1999;5:1805–1815.

159. Algar EM, Khromykh T, Smith SI, Blackburn DM, Bryson GJ, Smith PJ. A WT1 antisense oligonucleotide inhibits proliferation and induces apoptosis in myeloid leukaemia cell lines. Oncogene 1996;12:1005–1014.

160. Morgenbesser SD, Williams BO, Jacks T, DePinho RA. p53-dependent apoptosis produced by RB-deficiency in the developing mouse lens. Nature 1994;371:72–74.

161. Guo Z, Yikang S, Yoshida H, Mak TW, Zacksenhaus E. Inactivation of the retinoblastoma tumor suppressor induces apoptosis protease-activating factor-1 dependent and independent apoptotic pathways during embryogenesis. Cancer Res 2001;61:8395–8400.

162. Radhakrishnan SK, Feliciano CS, Najmabadi F, et al. Constitutive expression of E2F-1 leads to p21-dependent cell cycle arrest in S phase of the cell cycle. Oncogene 2004;23:4173–4176.

163. Nahle Z, Polakoff J, Davuluri RV, et al. Direct coupling of the cell cycle and cell death machinery by E2F. Nat Cell Biol 2002;4:859–864.

164. Irwin M, Marin MC, Phillips AC, et al. Role for the p53 homologue p73 in E2F-1–induced apoptosis. Nature 2000;407:645–648.

165. Pennaneach V, Barbier V, Regazzoni K, Fotedar R, Fotedar A. RB inhibits E2F-1–induced cell death in a LXCXE-dependent manner by active repression. J Biol Chem 2004;279:23,376–23,383.

166. Dahiya A, Gavin MR, Luo RX, Dean DC. Role of the LXCXE binding site in RB function. Mol Cell Biol 2000;20:6799–6805.

167. Dick FA, Dyson N. pRB contains an E2F1-specific binding domain that allows E2F1-induced apoptosis to be regulated separately from other E2F activities. Mol Cell 2003;12:639–649.

168. Dong YB, Yang HL, Elliott MJ, et al. Adenovirus-mediated E2F-1 gene transfer efficiently induces apoptosis in melanoma cells. Cancer 1999;86:2021–2033.

169. Dong YB, Yang HL, Elliott MJ, McMasters KM. Adenovirus-mediated E2F-1 gene transfer sensitizes melanoma cells to apoptosis induced by topoisomerase II inhibitors. Cancer Res 2002;62: 1776–1783.

170. Gray N, Detivaud L, Doerig C, Meijer L. ATP-site directed inhibitors of cyclin-dependent kinases. Curr Med Chem 1999;6:859–875.

171. Hajduch M, Havlieek L, Vesely J, Novotny R, Mihal V, Strnad M. Synthetic cyclin dependent kinase inhibitors. New generation of potent anti-cancer drugs. Adv Exp Med Biol 1999;457:341–353.

172. Burdette-Radoux S, Tozer RG, Lohmann RC, et al. Phase II trial of flavopiridol, a cyclin dependent kinase inhibitor, in untreated metastatic malignant melanoma. Invest New Drugs 2004;22:315–322.

173. Luo J, Manning BD, Cantley LC. Targeting the PI3K-Akt pathway in human cancer: rationale and promise. Cancer Cell 2003;4:257–262.

174. Karasarides M, Chiloeches A, Hayward R, et al. B-RAF is a therapeutic target in melanoma. Oncogene 2004;64:2338–2342.

175. Lee JT, McCubrey JA. BAY-43-9006 Bayer/Onyx. Curr Opin Investig Drugs 2003;4:757–763.

176. Kaelin WG Jr. Gleevec: prototype or outlier? Sci STKE 2004;2004:e12.

177. Kaelin WG Jr. E2F1 as a target: promoter-driven suicide and small molecule modulators. Cancer Biol Ther 2003;2:S48–S54.

178. Parr MJ, Manome Y, Tanaka T, et al. Tumor-selective transgene expression in vivo mediated by an E2F-responsive adenoviral vector. Nature Med 1997;3:1145–1149.

179. Johnson L, Shen A, Boyle L, et al. Selectively replicating adenoviruses targeting deregulated E2F activity are potent, systemic antitumor agents. Cancer Cell 2002;1:325–337.

180. Jakubczak JL, Ryan P, Gorziglia M, et al. An oncolytic adenovirus selective for retinoblastoma tumor suppressor protein pathway-defective tumors: dependence on E1A, the E2F-1 promoter, and viral replication for selectivity and efficacy. Cancer Res 2003;63:1490–1499.

181. Tsukuda K, Wiewrodt R, Molnar-Kimber K, Jovanovic VP, Amin KM. An E2F-responsive replication-selective adenovirus targeted to the defective cell cycle in cancer cells: potent antitumoral efficacy but no toxicity to normal cell. Cancer Res 2002;62:3438–3447.

182. Lee C, Chang JH, Lee HS, Cho Y. Structural basis for the recognition of the E2F transactivation domain by the retinoblastoma tumor suppressor. Genes Dev 2002;16:3199–3212.

183. Xiao B, Spencer J, Clements A, et al. Crystal structure of the retinoblastoma tumor suppressor protein bound to E2F and the molecular basis of its regulation. Proc Natl Acad Sci U S A 2003;100: 2363–2368.

184. Cam H, Dynlacht BD. Emerging roles for E2F: Beyond the G1/S transition and DNA replication. Cancer Cell 2003;3:311–316.

14 Melanoma Development and Pigment Cell Transformation

Claudia Wellbrock

CONTENTS

Summary

The unique nature of a melanocyte is based on its capacity to respond to ultraviolet (UV) radiation with the production of melanin-containing melanosomes, which subsequently are transferred to adjacent keratinocytes to deliver a protective shield. Besides the specific expression of some melanogenesis-related genes, a melanocyte is equipped with an elevated level of antiapoptotic activities, which seems to enhance the threshold for UV-induced apoptosis in this cell type. A further response to UV exposure of the skin is the induction of mitogenic activities and a subsequent increase in the number of melanocytes, which is reflected in the existence of acquired nevi. Melanocytes originate from cells with a high migratory activity and they can react to UV radiation by migration into deeper dermal layers of the skin. Thus, because antiapoptotic, mitogenic, and migratory activities can easily be induced in a melanocyte, it is a sensitive target for factors disturbing its physiological homeostasis and it might also explain why the transformation of melanocytes leads to such highly aggressive tumor cells.

The coordinated balance of differentiation, proliferation, and apoptosis is a prerequisite for the maintenance of cellular homeostasis. Understanding the signaling pathways and molecules involved in the regulation of melanocyte biology and finding the factors that lead to deregulation and ultimately to the transformation of a pigment cell will help in understanding melanoma development. Today, more and more pigment cell-specific-signaling pathways, whose relevance is also reflected in the genetics of melanoma, have been discovered. In the following chapter, some of the signaling pathways that are important for physiological processes in melanocytes, and which have been shown to be deregulated in melanoma cells, are discussed.

Key Words: Signaling pathways; B-RAF; ERK; MITF; Brn-2; osteopontin; Src kinases; Fyn; PI3-kinase; AKT.

From: *From Melanocytes to Melanoma: The Progression to Malignancy*
Edited by: V. J. Hearing and S. P. L. Leong © Humana Press Inc., Totowa, NJ

PHYSIOLOGICAL SIGNALING IN NORMAL MELANOCYTES

UV-Induced Pigmentation: "Terminal" Differentiation

Melanocytes originate from neural crest–derived progenitors that migrate to the skin during embryonic development. Once it arrives at its destination, a mature melanocyte functions as a highly specialized cell to protect the skin from damage caused by ultraviolet (UV) radiation. In the skin, a melanocyte is the target of a variety of signals emitted by its microenvironment. In this scenario, keratinocytes play an important role, because they express and secret specific paracrine-acting factors that modulate the physiology of the melanocyte (1). One of these factors is the α-melanocyte-stimulating hormone (α-MSH), which binds to the melanocortin-1 receptor (MC1R), a G protein-coupled receptor located in the plasma membrane of melanocytes (2). Stimulation of MC1R leads to upregulation of intracellular cAMP levels in melanocytes and activates cellular signaling, finally inducing melanogenesis (3).

The key factors involved in melanogenesis that also represent the main pigment cell differentiation markers are tyrosinase and tyrosinase-related proteins 1 and 2 (TYRP-1 and DCT). Expression of *tyrosinase* as well as *TYRP-1* is predominantly regulated by the *microphthalmia*-associated transcription factor (MITF) (4–6). The *MITF* gene itself is a target of cAMP signaling induced by α-MSH, and stimulation of the receptor leads to a fast but transient upregulation of the transcription factor (7,8). Other factors acting in UV-induced melanogenesis by increasing *tyrosinase* expression or by upregulating melanocyte markers are endothelin-1 (ET-1), which binds to the G protein-coupled endothelin receptor (EDNRB) (9,10), and stem cell factor (SCF), which binds to the receptor tyrosine kinase, KIT (11). In addition, UV irradiation can directly induce *tyrosinase* expression through the stress-activated MAP kinase, p38, and the transcription factor, USF-1, which binds to the *tyrosinase* promoter (12), but p38 has also been shown to be involved in α-MSH-induced melanin production (13).

Nevi Formation—Proliferation and Senescence

An important aspect of the UV response in the skin is that "UV-activated" keratinocytes express and secrete a series of factors acting synergistically to enhance the number of melanocytes, thereby functioning as mitogens.

How melanocytes increase in number after UV irradiation and which cells respond to mitogens is still a matter of debate. Because UV stimulation triggers terminal differentiation of melanocytes, the questions are whether and how terminally differentiated melanocytes in the skin can reenter the cell cycle and proliferate.

One explanation for the mitogenic response of melanocytes is based on the idea that a reservoir of precursor melanocytes exists in the skin. Melanocyte precursor cells have been identified histologically in human skin as cells that do not express the differentiation marker TYRP-1, but are positive for the melanocyte marker, KIT (14); such KIT(+) precursor cells were also identified in mouse skin (15). KIT plays an essential role during melanocyte development, in which it is expressed by melanocyte progenitors. Activation of this receptor by SCF (also called mast cell growth factor, MGF) stimulates a weak proliferation of mature melanocytes in vitro as well as in vivo (11,16,17).

Many in vitro studies using cultured human melanocytes have also shown that other factors, such as ET-1 or the basic fibroblast growth factor (bFGF) can act as weak mitogens on melanocytes as single factors (16,18), but that the combination of these factors dramatically increases the response *(19,20)*. Even more striking is the fact that α-MSH does not provoke any growth signal, *per se*, but it significantly enhances melanocyte proliferation induced by bFGF or ET-1 *(18,21)*. Thus, the requirement of a synergistic action of different growth factors for a physiologically relevant mitogenic response seems to be a general principle in melanocyte proliferation. However, an understanding of how this synergistic stimulation of membrane-bound receptors results in a coordinated activation of different intracellular pathways and how it is reflected in the intracellular signaling of melanocytes is just beginning to emerge.

It is thought that one result of the mitogenic response of melanocytes is the formation of nevi *(22,23)*. The variety and individuality of different types of nevi suggests that each nevus originates from one single cell and, thus, might represent a clonal expansion of one melanocyte. In general the melanocytes in a nevus (nevus cells) differ little in their microscopic appearance from normal melanocytes, but they can start to express growth factors that are not expressed by normal melanocytes, which is reflected in vitro by a reduced growth factor dependence in culture *(1,24)*. In vivo, nevus cells stop proliferating at a certain stage to create a defined population of pigment cells that form a mole. This formation of nevi most obviously is controlled by the cell cycle inhibitor, CDKN2A/p16[INK4A], because defects in *CDKN2A* expression in humans correlate with an increased number of moles and a higher risk of these moles to give rise to a melanoma *(25)*. This might be explained by the fact that, in melanocytes, p16[INK4A] is required for replicative senescence (loss of ability to proliferate after a limited number of divisions) and, thus, the presence of an active p16 protein in a population of proliferating melanocytes would guarantee an ultimate limitation in cell division, resulting in the formation of a nevus *(23)*.

UV Protection and Escape: Survival and Migration

During embryonic development, stimulation of KIT by SCF is essential for cell survival, and mutations in either gene in mice or in humans result in pigmentation defects caused by the loss of neural crest-derived melanocytes *(26–28)*. For mature melanocytes in the skin, the presence of nerve growth factor (NGF) is essential; it prevents apoptosis after UV irradiation through upregulation of the antiapoptotic factor, BCL-2 *(29)*. Recently, α-MSH was also found to act as "protection" factor for UV-induced apoptosis in epidermal melanocytes *(30)*.

Survival signals are also important for the regulation of the physiological localization of melanocytes. Under physiological conditions, mature melanocytes are restricted to the epidermis and they undergo apoptosis in a dermal environment and in the absence of survival factors provided by epidermal keratinocytes *(31)*. Dermal nevus cells, however, are able to survive in the absence of keratinocytes, and one factor that contributes to keratinocyte-independent survival is bFGF, which is frequently expressed by nevus cells but not by melanocytes *(32,33)*.

Survival is also dependent on the presence of cell-surface molecules that regulate the contact between the cells and the extracellular matrix (ECM). The large family of integrin receptors can mediate such interactions, and the specific expression of integrins in melanocytes defines their location in the epidermis *(34)*. However, UV exposure can influence integrin expression in melanocytes *(35)*, and a different integrin function is observed in nevus cells *(36)*. Because integrins are involved in migration, an altered integrin function might enable melanocytes to invade the dermis, a process that is observed in response to UV irradiation *(37)*.

DEREGULATED SIGNALING IN TRANSFORMED MELANOCYTES

Factors and Receptors

Because growth signals are transmitted through growth factor receptors, their correct spatial and temporal expression and activation is a critical factor in growth control. Overexpression, activating mutations, and autocrine stimulation are mechanisms of nonphysiological receptor activation found frequently in transformed cells *(38)*. The predominant mechanism of deregulated growth receptor activation in human melanoma is based on autocrine stimulation, with activation of the receptors for bFGF being the most common incident *(1)*. Melanoma cells are notorious for the deregulated expression of growth factors and cytokines, and, in addition to bFGF, they produce a panel of other factors, including platelet-derived growth factor, transforming growth factors-α and -β, hepatocyte growth factor (HGF), and the interleukins (IL)-6, IL-8, and IL-10 *(1)*. Just recently, heregulin, a ligand for the epidermal growth factor receptor (EGFR) family, was identified as an autocrine-acting factor. Heregulin stimulates growth of melanoma cells through EGFR2 (HER2) and EGFR3 (HER3), and activation of these receptor tyrosine kinases by heregulin also triggers melanocyte proliferation *(39)*.

For several other receptor tyrosine kinases, such as EGFR (HER1); the platelet-derived growth factor receptor; and the HGF receptor, c-Met; increased expression has been correlated with melanoma development and progression *(1)*. On the other hand, the expression of KIT, which, as mentioned earlier, plays a crucial role in embryonic pigment cell development and which stimulates proliferation in melanocytes, is lost in melanoma cells in later stages of the disease *(40,41)*. Re-expression of KIT in metastatic melanoma cells reduces their tumorigenicity and induces apoptosis *(42,43)*, suggesting that melanoma cells cannot tolerate the interference of KIT-induced signals with their tumor cell-specific intracellular signaling.

In *Xiphophorus* hybrid fish, an animal model for melanoma, the pigment cell-specific expression of the EGFR-related receptor, Xmrk, induces the formation of hereditary melanoma, clearly demonstrating the capacity of receptor tyrosine kinases to induce pigment cell transformation *(44)*. The oncogenic function of the Xmrk receptor is generated by mutations leading to constitutive activation of this receptor *(45,46)*. However, in human melanoma, activating mutations seem not to be a general cause for deregulated receptor activation, because, in contrast to other cancer types, such as breast or thyroid cancer, no characteristic mutations in receptor tyrosine kinase genes are known thus far to be correlated with the development of this cancer.

In contrast, germline mutations in the *MC1R* gene are found frequently to be associated with an increased risk of melanoma *(47)*. However, because all mutations in the MC1R identified thus far predominantly result in the loss of receptor function but not activation *(30,48)*, the increased risk of melanoma development seems to be rather caused by the fact that carriers of these mutated receptors have a reduced protection from UV-induced DNA damage as a result of a modified melanogenesis.

During the development and progression of melanoma, adhesion receptors, such as cadherins and integrins, which mediate cell–cell contact or interaction with the ECM, show a characteristic change in their expression pattern. A very early event found already in benign nevi is the downregulation of E-cadherin and the upregulation of N-cadherin expression *(24)*. This enables pigment cells to escape the growth control imposed by keratinocytes and to establish contacts with fibroblasts. The transition from RGP to VGP melanoma cells is characterized by enhanced expression of the integrin, $\alpha_v\beta_3$, which is caused by an upregulation of the β_3 subunit *(49)*. $\alpha_v\beta_3$ mediates the cellular contact to dermal collagen and induces important survival signals.

Pathways

THE RAS/RAF/MEK/ERK PATHWAY

The RAF/MEK/ERK serine threonine kinase cascade is involved in the regulation of cell growth, survival, and differentiation, and it is activated by many different membrane-bound receptors, including receptor tyrosine kinases and G protein-coupled receptors *(50)*. Stimulation of these receptors leads to the activation of the small G protein, RAS (*see* Fig. 1), the upstream activator of the family of RAF kinases, which consists of A-RAF, B-RAF, and C-RAF. All three RAF kinases can activate MEK, which, in turn, activates ERK. Recently, the RAS/RAF/MEK/ERK pathway has gained much attention in the melanoma field because B-RAF was found to possess oncogenic mutations in approx 60% of cutaneous melanoma *(51)*.

In the biology of a melanocyte and in the establishment of melanoma, the RAF/MEK/ERK pathway plays a crucial role because it is involved in both proliferation and differentiation (*see* Fig. 1). Stimulation of growth receptors, such as KIT, HER2, and the FGF or HGF receptor, results in activation of MEK and ultimately in the phosphorylation and activation of ERK *(19,39)*. Importantly, a single growth factor alone, which has a weak mitogenic effect on melanocytes, induces an ERK activation that almost returns to basal level within 30 min. On the other hand, synergistic action of several factors, which stimulates significant proliferation of melanocytes in vitro, leads to a much stronger and prolonged activation of ERK *(16,19,20)*. Because this suggests that a prolonged activation of ERK is correlated with melanocyte proliferation, it seems not surprising that constitutive ERK activation is also found in the majority of human melanoma cell lines and that inhibition of ERK activation in melanoma cells completely blocks proliferation *(52,53)*. Furthermore, activated ERK is detectable in more than 90% of cutaneous melanomas *(54)* and was found in 100% of *Xiphophorus* melanomas *(55)*.

The connection between constant high ERK activation levels and pigment cell transformation is reasonable, given the recent identification of B-RAF mutations in melanoma, because the most predominant mutation, at codon 599, converts B-RAF into an extremely strong activator of MEK and ERK *(51)*. Expression of this B-RAF mutant ([V599E]B-RAF) in mouse immortal melanocytes induces constitutive activation of ERK, suppression of differentiation, and transformation *(56)*. The proliferation of these cells is absolutely dependent on MEK/ERK signaling, because its inhibition completely blocks cell cycle progression. The potency of MEK to trigger constitutive activation of ERK and to transform melanocytes has also been demonstrated in mouse immortal melanocytes expressing a constitutively active version of MEK *(56,57)*. It is, however, important to mention that the ability of constitutively active B-RAF, MEK, or ERK to transform melanocytes is most likely the result of the absence of the cell cycle inhibitor, p16[INK4A], because all cell lines used for the experiments described above were deficient for functional p16[INK4A]. The requirement of p16[INK4A] deficiency for at least RAS-induced melanocyte transformation has been shown in p16[INK4A]-null mice; although the overexpression of oncogenic RAS in melanocytes of transgenic mice only results in a hyperproliferative phenotype without evidence of transformation *(58)*, p16[INK4A]-null mice develop melanoma when oncogenic RAS is expressed in melanocytes *(59)*. Because

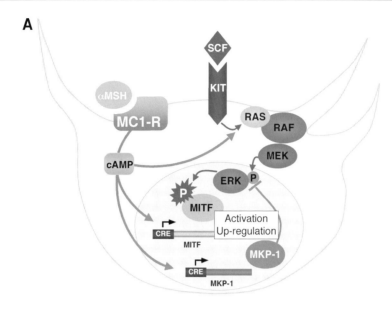

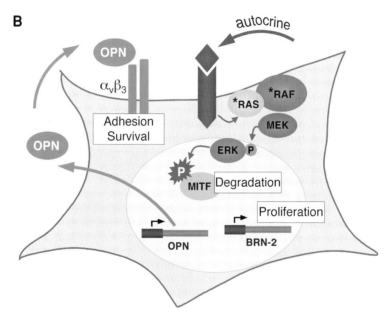

Fig. 1. Transient vs sustained ERK activation. **(A)** α-MSH stimulation of MC1-R leads to activation of ERK through RAS, B-RAF, and MEK. SCF activation of KIT stimulates RAS, but it is not known which RAF isoform activates MEK, finally leading to ERK activation. Both receptors induce a transient activation of ERK. Transient ERK activation in melanocytes induced by either α-MSH or SCF results in upregulation and activation of MITF, respectively. This leads to increased expression of melanogenesis-related genes and stimulates differentiation. cAMP-induced MKP-1 expression results in dephosphorylation of ERK within 1 h. **(B)** Sustained ERK activation in melanoma cells can be the result of either autocrine growth factor receptor stimulation or the presence of either mutated RAS or B-RAF (*RAS; *RAF). Constitutive activation of ERK results in degradation of MITF and upregulation of *Brn-2* and *OPN* expression. Brn-2 is important for melanoma cell proliferation and OPN expression results in an altered adhesion and survival behavior, thereby contributing to the metastatic potential of the cells.

nevus cells express functional p16^{INK4A}, this might explain the existence of B-RAF mutations in nevi (60) without any indications of cellular transformation.

Given that the activation of the MEK/ERK pathway is so evidently linked to proliferation, it seems rather surprising that the pathway is also induced by α-MSH (61) and, thus, by intracellular cAMP levels (Fig. 1A), which also upregulate the differentiation markers tyrosinase, TYRP1, and DCT (62), and consequently, induce differentiation. It should be mentioned, however, that the cAMP-induced activation of ERK in melanocytes is very weak and transient and lasts a maximum of 30 min (63). This might explain the finding that inhibition of constitutive MEK activity in B16 mouse melanoma cells triggers induction of tyrosinase expression, because the MEK inhibition in these cells resulted in reduced and rather weak ERK activation (64). Activation of the tyrosinase promoter as a result of MEK inhibition was also observed in Xiphophorus melanoma cells, suggesting that the same mechanism applies (65). Taken together, these observations suggest a mechanism in which a reduced and rather weak activation of the MEK/ERK kinases is connected with differentiation, whereas sustained activation leads to pigment cell proliferation and transformation.

This hypothesis has been tested in an inducible system using the Xiphophorus Xmrk receptor expressed in mouse melanocytes. Activation of the growth factor receptor in these melanocytes led to complete suppression of differentiation, enhanced proliferation, and induction of a depigmented transformed phenotype over a period of 6 d (63). Importantly, this was correlated with a sustained strong activation of ERK. Moreover, modulation of the receptor, which induced downstream signaling that resulted in a weaker and more transient activation of ERK also resulted in reduced growth and redifferentiation. These results clearly demonstrate that the concept of transient vs sustained ERK activation as a major influence on cell fate also applies to melanocytes, but this raises the question: What are the cellular consequences of constant ERK activation and why is ERK signaling such a sensitive trigger for either proliferation or differentiation?

The Microphthalmic-Associated Transcription Factor MITF. A major regulator of differentiation in melanocytes, which controls the expression of the melanogenesis components tyrosinase, TYRP1, and DCT, is the transcription factor, MITF (3,66).

MITF is regulated through the MEK/ERK pathway by phosphorylation on two sites, serine 73 (S73) and serine 409 (S409). ERK directly phosphorylates S73, whereas S409 becomes phosphorylated by the ERK substrate, RSK-1 (67,68). Phosphorylation of S73 increases the transcriptional activity of MITF by twofold to threefold (67), but phosphorylation of S73 also triggers ubiquitination of MITF (69), which induces the degradation of the phosphorylated form within 2–3 h (68). Accordingly, it was demonstrated that mutation of S73 to alanine is sufficient to prevent ubiquitination, ultimately leading to the stabilization of MITF (69). Although mutation of S409 to alanine was shown to also contribute to the stabilization of MITF (68), it is not known yet whether phosphorylation of S409 is involved in the ubiquitination process.

Stimulation of KIT in melanocytes induces ERK-mediated phosphorylation of MITF (68) (Fig. 1A) and it is assumed that this regulates KIT-induced tyrosinase expression (70). Because the activation of ERK induced by KIT returns to basal levels within 30 min (16,19,20), stimulation of KIT would result in a transient phosphorylation, activation, and consequently, ubiquitination of MITF, resulting in degradation of phosphorylated MITF. In summary, KIT stimulation would induce a short-lived peak of active MITF (Fig. 1A). However, the facts that the KIT-induced ERK activation is very transient and that MITF basal expression ensures constant *de novo* synthesis suggest that the total level of MITF would not be significantly affected over a longer period. This would explain the observation that KIT stimulation only leads to total MITF degradation when the *de novo* synthesis is inhibited *(68)*.

A similar situation is found for α-MSH-induced cAMP signaling (Fig. 1A). Because the activation of ERK induced by MC1R is also very transient, no significant degradation is observed after MSH stimulation of melanocytes *(7)*. Moreover, MITF expression is induced by cAMP (Fig. 1A), thus, the net effect is an increase in the protein amount up to 24 h *(7)*, which obviously has a more significant effect on *tyrosinase* expression than a short-lived activation through phosphorylation in the early phase of MSH stimulation. The fact that cAMP-induced activation of ERK lasts not longer than 30 min is the result of the cAMP-induced expression of MKP-1, an ERK-specific phosphatase (Fig. 1A). MKP-1 has been shown to lead to ERK dephosphorylation in melanocytes, and inhibition of MKP-1 expression results in prolonged ERK activation induced by cAMP *(63)*.

Strikingly, the prolonged activation of ERK in melanocytes results in complete MITF degradation, which coincides with the absence of tyrosinase and results in a depigmented phenotype. This has been observed in the Xmrk-inducible melanocyte system *(63)* and is also found in RAS-, B-RAF-, or MEK-transformed melanocytes in culture (*see* Fig. 1B).

Thus, the presence, the short-term phosphorylation, and the upregulation of MITF is clearly linked to the differentiated phenotype of melanocytes, whereas it seems that melanocyte transformation is linked to MITF long-term phosphorylation and degradation. This seems striking because expression of the MITF protein has been described in various melanoma biopsies *(71)*, and although this might reflect the influence of the tissue context acting on the melanoma cells in vivo, the MITF protein can still be found frequently in melanoma cell lines, even if they express a mutated B-RAF and thus have a constitutively active ERK. This suggests that MITF is differently regulated in melanoma cells with a high basal ERK activity than in melanocytes with a low basal ERK activity, an aspect that has not been examined thus far. It is also not clear yet what the function of MITF in melanoma cells is. On one hand, re-expression of MITF in melanoma cells and transformed melanocytes results in reduced tumorigenicity, which suggests that MITF counteracts melanoma cell growth *(72)*. On the other hand, MITF has been described as an important downstream factor in β-catenin-mediated melanoma cell growth, thereby acting as a survival factor *(73)*, which might be a result of the fact that it can induce *BCL-2* expression in melanoma cells *(74)*. Thus, because MITF is clearly an important differentiation factor but, on the other hand, has the potential of also acting as a survival factor for melanoma cells, its correct function in pigment cells seems to be a critical issue in the physiology of a melanocyte. Because in melanocytes regulation of MITF by the MEK/ERK pathway has an important impact on its stability, this might explain why a transient vs a sustained activation of ERK has such a powerful influence on the fate of a melanocyte.

The POU-Domain Transcription Factor Brn-2. Another consequence of strong constitutive ERK activation in pigment cells is the upregulation of the POU-domain transcription factor, Brn-2 (Fig. 1B). Brn-2 is not expressed in normal melanocytes but it is detectable in melanoma cells *(75,76)* and the specific downregulation of Brn-2 in melanoma cells affects their proliferation and tumorigenicity *(76–78)*. Brn-2 expression is also high in melanoblasts but is downregulated when these cells differentiate into mature melanocytes *(79)*, indicating that it counteracts differentiation. Accordingly,

Brn-2 expression can be induced in melanocytes by growth factors, such as bFGF or SCF *(79)*. However, significant Brn-2 expression requires synergistic action of these factors, which, as mentioned earlier, leads to prolonged activation of ERK. The requirement of ERK activation for Brn-2 expression was shown in the Xmrk-inducible melanocyte system *(77)*. Because the Xmrk receptor produces a strong and sustained activation of ERK, Brn-2 expression becomes upregulated after stimulation of the receptor and the expression level increases even further during the Xmrk-induced melanocyte transformation. However, when MEK is inhibited during receptor activation, Brn-2 expression cannot be induced. The relevance of MEK/ERK activation is also seen in RAS- as well as in B-RAF- or MEK-transformed melanocytes, in which Brn-2 expression is constantly detectable *(77)*. This is in accordance with the finding that oncogenic B-RAF mutants activate the *Brn-2* promoter and in oncogenic B-RAF-expressing melanoma cells, B-RAF downregulation results in loss of Brn-2 expression. In summary, this makes Brn-2 one of the first B-RAF downstream targets identified that is linked to pigment cell transformation. In the future, it will be important to identify the genes that are regulated by Brn-2 in melanoma cells, because they most likely are involved in the development of malignant melanoma.

The Secreted Factor Osteopontin. Osteopontin (*opn*) is another gene that is downstream of MEK/ERK signals in pigment cells (Fig. 1B). This gene encodes a secreted glycoprotein that acts as a cell attachment, survival, and growth factor and is involved in the tumorigenicity and the metastatic potential of melanoma cells *(80,81)*.

In mouse melanocytes, activation of growth factor receptors, such as the FGF receptor or the Xmrk receptor, induce *opn* expression, which is completely blocked when MEK is inhibited *(82)*. Expression of OPN enables melanocytes to grow and survive in a dermal environment, such as collagen, a behavior found to be characteristic for bFGF-expressing nevus cells *(31)*. Human melanoma cell lines frequently show constitutive expression of OPN, and blocking OPN-mediated interactions of the cells in three-dimensional collagen gels stimulates apoptosis *(82)*. Thus, OPN seems to act as an adhesion and survival factor for pigment cells in the dermal connective tissue.

The integrin $\alpha_v\beta_3$, known to be involved in melanoma cell survival and growth *(83)*, has been identified as an OPN receptor in murine melanocytes and OPN, once expressed by the melanocytes, can bind to the integrin in an autocrine way *(82)* (Fig. 1B). In B16 mouse melanoma cells, stimulation of $\alpha_v\beta_3$ by OPN leads to the upregulation of matrix metalloproteinases and enhanced migratory and invasive behavior of the cells, thus, inducing a metastatic phenotype *(80)*. B16 melanoma cells injected into OPN-deficient mice show a reduced capacity to metastasize compared with their metastatic potential in wild-type mice *(81)*. Thus, the expression and production of OPN by melanocytes as a result of active ERK signaling might be a crucial step in establishing cells that can give rise to metastatic melanoma, and indicates that the MEK/ERK pathway is also involved in processes linked to melanoma progression.

SRC KINASES

The tyrosine kinases of the Src family are known for their transforming potential and have been implicated in the cellular signaling induced by various types of receptors *(84)*. Although the first studies on the role of Src kinases in melanoma were performed more than 20 yr ago *(85)*, our current knowledge about the function of these kinases in melanoma development is still restricted. The basal activity of Src kinases in melanocytes was found to be approx 50-fold lower than in melanoma cells, and Src kinases have been shown to act as relevant downstream factors of FGF receptor-induced melanoma cell growth and tumorigenicity *(86)*. Furthermore, stimulation of human melanocytes with bFGF or HGF results in activation of Src kinases *(86)*. The proliferation of *Xiphophorus* melanoma cells is completely blocked in the presence of an Src-kinase inhibitor *(87)*, and a similar effect can be observed in Xmrk-transformed melanocytes *(63)*.

Although early studies on Src kinases in melanoma focused on Src itself, further analyses revealed that Yes and Fyn, rather than Src, may be relevant in melanoma cells. Enhanced expression of Yes was detected in melanoma cell lines *(88)* and enhanced Yes kinase activity seems to correlate with the potential of melanoma cells to metastasize to the brain *(89)*. Fyn was identified as a substrate of Xmrk in *Xiphophorus* melanoma cells and its phosphorylation and activity is highly upregulated in later stages of *Xiphophorus* melanoma *(90,91)*.

A striking role for Fyn was found in the Xmrk-inducible mouse melanocyte system, in which the phosphorylation and activity of Fyn is upregulated during transformation *(63)*. Inhibition of Fyn in the transformed melanocytes leads to redifferentiation, which is accompanied by re-expression of tyrosinase and MITF. This effect could be linked to the stabilization of the MITF protein based on suppression of constitutive ERK activation, and it indicated that Fyn can contribute to constitutive ERK activation. Further analyses revealed that Fyn can prevent dephosphorylation of ERK by suppressing the expression of the ERK-specific phosphatase, MKP-1 (Fig. 2). However, thus far, nothing is known about the regulation of *MKP-1* expression by Src kinases and it remains to be resolved if it is a direct or indirect effect on the *MKP-1* promoter.

Recently, Fyn, but not Scr or Yes, was identified as a Src kinase whose kinase activity was strongly upregulated in highly metastatic derivatives of K-1735 mouse melanoma cells *(92)*. In these cells, Fyn constitutively binds to the cytoskeleton-associated protein, Cortactin (Fig. 2), which shows increased tyrosine phosphorylation in the metastatic K-1735 clones. Both the tyrosine phosphorylation of Cortactin and the motility of the metastatic melanoma cells were inhibited by an Src-kinase inhibitor, which suggests a role for Fyn in processes associated with metastasis.

Thus, Fyn not only acts in early stages of pigment cell transformation by suppressing the differentiation and stimulating the proliferation of melanocytes, but also contributes to melanoma progression by enhancing cell motility and contributing to metastasis (Fig. 2).

PI3-Kinase/AKT Signaling

PI3-kinase is a lipid kinase that is involved in the regulation of motility, proliferation, and survival, but also in intracellular transport processes *(93)*. Active PI3-kinase produces the membrane lipid, PIP_3, which can induce further downstream signaling through protein kinase B (PKB/AKT; *see* Fig. 3). Inactivation of PIP_3-induced signaling occurs through its de-phosphorylation, and this is brought about by the phosphatase, PTEN. PTEN displays loss-of-function mutations in 5–20% of melanoma in later stages, resulting in constitutive activation of AKT *(94)*. Strikingly, mutations in RAS and PTEN are mutually exclusive, suggesting that PI3-kinase and RAS signaling are functionally overlapping in melanoma cells *(95)*. B-RAF, on the other hand, is suggested to cooperate with PTEN, because B-RAF and PTEN mutations were identified in the same tumors *(96)*.

In melanocytes, active PI3-kinase is crucial for the trafficking of TYRP1 to the melanosome *(97)* and PI3-kinase becomes activated by c-Met and seems to play a role in HGF-mediated motility *(98)*. Forced autocrine expression of HGF in normal melano-

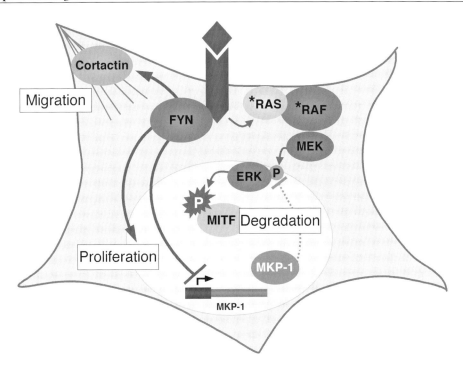

Fig. 2. Activation of the Src kinase, Fyn, in melanoma cells. The Src kinase, Fyn, is associated with growth factor receptors and exhibits enhanced kinase activity in melanoma cells. Fyn binds and phosphorylates the actin assembly activator, Cortactin. It is connected to the cytoskeleton and is involved in the regulation of integrin-mediated migration. Through inhibition of *MKP-1* expression, Fyn protects ERK from dephosphorylation and ensures constitutive activation of ERK. This results not only in MITF degradation but also in cell cycle progression.

cytes results in constitutive activation of PI3-kinase through c-Met, and, in HGF-expressing melanoma cells, PI3-kinase is constitutively active *(98)*. In these cells, PI3-kinase contributes to c-Met-induced downregulation of E-cadherin (Fig. 3), which is a crucial step for melanocytes and melanoma cells to escape the growth control mediated by epidermal keratinocytes. PI3-kinase also plays a role in integrin β_1-mediated migration *(99)* and N-cadherin-mediated adhesion *(100)* of melanoma cells, which points to a significant role for this kinase in pigment cell motility.

Whereas active PI3-kinase is necessary for melanocyte motility, inhibition correlates with pigment cell differentiation; α-MSH inhibits PI3-kinase through cAMP, and PI3-kinase inhibitors can induce tyrosinase expression in B16 mouse melanoma cells *(101)*. A link for this observation is provided by the fact that the affinity of MITF to the tyrosinase promoter is regulated by phosphorylation of serine 298 through the glycogen-synthase kinase, GSK-3β *(102,103)*. Because GSK-3β activity is inhibited by AKT (Fig. 3), inhibition of PI3-kinase results in stimulation of GSK-3β and, ultimately, activation of the MITF DNA-binding activity. Recently, inhibition of PI3-kinase was shown to also result in transcriptional upregulation of MITF, which, however, seems to be independent of GSK-3β *(103,104)*.

Because an active PI3-kinase is linked to suppression of differentiation (Fig. 3), it seems not surprising that, in human melanoma, PI3-kinase is constitutively active, which

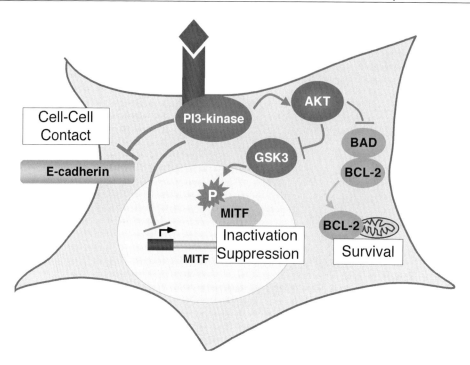

Fig. 3. PI3-kinase and AKT signaling in melanoma cells. PI3-kinase becomes activated by growth factor receptors, such as c-Met, and, through PIP_3 and PDK-1, it stimulates AKT activation. In the absence of the PIP_3-phosphatase, PTEN, AKT stays constitutively active. Constitutively active AKT induces antiapoptotic signaling by phosphorylating and thereby, inhibiting, the proapoptotic factor, BAD. This results in the release and activation of the antiapoptotic factor BCL-2 at the mitochondria. Active AKT also inhibits GSK-3β, which prevents phosphorylation of MITF on S298, which results in a reduced DNA-binding activity of MITF. In addition, constitutively active PI3-kinase suppresses MITF expression and contributes to E-cadherin downregulation.

is reflected by constitutive activation of AKT *(105)*. Constitutive activation of PI3-kinase is also found in *Xiphophorus* and it is correlated with melanoma progression, being much higher in late stages of melanoma development *(106)*. Inhibition of PI3-kinase activity in *Xiphophorus* melanoma cells completely blocks proliferation, and also, in human melanoma cells, the inhibition of PI3-kinase signaling by expression of PTEN results in growth inhibition *(107)*. Although this points to a role of PI3-kinase in melanoma cell proliferation, it is not clear yet if PI3-kinase contributes to mitogenic signaling in melanocytes.

The PI3-kinase downstream target, AKT, plays an important role in cell survival, because it can inactivate the proapoptotic protein, BAD, and induce further events to suppress apoptosis *(108)* (Fig. 3). A variety of studies have shown that activation of AKT is crucial for melanoma cell survival and that AKT inhibition renders melanoma cells more sensitive to apoptosis inducers *(100,109,110)*.

CONCLUSIONS AND PERSPECTIVES

The majority of intracellular signaling pathways are not only activated by growth or differentiation factors but can also be regulated by cell–cell and cell–ECM interactions, as well as by other extracellular stimuli, such as physical or mechanical stress. The concurrent activation of various pathways results in a complex signaling network, ultimately influencing cell cycle events, the cellular architecture, and the behavior of a cell.

The pathways described in this chapter represent only a part of the signaling network that regulates the biology of a melanocyte and that is implicated in melanocyte transformation. Other pathways, such as Wnt signaling through β-catenin, the activation of Rho kinases, or cytokine-induced JAK/STAT signaling have also been found to be deregulated in melanoma cells, but little is known about their physiological role in normal melanocytes. Importantly, although each individual signaling pathway seems to have a strong influence on the homeostasis of a melanocyte, more than one pathway needs to be deregulated before the establishment of a fully malignant phenotype.

To understand the mechanisms underlying pigment cell transformation and melanoma development it is, therefore, not only important to study the intracellular signaling events in pigment cells but also to uncover the role individual pathways are playing in different stages of melanoma development. This will help to identify pigment cell-specific factors critical for melanoma cell growth and survival, which is a prerequisite for the development of new, more specific, and more potent drugs that are able to interfere with the destructive nature of melanoma cells.

REFERENCES

1. Lazar-Molnar E, Hegyesi H, Toth S, Falus A. Autocrine and paracrine regulation by cytokines and growth factors in melanoma. Cytokine 2000;12:547–554.
2. Luger TA, Scholzen T, Grabbe S. The role of alpha-melanocyte-stimulating hormone in cutaneous biology. J Investig Dermatol Symp Proc 1997;2:87–93.
3. Busca R, Ballotti R. Cyclic AMP a key messenger in the regulation of skin pigmentation. Pigment Cell Res 2000;13:60–69.
4. Bentley NJ, Eisen T, Goding CR. Melanocyte-specific expression of the human tyrosinase promoter: activation by the microphthalmia gene product and role of the initiator. Mol Cell Biol 1994;14: 7996–8006.
5. Bertolotto C, Bille K, Ortonne JP, Ballotti R. Regulation of tyrosinase gene expression by cAMP in B16 melanoma cells involves two CATGTG motifs surrounding the TATA box: implication of the microphthalmia gene product. J Cell Biol 1996;134:747–755.
6. Yavuzer U, Keenan E, Lowings P, Vachtenheim J, Currie G, Goding CR. The Microphthalmia gene product interacts with the retinoblastoma protein in vitro and is a target for deregulation of melanocyte-specific transcription. Oncogene 1995;10:123–134.
7. Bertolotto C, Abbe P, Hemesath TJ, et al. Microphthalmia gene product as a signal transducer in cAMP-induced differentiation of melanocytes. J Cell Biol 1998;142:827–835.
8. Price ER, Horstmann MA, Wells AG, et al. alpha-Melanocyte-stimulating hormone signaling regulates expression of microphthalmia, a gene deficient in Waardenburg syndrome. J Biol Chem 1998;273:33,042–33,047.
9. Imokawa G, Miyagishi M, Yada Y. Endothelin-1 as a new melanogen: coordinated expression of its gene and the tyrosinase gene in UVB-exposed human epidermis. J Invest Dermatol 1995;105:32–37.
10. Tada A, Suzuki I, Im S, et al. Endothelin-1 is a paracrine growth factor that modulates melanogenesis of human melanocytes and participates in their responses to ultraviolet radiation. Cell Growth Differ 1998;9:575–584.
11. Grichnik JM, Burch JA, Burchette J, Shea CR. The SCF/KIT pathway plays a critical role in the control of normal human melanocyte homeostasis. J Invest Dermatol 1998;111:233–238.
12. Galibert MD, Carreira S, Goding CR. The Usf-1 transcription factor is a novel target for the stress-responsive p38 kinase and mediates UV-induced Tyrosinase expression. Embo J 2001;20: 5022–5031.
13. Smalley K, Eisen T. The involvement of p38 mitogen-activated protein kinase in the alpha-melanocyte stimulating hormone (alpha-MSH)–induced melanogenic and anti-proliferative effects in B16 murine melanoma cells. FEBS Lett 2000;476:198–202.

14. Grichnik JM, Ali WN, Burch JA, et al. KIT expression reveals a population of precursor melanocytes in human skin. J Invest Dermatol 1996;106:967–971.

15. Kawaguchi Y, Mori N, Nakayama A. Kit(+) melanocytes seem to contribute to melanocyte proliferation after UV exposure as precursor cells. J Invest Dermatol 2001;116:920–925.

16. Imokawa G, Yada Y, Kimura M. Signalling mechanisms of endothelin-induced mitogenesis and melanogenesis in human melanocytes. Biochem J 1996;314:305–312.

17. Hachiya A, Kobayashi A, Ohuchi A, Takema Y, Imokawa G. The paracrine role of stem cell factor/c-kit signaling in the activation of human melanocytes in ultraviolet-B-induced pigmentation. J Invest Dermatol 2001;116:578–586.

18. De Luca M, Siegrist W, Bondanza S, Mathor M, Cancedda R, Eberle AN. Alpha melanocyte stimulating hormone (alpha MSH) stimulates normal human melanocyte growth by binding to high-affinity receptors. J Cell Sci 1993;105(Pt 4):1079–1084.

19. Bohm M, Moellmann G, Cheng E, et al. Identification of p90RSK as the probable CREB-Ser133 kinase in human melanocytes. Cell Growth Differ 1995;6:291–302.

20. Imokawa G, Kobayasi T, Miyagishi M. Intracellular signaling mechanisms leading to synergistic effects of endothelin-1 and stem cell factor on proliferation of cultured human melanocytes. Crosstalk via trans-activation of the tyrosine kinase c-kit receptor. J Biol Chem 2000;275:33,321–33,328.

21. Swope VB, Medrano EE, Smalara D, Abdel-Malek ZA. Long-term proliferation of human melanocytes is supported by the physiologic mitogens alpha-melanotropin, endothelin-1, and basic fibroblast growth factor. Exp Cell Res 1995;217:453–459.

22. Bastian BC. Understanding the progression of melanocytic neoplasia using genomic analysis: from fields to cancer. Oncogene 2003;22:3081–3086.

23. Bennett DC. Human melanocyte senescence and melanoma susceptibility genes. Oncogene 2003;22:3063–3069.

24. Meier F, Satyamoorthy K, Nesbit M, et al. Molecular events in melanoma development and progression. Front Biosci 1998;3:D1005–D1010.

25. Hayward N. New developments in melanoma genetics. Curr Oncol Rep 2000;2:300–306.

26. Witte ON. Steel locus defines new multipotent growth factor. Cell 1990;63:5,6.

27. Manova K, Bachvarova RF. Expression of c-kit encoded at the W locus of mice in developing embryonic germ cells and presumptive melanoblasts. Dev Biol 1991;146:312–324.

28. Fleischman RA. From white spots to stem cells: the role of the Kit receptor in mammalian development. Trends Genet 1993;9:285–290.

29. Zhai S, Yaar M, Doyle SM, Gilchrest BA. Nerve growth factor rescues pigment cells from ultraviolet-induced apoptosis by upregulating BCL-2 levels. Exp Cell Res 1996;224:335–343.

30. Kadekaro AL, Kanto H, Kavanagh R, Abdel-Malek ZA. Significance of the melanocortin 1 receptor in regulating human melanocyte pigmentation, proliferation, and survival. Ann N Y Acad Sci 2003;994:359–365.

31. Alanko T, Rosenberg M, Saksela O. FGF expression allows nevus cells to survive in three-dimensional collagen gel under conditions that induce apoptosis in normal human melanocytes. J Invest Dermatol 1999;113:111–116.

32. Ahmed NU, Ueda M, Ito A, Ohashi A, Funasaka Y, Ichihashi M. Expression of fibroblast growth factor receptors in naevus-cell naevus and malignant melanoma. Melanoma Res 1997;7:299–305.

33. Ueda M, Funasaka Y, Ichihashi M, Mishima Y. Stable and strong expression of basic fibroblast growth factor in naevus cell naevus contrasts with aberrant expression in melanoma. Br J Dermatol 1994;130:320–324.

34. Hara M, Yaar M, Tang A, Eller MS, Reenstra W, Gilchrest BA. Role of integrins in melanocyte attachment and dendricity. J Cell Sci 1994;107(Pt 10):2739–2748.

35. Neitmann M, Alexander M, Brinckmann J, Schlenke P, Tronnier M. Attachment and chemotaxis of melanocytes after ultraviolet irradiation in vitro. Br J Dermatol 1999;141:794–801.

36. Mengeaud V, Grob JJ, Bongrand P, et al. Adhesive and migratory behaviors of nevus cells differ from those of epidermal melanocytes and are not linked to the histological type of nevus. J Invest Dermatol 1996;106:1224–1229.

37. Bacharach-Buhles M, Lubowietzki M, Altmeyer P. Dose-dependent shift of apoptotic and unaltered melanocytes into the dermis after irradiation with UVA 1. Dermatology 1999;198:5–10.

38. Rodrigues GA, Park M. Oncogenic activation of tyrosine kinases. Curr Opin Genet Dev 1994;4:15–24.

39. Stove C, Stove V, Derycke L, Van Marck V, Mareel M, Bracke M. The heregulin/human epidermal growth factor receptor as a new growth factor system in melanoma with multiple ways of deregulation. J Invest Dermatol 2003;121:802–812.

40. Montone KT, van Belle P, Elenitsas R, Elder DE. Proto-oncogene c-kit expression in malignant melanoma: protein loss with tumor progression. Mod Pathol 1997;10:939–944.

41. Baldi A, Santini D, Battista T, et al. Expression of AP-2 transcription factor and of its downstream target genes c-kit, E-cadherin and p21 in human cutaneous melanoma. J Cell Biochem 2001;83:364–372.

42. Huang S, Luca M, Gutman M, et al. Enforced c-KIT expression renders highly metastatic human melanoma cells susceptible to stem cell factor-induced apoptosis and inhibits their tumorigenic and metastatic potential. Oncogene 1996;13:2339–2347.

43. Huang S, Jean D, Luca M, Tainsky MA, Bar-Eli M. Loss of AP-2 results in downregulation of c-KIT and enhancement of melanoma tumorigenicity and metastasis. Embo J 1998;17:4358–4369.

44. Wittbrodt J, Adam D, Malitschek B, et al. Novel putative receptor tyrosine kinase encoded by the melanoma- inducing Tu locus in Xiphophorus. Nature 1989;341:415–421.

45. Dimitrijevic N, Winkler C, Wellbrock C, et al. Activation of the Xmrk proto-oncogene of Xiphophorus by overexpression and mutational alterations. Oncogene 1998;16:1681–1690.

46. Gomez A, Wellbrock C, Gutbrod H, Dimitrijevic N, Schartl M. Ligand-independent dimerization and activation of the oncogenic xmrk receptor by two mutations in the extracellular domain. J Biol Chem 2001;276:3333–3340.

47. Palmer JS, Duffy DL, Box NF, et al. Melanocortin-1 receptor polymorphisms and risk of melanoma: is the association explained solely by pigmentation phenotype? Am J Hum Genet 2000;66:176–186.

48. Scott MC, Wakamatsu K, Ito S, et al. Human melanocortin 1 receptor variants, receptor function and melanocyte response to UV radiation. J Cell Sci 2002;115:2349–2355.

49. Seftor RE. Role of the beta3 integrin subunit in human primary melanoma progression: multifunctional activities associated with alpha(v)beta3 integrin expression. Am J Pathol 1998;153: 1347–1351.

50. Chang F, Steelman LS, Shelton JG, et al. Regulation of cell cycle progression and apoptosis by the Ras/Raf/MEK/ERK pathway (Review). Int J Oncol 2003;22:469–480.

51. Davies H, Bignell GR, Cox C, et al. Mutations of the BRAF gene in human cancer. Nature 2002;417:949–954.

52. Satyamoorthy K, Li G, Gerrero MR, et al. Constitutive mitogen-activated protein kinase activation in melanoma is mediated by both BRAF mutations and autocrine growth factor stimulation. Cancer Res 2003;63:756–759.

53. Kortylewski M, Heinrich PC, Kauffmann ME, Bohm M, MacKiewicz A, Behrmann I. Mitogen-activated protein kinases control p27/Kip1 expression and growth of human melanoma cells. Biochem J 2001;357:297–303.

54. Cohen C, Zavala-Pompa A, Sequeira JH, et al. Mitogen-activated protein kinase activation is an early event in melanoma progression. Clin Cancer Res 2002;8:3728–3733.

55. Wellbrock C, Schartl M. Multiple binding sites in the growth factor receptor Xmrk mediate binding to p59fyn, GRB2 and Shc. Eur J Biochem 1999;260:275–283.

56. Wellbrock C, Ogilvie L, Hedley D, et al. V599EB-RAF is an Oncogene in Melanocytes. Cancer Res 2004;64:2338–2342.

57. Govindarajan B, Bai X, Cohen C, et al. Malignant transformation of melanocytes to melanoma by constitutive activation of mitogen-activated protein kinase kinase (MAPKK) signaling. J Biol Chem 2003;278:9790–9795.

58. Powell MB, Hyman P, Bell OD, et al. Hyperpigmentation and melanocytic hyperplasia in transgenic mice expressing the human T24 Ha-ras gene regulated by a mouse tyrosinase promoter. Mol Carcinog 1995;12:82–90.

59. Chin L, Pomerantz J, Polsky D, et al. Cooperative effects of INK4a and ras in melanoma susceptibility in vivo. Genes Dev 1997;11:2822–2834.

60. Pollock PM, Harper UL, Hansen KS, et al. High frequency of BRAF mutations in nevi. Nat Genet 2003;33:19–20.

61. Busca R, Abbe P, Mantoux F, et al. Ras mediates the cAMP-dependent activation of extracellular signal-regulated kinases (ERKs) in melanocytes. Embo J 2000;19:2900–2910.

62. Bertolotto C, Busca R, Abbe P, et al. Different cis-acting elements are involved in the regulation of TRP1 and TRP2 promoter activities by cyclic AMP: pivotal role of M boxes (GTCATGTGCT) and of microphthalmia. Mol Cell Biol 1998;18:694–702.

63. Wellbrock C, Weisser C, Geissinger E, Troppmair J, Schartl M. Activation of p59(Fyn) leads to melanocyte dedifferentiation by influencing MKP-1–regulated mitogen-activated protein kinase signaling. J Biol Chem 2002;277:6443–6454.

64. Englaro W, Bertolotto C, Busca R, et al. Inhibition of the mitogen-activated protein kinase pathway triggers B16 melanoma cell differentiation. J Biol Chem 1998;273:9966–9970.

65. Delfgaauw J, Duschl J, Wellbrock C, Froschauer C, Schartl M, Altschmied J. MITF-M plays an essential role in transcriptional activation and signal transduction in Xiphophorus melanoma. Gene 2003;320:117–126.

66. Goding CR. Mitf from neural crest to melanoma: signal transduction and transcription in the melanocyte lineage. Genes Dev 2000;14:1712–1728.

67. Hemesath TJ, Price ER, Takemoto C, Badalian T, Fisher DE. MAP kinase links the transcription factor Microphthalmia to c-Kit signalling in melanocytes. Nature 1998;391:298–301.

68. Wu M, Hemesath TJ, Takemoto CM, et al. c-Kit triggers dual phosphorylations, which couple activation and degradation of the essential melanocyte factor Mi. Genes Dev 2000;14:301–312.

69. Xu W, Gong L, Haddad MM, et al. Regulation of microphthalmia-associated transcription factor MITF protein levels by association with the ubiquitin-conjugating enzyme hUBC9. Exp Cell Res 2000;255:135–143.

70. Price ER, Ding HF, Badalian T, et al. Lineage-specific signaling in melanocytes. C-kit stimulation recruits p300/CBP to microphthalmia. J Biol Chem 1998;273:17,983–17,986.

71. King R, Weilbaecher KN, McGill G, Cooley E, Mihm M, Fisher DE. Microphthalmia transcription factor. A sensitive and specific melanocyte marker for Melanoma Diagnosis. Am J Pathol 1999;155:731–738.

72. Selzer E, Wacheck V, Lucas T, et al. The melanocyte-specific isoform of the microphthalmia transcription factor affects the phenotype of human melanoma. Cancer Res 2002;62:2098–2103.

73. Widlund HR, Horstmann MA, Price ER, et al. Beta-catenin-induced melanoma growth requires the downstream target Microphthalmia-associated transcription factor. J Cell Biol 2002;158: 1079–1087.

74. McGill GG, Horstmann M, Widlund HR, et al. Bcl2 regulation by the melanocyte master regulator Mitf modulates lineage survival and melanoma cell viability. Cell 2002;109:707–718.

75. Eisen T, Easty DJ, Bennett DC, Goding CR. The POU domain transcription factor Brn-2: elevated expression in malignant melanoma and regulation of melanocyte-specific gene expression. Oncogene 1995;11:2157–2164.

76. Thomson JA, Murphy K, Baker E, et al. The brn-2 gene regulates the melanocytic phenotype and tumorigenic potential of human melanoma cells. Oncogene 1995;11:691–700.

77. Goodall J, Wellbrock C, Dexter TJ, Roberts K, Marais R, Goding CR. The Brn-2 transcription factor links activated BRAF to melanoma proliferation. Mol Cell Biol 2004;24:2923–2931.

78. Goodall J, Martinozzi S, Dexter TJ, et al. Brn-2 expression controls melanoma proliferation and is directly regulated by beta-catenin. Mol Cell Biol 2004;24:2915–2922.

79. Cook AL, Donatien PD, Smith AG, et al. Human melanoblasts in culture: expression of BRN2 and synergistic regulation by fibroblast growth factor-2, stem cell factor, and endothelin-3. J Invest Dermatol 2003;121:1150–1159.

80. Philip S, Bulbule A, Kundu GC. Osteopontin stimulates tumor growth and activation of promatrix metalloproteinase-2 through nuclear factor-kappa B-mediated induction of membrane type 1 matrix metalloproteinase in murine melanoma cells. J Biol Chem 2001;276:44,926–44,935.

81. Nemoto H, Rittling SR, Yoshitake H, et al. Osteopontin deficiency reduces experimental tumor cell metastasis to bone and soft tissues. J Bone Miner Res 2001;16:652–659.

82. Geissinger E, Weisser C, Fischer P, Schartl M, Wellbrock C. Autocrine stimulation by osteopontin contributes to antiapoptotic signalling of melanocytes in dermal collagen. Cancer Res 2002;62: 4820–4828.

83. Petitclerc E, Stromblad S, von Schalscha TL, et al. Integrin alpha(v)beta3 promotes M21 melanoma growth in human skin by regulating tumor cell survival. Cancer Res 1999;59:2724–2730.

84. Abram CL, Courtneidge SA. Src family tyrosine kinases and growth factor signaling. Exp Cell Res 2000;254:1–13.

85. Schartl M, Barnekow A, Bauer H, Anders F. Correlations of inheritance and expression between a tumor gene and the cellular homolog of the Rous sarcoma virus-transforming gene in Xiphophorus. Cancer Res 1982;42:4222–4227.

86. Yayon A, Ma YS, Safran M, Klagsbrun M, Halaban R. Suppression of autocrine cell proliferation and tumorigenesis of human melanoma cells and fibroblast growth factor transformed fibroblasts by a kinase-deficient FGF receptor 1: evidence for the involvement of Src-family kinases. Oncogene 1997;14:2999–3009.

87. Wellbrock C, Gomez A, Schartl M. Signal transduction by the oncogenic receptor tyrosine kinase Xmrk in melanoma formation of Xiphophorus. Pigment Cell Res 1997;10:34–40.

88. Loganzo F, Dosik JS, Zhao Y, et al. Elevated expression of protein tyrosine kinase c-Yes, but not c-Src, in human malignant melanoma. Oncogene 1993;8:2637–2644.

89. Marchetti D, Parikh N, Sudol M, Gallick GE. Stimulation of the protein tyrosine kinase c-Yes but not c-Src by neurotrophins in human brain-metastatic melanoma cells. Oncogene 1998;16:3253–3260.

90. Wellbrock C, Lammers R, Ullrich A, Schartl M. Association between the melanoma-inducing receptor tyrosine kinase Xmrk and src family tyrosine kinases in Xiphophorus. Oncogene 1995;10: 2135–2143.

91. Wellbrock C, Schartl M. Activation of phosphatidylinositol 3-kinase by a complex of p59fyn and the receptor tyrosine kinase Xmrk is involved in malignant transformation of pigment cells. Eur J Biochem 2000;267:3513–3522.

92. Huang J, Asawa T, Takato T, Sakai R. Cooperative roles of Fyn and cortactin in cell migration of metastatic murine melanoma. J Biol Chem 2003;278:48,367–48,376.

93. Fukui Y, Ihara S, Nagata S. Downstream of phosphatidylinositol-3 kinase, a multifunctional signaling molecule, and its regulation in cell responses. J Biochem (Tokyo) 1998;124:1–7.

94. Wu H, Goel V, Haluska FG. PTEN signaling pathways in melanoma. Oncogene 2003;22:3113–3122.

95. Tsao H, Zhang X, Fowlkes K, Haluska FG. Relative reciprocity of NRAS and PTEN/MMAC1 alterations in cutaneous melanoma cell lines. Cancer Res 2000;60:1800–1804.

96. Tsao H, Goel V, Wu H, Yang G, Haluska FG. Genetic interaction between NRAS and BRAF mutations and PTEN/MMAC1 inactivation in melanoma. J Invest Dermatol 2004;122:337–341.

97. Chen H, Salopek TG, Jimbow K. The role of phosphoinositide 3-kinase in the sorting and transport of newly synthesized tyrosinase-related protein-1 (TRP-1). J Investig Dermatol Symp Proc 2001;6:105–114.

98. Li G, Schaider H, Satyamoorthy K, Hanakawa Y, Hashimoto K, Herlyn M. Downregulation of E-cadherin and Desmoglein 1 by autocrine hepatocyte growth factor during melanoma development. Oncogene 2001;20:8125–8135.

99. Hodgson L, Henderson AJ, Dong C. Melanoma cell migration to type IV collagen requires activation of NF-kappaB. Oncogene 2003;22:98–108.

100. Li G, Satyamoorthy K, Herlyn M. N-cadherin-mediated intercellular interactions promote survival and migration of melanoma cells. Cancer Res 2001;61:3819–3825.

101. Busca R, Bertolotto C, Ortonne JP, Ballotti R. Inhibition of the phosphatidylinositol 3-kinase/p70(S6)-kinase pathway induces B16 melanoma cell differentiation. J Biol Chem 1996;271:31,824–31,830.

102. Takeda K, Takemoto C, Kobayashi I, et al. Ser298 of MITF, a mutation site in Waardenburg syndrome type 2, is a phosphorylation site with functional significance. Hum Mol Genet 2000;9:125–132.

103. Khaled M, Larribere L, Bille K, et al. Glycogen synthase kinase 3beta is activated by cAMP and plays an active role in the regulation of melanogenesis. J Biol Chem 2002;277:33,690–33,697.

104. Khaled M, Larribere L, Bille K, Ortonne JP, Ballotti R, Bertolotto C. Microphthalmia associated transcription factor is a target of the phosphatidylinositol-3–kinase pathway. J Invest Dermatol 2003;121:831–836.

105. Dhawan P, Singh AB, Ellis DL, Richmond A. Constitutive activation of Akt/protein kinase B in melanoma leads to up-regulation of nuclear factor-kappaB and tumor progression. Cancer Res 2002;62:7335–7342.

106. Wellbrock C, Fischer P, Schartl M. PI3-kinase is involved in mitogenic signaling by the oncogenic receptor tyrosine kinase Xiphophorus melanoma receptor kinase in fish melanoma. Exp Cell Res 1999;251:340–349.

107. Stewart AL, Mhashilkar AM, Yang XH, et al. PI3 kinase blockade by Ad-PTEN inhibits invasion and induces apoptosis in RGP and metastatic melanoma cells. Mol Med 2002;8:451–461.

108. Franke TF, Hornik CP, Segev L, Shostak GA, Sugimoto C. PI3K/Akt and apoptosis: size matters. Oncogene 2003;22:8983–8998.

109. Stahl JM, Cheung M, Sharma A, Trivedi NR, Shanmugam S, Robertson GP. Loss of PTEN promotes tumor development in malignant melanoma. Cancer Res 2003;63:2881–2890.

110. Ivanov VN, Hei TK. Arsenite treatment sensitizes human melanomas to apoptosis via TNF-mediated pathway. J Biol Chem 2004;279:22,747–22,758.

15 The Biology and Genetics of Melanoma

Norman E. Sharpless and Lynda Chin

Summary

Like all human malignancies, the incidence of melanoma reflects the interaction of genetic predisposition with environmental exposures. Melanoma is perhaps unusual in this regard, however, in that in no other common tumor type is there such an advanced understanding of both the underlying environmental and genetic factors. The majority of melanoma occurs in the setting of a common environmental exposure: ultraviolet irradiation. Likewise, several congenital melanoma-prone genetic conditions have been identified, including germline polymorphisms that attenuate cell cycle regulation, that decrease skin pigmentation, that hamper DNA repair, and that impair melanocytic differentiation. Lastly, the large majority of sporadic melanomas share 2 classes of acquired mutations: those affecting RAS–RAF signaling and those that target the *INK4a/ARF* locus on chromosome 9p21. This well-developed comprehension of both the environmental and genetic causes of this disease has allowed for the generation of sophisticated in vitro and murine models, which have reinforced and furthered our understanding of the development of this cancer. This chapter reviews decades' worth of genetic and biologic insights from the study of these models, and their contribution to our understanding of the pathogenesis of melanoma. A review of this work also makes obvious the continued challenges in the field: to use our hard-earned molecular comprehension of this disease to elucidate the disturbing clinical features of melanoma; namely, an intense therapeutic resistance and proclivity for early metastasis. The present ability to study faithful murine melanoma models, coupled with advances in rational drug design, has generated optimism for the development of effective prevention and screening programs, as well as successful targeted therapeutics in the near future.

Key Words: Melanocyte; melanoma; mouse model; RB; cdkn2a; melanocortin receptor (MC1R).

From: *From Melanocytes to Melanoma: The Progression to Malignancy*
Edited by: V. J. Hearing and S. P. L. Leong © Humana Press Inc., Totowa, NJ

INTRODUCTION

Melanoma arises from the malignant transformation of the pigment-producing cells, melanocytes (Fig. 1), and has a strong familial component. In the 1820s, William Norris, a general practitioner, reported a familial predisposition for melanoma, particularly in individuals with light-colored hair and pale complexions *(1)*. Now, almost two centuries later, we are gaining insights into the genetic and environmental factors driving its pathogenesis.

The incidence of melanoma is influenced by genetic factors (including pigmentation) and geographical parameters, such as latitude and altitude *(2)*, an observation that suggested a causal role for ultraviolet (UV) light in melanoma development. Indeed, the current rise in melanoma incidence can be explained in part by altered patterns of sun exposure, relating to increased popularity of sun tanning and the relative ease of global travel or migration of fair-skinned individuals to more sun-intensive regions *(3)*. Conversely, the declining trend in recent years of melanoma incidence in Australia has been attributed to education resulting in reduced sun exposure *(4)*. Other genetically determined host factors—such as fair skin complexion, red hair, multiple benign or dysplastic nevi—have also been associated with increased melanoma risk, although our entire understanding of their genetic basis is less advanced.

Although curable at early stage, advanced melanoma is among the most treatment-refractory of human malignancies and therapy for advanced disease remains largely palliative. Therefore, prevention and early detection currently remain the most effective measures. We believe, however, that the convergence of technologies, model systems, and mechanistic insights has the potential to dramatically alter this clinical picture. The genetic changes in the melanoma genome are being identified through genomics, the relevance and importance of which are being validated by somatic cell genetics and in refined mouse models. These efforts should lead to the identification of rational targets for drug development and biomarkers for disease monitoring, which should impact positively on the clinical course of the disease.

GENETICS OF HERITABLE MELANOMA PREDISPOSITION

Inherited cancer syndromes have often shed light on the genetic lesions that govern the genesis of both familial and sporadic forms of the disease (*see also* Chapter 10). Familial melanomas, which represent approx 8–12% of all melanoma cases *(5)*, are an excellent case in point. Linkage analysis studies of large melanoma kindreds culminated in the identification of two susceptibility alleles—*inhibitor of cyclin-dependent kinase-4 (INK4)/alternative reading frame* (*ARF*) and *cyclin-dependent kinase-4* (*CDK4*)—the products of which are known components of potent tumor-suppression pathways. More recently, *melanocortin-1 receptor* (*MC1R*) polymorphic variants have been associated with red hair, fair skin, sun sensitivity, increased freckling, and melanoma. It is unclear at present whether the increase in melanoma of these patients results entirely from increased UV sensitivity or other alterations in melanocyte biology associated with altered melanocortin signaling (*see also* Chapters 18 and 19).

The INK4a/ARF Locus at Chromosome 9p21

The *INK4a/ARF* locus (also called the *CDKN2a* gene) on chromosome 9p21 was identified by its frequent homozygous deletion in cancer cell lines of many different

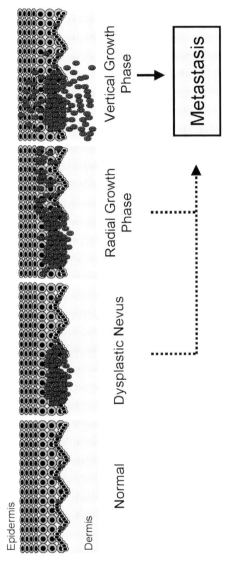

Epidermis

Dermis

Normal   Dysplastic Nevus   Radial Growth   Vertical Growth
                                          Phase   Phase

Metastasis

Fig. 1. Mutated melanocytes give rise to melanoma. Melanocytes are pigment-synthesizing cells of neural crest lineage, illustrated in red (*169*). Melanocytes migrate to the skin during development and are normally confined to the basal layer of the epidermis in a nonrandom pattern, sending out arborizing dendritic processes that contact keratinocytes in basal and superficial layers of the skin (*170*). Each melanocyte transfers pigment-containing melanosomes via these dendrites to approx 36 basal and suprabasal keratinocytes (the so-called epidermal melanin unit). Once with n the keratinocytes, the pigment protects the skin by absorbing and scattering harmful solar radiation (*170*). It is now appreciated that the proliferation, dendricity, and melanization of melanocytes are subject to regulation by neighboring basal keratinocytes, providing biological relevance to this highly ordered anatomical configuration (*171*).

Melanomas are classified histologically according to their location and stage of progression. Five distinct stages have been proposed in the evolution of melanoma, on the basis of such histological criteria as: common acquired and congenital nevi without dysplastic changes; dysplastic nevus with structural and architectural atypia; radial growth phase (RGP) melanoma; vertical growth phase (VGP) melanoma; and metastatic melanoma. As the presumed precursor to melanoma, both benign and dysplastic nevi are characterized by disruption of the epidermal melanin unit, leading to increased numbers of melanocytes in relation to keratinocytes. These precursor lesions progress to *in situ* melanoma, which grow laterally and remain largely confined to the epidermis, therefore, this stage is defined as the RGP. This is in contrast to the vertical growth phase (VGP) melanoma, which invades the upper layer of the epidermis and beyond and penetrates into the underlying dermis and subcutaneous tissue through the basement membrane, forming expansile nodules of malignant cells. It is believed that the transition from radial to vertical growth phases is the crucial step in the evolution of melanoma that presages the acquisition of metastatic potential and poor clinical outcome. Consistent with that, the total thickness/height of a primary melanoma lesion is still one of the most predictive parameters for metastatic disease and adverse clinical outcome (*172*). Correlating to these histological pictures, RGP melanoma cells remain dependent on exogenous growth factors supplied by surrounding keratinocytes, are incapable of anchorage-independent growth, are not tumorigenic in immunodeficient mice, and do not metastasize in patients. In contrast, VGP melanoma cells have completely escaped from keratinocyte control and established close communicative networks with fibroblasts; acquire growth factor- and anchorage-independent growth; are tumorigenic in animals; and are highly metastatic, both in patients and in experimental animal models (*171*).

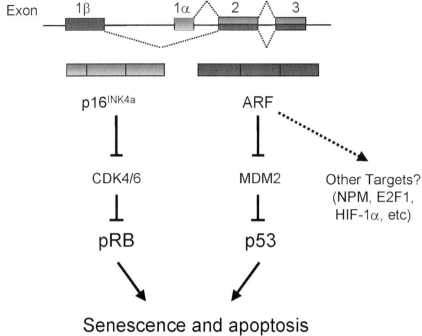

Fig. 2. The *INK4a/ARF* locus at chromosome 9p21. The 9p21 locus has a highly unusual genomic organization. The *INK4a/ARF* locus contains two upstream exons, 1α and 1β. These two exons are driven by separate promoters, which result in alternative transcripts that share common downstream exons 2 and 3. Although a common acceptor site in the second exon is used by both first exons, the open reading frames remain distinct in the shared exon 2, and result in two distinct protein products. The transcript initiated from the proximal promoter (1α) encodes p16^INK4a *(12)*, the founding member of the INK4 family proteins. The second transcript, initiated from the upstream exon 1β, encodes ARF (alternative reading frame) *(11)*. By inhibiting CDK4/6-cyclin D-mediated hyperphosphorylation of RB, p16^INK4a ensures that RB remains in complex with the E2F transcription factor *(173)*. These RB–E2F complexes recruit histone deacetylase to promote and repress transcription of target genes, leading to G1 arrest *(174)*. In the absence of inhibition by p16^INK4a, CDK4/6–cyclin D phosphorylates RB, which results in the release of E2F. E2F then activates genes necessary for progression into S phase *(173)*. ARF functions as a potent growth suppressor *(11,175)*, blocks oncogenic transformation, and sustains p53-dependent apoptosis in RB-null cells that have re-entered the cell cycle in vivo *(14)* or in the setting of hyperproliferative oncogenic signals *(176–178)*. Biochemically, ARF stabilizes and enhances p53 levels by blocking MDM2-mediated p53 ubiquitylation and degradation *(13–16)*. Several MDM2-independnet targets for ARF have been recently suggested.

types *(6,7)*. It was designated as the familial melanoma locus because mutations of this gene were found to cosegregate with melanoma susceptibility in familial melanoma kindreds *(8,9)*. This locus has an unusual and complex genomic organization (Fig. 2) *(10,11)*, encoding two distinct tumor suppressor proteins, p16^INK4a and ARF (also known as p14^ARF in humans, or p19^ARF in mice). The proteins are encoded by open reading frames with distinct promoters and first exons (1α for p16^INK4a and 1β for ARF), but splice to a common second exon. The shared portions of the *p16^INK4a* and *ARF* mRNAs are translated in different reading frames, and therefore the proteins are not isoforms and do not share any amino acid homology. Although the encoding of proteins in nonoverlapping reading frames is common in bacteria and viruses, such a genomic organization is practically unique in mammals.

p16^{INK4a}, the founding member of the INK4 family of proteins, inhibits CDK4/6-mediated phosphorylation and inactivation of retinoblastoma (RB) (Fig. 2) *(12)*. The ARF product of the locus *(11)* inhibits MDM2-mediated ubiquitination and subsequent degradation of p53 (Fig. 2) *(13–16)*. Therefore, the two products of the *INK4a/ARF* locus negatively regulate the pRB and p53 pathways, and their loss predisposes the development of melanoma. Interestingly, another member of the INK4 family of CDK inhibitors—*CDKN2B*, which encodes p15^{INK4b}—resides a short distance centromeric to exon 1β of the *INK4a/ARF* locus, still within the 9p21 locus *(7)*. Despite its relatedness to p16^{INK4a}, however, p15^{INK4b} does not seem to have a significant role in melanoma suppression.

p16^{INK4a}: Effector of Senescence

The presence of germline mutations that specifically target p16^{INK4a} in familial melanoma kindreds and melanoma-prone families *(8,9)* provide definitive evidence that this protein functions as a suppressor of melanoma formation in humans. Although melanoma-predisposing germline mutations have been found in all three exons of *INK4a*, the mutations of exon 1α, in particular, incriminate p16^{INK4a}, because these mutations do not alter ARF function or expression (reviewed in ref. *17*). The incidence of *p16^{INK4a}* mutations among melanoma-prone families ranges from 25–40%, and, moreover, 0.2–2% of sporadic melanoma patients (i.e., those lacking a family history) harbor occult germline *INK4a* mutations *(18,19)*. The recent association of melanoma with polymorphisms in both 5' and 3' untranslated regions of *INK4a* has expanded the range of 9p21-associated familial melanoma alleles to those that alter translation or possibly regulate message stability of p16^{INK4a} (and/or ARF; *see* page 269) *(20,21)*. Likewise, both promoter and splicing mutations of *INK4a* have also been associated with familial melanoma (reviewed in ref. *17*). Lastly, mice with specific p16^{INK4a} inactivation are modestly prone to carcinogen-induced and spontaneous melanoma *(22,23)*. In aggregate, these genetic data overwhelmingly support the notion that p16^{INK4a} is an important suppressor of melanoma formation in humans.

Although p16^{INK4a} loss appears to be a common feature of many, perhaps most, types of human cancer, the exquisite susceptibility of patients with germline inactivation of p16^{INK4a} to melanoma is not well understood. Patients with germline *INK4a* mutation also demonstrate an increased incidence of pancreatic adenocarcinoma, with suggested increases in susceptibility to glioblastoma, lung cancer, head and neck cancer, breast cancer, and myeloma *(24–34)*. In none of these other tumor types, however, has the association been nearly as clinically strong as it is with melanoma. This observation can be explained in several ways. It is possible that familial melanoma is a particularly remarkable clinical entity that is relatively obvious to clinicians, as opposed to familial clusters of more common tumors like breast, head and neck, or lung cancer. Additionally, it may be that other tumor types can inactivate the p16^{INK4a}–cyclin D–CDK4/6–RB pathway in numerous ways, whereas melanoma has a particular biochemical requirement for p16^{INK4a} loss. Although novel biochemical activities of p16^{INK4a} in melanocytes have been suggested *(35,36)*, genetic evidence suggest that the p16^{INK4a}–cdk4/6–RB pathway is the principal target in melanoma. For example, cdk6 amplification appears epistatic with p16^{INK4a} loss in murine melanomas *(37)*, and familial melanoma also occurs in humans with activating mutations of CDK4 or inactivating lesions of RB. Lastly, because these carriers are heterozygous for mutant *INK4a*, it may be that UV light is a particularly effective mechanism for mutating the remaining wild-type allele as opposed to other types of carcinogen exposure. This notion is consistent with the observation that the penetrance of melanoma in individuals that are heterozygous for mutant *INK4a* depends highly on the latitude (and therefore sun exposure) at which the kindred resides *(38)*.

CDK4: Proliferative Kinase

Given the finding of the importance of p16[INK4a] in family melanoma, it is not surprising that germline mutations of other components of the p16[INK4a]–RB pathway are also associated with familial melanoma. In particular, germline mutations of *CDK4*, an RB-kinase that is inhibited by p16[INK4a] (Fig. 2), have been identified in melanoma-prone kindreds *(39–42)*. These mutations, which are a rare cause of familial melanoma, target a conserved arginine residue (Arg24) and render the mutant protein insensitive to inhibition by the INK4 class of cell cycle inhibitors. The crystal structure of the p16[INK4a]–CDK6 heterodimer has revealed that this residue (conserved between CDK4 and CDK6) is crucial for the binding of p16[INK4a] to CDK6 and such substitutions perturb this crucial physical association *(43)*. Melanomas from patients harboring these germline *CDK4* mutations do not demonstrate p16[INK4a] inactivation (a frequent event in sporadic melanoma), suggesting that p16[INK4a] inactivation and CDK4 overactivation are epistatic in terms of melanoma progression. This hypothesis is in accordance with the indistinguishable clinical impact of germline *INK4a* and *CDK4* mutations, manifesting with similar mean age of melanoma diagnosis, mean number of melanomas, and number of nevi *(44)*. Consistent with the human data, Barbacid and colleagues have shown that mice with a mutant form of *Cdk4* (Arg24Cys) "knocked-in" to the wild-type locus were highly susceptible to melanoma formation after carcinogen treatment *(45)*. As the human genetic data would predict, melanomas arising in this genetic background do not show p16[INK4a] inactivation. In aggregate, these data provide strong biochemical evidence for the relevance of CDK4 kinase activity and its regulation by p16[INK4a] in familial melanoma.

Retinoblastoma: Cell Cycle Regulator

Although less commonly associated with familial melanoma than with hereditary retinoblastoma, patients with germline inactivation of RB are predisposed to melanoma *(46–49)*. In patients who are cured of bilateral retinoblastoma, the estimates of the increase in lifetime risk of melanoma range from 4- to 80-fold *(48,49)*. These tumors do not necessarily occur in skin associated with radiotherapy treatment ports of the retinoblastoma, and likewise the excess incidence of melanoma in these cohorts has not been reduced by the practice of decreasing radiotherapy for retinoblastoma. In contrast, the lifetime risk of sarcoma in retinoblastoma survivors has markedly decreased in the setting of less primary treatment radiotherapy, suggesting that the bulk of sarcoma risk in these patients is treatment-related. Therefore, the increased risk of melanoma in patients who survive bilateral retinoblastoma appears to result from the stochastic loss of the remaining wild-type allele in these patients. These data provide further evidence that RB mediates the antitumor activity of p16[INK4a] and the tumor-promoting effects of mutant CDK4 in melanoma.

ARF: The Other Tumor Suppressor at CDKN2A

Although *INK4a* is a definitive melanoma susceptibility gene, the fact that a significant proportion of familial cases segregating with 9p21 markers do not possess germline mutations targeting *INK4A* raises the possibility that the 9p21 locus harbors additional melanoma susceptibility gene(s). Because mutations in *INK4a/ARF* frequently eliminate both p16[INK4a] and ARF in melanoma (reviewed in ref. *50*), ARF has emerged as a prime candidate. Indeed, somatic mutations have been described in human melanomas that exclusively affect the *ARF* coding sequence in the shared exon 2 *(51,52)*, and ARF-specific exon 1β deletion has been identified in two metastatic melanoma cell lines *(53)*. Most significant is the report of two cases of ARF-specific germline mutations in human melanoma patients. In one case, a family in which four members developed melanoma was shown to harbor a 14-kb deletion encompassing the *ARF*-coding exon 1β in the germline. This deletion apparently spared the *INK4A* and *INK4B* genes and was mapped to 2.7 kb upstream of known promoter elements critical for *INK4A* expression, consistent with an ARF-specific event *(54)*. In another case, a patient with multiple melanomas was found to harbor a germline 16-bp insertion in exon 1β, generating a frame-shift mutant of ARF with impaired cell cycle arrest profile *(55)*. Although these germline alterations do not affect the known anatomy of *INK4A* genomic structure and would not be predicted to affect p16[INK4a] expression, the lack of definitive and rigorous demonstration of *INK4A* functional intactness continues to preclude the designation of ARF as a *bona fide* 9p21 melanoma suppressor, independent of *INK4A*. Fortunately, the evolutionary conservation of the peculiar genomic organization of 9p21 locus (Fig. 2) in mammals *(11,56–60)* provided an opportunity to exploit mouse genetics to address more directly the specific contributions of p16[INK4a] and ARF in melanoma suppression.

Additionally, ARF has been considered a good candidate as a suppressor for melanoma because of a peculiar feature of this tumor type: a lack of p53 inactivation. In contrast to most human tumors, p53 loss is unusual in melanoma *(61,62)*; although clearly p53 responses to oncogenic stress and DNA damage are attenuated in this disease. Therefore, it has been tempting to speculate that ARF loss can serve as the "p53-pathway" lesion in this tumor type, but perhaps not in other types of cancer. If true, this explains another interesting feature of melanoma: the high frequency of 9p21 deletion as opposed to other mechanisms of p16[INK4a] loss, such as promoter methylation or point mutation. These latter mechanisms only target p16[INK4a], and are more common in tumors, such as nonsmall cell lung cancer, in which direct p53 inactivation occurs. Perhaps in melanoma, therefore, simultaneous inactivation of p16[INK4a] and ARF is particularly effective in cooperating in melanoma formation, whereas other p53-related barriers are more significant in other nascent tumor types. Similar logic would apply to glioblastoma, another tumor type in which dual inactivation of p16[INK4a] and ARF through 9p21 loss is very common, and this lesion predicts a worse prognosis than p53 inactivation (reviewed in ref. *63*).

MC1R: Determinant of Red Hair Color Phenotype

Pigmentary traits such as red hair, fair complexion, the inability to tan and a tendency to freckle (red hair color [RHC] phenotype), have been shown to act as independent risk factors for all skin cancers, including melanoma (*see* Chapters 6 and 20). The human MC1R is a seven-transmembrane G protein-coupled receptor (GPCR) that is expressed on epidermal melanocytes. The MC1R ligand is melanocyte-stimulating hormone

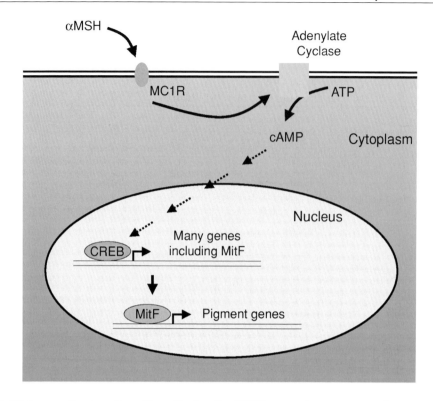

Fig. 3. Melanocortin signaling. The effects of α-MSH on melanocyte growth are mediated through upregulation of the cAMP pathway by the melanocortin receptor, MC1R, a G protein-coupled receptor (GPCR) that is present on melanocytes. Heterotrimeric G protein complexes that lie downstream of MC1R stimulate the intracellular messenger adenylyl cyclase (AC). AC, in turn, catalyzes the conversion of cytoplasmic ATP to cyclic AMP (cAMP), leading to increased intracellular cAMP. Increased intracellular cAMP acts as the second messenger, activating protein kinase A (PKA), which then translocates to the nucleus, where it phosphorylates the CREB (cAMP-responsive element binding protein) family of transcription factors. Phosphorylated CREB proteins induce expression of genes containing consensus CRE (cAMP-responsive element) sequences in their promoters (5'-TGACCTCA-3').

Although they respond in a cAMP-dependent manner, certain promoters of pigmentary genes, such as *tyrosinase TRP*-1 (tyrosinase-related protein-1) and *DCT* (dopachrome tautomerase), do not contain CRE consensus domains. Instead, their transcriptional activity is regulated by the basic helix-loop-helix (bHLH) transcription factor, MITF, which is important for the development of melanocytes *(179)*. The identification of a CRE consensus domain in the promoter of MITF provides the mechanistic link between the melanogenic effect of α-MSH signaling and the cAMP-dependent regulation of pigmentary genes *(179,180)*. The observation that the cAMP response of MITF is restricted to melanocytic cells *(181,182)*, however, indicates that additional lineage-specifying regulators of MITF activity have yet to be identified.

(MSH), a pituitary-derived hormone, and together these molecules regulate microphthalmia (MitF) and other key determinants of pigmentation (Fig. 3). MC1R is highly polymorphic in human populations, and allelic variation at this locus accounts, in large measure, for the variation in pigment phenotypes and skin phototypes in humans *(64,65)*. Three common variants of MC1R (R151C, R160W, and D294H) have been associated with the RHC phenotype *(66–71)*. Carrying a single RHC MC1R variant has been shown to significantly diminish the ability of the epidermis to respond to damage by UV *(68,71,72)*, presumably leading to increased melanoma risk *(69,72)*.

The mechanistic basis of the association between pigmentary traits and MC1R polymorphisms lies with the regulation of melanin synthesis by MSH–MC1R (covered further in Chapters 5, 18, and 19). MC1R variants may act to shift the balance of pheomelanin and eumelanin, increasing the relative amount of pheomelanin in skin. In addition to its diminished UV-protective capacity, pheomelanin produces metabolites that are believed to be mutagenic and cytotoxic *(73)*, which could further contribute to increased cancer risk. Along these lines, cell culture-based studies have shown that primary human melanocytes harboring RHC variants of MC1R demonstrate a pronounced increase in sensitivity to UV-induced cytotoxicity *(74)*. However, the fact that RHC MC1R variants are associated with increased melanoma risk in individuals with dark/olive complexions *(69,72,75)* suggests that they have additional pigment-independent effect(s) on melanoma risk.

Consistent with this hypothesis, several studies have shown that the impact of MC1R variants on melanoma risk can not be entirely attributed to its effect on skin type alone and that MC1R variants dramatically modify the penetrance of mutations at the *INK4a/ARF* locus *(71,75,76)*. In an Australian study of 15 familial melanoma kindreds, Hayward and colleagues showed that the presence of a single MC1R variant significantly increased the penetrance of *INK4a/ARF* mutation from 50 to 84%, and this increase was accompanied by a decrease in the mean age of onset from 58 yr to 37 yr *(71)*. In a separate study of Dutch melanoma families, Gruis and colleagues also found an increase in the penetrance of *INK4a/ARF* heterozygosity from 18 to 35% or 55%, in those with one or two MC1R variant alleles, respectively *(76)*. Both of these studies showed that the effect of MC1R on penetrance of the *INK4a/ARF* locus is primarily contributed by the common RHC variants. The molecular basis of this gene–gene interaction on melanoma risk will no doubt be the focus of future biochemical and genetic studies. This and other potential modifiers of melanoma risks have been reviewed recently *(77)*.

Xeroderma Pigmentosum and Other Defects of DNA Repair

Although more strongly associated with keratinocytic skin tumors, the xeroderma pigmentosum photosensitivity syndromes are also associated with melanoma, particularly in children. This increased incidence likely results from an increase in UV-associated DNA damage to melanocytes, although the molecular targets for UV-induced damage in xeroderma pigmentosum patients are not clear. *See* Chapter 16 for further details.

PATHWAYS TARGETED BY SOMATIC MUTATIONS IN MELANOMA

Despite their important roles in melanoma predisposition, the aforementioned mutations account for only a proportion of familial and sporadic melanomas, indicating that additional melanoma relevant genes likely exist. Detailed molecular analyses of human melanoma samples or cell lines have implicated many additional genes, primarily on the basis of altered patterns of expression. For most of these candidates, direct genetic evidence supporting their role in melanoma pathogenesis has not yet been obtained. However, for a handful of these genes and their pathways, mounting experimental data exist in support of their relevance.

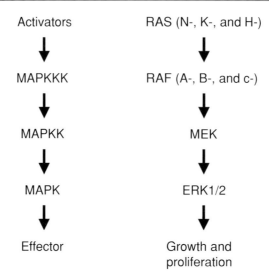

Fig. 4. Activation of the MAPK-signaling pathway. A simplified MAPK-signaling module is illustrated here with the RAS–RAF–MEK–ERK pathway. RTKs, such as HGF/SF, activate, among other targets, RAS family members, such as K-RAS and N-RAS. In melanoma, mutation of B-RAF, which is a MAPK kinase kinase, appears epistatic in oncogenic terms to RAS mutation. RAF, in turn, phosphorylates MAP kinases, such as the MEK family, which, in turn, phosphorylate ERKs (MAPK). Activated MAPK (phospho-ERK) then induces growth by a number of mechanisms, including alterations of transcription factor binding. Of note, this same signaling pathway appears to be responsible for the Ets-1-dependent induction of the *p16^INK4a* tumor suppressor gene *(183,184)*, suggesting the need for p16^INK4a inactivation is closely associated with RAS or RAF mutation in melanoma.

The genetic equivalence of N-RAS and B-RAF mutations in melanoma formation is surprising, because RAS activation induces other activities thought to be important for oncogenesis. For example, a recent study concluded that the Rho–GDP downstream effector arm is the primary mediator of the transforming activity of RAS in human fibroblasts, embryonic kidney epithelial cells, and astrocytes, whereas the Raf–MAPK pathway is more important in mouse fibroblasts or NIH3T3 cells *(185)*. In human melanoma, however, large-scale sequencing efforts have demonstrated that B-RAF mutations are present in a large proportion of human melanocytic and melanoma lesions, and that B-RAF and N-RAS are mutually exclusive mutations in these neoplasms. It is likely, therefore, that the downstream effectors of the transforming activity of RAS is context- and cell-type dependent.

Mitogen-Activated Protein Kinase Signaling Cascade

In the melanocytic lineage, proliferation, differentiation, and survival are tightly regulated and require synergistic paracrine stimulation by growth factors that signal from both heterotrimeric GPCRs (e.g., α-MSH) and receptor tyrosine kinases (RTKs, e.g., c-MET) *(78–82)*. The mitogen-activated protein kinase (MAPK) pathway appears able to transduce and integrate converging signals from both RTKs and GPCRs and, therefore, this may explain the frequent mutation of members of this signaling pathway in melanoma, because activating mutations in RAS or RAF might mimic mitogenic signals from both pathways.

The MAPKs are part of a system of kinases that translate a plethora of extracellular signals into diverse cellular responses (Fig. 4). In mammalian cells, there are at least four distinct signaling levels—activator, MAPK kinase kinase (MKKK), MAPK kinase, and

MAPK— each comprised of multiple members. The multiplicity of substrates at each sequential steps of physical interactions not only confers specificity to the ultimate cellular responses, but also serves to amplify the signals (reviewed in refs. *83* and *84*). Although the pathway can respond to a variety of stimuli, leading to various biological outcomes, including growth or growth arrest, for the purposes of melanoma formation, the most relevant signaling appears to be a mitogenic response to extracellular ligands that activate RAS.

RTKs are activated by interaction with a ligand, such as hepatocyte growth factor (HGF); or, in tumorigenesis, sometimes via an activating mutation, such as in epidermal growth factor receptor. After binding of ligands, receptor dimerization triggers the intrinsic tyrosine kinase activity of the receptor. This event is followed by autophosphorylation of specific tyrosine residues on the intracellular portion of the receptor. These phosphorylated tyrosine residues then bind the sequence homology 2 domains of adaptor proteins, such as GRB2. Such a complex formation recruits guanine exchange factors, such as son of sevenless, a cytosolic protein, into close proximity to RAS on the plasma membrane. Like other G proteins, RAS (H-RAS, N-RAS, and K-RAS) cycles between the GDP-bound inactive form and the GTP-bound active form. In the quiescent state, RAS exists in the GDP-bound form. The binding of son of sevenless to RAS causes a change in the RAS conformation and leads to the dissociation of GDP and binding of GTP. GTP-bound RAS is the activator of this signaling module. Although intimate cross talk between RTK and GPCR signaling no doubt exists at multiple levels (reviewed in ref. *85*), RAS activation has also been linked to GPCR signaling through cAMP via an as-yet poorly understood mechanism *(86)*. Therefore, in terms of tumorigenesis, oncogenic activation of RAS or RAF may be able to obviate the need for extracellular signals from both RTKs and GPCRs.

RAS activation in turn activates the RAF family of serine/threonine kinases—c-RAF, B-RAF, and A-RAF—known as MKKKs (Fig. 4). RAF then phosphorylates the MAPK kinase, MEK (also known as MKK1), which subsequently phosphorylates and activates the MAPKs, extracellular-regulated kinase 1 and 2 (ERK1 and ERK2). The ERKs translocate to the nucleus and regulate gene expression by phosphorylating a number of substrates involved in growth and cell division, such as S6 Kinase *(87)* and ETS1/2 *(88)*. It is worth noting that, although this cascade is classically thought of as being potently mitogenic, RAS and RAF also activate p16^{INK4a} transcription in an ETS1/2-dependent manner. Moreover, Spitz nevi with H-RAS amplification demonstrate high expression of p16^{INK4a} *(89)*, suggesting that progression of this melanocytic lesion is restrained by RB hypophosphorylation. Therefore, p16^{INK4a} inactivation may be a necessary event for the expression of the progrowth activity of RAS/RAF activation, explaining the frequent coexistence of these two lesions in melanoma.

Although not detected with high frequency, activating mutations of *RAS* in melanoma have been identified at a consistent, albeit low, incidence of 10–15%. In particular, activating *N-RAS* mutations have been correlated with nodular lesions and sun exposure *(90,91)*. Recent studies have reported that as many as 56% of congenital nevi *(92)*, 33% of primary, and 26% of metastatic clinical melanoma samples *(93)* harbor activating *N-RAS* point mutations. Interestingly, *N-RAS* mutations are rarely found in dysplastic nevi *(90,94,95)*, which could indicate that two distinct evolutionary paths to melanoma exist, from benign and dysplastic nevi. In the case of *H-RAS*, Bastian and colleagues have reported that chromosome 11p, where *H-RAS* resides, is occasionally amplified, and that this amplified *H-RAS* allele possesses oncogenic point mutations in Spitz nevi *(96)*. Transgenic studies in mice have shown that activated *H-RAS* mutations in melanocytes can lead to aberrant proliferation *(97)* and transformation, particularly in cooperation with inactivating mutations in tumor suppressors, such as $p16^{INK4a}$, $p19^{ARF}$, or *Trp53* *(98–100)*. These genetic data in the mouse, together with observations in human samples, have established an important role for the RAS-signaling pathway in melanoma genesis.

Recent genome-based, high-throughput sequencing efforts have identified activating *B-RAF* in as many as 60% of human melanoma samples and cell lines *(101)*. Importantly, these point mutations clustered in specific regions of biochemical importance, and 80% of them resulted in a single phosphomimetic substitution in the kinase activation domain (V599E) that is known to confer constitutive activation of B-RAF. On the genetic level, it is also reassuring to observe that the *B-RAF* V599E and *N-RAS* activated alleles are mutually exclusive, consistent with the view that these mutants are functionally equivalent in transformation *(101,102)*. More recently, *B-RAF* mutations have also been shown to be common in benign and dysplastic nevi *(103)*, which supports the observation that activation of ERKs is an early event in melanoma progression *(104)*. The finding of BRAF mutations in both benign and malignant melanocytic lesions points to its potential initiating role in transformation and to the need for additional cooperating genetic events to achieve full malignancy. Given these additional genetic events, it will therefore be important to assess the role of BRAF in maintenance of established melanoma in the appropriate context.

In addition to upstream RTK dimerization, there is evidence linking ERK activation to GPCR signaling, although the precise molecular steps have not been established *(85)*. A model of GPCR signaling to ERKs in melanocytes has been recently proposed, based on studies in B16 melanoma cells in culture, which implicate a novel melanocyte-specific RAS guanine exchange factor that activates RAS–RAF–ERKs in a cAMP-dependent and PKA-independent manner in response to α-MSH *(86)*. The relevance of this model remains to be validated in vivo.

HGF/Scatter Factor–MET Signaling

HGF/scatter factor (SF) executes its actions through its tyrosine kinase receptor, c-MET *(105)*, which is present on epithelial cells and melanocytes *(105)*. Although HGF normally acts in a paracrine manner, autocrine activation of HGF–MET has been demonstrated in transformed cells and tumors (reviewed in ref. *106*), including melanoma *(107)*. In addition to stimulating proliferation and motility of melanocytes in culture *(108)*, HGF has been shown to disrupt adhesion between melanocytes and keratinocytes via downregulation of E-cadherin and Desmoglein 1. The resultant decoupling of melanocytes from keratinocytes is thought to be permissive for scattering *(107)*. Additionally, HGF–MET activation has been implicated in melanoma progression. Increased c-MET expression has been observed in metastatic melanoma *(109)*, and gain of the 7q33–qter locus, where c-MET resides, seems to be a late event in melanoma progression *(110,111)*. Correspondingly, studies of mouse melanoma cells in explant models have shown that expression of c-Met, or Met RTK activity, are correlated with metastasis *(112)*.

Some of the most compelling data supporting aberrant HGF–MET signaling in melanoma pathogenesis derives from transgenic mice, in which the constitutive and ubiquitous expression of HGF *(113)* induces the development of various tumors, including melanoma. Although this model shows low penetrance and long latency, 20% of these melanoma-bearing mice develop distant metastasis *(113)*, which is thought to require autocrine activation of c-Met *(113)*. This is in contrast to melanocyte-specific *H-RAS* transgenic animals on a *Ink4a/Arf*$^{-/-}$ background, which developed cutaneous melanoma with much higher penetrance and shorter latency, but without metastasis *(98)*, further supporting a role for MET signaling in tumor progression.

The PTEN Tumor Suppressor

Loss of heterozygosity (LOH) and chromosomal rearrangements spanning 10q24–26 have been observed frequently in a wide spectrum of cancers, including melanoma. Human melanomas have been shown to sustain 10q LOH in approx 30–50% of cases (reviewed in ref. *114*). The region of deletion is often large, thus is capable of eliminating several *bona fide* tumor suppressors, which include the Myc antagonist, MXI1, and the phosphatase, PTEN.

PTEN encodes a negative regulator of the phosphatidylinositol 3-kinase (PI3K)/AKT-signaling pathway, which conveys potent cell proliferation and survival signals *(115)*. It was identified as the 10q tumor suppressor through homozygous deletion mapping in gliomas and breast tumors *(116–118)*. In melanoma, allelic loss or mutations of *PTEN* have been described in 5–15% of uncultured melanoma specimens and metastases, as well as in 30–40% of established melanoma cell lines *(119,120)*. Moreover, ectopic expression of PTEN in *PTEN*-deficient melanoma cells was able to suppress growth *(121)*, tumorigenicity, and metastasis *(122)*.

Germline heterozygous *PTEN* mutations in humans are associated with three clinically related, dominantly inherited cancer syndromes: Cowden disease, Lhermitte-Duclos disease, and Bannayan-Zonana syndrome *(123–125)*. In the mouse, *Pten* nullizygosity results in early embryonic death (*circa* d 6.5–7.5), whereas heterozygotes survive into adulthood but succumb to a wide spectrum of tumor types that is variably altered by the specific *Pten* mutation and/or genetic background *(126–129)*. Cutaneous melanoma was not observed in mice mutated for *Pten* alone, but was manifested at low frequency in *Pten*$^{+/-}$, *Ink4a/Arf*$^{+/-}$ mice *(129)*, confirming their collaborative interactions in melanoma formation.

Although *PTEN* is a *bona fide* tumor suppressor of 10q24, the existence of additional melanoma suppressors has been inferred by the fact that only 5–15% of uncultured melanoma specimens and metastases harbor *PTEN* mutation or allelic loss, compared with 30–50% of human melanomas with LOH of the 10q region, and that reintroduction of *PTEN* into such melanoma cells seems to have no growth-suppressive effect *(121)*. The Myc antagonist, *MXI1*, is a strong candidate for this, because *Myc* is amplified or overexpressed in *RAS*-induced *Trp53*-deficient melanomas in mouse *(99)*, and the *Mxi1*-deficient mice are moderately predisposed to cancer *(130)*. A role for Mxi1 in melanoma genesis in mice and humans has not, however, been rigorously evaluated.

LKB1: Regulator of Amp Kinase

Patients with the Peutz Jeghers syndrome demonstrate abnormal areas of hyperpigmentation of the bowel, oral mucosa, and lips. Most patients with this syndrome harbor inactivating mutations of a serine/threonine kinase, LKB1, of unknown function. This syndrome is associated with an increase in colonic polyps, colon cancer, and pancreatic cancer, but these patients do not appear to be at markedly increased risk for melanoma.

Sporadic mutations of *LKB1*, however, have been reported in series of melanoma, suggesting that LKB1 may have some tumor suppressor properties in melanocytes *(131,132)*. The observations that sporadic tumors harbor *LKB1* lesions, whereas germline mutations do not seem to increase the incidence of melanoma, are hard to reconcile. It is possible that *LKB1* mutations provide only a low-penetrance melanoma-prone condition (e.g., that requires significant UV exposure for manifestation) and this association has eluded investigators of this complex familial syndrome with variable expressivity. Experiments from *Lkb1*-deficient animals, however, suggest another likely explanation *(99)*. Cells from *Lkb1*-deficient embryos demonstrated a reduced susceptibility to RAS-mediated transformation, leading to the speculation that LKB1 has both tumor suppressor and oncogenic activity depending on genetic context. These data suggest the intriguing possibility that an *LKB1* mutation in an otherwise normal cell produces abnormal melanocyte differentiation but does not lead to melanoma and may in fact be antiproliferative, whereas the same mutation in the setting of other established oncogenic events does facilitate transformation. This hypothesis of conditional tumor suppressor activity awaits further elucidation of the biochemical tumor-relevant activities of LKB1.

GENETIC DISSECTION OF PATHWAYS IN MICE

The effort to understand human melanoma has been bolstered by the development of murine models of melanoma. These animal models have helped to determine the relative contributions of p53, p16^{INK4a}, and ARF to the prevention of RAS-induced melanoma, have aided in the identification of molecular UV targets in melanoma, and have provided a platform for high-throughput genomic analysis of this tumor type. For example, to study the role of *INK4a/ARF* loss in 9p21-mediated melanoma suppression, a conventional gene targeting approach was used to delete exons 2 and 3 of the *Ink4a/Arf* locus in the mouse germline, generating a mutant mouse that is null for both p16^{INK4a} and Arf *(133)*. These mice succumbed to fibrosarcomas and lymphomas with high frequency *(133)* and became highly prone to cutaneous melanomas with short latency when combined with an activated *H-RAS* mutation in their melanocytes (*Tyr-RAS$^+$*) *(98)*. Moreover, melanomas that arose in *Tyr-RAS$^+$*, *Ink4a/Arf$^{+/-}$* animals exhibited LOH in the remaining wild-type allele. The extent of LOH varied among tumors, but always included the second exon, thereby targeting both p16^{INK4a} and ARF, and suggesting that inactivation of both was necessary for tumor progression.

Likewise, murine models have been used to address the pathogenetic relevance of p53 pathway inactivation in melanoma. This topic has been controversial because numerous melanoma surveys have reported an absence or very low incidence of point mutation or allelic loss of *TP53* in surgical specimens of primary and metastatic melanomas (reviewed in ref. *134*). An early mouse modeling study by Mintz and colleagues, however, showed that expression of SV40 T antigen (which inactivates both RB and p53) generated a highly penetrant and aggressive melanoma phenotype *(135)*, suggesting involvement of the p53 pathway in melanoma pathogenesis. More direct evidence was later provided by the demonstration that *Tyr-RAS$^+$*, *Trp53$^{-/-}$* mice readily developed cutaneous melanomas *(99)*. LOH analysis of *Trp53* in melanomas that had arisen from *Tyr-RAS$^+$*, *Trp53$^{+/-}$* mice showed loss of the wild-type *Trp53* allele and retention of Arf *(99,134)*. These data, therefore, would suggest that either ARF or p53 inactivation can cooperate with other genetic lesions to promote melanoma formation, but that the lesions are functionally equivalent. In human melanoma, ARF loss is likely favored over p53 deletion, because the former often occurs with concomitant p16^{INK4a} loss by 9p21 deletion.

It is interesting to note that in contrast to *Tyr-Ras*$^+$, *Arf*$^{-/-}$ melanomas, in which p16^{INK4a} is lost in 50% of cases, *Tyr-Ras*$^+$, *Trp53*$^{-/-}$ melanomas almost always retain functional p16^{INK4a}. The RB pathway is, instead, inactivated via Myc amplification and overexpression *(99)*. c-Myc can bypass the G1 block conferred by p16^{INK4a}, in part, because of its ability to regulate G1 molecules that operate parallel to and downstream of p16^{INK4a} (reviewed in ref. *136*). Consistent with this, MYC overexpression *(137)* and increased copy number *(138)* have been described in human melanomas. The basis for this difference in preference of pRB pathway lesions between Arf- and p53-null mice is unknown. In other murine systems, however, it is clear that Myc overexpression can cooperate with Arf loss *(139)*, whereas p16^{INK4a} loss can cooperate with that of p53 *(140)*. Thus, despite our current lack of understanding regarding these combinations of genetic lesions in melanoma, data from these studies support the idea that both the RB and p53 pathways are important in melanoma suppression.

The contribution of p16^{INK4a} vs Arf in melanoma suppression has also been compared more directly using specific knockout for the two products of the *Ink4a/Arf* locus. Interestingly, animals specifically deficient for p16^{INK4a} demonstrate a low frequency of melanoma spontaneously or after carcinogen treatment with 7,12-dimethylbenz-anthracene (DMBA) *(22,23,140)*. Moreover, melanoma susceptibility imparted by p16^{INK4a} deficiency is significantly enhanced in the setting of *Arf* haploinsufficiency *(23)*, arguing for contribution from Arf in *Ink4a/Arf*-mediated melanoma suppression. When crossed onto the melanoma-prone *Tyr-RAS* transgenic allele, either p16^{INK4a} or Arf loss facilitated melanoma formation *(100)*. Notably, RB pathway lesions were encountered in melanomas from *Tyr-RAS*$^+$, *Arf*$^{-/-}$ mice, and p53 pathway lesions were detected in *Tyr-RAS*$^+$, *Ink4a*$^{-/-}$ melanomas. Such molecular profiles provide evidence that both products of the *Ink4a/Arf* locus have prominent roles in melanoma suppression in vivo, and this shared function may underlie the need for coordinated regulation, which might explain in some manner their intimate and evolutionarily conserved genomic arrangement *(17)*.

In conclusion, the combined experimental weight of the mouse and human genetic data strongly support the view that loss of ARF, and hence the p53 pathway, is involved in melanoma pathogenesis, and that ARF functions as a *bona fide* melanoma suppressor in vivo. Furthermore, the genetic data in the mouse provide a rational explanation for the low incidence of *TP53* mutations in human melanoma, given the frequent and early loss of *INK4a/ARF (50)* and the functional link between ARF and p53 *(13–16)* (Fig. 2).

THE GENE–ENVIRONMENT INTERFACE

The link between sun exposure and skin cancer, including melanoma, has long been recognized. It has been hypothesized on the basis of migration studies *(141)* that childhood may be a particularly susceptible time for sun damage *(142)* and that intense intermittent UV exposure associated with sunburn early in life confers the highest risk for melanoma development later in life *(2,143)*. This compelling epidemiological link between UV and melanoma risk is supported further by observations that UV can directly induce melanocytic lesions and melanoma in human skin grafts *(144,145)* and in neonatal mice (described on page 278).

The molecular basis of UV's cancer-promoting effects has been the focus of significant investigation and several mechanisms have been suggested, including that UV acts as a mutagen, a mitogen *(3)*, an inducer of tumor-promoting paracrine factors *(146)*, and an attenuator of antitumor immune surveillance *(147)*. Although the role for UV as a global mutagen would seem most appealing, the molecular targets have been elusive. The search for UV targets often relies on the identification of "UV-signature" mutations—represented as C→T or CC→TT base substitutions at dipyrimidine sites that result from the repair of cyclobutane pyrimidine dimers (CPDs) and 6-4 photoproducts induced by UVB. For example, the finding of C→T transitions in the *INK4a/ARF* locus in human melanoma samples *(7,148,149)* raised the possibility that p16^{INK4a} could be a target in humans, although others have reported similar mutation bias in gliomablastoma *(150)*. Although thought to be uncommon, UV also has the capacity to induce other types of damage, including protein–DNA cross-links; oxidative base damage; single-strand breaks *(151)*; chromosomal aberrations that are classically associated with double-strand breaks, such as deletion *(152)*; as well as epigenetic changes, such as altered methylation that can lead to increased mutation rates *(153)*. Given UV's broad actions, the identification of targeted genes/pathways and the relevance of each mechanism to melanoma development will require a multipronged approach that includes genomics and genetic model systems. Recently, genetically defined mouse models have proven useful in advancing our understanding of how this complex environmental mutagen promotes melanoma formation.

In the *Hgf* transgenic model, Merlino and colleagues showed that a single episode of mild sunburn during the neonatal period dramatically increases melanoma risk *(154)*. This result is in contrast to the development of nonmelanoma skin cancers in adult *Hgf* transgenic mice that are chronically exposed to UV *(155)*. Moreover, UV profoundly accelerated melanoma development with respect to both incidence and latency in *Hgf⁺*, *Ink4a/Arf⁻/⁻* mice *(156)*. To gain insight into UV's molecular targets, the effect of UV on melanoma incidence and latency was examined in *Tyr-RAS⁺* mice that were deficient for either p16^{INK4a} or Arf. After a single erythrogenic dose of UV on postnatal d 1, accelerated melanoma formation was observed exclusively in the *Tyr-RAS⁺*, *Arf⁻/⁻* animals *(37)*. These UV-induced *Tyr-RAS⁺*, *Arf⁻/⁻* melanomas exhibited genetic lesions in the pRB pathway as expected; however, the spectrum of those RB pathway lesions was different from those observed in the spontaneous *Tyr-RAS⁺*, *Arf⁻/⁻* melanomas. Whereas p16^{INK4a} inactivation is observed in 50% of spontaneous and 25% of UV-induced melanomas, amplification of *Cdk6* was present in 50% of the UV-induced melanomas. Loss of p16^{INK4a} and *Cdk6* amplification were mutually exclusive in the UV-induced melanomas. This pattern of mutations raises the possibility that components of the RB pathway are targets of UV's mutagenic actions, a hypothesis that is supported by the complete lack of cooperation between UV and p16^{INK4a} deficiency in the *Tyr-RAS⁺*, *p16$^{INK4a-/-}$* model *(37)*. In genetic terms, UV exposure and p16^{INK4a} loss, therefore, appear to be epistatic, at least in this *Ras*-driven murine model.

TUMOR MAINTENANCE GENES AS RATIONAL THERAPEUTIC TARGETS

The success of the selective tyrosine kinase inhibitor, imatinib (Gleevec), in the treatment of chronic myelogenous leukemia (CML) and gastrointestinal stromal tumors has validated the concept of molecularly targeted cancer therapy *(157,158)*. The cancer research community has been galvanized into the pursuit of molecular targets against which small-molecule inhibitors will be effective. Although such plausible targets are abundant in this genomics era, the imatinib experience has also brought into focus several current and future challenges, such as the problem of drug resistance *(159)*, which occurs even to imatinib in CML, which harbors relative genetic simplicity compared with solid tumors. Likewise, the imatinib paradigm underscores the importance of choosing "druggable" targets; that is, molecules whose tumor-promoting activity can be inhibited by a bioavailable small molecule. Lastly, an enormous challenge will be to select those promising targets that not only promote or are associated with tumor progression, but also are indeed essential for tumor maintenance, such as BCR-ABL in CML.

The concept of tumor maintenance stems from the observation that advanced malignancy represents the phenotypic end point of many successive genetic lesions and the established tumor is maintained and sustained through complex and poorly understood host–tumor interactions. Thus, the numerous and diverse genetic changes that accompany tumor development raise questions regarding whether a causal genetic alteration is still required for maintenance of viability of the established tumor. The development of inducible oncogene-transgenic models that permit extinction of oncogene activity in established tumors has been useful for validating targets, because it allows oncogenes that are important for tumor maintenance, as opposed to initiation, to be identified *(160)*. Using such a model, activated RAS has been shown to play not only a causal role in melanoma genesis, but also an essential role in the maintenance of established melanoma *(161)*.

Employing the tetracycline regulatory system, an inducible version of the *Tyr-RAS⁺*, *Ink4a/Arf⁻/⁻* melanoma model (*Tyr-rtTA⁺*, *Tet-RAS⁺*, *Ink4a/Arf⁻/⁻*) has been generated, whereby expression of the oncogenic lesion RAS can be regulated in a tissue-specific and developmental stage-specific manner *(161)*. In this system, postnatal activation of transgenic RAS expression via doxycycline drinking water leads to development of cutaneous melanomas that are phenotypically and clinically similar to those observed in the original *Tyr-RAS⁺*, *Ink4a/Arf⁻/⁻* model. Importantly, by conventional and array-based CGH analysis, these RAS-activated *Ink4a/Arf⁻/⁻* melanoma cells harbor secondary genomic changes, including gains and losses in regions syntenic to chromosomal alterations in human melanoma (*99*; L. Chin, unpublished observation). When adapted to culture, the presence or absence of doxycycline (e.g., with or without activated RAS, respectively) did not significantly influence the subconfluent growth rates of multiple independently derived melanoma cell lines in both high- and low-serum conditions. In contrast, regulation of activated RAS expression in vivo is associated with striking phenotypic changes in established tumors. When these doxycycline-treated *Tyr-rtTA⁺*, *Tet-RAS⁺*, *Ink4a/Arf⁻/⁻* mice bearing a single or multiple independent primary melanomas were withdrawn from doxycycline administration, established melanomas (0.5–1.5 cm in diameter) rapidly regressed to barely detectable or undetectable masses with only residual scattered tumor foci on microscopic examination within 10–14 d. In other words, removal of activated RAS in an established melanoma harboring many other irreversible genomic alterations resulted in tumor regression, a remarkable finding that attests to the essential role of RAS activation in tumor maintenance.

With the capacity to regulate activated RAS in established primary or explanted melanomas in vivo, this inducible oncogene-transgenic model system provides an opportunity to examine the roles of host–tumor interactions in tumor maintenance. For example, a well-known aspect of host–tumor interaction involves angiogenic support.

Analysis of regressing *Tyr-rtTA*[+], *Tet-RAS*[+], *Ink4a/Arf* [-/-] tumors was highlighted by dramatic activation of apoptosis in the tumor cell compartment as well as host-derived endothelial cells. The finding of endothelial cell apoptosis would suggest that vascular integrity of the tumor is compromised when RAS expression is downregulated, and that sustained activated RAS expression may be required for the critical host–tumor symbiotic interaction that sustains stable tumor vasculature. Previous cell culture-based studies have shown that oncogenic K- and H-RAS can stimulate expression of VEGF *(162–164)*, one of the most potent endothelial cell survival factors. These in vitro data would imply that activated RAS might maintain the tumor vasculature through enhanced VEGF gene expression. However, preliminary data from this in vivo model underscores the complexity of the RAS–VEGF angiogenesis link. Specifically, although a decline in VEGF mRNA and protein was associated with a decrease in RAS activity after doxycycline withdrawal in cell culture, an initial increase in VEGF was observed in vivo after doxycycline withdrawal *(161)*. These rising levels of VEGF are coincident with the initial stages of regression and tumor collapse and, thus, point to RAS-independent mechanisms of VEGF stimulation, such as that induced by tumor hypoxia *(165–168)*. Furthermore, enforced VEGF expression failed to "rescue" or reverse the tumor regression phenotype and associated vascular collapse after doxycycline withdrawal, conclusively establishing that VEGF is not sufficient for tumor maintenance. Given the pleiotropic effects of activated RAS and its importance in such a wide variety of human cancers, it is not surprising that its role in maintenance of established melanomas extends beyond VEGF and likely extends beyond the process of tumor angiogenesis.

This in vivo inducible model can serve as an ideal system in which additional aspects of host–tumor symbiosis can be uncovered. In addition to angiogenesis, these aspects may include immune surveillance, extracellular matrix degradation or other yet to be identified processes that are essential for the maintenance of established melanomas or other solid tumors in their natural settings. The elucidation of the biological function of a maintenance gene in tumor maintenance, such as that described for RAS, offers not only critical knowledge that can guide therapeutic development against RAS, but also a rational approach to design a synergistic regimen.

CONCLUSIONS AND PERSPECTIVES

The challenges that face the melanoma research community are formidable and require that we translate the growing body of genetic and biochemical information concerning the disease and its relation with other genetic lesions and cellular/environmental factors into effective preventive and therapeutic measures. The activated *B-RAF* allele would represent one such translational opportunity, particularly because RAF inhibitors are in clinical trials at present. However, it is worth noting that the role for *B-RAF* mutations in melanoma maintenance is not yet established. Development of inducible melanoma models driven by activated B-RAF would not only enable the assessment of its role in maintenance, but also provide insights into its biological function in the maintenance process. This genotype–phenotype information should lead to morphological and molecular surrogates of drug efficacy, that is, biomarkers that might guide the design and evaluation of small-molecule inhibitors in preclinical and clinical phases of drug development. Finally, the genotype–phenotype correlation and a better understanding of the cooperative events in tumorigenesis should provide additional strategies for combination therapy—it should be anticipated that resistance to RAF inhibitors would emerge in the setting of monotherapy. The good news is that comprehensive genomic, genetic, and phenotypic analyses of human samples and refined mouse models will provide molecular insights into mechanism of drug resistance. Coupled with rational drug development programs, it is reasonable to anticipate that alterative therapeutics for resistant tumors and synergistic combination therapies will emerge in the near future. Beyond *B-RAF*, many genetic lesions that are important to melanoma genesis, progression, and maintenance remain to be discovered, and genomic technologies will greatly enhance our ability to identify these genes. Tumor maintenance assays in inducible melanoma models will permit a more precise selection of maintenance targets for drug development.

Regarding the role of UV in melanoma genesis, the confirmation of the RB pathway as a primary target for inactivation in humans is a first step toward molecularly dissecting the mechanism of action of UV. The findings in the mouse indicates that there is great prognostic potential in assaying RB pathway status in pigmented lesions among individuals with significant UV exposure history or with constitutive predisposition to UV sensitivity. Furthermore, the delineation of UV's molecular targets can also open new opportunities for evaluation and development of effective sun protection measures. Although there is progress and hope on the horizon, it is likely that an effective therapeutic regimen for advanced melanoma will require a sustained effort. Therefore, improved prevention and early diagnosis may well have the most significant clinical impact on this disease in the near term.

ACKNOWLEDGMENTS

This work was supported in part by grants from the NIH to N.E.S. (K08 CA090679) and L.C. (RO1 CA93947; U01 CA84313). N.E.S. is a Sidney Kimmel Foundation Scholar in Cancer Research, and L.C. is a Charles E. Culpeper Scholar.

REFERENCES

1. Norris W. A case of fungoid disease. Edinburgh Medicine and Surgery, 1820;16:562–565.
2. Armstrong BK, Kricker A. The epidemiology of UV induced skin cancer. J Photochem Photobiol B 2001;63(1-3):8–18.
3. Gilchrest BA, Eller MS, Geller AC, Yaar M. The pathogenesis of melanoma induced by ultraviolet radiation. N Engl J Med 1999;340(17):1341–1348.
4. Marrett LD, Nguyen HL, Armstrong BK. Trends in the incidence of cutaneous malignant melanoma in New South Wales, 1983–1996. Int J Cancer 2001;92(3):457–462.
5. Fountain JW, Bale SJ, Housman DE, Dracopoli NC. Genetics of melanoma. Cancer Surv 1990;9(4):645–671.
6. Nobori T, Miura K, Wu DJ, Lois A, Takabayashi K, Carson DA. Deletions of the cyclin-dependent kinase-4 inhibitor gene in multiple human cancers. Nature 1994;368:753–756.
7. Kamb A, Gruis NA, Weaver-Feldhaus J, et al. A cell cycle regulator potentially involved in genesis of many tumor types. Science 1994;264(5157):436–440.
8. Hussussian CJ, Struewing JP, Goldstein AM, et al. Germline p16 mutations in familial melanoma. Nat Genet 1994;8(1):15–21.
9. Kamb A, Shattuck-Eidens D, Eeles R, et al. Analysis of the p16 gene (CDKN2) as a candidate for the chromosome 9p melanoma susceptibility locus. Nat Genet 1994;8(1):23–26.
10. Kamb A. Cell-cycle regulators and cancer. Trends Genet 1995;11(4):136–140.
11. Quelle DE, Zindy F, Ashmun RA, Sherr CJ. Alternative reading frames of the INK4a tumor suppressor gene encode two unrelated proteins capable of inducing cell cycle arrest. Cell 1995;83(6):993–1000.

12. Serrano M, Hannon GJ, Beach D. A new regulatory motif in cell-cycle control causing specific inhibition of cyclin D/CDK4. Nature 1993;366(6456):704–707.

13. Kamijo T, Weber JD, Zambetti G, Zindy F, Roussel MF, Sherr CJ. Functional and physical interactions of the ARF tumor suppressor with p53 and Mdm2. Proc Natl Acad Sci USA, 1998;95: 8292–8297.

14. Pomerantz J, Schreiber-Agus N, Liegeois NJ, et al. The Ink4a tumor suppressor gene product, p19Arf, interacts with MDM2 and neutralizes MDM2's inhibition of p53. Cell 1998;92(6):713–723.

15. Stott FJ, Bates S, James MC, et al. The alternative product from the human CDKN2A locus, p14(ARF), participates in a regulatory feedback loop with p53 and MDM2. EMBO J 1998;17:5001–5014.

16. Zhang Y, Xiong Y, Yarbrough WG. ARF promotes MDM2 degradation and stabilizes p53: ARF-INK4a locus deletion impairs both the Rb and p53 tumor suppression pathways. Cell 1998;92(6): 725–734.

17. Sharpless NE. INK4a/ARF: a multifunctional tumor suppressor locus. Mutat Res 2004, in press.
Au: Please update publication information for Ref. 17, if known.

18. Aitken J, Welch J, Duffy D, et al. CDKN2A variants in a population-based sample of Queensland families with melanoma. J Natl Cancer Inst 1999;91(5):446–452.

19. Tsao H, Zhang X, Kwitkiwski K, Finkelstein DM, Sober AJ, Haluska FG. Low prevalence of germline CDKN2A and CDK4 mutations in patients with early-onset melanoma. Arch Dermatol 2000; 136(9):1118–1122.

20. Liu L, Dilworth D, Gao L, et al. Mutation of the CDKN2A 5′ UTR creates an aberrant initiation codon and predisposes to melanoma. Nat Genet 1999;21(1):128–132.

21. Kumar R, Smeds J, Berggren P, et al. A single nucleotide polymorphism in the 3′ untranslated region of the CDKN2A gene is common in sporadic primary melanomas but mutations in the CDKN2B, CDKN2C, CDK4 and p53 genes are rare. Int J Cancer 2001;95(6):388–393.

22. Sharpless NE, Bardeesy N, Lee KH, et al. Loss of p16Ink4a with retention of p19Arf predisposes mice to tumorigenesis. Nature 2001;413(6851):86–91.

23. Krimpenfort P, Quon KC, Mooi WJ, Loonstra A, Berns A. Loss of p16Ink4a confers susceptibility to metastatic melanoma in mice. Nature 2001;413(6851):83–86.

24. Yarbrough WG, Aprelikova O, Pei H, Olshan AF, Liu ET. Familial tumor syndrome associated with a germline nonfunctional p16INK4a allele. J Natl Cancer Inst 1996;88(20):1489–1491.

25. Hruban RH, Petersen GM, Goggins M, et al. Familial pancreatic cancer. Ann Oncol 1999; 10(suppl 4):6–73.

26. Vasen HF, Gruis NA, Frants RR, van Der Velden PA, Hille ET, Bergman W. Risk of developing pancreatic cancer in families with familial atypical multiple mole melanoma associated with a specific 19 deletion of p16 (p16-Leiden). Int J Cancer 2000;87(6):809–811.

27. Whelan AJ, Bartsch D, Goodfellow PJ. A familial syndrome of pancreatic cancer and melanoma in the CDKN2 tumor-suppressor gene. N Engl J Med 1995;333:975–977.

28. Bahuau M, Viduad D, Jenkins R, et al. Germ-line deletion involving the ink4 locus in familial proneness to melanoma and nervous system tumors. Cancer Res 1998;58:2298–2303.

29. Tachibana I, Smith JS, Sato K, Hosek SM, Kimmel DW, Jenkins RB. Investigation of germline PTEN, p53, p16(INK4A)/p14(ARF), and CDK4 alterations in familial glioma. Am J Med Genet 2000;92(2):136–141.

30. Dilworth D, Liu L, Stewart AK, Berenson JR, Lassam N, Hogg D. Germline CDKN2A mutation implicated in predisposition to multiple myeloma. Blood 2000;95(5):1869–1871.

31. Oldenburg RA, de Vos tot Nederveen Cappel WH, van Puijenbroek M, et al. Extending the p16-Leiden tumour spectrum by respiratory tract tumours. J Med Genet 2004;41(3):e31.

32. Borg A, Sandberg T, Nilsson K, et al. High frequency of multiple melanomas and breast and pancreas carcinomas in CDKN2A mutation-positive melanoma families. J Natl Cancer Inst 2000;92(15): 1260–1266.

33. Lal G, Liu L, Hogg D, Lassam NJ, Redston MS, Gallinger S. Patients with both pancreatic adenocarcinoma and melanoma may harbor germline CDKN2A mutations. Genes Chromosomes Cancer 2000;27(4):358–361.

34. Bartsch DK, Sina-Frey M, Lang S, et al. CDKN2A germline mutations in familial pancreatic cancer. Ann Surg 2002;236(6):730–737.

35. Fahraeus R, Lane DP. The p16(INK4a) tumour suppressor protein inhibits alphavbeta3 integrin-mediated cell spreading on vitronectin by blocking PKC-dependent localization of alphavbeta3 to focal contacts. EMBO J 1999;18(8):2106–2118.

36. Wolff B, Naumann M. INK4 cell cycle inhibitors direct transcriptional inactivation of NF-kappaB. Oncogene, 1999;18(16):2663–2666.

37. Kannan K, Sharpless NE, Xu J, O'Hagan RC, Bosenberg M, Chin L. Components of the Rb pathway are critical targets of UV mutagenesis in a murine melanoma model. Proc Natl Acad Sci USA 2003;100(3):1221–1225.

38. Bishop DT, Demenais F, Goldstein AM, et al. Geographical variation in the penetrance of CDKN2A mutations for melanoma. J Natl Cancer Inst 2002;94(12):894–903.

39. Wolfel T, Hauer M, Schneider J, et al. A p16INK4a-insensitive CDK4 mutant targeted by cytolytic T lymphocytes in a human melanoma. Science 1995;269(5228):1281–1284.

40. Zuo L, Weger J, Yang Q, et al. Germline mutations in the p16INK4a binding domain of CDK4 in familial melanoma. Nat Genet 1996;12(1):97–99.

41. Soufir N, Avril MF, Chompret A, et al. Prevalence of p16 and CDK4 germline mutations in 48 melanoma-prone families in France. The French Familial Melanoma Study Group. Hum Mol Genet 1998;7:209–216.

42. Tsao H, Benoit E, Sober AJ, Thiele C, Haluska FG. Novel mutations in the p16/CDKN2A binding region of the cyclin-dependent kinase-4 gene. Cancer Res 1998;58(1):109–113.

43. Russo AA, Tong L, Lee JO, Jeffrey PD, Pavletich NP. Structural basis for inhibition of the cyclin-dependent kinase Cdk6 by the tumour suppressor p16INK4a. Nature 1998;395(6699):237–243.

44. Goldstein AM, Struewing JP, Chidambaram A, Fraser MC, Tucker MA. Genotype-phenotype relationships in U.S. melanoma-prone families with CDKN2A and CDK4 mutations. J Natl Cancer Inst 2000;92(12):1006–1010.

45. Sotillo R, Garcia JF, Ortega S, et al. Invasive melanoma in Cdk4-targeted mice. Proc Natl Acad Sci USA 2001;98(23):13,312–13,317.

46. Draper GJ, Sanders BM, Kingston JE. Second primary neoplasms in patients with retinoblastoma. Br J Cancer 1986;53(5):661–671.

47. Sanders BM, Jay M, Draper GJ, Roberts EM. Non-ocular cancer in relatives of retinoblastoma patients. Br J Cancer 1989;60(3):358–365.

48. Fletcher O, Easton D, Anderson K, Gilham C, Jay M, Peto J. Lifetime risks of common cancers among retinoblastoma survivors. J Natl Cancer Inst 2004;96(5):357–363.

49. Eng C, Ponder BA. The role of gene mutations in the genesis of familial cancers. FASEB J 1993;7(10):910–919.

50. Ruas M, Peters G. The p16INK4a/CDKN2A tumor suppressor and its relatives. Biochim Biophys Acta 1998;1378(2):F115–F177.

51. Piccinin S, Doglioni C, Maestro R, et al. p16/CDKN2 and CDK4 gene mutations in sporadic melanoma development and progression. Int J Cancer 1997;74(1):26–30.

52. Straume O, Smeds J, Kumar R, Hemminki K, Akslen LA. Significant impact of promoter hypermethylation and the 540 C>T polymorphism of CDKN2A in cutaneous melanoma of the vertical growth phase. Am J Pathol 2002;161(1):229–237.

53. Kumar R, Sauroja I, Punnonen K, Jansen C, Hemminki K. Selective deletion of exon 1 beta of the p19ARF gene in metastatic melanoma cell lines. Genes Chromosomes Cancer 1998;23(3):273–277.

54. Randerson-Moor JA, Harland M, Williams S, et al. A germline deletion of p14(ARF) but not CDKN2A in a melanoma-neural system tumour syndrome family. Hum Mol Genet 2001;10(1):55–62.

55. Rizos H, Puig S, Badenas C, et al. A melanoma-associated germline mutation in exon 1beta inactivates p14ARF. Oncogene 2001;20(39):5543–5547.

56. Duro D, O Bernard, V Della Valle, R Berger, CJ Larsen. A new type of p16INK4/MTS1 gene transcript expressed in B-cell malignancies. Oncogene 1995;11(1):21–29.

57. Mao L, Merlo A, Bedi G, et al. A novel p16INK4a transcript. Cancer Res 1995;55:2995–2997.

58. Stone S, Jiang P, Dayananth P, et al. Complex structure and regulation of the p16(MTS1) locus. Cancer Res 1995;55:2988–2994.

59. Swafford DS, Middleton SK, Palmisano WA, et al. Frequent aberrant methylation of p16INK4a in primary rat lung tumors. Mol Cell Biol 1997;17(3):1366–1374.

60. Sherburn TE, Gale JM, Ley RD. Cloning and characterization of the CDKN2A and p19ARF genes from Monodelphis domestica. DNA Cell Biology 1998;17(11):975–981.

61. Castresana JS, Rubio MP, Vazquez JJ, et al. Lack of allelic deletion and point mutation as mechanisms of p53 activation in human malignant melanoma. Int J Cancer 1993;55(4):562–565.

62. Zerp SF, van Elsas A, Peltenburg LT, Schrier PI. p53 mutations in human cutaneous melanoma correlate with sun exposure but are not always involved in melanomagenesis. Br J Cancer 1999;79(5-6):921–926.

63. Maher EA, Furnari FB, Bachoo RM, et al. Malignant glioma: genetics and biology of a grave matter. Genes Dev 2001;15(11):1311–1333.

64. Valverde P, Healy E, Jackson I, Rees JL, Thody AJ. Variants of the melanocyte-stimulating hormone receptor gene are associated with red hair and fair skin in humans. Nat Genet 1995;11(3):328–330.

65. Sturm RA. Skin colour and skin cancer—MC1R, the genetic link. Melanoma Res 2002;12(5):405–416.

66. Box NF, Wyeth JR, O'Gorman LE, Martin NG, Sturm RA. Characterization of melanocyte stimulating hormone receptor variant alleles in twins with red hair. Hum Mol Genet 1997;6(11):1891–1897.

67. Smith R, Healy E, Siddiqui S, et al. Melanocortin 1 receptor variants in an Irish population. J Invest Dermatol 1998;111(1):119–122.

68. Flanagan N, Healy E, Ray A, et al. Pleiotropic effects of the melanocortin 1 receptor (MC1R) gene on human pigmentation. Hum Mol Genet 2000;9(17):2531–2537.

69. Palmer JS, Duffy DL, Box NF, et al. Melanocortin-1 receptor polymorphisms and risk of melanoma: is the association explained solely by pigmentation phenotype? Am J Hum Genet 2000;66(1):176–186.

70. Bastiaens M, ter Huurne J, Gruis N, et al. The melanocortin-1-receptor gene is the major freckle gene. Hum Mol Genet 2001;10(16):1701–1708.

71. Box NF, Duffy DL, Chen W, et al. MC1R genotype modifies risk of melanoma in families segregating CDKN2A mutations. Am J Hum Genet 2001;69(4):765–773.

72. Healy E, Flannagan N, Ray A, et al. Melanocortin-1-receptor gene and sun sensitivity in individuals without red hair. Lancet 2000;355(9209):1072–1073.

73. Harsanyi ZP, Post PW, Brinkmann JP, Chedekel MR, Deibel RM. Mutagenicity of melanin from human red hair. Experientia 1980;36(3):291–292.

74. Scott MC, Wakamatsu K, Ito S, et al. Human melanocortin 1 receptor variants, receptor function and melanocyte response to UV radiation. J Cell Sci 2002;115(Pt 11):2349–2355.

75. Kennedy C, ter Huurne J, Berkhout M, et al. Melanocortin 1 receptor (MC1R) gene variants are associated with an increased risk for cutaneous melanoma which is largely independent of skin type and hair color. J Invest Dermatol 2001;117(2):294–300.

76. van der Velden PA, Sandkuijl LA, Bergman W, et al. Melanocortin-1 receptor variant R151C modifies melanoma risk in Dutch families with melanoma. Am J Hum Genet 2001;69(4):774–779.

77. Hayward NK. Genetics of melanoma predisposition. Oncogene 2003;22:3053–3062.

78. Imokawa G, Yada Y, Miyagishi M. Endothelins secreted from human keratinocytes are intrinsic mitogens for human melanocytes. J Biochem 1992;267(34):24,675–24,680.

79. Gilchrest BA, Park HY, Eller MS, Yaar M. Mechanisms of ultraviolet light-induced pigmentation. Photochem Photobiol 1996;63(1):1–10.

80. Tada A, Suzuki I, Im S, et al. Endothelin-1 is a paracrine growth factor that modulates melanogenesis of human melanocytes and participates in their responses to ultraviolet radiation. Cell Growth and Differentiation 1998;9(7):575–584.

81. Nesbit M, Nesbit HK, Bennett J, et al. Basic fibroblast growth factor induces a transformed phenotype in normal human melanocytes. Oncogene 1999;18(47):6469–6476.

82. Dupin E, Le Douarin NM. Development of melanocyte precursors from the vertebrate neural crest. Oncogene 2003;22:3016–3023.

83. Chang L, Karin M. Mammalian MAP kinase signalling cascades. Nature 2001;410(6824):37–40.

84. Johnson GL, Lapadat R. Mitogen-activated protein kinase pathways mediated by ERK, JNK, and p38 protein kinases. Science 2002;298(5600):1911–1912.

85. Lowes VL, Ip NY, Wong YH. Integration of signals from receptor tyrosine kinases and G protein-coupled receptors. Neurosignals 2002;11(1):5–19.

86. Busca R, Abbe P, Mantoux F, et al. Ras mediates the cAMP-dependent activation of extracellular signal-regulated kinases (ERKs) in melanocytes. EMBO J 2000;19(12):2900–2910.

87. Crews CM, Alessandrini AA, Erikson RL. Mouse Erk-1 gene product is a serine/threonine protein kinase that has the potential to phosphorylate tyrosine. Proc Natl Acad Sci USA 1991;88(19): 8845–8849.

88. Paumelle R, Tulasne D, Kherrouche Z, et al. Hepatocyte growth factor/scatter factor activates the ETS1 transcription factor by a RAS-RAF-MEK-ERK signaling pathway. Oncogene 2002;21(15): 2309–2319.

89. Maldonado JL, Timmerman L, Fridlyand J, Bastian BC. Mechanisms of cell-cycle arrest in Spitz nevi with constitutive activation of the MAP-kinase pathway. Am J Pathol 2004;164(5):1783–1787.

90. Jafari M, Papp T, Kirchner S, et al. Analysis of ras mutations in human melanocytic lesions: activation of the ras gene seems to be associated with the nodular type of human malignant melanoma. Journal of Cancer Research and Clinical Oncology 1995;121(1):23–30.

91. van Elsas A, Zerp SF, van der Flier S, et al. Relevance of ultraviolet-induced N-ras oncogene point mutations in development of primary human cutaneous melanoma. Am J Pathol 1996;149(3): 883–893.

92. Papp T, Pemsel H, Zimmermann R, Bastrop R, Weiss DG, Schiffmann D. Mutational analysis of the N-ras, p53, p16INK4a, CDK4, and MC1R genes in human congenital melanocytic naevi. J Med Genet 1999;36(8):610–614.

93. Demunter A, Stas M, Degreef H, De Wolf-Peeters C, van den Oord JJ. Analysis of N- and K-ras mutations in the distinctive tumor progression phases of melanoma. J Invest Dermatol 2001;117(6): 1483–1489.

94. Albino AP, Nanus DM, Mentle IR, et al. Analysis of ras oncogenes in malignant melanoma and precursor lesions: correlation of point mutations with differentiation phenotype. Oncogene 1989;4(11):1363–1374.

95. Papp T, Pemsel H, Rollwitz I, et al. Mutational analysis of N-ras, p53, CDKN2A (p16(INK4a)), p14(ARF), CDK4, and MC1R genes in human dysplastic melanocytic naevi. J Med Genet 2003;40(2):E14.

96. Bastian BC, M Kashani-Sabet, H Hamm, et al. Gene amplifications characterize acral melanoma and permit the detection of occult tumor cells in the surrounding skin. Cancer Res 2000;60(7): 1968–1973.

97. Powell MB, Hyman P, Bell OD, et al. Hyperpigmentation and melanocytic hyperplasia in transgenic mice expressing the human T24 Ha-ras gene regulated by a mouse tyrosinase promoter. Mol Carcinog 1995;12(2):82–90.

98. Chin L, Pomerantz J, Polsky D, et al. Cooperative effects of INK4a and ras in melanoma susceptibility in vivo. Genes Dev 1997;11(21):2822–2834.

99. Bardeesy N, Bastian BC, Hezel A, Pinkel D, DePinho RA, Chin L. Dual inactivation of RB and p53 pathways in RAS-induced melanomas. Mol Cell Biol 2001;21(6):2144–2153.

100. Sharpless NE, Kannan K, Xu J, Bosenberg MW, Chin L. Both products of the mouse Ink4a/Arf locus suppress melanoma formation in vivo. Oncogene 2003;22(32):5055–5059.

101. Davies H, Bignell GR, Cox C, et al. Mutations of the BRAF gene in human cancer. Nature 2002;417(6892):949–954.

102. Rajagopalan H, Bardelli A, Lengauer C, Kinzler KW, Vogelstein B, Velculescu VE. Tumorigenesis: RAF/RAS oncogenes and mismatch-repair status. Nature 2002;418(6901):934.

103. Pollock PM, Harper UL, Hansen KS, et al. High frequency of BRAF mutations in nevi. Nat Genet 2003;33(1):19–20.

104. Cohen C, Zavala-Pompa A, Sequeira JH, et al. Mitogen-activated protein kinase activation is an early event in melanoma progression. Clin Cancer Res 2002;8(12):3728–3733.

105. Bottaro DP, Rubin JS, Faletto DL, et al. Identification of the hepatocyte growth factor receptor as the c-met proto-oncogene product. Science 1991;251:802–804.

106. Vande Woude GF, Jeffers M, Cortner J, Alvord G, Tsarfaty I, Resau J. Met-HGF/SF: tumorigenesis, invasion and metastasis. Ciba Found Symp 1997;212:119–130; discussion 130–132, 148–154.

107. Li G, Schaider H, Satyamoorthy K, Hanakawa Y, Hashimoto K, Herlyn M. Downregulation of E-cadherin and Desmoglein 1 by autocrine hepatocyte growth factor during melanoma development. Oncogene. 2001;20(56):8125–8135.

108. Halaban R, Rubin JS, Funasaka Y, et al. Met and hepatocyte growth factor/scatter factor signal transduction in normal melanocytes and melanoma cells. Oncogene 1992;7:2195–2206.

109. Natali PG, Nicotra MR, Di Renzo MF, et al. Expression of the c-Met/HGF receptor in human melanocytic neoplasms: demonstration of the relationship to malignant melanoma tumour progression. Br J Cancer 1993;68:746–750.

110. Wiltshire RN, Duray P, Bittner ML, et al. Direct visualization of the clonal progression of primary cutaneous melanoma: application of tissue microdissection and comparative genomic hybridization. Cancer Res 1995;55(18):3954–3957.

111. Bastian BC, LeBoit PE, Hamm H, Brocker EB, Pinkel D. Chromosomal gains and losses in primary cutaneous melanomas detected by comparative genomic hybridization. Cancer Res 1998;58:2170–2175.

112. Rusciano D, Lorenzoni P, Burger MM. Expression of constitutively activated hepatocyte growth factor/scatter factor receptor (c-met) in B16 melanoma cells selected for enhanced liver colonization. Oncogene 1995;11:1979–1987.

113. Otsuka T, Takayama H, Sharp R, et al. c-Met autocrine activation induces development of malignant melanoma and acquisition of the metastatic phenotype. Cancer Res 1998;58(22):5157–5167.

114. Wu H, Goel V, Haluska FG. PTEN signaling pathways in melanoma. Oncogene 2003;22:3113–3122.
115. Stambolic V, Suzuki A, de la Pompa JL, et al. Negative regulation of PKB/Akt-dependent cell survival by the tumor suppressor PTEN. Cell 1998;95(1):29–39.
116. Li J, Yen C, Liaw D, et al. PTEN, a putative protein tyrosine phosphatase gene mutated in human brain, breast, and prostate cancer [see comments]. Science 1997;275:1943–1947.
117. Steck PA, Pershouse MA, Jasser SA, et al. Identification of a candidate tumour suppressor gene, MMAC1, at chromosome 10q23.3 that is mutated in multiple advanced cancers. Nat Genet 1997;15(4):356–362.
118. Li DM, Sun H. TEP1, encoded by a candidate tumor suppressor locus, is a novel protein tyrosine phosphatase regulated by transforming growth factor beta. Cancer Res 1997;57(11):2124–2129.
119. Guldberg P, thor Straten P, Birck A, Ahrenkiel V, Kirkin AF, Zeuthen J. Disruption of the MMAC1/PTEN gene by deletion or mutation is a frequent event in malignant melanoma. Cancer Res 1997;57:3660–3663.
120. Teng DH, Hu R, Lin H, et al. MMAC1/PTEN mutations in primary tumor specimens and tumor cell lines. Cancer Res 1997;57(23):5221–5225.
121. Robertson GP, Furnari FB, Miele ME, et al. In vitro loss of heterozygosity targets the PTEN/MMAC1 gene in melanoma. Proc Natl Acad Sci USA 1998;95(16):9418–9423.
122. Hwang PH, Yi HK, Kim DS, Nam SY, Kim JS, Lee DY. Suppression of tumorigenicity and metastasis in B16F10 cells by PTEN/MMAC1/TEP1 gene. Cancer Lett 2001;172(1):83–91.
123. Liaw D, Marsh DJ, Li J, et al. Germline mutations of the PTEN gene in Cowden disease, an inherited breast and thyroid cancer syndrome. Nat Genet 1997;16(1):64–67.
124. Marsh DJ, Dahia PL, Zheng Z, et al. Germline mutations in PTEN are present in Bannayan-Zonana syndrome. Nat Genet 1997;16(4):333–334.
125. Nelen MR, van Staveren WC, Peeters EA, et al. Germline mutations in the PTEN/MMAC1 gene in patients with Cowden disease. Hum Mol Genet 1997;6(8):1383–1387.
126. Di Cristofano A, Pesce B, Cordon-Cardo C, Pandolfi PP. Pten is essential for embryonic development and tumour suppression. Nat Genet 1998;19(4):348–355.
127. Podsypanina K, Ellenson LH, Nemes A, et al. Mutation of Pten/Mmac1 in mice causes neoplasia in multiple organ systems. Proc Natl Acad Sci USA 1999;96(4):1563–1568.
128. Suzuki A, de la Pompa JL, Stambolic V, et al. High cancer susceptibility and embryonic lethality associated with mutation of the PTEN tumor suppressor gene in mice. Curr Biol 1998;8(21):1169–1178.
129. You MJ, Castrillon DH, Bastian BC, et al. Genetic analysis of Pten and Ink4a/Arf interactions in the suppression of tumorigenesis in mice. Proc Natl Acad Sci USA 2002;99(3):1455–1460.
130. Schreiber-Agus N, Meng Y, Hoang T, et al. Role of Mxi1 in ageing organ systems and the regulation of normal and neoplastic growth. Nature 1998;393(6684):483–487.
131. Rowan A, Bataille V, MacKie R, et al. Somatic mutations in the Peutz-Jegners (LKB1/STKII) gene in sporadic malignant melanomas. J Invest Dermatol 1999;112(4):509–511.
132. Guldberg P, thor Straten P, Ahrenkiel V, Seremet T, Kirkin AF, Zeuthen J. Somatic mutation of the Peutz-Jeghers syndrome gene, LKB1/STK11, in malignant melanoma. Oncogene 1999;18(9):1777–1780.
133. Serrano M, Lee H, Chin L, Cordon-Cardo C, Beach D, DePinho RA. Role of the INK4a locus in tumor suppression and cell mortality. Cell 1996;85(1):27–37.
134. Yang FC, Merlino G, Chin L. Genetic dissection of melanoma pathways in the mouse. Semin Cancer Biol 2001;11(3):261–268.
135. Bradl M, Klein-Szanto A, Porter S, Mintz B. Malignant melanoma in transgenic mice. Proc Natl Acad Sci USA 1991;88(1):164–168.
136. Dang CV. c-Myc target genes involved in cell growth, apoptosis, and metabolism. Mol Cell Biol 1999;19(1):1–11.
137. Ross DA, Wilson GD. Expression of c-myc oncoprotein represents a new prognostic marker in cutaneous melanoma. Br J Surg 1998;85(1):46–51.
138. Kraehn GM, Utikal J, Udart M, et al. Extra c-myc oncogene copies in high risk cutaneous malignant melanoma and melanoma metastases. Br J Cancer 2001;84(1):72–79.
139. Schmitt CA, McCurrach ME, de Stanchina E, Wallace-Brodeur RR, Lowe SW. INK4a/ARF mutations accelerate lymphomagenesis and promote chemoresistance by disabling p53. Genes Dev 1999;13(20):2670–2677.
140. Sharpless NE, Alson S, Chan S, Silver DP, Castrillon DH, DePinho RA. p16INK4a and p53 deficiency cooperate in tumorigenesis. Cancer Res 2002;62:2761–2765.

141. Holman CD, Armstrong BK. Cutaneous malignant melanoma and indicators of total accumulated exposure to the sun: an analysis separating histogenetic types. J Natl Cancer Inst 1984;73(1):75–82.

142. Autier P, Dore JF. Influence of sun exposures during childhood and during adulthood on melanoma risk. EPIMEL and EORTC Melanoma Cooperative Group. European Organisation for Research and Treatment of Cancer. Int J Cancer 1998;77(4):533–537.

143. Whiteman DC, Whiteman CA, Green AC. Childhood sun exposure as a risk factor for melanoma: a systematic review of epidemiologic studies. Cancer Causes Control 2001;12(1):69–82.

144. Atillasoy ES, Seykora JT, Soballe PW, et al. UVB induces atypical melanocytic lesions and melanoma in human skin. Am J Pathol 1998;152(5):1179–1186.

145. Berking C, Takemoto R, Binder RL, et al. Photocarcinogenesis in human adult skin grafts. Carcinogenesis 2002;23(1):181–187.

146. Jamal S, Schneider RJ. UV-induction of keratinocyte endothelin-1 downregulates E-cadherin in melanocytes and melanoma cells. J Clin Invest 2002;110(4):443–452.

147. Donawho CK, Kripke ML. Evidence that the local effect of ultraviolet radiation on the growth of murine melanomas is immunologically mediated. Cancer Res 1991;51(16):4176–4181.

148. Pollock PM, Pearson JV, Hayward NK. Compilation of somatic mutations of the CDKN2 gene in human cancers: non-random distribution of base substitutions. Genes Chromosomes Cancer 1996;15(2):77–88.

149. Peris K, Chimenti S, Fargnoli MC, Valeri P, Kerl H, Wolf P. UV fingerprint CDKN2a but no p14ARF mutations in sporadic melanomas. J Invest Dermatol 1999;112(5):825–826.

150. Kyritsis AP, Zhang B, Zhang W, et al. Mutations of the p16 gene in gliomas. Oncogene 1996; 12(1):63–67.

151. de Gruijl FR, van Kranen HJ, Mullenders LH. UV-induced DNA damage, repair, mutations and oncogenic pathways in skin cancer. J Photochem Photobiol B 2001;63(1-3):19–27.

152. Horiguchi M, Masumura KI, Ikehata H, Ono T, Kanke Y, Nohmi T. Molecular nature of ultraviolet B light-induced deletions in the murine epidermis. Cancer Res 2001;61(10):3913–3918.

153. Jones PA, Baylin SB. The fundamental role of epigenetic events in cancer. Nat Rev Genet 2002;3(6):415–428.

154. Noonan FP, Recio JA, Takayama H, et al. Neonatal sunburn and melanoma in mice. Nature 2001;413(6853):271–272.

155. Noonan FP, Otsuka T, Bang S, Anver MR, Merlino G. Accelerated ultraviolet radiation-induced carcinogenesis in hepatocyte growth factor/scatter factor transgenic mice. Cancer Res 2000; 60(14):3738–3743.

156. Recio JA, Noonan FP, Takayama H, et al. Ink4a/arf deficiency promotes ultraviolet radiation-induced melanomagenesis. Cancer Res 2002;62(22):6724–6730.

157. Druker BJ, Talpaz M, Resta DJ, et al. Efficacy and safety of a specific inhibitor of the BCR-ABL tyrosine kinase in chronic myeloid leukemia. N Engl J Med 2001;344(14):1031–1037.

158. Demetri GD, von Mehren M, Blanke CD, et al. Efficacy and safety of imatinib mesylate in advanced gastrointestinal stromal tumors. N Engl J Med 2002;347(7):472–480.

159. Gorre ME, Mohammed M, Ellwood K, et al. Clinical resistance to STI-571 cancer therapy caused by BCR-ABL gene mutation or amplification. Science 2001;293(5531):876–880.

160. Felsher DW. Cancer revoked: oncogenes as therapeutic targets. Nat Rev Cancer 2003;3(5):375–380.

161. Chin L, Tam A, Pomerantz J, et al. Essential role for oncogenic Ras in tumour maintenance. Nature 1999;400(6743):468–472.

162. Rak J, Mitsuhashi Y, Bayko L, et al. Mutant ras oncogenes upregulate VEGF/VPF expression: implications for induction and inhibition of tumor angiogenesis. Cancer Res 1995;55(20): 4575–4580.

163. Arbiser JL, Moses MA, Fernandez CA, et al. Oncogenic H-ras stimulates tumor angiogenesis by two distinct pathways. Proc Natl Acad Sci USA 1997;94(3):861–866.

164. Okada F, Rak JW, Croix BS, et al. Impact of oncogenes in tumor angiogenesis: mutant K-ras up-regulation of vascular endothelial growth factor/vascular permeability factor is necessary, but not sufficient for tumorigenicity of human colorectal carcinoma cells. Proc Natl Acad Sci USA 1998;95(7):3609–3614.

165. Shweiki D, Itin A, Soffer D, Keshet E. Vascular endothelial growth factor induced by hypoxia may mediate hypoxia-initiated angiogenesis. Nature 1992;359(6398):843–845.

166. Goldberg MA, Schneider TJ. Similarities between the oxygen-sensing mechanisms regulating the expression of vascular endothelial growth factor and erythropoietin. J Biol Chem. 1994;269(6): 4355–4359.

167. Mukhopadhyay D, Tsiokas L, Zhou XM, Foster D, Brugge JS, Sukhatme VP. Hypoxic induction of human vascular endothelial growth factor expression through c-Src activation. Nature 1995; 375(6532):577–581.

168. Mazure NM, Chen EY, Yeh P, Laderoute KR, Giaccia AJ. Oncogenic transformation and hypoxia synergistically act to modulate vascular endothelial growth factor expression. Cancer Res 1996;56(15):3436–3440.

169. Bennett DC. Genetics, development, and malignancy of melanocytes. Int Rev Cytol 1993; 146:191–260.

170. Jimbow K, Quevedo J, Fitzpatrick T, Szabo G. Biology of melanocytes. In: Austen K, ed. Dermatology in General Medicine. McGraw-Hill, New York, NY: 1993, pp. 261–289.

171. Hsu MY, Meier F, Herlyn M. Melanoma development and progression: a conspiracy between tumor and host. Differentiation 2002;70(9-10):522–536.

172. Balch CM, Soong SJ, Gershenwald JE, et al. Prognostic factors analysis of 17,600 melanoma patients: validation of the American Joint Committee on Cancer melanoma staging system. J Clin Oncol 2001;19(16):3622–3634.

173. Sherr CJ, Roberts JM. CDK inhibitors: positive and negative regulators of G1-phase progression. Genes Dev 1999;13(12):1501–1512.

174. DePinho RA. Transcriptional repression: the cancer-chromatin connection. Nature 1998; 391:533–536.

175. Quelle DE, Cheng M, Ashmun RA, Sherr CJ. Cancer-associated mutations at the INK4a locus cancel cell cycle arrest by p16INK4a but not by the alternative reading frame protein p19ARF. Proc Natl Acad Sci USA, 1997;94(2):669–673.

176. de Stanchina E, McCurrach ME, Zindy F, et al. E1A signaling to p53 involves the p19(ARF) tumor suppressor. Genes Dev 1998;12:2434–2442.

177. Zindy F, Eischen CM, Randle DH, et al. Myc signaling via the ARF tumor suppressor regulates p53-dependent apoptosis and immortalization. Genes Dev 1998;12:2424–2433.

178. Radfar A, Unnikrishnan I, Lee HW, DePinho RA, Rosenberg N. p19(Arf) induces p53-dependent apoptosis during abelson virus-mediated pre-B cell transformation. Proc Natl Acad Sci USA 1998;95(22):13,194–13,199.

179. Wildlund HR, Fisher DE. Microphthalamia-associated transcription factor: a critical regulator of pigment cell development and survival. Oncogene 2003;22:3035–3041.

180. Busca R, Ballotti R. Cyclic AMP a key messenger in the regulation of skin pigmentation. Pigment Cell Res 2000;13(2):60–69.

181. Bertolotto C, Abbe P, Hemesath TJ, et al. Microphthalmia gene product as a signal transducer in cAMP-induced differentiation of melanocytes. J Cell Biol 1998;142(3):827–835.

182. Price ER, Horstmann MA, Wells AG, et al. alpha-Melanocyte–stimulating hormone signaling regulates expression of microphthalmia, a gene deficient in Waardenburg syndrome. J Biol Chem 1998;273(49):33,042–33,047.

183. Ohtani N, Zebedee Z, Huot TJ, et al. Opposing effects of Ets and Id proteins on p16INK4a expression during cellular senescence. Nature 2001;409(6823):1067–1070.

184. Zhu J, Woods D, McMahon M, Bishop JM. Senescence of human fibroblasts induced by oncogenic Raf. Genes Dev 1998;12(19):2997–3007.

185. Hamad NM, Elconin JH, Karnoub AE, et al. Distinct requirements for Ras oncogenesis in human versus mouse cells. Genes Dev 2002;16(16):2045–2057.

16

The Biology of Xeroderma Pigmentosum

Insights Into the Role of Ultraviolet Light in the Development of Melanoma

James E. Cleaver

CONTENTS

Summary

Exposure to solar ultraviolet (UV) light is a risk factor for the induction of melanoma, but the precise mechanism remains unclear. The increased incidence of the disease in xeroderma pigmentosum patients, whose cells cannot repair DNA damage caused by defects in nucleotide excision repair, demonstrates that UV-induced DNA damage and mutagenesis can plan a role in melanoma. I propose, therefore, that solar exposure in the UVA and UVB range produces a mixture of DNA photoproducts, some being typical pyrimidine dimers and others the result of photosensitizing reactions with melanin precursors that produce DNA damage that requires the nucleotide excision repair or base excision repair pathways. Not all of these damages necessarily produce typical UV-specific mutations in target genes; the association of melanoma induction with acute burns suggests that high UV doses can overwhelm intracellular anti-oxidant defense mechanisms to produce DNA damage. The progression of melanomas is additionally enhanced by early deletions involving one or more of the nucleotide excision repair (NER) genes that leads to enhanced genomic instability.

Key Words: Ultraviolet (UV) light; DNA damage; DNA repair; nucleotide excision repair; transcription-coupled repair; base excision repair; excision; polymerase; low fidelity; mutation.

From: *From Melanocytes to Melanoma: The Progression to Malignancy*
Edited by: V. J. Hearing and S. P. L. Leong © Humana Press Inc., Totowa, NJ

INTRODUCTION AND HYPOTHESIS

The incidence of melanoma has been increasing worldwide over many decades *(1)*. The reasons for the increased incidence of melanoma are varied, and include increased ultraviolet (UV) exposure, changing leisure activities, change in clothing, environmental factors, and changes in the histological criteria for diagnosing melanoma *(2)*. The role of sun exposure in melanoma induction remains difficult to explain in molecular detail. Melanoma develops from the malignant transformation of melanocytes located in the epidermis, dermis, or mucosa, often occurring in pigmented nevi rather than in isolated melanocytes. Several important genes that act at early stages of melanoma induction have been identified, including *p16* and *B-RAF*. However, the precise molecular mechanisms that result in mutagenesis of these genes is still a mystery. Excessive sun exposure may predispose a susceptible individual to the development of melanoma, but the link between UV exposure and melanoma is not as strong as in squamous cell carcinomas, in which p53 mutations with a UV signature are seen *(3)*. Evidence is strong in studies with the marsupial, *Monodelphis*, and the platyfish, *Xiphophorus*, that typical UV photoproducts can initiate melanomas *(4,5)*. Recently developed mouse models also demonstrate that neonatal UV exposure can cause melanoma development *(6–8)*. Some of these studies also indicate that the wavelengths for melanoma induction can involve longer UVA wavelengths than for nonmelanoma skin cancers *(9)*. Intermittent exposure and exposure in an individual's early years apparently play a greater role than chronic exposure or exposures in later life. For example, the greatest increases in incidence of melanomas are seen on the lower extremities in women and the trunk in men *(2)*. Severe sunburns in childhood or sun exposure in sunny locales during childhood also increase the risk of melanoma *(10,11)*. Melanomas are also more common in light-skinned individuals, particularly those with red or blond hair who freckle easily *(12,13)*. There is an association between the risk of developing melanoma and having specific mutations in the melanocortin-1 receptor *(12)*, which plays a key role in determining the type of melanin produced in melanocytes, eumelanin or pheomelanin. One of the stronger examples of a major role for UVB exposure in melanoma is the increased incidence of the disease in xeroderma pigmentosum (XP) patients who cannot repair UVB damage because of defects in nucleotide excision repair (NER) *(14)*. However, even here, the distribution of melanomas over the body resembles that in the normal population, and is not on the commonly exposed regions of the skin. Taken together, these data suggest that UV does indeed play a role in the development of melanoma, although its exact role is not completely understood. Therefore, I propose the following simple, testable hypothesis for the role of solar exposure in melanoma induction: solar exposure in the UVA and UVB range produces a mixture of DNA photoproducts, some being typical pyrimidine dimers and others the result of photosensitizing reactions with melanin precursors that produce DNA damage that requires the NER or base excision repair (BER) pathways. Not all of these damages necessarily produce typical UV-specific mutations in target genes; the association of melanoma induction with acute burns suggests that high UV doses are required to overwhelm intracellular antioxidant defense mechanisms. The progression of melanomas is additionally enhanced by early deletions involving one or more of the NER genes that leads to enhanced genomic instability.

This chapter will expand on this hypothesis and will discuss various mechanisms of DNA damage and repair and evidence from XP and other animal models for the induction of melanoma by solar exposure.

Table 1
Human Exinuclease Efficiency

Substrate	Cleavage	Alternative pathway
[6-4]photoproduct	3–4%	
T=T dimer	3–4%	
AP site	3.9, 5%	BER
*Cis*Pt	3.3%	
T-HMT mono	1%	
O-6-mG	0.1%	Transferase
N-6-mA	0.06%	BER
G*-A mismatch	0.2%	MMR
G-A* mismatch	0.1%	MMR

This table represents the approximate cleavage efficiency using cell-free extracts active for NER on synthetic substrates containing various lesions *(17)*. The cleavage efficiency on T=T dimers represents the maximum activity of the NER extract when assayed in vitro.

UV DAMAGE

Types of Damage Repaired by NER

DNA damage can involve a very large variety of different kinds of chemical- and radiation-induced alterations in DNA bases and polynucleotide chains. In an approximate sense, one can classify DNA damage according to which kind of DNA repair system is required for its repair. Large adducts, such as those produced by solar exposure (UVB and UVC), require excision of single-stranded regions of DNA by the NER system *(15,16)*. Other kinds of damage, involving smaller modifications to DNA bases (alkylation) or DNA breakage, require a different suite of enzymes, many of which are involved with immunoglobulin rearrangements and neurodegeneration. The distinctions between the various repair systems are not absolute, however, and there are overlaps in the substrate specificity of these various repair systems and variations in the efficiencies and sites of action on DNA in differing metabolic states (Table 1).

The NER system recognizes and repairs DNA damage that consists of photoproducts produced by UV light and large DNA adducts produced by carcinogenic chemicals (Fig. 1) *(15,16)*. The most important wavelengths of UV are those in the UVC (240–280 nm) and the UVB (280–320 nm) ranges, which are strongly absorbed by nucleic acids. The photoproducts include the cyclobutane [5-5], [6-6] pyrimidine dimers (CPDs) and the [6-4] pyrimidine pyrimidinone dimers ([6-4]PDs) that involve both T and C pyrimidines. The [6-4]PD can further photoisomerase to the Dewar photoproduct at longer UV wavelengths, and cytosine in dimers has an increased propensity to deaminate, contributing a C to thymine T mutagenesis. Chemical adducts include those produced by *N*-acetoxy-*N*-acetyl aminofluorene (AAAF), benzo(a)pyrene, aflatoxin, photoactivated psoralens, and *cis*-platinum. An oxidative purine product, 5',8-purine cyclodeoxynucleoside, which may accumulate in neurological tissue, also requires the NER system for repair. The NER system can even recognize DNA triplexes formed by the binding of short oligonucleotides to double-stranded DNA.

Other damage that would not, *a priori*, be expected to require the NER system can be recognized and cleaved, including apurinic sites, alkylated bases, and mismatches *(17)*. The efficiency with which some of these substrates are repaired, especially for mis-

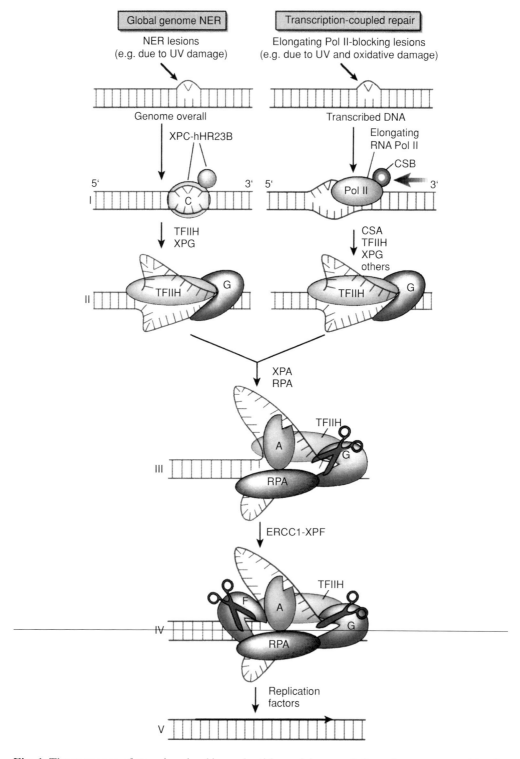

Fig. 1. The sequence of steps involved in nucleotide excision repair from damage recognition by global genome repair (GGR) or transcription coupled repair (TCR) mechanisms (I), DNA unwinding (II), verification (III), excision (III, IV), and polymerization and ligation (V). (Reproduced from ref. *16*, with permission from Macmillan Publishers.)

matched bases, is weak, and consequently, NER is only a backup mechanism for other kinds of repair (Table 1).

Types of Damage Repaired by BER

DNA can be damaged by hydrolysis, deamination, oxidative reactions, or alkylations that occur as the result of naturally occurring intracellular oxidative metabolism, as well as from external ionizing radiation, UV light, carcinogens, and alkylating agents *(18,19)*. These processes create singly modified DNA bases and can cause base loss leading to the production of apurinic/apyrimidinic sites. The single modified bases include uracil and thymine, produced by deamination of cytosine and 5-methylcytosine, respectively; 8-oxoguanine and other oxidized purines; thymine glycol; cytosine hydrate; 3-methyladenine; 7-methylguanine; and others. DNA adducts can also be produced from oxidative products of dopamine and other neurotransmitters *(20,21)* and ischemic brain damage *(22)*. Mitochondrial DNA is especially at risk from oxidative damage, containing approx eight 8-oxoguanine residues per DNA molecule under steady-state conditions, even in absence of additional irradiation, which is significantly greater than the nuclear level *(23,24)*.

Processes such as lipid peroxidation in nuclei and cytoplasm can be augmented by UV irradiation. Exocyclic DNA base adducts generated from lipid peroxidation byproducts have been characterized. The most abundant of these appears to be the exocyclic pyrimidopurinone, M_1G, which is generated by reaction between a G residue in DNA and the lipid peroxidation product, malondialdehyde *(25)*, and undergoes decomposition to a secondary ring-opened derivative. Lipid peroxidation may also yield acrolein and crotonaldehyde, which are readily metabolized to epoxides that can generate exocyclic etheno modifications of DNA bases.

These classes of damaged bases all have recognition steps that require specific glycosylases to remove the base, and the pathways then converge on common excision steps.

DNA Damage Associated With Melanin: Protection and Photosensitization

Melanin, when distributed uniformly in keratinocytes in the skin, generally acts as a photoprotector and reduces the amount of pyrimidine dimers and [6-4] photoproducts in DNA *(26)*. Melanin in nevi, however, is in a different state from that in normal melanocytes, and may be involved in oxidative reactions from UVA exposure that cause additional DNA damage *(27,28)*. Some of the melanin precursors, L-DOPA for example, can be oxidized to form DNA-damaging products, and the reaction is enhanced by tyrosinase and inhibited by antioxidants *(29,30)*. The combination of UV exposure; eumelanin and pheomelanin; endogenous photosensitizers; and antioxidants can result in complex outcomes in terms of DNA damage. In one summary, different photoprotection and photosensitizing effects of melanin were noted with UVB and UVA, respectively *(31)*. One possible reason for the prominence of acute burns in increasing melanoma risk could be the saturation of endogenous photoprotection by high UVA doses.

DNA REPAIR MECHANISMS

Clinical Consequences of NER Deficiencies: Cancer

XP is a multigenic, multiallelic autosomal recessive disease that occurs with a frequency in the United States of approx 1 in 250,000. Higher incidence is seen in Japan and the Mediterranean and possibly in Central American areas *(32)*. Heterozygotes are unaffected, but homozygotes have severe sun sensitivity that leads to progressive degeneration of sun-exposed regions of the skin and eyes, usually leading to various forms of cutaneous malignancy (melanoma and nonmelanoma) *(14,33)*. The disease begins in early life with the first exposures to sunlight, the median age of onset being 1–2 yr of age, with skin rapidly exhibiting the signs associated with years of sun exposure. Pigmentation is patchy, and skin shows atrophy and telangiectasia with development of basal and squamous cell carcinomas and melanomas. Cancer incidence for those individuals under 20 yr of age is 2000 times that seen in the general population.

The nonmelanoma skin cancers that develop in XP patients contain mutations in *p53* for squamous carcinomas *(34)* or *patched*, for basal-cell carcinomas *(35)* that are mainly C to T transitions at dipyrimidine sequences, characteristic of the UV photoproducts that are the substrates for NER *(17)*. Melanomas are also found at higher frequency in XP patients, with a similar body distribution to melanomas in non-XP patients *(33)*, and a limited number of melanomas have been analyzed for mutations in selected genes.

One study of 20 melanomas in XP-C and XP-V patients showed that the majority were lentigo malignant melanomas typical of those seen in older normal patients *(36)*. Mutations were found in the *p53* gene at increased frequency (60%) in XP-C melanomas but not in those from XP-V patients (10%). The mutations in XP-C melanomas were CC to TT or C to T, arising from photoproducts in the nontranscribed strand, characteristic of UV and of the repair deficiency of XP-C. One possible way to reconcile these observations with those in the general population would be to suggest that the repair deficiency in XP patients increases the relative importance of UVB-induced pyrimidine dimers over nondimer UVA-induced photoproducts. XP melanomas would then show a greater number of tumors with UVB-signature mutations than the normal population. Of particular interest will be analysis of mutations in the *BRAF* gene in XP melanomas to compare with those reported for the general population, in which the mutations are not of the UVB type *(37)*.

NER Mechanisms

Large DNA adducts, especially those produced by UVB exposure, are repaired by an excision process that removes a large, 27–29 nucleotide-long oligonucleotide (Fig. 1) *(15,16)*. This requires a complex set of recognition factors, excision nucleases, and polymerization. There are two major damage mechanisms, depending on the location of damage in either transcriptionally silent or actively transcribed regions of the genome. These give rise to the pathways called global genome repair (GGR) and transcription-coupled repair (TCR).

RECOGNITION OF DAMAGE IN TRANSCRIPTIONALLY SILENT REGIONS OF THE GENOME

The damage recognition factors required for GGR are two sets of DNA binding proteins: the XPC/H23B *(38,39)* and XPE (DDB1/DDB2) heterodimers *(40)* (Fig. 2). The XPC/HR23B complex is the earliest damage detector to initiate NER in nontranscribed DNA, with highest affinity for the [6-4]PD. Recognition of cyclobutane dimers is more difficult and requires the combined action of the XPC and XPE protein complexes *(41)*. The DNA binding proteins are transcriptionally regulated by p53 and increase expression after UV irradiation *(42–44)*. In mice, XPE is not functional because the promoter of the DDB2 (p48) component has a mutation in the p53 recognition sequence *(40)*.

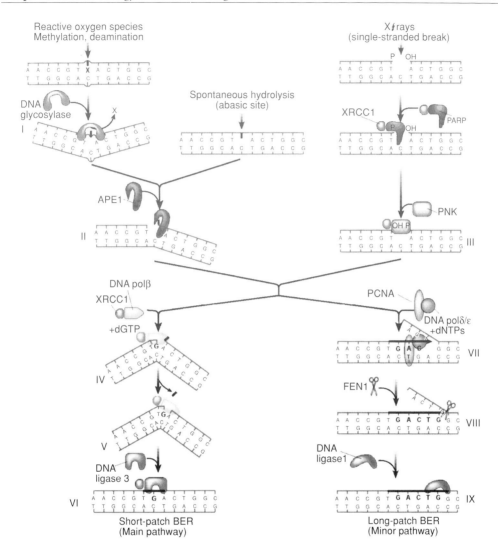

Fig. 2. The sequence of steps involved in base excision repair from damage recognition by a battery of glycosylases, followed by the two branches of short-patch and long-patch pathways. (Reproduced from ref. *16*, with permission from Macmillan Publishers.)

The complete excision process on a purified DNA substrate can be carried out in vitro using a minimal set of recombinant proteins: replication protein A (RPA), XPA, TFIIH (6 subunit core of XPB, XPD, p44, p34, p52, p62; and 3 subunit kinase, CAK), XPC, HR23B, XPG, ERCC1, and XPF *(45)*. CAK appears to act as a negative regulator, and inhibition of phosphorylation stimulates repair. These individual factors of NER associate sequentially and independently on UV photoproducts, in vivo, without preassembly of a "repairosome" complex *(46)*.

RECOGNITION OF DAMAGE IN ACTIVELY TRANSCRIBED REGIONS OF THE GENOME

CPDs are excised more rapidly from actively transcribed genes, especially from the DNA strand used as the template for transcription *(47,48)*. Excision is slow in the promoter regions and increases immediately after the ATG start site for transcription. The initial damage recognition mechanism for TCR may be the stalled RNA polymerase (Pol II), itself *(49)*, although a potentially large number of gene products, especially the components of the transcription factor TFIIH, play a role in repair of transcriptionally active genes. The blocked RNA Pol II masks damaged sites and must be removed, or backed off, to alleviate the arrested transcription and provide access for repair enzymes. The processes that alleviate the arrested RNA Pol II enhance the overall accessibility of the damaged site and permit more rapid repair than in nontranscribed regions of the genome. Persistently blocked RNA Pol II can be a signal for UV-induced apoptosis *(50)* that may involve signal transduction via the mismatch repair system *(51)*.

Cells from Cockayne Syndrome (CS) patients are specifically defective in TCR *(52)*. The excision of DNA photoproducts from total genomic DNA of CS cells is normal, but repair of transcriptionally active genes is reduced *(52)*. Two CS genes, *CSA* and *CSB*, are involved specifically in TCR. CSA contains WD-repeat motifs that are important for protein–protein interactions *(53)*. CSB contains an ATPase, helicase motifs, and a nucleotide-binding domain, but only the latter is essential for TCR, and CSB does not function as a helicase *(54,55)*. Cells lacking either CSA or CSB are unable to ubiquitinate the C-terminal domain of RNA Pol II *(56)*. CS patients are photosensitive but do not show increased skin carcinogenesis *(57)*, unlike mice with inactivated *Xpc* or *Csb* genes that both show increased skin carcinogenesis from UV light or chemical carcinogens *(58)*.

THE CORE EXCISION PROCESS COMMON TO GGR AND TCR

The damaged site is unwound by the 3'-5' (XPB) and 5'-3' (XPD) helicases of TFIIH in concert with XPG, and then stabilized by the XPA–RPA binding complex that replaces the XPC and XPE binding proteins *(59)* (Fig. 2). The basal transcription factor, TFIIH, which is involved in transcription initiation and elongation, plays a major role in remodeling the damaged regions for excision to occur after damage recognition by TCR and GGR *(60,61)*. The XPB and D components of TFIIH and CSB interact with p53, suggesting a role for p53 in regulation of TCR *(62,63)*.

XPA binds to both the damaged and the undamaged strand, but RPA binds mainly to the undamaged strand *(59)*. XPA acts as a foundation on which other components of the NER process subsequently assemble. XPA binds to the p34 subunit of RPA through its *N*-terminal region and to the p70 subunit through a central portion in exon IV, as well as to many other NER components, including: ERCC1, TFIIH, XPC, XPG, and DNA itself *(61)*. The final stable complex that remains at the damaged site is unclear, but a subset of these components acts as an assembly point for the XPG *(64)* and ERCC1/XPF *(65)* nucleases that cut the damaged strand 3' and 5' to the damaged site.

The excision process involves removal of an oligonucleotide, 27–29 nucleotides long, containing the photoproduct as a result of cleavages 5 nucleotides on the 3' side of the photoproduct, and 24 nucleotides on the 5' side *(17)*. The structure-specific cleavage pattern is determined by binding of RPA to the unwound damaged site, and the excised fragment is close in size to the footprint of RPA on DNA *(59,66)*. Slight variations in the precise sites of cleavage result in the removal of variable fragments between 27 and 29 nucleotides. The XPG nuclease cleaves first on the 3' side of the damage and interacts with the XPC-HR23B complex and with TFIIH *(61)*; the XPF-ERCC1 heterodimer cleaves subsequently on the 5' side of the damaged site *(67)*. XPA serves as an anchor for the 5' nuclease through binding to ERCC1 *(68)*.

The XPG nuclease has a particularly complex range of activities, and mutations in XPG are associated with both XP and CS diseases *(69)*. XPG is an endonuclease in the FEN-1 family that is capable of strand-specific cleavage of a range of DNA substrates that may arise during DNA replication, repair, and recombination *(66,70)*. The XPG gene product also interacts with RNA pol II and facilitates efficient transcription elongation *(71)*, thereby providing an explanation for the complex symptoms of some XPG patients who show both XP and CS symptoms. XPG is also a cofactor required for the activity of thymine glycosylase *(nth* gene) and is thereby linked to repair of oxidative damage *(72)*.

The excised region is replaced by the action of a complex similar to that involved in normal DNA replication *(73)*. Proliferating cell nuclear antigen (PCNA) is loaded onto the DNA by the 5 subunit Replication Factor C complex, which then anchors the replicative DNA polymerases, Pol-δ or Pol-ε. Damage to cells usually activates p53, which then transactivates p21 and inhibits DNA synthesis by binding to PCNA, which would inhibit repair synthesis. In the particular case of UV damage, p21 transcription is still increased but the protein is secondarily degraded, thereby releasing the potential inhibition of PCNA-directed repair synthesis *(74)*. The final closure of the repaired site occurs with DNA ligase I *(73)*.

REPAIR DEFICIENCIES ASSOCIATED WITH MELANOMA

Direct measurement of pyrimidine dimers in UV-damaged DNA from patients with melanoma has not shown any specific deficiencies of excision repair associated with disease *(75,76)*. No consistent differences could be detected in the cell cycle response to UV irradiation of cells from carriers and noncarriers of hereditary melanoma risk factors *(77)*. One report found defective induction of the damage-responsive gene, *GADD45*, by ionizing radiation in a set of melanoma cells, but the relationship of this gene to UV repair is still unclear *(78)*. An association between polymorphisms in the repair gene *XRCC3* and melanoma was claimed *(79)* but later challenged *(80)*.

One study using reactivation of an irradiated episomal vector to assay for repair claimed a reduced repair capacity in patients with high risk for melanoma *(81)*, especially those with additional risk factors *(82)*. An enhanced repair was observed in metastatic melanoma cells using the same assay *(83)*. These studies, however, measured only residual gene activity at a single UV dose to the extracellular plasmid. Because the residual activity is an exponential function of UV dose, and not linearly related to the excision repair capacity of the host cells, this measure of DNA repair capacity exaggerates possible differences in repair. The small differences reported might therefore be less significant than first thought, and contrast to the direct measures of photoproduct excision that did not detect differences associated with melanoma *(75,76)*.

Base Excision Repair

Base damage, from endogenous or exogenous sources, is repaired mainly by the BER system. BER, in its simplest form (Fig. 2), consists of one or more glycosylases that remove damaged bases by cleavage of the deoxyribose–base bond, leaving an abasic site, which is subsequently cleaved by apurinic/apyrimidinic endonuclease (AP endo), and the deoxyribose residue is removed by polymerase-β *(16,84)*. The resulting single-base gap is filled in by DNA polymerase-β and ligase. Single-strand breaks, which are produced by free radicals, ionizing radiation, and long wavelength UV, are also repaired by the BER pathway *(85)*.

BER repairs a wide range of singly modified bases, many of which can be created by reactive oxygen and nitrogen intermediates of normal cell metabolism *(19,86)*. Consequently, there are numerous DNA glycosylases with various substrate specificities directed against these modified bases. These include uracil glycosylase, 8-hydroxyguanine glycosylase, and many others *(86,87)*. Two bases formed by reactive products of lipid peroxidation, etheno-A and etheno-C, are excised efficiently by DNA glycosylases *(88)*, which strongly suggests that generation of such adducts occurs at sufficiently high rates in vivo to endanger genomic stability. Because of the variety of possible substrates and the number of different glycosylases, it is not surprising that defects in individual glycosylases do not cause lethality in mice *(89–91)*. Later stages of repair that are common to most of the base lesions are, in contrast, lethal when interrupted in knockout mice.

The BER system acts through multicomponent protein complexes, and at least two major forms of BER can be categorized based on their substrates and enzymatic mechanisms. The short-patch form involves insertion of one to two nucleotides by polymerase-β, and sealing this patch involves either ligase I or ligase III. BER of uracil can be carried out in testis cell extracts that have been partially purified, that contain uracil DNA glycosylase, AP endo, polymerase β, and ligase I *(92)*. The long-patch form involves insertion of longer patches by the action of PCNA, FEN-1 nuclease, and polymerases-α or -δ *(91,93)*. Short-patch BER appears to account for up to 80% of repair in vitro *(94)*.

XRCC1 is a critically important protein in short-patch BER that coordinates the later stages of repair *(85)*. DNA ligase III and XRCC1 are strongly associated, and ligase III is unstable in the absence of XRCC1 and loses activity *(85)*. XRCC1 interacts with DNA ligase III and PARP through regions known as BRCT domains, found in several repair enzymes *(85)*. In mammalian cells, the ligase III interaction is only required during BER in noncycling cells, and, during the cell cycle, XRCC1 plays a role in recombination and DNA replication *(95)*.

Defects in enzymes that are involved in the intermediate stages of repair that are common to all base lesions, such as AP endo *(96)*, DNA polymerase-β *(97)*, XRCC1 *(98)*, and ligase I *(99,100)* are, however, lethal during embryogenesis. Embryo lethality in these animals could be because all base damage requires these enzymes, and deficiencies result in the accumulation of repair intermediates or single-strand breaks. Embryo lethality is expressed at the time of rapid increase in the rate of cell division and differentiation during gastrulation or later *(99,101)*. A putative role for XRCC1 in recombination *(102)* could be an alternative cause of embryo lethality, by analogy with Rad51, and other recombinational genes *(103)*.

The observation of a longer UVA component for melanoma induction *(27,28)* suggests that solar exposure could act in part through oxidative photochemical reactions that would require the BER pathways. These would not result in typical UV mutation spectra in affected genes in melanomas, and mechanisms would be more difficult to identify.

REPLICATION OF DAMAGED DNA

NER can remove DNA damage before DNA replication begins, and consequently plays a major role in reducing the amount of damage that becomes fixed as mutations during replication *(104)*. DNA photoproducts, however, are blocks to the replicative DNA polymerases, polymerase-α, -δ, and -ε (Pol-α, -δ, and -ε) that cannot accommodate large distortions, such as DNA photoproducts or adducts in their active sites *(105,106)*. Replicative bypass of these photoproducts is achieved instead by damage-specific, class-Y polymerases with relaxed substrate specificity *(107)*.

Three class-Y polymerase genes have been identified in the mammalian genome, *Pol-η, -ι*, and *-κ. Pol-η* and *-ι* are close homologs, unique to mammalian cells, and only a single *Pol- h* gene is found in yeast *(107)*. Mutations in Pol-η are found in certain XP patients (XP variants), but their clinical symptoms of elevated skin cancer are not easily distinguished from those seen in the NER-defective patients *(108)*. Pol-η has a poorer capacity for replication of UV damage than Pol-κ, and Pol-κ has the poorest; but their relative efficiencies may differ for other kinds of chemical adducts *(109–111)*. Pol-η acts distributively to extend nascent DNA chains by one or two bases across from CPDs, and the inserted bases may be edited by a separate exonuclease. The apparent base specificity of Pol-η and Pol-ι indicates that Pol-η may exercise a preference for replicating T-containing photoproducts accurately; Pol-ι a preference for C-containing sites. Pol-η can therefore insert adenines across from thymine-containing photoproducts, resulting in accurate replication of a T-T CPD. Pol-ι can insert guanines across from cytosine-containing photoproducts, resulting in accurate replication of a T-C CPD or [6-4]PD. Chain extension then requires the activity of Pol-ζ or Pol-κ that can extend the nascent chain from a terminal mispaired base and then restore normal DNA replication *(112–115)*.

The class-Y polymerases have larger active sites that allow them to read through noninformative sequence information resulting from DNA damage, and can, in particular, accommodate the dipyrimidine photoproduct within the active site *(116,117)*. Consequently, these polymerases have high error rates, of the order of 1% or more when assayed in vitro *(118–120)*, which must be controlled in vivo, otherwise the results would be catastrophic to the cells. Mechanisms of regulation could involve sequestering polymerases in locations away from the replication forks under normal conditions, and specific translocation after DNA damage occurs. Pol-η is uniformly distributed in the nucleus, and excluded from the replication fork until replication is stalled by UV damage *(121,122)*. Pol-η then traffics into the nucleus and accumulates with a large number of other proteins in microscopically visible foci at the replication fork. This requires specific sequence motifs in the protein for translocation and for binding to PCNA *(121,123)*. Displacement of the replicative polymerases, and increased binding of the bypass polymerases, by mono-ubiquitination and SUMO modification of PCNA appears to be one way that access is provided for Pol-η and -ζ *(124)*.

UV-INDUCED MUTAGENESIS

Mutations are produced by a series of enzymatic processes. Damaged sites in DNA are processed to reduce their toxic effects at the expense of their precise nucleotide sequence. The mutation frequency from UV at a particular site depends on the particular photoproduct, the flanking sequences, the strand that contains the photoproduct (transcribed or nontranscribed) the efficiency of NER at that site, and the cell's capacity to replicate the photoproduct. Secondary effects depend on cell cycle checkpoints, promoter binding, and other cellular and tissue levels of regulation. The photochemistry of DNA, however, leaves a characteristic footprint on the mutation spectrum. In general, UV-induced mutations occur at dipyrimidine sites, particularly the 3'C of a TC or CC site because of increased deamination of C within a photoproduct. Tandem mutations occurring at both Cs of a CC site are distinctive signs that UV was the causative agent of a mutation (125).

The relative contributions of the two major classes of photoproduct has been determined by enzymatic photoreactivation of episomal plasmids before transfection into cultured cells, which reverses pyrimidine dimers but not [6-4]PPs (126,127). Photoreactivation reduced the mutation frequency in normal cells by 75% and in XP-A cells by 90%. CPDs occurring at dipyrimidine sites containing at least one cytosine base are the predominant mutagenic lesions induced in human cells and the [6-4]PPs at these sites accounted for only approx 10% of the mutations (126).

The frequencies of CPDs and [6-4]PPs at individual dipyrimidine sites does not correlate directly with mutation frequency, suggesting that although the presence of UV-induced photoproducts are required for mutagenesis, the frequency of mutagenesis is determined by additional factors. A comparison of photoproduct yields, rates of repair, and mutations in the *PGK1*, *ras*, and *p53* genes has shown that regions of high UV-induced mutation can be caused by either or both high photoproduct yield and/or low repair (128–131). In XP-C mice, squamous cell carcinomas induced by UV show a high incidence of a particular mutation, T122L, in the *p53* gene (132). UV-induced mutations in the *p53* gene, for example, are important in development of squamous cell carcinomas and may arise at DNA repair "coldspots," sites of low repair, rather than photoproduct "hotspots" (3). A determining factor in mutagenesis, therefore, appears to be the persistence of damage during DNA replication, by a combination of rates of formation and rates of repair.

Mutation frequencies from UV damage are increased in cells that lack NER capacity (133) or that lack the class-Y polymerase Pol-η (134), but is reduced in cells that lack a functional polymerase Pol-ζ or deoxycytidyl transferase hRev1p (135,136). The yield of mutations in XPA-deficient cells is increased and the spectrum shifted to different "hotspots" and a lower ratio of transitions to deletions (137); the bias toward mutations in the transcribed strand was greater than for wild-type controls, and characteristic CC to TT tandem mutations could be detected in a transgene, *rpsL* (138). Because of the strand specificity of repair, there is a bias between mutations in the coding and the noncoding strands of expressed genes that differs according to the NER capacity of the cells (139,140). In mice with normal NER bearing a transfected *gpt* gene, UVB induced a higher mutation rate in the epidermis than the dermis (141). The majority of the mutations were transitions at dipyrimidine sites, including tandem mutations, with a strong bias toward mutations in the template strand of the *gpt* gene (141).

UVB can also cause deletions, though these are much less prominent than from ionizing radiation, where the major damage involves direct DNA breakage. In one study, UVB irradiation of the epidermis of mice with normal NER produced large deletions that were approx 75-fold less frequent than point mutations (142). The junctions of the deletions contained short regions of homology that are characteristic of those produced by nonhomologous endjoining reactions.

TARGET PATHWAYS IN MELANOMA

Approximately 5–12% of patients who develop melanomas have one or more first-degree relatives with melanoma, suggestive of an autosomal dominant inheritance (143). Familial melanoma cases are generally diagnosed at an earlier age with thinner tumors and an increased frequency of multiple tumors *(144–146)*. Genes that have been identified as important in melanoma include *CDKN2A, cyclin-dependent kinase 4 (CDK4), BRAF, PTEN*, and the p53, RB, and mdm2 pathways *(37,147–149)*.

Two major melanoma predisposition genes, *CDKN2A* and *CDK4*, have been identified *(143)*. *CDKN2A* is a located on the short arm of chromosome 9 (9p21) and functions as a tumor suppressor gene encoding two different proteins, p16 and p14^{ARF} *(150,151)*. The p16 protein is encoded from exons 1α, 2, and 3 of *CDKN2A* and functions as a cell cycle regulatory protein that inhibits the activity of cyclin D1–CDK4/6 complex. The expression of p16 is upregulated by UV exposure *(152)*. A deficiency of murine p19^{ARF} (the mouse homolog of p14^{ARF}) allows a strong acceleration of melanoma development *(149)*. The loss of chromosome 9p, the site of the *p16* gene, is frequent in primary melanoma and occurs early in tumor progression *(153)*. The p16 protein acts as a negative regulator of growth by arresting cells at the G1 phase of the cell cycle. P14^{ARF} is formed from alternative reading frames. It acts via p53 to induce cell cycle arrest and apoptosis. CDK4 is found on the long arm of chromosome 12 (12q13). It seems to function as an oncogene that is resistant to the normal physiological function of p16.

BRAF, a cytoplasmic serine/threonine kinase regulated by *RAS*, has recently been identified as an important gene mutated in melanoma, although the mutations that have been identified do not contain characteristic UV-induced signatures *(37)*.

Despite considerable progress in understanding many of the pathways that become dysregulated in melanoma, the precise targets for UV-induced mutation and dysregulation of signal transduction remain to be identified.

ANIMAL MODELS FOR MELANOMA

Mouse models for melanoma have been limited because of differences in melanocyte location and distribution in mouse skin as compared with human. Several other animal models have therefore been used for investigating the role of solar exposure, especially the opossum *Monodelphus domestica (4)* and the species of the fish genus *Xiphophorus (5)*. These two animals retain active photolyase enzymes that monomerize pyrimidine dimers, unlike mammals that lack this repair system. A photolyase binds to pyrimidine dimers and, after illumination with visible light, the 5-5 and 6-6 bonds of the dimer revert to the 5-6 double bonds of the pyrimidine rings, eliminating the photoproduct. These experiments have shown that DNA photoproducts induced by UVB can be reversed and the induction of melanomas reduced accordingly *(4,5)*. In both *Monodelphus domestica* and *Xiphophorus*, melanoma can also be induced by UVA wavelengths *(9)*.

The mouse models that have shown promise have tended to be genetically engineered to increase the melanocyte distribution in the upper skin and produce a population of cells at risk, as well as to manipulate pathways known to be relevant to melanoma *(6,7)*. The HGF/SF strain of transgenic mice, for examples, expresses hepatocyte growth factor and melanocytes are distributed in a similar fashion to human skin. In these animals, a single acute dose of UV to neonatal animals induces melanomas, consistent with the epidemiological evidence that early exposures to sunburn is a melanoma risk factor *(8)*.

A series of DNA-repair deficient mouse strains have been developed in which the *XP* or *CS* genes have been knocked out *(103)*. The XP knockouts, in general, exhibit increased cancer rates from treatment with UVB or chemical carcinogens, as expected from their human counterparts *(58)*. Xpa, Xpc, Csa, and Csb knockouts, for example, are very sensitive to skin-cancer induction *(58,138,154–156)*. The *XPB* and *XPD* genes are part of the essential transcription factor, TFIIH, and, thus, homozygous knockouts are lethal very early in embryonic cell division *(157)*. Specific mutations that result in viable Xpd mice have, however, been made. Mice with a human TTD mutation in the *Xpd* gene have many of the same symptoms as TTD patients, but are sensitive to increased UV-induced skin cancer and age prematurely, although TTD patients do not exhibit a corresponding increase in cancer *(158)*. None of these repair-deficient mouse strains have yet been used to develop melanoma, but crosses between an Xpa knockout and some of the other mouse models for melanoma could be informative.

CONCLUSIONS AND PERSPECTIVES

UV exposure is linked to melanoma induction both from epidemiological studies and animal models, and from the observations of XP patients. However, mysteries remain. The exact wavelengths of UV that are causative remain controversial and additional photoproducts to the pyrimidine dimers need to be identified. Anecdotal observations that some XP patients develop multiple melanomas, whereas others develop predominantly squamous cell carcinomas or basal-cell carcinomas indicate that additional genetic factors may be important modifiers of melanoma induction. Mouse strains that combine increased melanoma induction with DNA repair deficiencies would be very helpful in understanding the role of UV exposure.

REFERENCES

1. Setlow RB, Woodhead AD. Temporal changes in the incidence of malignant melanoma: explanation from action spectra. Mutat Res 1994;307:365–374.
2. Freedberg IM, Eisen AZ, Wolff K, et al. Fitzpatrick's Dermatology in General Medicine. Vol. I & II. McGraw-Hill Health Professional Division, New York, NY: 1999.
3. Ziegler A, Jonason AS, Leffell DJ, et al. Sunburn and p53 in the onset of skin cancer. Nature 1994;372:773–776.
4. Ley RD, Reeve VF, Kusewitt DF. Photobiology of Monodelphis domestica. Dev Comp Immunol 2000;24:503–516.
5. Setlow RB, Woodhead AD, Grist E. Animal model for ultraviolet radiation-induced melanoma: platyfish-swordtail hybrid. Proc Natl Acad Sci USA 1989;86:8922–8926.
6. Jhappan C, Noonan FP, Merlino G. Ultraviolet radiation and cutaneous malignant melanoma. Oncogene 2003;22:3099–3112.
7. Merlino G, Noonan FP. Modeling gene-environment interactions in malignant melanoma. Trends in Molec Med 2003;9:102–108.
8. Noonan FP, Recio JA, Takayama H, et al. Neonatal sunburn and melanoma in mice. Nature 2001;413:271–272.
9. Wang SQ, Setlow RB, Berwick M, et al. Ultraviolet A and melanoma: a review. J Amer Acad Dermatol 2001;44:837–846.
10. Kaskel P, Sander S, Kron M, Kind P, Peter RU, Krahn G. Outdoor activities in childhood: a protective factor for cutaneous melanoma? Results of a case-control study in 271 matched pairs. Br J Dermatol 2001;145:602–609.
11. Pfahlberg A, Schneider D, Kolmel KF, Gefeller O. [Ultraviolet exposure in childhood and in adulthood: which life period modifies the risk of melanoma more substantially?] German. Soz Praventivmedicin 2000;45:119–124.
12. Schaffer JV, Bolognia JL. The melanocortin-1 receptor: red hair and beyond. Arch Dermatol 2001;137:1477–1485.
13. Garbe C, Buttner P, Weiss J, et al. Risk factors for developing cutaneous melanoma and criteria for identifying persons at risk: multicenter case-control study of the Central Malignant Melanoma Registry of the German Dermatological Society. JInvest Dermatol 1994;102:695–699.
14. Kraemer KH, Lee MM, Andrews AD, Lambert WC. The role of sunlight and DNA repair in melanoma and nonmelanoma skin cancer. The xeroderma pigmentosum paradigm. Arch Dermatol 1994;130:1018–1021.

15. Wood RD, Mitchell M, Sgouros J, Lindahl T. Human DNA repair genes. Science 2001;291: 1284–1289.
16. Hoeijmakers JH. Genome maintenance mechanisms for preventing cancer. Nature 2001; 411:366–374.
17. Huang JC, Hsu DS, Kazantsev A, Sancar A. Substrate spectrum of human excinuclease: repair of abasic sites, methylated bases, mismatches, and bulky adducts. Proc Natl Acad Sci USA 1994;91:12,213–12,217.
18. Lindahl T. Instability and decay of the primary structure of DNA. Nature 1993;362:709–715.
19. Wiseman H, Halliwell B. Damage to DNA by reactive oxygen and nitrogen species: role in inflammatory disease and progression to cancer. Biochem J 1996;313:17–29.
20. Levay G, Bodell WJ. Detection of dopamine-DNA adducts: potential role in Parkinson's disease. Carcinogenesis 1993;14:1241–1245.
21. Levay G, Ye Q, Bodell WJ. Formation of DNA adducts and oxidative base damage by copper mediated oxidation of dopamine and 6-hydroxydopamine. ExpNeurol 1997;146:570–574.
22. Chan PK. Role of oxidants in ischemic brain damage. Stroke 1996;27:1124–1129.
23. Driggers WJ, Grishko VI, LeDoux SP, Wilson GL. Defective repair of oxidative damage in the mitochondrial DNA of a xeroderma pigmentosum group A cell line. Cancer Res 1996;56:1262–1266.
24. Driggers WJ, Holmquist GP, LeDoux SP, Wolson GL. Mapping frequencies of endogenous oxidative damage and the kinetic response to oxidative stress in a region of rat mtDNA. Nucleic Acids Res 1997;25:4362–4369.
25. Fink SP, Reddy GR, Marnett LJ. Mutagenicity in Escherichia coli of the major DNA adduct derived from the endogenous mutagen malondialdehyde. Proc Natl Acad Sci USA 1997;94:8652–8657.
26. Tadokoro T, Kobayashi N, Zmudzka BZ, et al. UV-induced DNA damage and melanin content in human skin differing in racial/ethnic origin. FASEB 2003;17:1177–1179.
27. Kvam E, Tyrell RM. The role of eumelanin in the induction of oxidative DNA base damage by ultraviolet A irradiation of DNA or melanoma cells. J Invest Dermatol 1999;113:209–213.
28. Marrot L, Belaidi JP, Meunier JR, Perez P, Agapakis-Causse C. The human melanocyte as a particular target for UVA radiation and an endpoint for photoprotection assessment. Photochem Photobiol 1999;69:686–693.
29. Husain S, Hadi SM. DNA breakage by L-DOPA and Cu(II): breakage by melanin and bacteriophage inactivation. Mutat Res 1998;397:161–168.
30. Stokes AH, Brown BG, Lee CK, Doolittle DJ, Vrana KE. Tyrosinase enhances the covalent modification of DNA by dopamine. Brain Res Mol Brain Res 1996;42:167–170.
31. Hill HZ, Hill GJ. UVA, pheomelanin and the carcinogenic response. Pigment Cell Res 2000; 13(suppl 8):140–144.
32. Cleaver JE, Kraemer KH. Xeroderma pigmentosum and Cockayne Syndrome. In: Scriver CR, Beaudet AL, Sly WS, Valle D, eds. The Metabolic and Molecular Bases of Inherited Disease. Vol. III. McGraw-Hill, New York, NY: 1995, pp. 4393–4419.
33. Kraemer KH, Lee MM, Andrews AD, Lambert WC. The role of sunlight and DNA repair in melanoma and nonmelanoma skin cancer. The xeroderma pigmentosum paradigm. Arch Dermatol 1994;130:1018–1021.
34. Giglia G, Dumaz N, Drougard C, Avril MF, Daya-Grosjean L, Sarasin A. p53 mutations in skin and internal tumors of xeroderma pigmentosum patients belonging to the complementation group C. Cancer Res 1998;58:4402–4409.
35. Bodak N, Queille S, Avril MF, et al. High levels of patched gene mutations in basal-cell carcinomas from patients with xeroderma pigmentosum. Proc Natl Acad Sci USA 1999;96:5117–5122.
36. Spatz A, Giglia-Mari G, Benhamou S, Sarasin A. Association between DNA repair-deficiency and high level of p53 mutations in melanoma of xeroderma pigmentosum. Cancer Res 2001;61: 2480–2486.
37. Davies H, Bignell GR, Cox C, et al. Mutations of the BRAF gene in human cancer. Nature 2002;417:949–954.
38. Sugasawa K, Ng JMY, Masutani C, et al. Xeroderma pigmentosum group C protein complex is the initiator of global nucleotide excision repair. Mol Cell 1998;2:223–232.
39. Masutani C, Sugasawa K, Yanagisawa J, et al. Purification and cloning of a nucleotide excision repair complex involving the xeroderma pigmentosum group C protein and a human homologue of yeast RAD23. EMBO J 1994;13:1831–1843.
40. Tang J, Chu G. Xeroderma pigmentosum complementation group E and UV-damaged DNA-binding protein. DNA Repair 2002;1:601–616.

41. Fitch ME, Nakajima S, Yasui A, Ford JM. In vivo recruitment of XPC to UV-induced cyclobutane pyrimidine dimers by the DDB2 gene product. J Biol Chem 2003;276:46,909–46,910.
42. Hwang BJ, Ford JM, Hanawalt PC, Chu G. Expression of the p48 xeroderma pigmentosum gene is p53-dependent and is involved in global genome repair. Proc Natl Acad Sci USA 1999;96:424–428.
43. Tan T, Chu G. p53 Binds and activates the xeroderma pigmentosum DDB2 gene in humans but not mice. Mol Cell Biol 2002;22:3247–3254.
44. Nichols AF, Itoh T, Graham JA, Lui W, Yamaizumi M, Linn S. Human damage-specific DNA binding protein p48. Characterization of XPE mutations and regulation following UV irradiation. J Biol Chem 2001;275:21,422–21,428.
45. Wakasugi M, Sancar A. Assembly, subunit composition, and footprint of human DNA repair excision nuclease. Proc Natl Acad Sci USA 1998;95:6669–6674.
46. Volker M, Mone MJ, Karmakar P, et al. Sequential assembly of the nucleotide excision repair factors in vivo. MolCell 2001;8:213–224.
47. Bohr V. DNA repair fine structure and its relations to genomic instability. Carcinogenesis 1995;16:2885–2892.
48. Mellon I, Spivak G, Hanawalt PC. Selective removal of transcription-blocking DNA damage from the transcribed strand of the mammalian DHFR gene. Cell 1987;51:241–249.
49. Lee KB, Wang D, Lippard SJ, Sharp PA. Transcription-coupled repair and DNA damage-dependent ubiquitination of RNA polymerase II in vitro. Proc Natl Acad Sci USA 2002;99:4239–4244.
50. Ljungman M, Zhang F. Blockage of RNA polymerase as a possible trigger for u.v. light-induced apoptosis. Oncogene 1996;13:823–831.
51. Mellon I, Rajpal DK, Koi M, Boland CR, Champe GN. Transcription-coupled repair deficiency and mutations in mismatch repair genes. Science 1996;272:557–560.
52. Venema J, Mullenders LH, Natarajan AT, Zeeland AAv, Mayne LY. The genetic defect in Cockyne syndrome is associated with a defect in repair of UV-induced DNA damage in transcriptionally active DNA. Proc Natl Acad Sci USA 1990;87:4707–4711.
53. Henning KA, Li L, Iyer N, et al. The Cockayne syndrome group A gene encodes a WD repeat protein that interacts with the CSB protein and a subunit of RNA polymerase II, TFIIH. Cell 1995;82: 555–564.
54. Selby CP, Sancar A. Human transcription-repair coupling factor CSB/ERCC6 is a DNA-stimulated ATPase but is not a helicase and does not disrupt the ternary transcription complex of stalled RNA polymerase II. J Biol Chem 1997;272:1885–1890.
55. Citterio E, Rademakers S, van der Horst GT, van Gool AJ, Hoeijmakers JHJ, Vermeulen W. Biochemical and biological characterization of wild-type and ATPase-deficient Cockayne syndrome B repair protein. J Biol Chem 1998;273:11,844–11,851.
56. Bregman DB, Halaban R, van Gool AJ, Henning KA, Friedberg EC, Warren SL. UV-induced ubiquitination of RNA polymerase II: a novel modification deficient in Cockayne syndrome cells. Proc Natl Acad Sci USA 1996;93:11,586–11,590.
57. Nance MA, Berry SA. Cockayne syndrome:review of 140 cases. Amer J Med Genet 1992;42:68–84.
58. Berg RJ, Rebel H, van der Horst GT, et al. Impact of global genome repair versus transcription-coupled repair on ultraviolet carcinogenesis in hairless mice. Cancer Res 2000;60:2858–2863.
59. Hermanson-Miller IL, Turchi JJ. Strand-specific binding of RPA and XPA to damaged duplex DNA. Biochemistry 2002;41:2402–2408.
60. Schaeffer L, Roy R, Humbert S, et al. DNA repair helicase: a component of BTF2 (TFIIH) basic transcription factor. Science 1993;260:58–63.
61. Araujo SJ, Nigg EA, Wood RD. Strong functional interactions of TFIIH with XPC and XPG in human DNA nucleotide excision repair, without a preassembled repairosome. Mol Cell Biol 2001;21: 2281–2291.
62. Wang XW, Yeh H, Schaeffer L, et al. p53 modulation of TFIIH associated nucleotide excision repair activity. Nat Genet 1995;10:188–195.
63. Wang XW, Vermeulen W, Coursen JD, et al. The XPB and XPD DNA helicases are components of the p53-mediated apoptosis pathway. Genes Dev 1996;10:1219–1232.
64. O'Donovan A, Davies AA, Moggs JG, West SC, Wood RD. XPG endonuclease makes the 3' incision in human DNA nucleotide excision repair. Nature 1994;371:432–435.
65. Houtsmuller AB, Rademakers S, Nigg AL, Hoogstraten D, Hoeijmakers JH, Vermeulen W. Action of DNA repair endonuclease ERCC1/XPF in living cells. Science 1999;284:958–961.
66. Matsunaga T, Park CH, Bessho T, Mu D, Sancar A. Replication protein A confers structure-specific endonuclease activities to the XPF-ERCC1 and XPG subunits of human DNA repair excision nuclease. J Biol Chem 1996;271:11,047–11,050.

67. Batty DP, Wood RW. Damage recognition in nucleotide excision repair of DNA. Gene 2000; 241:193–204.
68. Saijo M, Kuraoka I, Masutani C, Hanoaka F, Tanaka K. Sequential binding of DNA repair proteins RPA and ERCC1 to XPA in vitro. Nucleic Acids Res 1996;24:4719–4724.
69. Nouspikel T, Lalle P, Leadon SA, Cooper PK, Clarkson SG. A common mutational pattern in Cockayne syndrome patients from xeroderma pigmentosum group G: implications for a second XPG function. Proc Natl Acad Sci USA 1997;94:3116–3121.
70. Lieber MR. The FEN-1 family of structure-specific nucleases in eukaryotic DNA replication, recombination and repair. Bioessays 1997;19:233–240.
71. Lee S-K, Yu S-L, Prakash L, Prakash S. Requirement of yeast RAD2, a homolog of human XPG gene, for efficient RNA polymerase II transcription: implications for Cockayne syndrome. Cell 2002;109:823–834.
72. Cooper PK, Nouspikel T, Clarkson SG, Leadon SA. Defective transcription coupled repair of oxidative base damage in Cockayne syndrome patients from XP group G. Science 1997;275:990–993.
73. Wood RD. Nucleotide excision repair in mammalian cells. J Biol Chem 1997;272:23,465–23,468.
74. Bendjennat M, Boulaire JRM, Jascur T, et al. UV irradiation triggers ubiquitin-dependent degradation of p21 WAF1 to promote DNA repair. Cell 2003;114:599–610.
75. Xu G, Snellman E, Bykov VJ, Jansen CT, Hemminki K. Cutaneous melanoma patients have normal repair kinetics of ultraviolet-induced DNA repair in skin in situ. J Invest Dermatol 2000;114:628–631.
76. Zhao C, Snellman E, Jansen CT, Hemminski K. In situ repair of cyclobutane pyrimidine dimers in skin and melanocytic nevi of cutaneous melanoma patients. Int J Cancer 2002;98:331–334.
77. Shannon JA, Kefford RF, Mann GJ. Responses to ultraviolet-B in cell lines form hereditary melanoma kindreds. Melanoma Res 2001;11:1–9.
78. Bae I, Smith ML, Sheikh MS, et al. An abnormality in the p53 pathway following gamma-irradiation in many wild-type p53 human melanoma lines. Cancer Res 1996;56:840–847.
79. Winsey SL, Haldar NA, Marsh HP, et al. A variant within the DNA repair gene XRCC3 is associated with the development of melanoma skin cancer. Cancer Res 2000;60:5612–5616.
80. Duan Z, Shen H, Lee JE, et al. DNA repair gene XRCC3 241Met variant is not associated with risk of cutaneous malignant melanoma. Cancer Epidemiol Biomarkers Prev 2002;11(10 Pt 1):1142–1143.
81. Landi MT, Baccarelli A, Tarone RE, et al. DNA repair, dysplastic nevi, and sunlight sensitivity in the development of cutaneous malignant melanoma. J Natl Cancer Inst 2002;94:94–101.
82. Wei Q, Lee JE, Gershenwald JE, et al. Repair of UV light-induced DNA damage and risk of cutaneous malignant melanoma. J Natl Cancer Inst 2003;95:308–315.
83. Wei Q, Cheng L, Xie K, Bucana CD, Dong Z. Direct correlation between DNA repair capacity and metastatic potential of K-1735 murinemelanoma cells. J Invest Dermatol 1997;108:3–6.
84. Singer B, Hang B. What structural features determine repair enzyme specificity and mechanisms in chemically modified DNA? 1997;10:713–723.
85. Caldecott KW. XRCC1 and DNA strand break repair. DNA Repair 2003;2:955–969.
86. Gros L, Saparbaev MK, Laval J. Enzymology of the repair of free radicals-induced DNA damage. Oncogene 2002;21:8905–8925.
87. Singer B, Hang B. What structural features determine repair enzyme specificity and mechanism in chemically modified DNA? Chem Res Toxicol 1997;10:713–732.
88. Saparbaev M, Langouet S, Privezentzev CV, et al. 1,N(2)-ethenoguanine, a mutagenic DNA adduct, is a primary substrate of Escherichia coli mismatch-specific uracil-DNA glycosylase and human alkylpurine-DNA-N-glycosylase. J Biol Chem 2002;277:26,987–26,993.
89. Engelward BP, Dreslin A, Christensen J, Huszar D, Kurahara C, Samson L. Repair-deficient 3-methyladenine DNA glycosylase homozygous mutant mouse cells have increased sensitivity to alkylation-induced chromosome damage and cell killing. EMBO J. 1996;15:945–952.
90. Hang B, Singer B, Margison GP, Elder RH. Targeted deletion of alkylpuring DNA-N-glycosylase in mice eliminates repair of 1,N6-ethenoadenine and hypoxanthine but not of 3,N4-ethenocytosine or 8-oxoguanine. Proc Natl Acad Sci USA 1997;94:12,869–12,874.
91. Wilson DM, Thompson LH. Life without DNA repair. Proc Natl Acad Sci USA 1997;94:12,758–12,760.
92. Sobol RW, Horton JK, Kuhn R, et al. Requirement of mammalian DNA polymerase-b in base-excision repair. Nature 1996;379:183–186.
93. Frosina G, Fortini P, Carrozzino F, et al. Two pathways for base excision repair in mammalian cells. J Biol Chem 1996;271:9573–9578.

94. Fortini P, Pascucci B, Parlanti E, Sobol RW, Wilson SW, Dogliotti E. Different DNA polymerases are involved in the short- and long-patch base excision repair in mammalian cells. Biochemistry 1998;37:3575–3580.

95. Moore DJ, Taylor RM, Clements P, Caldecott KW. Mutation of a BRCT domain selectively disrupts DNA single-strand break repair in noncycling Chinese hamster ovary cells. Proc Natl Acad Sci USA 2000;97:13,649–13,654.

96. Xanthoudakis S, Smeyne RJ, Wallace JD, Curran T. The redox/DNA repair protein, Ref-1, is essential for early embryonic development in mice. Proc Natl Acad Sci USA 1996;93:8919–8923.

97. Gu H, Marth JD, Orban PC, Mossmann H, Rajewsky K. Deletion of a DNA polymerase b gene segment in T cells using cell type-specific gene targeting. Science 1994;265:103–106.

98. Tebbs RS, Flannery M, Meneses JJ, et al. Requirement for the Xrcc1 DNA base excision repair gene during early mouse development. Dev Biol 1999;208:513–529.

99. Bentley D, Selfridge J, Millar JK, et al. DNA ligase I is required for fetal liver erythropoeisis but is not essential for mammalian cell viability. Nat Genet 1996;13:489–491.

100. Petrini JH, Xiao Y, Weaver DT. DNA ligase I mediates essential functions in mammalian cells. Mol Cell Biol 1995;15:4303–4308.

101. MacAuley A, Werb Z, Mirkes PE. Characterization of the unusually rapid cell cycles during rat gastulation. Development 1993;117:873–883.

102. Hoy CA, Fuscoe JC, Thompson LH. Recombination and ligation of transfected DNA in CHO mutant EM9, which has high levels of sister chromatid exchange. Mol Cell Biol 1987;7:2007–2011.

103. Friedberg EC, Meira LB, Cheo DL. Database of mouse strains carrying targeted mutations in genes affecting cellular responses ot DNA damage. Version 2. Mutation Res 1998;407:217–226.

104. Chen RH, Maher VM, McCormick JJ. Effect of excision repair by diploid human fibroblasts on the kinds and locations of mutations induced by (+/–)-7 beta,8 alpha-dihydroxy-9 alpha,10 alpha-epoxy-7,8,9,10-tetrahydrobenzo[a]pyrene in the coding region of the HPRT gene. Proc Natl Acad Sci USA. 1990;87:8680–8684.

105. Steitz TA. DNA polymerases: structural diversity and common mechanisms. J Biol Chem 1999; 274:17,395–17,398.

106. Hubscher U, Maga G, Spadari S. Eukaryotic DNA polymerases. Annu Rev Biochem 2002;71:133–163.

107. Ohmori H, Friedberg EC, Fuchs RPP, et al. The Y-family of DNA polymerases. Mol Cell 2001;8:7–8.

108. Broughton BC, Cordonnier A, Kleijer WJ, et al. Molecular analysis of mutations in DNA polymerase eta in xeroderma pigmentosum-variant patients. Proc Natl Acad Sci USA. 2002;99:815–820.

109. Huang X, Kolbanovskiy A, Wu X, et al. Effects of base sequence context on translesion synthesis past a bulky (+)-trans-anti-B[a]P-N2-dG lesion catalyzed by the Y-family polymerase pol kappa. Biochem 2003;42:2456–2466.

110. Rechkoblit O, Zhang Y, Guo D, et al. trans-Lesion synthesis past bulky benzo[a]pyrene diol epoxide N2-dG and N6-dA lesions catalyzed by DNA bypass polymerases. J Biol Chem 2002;277: 30,488–30,494.

111. Levine RL, Miller H, Grollman A, et al. Translesion DNA synthesis catalyzed by human pol eta and pol kappa across 1,N6-ethenodeoxyadenosine. J Biol Chem 2001;276:18,717–18,721.

112. Johnson RE, Washington MT, Haracska L, Prakash S, Prakash L. Eukaryotic polymerases i and z act sequentially to bypass DNA lesions. Nature 2000;406:1015–1019.

113. Woodgate R. Evolution of the two-step model for UV-mutagenesis. Mutation Res 2001;485:83–92.

114. Washington MT, Johnson RE, Prakash L, Prakash S. Human *DINB1*-encoded DNA polymerase k is a promiscuous extender of mispaired promer termini. Proc Natl Acad Sci USA 2002;99:1910–1914.

115. Haracska L, Prakash L, Prakash S. Role of human DNA polymerase kappa as an extender in translesion synthesis. Proc Natl Acad Sci USA 2002;99:16,000–16,005.

116. Trincao J, Johnson RE, Escalante CR, Prakash S, Prakash L, Aggarwal AK. Structure of the catalytic core of S. cerevisiae DNA polymerase h: implications for translesion synthesis. Mol Cell 2001; 8:417–426.

117. Ling H, Boudsocq F, Plosky BS, Woodgate R, Yang W. Replication of a cis-syn thymine dimer at atomic resolution. Nature 2003;424:1083–1087.

118. Johnson RE, Washington MT, Prakash S, Prakash L. Fidelity of human DNA polymerase h. J Biol Chem 2000;275:7447–7450.

119. Matsuda T, Bebenek K, Masutani C, Hanoaka F, Kunkel TA. Low fidelity DNA synthesis by human DNA polymerase eta. Nature 2000;404:1011–1013.

120. Tissier A, McDonald JP, Frank EG, Woodgate R. Pol iota, a remarkable error-prone human DNA polymerase. Genes Dev 2000;14:1642–1650.

121. Kannouche P, Fernandez de Henestrosa AR, Coull B, et al. Localization of DNA polymerases eta and iota to the replication machinery is tightly co-ordinated in human cells. EMBO J 2003;22:1223–1233.

122. Thakur M, Wernick M, Collins C, Limoli C, Crowley E, Cleaver JE. DNA polymerase h undergoes alternative splicing, protects against UV sensitivity and apoptosis, and suppresses Mre11-dependent recombination. Genes Chromosomes Cancer 2001;32:222–235.

123. Haracska L, Unk I, Johnson RE, et al. Stimulation of DNA synthesis activity of human DNA polymerase kappa by PCNA. Mol Cell Biol 2002;22:784–791.

124. Stelter P, Ulrich HD. Control of spontaneous and damage-induced mutagenesis by SUMO and ubiquitin conjugation. Nature 2003;425:188–191.

125. Douki T, Cadet J. Individual determination of the yield of the main UV-induced dimeric pyrimidine photoproducts in DNA suggests high mutagenicity of CC photoproducts. Biochemistry 2001;40: 2495–2501.

126. Brash DE, Seetharam S, Kraemer KH, Seidman MM, Bredberg A. Photoproduct frequency is not the major determinant of UV base substitution hot spots or cold spots in human cells. Proc Natl Acad Sci USA 1987;84:3782–3786.

127. Protic-Sabljic M, Tuteja N, Munson PJ, Hauser J, Kraemer KH, Dixon K. UV light-induced cyclobutane pyrimidine dimers are mutagenic in mammalian cells. Mol Cell Biol 1986;6:3349–3356.

128. Gao S, Drouin R, Holmquist GP. DNA repair rates mapped along the human PGK-1 gene at nucleotide resolution. Science 1994;263:1438–1440.

129. Tornaletti S, Pfeiffer GP. Slow repair of pyrimidine dimers at p53 mutation hotspots in skin cancer. Science 1994;263:1436–1438.

130. Tornaletti S, Rozek D, Pfeifer GP. Mapping of UV photoproducts along the human p53 gene. Ann N Y Acad Sci 1994;726:324–326.

131. Tormanen VT, Pfeifer GP. Mapping of UV photoproducts within ras proto-oncogenes in UV irradiated cells: correlation with mutations in human skin cancer. Oncogene 1992;7:1729–1736.

132. Reis AM, Cheo DL, Meira LB, et al. Genotype-specific Trp53 mutational analysis in ultraviolet B radiation-induced skin cancers in Xpc and Xpc Trp53 mutant mice. Cancer Res 2000;60:1571–1579.

133. Maher VM, Dorney DJ, Mendrake AL, Konze-Thomas B, McCormick JJ. DNA excision repair processes in human cells can eliminate the cytotoxic and mutagenic consequences of ultraviolet irradiation. Mutation Res 1979;62:311–323.

134. Wang YC, Maher VM, Mitchell DL, McCormick JJ. Evidence from mutation spectra that the UV hypermutability of xeroderma pigmentosum variant cells reflects abnormal error-prone replication on a template containing photoproducts. Mol Cell Biol 1993;13:4276–4283.

135. Gibbs PE, McGregor WG, Maher VM, Nisson P, Lawrence CW. A human homolog of the Saccharomyces cerevisiae REV3 gene, which encodes the catalytic subunit of DNA polymerase zeta. Proc Natl Acad Sci USA 1998;95:6876–6880.

136. Gibbs PE, Wang XD, Li Z, et al. The function of the human homolog of Saccharomyces cerevisiae REV1 is required for mutagenesis induced by UV light. Proc Natl Acad Sci USA 2000;97: 4186–4191.

137. King NM, Oakley GG, Medvedovic M, Dixon K. XPA protein alters the specificity of ultraviolet light-induced mutagenesis in vitro. Environ Mol Mutagen 2001;37:329–339.

138. Tanaka K, Kamiuchi S, Ren Y, et al. UV-induced skin carcinogenesis in xeroderma pigmentosum group A (XPA) gene-knockout mice with nucleotide excision repair-deficiency. Mutation Res 2001;477:31–40.

139. Kress S, Sutter C, Strickland PT, Mukhtar H, Schweizer J, Schwarz M. Carcinogen-specific mutational pattern in the p53 gene in ultraviolet B radiation-induced squamous cell carcinomas of mouse skin. Cancer Res 1992;52:6400–6403.

140. Dumaz N, Drougard C, Sarasin A, Daya-Grosjean L. Specific UV-induced mutation spectrum in the p53 gene of skin tumors from DNA-repair-deficient xeroderma pigmentosum patients. Proc Natl Acad Sci USA 1993;90:10,519–10,533.

141. Horiguchi M, Masumura K, Ikehata H, et al. UVB-induced gpt mutations in the skin of gpt delta transgenic mice. Environ Mol Mutagen 1999;34:72–79.

142. Horiguchi M, Masumura KI, Ikehata H, Ono T, Kanke Y, Nohmi T. Molecular nature of ultraviolet B light-induced deletions in the murine epidermis. Cancer Res 2001;61:3913–3918.

143. Goldstein AM, Tucker MA. Genetic epidemiology of cutaneous melanoma: a global perspective. Arch Dermatol 2001;137:1493–1496.

144. Barnhill RL, Roush GC, Titus-Ernstoff L, Ernstoff MS, Duray PH, Kirkwood JM. Comparison of nonfamilial and familial melanoma. Dermatology 1992;184:2–7.

145. Kopf AW, Hellman LJ, Rogers GS, et al. Familial malignant melanoma. JAMA 1986;256: 1915–1919.

146. Aitken JF, Duffy DL, Green A, Youl P, MacLennan R, Martin NG. Heterogeneity of melanoma risk in families of melanoma patients. American Journal Epidemiology 1994;140:961–973.

147. Bastian BC, Kashani-Sabet M, Hamm H, et al. Gene amplifications characterize acral melanoma and permit detection of occult tumor cells in the surrounding matrix. Cancer Res 2000;60:1968–1973.

148. Pollock PM, Trent JM. The genetics of cutaneous melanoma. Clinical Laboratory Medicine 2000;20:667–690.

149. Kannan K, Sharpless NE, Xu J, O'Hagan RC, Bosenburg M, Chin L. Components of the Rb pathway are critical targets of UV mutagenesis in a murine melanoma model. Proc Nat Acad Sci USA 2003;100:1221–1225.

150. Kamb A, Shattuck-Eidens D, Eeles R, et al. Analysis of the p16 gene (CDKN2) as a candidate for the chromosome 9p melanoma susceptibility locus. Nature Genet 1994;8:23–26.

151. Nobori T, Miura K, Wu DJ, Lois A, Takabayashi K, Carson DA. Deletions of the cyclin-dependent kinase-4 inhibitor gene in multiple human cancers. Nature 1994;368:753–756.

152. Pavey S, Conroy S, Russell T, Gabrielli B. Ultraviolet radiaiton induced p16 [CDKN2A] expression in human skin. Cancer Res 1999;59:4185–4189.

153. Bastian B, LeBoit PE, Hamm H, Brocker E-B, Pinkel D. Chromosomal gains and losses in primary cutaneous melanomas detected by comparative genome hybridization. Cancer Res 1998;58: 2170–2175.

154. Sands AT, Abuin A, Sanchez A, Conti CJ, Bradley A. High susceptibility to ultraviolet-induced carcinogenesis in mice lacking XPC. Nature 1995;377:162–165.

155. van der Horst GT, Meira L, Gorgels TG, et al. UVB radiation-induced cancer predisposition in Cockayne syndrome group A (Csa) mutant mice. DNA Repair 2002;1:143–157.

156. Wijnhoven SW, Kool HJ, van Oostrom CT, et al. The relationship between benzo[a]pyrene-induced mutagenesis and carcinogenesis in repair-deficient Cockayne syndrome group B mice. Cancer Res 2000;60:5681–5687.

157. de Boer J, Donker I, de Wit J, Hoeijmakers JHJ, Weeda G. Disruption of the mouse xeroderma pigmentosum group D DNA repair/basal transcription gene results in preimplantation lethality. Cancer Res 1998;58:89–94.

158. de Boer J, de Wit J, van Steeg H, et al. A mouse model for the basal transcription/DNA repair syndrome trichothiodystrophy. Mol Cell 1998;1:981–990.

17 Divergent Pathways to Cutaneous Melanoma

David C. Whiteman and Adèle C. Green

Summary

Cutaneous melanomas arise on all skin surfaces, but they do so at markedly different rates. Understanding the reasons behind site-specific differences in melanoma rates should help unravel some of the inconsistent findings reported from epidemiological studies and provide the basis for informed preventive activities. Although exposure to sunlight is generally accepted to determine the rate at which melanocytes at any particular anatomical site are transformed, there are also likely to be anatomical differences (within a host) and constitutional differences (among hosts) in the susceptibility of melanocytes to progress to neoplasia. The contributions of these competing causal factors (environmental, anatomical, and genetic) to the development of melanoma have not been collectively studied, yet this is necessary if deeper understanding of melanoma pathogenesis is to yield tangible public health benefits. Here, we review the literature for evidence of causal heterogeneity for melanoma and present the findings of a recent epidemiological study from Queensland, Australia.

Key Words: Melanoma; causality; sunlight; risk factor; occupation; nevus; solar keratosis.

OVERVIEW

A fundamental requirement for developing effective strategies to control melanoma is to better understand the causes of this disease. An implicit assumption behind most studies of cutaneous melanoma has been that all such tumors arise through the same developmental pathway. Thus, researchers have approached their analyses as if all cutaneous melanomas are caused by the same mix of environmental and genetic factors.

From: *From Melanocytes to Melanoma: The Progression to Malignancy*
Edited by: V. J. Hearing and S. P. L. Leong © Humana Press Inc., Totowa, NJ

When viewed afresh, there is little to justify this approach. For example, there is general acceptance that familial and sporadic melanomas have different causal pathways. That is, a very small proportion of melanomas arise as a result of inherited germline mutations in one of several tumor suppressor genes, whereas the vast majority of melanomas arise sporadically in the general population. Furthermore, melanomas of the eye *(1,2)*, and those arising on mucosal, subungual, or palmar/plantar surfaces *(3,4)* are also studied separately on the grounds that they have different origins. Even among cutaneous melanomas, several histological subtypes, lentigo maligna melanoma (LMM) and desmoplastic melanomas, are likewise considered to be distinct from other cutaneous melanomas *(5–7)*, and are usually considered by epidemiologists to be separate from more common histological types of cutaneous melanoma.

Thus, the precedent has long been set that melanocytic target cells may progress to malignancy through a multitude of pathways. This notion was first articulated in 1980 by Ackerman *(8)*, who speculated:

> *It would not be surprising ... if one day it were shown that the causes and pathogenesis of malignant melanomas at different anatomic sites and those that arise de novo, rather than in association with melanocytic nevi (MN), are very different.*

This provocative hypothesis was pursued by Green *(9)*, who put forward a theory of melanoma development grounded in a detailed examination of melanoma incidence across anatomical sites, with and without nevoid remnants.

Here, we review the evidence regarding the heterogeneity of melanoma development. We have not further considered ocular melanomas, or those of mucosal or subungual surfaces, but rather have restricted our examination to the origins of cutaneous melanomas. We have focused on the epidemiological literature, paying particular attention to studies comparing occurrence or risk factors for melanomas arising on different anatomical sites, supplemented with information from histological and molecular analyses of cutaneous melanomas and animal models. We conclude by describing the findings from a recent epidemiological study designed to test the hypothesis that melanomas arising at different anatomical sites develop through divergent causal pathways.

EPIDEMIOLOGICAL STUDIES

Epidemiological studies are of two types: descriptive studies, that compare patterns of melanoma occurrence across populations using routinely collected statistical data; and analytical studies that compare individual exposure data collected from people with and without melanoma. Epidemiological studies of both types have consistently pointed to a core of phenotypic and/or inherited factors that are associated with cutaneous melanoma, including:

- A large number of MN on the skin *(10–12)*.
- A family history of melanoma *(13)*.
- Fair skin that burns easily and does not tan *(14)*.
- A propensity to freckling *(14)*.
- Red hair.

The role of these factors in divergent causal pathways will be considered subsequently. Initial focus of this review is on the interaction between sunlight and melanoma at different anatomical sites.

Descriptive Epidemiological Studies

At the population level, the dual observations of markedly higher incidence of cutaneous melanoma among fair-skinned people compared with dark-skinned people, and the inverse gradient of increasing melanoma incidence with decreasing latitude are widely accepted. Moreover, the interpretation that these observations reflect population-wide differences in exposure and susceptibility to sunlight are not seriously disputed. The point of interest is whether the role of sun exposure in tumor development is uniform for all melanomas, or whether subsets of melanoma exist that have different associations with sunlight.

Melanoma Incidence at Anatomical Sites

Descriptive epidemiological studies report a crude excess of melanomas on the back and shoulders in men and the lower limb in women *(15–18)*. At first sight, these figures suggest that melanomas are overrepresented on sites not habitually exposed to the sun, and thus have been taken to indicate that intermittent exposure to sunlight is a more potent carcinogen than chronic exposure. To properly assess the relative rate of occurrence of melanoma at different anatomical sites to undergo malignant change, it is necessary to adjust for the surface areas of the sites being compared. When this is done, the incidence of melanoma is found to be highest on the ears (in men) and face (body sites habitually exposed to the sun) and next highest on the shoulders and back in men, and the shoulders, upper arms and back in women (sites usually with intermittent exposure to the sun) *(19)*. Negligibly low rates of melanoma are observed on body sites with very low levels of sun exposure, such as the buttocks and the female scalp *(15,20)*.

Considered in this way, it appears that the site-specific incidence of melanoma may simply reflect the cumulative solar dose experienced by each anatomical site. There are notable deviations from such an anticipated distribution, however, that defy a simple explanation based on exposure to sunlight alone. For example, the area-adjusted incidence of melanoma on the back and shoulders, although lower than the face, is still considerably higher than the dorsum of the hand, despite the back of the hand being habitually exposed to the sun.

Site-Specific Melanoma Incidence by Age

Houghton *(21)* first proposed that melanomas of the face might have a different relationship to sunlight compared with other sites, based on the observation that the melanomas of the trunk occur more commonly at younger ages than those of the head and neck *(16,22,23)*. Because LMM, the histological subtype associated with chronic solar exposure and older age, frequently occur on the face and account for a sizable proportion of melanomas at this site, any analysis that includes these lesions may lead to mistaken inferences regarding the etiology of facial melanomas. Few descriptive studies have explicitly excluded LMMs, yet this is necessary to validly interpret differences in the onset of cutaneous melanomas at different anatomical sites.

A detailed analysis of notifications to the British Columbia Cancer Registry calculated area-adjusted melanoma incidence for various anatomical sites, stratified by age at diagnosis, with LMMs reported separately. Among younger people (those less than 50 yr), the area-adjusted incidence of melanoma was more than threefold higher on "intermittently exposed body sites" (35–49 yr, 17.1×10^{-5} person-yr) than on "maximally exposed sites" (35–49 yr, 4.9×10^{-5} person-yr). Among older people, however, there was a shift in area-adjusted melanoma incidence. Although the incidence of melanoma on intermittently exposed sites was somewhat higher among older than younger people (50–64 yr, $25.4.1 \times 10^{-5}$ person-yr; >65 yr, 36.5×10^{-5} person-yr), the incidence of melanoma on maximally exposed sites was considerably higher (50–64 yr, 32.2×10^{-5} person-yr; >65 yr, 61.3×10^{-5} person-yr).

These interesting data have been widely interpreted as demonstrating different effects of intermittent and chronic sun exposure on melanoma development. Under this model, intermittent exposure to the sun is postulated to rapidly induce melanocytic tumors, whereas chronic exposure is postulated to cause slower tumor development. An alternative but equally plausible explanation is that melanocytes on the trunk are induced to malignant progression at a lower sun exposure threshold than melanocytes of the face, irrespective of the pattern of sun exposure. Indeed, both phenomena may occur, although descriptive studies cannot address this.

SITE-SPECIFIC MELANOMA INCIDENCE BY OCCUPATION

A subset of descriptive studies have used occupational records to infer the pattern and amount of sun exposure a person might have sustained during their adult life. Overall, these studies have tended to report that outdoor workers have lower risks of melanoma than indoor workers *(24–26)*, suggesting that chronic sun exposure is *not* associated with higher rates of melanoma.

When melanomas of the skin are assessed according to their anatomical location, however, outdoor workers consistently have a crude excess of melanomas on the face, ears, and neck, and a crude deficit of melanomas on the trunk *(27–30)*. In contrast, office workers typically have a higher incidence of melanoma on the trunk and a lower incidence of melanoma on the head and neck *(27,28)*.

Thus, occupational studies provide interesting insights into the site distribution of cutaneous melanoma; however, further analyses are required to unravel the complex relationships between anatomical site, sunlight, and melanoma. For example, none of the occupational studies to date have standardized melanoma incidence according to the area of each anatomical site, as has been done for most recent descriptive studies comparing site-specific incidence for melanoma *(15,20)*. When undertaken, such analyses would be expected to confirm the very high rates of melanoma at sun-exposed sites among outdoor workers, however, interest would focus on the comparisons of area-adjusted melanoma incidence between maximally and intermittently exposed sites among indoor workers. If indoor workers were found to have higher area-adjusted rates of melanoma on the face than on the trunk, then it raises interesting questions about the relative influence of intermittent and chronic exposures on melanoma development.

When interpreting descriptive data from occupational studies, it is also necessary to consider two further points, namely, the level of ambient solar radiation in the setting where the study was conducted *(31,32)*, and the likely patterns of recreational sun exposure among indoor and outdoor workers in that setting. Most occupational studies have been conducted in temperate climates in northern Europe or Canada, where outdoor workers are fully clothed for most working days of the year, even in summer. For outdoor workers in these environments, some body sites (such as the face) would be chronically exposed to sunlight, whereas their truncal melanocytes would be infrequently exposed to the sun. Indoor workers would clearly sustain lower solar doses to the face, however the solar dose sustained by their truncal melanocytes may actually exceed those of outdoor workers, depending on their recreational and vacation activities. A Danish study found that those who visited southern Europe for summer vacation received daily doses of solar radiation (measured at the wrist) up to sevenfold higher than those who remained in northern Europe *(33)*. Moreover, the travelers spent considerably more of their outdoor time in a bathing suit than those who remained in northern Europe. These data clearly demonstrate the importance of recreational activities in determining a person's total solar dose, particularly for indoor workers, and most particularly for anatomical sites that are infrequently exposed to the sun.

Details of recreational sun exposure are not collected in routine statistical data sets, nevertheless, some investigators have attempted to infer different patterns of recreational sun exposure using measures of social class *(25)*, or by separately analyzing office workers and other indoor workers on the assumption that vacations in sunny environments are more likely among those of higher social class. These approaches have yielded some interesting differences in melanomas incidence, and suggest that melanoma occurs more commonly among those of higher social class *(34–37)*.

In summary, occupational studies provide interesting insights into patterns of melanoma occurrence, and confirm that melanomas are distributed unequally across anatomical sites, but these studies do not resolve whether melanomas at different sites arise through different causal pathways. One methodological shortcoming of all descriptive studies is that they make inferences about sun exposure based on the site of melanoma, and cannot account for the large variation in sun exposure even within populations homogeneous for ambient solar irradiation *(31)*, or the presence of important phenotypic determinants of melanoma risk. These issues are addressed in analytical studies.

Analytical Epidemiological Studies

Numerous case–control studies have investigated the causes of melanoma in different populations *(14,38,39)*, although few have examined risk factors separately for subgroups of cutaneous melanomas. Early investigations into causal heterogeneity for melanoma focused on separate analyses by histological subtype of melanoma *(40)*. Although some statistically significant differences in risk were noted for some exposures, no consistent differences of biological relevance were observed.

More recently, several case–control studies have undertaken stratified analyses, in which cases were categorized according to the anatomical site of their melanoma. The relative risks of melanoma at each site were then estimated for various phenotypic risk factors, notably, numbers of nevi. For example, a case–control study nested within the Nurses' Health Study found that melanomas of the trunk and legs were associated with high nevus counts, but not melanomas of the arms *(41)*. The authors postulated that some degree of etiological heterogeneity by anatomic site might explain these differences. Similarly, a study in Connecticut reported that people with melanoma of the head and neck were threefold more likely to have 10 or more nevi on the arms compared with population controls. In contrast, those with melanomas on the trunk, arms, or legs were five to six times more likely than disease-free controls to have 10 or more nevi on the arms, although these differences were not statistically significant *(42)*. Other studies have also reported different levels of risk associated with nevus density for melanomas at different sites. Two German case–control studies reported that high nevus counts conferred substantially increased risks for melanoma of the trunk and legs, but were much less strongly associated with melanomas of the head and neck or arms *(43,44)*. A case–control study of cutaneous melanoma conducted in New South Wales, Australia, found that patients with head and neck melanomas had substantially fewer nevi and more solar keratoses than patients with melanoma of the trunk or legs (45). Taken together, the few case–control studies that have undertaken site-specific analyses have found reasonably consistent results. By collecting phenotypic data about individuals, these studies extend the findings of descriptive epidemiological studies and provide further evidence that melanomas arising at various anatomical sites have different relationships to established risk factors.

HISTOPATHOLOGY STUDIES

Given the consistent epidemiological evidence that people with numerous MN have significantly higher risks of melanoma than other people, the question arises whether nevi are precursors of melanoma or simply epidemiological risk markers. In attempting to answer this question, numerous groups have histologically evaluated melanoma tumor specimens for the presence or absence of contiguous neval remnants (hereafter, "MN + melanoma" and "MN – melanoma"). The findings are remarkably consistent, with most studies reporting approx 20–25% of cutaneous melanomas having histological evidence of a coexisting nevus (43,46–49). Moreover, all analyses to date have all found that MN + melanomas occur more commonly on the trunk than on the head and neck (43,49,50) (see Table 1).

Because head and neck melanomas occur at older ages than truncal melanoma, and because nevi overall are less prevalent with increasing age (51), it is possible that the association between MN + melanoma and anatomical site reflects confounding by age. However, the only study to have specifically addressed this issue (50) reported that the associations were similar among older and younger age-groups, and the investigators concluded that anatomical site was an independent predictor of MN + melanoma.

Only one study to date has separately compared MN + melanoma cases and MN – melanoma cases to a control group of people without melanoma (49) to test the hypothesis that these two groups of melanomas arise through different causal pathways. In addition to different anatomical distributions of the two groups, this study found that patients with MN + melanomas were eightfold more likely to have more than 30 nevi than controls, whereas patients with MN – melanomas were only threefold more likely to have more than 30 nevi. Further, MN + melanoma patients were nearly seven times more likely to report episodes of severe sunburn than controls, whereas MN – melanoma patients did not differ from controls in terms of their sunburn history.

These epidemiological observations suggest that melanomas with contiguous neval remnants differ from de novo melanomas in their association with some risk factors, and point to fundamentally different biological origins. This hypothesis has recently been explored using the tools of molecular biology (see Molecular Studies) to investigate the genetic profiles of MN + and MN – tumors.

ANIMAL STUDIES

Few animal species spontaneously develop melanomas, and melanomas that do arise in animals generally differ in their histopathological characteristics and behavior from human melanomas (52). Recently, however, susceptible strains of transgenic mice have

Table 1
Studies Reporting Melanomas Arising in Conjunction With Melanocytic Nevi

Study	Trunk MN+/all MN (%)	Head MN+/all MN (%)	All sites MN+/all MN (%)
Kruger (43)	24/88 (27%)	3/15 (20%)	42/200 (21%)
Skender-Kalnenas (50)	69/108 (64%)	13/45 (29%)	147/289 (51%)
Carli (49)	21/54 (39%)	0/6 (0%)	27/131 (21%)
Kaddu (48)	51/224 (23%)	21/125 (17%)	148/667 (22%)

been developed whose melanomas more closely approximate human tumors. Although mouse models potentially offer great promise for unlocking the genetic and environmental pathways to melanoma, their relevance to human melanoma is questionable.

To specifically test the hypothesis whether local factors influenced the susceptibility of anatomical sites to melanoma, Silvers and Mintz performed a series of skin-grafting experiments on the TYR-SV40E strain of mice (53). They showed that skin grafted from the snout of a mouse to the lateral trunk developed many more melanomas than skin grafted from the base of the tail or the dorsal body. They concluded that susceptibility to melanoma was determined, in part, by anatomical site. In the case of mice, it is speculated that growth factors in the follicles of vibrissae influence the development of melanomas, although data to support this are scarce. As far as we are aware, these interesting experiments have not been replicated.

Another animal model for human melanoma is the angora goat. A prevalence survey of 1731 angora goats in Queensland, Australia (54) reported that 2.2% had cutaneous melanomas, predominantly on hairless body sites, such as the ears. In contrast, 3.8% of goats had squamous cell carcinomas, and these were most common on the perineum, suggesting site-specific differences in cancer development. To further examine the effects of sunlight on melanocytic neoplasia in these animals, a trial was conducted in which 8 goats were shorn of their hair on one side only (54). After 9 mo, the investigators found significantly higher numbers of new melanocytic lesions on the shorn (sun-exposed) sites than those covered by hair. This animal model suggests that there is an interaction between sun exposure and anatomical site in melanocytic neoplasia.

MOLECULAR STUDIES

New methods for rapidly assessing genomic aberrations in large numbers of melanoma specimens provide opportunities for insights into causal mechanisms. If the hypothesis that sporadic cutaneous melanomas arise though different causal pathways is true, then melanomas would be expected to display different genetic profiles reflecting their different origins.

The genes that have been most closely examined for somatic mutations in sporadic human cutaneous melanomas are *NRAS*, *TP53*, *CDKN2A*, *PTEN*, and more recently, *BRAF*. Increasingly, it appears that the frequency and types of mutations in some of these genes is related to the amount of sun exposure received by the host and the anatomical site of the tumor.

TP53

The *TP53* tumor-suppressor gene was an early candidate for somatic mutation in cutaneous melanoma, given the finding that ultraviolet (UV)-specific mutations in *TP53* were commonly observed in nonmelanoma skin cancers and were associated with overexpression of the *P53* gene product in skin cancer cells *(55)*. Immunohistochemical studies subsequently reported *TP53* overexpression in between 20 and 40% of primary melanomas *(56–60)*, however, interest in this phenomenon waned when sequencing experiments revealed that few melanomas actually harbor mutations in the gene *(60–63)*.

The presence or absence of immunoreactivity for the p53 protein product provides a biological basis for distinguishing cases of melanoma. We previously conducted a molecular epidemiological study in which melanoma cases were categorized into p53-immunoreactive and p53-immunonegative lesions *(64)*. We found that patients with p53-immunoreactive melanomas were associated with a cluster of features, including sun-exposed anatomical location, a past history of nonmelanoma skin cancer, and a tendency to burn on exposure to the sun. In contrast, patients with p53-immunonegative melanomas were more likely to have numerous MN and dense freckling. No other epidemiological studies have separately compared p53-positive and p53-negative melanomas for the prevalence of risk factors, however, the predilection for p53-immunoreactive melanomas to occur at sun exposed sites has been confirmed in several series *(65,66)* but not in all series *(67,68)*.

CDKN2A

Another early candidate as a target for somatic mutation in sporadic primary melanoma was the *CDKN2A* tumor-suppressor gene. This gene encodes the cell cycle regulator, p16, which binds to and inhibits *CDK4* and *CDK6*, thereby repressing cell cycle progression from G1 to S phase. Interest in this gene followed from the finding that *CDKN2A* germline mutations were observed in 40% of affected cases with familial melanoma syndromes *(69,70)*. Although there is experimental evidence that mutations in *CDKN2A* play a causal role in familial melanoma, its role in sporadic melanoma is unclear. Immunohistochemical studies have been somewhat limited and have yielded conflicting results (reviewed in ref. *71*). The reported prevalence of p16 immunoreactivity in primary lesions ranges from less than 20% *(72)*, to more than 90% *(66,73,74)*. Such heterogeneity of effect almost certainly reflects different methodologies across studies as well as considerable variation in the selection of melanoma specimens for analysis. Although some investigations have focused solely on acral lentiginous melanomas *(72,75)*, others have investigated nodular melanomas *(66)*. Only one molecular epidemiological study has been performed to date *(71)*; it found weak evidence that *CDKN2A* expression was associated with some histological and clinical features of the tumors.

PTEN

The protein product of *PTEN* is a negative regulator of the PI3K/AKT–signaling pathway, which strongly promotes cellular proliferation and survival *(76)*. Germline mutations of *PTEN* cause Cowden syndrome, an autosomal dominant multiple hamartoma syndrome with a high risk of breast, thyroid, and endometrial cancers, and, possibly, melanoma *(77)*. Although *PTEN* is deleted or mutated in up to 57% of melanoma cell lines *(78–80)*, mutations or deletions have been detected at much lower rates (between 5 and 15%) in primary human melanomas *(78–81)*. It is not yet clear whether *PTEN* mutations in melanoma reflect exposure to sunlight or occur in a site-specific manner *(82)*.

MAPK Pathway

More compelling evidence of site-specific differences in somatic gene mutations in cutaneous melanoma has recently emerged from studying patterns of mutations in *NRAS* and *BRAF*, one oncogenes involved in the MAP kinase-signaling pathway *(83,84)*. Activating mutations within these genes are thought to stimulate melanocytes to proliferate through downstream signaling cascades involved in cell growth and mitosis *(83,85)*.

NRAS was the first gene in this pathway to be implicated as having a role in melanoma development. Overall, approx 15–20% of cutaneous melanomas carry mutations in the *NRAS* gene *(86,87)*, and several studies have reported that *NRAS* mutations are considerably more common among melanomas occurring on sites habitually exposed to the sun *(86–88)*. *NRAS* mutations in melanoma occur most frequently at codon 61, opposite a pyrimidine doublet, and are thus compatible with sunlight as a mutagenic agent *(86,88)*.

In contrast to the relatively low prevalence of *NRAS* mutations in cutaneous melanomas, *BRAF* mutations appear to be substantially more common in almost all series published to date. Estimates of prevalence vary, largely because cases have been collected opportunistically from diverse diagnostic centers and cannot reliably represent the population from which they arose, however, most investigators report *BRAF* mutations in 30–60% of melanomas *(89–94)*. To further explore determinants of *BRAF* mutations, Maldonado et al. performed analyses on cases of melanoma sampled from different anatomical sites *(95)*. They found *BRAF* mutations were significantly more common among melanomas arising on the trunk compared with melanomas arising on the face.

In all series to date, almost all *BRAF* mutations in cutaneous melanomas were T–A changes at residue 1796, resulting in an amino acid substitution of valine by glutamic acid at position 599 (*BRAF* V599E) *(85)*. This mutation is distinct from the characteristic dipyrimidine mutations associated with UV exposure (such as observed with *NRAS*), and suggests that some other mechanism underlies mutation of *BRAF*. Moreover, because melanomas harbor either *NRAS* or *BRAF* mutations exclusively, it appears that these are functionally equivalent alterations to the MAP kinase pathway arising through different mutagenic stimuli. *BRAF* mutations are also common in nevi, whereas *NRAS* mutations are rare *(96,97)*, further suggesting that mutations in each of these genes reflect different pathways to melanoma. The logical next step is to revisit the pathology studies to investigate whether *de novo* melanomas and those with contiguous neval remnants differ in their expression of mutant *NRAS* or *BRAF*.

Summary

Clearly, there is considerable heterogeneity among cutaneous melanomas in terms of molecular profiles. Increasing numbers of studies have reported investigations between somatic molecular expression and various predictive factors (such as sunlight exposure or anatomical site); however, most studies have suffered serious methodological flaws when viewed from an epidemiological perspective. For example, the studies have usually had very small numbers of cases (i.e., statistically underpowered to answer the

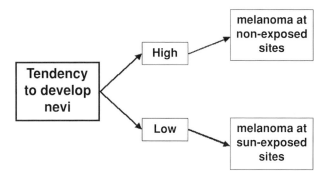

Fig. 1. The divergent pathway hypothesis for melanoma.

research question), have ascertained unrepresentative collections of melanoma tissue sourced from referral centers servicing disparate populations (i.e., high likelihood of biased patient selection), and, when presenting findings, have not addressed the role of confounding factors (such as age, ethnicity, occupation, and ambient sun exposure) that may all explain the phenomenon being reported. These shortcomings mean that most molecular studies to date are less informative than they might otherwise have been.

THE DIVERGENT PATHWAY HYPOTHESIS

The collected findings from studies across the research spectrum indicate that cutaneous melanomas may be categorized according to a variety of epidemiological, pathological, or molecular criteria, each of which provide some evidence for causal heterogeneity. These data are consistent with a model characterizing melanoma as a cancer arising from melanocytes through several causal pathways, depending on the site of the target cell, the constitution of the host, and the external environment.

We have proposed a model for the development of cutaneous melanoma that acknowledges differences in susceptibility to melanocytic neoplasia across individuals in the population, as well as differences in exposure to sunlight, the only known environmental cause. Our model assumes that the fundamental unit of risk (in epidemiological terms) is the individual human host, and that each individual can be broadly classified on the basis of the proliferative potential of their melanocytes.

In this model, people with an inherently low propensity for melanocyte proliferation (identified phenotypically by low nevus counts) require ongoing external stimulation in the form of chronic sun exposure sun to stimulate their melanocytes to proliferate (*see* Fig. 1). In contrast, among people having an inherently high propensity for melanocyte proliferation, we predict that sun exposure is required early in the process of melanoma development, after which point, inherited host factors supervene to drive tumor progression.

If the hypothesis is correct, then we predict that melanomas arising in the former group will occur on habitually sun-exposed body sites, such as the face, whereas melanomas arising in the latter group will develop on body sites with unstable melanocyte populations, such as the trunk. Such patients should also have few signs of solar damage, such as solar keratoses and keratinocyte cancers.

TESTING THE HYPOTHESIS

We recently tested the divergent pathway hypothesis for the development of melanoma in a population-based epidemiological study *(98)*, and summarize the methods and key findings here.

Methods

Briefly, patients were randomly selected from three prespecified groups of melanoma notifications to the Queensland Cancer Registry (a compulsory cancer registry), namely, superficial spreading or nodular melanomas of the trunk ($n = 154$) and head and neck ($n = 77$), or LMM ($n = 75$) (chosen as a "chronic sun-exposure control group" because the LMM subtype is widely accepted as being caused by chronic exposure to sunlight). Each participant completed a questionnaire asking about past sun exposure; details of their complexion and skin type; and details of previous treatment for solar keratoses, basal cell carcinomas, and squamous cell carcinomas. All participants underwent a clinical examination conducted by a single trained research nurse, who counted MN and solar keratoses unaware of study hypotheses.

We calculated exposure odds ratios (OR) to measure the association between phenotypic factors and each melanoma group; in all analyses, the referent group was patients with melanomas of the trunk.

Melanocytic Nevi and Cutaneous Melanoma by Site

People with melanomas of the head and neck were significantly less likely than those with melanomas of the trunk to have more than 60 nevi (OR, 0.3; 95% CI, 0.2–0.8), as were patients with LMM (OR, 0.3; 95% CI, 0.1–0.8). We observed similar associations with counts of large nevi and with self-reported numbers of nevi as a teenager. Because nevi are considerably less common among older people, and because of the propensity for both head and neck melanomas and LMM to develop at older ages, it was possible that the observed association was confounded by age. We conducted stratified analyses and found similar magnitude associations among people older and younger than 50 yr, indicating that confounding by age did not explain the observation.

Solar Keratoses and Melanoma by Site

Counts of solar keratoses were used as a marker of chronic solar exposure. In this sample of Queensland melanoma patients, 64% had at least one solar keratosis at interview (median = 4; range, 0–262). Patients with head and neck melanomas were more than three times as likely as patients with truncal melanomas to have one or more solar keratoses (OR, 3.7; 95% CI, 1.6–8.4). Again, there was a strong possibility of confounding by age for this association, because solar keratoses and melanomas of the head and neck both become more prevalent with increasing age. Further analyses stratified by age found similar strong associations among both younger (<50 yr) and older (>50 yr) patients. Patients with head and neck melanomas were also significantly more likely than patients with truncal melanoma to report a past history of having had skin lesions excised (presumably solar keratoses or keratinocyte cancers) (some vs none: OR, 2.9; 95% CI, 1.0–8.5; many vs none: OR, 4.2; 95% CI, 1.3–13.0).

Discussion

These data demonstrate that people who develop melanomas of the head and neck differ from people who develop melanomas of the trunk in terms of their prevalence of nevi and solar keratoses. From these findings, we infer support for the divergent pathway model for melanoma, which posits that the role of sunlight in the development of melanoma differs according to anatomical site of the target melanocyte and the constitution of the host.

All epidemiological studies are prone to error, and this was considered as a possible explanation for the findings. Recall bias (in which people with the disease of interest typically overreport their exposure to putative causal factors, whereas people without disease tend to underreport their exposure) could not explain these findings, because all study participants were diagnosed with melanoma (i.e., they were "cases" with disease) and were not told of the study aims. In addition, the counts of nevi and solar keratoses were all undertaken by a single nurse who was also not informed about the study hypotheses.

We were most concerned about possible confounding effects of age, because nevi become less common and solar keratoses become more common with advancing age, and both of these phenotypic factors were associated with melanoma. However, we adjusted for linear and nonlinear effects of age in all regression models, and also examined risk estimates for nevi and solar keratoses restricted to older and younger participants, respectively, and found risks of similar magnitude within both age strata. Thus, the effects of age are not likely to confound the results reported here.

Since these data were originally published, others have confirmed the findings presented here (99). We conclude that these data provide a critical test of the divergent pathway hypothesis, and when considered with the findings of epidemiological, molecular, and animal studies, support the existence of different pathogenic pathways to melanoma.

The divergent pathway model may go some way toward resolving apparent paradoxes in melanoma epidemiology. Although rates of melanoma in susceptible populations have long been known to vary with latitude (100), measures of individual sun exposure have been inconsistently associated with melanoma (101). Failure to separately consider the effects of sunlight on people with different propensities to develop melanoma is one explanation for the apparent paradox.

CONCLUSIONS AND PERSPECTIVES: WHERE TO FROM HERE?

This chapter has assembled considerable supportive evidence that melanocytes develop into melanomas through several different pathways, depending on the site of the target melanocyte and the genetic predisposition of the host. Further work is needed, however, if we are to better understand the magnitude of risks associated with environmental and phenotypic exposures in the different pathways.

At the level of descriptive epidemiology, it ought to be a simple matter to confirm that melanomas of the head and neck are more strongly associated with markers of chronic sun exposure, such as squamous cell carcinoma, than are melanomas of the trunk. Future studies of occupational cohorts that seek to compare site-specific melanoma incidence for indoor and outdoor workers must measure recreational sun exposure and also adjust for the area of anatomical sites. This should avoid mistaken inferences being drawn about patterns of sun exposure and melanoma occurrence.

The key finding that MN + melanomas differ from MN − melanomas needs to be confirmed in a well-designed study with appropriate sampling of prospectively ascertained cases. Moreover, the molecular profiles of these histologically distinctive groups need to be determined. Future studies in this area would ideally combine genetic and pathological information about lesions with epidemiological information about the risk factors of the host. One study has shown similar patterns of mutations in melanomas and contiguous neval, but such findings require confirmation in representative groups of tumor samples.

REFERENCES

1. Kricker A, Vajdic C, Armstrong B. Ocular melanoma and cutaneous melanoma. Int J Cancer 2003; 104:259.
2. Cree IA. Cell cycle and melanoma-two different tumours from the same cell type [editorial; comment]. J Pathol 2000;191:112–124.
3. Ridgeway CA, Hieken TJ, Ronan SG, Kim DK, Das Gupta TK. Acral lentiginous melanoma. Arch Surg 1995;130:88–92.
4. Green A, McCredie M, MacKie R, et al. A case-control study of melanomas of the soles and palms (Australia and Scotland). Cancer Causes Control 1999;10:21–25.
5. Cohen LM. Lentigo maligna and lentigo maligna melanoma. J Am Acad Dermatol 1995;33: 923–936.
6. Cox NH, Aitchison TC, Sirel JM, MacKie RM. Comparison between lentigo maligna melanoma and other histogenetic types of malignant melanoma of the head and neck. Scottish Melanoma Group. Br J Cancer 1996;73:940–944.
7. Deveraj VS, Moss ALH, Briggs JC. Desmoplastic melanoma: A clinico-pathological review. Br J Plastic Surgery 1992;45:595–598.
8. Ackerman AB. Malignant melanoma: a unifying concept. Hum Pathol 1980;11:591–595.
9. Green A. A theory of site distribution of melanomas: Queensland, Australia. Cancer Causes Control 1992;3:513–516.
10. Green A, MacLennan R, Siskind V. Common acquired naevi and the risk of malignant melanoma. Int J Cancer 1985;35:297–300.
11. Holly EA, Kelly JW, Shpall SN, Chiu SH. Number of melanocytic nevi as a major risk factor for malignant melanoma. J Am Acad Dermatol 1987;17:459–468.
12. Holman CD, Armstrong BK. Pigmentary traits, ethnic origin, benign nevi, and family history as risk factors for cutaneous malignant melanoma. J Natl Cancer Inst 1984;72:257–266.
13. Ford D, Bliss JM, Swerdlow AJ, et al. Risk of cutaneous melanoma associated with a family history of the disease. Int J Cancer 1995;62:377–381.
14. Bliss JM, Ford D, Swerdlow AJ, et al. Risk of cutaneous melanoma associated with pigmentation characteristics and freckling: systematic overview of 10 case-control studies. Int J Cancer 1995;62:367–376.
15. Osterlind A, Hou-Jensen K, Moller-Jensen O. Incidence of cutaneous malignant melanoma in Denmark 1978–1982. Anatomic site distribution, histologic types and comparison with non-melanoma skin cancer. Br J Cancer 1988;58:385–391.
16. Magnus K. Habits of sun exposure and risk of malignant melanoma: an analysis of incidence rates in Norway 1955–1977 by cohort,sex, age and primary tumor site. Cancer 1981;48:2329–2335.
17. Popescu NA, Beard CM, Treacy PJ, Winkelmann RK, O'Brien PC, Kurland LT. Cutaneous malignant melanoma in Rochester, Minnesota: trends in incidence and survivorship, 1950 through 1985. Mayo Clin Proc 1990;65:1293–1302.
18. Masback A, Westerdahl J, Ingvar C, Olsson H, Jonsson N. Cutaneous malignant melanoma in South Sweden 1965, 1975, and 1985. A histopathologic review. Cancer 1994;73:1625–1630.
19. Green A, MacLennan R, Youl P, Martin N. Site distribution of cutaneous melanoma in Queensland. Int J Cancer 1993;53:232–236.
20. Chen YT, Zheng T, Holford TR, Berwick M, Dubrow R. Malignant melanoma incidence in Connecticut (United States): time trends and age-period-cohort modeling by anatomic site. Cancer Causes Control 1994;5:341–350.
21. Houghton A, Flannery J, Viola MV. Malignant melanoma in Connecticut and Denmark. Int J Cancer 1980;25:95–104.

22. Bulliard J-L. Site-specific risk of cutaneous malignant melanoma and pattern of sun exposure in New Zealand. Int J Cancer 2000;85:627–632.

23. Teppo L, Pakkanen M, Hakulinsen T. Sunlight as a risk factor of malignant melanoma of the skin. Cancer 1978;41:2018–27.

24. Fincham SM, Hanson J, Berkel J. Patterns and risks of cancer in farmers in Alberta. Cancer 1992;69:1276–1285.

25. Lee JAH, Strickland D. Malignant melanoma: social status and outdoor work. Br J Cancer 1980;41:757–763.

26. Vagero D, Swerdlow AJ, Beral V. Occupation and malignant melanoma: a study based on cancer registration data in England and Wales and in Sweden. British Journal of Industrial Medicine 1990;47:317–324.

27. Beral V, Robinson N. The relationship of malignant melanoma, basal and squamous skin cancers to indoor and outdoor work. Br J Cancer 1981;44:886–891.

28. Vagero D, Ringback G, Kiviranta H. Melanoma and other tumours of the skin among office, other indoor workers and outdoor workers in Sweden 1961–1979. Br J Cancer 1986;53:507–512.

29. Linet MS, Malker HS, Chow WH, et al. Occupational risks for cutaneous melanoma among men in Sweden. J Occup Environ Med 1995;37:1127–35 PA Hospital Journal holding: 37(995)-42(2000);43(1)- Departmental Holdings holding: 37(1995)-42(2000);43(1)-.

30. Hakanson N, Floderus B, Gustavsson P, Feychting M, Hallin N. Occupational sunlight exposure and cancer incidence among Swedish construction workers. Epidemiology 2001;12:552–557.

31. Diffey BL, Gies HP. The confounding influence of sun exposure in melanoma. Lancet 1998;351: 1101–1102.

32. Elwood JM, Diffey BL. A consideration of ambient solar ultraviolet radiation in the interpretation of studies of the aetiology of melanoma. Melanoma Res 1993;3:113–122.

33. Thieden E, Agren MS, Wulf HC. Solar UVR exposures of indoor workers in a Working and a Holiday Period assessed by personal dosimeters and sun exposure diaries. Photodermatol Photoimmunol Photomed 2001;17:249–255.

34. Vagero D, Persson G. Risks, survival and trends of malignant melanoma among white and blue collar workers in Sweden. Soc Sci Med 1984;19:475–478.

35. Rimpela AH, Pukkala EI. Cancers of affluence: positive social class gradient and rising incidence trend in some cancer forms. Soc Sci Med 1987;24:601–606.

36. Faggiano F, Partanen T, Kogevinas M, Boffetta P. Socioeconomic differences in cancer incidence and mortality. IARC Sci Publ 1997:65–176.

37. Pearce N, Bethwaite P. Social class and male cancer mortality in New Zealand, 1984–7. NZ Med J 1997;110:200–202.

38. Elwood JM, Jopson J. Melanoma and sun exposure: an overview of published studies. Int J Cancer 1997;73:198–203.

39. Whiteman DC, Whiteman CA, Green AC. Childhood sun exposure as a risk factor for melanoma: a systematic review of epidemiologic studies. Cancer Causes Control 2001;12:69–82.

40. Holman CD, Armstrong BK. Cutaneous malignant melanoma and indicators of total accumulated exposure to the sun: an analysis separating histogenetic types. J Natl Cancer Inst 1984;73:75–82.

41. Weinstock MA, Colditz GA, Willett WC, Stampfer MJ, Bronstein BR, Mihm MC, et al. Moles and site-specific cutaneous malignant melanoma in women. J Natl Cancer Inst 1989;81:948–952.

42. Chen YT, Dubrow R, Holford TR, et al. Malignant melanoma risk factors by anatomic site: a case-control study and polychotomous logistic regression analysis. Int J Cancer 1996;67:636–643.

43. Kruger S, Garbe C, Buttner P, Stadler R, Guggenmoos-Holzmann I, Orfanos CE. Epidemiologic evidence for the role of melanocytic nevi as risk markers and direct precursors of cutaneous malignant melanoma. J Am Acad Dermatol 1992;26:920–926.

44. Rieger E, Soyer HP, Garbe C, et al. Overall and site-specific risk of malignant melanoma associated with nevus counts at different body sites: a multicenter case-control study of the German central malignant-melanoma registry. Int J Cancer 1995;62:393–397.

45. Bataille V, Sasieni P, Grulich A, et al. Solar keratoses: A risk factor for melanoma but negative association with melanocytic naevi. Int J Cancer 1998;78:8–12.

46. Urso C, Giannotti V, Reali UM, Giannotti B, Bondi R. Spatial association of melanocytic naevus and melanoma. Melanoma Res 1991;1:245–249.

47. Marks R, Dorevitch AP, Mason G. Do all melanomas come from "moles"? A study of the histological association between melanocytic naevi and melanoma. Australas J Dermatol 1990;31:77–80.

48. Kaddu S, Smolle J, Zenahlik P, Hofmann-Wellenhof R, Kerl H. Melanoma with benign melanocytic naevus components: reappraisal of clinicopathological features and prognosis. Melanoma Res 2002;12:271–278.

49. Carli P, Massi D, Santucci M, Biggeri A, Gianotti B. Cutaneous melanoma histologically associated with a nevus and melanoma de novo have a different profile of risk: results from a case-control study. J Am Acad Dermatol 1999;40:549–557.

50. Skender-Kalnenas TM, English DR, Heenan PJ. Benign melanocytic lesions: risk markers or precursors of cutaneous melanoma? J Am Acad Dermatol 1995;33:1000–1007.

51. Grulich AE, Bataille V, Swerdlow AJ, al. e. Naevi and pigmentary characteristics as risk factors for melanoma in a high-risk population: a case-control study in New South Wales, Australia. Int J Cancer 1996;67:485–491.

52. Merlino G, Noonan FP. Modeling gene-environment interactions in malignant melanoma. Trends Mol Med 2003;9:102–108.

53. Silvers WK, Mintz B. Differences in latency and inducibility of mouse skin melanomas depending on the age and anatomic site of the skin. Cancer Res 1998;58:630–602.

54. Green A, Neale R, Kelly R, et al. An animal model for human melanoma. Photochem Photobiol 1996;64:577–580.

55. Ziegler A, Jonason A, Simon J, Leffell D, Brash DE. Tumor suppressor gene mutations and photocarcinogenesis. Photochem Photobiol 1996;63:432–435.

56. Stretch JR, Gatter KC, Ralfkiaer E, Lane DP, Harris AL. Expression of mutant p53 in melanoma. Cancer Res 1991;51:5976–5979.

57. Lassam NJ, From L, Kahn HJ. Overexpression of p53 is a late event in the cevelopment of malignant melanoma. Cancer Res 1993;53:2235–2238.

58. Cristofolini M, Boi S, Girlando S, et al. p53 Protein Expression in Nevi and Melanomas. Arch Dermatol 1993;129:739–743.

59. Platz A, Ringborg U, Grafstrom E, Hoog A, Lagerlof B. Immunohistochemical analysis of the N-ras p21 and the p53 proteins in naevi, primary tumours and metastases of human cutaneous malignant melanoma: increased immunopositivity in hereditary melanoma. Melanoma Res 1995;5:101–106.

60. Sparrow LE, Soong R, Dawkins HJS, Iacopetta BJ, Heenan PJ. p53 gene mutation and expression in naevi and melanomas. Melanoma Res 1995;5:93–100.

61. Albino AP, Vidal MJ, McNutt NS, et al. Mutation and expression of the p53 gene in human malignant melanoma. Melanoma Res 1994;4:35–45.

62. Castresana JS, Rubio MP, Vazquez JJ, et al. Lack of allelic deletion and point mutation as mechanisms of p53 activation in human malignant melanoma. Int J Cancer 1993 1993;554:562–565.

63. Florenes VA, Oyjord T, Holm R, Borresen A-L, Nesland JM, Fodstad O. TP53 allele loss, mutations and expressions in malignant melanoma. Br J Cancer 1994;69:253–259.

64. Whiteman DC, Parsons PG, Green AC. p53 expression and risk factors for cutaneous melanoma: a case-control study. Int J Cancer 1998;77:843–848.

65. Kim YC, Lee MG, Cho SH, Lee JH, Lee DH, Ahn BK. The relation between p53 expression and physical site of melanoma: an immunohistochemical study. Br J Dermatol 2003;149:1299–1300.

66. Straume O, Akslen LA. Alterations and prognostic significance of p16 and p53 protein expression in subgroups of cutaneous melanoma. Int J Cancer 1997;74:535–539.

67. Ragnarsson-Olding BK, Karsberg S, Platz A, Ringborg UK. Mutations in the TP53 gene in human malignant melanomas derived from sun-exposed skin and unexposed mucosal membranes. Melanoma Res 2002;12:453–463.

68. Essner R, Kuo CT, Wang H, et al. Prognostic implications of p53 overexpression in cutaneous melanoma from sun-exposed and nonexposed sites. Cancer 1998;82:309–316.

69. Zuo L, Weger J, Yang Q, et al. Germline mutations in the p16INK4a binding domain of CDK4 in familial melanoma. Nat Genet 1996;12:97–99.

70. Pollock PM, Pearson JV, Hayward NK. Compilation of somatic mutations of the CDKN2 gene in human cancers: non-random distribution of base substitutions. Genes Chromosomes Cancer 1996;15:77–88.

71. Pavey SJ, Cummings MC, Whiteman DC, et al. Loss of p16 expression is associated with histological features of melanoma invasion. Melanoma Res 2002;12:539–547.

72. Wang YL, Uhara H, Yamazaki Y, Nikaido T, Saida T. Immunohistochemical detection of CDK4 and p16INK4 proteins in cutaneous malignant melanoma. Br J Dermatol 1996;134:269–275.

73. Keller-Melchior R, Schmidt R, Piepkorn M. Expression of the tumor suppressor gene product p16INK4 in benign and malignant melanocytic lesions. J Invest Dermatol 1998;110:932–928.

74. Radhi JM. Malignant melanoma arising from nevi, p53, p16, and Bcl-2: expression in benign versus malignant components. J Cutan Med Surg 1999;3:293–297.

75. Morita R, Fujimoto A, Hatta N, Takehara K, Takata M. Comparison of genetic profiles between primary melanomas and their metastases reveals genetic alterations and clonal evolution during progression. J Invest Dermatol 1998;111:919–924.

76. Paramio JM, Navarro M, Segrelles C, Gomez-Casero E, Jorcano JL. PTEN tumour suppressor is linked to the cell cycle control through the retinoblastoma protein. Oncogene 1999;18 (52): 7462–7468.

77. Nelen MR, Kremer H, Konings IB, et al. Novel PTEN mutations in patients with Cowden disease: absence of clear genotype-phenotype correlations. Eur J Hum Genet 1999;7:267–273.

78. Boni R, Vortmeyer AO, Burg G, Hofbauer G, Zhuang Z. The PTEN tumour suppressor gene and malignant melanoma. Melanoma Research 1998;8 (4):300–302.

79. Teng DH, Hu R, Lin H, Davis T, Iliev D, Frye C, et al. MMAC1/PTEN mutations in primary tumor specimens and tumor cell lines. Cancer Res 1997;57:5221–5.

80. Tsao H, Zhang X, Benoit E, Haluska FG. Identification of PTEN/MMAC1 alterations in uncultured melanomas and melanoma cell lines. Oncogene 1998;16:3397–3402.

81. Pollock PM, Walker GJ, Glendening JM, et al. PTEN inactivation is rare in melanoma tumours but occurs frequently in melanoma cell lines. Melanoma Res 2002;12:565–575.

82. Whiteman DC, Zhou X-P, Cummings MC, Pavey S, Hayward NK, Eng C. Nuclear PTEN expression and clincopathologic features in a population-based series of primary cutaneous melanoma. Int J Cancer 2002; 99:63–67.

83. Smalley KS. A pivotal role for ERK in the oncogenic behaviour of malignant melanoma? Int J Cancer 2003;104:527–532.

84. Pollock PM, Meltzer PS. Lucky draw in the gene raffle. Nature 2002;417:906–907.

85. Davies H, Bignell GR, Cox C, et al. Mutations of the BRAF gene in human cancer. Nature 2002;417:949–954.

86. van-'t-Veer LJ, Burgering BM, Versteeg R, et al. N-ras mutations in human cutaneous melanoma from sun-exposed body sites. Mol Cell Biol 1989;9:3114–3116.

87. van-Elsas A, Zerp SF, van-der-Flier S, et al. Relevance of ultraviolet-induced N-ras oncogene point mutations in development of primary human cutaneous melanoma. Am J Pathol 1996;149:883–893.

88. Jiveskog S, Ragnarsson-Olding B, Platz A, Ringborg U. N-ras mutations are common in melanomas from sun-exposed skin of humans but rare in mucosal membranes or unexposed skin. J Invest Dermatol 1998;111:757–761.

89. Reifenberger J, Knobbe CB, Sterzinger AA, et al. Frequent alterations of Ras signaling pathway genes in sporadic malignant melanomas. Int J Cancer 2004;109:377–384.

90. Dong J, Phelps RG, Qiao R, et al. BRAF oncogenic mutations correlate with progression rather than initiation of human melanoma. Cancer Res 2003;63:3883–3885.

91. Yazdi AS, Palmedo G, Flaig MJ, et al. Mutations of the BRAF gene in benign and malignant melanocytic lesions. J Invest Dermatol 2003;121:1160–1162.

92. Omholt K, Platz A, Kanter L, Ringborg U, Hansson J. NRAS and BRAF mutations arise early during melanoma pathogenesis and are preserved throughout tumor progression. Clin Cancer Res 2003;9:6483–6488.

93. Gorden A, Osman I, Gai W, et al. Analysis of BRAF and N-RAS mutations in metastatic melanoma tissues. Cancer Res 2003;63:3955–3957.

94. Kumar R, Angelini S, Hemminki K. Activating BRAF and N-Ras mutations in sporadic primary melanomas: an inverse association with allelic loss on chromosome 9. Oncogene 2003;22: 9217–9224.

95. Maldonado JL, Fridlyand J, Patel H, Jain AN, Busam K, Kageshita T, et al. Determinants of BRAF mutations in primary melanomas. J Natl Cancer Inst 2003;95:1878–1890.

96. Uribe P, Wistuba, II, Gonzalez S. BRAF mutation: a frequent event in benign, atypical, and malignant melanocytic lesions of the skin. Am J Dermatopathol 2003;25:365–370.

97. Papp T, Pemsel H, Zimmermann R, Bastrop R, Weiss DG, Schiffmann D. Mutational analysis of the N-ras, p53, p16INK4a, CDK4, and MC1R genes in human congenital melanocytic naevi. J Med Genet 1999;36:610–614.

98. Whiteman DC, Watt P, Purdie DM, Hughes MC, Hayward NK, Green AC. Melanocytic nevi, solar keratoses, and divergent pathways to cutaneous melanoma. J Natl Cancer Inst 2003;95:806–812.
99. Carli P, Palli D. Re: Melanocytic nevi, solar keratoses, and divergent pathways to cutaneous melanoma. J Natl Cancer Inst 2003;95:1801; author reply, 2.
100. Lancaster HO. Some geographical aspects of the mortality from melanoma in Europeans. Med J Aust 1956;1:1082–1087.
101. Armstrong BK. Epidemiology of malignant melanoma: intermittent or total accumulated exposure to the sun. J Dermatol Surg Oncol 1988;14:835–849.
102. Libow LF, Scheide S, DeLeo VA. Ultraviolet radiation acts as an independent mitogen for normal human melanocytes in culture. Pigment Cell Res 1988;1:397–401.
103. Stierner U, Rosdahl I, Augustsson A, Kagedal B. UVB irradiation induces melanocyte increase in both exposed and shielded human skin. J Invest Dermatol 1989;92:561–564.
104. Autier P, Boniol M, Severi G, et al. The body site distribution of melanocytic naevi in 6–7 year old European children. Melanoma Res 2001;11:123–131.

18

Pigmentation, DNA Repair, and Candidate Genes

The Risk of Cutaneous Malignant Melanoma in a Mediterranean Population

Maria Teresa Landi

Summary

This chapter summarizes the results of a case–control and a family study of melanoma we have conducted in a Mediterranean population of Southern Emilia-Romagna and Northern Marche regions of Italy. This area includes approx 1 million people, with a wide range of pigmentary phenotypes, who are often exposed to intense sun exposure in the popular sea resorts of the region. The role of pigmentation, DNA repair, and major candidate genes for melanoma has been investigated in this population and is discussed here. As the incidence and mortality of melanoma continue to increase in Southern European countries once considered at low risk for melanoma, a better comprehension of the etiology of this disease can have considerable clinical and preventive impact on melanoma.

Key Words: Mediterranean population; DNA repair; pigmentation; susceptibility genes; dysplastic nevi; familial aggregation; MC1R; CDKN2A.

BACKGROUND

The incidence and mortality of cutaneous malignant melanoma (CMM) in white people have rapidly increased in recent decades *(1–3)*. The world's highest rates of CMM are in Australia, where a largely Celtic population inhabits a subtropical zone *(4)*. In Western Europe, CMM rates tend to be lower in Southern countries *(5)*, in which high levels of ultraviolet (UV) radiation are present and relatively dark skin predominates (Fig. 1). In Eastern Europe, the gradient is opposite, with the highest rates in Southern regions *(6)*. In the United States, in the 1950 through 1969 study period, melanoma

From: *From Melanocytes to Melanoma: The Progression to Malignancy*
Edited by: V. J. Hearing and S. P. L. Leong © Humana Press Inc., Totowa, NJ

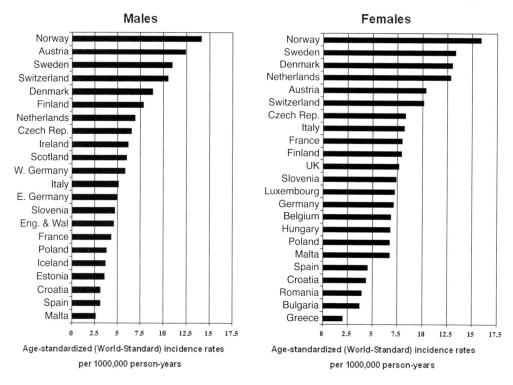

Fig. 1. Incidence rates of cutaneous malignant melanoma in Europe. Data from ref. *10.*

mortality rates showed a strong North–South gradient following UV intensity levels, but the gradient weakened in recent periods *(1)*. Thus, melanoma rates reflect the complex interplay of UV radiation levels in each geographic region, pigmentation characteristics and other host mechanisms of defense, sun exposure and sun-protection behaviors, geographic mobility of the population, and risk awareness and early detection.

Most studies on melanoma are from countries in which the fair skin type predominates. Although Mediterranean populations have been considered at low risk of CMM because of their relatively dark complexion, CMM incidence rates are steadily increasing in Italy, Spain, France, and former Yugoslavia *(7–9)*. According to the estimates for the year 2000 provided by the International Agency for Research on Cancer *(10)*, the Italian national age-adjusted incidence of CMM was 4.6 cases/100,000 person-yr for men and 5.5 cases/100,000 person-yr for women. Although these rates are lower than those of Australia or North America *(9)*, they demonstrate that CMM is a concern in the Italian population. Thus, we investigated the role of potential risk factors in the etiology of melanoma in a Mediterranean population of Italy. A number of host factors, such as pigmentation, UV-sensitivity, DNA repair, dysplastic nevi (DN), and candidate genes were measured in both a case–control and a family study of melanoma. This chapter summarizes the results of this work, and highlights our plans for future investigations.

STUDY SUBJECTS AND METHODS

We began our research with a case–control study including 183 incident melanoma cases and 179 healthy controls from Southern Emilia-Romagna and Northern Marche regions of Italy *(11)*. Study subjects included 87 male and 96 female cases with 89 male and 90 female controls. The age range was 17–77 yr. Controls were recruited mostly among spouses or close friends of the cases, and were frequency matched to cases by age and gender. Cases and controls were examined and recruited at the Bufalini Hospital of Cesena, Italy, which examines over 85% of melanoma cases of the area. Approximately 95% of cases and 83% of controls agreed to participate in the study.

A single dermatologist performed all skin examinations of the entire body, except the genital area. Multiple lightly pigmented macular lesions, commonly present on the face, upper back, and arms were defined as freckles. We classified the frequency of freckles by comparison with drawings describing patterns of distribution on a six-scale category. Nevi were pigmented macules or papules greater than 2 mm in diameter, and did not include freckles, lentigines, keratoses, and other pigmented lesions. A dysplastic nevus had to be approx 5 mm, be predominantly flat, and have at least two of the following criteria: variable pigmentation, indistinct borders, and irregular outline *(12)*. The dermatologist assessed the skin color of the inner part of the subjects' upper arm using a three-category scale, i.e., dark/olive, medium, and light; the eye color using a nine-category scale, i.e., black, dark brown, light brown, brown-green, green, blue-green, dark blue, light blue, and grey; and the hair color using a six-category scale, i.e., black, dark brown, light brown, reddish brown, blond, and red *(13)*.

A standardized in-person questionnaire was administered by trained interviewers, who asked questions on lifetime residential history, exposure to UVR, medical and family history of cancer and other diseases, smoking habits, drug consumption, skin reaction to the first half an hour of sun exposure, tanning ability, and sunscreen use. Tanning ability was ascertained through the following question: "After repeated and prolonged exposure to sunlight, your skin becomes:

1. Very tanned.
2. Medium tanned.
3. Hardly tanned.
4. Has tendency to peel.
5. Has absolutely no change."

The amount of lifetime sun exposure is notoriously very difficult to assess, and imprecision in reporting hours of exposure as well as recall bias are possible. Thus, in addition to the questionnaire information, we recorded the latitude, altitude, and proximity to the sea for each residence of at least 6 mo. We calculated an index of UVB exposure that takes into account latitude and altitude of each town using the following formula:

$$\text{UVB index} = [\exp(15.545 - (0.039 \times \text{latitude}) + (0.0001038 \times \text{altitude})\ 10,000],$$

in which altitude is measured in meters *(14)*. We computed a lifetime time-weighted UV-residence index for each subject.

MAJOR RISK FACTORS FOR MELANOMA

We first investigated whether the risk factors for melanoma in this Mediterranean population were similar to those identified in more fair-skinned individuals. We found that the major risk factors were similar: presence of DN (OR, 4.2; 95% CI, 2.4–7.4), low propensity to tan (OR, 2.4; 95% CI, 1.1–5.0), light eyes (OR, 2.4; 95% CI, 1.1–5.2), and

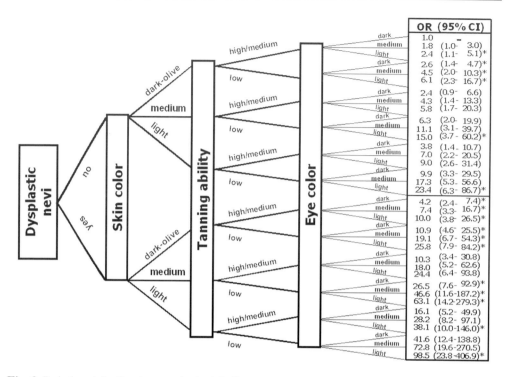

	OR	(95% CI)
dark	1.0	-
medium	1.8	(1.0- 3.0)
light	2.4	(1.1- 5.1)*
dark	2.6	(1.4- 4.7)*
medium	4.5	(2.0- 10.3)*
light	6.1	(2.3- 16.7)*
dark	2.4	(0.9- 6.6)
medium	4.3	(1.4- 13.3)
light	5.8	(1.7- 20.3)
dark	6.3	(2.0- 19.9)
medium	11.1	(3.1- 39.7)
light	15.0	(3.7- 60.2)*
dark	3.8	(1.4- 10.7)
medium	7.0	(2.2- 20.5)
light	9.0	(2.6- 31.4)
dark	9.9	(3.3- 29.5)
medium	17.3	(5.3- 56.6)
light	23.4	(6.3- 86.7)*
dark	4.2	(2.4- 7.4)*
medium	7.4	(3.3- 16.7)*
light	10.0	(3.8- 26.5)*
dark	10.9	(4.6- 25.5)*
medium	19.1	(6.7- 54.3)*
light	25.8	(7.9- 84.2)*
dark	10.3	(3.4- 30.8)
medium	18.0	(5.2- 62.6)
light	24.4	(6.4- 93.8)
dark	26.5	(7.6- 92.9)*
medium	46.6	(11.6-187.2)*
light	63.1	(14.2-279.3)*
dark	16.1	(5.2- 49.9)
medium	28.2	(8.2- 97.1)
light	38.1	(10.0-146.0)*
dark	41.6	(12.4-138.8)
medium	72.8	(19.6-270.5)
light	98.5	(23.8-406.9)*

Fig. 2. Relative risk of melanoma in the Mediterranean population of Southern Emilia-Romagna and Northern Marche regions of Italy caused by the combination of multiple risk factors (from ref. *11*). ORs and 95% CI are adjusted for age and gender in multivariable logistic regression analysis. Asterisks indicate extrapolated data.

light skin color (OR, 4.1; 95% CI, 1.4–12.1) were the strongest risk factors *(11)*. Intriguingly, glucocorticoid-based therapy appeared to be protective against melanoma in this population (OR, 0.39; 95% CI, 0.20–0.74). The degree of protection increased with treatment duration and was not associated with reason for treatment or route of administration *(15)*.

We constructed a flow chart to describe the relative risk associated with the combinations of three-scale skin color (dark/olive, medium, or light), three-scale eye color (dark, medium, or light), two-scale propensity to tan (high/medium or low), and the presence of DN (yes or no), after adjustment for age and gender (Fig. 2). We computed OR for the combination of individual risk factors using the corresponding linear combinations of coefficients estimated by the logistic model. We used the categories at lowest risk for CMM (i.e., no DN, dark/olive skin color, high/medium propensity to tan, and dark eye color) as the reference category. The risk ranged between 1- and almost 100-fold, depending on how these factors were combined in the subjects. The chart can be easily used to identify subjects who would most benefit from preventive measures in Mediterranean populations.

In our study subjects, melanoma lesions were frequently at an advanced stage. Interestingly, individuals with light skin color and low propensity to tan and subjects who experienced sunburns with blistering had generally thicker CMM lesions *(11)*. One possible explanation is that these subjects are not aware that they are at high risk for

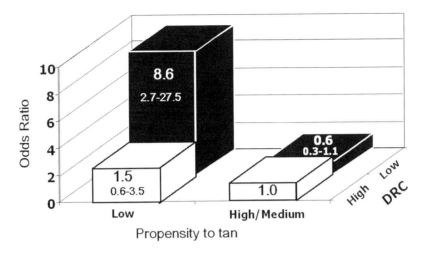

Fig. 3. Risk of cutaneous malignant melanoma in the Mediterranean population of Southern Emilia-Romagna and Northern Marche regions of Italy by DNA repair capacity and tanning ability after prolonged sun exposure (from ref. 20). In the columns are indicated the ORs and 95% CI adjusted for age, gender, cell viability, and storage length in multivariable logistic regression analysis. DRC, DNA repair capacity above or below the median value in control subjects, after 254 nm UV-irradiation at 350 J/m².

melanoma, and consequently do not seek dermatological examinations until their lesion is large. Subjects with DN or many nevi are possibly more aware of their at-risk condition, and, in fact, had generally thinner CMM lesions. In addition, subjects who spend long times under the sun in bathing suits are more likely to be observed by other people, who may notice and call the attention to suspicious skin lesions at an early stage. In fact, high number of hours of sun exposure, particularly during childhood, was associated with thinner CMM lesions.

Role of DNA Repair

UVR induces damage to DNA (16), which can be repaired by nucleotide excision repair (17) and other repair pathways. Melanin, mainly the dark pigment, eumelanin, abundant in dark skin, serves as a physical barrier that reduces the penetration of UV through the epidermis. Fair skin has low eumelanin content and higher relative amount of pheomelanin, the red-yellow pigment, and consequently has reduced photoprotection against UV damage. Irradiation of pheomelanin results in the generation of free radicals, which may further contribute to DNA damage (18), which can be repaired by the base excision repair. We explored whether the capacity to repair UV-damaged DNA, as measured by the host-cell reactivation assay (19) in lymphocytes, was associated with the risk of CMM in this population. We found no statistically significant association between melanoma risk and DNA repair capacity (DRC) overall (20). However, DRC strongly influenced CMM risk in those individuals with low tanning ability. Subjects with a low tanning response after prolonged sun exposure and low DRC had a higher relative risk for CMM (OR, 8.6; 95% CI, 2.7–27.5) than those with higher tanning ability and high DRC (Fig. 3). CMM may be caused by intermittent exposure of nonacclimatized white skin to sunlight, which may result in repeated burning (21–23). In contrast, continuous sun exposure able to induce persistent tanning in those who tan well may be somewhat protective against melanoma *(24)*. CMM relative risk may increase proportionally to the dose received by nontanned skin *(23)* and to the capacity of that skin to repair sunlight-induced DNA damage.

We also found that subjects with DN and low DRC had a higher relative risk (OR, 6.7; 95% CI, 2.4–18.6) than those lacking DN and with high DRC *(20)*. Early studies suggested that individuals with DN may have high genomic instability *(25–27)*. The accumulating mutations in subjects with high genomic instability may continuously induce DNA repair activity. Subjects with DN and low inducible DNA repair activity may accumulate mutations, which consequently can increase their risk of melanoma.

We investigated the genetic basis for these findings by analyzing a series of polymorphisms in genes involved in DNA repair. Among the nucleotide excision repair, the first analysis was based on the Asp312Asn and Lys751Gln SNPs of *XPD* (MIM 126340).

As with the results based on DRC, we found no significant association between *XPD* polymorphisms and melanoma risk. However, *XPD* variants were associated with increased risk in older (>50 yr) subjects (OR, 3.4; 95% CI, 1.6–7.3 for 312Asn; OR, 2.3; 95% CI, 1.1–4.9 for 751Gln). The 751Gln allele was associated with CMM risk among subjects with no DN and poor tanning ability *(28)*. We also found that there was a 19% reduction in DRC per copy of the variant R415Q of the *ERCC4* (or *XPF*) gene (MIM 133520) (*p* = 0.03, after appropriate adjustment). More SNPs are in the pipeline for the analysis.

Pigmentation and UV Sensitivity

Given the relevance of pigmentation in the association with melanoma risk, we decided to obtain more accurate measurements of pigmentary traits and skin reaction to sun exposure, along with the Fitzpatrick scale and other traditionally assessed risk factors. In fact, imprecise assessment of pigmentation and sun exposure and potentially differential reporting between cases and controls can bias the results. For example, sun sensitivity as assessed by ability to tan, but not by hair color, was subject to recall bias in one study *(24)*. However, another work found that reporting of tanning and burning was less biased than that of sunbathing in childhood and adulthood, and possibly of freckling in childhood *(29)*.

We measured skin color on the buttock with a Minolta CR-300 colorimeter. This is a reflectance spectrophotometer measuring reflected light in the visible spectrum (range, 400–700 nm). It also works as a tristimulus chromameter, recording colors in a three-dimensional space, Commission International d'Eclairge 1976 L*a*b* color space (CIELAB) *(30–33)*. Under standardized conditions, when the distortion of instrument readings is minimal, this method shows high reproducibility *(31)* and correlation with measurements based on direct ascertainment of pigmentary chromophores *(30,34)*. Every color in this system can be described by a combination of L*, a*, and b* coordinates *(35,36)*; in which L* is the total quantity of light reflected or brightness that can be described as light, dark, and so on, a* represents color ranging from red (positive values) to green (negative values), and b* represents color ranging from blue (negative values) to yellow (positive values). The a* and b* coordinates could be converted into polar coordinates *(31,36)*, defined as hue angle,

$$h^{\underline{o}} = \arctan(b^*/a^*)$$

and chroma, often referred to as saturation of color,

$$C = [(a^*)^2 + (b^*)^2]^{1/2}.$$

Hue refers to the basic color of an object in which $0°C$ represents red and $90°C$ represents yellow. The hue angle in our population ranged from $43°C$ to $82°C$. Chroma describes the intensity of color, with higher chroma indicating greater intensity. The instrument was white calibrated and turned on at least 15 min before each set of measurements. Measurements were taken by a single dermatologist after 15 min acclimatization in a room with air conditioning at $19–20°C$. Before the measurements, subjects were put in horizontal position to avoid orthostatic effects influencing skin color. During measurement, the measuring head was held steady, perpendicular to the skin surface. Special care was taken not to apply excessive pressure on the head of the instrument to avoid venous congestion that could artificially distort the measurements *(31)*. Measurements of L*, a*, and b* were repeated three times consecutively and averaged. The a* and b* values were then re-expressed as hue and chroma. Skin sensitivity to UV radiation was assessed by measurement of minimal erythema dose (MED). Skin was irradiated with simulated solar radiation from an artificial UV source (IL 1700, Blue-Point, Germany), and measured by an International Light detector (SED240/SCS280/W head model, Newburyport, MA) equipped with a cousin response diffuser. A spectroradiometer (FLYBY, s.r.l., SpectraMED, Livorno, Italy) was used to characterize the spectral features of the UV lamp radiation, which extended from 290 to 440 nm (i.e., covering the whole UV solar spectrum reaching the earth's surface) and to evaluate the erythemal effective irradiance at skin surface, which resulted in 1.65 mW/cm^2. Depending on the subjects' constitutive skin color, a suberythemal UV dose (in the order of 10–20 mJ/cm^2) and additional incremental doses comparable with biological exposures to sunlight *(37)* were administered by a single nurse on a very small area of the buttock skin. Each area of irradiation was circled with a fine-point waterproof permanent black marker. In particular, for skin types very sensitive to UV, the dose ranged between 15 and 67 mJ/cm^2, whereas, for individuals with darker skin, the dose ranged between 21 and 108 mJ/cm^2. Incremental doses of UV radiation were as follows: 15/21, 27, 40, 54, 67, and 94/108 mJ/cm^2. Subjects returned to the hospital the following day, so that the marked skin areas could be checked. The MED was defined as the lowest dose of radiation that produced the minimum noticeable (by visual inspection of nurse) reddening of the skin 24 h after the exposure.

Except for skin color, brightness of the skin, as determined by L*, hue, chroma, and MED were generally unrelated to age, sex, and host characteristics, such as eye color, hair color, freckling, presence of DN, and number of nevi *(38)*. In contrast, the instrumental measurements differed markedly by skin color. As expected, higher values of L* and hue, and lower values of chroma and MED were associated with light skin color, and with a self-reported propensity to severe burn or blister, and an inability to tan. L* and chroma were related to recreational sun exposure, but hue and MED were not. L*, and, to a lesser extent, MED, were the strongest predictors of CMM risk: ORs for CMM increased significantly with increasing levels of L* and decreasing levels of MED, although the latter trend was not monotonic (Table 1). Using the continuous measurement values, we calculated that there was a 20% increased melanoma risk per unit of skin brightness (OR, 1.20; 95% CI, 1.12–1.30), and a 24% increase risk per 10 units of MED (OR, 1.24; 95% CI, 1.07–1.43). This association persisted, although attenuated, after

Table 1
Risk of Cutaneous Malignant Melanoma
by Instrumental Measurements of Skin Color and UV Sensitivity

	Cases n = 183[a]	Controls n = 179[a]	OR[b]	95% CI[b]
Skin brightness (L*)				
70.0	30	54	1.00	Ref.
>70.0– 72.3	37	52	1.30	0.70–2.41
>72.3– 74.0	52	40	2.19	1.18–4.08
>74	64	30	4.35	2.29–8.27
Minimal Erythema Dose (MED)				
>40	38	59	1.00	Ref.
>33.0– 40.0	51	39	2.22	1.22–4.03
>26.0– 33.0	47	42	1.90	1.04–3.46
26.0	45	36	2.11	1.14–3.91

[a]Numbers may not add up to column totals because of missing data.
[b]ORs and 95% CI are adjusted for age and gender in multivariable logistic regression analysis (from ref. *38*).

adjustment for pigmentation characteristics and DN, and was stronger in subjects with the highest number of cumulative hours of sun exposure *(38)*. Further, these effects largely persisted after adjustments for phenotypic or sun-related factors. Thus, there are elements of the pigmentary trait that are not captured well if we limit our assessment to the phenotypic observation of pigmentation.

To further explore the role of pigmentation on melanoma risk and its interaction with DNA repair or sun exposure, we sequenced the melanocortin-1 receptor gene (*MC1R*, MIM 155555) in this population. MC1R is involved in the regulation of pigmentation. Specific *MC1R* variants have been associated with red hair phenotype, freckling, and poor tanning ability *(39–44)*. Interestingly, *MC1R* variant alleles have also been associated with increased risk for melanoma, after adjustment for pigmentation phenotype. In one study, this association was stronger in subjects with darker skin color *(42)*. In our population, sequencing of *MC1R* revealed the presence of 51 variants, 11 of which were synonymous. The variant alleles previously reported to be associated with red hair and possibly melanoma risk, including R151C, D294H, and R160W *(45)*, were present in 9.4%, 3.5%, and 5.3% of the controls, and in 23.6%, 6.7%, and 5.5% of the cases, respectively. The variants were associated, although not consistently, with light pigmentation and freckling. Individuals with any *MC1R* variant, "red hair" variants, or multiple *MC1R* variants were at increased risk of melanoma. This association was stronger in subjects with darker phenotype, and persisted after adjustment for the pigmentation characteristics as assessed by the physician or self-reported. We did not find interaction between *MC1R* variants and DNA repair or hours of sun exposure in the association with melanoma risk. We are now extending the analysis to other pigmentation genes and larger number of subjects to explore the role of pigmentation and its interaction with other host factors in this Mediterranean population.

Familial Aggregation

To complement the case–control study and to take advantage of a different approach of examining genetic and environmental determinants of melanoma, we also conducted a family study of melanoma-prone families from the same North-Eastern region of Italy. We measured melanoma familial aggregation in this area using data from 589 incident melanoma cases examined at the Bufalini Hospital from 1994 to 1999. Approximately 5% of melanoma cases reported a first-degree relative with melanoma, but only 3.4% of melanomas in relatives were histologically confirmed *(46)*. Of these, only 2.5% were in first-degree relatives, showing that familial aggregation of melanoma in the area is quite rare.

Familial aggregation may occur because family members share environmental factors (such as excessive sun exposure) or common genetic factors (such as strongly penetrant melanoma susceptibility alleles). Worldwide studies of melanoma-prone families have demonstrated linkage to at least two chromosome loci and identified candidate genes that account for approx 25% of melanoma kindreds worldwide. The major melanoma susceptibility gene identified to date is cyclin-dependent kinase inhibitor 2a (*CDKN2A*), a tumor suppressor gene located on chromosome 9p21 (MIM 600160) *(47–48)*. *CDKN2A* encodes two distinct proteins translated in alternative reading frames from alternatively spliced transcripts. The α-transcript, which comprises exons 1α, 2, and 3, encodes a low molecular weight protein, p16, or p16INK4a. The p16 protein binds to the cyclin-dependent kinases, CDK4 and CDK6, and inhibits their ability to phosphorylate the retinoblastoma protein, and thereby controls passage through the G1 checkpoint of the cell cycle *(49–50)*. The smaller α-transcript, which comprises exons 1, 2, and 3, encodes the alternative protein product, p14[ARF] which acts through the p53 pathway to induce cell cycle arrest or apoptosis *(51–52)*. Most *CDKN2A* mutations that segregate with disease through melanoma-prone families affect p16, and may or may not alter p14[ARF]. Such mutations have also been associated with increased risk of pancreatic and breast carcinomas *(53–57)*. In contrast, mutations that affect only p14[ARF] and not p16 are much less common *(58–60)*. The corresponding families may display a different spectrum of malignancy that includes melanoma and neural tumors *(58–59)*. Even in the absence of detected mutations in the coding regions of the *CDKN2A* gene, many melanoma-prone families appear to be linked to the 9p21 locus, suggesting the presence of noncoding *CDKN2A* mutations or the presence of another susceptibility gene at this locus *(61)*.

Rare somatic mutations have also been reported in the related *CDKN2B* gene, which, in addition to being codeleted along with the *CDKN2A* gene in a number of cancers, is occasionally targeted independently in tumors, including melanoma *(62–63)*. *CDKN2B* encodes p15[INK4b] and is located 40 kb centromeric to the *CDKN2A* gene *(62)*. An additional susceptibility gene for melanoma, accounting for a very limited number of melanoma kindreds, is *CDK4* (MIM 12829), located on chromosome 12q14. Activating mutations of the *CDK4* gene, specifically Arg24Cys or Arg24His *(64–65)* have been found in few families *(66–67)*. In addition, a Ser52Asn variant of uncertain significance was found in a kindred that also bore a *CDKN2A* mutation *(68)*. No Italian families have been shown to carry mutations in *CDK4*.

To date, we recruited 61 families with two or more melanoma cases. Melanoma clinical characteristics in these Italian families are generally similar to those seen in more fair-skinned populations, except for a higher proportion of nodular melanomas and invasive lesions *(12)*. As in other melanoma-prone families worldwide, cases with DN, multiple primary melanomas, or pancreatic cancer are present in these families.

In the first 55 families enrolled, we sequenced the *CDKN2A* (including the exon 1β of the p14^{ARF} protein), *CDKN2B*, and *CDK4* genes to verify whether a mutation in one or more of these genes segregate with melanoma in these families. In addition, in the melanoma families with multiple breast cancer cases and in those with multiple gastric cancer cases we also sequenced the breast cancer 2 (*BRCA2*) and cadherin 1 (*CDH1*) genes, respectively. Mutations or altered expression of the *CDH1* gene (MIM *192090), on chromosome 16q22.1, have been associated with inherited diffuse gastric cancer *(69)*. *BRCA2* gene (MIM *600185), on chromosome 13q12.3, is a known susceptibility gene for breast cancer *(70)* and melanoma *(71)*. We found only four mutations (7%) in the *CDKN2A* gene in seven different members of four families, and no other mutations in any other candidate gene *(72)*. This is unusual, because in other Italian families with similar number of cases, similar average age at onset and clinical characteristics, the frequency of *CDKN2A* mutations was overall 33% *(57,73–76)*. Thus, in this Italian subpopulation, either noncoding susceptibility alleles of *CDKN2A* that we cannot detect using current methods exist, or germline alterations of additional gene(s) play an important role in melanoma predisposition.

Three of the *CDKN2A* mutations identified, which determine the amino acid changes G101W, R24P, and S56I, have already been found in many families, including Italians *(73,75,76)*. The fourth potentially disease-related mutation we found was a novel T to C transition at basepair 194 of exon 2, which results in a missense mutation L65P in p16 and a silent mutation A79A in p14 ^{ARF}. This mutation was present in a family with one pancreatic cancer case and four melanoma cases, one of whom had two primary melanomas. We analyzed the changes in the tertiary structure of the p16 protein caused by the novel L65P mutation, using publicly available web services. Leu65Pro (Fig. 4) is at the last residue position in helix 6 and, thus, could shorten the helix and disrupt secondary structure. Both the FOLD-X calculations (ddG = 5.11 kcal/mol) *(77)*, and the PoPMuSiC calculations (ddG = 1.38 kcal/mol) *(78)* revealed a difference in folding energy between the mutant and wild-type protein, but the PolyPhen predictions *(79)*, based on alignment, failed to predict this mutation to be disruptive on protein function (the Leucine at position 65 is not highly conserved in mammals) *(72)*. To confirm the conclusions derived from protein modeling, we elected to test the interaction of the L65P mutant to CDK4 by means of a yeast two-hybrid system. We expressed the mutant and wild-type cDNA sequences in the presence or absence of CDK4 and measured their corresponding interactions by means of a liquid β-galactosidase assay, using a modification of the method of Miller *(80)*. In repeated experiments, we observed a significant decrease of approx 50% in the binding of L65P with CDK4, compared with the wild-type p16 at both 30°C ($p = 0.002$) and 37°C ($p = 0.009$; *t*-test) *(72)* (Fig. 5). In contrast to other p16 missense mutations *(81)*, the L65P mutant does not demonstrate any strong temperature dependence on binding of CDK4.

Given the low frequency of mutations in the known candidate genes in these families, we decided to perform a genome-wide scan to identify loci possibly linked with melanoma. We began with the analysis of chromosomes 1 and 9 to verify linkage with previously identified loci. A recent publication from the Melanoma Genetics Consortium, an international group of melanoma researchers who investigate factors related to

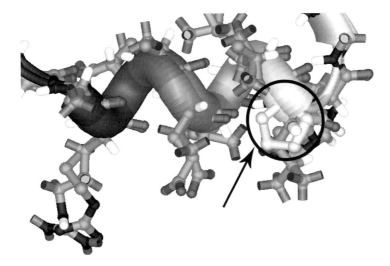

Fig. 4. Structural model of the leucine to proline substitution at position 65 of p16 (from ref. *72*). The model shows that the proline amino acid (indicated by the arrow), differently from the leucine (behind the proline), no longer makes hydrogen atoms available to the surface of the protein, possibly affecting the ability of this protein to complex or bind with its ligand. Please *see* color insert following p. 430.

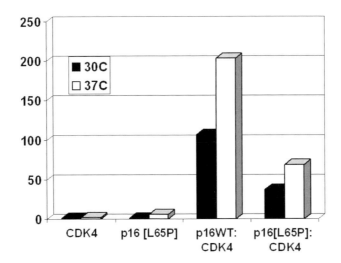

Fig. 5. Binding of p16 with CDK4 protein in a yeast two-hybrid system. Quantitative analysis of β-galactosidase activity was performed using a liquid β-galactosidase assay. Columns 1–4 show CDK4 and p16 proteins with no binding; columns 5 and 6 and columns 7 and 8 show CDK4 binding with wild-type and mutant (L65P) p16, respectively (from ref. *72*). The listed values represent the mean of at least 28 separate assays performed at 30°C or 20 separate assays performed at 37°C. Statistically significant differences ($\alpha = 0.05$) were observed between the WT variant and the L65P mutant at both 30°C ($p = 0.002$) and at 37°C ($p = 0.009$).

the inheritance of an increased risk of melanoma *(60,82)*, has provided evidence for a novel susceptibility locus for melanoma within chromosome band 1p22 *(83)*. Previous studies have suggested that 1p36 may harbor a susceptibility gene(s) *(84)*. In addition, only about a third of 9p21-linked families carry mutations in *CDKN2A*. Thus, other candidate gene(s) may be located on 9p21. We conducted linkage analysis of chromosome 1 in 47 informative families and chromosome 9 in 46 families, with 31 and 20 diallelic microsatellite markers, respectively. We performed both two-point and multipoint linkage analyses under a dominant model with 50% penetrance, consistent with the inheritance pattern for *CDKN2A* in European families *(60)* and similar to the reported 1p linkage studies *(83–85)*. There was no evidence for linkage of melanoma susceptibility to markers on chromosome 1 or 9 in either the parametric or nonparametric analyses. There was no significant evidence for genetic heterogeneity *(72)*. Thus, critical genes responsible for the inheritance of a susceptibility to develop melanoma among family members in this Italian population have yet to be identified.

CONCLUSIONS AND PERSPECTIVES

Melanoma etiology is complex, involving both heterogeneous genetic and environmental components *(82)*. As we have seen, pigmentation has a crucial role in CMM development, but phenotypic pigmentation *per se* cannot always predict susceptibility to melanoma. Sun exposure, particularly if intermittent and acute on untanned skin may strongly increase melanoma risk, particularly if subjects have a reduced capacity to repair UV-induced DNA damage. The DNA repair system is complex and extremely versatile; many proteins in the system may have different and overlapping functions, they can interact with one another in a coordinated process under different physiological conditions, and are inducible by UV irradiation and other environmental factors. Thus, it is unlikely that the identification of some polymorphisms in a few DNA repair genes can be sufficient to depict the role of DNA repair in the etiology of melanoma. Moreover, subjects often carry multiple common melanocytic nevi and atypical or DN *(86)*, which have been recognized as precursors of melanoma, but development of melanoma through pathways that do not include nevi formation are likely, and they may be linked to different genes *(87)*. As for the family history of melanoma, the known susceptibility genes explain only approx 25% of familial melanoma world wide, and the frequency of *CDKN2A* mutations in familial melanoma varies according to the number of cases in the families, the presence of multiple melanomas in the same patient *(67–68)*, the history of pancreatic cancer cases in the family *(53)*, and their geographical location *(60,88)*. Even the average lifetime risk conferred by *CDKN2A* mutations shows significant variation between regions, with the lowest penetrance in the Southern European countries *(60)*. Moreover, *MC1R* variants may act as modifiers of the *CDKN2A* gene penetrance *(89–90)* in the families. Clearly, to explore such a complex pattern, a very large study population is required, possibly taking advantage of different methodological approaches (e.g., association and linkage studies), and comparing different populations (e.g., populations at higher risk given the light pigmentation and intense sun exposure, with those with darker pigment or those with no DN). Collaboration with different investigators is crucial for an appropriate approach to the understanding and possibly prevention of such lethal disease. We are continuing our research on melanoma in both sporadic and familial cases from the area in collaboration with other groups. DNA repair, pigmentation, and other candidate genes are being explored, while genome-wide scanning of Mediterranean families proceed. Many melanoma cases identified in our study were advanced in stage. This suggests that this population does not generally appreciate the risk for melanoma. The magnitude of risk associated with the combination of DN and light pigmentation shows the need for frequent screenings, particularly of at-risk subjects, and for public health campaigns against unprotected sun exposure in this population. As the incidence and mortality of melanoma continue to increase, particularly in Southern European countries, such as Italy, identification of novel genes may also have considerable clinical impact on melanoma.

ACKNOWLEDGMENTS

We are indebted to the study participants, without whom our study could not be done. Among the many investigators that made this research possible, we thank Drs. Donato Calista, Paola Minghetti, Daniela Capirossi, Arrigo Bondi, Giorgio Landi, and Fabio Arcangeli of the Bufalini Hospital, Cesena, Italy for the clinical examination and recruitment of all patients; Drs. Alisa Goldstein, Monica Ter-Minassian, Alina Brenner, and Peggy Tucker, NCI, Bethesda, MD and Andrea Baccarelli and Pier Alberto Bertazzi, EPOCA, University of Milan, Milan, Italy for their collaborative effort in the study design and analyses of the data. For all the genetic and functional analyses reported, we are grateful to Drs. David Hogg and Ron Agatep, University of Toronto, Toronto, CA; Dr. Peter Kanetsky, University of Pennsylvania, Philadelphia, PA; Drs. Jeffrey Struewing, Robert Steighner, Brian Staats, Bert Gold, William Modi, Shirley Tsang, and David Munroe, NCI, Gaithersburg and Frederick, MD; and Drs. Lawrence Grossman and Mohammad Hedayati, The Johns Hopkins University, Baltimore, MD.

REFERENCES

1. Jemal A, Devesa SS, Fears TR, Hartge P. Cancer surveillance series: changing patterns of cutaneous malignant melanoma mortality rates among whites in the United States. J Natl Cancer Inst 2000; 92(10):811–818.
2. Dennis LK. Analysis of the melanoma epidemic, both apparent and real: data from the 1973 through 1994 surveillance, epidemiology, and end results program registry. Arch Dermatol 1999; 135(3):275–280.
3. Serraino D, Fratino L, Gianni W, Campisi C, Pietropaolo M, Trimarco G et al. Epidemiological aspects of cutaneous malignant melanoma (review). Oncol Rep 1998; 5(4):905–909.
4. Marrett LD, Nguyen HL, Armstrong BK. Trends in the incidence of cutaneous malignant melanoma in New South Wales, 1983–1996. Int J Cancer 2001; 92(3):457–462.
5. Ferlay J, Bray S, Sankila R, Parkin D. EUCAN: cancer incidence, mortality and prevalence in the European Union 1996. Version 3.1 ed. Lyon: IARC Press, 1999.
6. de Vries E, Boniol M, Dore JF, Coebergh JW. Lower incidence rates but thicker melanomas in Eastern Europe before 1992: a comparison with Western Europe. Eur J Cancer 2004; 40(7):1045–1052.
7. Muir C, Waterhouse J, Mack T, Powell J, Whelan S. Cancer incidence in five continents. 1 ed. Lyon: IARC Press, 1987.
8. Parkin D, Muir C, Whelan S, Gao Y, Ferlay J, Powell J. Cancer incidence in five continents. 2 ed. Lyon: IARC Press, 1992.
9. Parkin D, Whelan S, Ferlay J, Raymond L, Young J. Cancer Incidence in Five Continents. Vol VII. Lyon, France: International Agency for Research on Cancer, 1997.
10. Ferlay J, Bary S, Pisani P, Parkin D. GLOBOCAN 2000: Cancer incidence, mortality and prevalence worldwide. Version 1 ed. Lyon: IARC Press, 2001.
11. Landi MT, Baccarelli A, Calista D, Pesatori A, Fears T, Tucker MA et al. Combined risk factors for melanoma in a Mediterranean population. Br J Cancer 2001; 85(9):1304–1310.
12. Landi MT, Calista D, Landi G, Bernucci I, Bertazzi PA, Clark WH, Jr. et al. Clinical characteristics of 20 Italian melanoma-prone families. Arch Dermatol 1999; 135(12):1554–1555.
13. Cristofolini M, Franceschi S, Tasin L, Zumiani G, Piscioli F, Talamini R et al. Risk factors for cutaneous malignant melanoma in a northern Italian population. Int J Cancer 1987; 39(2):150–154.

14. Scotto J, Fears T, Fraumeni JJr. Solar radiation. In: Schottenfeld D, Fraumeni JF Jr., editors. Cancer epidemiology and prevention. New York: Oxford University Press, 1996: 355–372.

15. Landi MT, Baccarelli A, Calista D, Fears TR, Landi G. Glucocorticoid use and melanoma risk. Int J Cancer 2001; 94(2):302–303.

16. Langley RG, Sober AJ. A clinical review of the evidence for the role of ultraviolet radiation in the etiology of cutaneous melanoma. Cancer Invest 1997; 15(6):561–567.

17. Bohr VA. DNA repair fine structure and its relations to genomic instability. Carcinogenesis 1995; 16(12):2885–2892.

18. Kadekaro AL, Kanto H, Kavanagh R, Abdel-Malek ZA. Significance of the melanocortin 1 receptor in regulating human melanocyte pigmentation, proliferation, and survival. Ann N Y Acad Sci 2003; 994:359–365.

19. Athas WF, Hedayati MA, Matanoski GM, Farmer ER, Grossman L. Development and field-test validation of an assay for DNA repair in circulating human lymphocytes. Cancer Res 1991; 51(21):5786–5793.

20. Landi MT, Baccarelli A, Tarone RE, Pesatori A, Tucker MA, Hedayati M et al. DNA repair, dysplastic nevi, and sunlight sensitivity in the development of cutaneous malignant melanoma. J Natl Cancer Inst 2002; 94(2):94–101.

21. Elwood JM, Jopson J. Melanoma and sun exposure: an overview of published studies. Int J Cancer 1997; 73(2):198–203.

22. MacKie RM. Incidence, risk factors and prevention of melanoma. Eur J Cancer 1998; 34(suppl 3):S3–S6.

23. Armstrong B, English D. Cutaneous malignant melanoma. In: Schottenfeld D, Fraumeni JJr, editors. CAncer epidemilogy and prevention. New York: Oxford University Press, 1996: 1282–1312.

24. Weinstock MA, Colditz GA, Willett WC, Stampfer MJ, Bronstein BR, Mihm MC, Jr. et al. Melanoma and the sun: the effect of swimsuits and a "healthy" tan on the risk of nonfamilial malignant melanoma in women. Am J Epidemiol 1991; 134(5):462–470.

25. Hansson J, Loow H. Normal reactivation of plasmid DNA inactivated by UV irradiation by lymphocytes from individuals with hereditary dysplastic naevus syndrome. Melanoma Res 1994; 4(3):163–167.

26. Perera MI, Um KI, Greene MH, Waters HL, Bredberg A, Kraemer KH. Hereditary dysplastic nevus syndrome: lymphoid cell ultraviolet hypermutability in association with increased melanoma susceptibility. Cancer Res 1986; 46(2):1005–1009.

27. Seetharam S, Waters HL, Seidman MM, Kraemer KH. Ultraviolet mutagenesis in a plasmid vector replicated in lymphoid cells from patient with the melanoma-prone disorder dysplastic nevus syndrome. Cancer Res 1989; 49(21):5918–5921.

28. Baccarelli A, Calista D, Minghetti P, Marinelli B, Albetti B, Tseng T et al. XPD gene polymorphism and host characteristics in the association with cutaneous malignant melanoma risk. Br J Cancer 2004; 90(2):497–502.

29. Cockburn M, Hamilton A, Mack T. Recall bias in self-reported melanoma risk factors. Am J Epidemiol 2001; 153(10):1021–1026.

30. Takiwaki H. Measurement of skin color: practical application and theoretical considerations. J Med Invest 1998; 44(3-4):121–126.

31. Fullerton A, Fischer T, Lahti A, Wilhelm KP, Takiwaki H, Serup J. Guidelines for measurement of skin colour and erythema. A report from the Standardization Group of the European Society of Contact Dermatitis. Contact Dermatitis 1996; 35(1):1–10.

32. Andreassi L, Flori L. Practical applications of cutaneous colorimetry. Clin Dermatol 1995; 13(4):369–373.

33. Kollias N. The physical basis of skin color and its evaluation. Clin Dermatol 1995; 13(4):361–367.

34. Takiwaki H, Overgaard L, Serup J. Comparison of narrow-band reflectance spectrophotometric and tristimulus colorimetric measurements of skin color. Twenty-three anatomical sites evaluated by the Dermaspectrometer and the Chroma Meter CR-200. Skin Pharmacol 1994; 7(4):217–225.

35. Billmeyer F, Saltzman M. Principles of color technology. New York: Wiley-Interscience, 1981.

36. Weatherall IL, Coombs BD. Skin color measurements in terms of CIELAB color space values. J Invest Dermatol 1992; 99(4):468–473.

37. Bataille V, Bykov VJ, Sasieni P, Harulow S, Cuzick J, Hemminki K. Photoadaptation to ultraviolet (UV) radiation in vivo: photoproducts in epidermal cells following UVB therapy for psoriasis. Br J Dermatol 2000; 143(3):477–483.

38. Brenner AV, Lubin JH, Calista D, Landi MT. Instrumental measurements of skin color and skin ultraviolet light sensitivity and risk of cutaneous malignant melanoma: a case-control study in an Italian population. Am J Epidemiol 2002; 156(4):353–362.

39. Valverde P, Healy E, Jackson I, Rees JL, Thody AJ. Variants of the melanocyte-stimulating hormone receptor gene are associated with red hair and fair skin in humans. Nat Genet 1995; 11(3):328–330.

40. Box NF, Wyeth JR, O'Gorman LE, Martin NG, Sturm RA. Characterization of melanocyte stimulating hormone receptor variant alleles in twins with red hair. Hum Mol Genet 1997; 6(11):1891–1897.

41. Smith R, Healy E, Siddiqui S, Flanagan N, Steijlen PM, Rosdahl I et al. Melanocortin 1 receptor variants in an Irish population. J Invest Dermatol 1998; 111(1):119–122.

42. Palmer JS, Duffy DL, Box NF, Aitken JF, O'Gorman LE, Green AC et al. Melanocortin-1 receptor polymorphisms and risk of melanoma: is the association explained solely by pigmentation phenotype? Am J Hum Genet 2000; 66(1):176–186.

43. Flanagan N, Healy E, Ray A, Philips S, Todd C, Jackson IJ et al. Pleiotropic effects of the melanocortin 1 receptor (MC1R) gene on human pigmentation. Hum Mol Genet 2000; 9(17):2531–2537.

44. Bastiaens M, ter Huurne J, Gruis N, Bergman W, Westendorp R, Vermeer BJ et al. The melanocortin-1–receptor gene is the major freckle gene. Hum Mol Genet 2001; 10(16):1701–1708.

45. Sturm RA. Skin colour and skin cancer - MC1R, the genetic link. Melanoma Res 2002; 12(5):405–416.

46. Calista D, Goldstein AM, Landi MT. Familial melanoma aggregation in north-eastern Italy. J Invest Dermatol 2000; 115(4):764–765.

47. Kamb A, Shattuck-Eidens D, Eeles R, Liu Q, Gruis NA, Ding W et al. Analysis of the p16 gene (CDKN2) as a candidate for the chromosome 9p melanoma susceptibility locus. Nat Genet 1994; 8(1):23–26.

48. Nobori T, Miura K, Wu DJ, Lois A, Takabayashi K, Carson DA. Deletions of the cyclin-dependent kinase-4 inhibitor gene in multiple human cancers. Nature 1994; 368(6473):753–756.

49. Serrano M, Hannon GJ, Beach D. A new regulatory motif in cell-cycle control causing specific inhibition of cyclin D/CDK4. Nature 1993; 366(6456):704–707.

50. Serrano M, Gomez-Lahoz E, DePinho RA, Beach D, Bar-Sagi D. Inhibition of ras-induced proliferation and cellular transformation by p16INK4. Science 1995; 267(5195):249–252.

51. Zhang Y, Xiong Y, Yarbrough WG. ARF promotes MDM2 degradation and stabilizes p53: ARF-INK4a locus deletion impairs both the Rb and p53 tumor suppression pathways. Cell 1998; 92(6):725–734.

52. Pomerantz J, Schreiber-Agus N, Liegeois NJ, Silverman A, Alland L, Chin L et al. The Ink4a tumor suppressor gene product, p19Arf, interacts with MDM2 and neutralizes MDM2's inhibition of p53. Cell 1998; 92(6):713–723.

53. Goldstein AM, Fraser MC, Struewing JP, Hussussian CJ, Ranade K, Zametkin DP et al. Increased risk of pancreatic cancer in melanoma-prone kindreds with p16INK4 mutations. N Engl J Med 1995; 333(15):970–974.

54. Borg A, Sandberg T, Nilsson K, Johannsson O, Klinker M, Masback A et al. High frequency of multiple melanomas and breast and pancreas carcinomas in CDKN2A mutation-positive melanoma families. J Natl Cancer Inst 2000; 92(15):1260–1266.

55. Rulyak SJ, Brentnall TA, Lynch HT, Austin MA. Characterization of the neoplastic phenotype in the familial atypical multiple-mole melanoma-pancreatic carcinoma syndrome. Cancer 2003; 98(4):798–804.

56. Vasen HF, Gruis NA, Frants RR, Der Velden PA, Hille ET, Bergman W. Risk of developing pancreatic cancer in families with familial atypical multiple mole melanoma associated with a specific 19 deletion of p16 (p16-Leiden). Int J Cancer 2000; 87(6):809–811.

57. Ghiorzo P, Ciotti P, Mantelli M, Heouaine A, Queirolo P, Rainero ML et al. Characterization of ligurian melanoma families and risk of occurrence of other neoplasia. Int J Cancer 1999; 83(4):441–448.

58. Randerson-Moor JA, Harland M, Williams S, Cuthbert-Heavens D, Sheridan E, Aveyard J et al. A germline deletion of p14(ARF) but not CDKN2A in a melanoma-neural system tumour syndrome family. Hum Mol Genet 2001; 10(1):55–62.

59. Rizos H, Puig S, Badenas C, Malvehy J, Darmanian AP, Jimenez L et al. A melanoma-associated germline mutation in exon 1beta inactivates p14ARF. Oncogene 2001; 20(39):5543–5547.

60. Bishop DT, Demenais F, Goldstein AM, Bergman W, Bishop JN, Bressac-de Paillerets B et al. Geographical variation in the penetrance of CDKN2A mutations for melanoma. J Natl Cancer Inst 2002; 94(12):894–903.

61. Loo JC, Liu L, Hao A, Gao L, Agatep R, Shennan M et al. Germline splicing mutations of CDKN2A predispose to melanoma. Oncogene 2003; 22(41):6387–6394.

62. Platz A, Ringborg U, Lagerlof B, Lundqvist E, Sevigny P, Inganas M. Mutational analysis of the CDKN2 gene in metastases from patients with cutaneous malignant melanoma. Br J Cancer 1996; 73(3):344–348.

63. Glendening JM, Flores JF, Walker GJ, Stone S, Albino AP, Fountain JW. Homozygous loss of the p15INK4B gene (and not the p16INK4 gene) during tumor progression in a sporadic melanoma patient. Cancer Res 1995; 55(23):5531–5535.

64. Wolfel T, Hauer M, Schneider J, Serrano M, Wolfel C, Klehmann-Hieb E et al. A p16INK4a-insensitive CDK4 mutant targeted by cytolytic T lymphocytes in a human melanoma. Science 1995; 269(5228):1281–1284.

65. Brotherton DH, Dhanaraj V, Wick S, Brizuela L, Domaille PJ, Volyanik E et al. Crystal structure of the complex of the cyclin D-dependent kinase Cdk6 bound to the cell-cycle inhibitor p19INK4d. Nature 1998; 395(6699):244–250.

66. Zuo L, Weger J, Yang Q, Goldstein AM, Tucker MA, Walker GJ et al. Germline mutations in the p16INK4a binding domain of CDK4 in familial melanoma. Nat Genet 1996; 12(1):97–99.

67. Soufir N, Avril MF, Chompret A, Demenais F, Bombled J, Spatz A et al. Prevalence of p16 and CDK4 germline mutations in 48 melanoma-prone families in France. The French Familial Melanoma Study Group. Hum Mol Genet 1998; 7(2):209–216.

68. Holland EA, Schmid H, Kefford RF, Mann GJ. CDKN2A (P16(INK4a)) and CDK4 mutation analysis in 131 Australian melanoma probands: effect of family history and multiple primary melanomas. Genes Chromosomes Cancer 1999; 25(4):339–348.

69. Suriano G, Oliveira C, Ferreira P, Machado JC, Bordin MC, de Wever O et al. Identification of CDH1 germline missense mutations associated with functional inactivation of the E-cadherin protein in young gastric cancer probands. Hum Mol Genet 2003; 12(5):575–582.

70. Wooster R, Bignell G, Lancaster J, Swift S, Seal S, Mangion J et al. Identification of the breast cancer susceptibility gene BRCA2. Nature 1995; 378(6559):789–792.

71. The Breast Cancer Linkage Consortium. Cancer risks in BRCA2 mutation carriers. J Natl Cancer Inst 1999; 91:1310–1316.

72. Landi MT, Goldstein AM, Tsang S, Munroe D, Modi WS, Ter-Minassian M et al. Genetic susceptibility in familial melanoma from North Eastern Italy. J Med Genet 2004; 41:557–566.

73. Mantelli M, Barile M, Ciotti P, Ghiorzo P, Lantieri F, Pastorino L et al. High prevalence of the G101W germline mutation in the CDKN2A (P16(ink4a)) gene in 62 Italian malignant melanoma families. Am J Med Genet 2002; 107(3):214–221.

74. Ciotti P, Struewing JP, Mantelli M, Chompret A, Avril MF, Santi PL et al. A single genetic origin for the G101W CDKN2A mutation in 20 melanoma-prone families. Am J Hum Genet 2000; 67(2):311–319.

75. Fargnoli MC, Chimenti S, Keller G, Soyer HP, Dal P, V, Hofler H et al. CDKN2a/p16INK4a mutations and lack of p19ARF involvement in familial melanoma kindreds. J Invest Dermatol 1998; 111(6): 1202–1206.

76. Della Torre G, Pasini B, Frigerio S, Donghi R, Rovini D, Delia D et al. CDKN2A and CDK4 mutation analysis in Italian melanoma-prone families: functional characterization of a novel CDKN2A germ line mutation. Br J Cancer 2001; 85(6):836–844.

77. Guerois R, Nielsen JE, Serrano L. Predicting changes in the stability of proteins and protein complexes: a study of more than 1000 mutations. J Mol Biol 2002; 320(2):369–387.

78. Gilis D, Rooman M. PoPMuSiC, an algorithm for predicting protein mutant stability changes: application to prion proteins. Protein Eng 2000; 13(12):849–856.

79. Sunyaev S, Lathe W, III, Bork P. Integration of genome data and protein structures: prediction of protein folds, protein interactions and "molecular phenotypes" of single nucleotide polymorphisms. Curr Opin Struct Biol 2001; 11(1):125–130.

80. Miller JF. Assay of β-galactosidase. Experiments in Molecular Genetics. Cold Spring Harbour: Cold Spring Harbour Press, 1972: 352–355.

81. Monzon J, Liu L, Brill H, Goldstein AM, Tucker MA, From L et al. CDKN2A mutations in multiple primary melanomas. N Engl J Med 1998; 338(13):879–887.

82. Kefford RF, Newton Bishop JA, Bergman W, Tucker MA. Counseling and DNA testing for individuals perceived to be genetically predisposed to melanoma: A consensus statement of the Melanoma Genetics Consortium. J Clin Oncol 1999; 17(10):3245–3251.

83. Gillanders E, Hank Juo SH, Holland EA, Jones M, Nancarrow D, Freas-Lutz D et al. Localization of a novel melanoma susceptibility locus to 1p22. Am J Hum Genet 2003; 73(2):301–313.

84. Bale SJ, Dracopoli NC, Tucker MA, Clark WH, Jr., Fraser MC, Stanger BZ et al. Mapping the gene for hereditary cutaneous malignant melanoma-dysplastic nevus to chromosome 1p. N Engl J Med 1989; 320(21):1367–1372.

85. Goldstein AM, Dracopoli NC, Ho EC, Fraser MC, Kearns KS, Bale SJ et al. Further evidence for a locus for cutaneous malignant melanoma-dysplastic nevus (CMM/DN) on chromosome 1p, and evidence for genetic heterogeneity. Am J Hum Genet 1993; 52(3):537–550.

86. Greene MH. The genetics of hereditary melanoma and nevi. 1998 update. Cancer 1999; 86(suppl 11):2464–2477.

87. Goldstein AM, Goldin LR, Dracopoli NC, Clark WH, Jr., Tucker MA. Two-locus linkage analysis of cutaneous malignant melanoma/dysplastic nevi. Am J Hum Genet 1996; 58(5):1050–1056.

88. Goldstein AM, Falk RT, Fraser MC, Dracopoli NC, Sikorski RS, Clark WH, Jr. et al. Sun-related risk factors in melanoma-prone families with CDKN2A mutations. J Natl Cancer Inst 1998; 90(9):709–711.

89. van der Velden PA, Sandkuijl LA, Bergman W, Pavel S, van Mourik L, Frants RR et al. Melanocortin-1 receptor variant R151C modifies melanoma risk in Dutch families with melanoma. Am J Hum Genet 2001; 69(4):774–779.

90. Box NF, Duffy DL, Chen W, Stark M, Martin NG, Sturm RA et al. MC1R genotype modifies risk of melanoma in families segregating CDKN2A mutations. Am J Hum Genet 2001; 69(4):765–773.

19 Low-Penetrance Genotypes, Pigmentation Phenotypes, and Melanoma Etiology

Peter A. Kanetsky and Timothy R. Rebbeck

CONTENTS

OVERVIEW
CANDIDATE GENES
INTERACTION OF PIGMENT GENES
CONCLUSIONS AND PERSPECTIVES
REFERENCES

Summary

The etiology of melanoma involves the interplay of numerous factors, including sun exposure and genetic predisposition. This chapter highlights the current state of knowledge about the impact of genomic sequence variation in genes involved in cutaneous pigmentation. A brief background of the pigmentation pathway is presented in the context of candidate susceptibility genes in molecular epidemiological studies. Candidate genes include the melanocortin-1 receptor (*MC1R*), agouti-signaling protein (*ASIP*), and *P* gene. For each gene, known associations with pigmentation phenotypes and melanoma etiology are presented. Other candidate susceptibility genes considered are tyrosinase (*TYR*), tyrosinase-related protein 1 (*TYRP1*), and dopachrome tautomerase (*DCT*; or, alternatively, tyrosinase-related protein 2 [*TYRP2*]).

Key Words: Genetic susceptibility; polymorphisms; minor genes; cutaneous pigmentation; melanoma.

OVERVIEW

The etiology of melanoma is complex and results from an intricate combination of exogenous exposures and genetics. A multifactorial model of melanoma etiology is exemplified by the observation that not all people who receive elevated exposure to sunlight or who carry genetic mutations in melanoma predisposition genes (i.e., cyclin-dependent inhibitor 2 [*CDKN2A*] or cyclin-dependent kinase 4 [*CDK4*]) will develop melanoma. Thus, exposures or genotypes alone may be necessary but not sufficient to cause melanoma.

Candidate melanoma susceptibility genes can be identified based on biologically plausible pathways associated with melanoma itself, with phenotypic traits that can be linked to melanoma, or with exposures that can be related to the development of mela-

From: *From Melanocytes to Melanoma: The Progression to Malignancy*
Edited by: V. J. Hearing and S. P. L. Leong © Humana Press Inc., Totowa, NJ

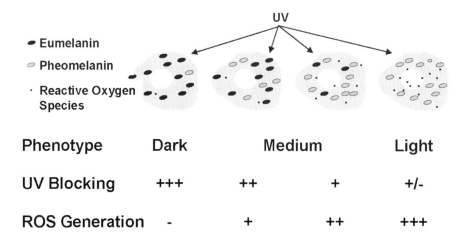

Fig. 1. Model for melanogenesis and pigmentation under UV exposure.

noma. For example, genes involved in DNA damage recognition and repair are logical candidate melanoma susceptibility genes because they help maintain genomic integrity in response to the damaging effects of ultraviolet (UV) exposure to the skin. Because melanoma is a cancer of the melanocyte and is strongly associated with pigmentation phenotypes, another set of candidate melanoma susceptibility genes is the set that determines pigmentation phenotypes.

As shown in Fig. 1, two complementary mechanisms coupled to the synthesis of melanins can be associated with melanoma risk. It is well established that individuals with dark pigmentation phenotypes have a decreased risk of melanoma (1). These individuals have a higher relative proportion of eumelanin than pheomelanin and are capable of blocking UV irradiation from reaching DNA in the melanocyte. Conversely, individuals with fair complexion and light or red hair color may have poorer UV blocking capacity related to the predominance of pheomelanins over eumelanins, and, as such, may be at greater risk of somatic mutation caused by sun exposure (2).

Not only are darkly pigmented individuals more proficient at blocking UV irradiation from reaching DNA in the melanocyte, but these individuals may also generate fewer reactive oxygen species in the process of eumelanin synthesis (2,3). In contrast, the synthesis of pheomelanin that predominates in individuals with fair complexions appears to produce higher levels and different types of potentially damaging bioactive intermediate compounds (e.g., reactive oxygen species). These compounds may in turn result in higher levels of oxidative stress in the context of pheomelanogenesis than in the context of eumelanogenesis (4,5). It is plausible, therefore, that melanoma results from DNA damage tied to the combination of a decreased ability to effectively block UV exposure and an increased induction of reactive oxygen species generated as a byproduct of melanin synthesis.

Melanin Synthesis in Humans

The biochemical processes involved in the initial steps of melanin synthesis are known and are offered in abbreviated form in Fig. 2. Briefly, melanin synthesis commences with the binding of the melanocyte-stimulating hormone (α-MSH) to the melanocyte-stimu-

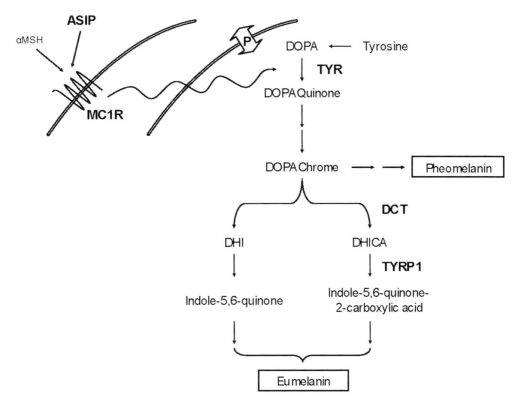

Fig. 2. Overview of melanogenesis.

lating hormone receptor (alternatively known and hereinafter referred to as the melanocortin-1 receptor [MC1R]). The subsequent signaling cascade acting through the secondary messenger adenylate cyclase results in the upregulation of tyrosinase. The initiation of these events produces a series of spontaneous and catalytic reactions involving other proteins, including tyrosinase-related protein (TYRP)-1 and dopachrome tautomerase (DCT). The downstream effect of this signaling process is the production of brown/black eumelanin.

Alternatively, agouti-signaling protein (ASIP) can also bind to MC1R. Although the specific role of ASIP in human pigmentation remains to be determined, investigation of murine agouti has determined that binding of this ligand blocks the α-MSH-signaling cascade and thus prevents the effective production of eumelanin *(6–8)*. Binding of agouti is associated with the production of red/yellow pheomelanin.

CANDIDATE GENES

Knowledge of melanin synthesis can help guide the selection of biologically plausible candidate susceptibly genes for melanoma. Here, we focus on the so-called low-penetrance variants of genes that may confer a small to moderate elevated risk of melanoma when mutated. These low-penetrance variants are not linked to known clinical syndromes involving melanoma and are polymorphic (i.e., alleles being observed in greater than 1% of the general population). Candidate low-penetrance genes and gene variants can be identified by applying selection criteria that optimize the likelihood of choosing a genetic variant that impacts the function of the gene product. For example, the following selection guidelines can be applied:

1. Plausibility. Genes that encode products with biochemical or physiological activities that have a plausible role in the pathobiology of melanoma are considered.
2. Genotype–phenotype relationship. Among biologically plausible biomarkers, genetic polymorphisms with relationships to biochemical or physiological traits that have been well characterized and are known to be associated with melanoma susceptibility are given first consideration. Genetic polymorphisms with well-characterized relationships to biochemical or physiological traits that have no established role in melanoma susceptibility are given lower priority. Anonymous DNA markers (e.g., those that do not encode or regulate any known phenotype) are considered with lowest priority.
3. Polymorphic characteristic. When two markers are available and are equally plausible by the first two criteria, the more highly polymorphic marker is chosen for analysis. A more highly polymorphic marker will, in general, provide better statistical power to detect significant genotype–disease associations. Markers without known polymorphisms were not considered.

Using these criteria and our knowledge of melanin synthesis, a number of candidate melanoma susceptibility genes and low-penetrance variants in these genes can be identified. Information about these genes and variants, and their association with pigmentation characteristics and melanoma, is presented.

MC1R (OMIM 155555; Chromosome 16q24.3)

As described in "Melanin Synthesis in Humans" and in Fig. 2, the binding of α-MSH to the MC1R initiates a signaling path that ultimately results in production of eumelanin through the upregulation of several genes involved in melanogenesis. The human *MC1R* gene was cloned and mapped in the early 1990s and is the human homolog to the mammalian *extension* locus *(9,10)*. The gene consists of a one-exon coding region 954 nucleotides in length, and produces a 317-amino-acid protein product.

Natural Variation in MC1R

Studies among people of northwestern European descent have demonstrated that *MC1R* is highly polymorphic *(11)*. Natural variation at this locus also has been observed among people of African and Asian descent; however, these studies tend to be limited in scope *(11–17)*. The total number of *MC1R* polymorphisms in the published literature approaches 40 (reviewed in ref. *18*). There is substantial variability in the frequency and distribution of *MC1R* variants across population groups, although, within populations groups the frequency and distribution of *MC1R* variants is much more consistent.

A substantial number of nonsynonymous variants in *MC1R* that potentially affect receptor function have been described in populations of Northwestern European descent (reviewed in ref. *18*). In populations of African descent, synonymous changes that affect only the primary nucleotide sequence, but not the secondary amino acid sequence, are the norm. Recently, however, nonsynonymous variants have been reported among normally pigmented sub-Saharan and San populations *(17)* and among selected Jamaicans with "rust-colored" complexions *(16)*.

Considering the numerous nonsynonymous *MC1R* polymorphisms noted in the literature, only a portion occur at a frequency great enough to make them useful for

Table 1

Selected Variants in Melanoma Candidate Susceptibility Genes and Associations With Pigmentation Phenotypes and Melanoma

Gene	Region	Nucleotide change	Amino acid change	Association with pigmentation phenotypes[a]	Association with melanoma etiology[a]
Melanocortin-1 receptor (MC1R)	Exon 1	g.178T>G	Val60Leu	Red hair color, Blonde hair color, weakly Light skin complexion Freckling	Yes
MC1R	Exon 1	g.252C>A	Asp84Glu	Red hair color, strongly Blonde hair color Light skin complexion Freckling	Yes
MC1R	Exon 1	g.274G>A	Val92Met	Red hair color Light skin complexion Freckling	Yes[b]
MC1R	Exon 1	g.425G>A	Arg142His	Red hair color Light skin complexion	No[c]
MC1R	Exon 1	g.451C>T	Arg151Cys	Red hair color, strongly Blonde hair color Light skin complexion Freckling	Yes
MC1R	Exon 1	g.464T>C	Ile155Trp	Blonde hair color Light skin complexion	N/A[d]
MC1R	Exon 1	g.478C>T	Arg160Trp	Red hair color, strongly Blonde hair color, weakly Light skin complexion Freckling	Yes
MC1R	Exon 1	g.488G>A	Arg163Gln	Light skin complexion	Yes[b]
MC1R	Exon 1	g.880G>C	Asp294His	Red hair color, strongly Blonde hair color Light skin complexion Freckling	Yes

(continued)

351

Table 1 (*Continued*)

Selected Variants in Melanoma Candidate Susceptibility Genes and Associations With Pigmentation Phenotypes and Melanoma

Gene	Region	Nucleotide change	Amino acid change	Association with pigmentation phenotypes[a]	Association with melanoma etiology[a]
Agouti Signaling Protein (ASIP)	3'-UTR	g.8818A>G	—	Dark hair color Dark eye color	No
P gene	Exon 7	c.770A>C	Asp257Ala	N/A	N/A
P gene	Exon 9	c.913C>T	Arg305Trp	Dark eye color (vs blue)	N/A
P gene	Exon 13	c.1256G>A	Arg419Gln	Green/hazel eye color	N/A
P gene	Exon 13	c.1320G>C	Leu440Phe	N/A	N/A
P gene	Exon 18	c.1844A>	His615Arg	N/A	N/A
P gene	Exon 21	c.2165T>G	Ile722Thr	N/A	N/A
Tyrosinase (TYR)	Exon 1	c.575A>C	Tyr192Ser	N/A	N/A
TYR	Exon 4	c.1205G>A	Arg402Gln	N/A	N/A

[a]Unless otherwise noted, associations are for heterozygous carriage of variant.
[b]Statistically significant association noted only for homozygous or compound heterozygous (i.e., with another *MC1R* variant) carriage.
[c]Because of the rarity of this variant, the power to detect associations with heterozygous carriage is limited; a suggestive association with homozygous or compound heterozygous carriage is noted in ref. *31*.
[d]N/A, not applicable; association not studied to date.

352

epidemiological studies that explain variability in human pigmentation or of melanoma etiology (Table 1). Among healthy populations of Northern European ancestry, four nonsynonymous variants are consistently found at a frequency of greater than 5%: V60L, V92M, R151C, and R160W. An additional five variants, D84E, R142H, I155T, R163Q, and D294H, occur at a frequency between 1 and 5% in these sample populations. The remaining variants in *MC1R* occur at a frequency of less than 1%. Although these are potentially interesting and may contribute to pigmentation and melanoma etiology, they account for only a small proportion of the total genetic variation in *MC1R*.

Most, but not all, *MC1R* variants reported to date result from single nucleotide changes. Some have been experimentally shown to compromise the quantity of α-MSH-induced cyclic adenosine monophosphate (cAMP) production *(19,20)*. Other experimental studies have demonstrated that sequence variants in *MC1R* can alter protein function in vitro, expression of pigmentation in the mouse and primary human melanocyte cell lines, and in vivo response to UV radiation *(21–23)*. However, definitive information about the functional significance of most *MC1R* variants from basic science investigations is not available.

Recently, an *in silico* approach was used in an attempt to predict *MC1R* variants that may be more likely to affect native receptor function. Using publicly available sorting intolerant from tolerant software *(24,25)*, a comparison of MC1R protein sequences across species was made *(26)*. The underlying assumption for these analyses is that amino acid positions that are important to the native biological functioning of the protein should be conserved across the protein family and/or across evolutionary history. Results from the sorting intolerant from tolerant analysis showed that a predicted 65% of amino acid residues in MC1R are to be conserved. Among the nine most frequently occurring nonsynonymous MC1R variants, D84E, R142H, R151C, I155T, R160W, and D294H were predicted to be intolerant (i.e., putatively functional) substitutions, whereas the V60L, V92M, and R163Q variants were predicted to be tolerant (i.e., putatively nonfunctional) substitutions.

ASSOCIATION OF MC1R VARIANTS WITH CUTANEOUS PHENOTYPES

The relationship between *MC1R* variants and pigmentation phenotypes (for melanoma etiology, *see* "Association of *MC1R* Variants With Cutaneous Melanoma") among white populations has been extensively studied, and an aggregation of the results of these investigations are available from a number of reviews *(18,27–29)*. We briefly summarize these associations here.

Hair Color, Skin Type, and Freckling. The first epidemiological evidence indicating that *MC1R* contributed to human pigmentation came from a small study in the United Kingdom showing an association between *MC1R* variants and red hair color and fair skin type *(30)*. Subsequent results from many studies have supported the association of *MC1R* variants and red hair color. The R151C, R160W, and D294H variants, which have become known as the "red hair color" variants have consistently demonstrated very strong associations with this phenotype, with associations most evident among those individuals who carry two or more *MC1R* variants *(31–36)*. Carriage of other select *MC1R* variants also has been associated with red hair color, although less strongly than that of carriage of the "red hair color" variants. Recently, Sturm et al. demonstrated that the D84E variant is also strongly associated with red hair color and that carriage of any one of the D84E, R151C, R160W, or D294H variant *MC1R* alleles resulted in a greater than 60-fold increased risk of red hair color (odd ratio [OR], 63.3; 95% confidence interval [CI], 31.9–140), although only a 40% increased risk of blonde hair color (OR, 1.4; 95% CI, 1.2–1.8) *(36,37)*.

Similarly, the association of *MC1R* variants with skin type first noted by Valverde et al. has been consistently demonstrated across several studies. Not surprisingly, individuals with fair complexions carry a greater proportion of *MC1R* variants, including the "red hair color" variants *(31–33,35)*. Carriage of these variants is generally thought to be independent of ethnicity or hair color *(31,32)*. Sturm et al. noted that *MC1R* variants contributed to skin reflectance in an additive manner; the D84E, R151C, R160W, and D294H variants added, on average, 1.9%, and the V60L, V92M, and R163Q added, on average, 0.9% to skin reflectance measurements above that observed among people carrying two copies of the *MC1R* consensus sequence *(36,37)*.

MC1R variants are associated with freckling, including solar lentigines and childhood freckling *(38)*. Although most other studies have not separated out lentigines from ephelides in childhood, the associations with freckling have been observed across various study populations *(26,32,33)*. *MC1R* variants have also been associated with the number of body sites on which freckling occurred *(35)*. Sturm et al. observed a positive association between increasing composite freckling scores and carriage of *MC1R* variants, with carriage of two of the D84E, R151C, R160W, or D294H variants associated with the most extreme frecklers *(36,37)*.

Eye Color. Because eye color is correlated with other pigmentation phenotypes, such as skin type and hair color, it may be expected that an association exists between this characteristic trait and *MC1R* variants. However, data from several studies have not demonstrated such a main effect *(31,32)*. One smaller study did find an association with carriage of the "red hair color" variants and light eye color, although adjustment for other correlated pigmentation phenotypes was not undertaken *(26)*.

ASSOCIATION OF *MC1R* VARIANTS WITH CUTANEOUS MELANOMA

The first published report of an MC1R–melanoma association came from a small study in the United Kingdom *(39)*. Subsequently, the association of *MC1R* variants with melanoma has been demonstrated in two larger, better-designed epidemiological studies set in Australia *(32)* and the Netherlands *(40)*. Elevated risk of melanoma was related not only to the absolute number of *MC1R* variants carried, but also to carriage of specific *MC1R* variants. People with melanoma were over twofold more like to carry variants than were healthy controls; and melanoma cases were more likely to carry the R151C, R160W, and D294H variants. Importantly, the association between *MC1R* variants and melanoma outcomes remained statistically significant even after adjustment for pigmentation phenotypes. The association between *MC1R* variants and melanoma was shown to be stronger among people with darker skin types that among those with lighter skin types *(32)*.

MC1R variants are also modifiers of age of onset of melanoma within melanoma-prone families. Results from two studies demonstrate a significantly younger age at diagnosis of melanoma among those family members who carry both a mutation in *CDKN2A* and one of the R151C, R160W, or D294H variants in *MC1R* *(41,42)*.

ASSOCIATION OF **MC1R** VARIANTS WITH UVEAL MELANOMA

In great contrast to the consistent finding of a significant association between *MC1R* variants and cutaneous melanoma, *MC1R* does not appear to be associated with the development of uveal melanoma. Two case–control studies found no differences in the frequency of or total carriage of *MC1R* variants comparing people with uveal melanoma with control subjects free of cancer *(43,44)*.

ASIP (OMIM No. 600201; Chromosome 20q11.2)

Most of what is known about the functional and mechanistic action of ASIP on the human pigmentation process has been gleaned from studies of its murine homolog, agouti. In mice, expression of *agouti* in the hair follicle results in deposition of a band of pheomelanin on a background of a eumelanin-colored hair shaft *(45,46*; reviewed in ref. *47)*. The binding of agouti to MSH-receptor (R) prevents downstream signaling through cAMP that is otherwise initiated by the binding of α-MSH to its receptor. The result is an effective downregulation of synthesis of eumelanin and a net increase in synthesis of pheomelanin *(6–8)*. The introduction of agouti to murine melanocyte cell lines has been linked to the downregulation of several genes important to the production of eumelanin, including *TYR* and *TYRP2 (48)*. In contrast to α-MSH-mediated signaling via cAMP, agouti signaling is hypothesized to occur via the regulation of microphthalmia and initiation transcription factors *(49)*.

Nucleotide sequence variation in *agouti* and the concomitant effects on mouse coat colors have been extensively studied and further provide a strong basis for regarding this locus as a candidate gene in humans for pigmentation regulation and melanoma etiology. Recessive mutations in *agouti* are associated with varied patterns of darkened coat colors, whereas dominant mutations, a consequence of the splicing of the agouti promoter region to an alternative and ubiquitously expressed promoter, result in mice with yellow coats *(50–52*; reviewed in ref. *53)*. The specific genetic sequence variants associated with phenotypic expression of darkened coat colors have been documented in nearly all gene regions of *agouti*, including coding, intronic, and regulatory regions.

The identification of the human *ASIP* demonstrated a very high identity to *agouti* both at the transcriptional and translational levels *(54,55)*. In human melanoma cell lines in which ASIP was overexpressed, expression of pigmentation genes known to be modulated by agouti in murine models were not found to be upregulated or downregulated at the transcriptional level, although *TYRP1* was downregulated at the translational level *(56)*. Still, compared with the known contributions of *agouti* in determining murine coat color, the specific involvement of *ASIP* in human pigmentation has not yet been clearly elucidated.

Natural Variation in *ASIP*

Resequencing efforts to characterize *ASIP* have been undertaken in several different population groups, including people of northwestern European descent, African Americans, Pima Indians, Spanish Basque, Hispanic, Apache, and Australian Aboriginal *(57–59)*. However, for all population groups, with the exception of people of northwestern European ancestry, the number of alleles resequenced has been relatively small. In contrast to *MC1R*, which is highly polymorphic at the nucleotide level, *ASIP* has a highly conserved primary nucleotide sequence with very little natural variation. No evidence of genetic variation has been reported in the *ASIP* coding exons. Two reports, however, documented the existence of a polymorphism in the 3'-untranslated region (UTR) region of *ASIP*, an A to G substitution (g.8818A>G) at a position 25 basepairs downstream of the TGA termination codon *(58,59)*.

ASSOCIATIONS OF *ASIP* VARIANTS WITH PIGMENTATION PHENOTYPES AND MELANOMA

An indication of the potential contribution of the *ASIP* g.8818A>G polymorphism to human pigmentation can be drawn from observations of differing frequency of the g.8818G allele across population groups of dissimilar skin types. In one report, a statistically significant difference in the G-allele frequency was noted among people of northwestern European (0.12), northeastern Asian (0.28), African-American (0.62), and West African (0.80) descent *(60)*. Other reports, however, note somewhat different frequencies for the g.8818G allele among African Americans (0.20), whites (0.015), Asians (0.25), and Koreans (0.12) *(59,61)*. Some of the apparent differences may be caused, in part, by the limited numbers of individuals genotyped in the African-American and white sample populations and the selection of white individuals to overrepresent people with red or blond hair color in some studies but not others. These comparisons of allele or genotype frequencies across whole populations are limited, however, by the lack of a measure of pigmentation phenotype at the individual level.

One investigation has examined associations of the *ASIP* g.8818A>G polymorphism pigmentation phenotypes using individual data *(58)*. This study set in Philadelphia demonstrated that people who were heterozygous or homozygous carriers of the g.8818G allele were more likely to report having naturally occurring dark hair color at the age of 18 (OR, 1.8; 95% CI, 1.2–2.8) and dark eye color (OR, 1.9; 95% CI, 1.3–2.8) compared with people who were homozygous carriers of the g.8818A allele and after adjustment for age, sex, presence of clinically apparent dysplastic nevi, and melanoma status. An allele dosage association was apparent, although not statistically significant, likely related to the reduced frequency (0.12) of the g.8818G allele in this population and the small numbers of homozygous carriers. The observed relationship between the G allele and dark hair color may explain the disparate allele frequency observed among people of European descent by Kanetsky et al. (0.12) compared with that of Voisey et al. (0.015). Because the Voisey et al. study included whites selected for lighter hair color, the observed decreased frequency of the G allele is consistent with the hypothesized effect of *ASIP* on pigmented phenotypes *(59)*.

Kanetsky et al. also evaluated the association of g.8818G with other pigmentation phenotypes, including skin reaction to acute sun exposure, skin reaction to chronic sun exposure, eye color, and freckling *(58)*. However, no association with the *ASIP* g.8818A>G polymorphism was found, except for an approximate doubling of the probability of having brown eye color among individuals who carried at least one variant allele (OR, 1.9; 95% CI, 1.3–2.8). Also examined was the association of the *ASIP* g.8818A>G polymorphism with melanoma etiology *(58)*. In a comparison of 423 case subjects with melanoma and 147 healthy controls without a history of melanoma, no difference in the proportion of people who carried the g.8818G allele was noted (OR, 0.97; 95% CI, 0.62–1.5).

Because the 3'-UTR domains of primary *ASIP* transcripts have been shown to be critical to *ASIP* messenger (m)RNA stability (reviewed in ref. *62*), a proposed functional mechanism for the effects of the g.8818G allele is early destabilization and early degradation of *ASIP* mRNA transcript. Reduction in the level of *ASIP* could hinder the antagonism of α-MSH-mediated signaling through MSH-R, leading ultimately to a bias toward eumelanin synthesis and away from production of pheomelanin. Mechanistic investigation into the functional significance of this polymorphism and whether the G allele affects mRNA stability is necessary to corroborate the epidemiological findings.

Additionally, it remains possible that sequence variation in other noncoding domains of *ASIP*, e.g., the promoter or intronic regions, may be associated with human pigmentation or disease risk.

P Protein (MIM 203200; Chromosome 15q11.2-q12)

The phenotypic effects of mutations in the murine *p protein* gene, also known as *pink-eyed dilution*, on coat colors have been known for years and are the result of reduced levels of eumelanin production in melanocytes (reviewed in ref. *47,63*). Mutations in the human homolog, *P gene*, result in oculocutaneous albinism (OCA) type 2 and other phenotypes that confer eye hypopigmentation.

Although P protein is known to be an integral melanosomal membrane protein *(64,65)*, its specific biological function remains uncertain. The hypothesized roles of P protein include a protein transport system *(66)*, perhaps involved with trafficking of the enzyme tyrosinase *(67)*, or a regulator of melanosomal pH through the transport of ions *(68,69)*. Even without a known definitive functional mechanism for this protein, it appears that altered function of the P protein affects tyrosine bioavailability or function in the melanosome, which is reflected in altered pigmentation characteristics.

NATURAL VARIATION IN *P Gene*

More than 40 sequence variants have been reported in the *P gene* from among diverse populations, including African Americans *(70,71)*, African Blacks *(67,70,72,73)*, whites *(67,74,75)*, Asians *(67,76,77)*, and Native American Navajo *(78)*. However, characterization of nucleotide changes in this locus has occurred almost exclusively in selected populations of people who exhibit clinical OCA. Therefore, the reported frequency and distribution of *P gene* variants are not readily generalized to the population level.

Many of the detected variants in the *P gene* are present in people with severe pigmentation phenotype and are observed at a low prevalence in the general population. However, an abundance of common genetic variants has been identified from genetic screenings of individuals with OCA2 and includes both nonsynonymous and synonymous variants *(66,72)*. In contrast to other identified variants in *P gene*, these are low-penetrance variants not believed to cause frank albinism because of their lack of associated amino acid substitution, location outside of the P protein transmembrane regions, possible linkage disequilibrium with other known variants in *P gene*, or increased frequency in otherwise normally pigmented people *(72)*. Table 1 details the low-penetrance nonsynonymous variants that form the heart of the discussion in the following section; synonymous variants are not included.

ASSOCIATIONS OF *P GENE* VARIANTS WITH PIGMENTATION PHENOTYPES AND MELANOMA

Sequence variants that severely disrupt the native function of P protein are responsible for tyrosinase-positive OCA2 *(79)*, which is the most common type of albinism in the world *(80,* reviewed in ref. *81)*. Variants in *P gene* are also associated with the closely related brown OCA and other clinical syndromes involving hypopigmentation of the skin, hair, and eyes, such as Prader-Willi and Angelman syndromes *(74,82)*. We focus here on known variants in *P gene* predicated to be low-penetrance variants.

A study investigated the association of two *P gene* variants, Arg305Trp and Arg419Gln, and pigmentation phenotypes among people of European ancestry living in Philadelphia *(83)*. No participant demonstrated clinical syndromes that included systemic pigmentation abnormalities; however, the target study population consisted of people with melanoma, dysplastic nevi, and healthy controls. There was an increased proportion of the 305Trp allele in individuals who reported having brown or black eyes compared with those with lighter eyes ($p < 0.001$), and an increased proportion of the 419Gln allele in individuals reporting having green or hazel eyes compared with others ($p < 0.001$). An increased frequency in multivariant carriage of both the 305Trp and 419Gln alleles was found among individuals reporting non-blue eyes compared with those reporting blue or gray eyes ($p < 0.001$). All associations with eye color remained statistically significant after adjustment for the presence of melanoma and of clinically apparent dysplastic nevi. The Arg305Trp and Arg419Gln were in linkage equilibrium with one another, indicating the possibility that both variants could independently influence eye color. Duffy et al. confirmed that these same variants were associated with eye color *(37)*. These results confirm the suggestion of Eiberg and Mohr that the *P gene* is an eye color-determining locus *(84)*. Four other previously characterized non-synonymous variants in the *P gene* that were not associated with frank clinical pigmentation syndromes, Asp257Ala, Leu440Phe, His615Arg, and Ile722Thr *(67,85)* were not examined in these investigations. Previous reports demonstrated that the His615Arg was not polymorphic in whites *(67)*, and, among 312 individuals genotyped for Leu440Phe by Rebbeck et al., only two subjects were found to be carriers of the 440Phe variant *(83)*.

Rebbeck et al. also evaluated whether the Arg305Trp and Arg419Gln *P gene* variants were associated with natural hair color at age 18 *(83)*. They found a borderline statistically significant difference in the proportion of individuals with the Arg305Trp variant in individuals with red or blond hair color (9.4%) compared with people with brown or black hair color (16.0%; $p = 0.041$). However, unlike the association with eye color, the association with hair color lost significance after further adjustment for disease status. No studies to date have been published on *P gene* variation and melanoma outcomes.

Other Melanogenesis Candidate Genes

A number of additional genes linked to human pigmentation synthesis are also good candidates for studies of melanoma etiology. None of these genes has been studied in the context of low-penetrance susceptibility to melanoma or human pigmentation phenotypes.

Tyrosinase (TYR; OMIM No. 606933; Chromosome 11q14-q21)

The tyrosinase *(TYR)* gene is a central checkpoint in melanogenesis (reviewed in ref. *86)*. It has a multiple functions at various steps in melanogenesis, including the hydroxylation of L-tyrosine to 3,4-DOPA, the oxidation of DOPA to DOPAquinone *(87)* and the oxidation of 5,6-dihydroxyindole to 5,6-dihydroxyquinone *(88)*. More than 60 alleles, including nonsynonymous changes, nonsense mutations, insertions, deletions, and splice site variants, have been identified in *TYR* that are associated with OCA1 *(80,88,89)*. A small number of polymorphisms not associated with albinism have also been reported, including two coding region nonsynonymous changes, Y192S *(92)* and R402Q *(88)*. The association of these variants with human pigmentation and melanoma etiology is not known.

TYR-Related Protein 1 (TYRP1; OMIM No. 115501; Chromosome 9p23)

The *TYRP1* gene is structurally and functionally related to *TYR*. TYRP1 converts 5,6-dihydroxyindole-2 carboxylic acid (DHICA) to indole-5,6-quinone-2-carboxylic acid, and has been shown to stimulate tyrosinase activity in melanogenesis *(93)*. *TYRP1* has also been implicated in the determination of the eumelanin/pheomelanin ratio and in the production of "brown" vs "black" melanin *(94)*. Because *TYRP1* function is realized downstream in the melanogenesis pathway, its effects do not lead to a loss of eumelanin, but instead to a change in the amount of character of eumelanin *(81)*.

Mutations resulting in severe disruption of native TYRP1 function have been identified as causative of OCA3 also known as "brown" or "rufous" albinism *(95)*. This autosomal recessive trait is explained by a reduction in tyrosine hydroxylase activity induced by the absence of TYRP1 regulation of tyrosinase *(96)*. The screening of healthy people with normal pigmentation demonstrated a lack of nonsynonymous changes in the exon regions of *TYRP1 (97)*. However, a small number of synonymous polymorphisms, as well as other alterations occurring in the intron and 3'-UTR regions of *TYRP1* have been detected *(91,95,97,98)*. The functional significance on protein function for these noncoding region polymorphisms remains to be elucidated.

DOPACHROME TAUTOMERASE (OMIM No. 191275; CHROMOSOME 13q31-q32; ALTERNATIVELY, TYROSINASE-RELATED PROTEIN 2, TYRP2)

Dopachrome tautomerase (DCT) is responsible for DCT activity in melanogenesis, and is homologous to the mouse slaty locus *(99,100)*. Although *DCT* represents a strong candidate melanoma gene, no germline variants in the human *DCT* gene have been reported to date. Therefore, its relevance to human melanoma or pigmentation phenotypes is unknown.

INTERACTION OF PIGMENT GENES

To date, studies evaluating the role of candidate pigmentation genes in pigmentation or melanoma susceptibility have generally studied each gene in isolation. Because it is anticipated that these genes will interact with one another and with UV exposures to produce pigmentation phenotypes and melanoma risk, the results of candidate gene studies to date can only be interpreted as a main effect of the gene polymorphism independent of other factors. It is clear, however, that this model of susceptibility, highlighting the effects of single low-penetrance genes in isolation is not likely to correctly represent the contribution of these loci to human pigmentation or melanoma risk. Rather, a host of genetic factors likely underlies genetic susceptibility to melanoma, implying that gene–environment and gene–gene interaction may be key to elucidating human pigmentation or melanoma susceptibility. Still, few epidemiological studies have formally addressed the notion of gene–gene interactions, in part because these studies require large sample sizes to insure adequate power to detect differences between groups.

A small number of studies have explored the interactions of *MC1R* and *P gene* and the interaction of *MC1R* and *ASIP*. In a study of 184 Tibetans, the association between three *MC1R* (R67Q, V92M, and R163Q) and two *P gene* variants (Gly780Gly and IVS13-15) and pigmentation quantitatively measured using a reflectometer was investigated *(13)*. There were no noted main effects of these variants. However, in combination, an association between pigmentation level and carriage of both the V92M and IVS13-15 variants was noted.

Additional evidence of the interaction between *MC1R* and *P gene* comes from an observation among a small number of people with OCA2 who exhibit an atypical red hair color rather than the traditional white or blond hair *(101)*. Among six individuals with demonstrated OCA2 phenotypes caused by inherited *P gene* mutations who had red hair color that persisted past birth, five also carried variants in *MC1R*. Although three of the five were compound heterozygotes for variants known to be associated with red hair color, two carried other variants. Neither of the two OCA2 individuals whose hair color darkened from red after birth carried variants in *MC1R*. These data suggest that *MC1R* may act to modify the effects of mutations in *P* gene that cause otherwise classical OCA2 phenotypes. Complementary to this finding, Duffy et al. noted that the *P* 305Trp allele acts as a modifier of *MC1R* penetrance for red hair *(37)*. Among people who were homozygous carriers for the "red hair color" *MC1R* variants (here including also the D84E variant), those who carried one copy of the *P* 305Trp were less likely to have red hair color compared with people who carried two copies of the *P* 305Trp (25% vs 71%, respectively).

This group also investigated the interaction of *MC1R* and OCA2 alleles on skin type and freckling *(36,37)*. Using a genetic marker (D15S165) tightly linked to the OCA2 locus and reported eye color, individuals were assigned to OCA2 *B/B*, *B/b*, or *b/b* genotype groups, for which greater than 97% of people with blue eyes were predicted to be *b/b*. Among the *b/b* group, more individuals had a fair complexion compared with the *B/B* or *B/b* groups, and this difference became further delineated after consideration for carriage of one of the D84E, R151C, R160W, or D294H *MC1R* alleles *(36,37)*. A somewhat similar association was noted for freckling, for which the *b/b* genotype increased composite freckling scores among people carrying one of the D84E, R151C, R160W, or D294H *MC1R* alleles, although the *b/b* genotype did not appear to contribute to freckling scores among those who either carried two copies of the *MC1R* consensus allele (lowest freckling scores) or two copies of one of the D84E, R151C, R160W, or D294H *MC1R* alleles (highest freckling scores) *(36,37)*.

CONCLUSIONS AND PERSPECTIVES

There is consistent epidemiological evidence that genes involved in melanogenesis represent good candidates for explaining genetic variation in human pigmentation phenotypes and melanoma risk. The frequency of genetic variants involved in melanogenesis differs significantly by ethnicity, which may be a surrogate measure for pigmentation phenotypes. *MC1R* has been consistently and strongly associated with cutaneous pigmentation phenotypes, as well as melanoma susceptibility. The *P gene* is associated with eye color and other pigmentation phenotypes. *ASIP* is a likely factor contributing to certain phenotypic traits, including hair color and skin type. Despite this initial evidence, substantial additional research is required in a number of areas. First, molecular and genetic epidemiological studies must be undertaken to characterize inherited genetic variation in these candidate genes in well-characterized population samples. Second, well-designed, adequately powered association studies must be undertaken to characterize the association of these genes with pigmentation phenotypes and melanoma risk. In addition, these studies must consider interactions among these genes, as well as among genes and UV exposures. Finally, characterization of the functional significance of variants in these genes is required to allow an improved interpretation of epidemiological associations, and to elucidate the underlying mechanisms that explain these associations. Despite the substantial amount of research that lies ahead, there is sufficient evidence at this point to conclude that inherited variation in *MC1R*, *ASIP*, *P gene*, and probably other genes involved in melanogenesis are causatively involved in human pigmentation and melanoma etiology.

REFERENCES

1. Holman CD, Armstrong BK. Pigmentary traits, ethnic origin, benign nevi, and family history as risk factors for cutaneous malignant melanoma. J Nl Cancer Inst 1984;72:257–266.
2. Chedekel MR, Smith SK, Post PW, Pokora A, Vessell DL. Photodestruction of pheomelanin: role of oxygen. Proc Natl Acad Sci USA 1978;75:5395–5399.
3. Harsanyi ZP, Post PW, Brinkmann JP, Chedekel MR, Deibel RM. Mutagenicity of melanin from human red hair. Experientia 1980;36:291–292.
4. Persad S, Menon IA, Haberman HF. Comparison of the effects of UV-visible irradiation of melanins and melanin-hematoporphyrin complexes from human black and red hair. Photochem Photobiol 1983;37:63–68.
5. Sealy RC, Hyde JS, Felix CC, et al. Novel free radicals in synthetic and natural pheomelanins: distinction between dopa melanins and cysteinyldopa melanins by ESR spectroscopy. Proc Natl Acad Sci USA 1982;79:2885–2889.
6. Lu D, Willard D, Patel IR, et al. Agouti protein is an antagonist of the melanocyte-stimulating–hormone receptor. Nature 1994;371:799–802.
7. Suzuki I, Tada A, Ollmann MM, et al. Agouti signaling protein inhibits melanogenesis and the response of human melanocytes to alpha-melanotropin. J Invest Dermatol 1997;108:838–842.
8. Yang YK, Ollmann MM, Wilson BD, et al. Effects of recombinant agouti-signaling protein on melanocortin action. Mol Endocrinol 1997;11:274–280.
9. Gantz I, Yamada T, Tashiro T, et al. Mapping of the gene encoding the melanocortin-1 (alpha-melanocyte stimulating hormone) receptor (MC1R) to human chromosome 16q24.3 by fluorescence in situ hybridization. Genomics 1994;19:394–395.
10. Mountjoy KG, Robbins LS, Mortrud MT, Cone RD. The cloning of a family of genes that encode the melanocortin receptors. Science 1992;257:1248–1251.
11. Harding RM, Healy E, Ray AJ, et al. Evidence for variable selective pressures at MC1R. Am J Hum Genet 2000;66:1351–1361.
12. Yao YG, Lu XM, Luo HR, Li WH, Zhang YP. Gene admixture in the silk road region of China: evidence from mtDNA and melanocortin 1 receptor polymorphism. Genes Genet Syst 2000; 75:173–178.
13. Akey JM, Wang H, Xiong M, et al. Interaction between the melanocortin-1 receptor and P genes contributes to inter-individual variation in skin pigmentation phenotypes in a Tibetan population. Hum Genet 2001;108:516–520.
14. Peng S, Lu XM, Luo HR, Xiang-Yu JG, Zhang YP. Melanocortin-1 receptor gene variants in four Chinese ethnic populations. Cell Res 2001;11:81–84.
15. Rana BK, Hewett-Emmett D, Jin L, et al. High polymorphism at the human melanocortin 1 receptor locus. Genetics 1999;151:1547–1557.
16. McKenzie CA, Harding RM, Tomlinson JB, Ray AJ, Wakamatsu K, Rees JL. Phenotypic expression of melanocortin-1 receptor mutations in Black Jamaicans. Journal of Investigative Dermatology 2003;121:207–208.
17. John PR, Makova K, Li WH, Jenkins T, Ramsay M. DNA polymorphism and selection at the melanocortin-1 receptor gene in normally pigmented southern African individuals. Ann NY Acad Sci 2003;994:299–306.
18. Sturm RA, Teasdale RD, Box NF. Human pigmentation genes: identification, structure and conse-quences of polymorphic variation. Gene 2001;277:49–62.
19. Schioth HB, Phillips SR, Rudzish R, Birch-Machin MA, Wikberg JE, Rees JL. Loss of function mutations of the human melanocortin 1 receptor are common and are associated with red hair. Biochem Biophys Res Commun 1999;260:488–491.
20. Frandberg PA, Doufexis M, Kapas S, Chhajlani V. Human pigmentation phenotype: a point mutation generates nonfunctional MSH receptor. Biochem Biophys Res Commun 1998;245:490–492.
21. Healy E, Jordan SA, Budd PS, Suffolk R, Rees JL, Jackson IJ. Functional variation of MC1R alleles from red-haired individuals. Hum Mol Genet 2001;10:2397–2402.
22. Leonard JH, Marks LH, Chen W, et al. Screening of human primary melanocytes of defined melanocortin-1 receptor genotype: pigmentation marker, ultrastructural and UV-survival studies. Pigment Cell Res 2003;16:198–207.
23. Flanagan N, Ray AJ, Todd C, Birch-Machin MA, Rees JL. The relation between melanocortin 1 receptor genotype and experimentally assessed ultraviolet radiation sensitivity. J Invest Dermatol 2001;117:1314–1317.

24. Ng PC, Henikoff S. Predicting deleterious amino acid substitutions. Genome Res 2001;11:863–874.

25. Ng PC, Henikoff S. Accounting for human polymorphisms predicted to affect protein function. Genome Res 2002;12:436–446.

26. Kanetsky PA, Ge F, Najarian D, et al. Assessment of polymorphic variants in the melanocortin-1 receptor gene with cutaneous pigmentation using an evolutionary approach. Cancer Epidemiol Biomarkers Prev 2004;13:808–819.

27. Hayward NK. Genetics of melanoma predisposition. Oncogene 2003;22:3053–3062.

28. Sturm RA. Skin colour and skin cancer—MC1R, the genetic link. Melanoma Res 2002;12:405–416.

29. Rees JL, Birch-Machin M, Flanagan N, Healy E, Phillips S, Todd C. Genetic studies of the human melanocortin-1 receptor. Ann NY Acad Sci 1999;885:134–142.

30. Valverde P, Healy E, Jackson I, Rees JL, Thody AJ. Variants of the melanocyte-stimulating hormone receptor gene are associated with red hair and fair skin in humans [see comments]. Nat Genet 1995;11:328–330.

31. Bastiaens MT, ter Hunne JA, Kielich C, et al. Leiden Skin Cancer Study Team. Melanocortin-1 receptor gene variants determine the risk of nonmelanoma skin cancer independently of fair skin and red hair. Am J Hum Genet 2001;68:884–894.

32. Palmer JS, Duffy DL, Box NF, et al. Melanocortin-1 receptor polymorphisms and risk of melanoma: is the association explained solely by pigmentation phenotype? Am J Hum Genet 2000;66:176–186.

33. Smith R, Healy E, Siddiqui S, et al. Melanocortin 1 receptor variants in an Irish population. J Invest Dermatol 1998;111:119–122.

34. Box NF, Wyeth JR, O'Gorman LE, Martin NG, Sturm RA. Characterization of melanocyte stimulating hormone receptor variant alleles in twins with red hair. Hum Mol Genet 1997;6:1891–1897.

35. Flanagan N, Healy E, Ray A, et al. Pleiotropic effects of the melanocortin 1 receptor (MC1R) gene on human pigmentation. Hum Mol Genet 2000;9:2531–2537.

36. Sturm RA, Duffy DL, Box NF, et al. The role of melanocortin-1 receptor polymorphism in skin cancer risk phenotypes. Pigment Cell Res 2003;16:266–272.

37. Duffy DL, Box NF, Chen W, et al. Interactive effects of MC1R and OCA2 on melanoma risk phenotypes. Hum Mol Genet 2004;13:447–461.

38. Bastiaens M, ter Huurne J, Gruis N, et al. The melanocortin-1 receptor gene is the major freckle gene. Hum Mol Genet 2001;10:1701–1708.

39. Valverde P, Healy E, Sikkink S, et al. The Asp84Glu variant of the melanocortin 1 receptor (MC1R) is associated with melanoma. Hum Mol Genet 1996;5:1663–1666.

40. Kennedy C, ter Huurme J, Berkhout M, et al. Melanocortin 1 receptor (MCR1) gene variants are associated with an increased risk for cutaneous melanoma which is largely independent of skin type and hair color. J Invest Dermatol 2001;117:294–300.

41. Box NF, Duffy DL, Chen W, et al. Mc1r genotype modifies risk of melanoma in families segregating cdkn2a mutations. Am J Hum Genet 2001;69:765–773.

42. van Der Velden PA, Sandkuijl LA, Bergman W, et al. Melanocortin-1 receptor variant r151c modifies melanoma risk in dutch families with melanoma. Am J Hum Genet 2001;69:774–779.

43. Metzelaar-Blok JA, ter Huurne JA, Hurks HM, Keunen JE, Jager MJ, Gruis NA. Characterization of melanocortin-1 receptor gene variants in uveal melanoma patients. Invest Ophthalmol Vis Sci 2001;42:1951–1954.

44. Hearle N, Humphreys J, Damato BE, et al. Role of MC1R variants in uveal melanoma. Br J Cancer 2003;89:1961–1965.

45. Miller MW, Duhl DM, Vrieling H, et al. Cloning of the mouse agouti gene predicts a secreted protein ubiquitously expressed in mice carrying the lethal yellow mutation. Genes Dev 1993;7:454–467.

46. Bultman SJ, Michaud EJ, Woychik RP. Molecular characterization of the mouse agouti locus. Cell 1992;71:1195–1204.

47. Silvers WK. The Coat Colors of Mice: A Model for Mammalian Gene Action. Springer-Verlag, New York, NY: 1979, pp. 6–44.

48. Furumura M, Sakai C, Potterf SB, Vieira WD, Barsh GS, Hearing VJ. Characterization of genes modulated during pheomelanogenesis using differential display. Proc Natl Acad Sci USA 1998;95:7374–7378.

49. Furumura M, Potterf SB, Toyofuku K, Matsunaga J, Muller J, Hearing VJ. Involvement of ITF2 in the transcriptional regulation of melanogenic genes. J Biol Chem 2001;276:28,147–28,154.

50. Bultman SJ, Klebig ML, Michaud EJ, Sweet HO, Davisson MT, Woychik RP. Molecular analysis of reverse mutations from nonagouti (a) to black-and- tan (a(t)) and white-bellied agouti (Aw) reveals alternative forms of agouti transcripts. Genes Dev 1994;8:481–490.

51. Hustad CM, Perry WL, Siracusa LD, et al. Molecular genetic characterization of six recessive viable alleles of the mouse agouti locus. Genetics 1995;140:255–265.

52. Duhl DM, Stevens ME, Vrieling H, et al. Pleiotropic effects of the mouse lethal yellow (Ay) mutation explained by deletion of a maternally expressed gene and the simultaneous production of agouti fusion RNAs. Development 1994;120:1695–1708.

53. Siracusa LD. The agouti gene: turned on to yellow. Trends Genet 1994;10:423–428.

54. Kwon HY, Bultman SJ, Loffler C, et al. Molecular structure and chromosomal mapping of the human homolog of the agouti gene. Proc Natl Acad Sci USA 1994;91:9760–9764.

55. Wilson BD, Ollmann MM, Kang L, Stoffel M, Bell GI, Barsh GS. Structure and function of ASP, the human homolog of the mouse agouti gene. Hum Mol Genet 1995;4:223–230.

56. Voisey J, Kelly G, Van Daal A. Agouti signal protein regulation in human melanoma cells. Pigment Cell Res 2003;16:65–71.

57. Norman RA, Permana P, Tanizawa Y, Ravussin E. Absence of genetic variation in some obesity candidate genes (GLP1R, ASIP, MC4R, MC5R) among Pima indians. Int J Obes Relat Metab Dis 1999;23:163–165.

58. Kanetsky PA, Swoyer J, Panossian S, Holmes R, Guerry D, Rebbeck TR. A polymorphism in the agouti signaling protein gene is associated with human pigmentation. Am J Hum Genet 2002;70:770–775.

59. Voisey J, Box NF, van Daal A. A polymorphism study of the human Agouti gene and its association with MC1R. Pigment Cell Res 2001;14:264–267.

60. Zeigler-Johnson C, Panossian S, Gueye SM, Jalloh M, Ofori-Adjei D, Kanetsky PA. Population differences in the frequency of the agouti signaling protein g.8818A>G polymorphism. Pigment Cell Res 2004;17:185–187.

61. Na GY, Lee KH, Kim MK, Lee SJ, Kim DW, Kim JC. Polymorphisms in the melanocortin-1 receptor (MC1R) and agouti signaling protein (ASIP) genes in Korean vitiligo patients. Pigment Cell Res 2003;16:383–387.

62. Ross J. mRNA stability in mammalian cells. Microbiol Rev 1995;59:423–450.

63. Gardner JM, Nakatsu Y, Gondo Y, et al. The mouse pink-eyed dilution gene: association with human Prader-Willi and Angelman syndromes. Science 1992;257:1121–1124.

64. Rinchik EM, Bultman SJ, Horsthemke B, et al. A gene for the mouse pink-eyed dilution locus and for human type II oculocutaneous albinism. Nature 1993;361:72–76.

65. Rosemblat S, Durham-Pierre D, Gardner JM, Nakatsu Y, Brilliant MH, Orlow SJ. Identification of a melanosomal membrane protein encoded by the pink-eyed dilution (type II oculocutaneous albinism) gene. Proc Natl Acad Sci USA 1994;91:12,071–12,075.

66. Manga P, Boissy RE, Pifko-Hirst S, Zhou BK, Orlow SJ. Mislocalization of melanosomal proteins in melanocytes from mice with oculocutaneous albinism type 2. Exp Eye Res 2001;72:695–710.

67. Lee ST, Nicholls RD, Jong MT, Fukai K, Spritz RA. Organization and sequence of the human P gene and identification of a new family of transport proteins. Genomics 1995;26:354–363.

68. Puri N, Gardner JM, Brilliant MH. Aberrant pH of melanosomes in pink-eyed dilution (p) mutant melanocytes [see comment]. J Invest Dermatol 2000;115:607–613.

69. Brilliant MH. The mouse p (pink-eyed dilution) and human P genes, oculocutaneous albinism type 2 (OCA2), and melanosomal pH. Pigment Cell Res 2001;14:86–93.

70. Durham-Pierre D, Gardner JM, Nakatsu Y, et al. African origin of an intragenic deletion of the human P gene in tyrosinase positive oculocutaneous albinism. Nat Genet 1994;7:176–179.

71. Lee ST, Nicholls RD, Schnur RE, et al. Diverse mutations of the P gene among African-Americans with type II (tyrosinase-positive) oculocutaneous albinism (OCA2). Hum Mol Genet 1994;3:2047–2051.

72. Kerr R, Stevens G, Manga P, et al. Identification of P gene mutations in individuals with oculocutaneous albinism in sub-Saharan Africa. [Erratum appears in Hum Mutat 2000;16(1):following 86]. Hum Mutat 2000;15:166–172.

73. Puri N, Durbam-Pierre D, Aquaron R, Lund PM, King RA, Brilliant MH. Type 2 oculocutaneous albinism (OCA2) in Zimbabwe and Cameroon: distribution of the 2.7-kb deletion allele of the P gene. Hum Genet 1997;100:651–656.

74. Spritz RA, Lee ST, Fukai K, et al. Novel mutations of the P gene in type II oculocutaneous albinism (OCA2). Hum Mutat 1997;10:175–177.

75. Passmore LA, Kaesmann-Kellner B, Weber BH. Novel and recurrent mutations in the tyrosinase gene and the P gene in the German albino population. [Erratum appears in Hum Genet 2001 Apr;218(4):208]. Hum Genet 1999;105:200–210.

76. Suzuki T, Miyamura Y, Tomita Y. High frequency of the Ala481Thr mutation of the P gene in the Japanese population. Am J Med Genet 2003;118A:402–403.

77. Suzuki T, Miyamura Y, Matsunaga J, et al. Six novel P gene mutations and oculocutaneous albinism type 2 frequency in Japanese albino patients. J Invest Dermatol 2003;120:781–783.
78. Yi Z, Garrison N, Cohen-Barak O, et al. A 122.5-kilobase deletion of the P gene underlies the high prevalence of oculocutaneous albinism type 2 in the Navajo population. Am J Hum Genet 2003;72:62–72.
79. Ramsay M, Colman MA, Stevens G, et al. The tyrosinase-positive oculocutaneous albinism locus maps to chromosome 15q11.2-q12. Am J Hum Genet 1992;51:879–884.
80. Lee ST, Nicholls RD, Bundey S, Laxova R, Musarella M, Spritz RA. Mutations of the P gene in oculocutaneous albinism, ocular albinism, and Prader-Willi syndrome plus albinism. N Engl J Med 1994;330:529–534.
81. Oetting WS, King RA. Molecular basis of albinism: mutations and polymorphisms of pigmentation genes associated with albinism. Hum Mutat 1999;13:99–115.
82. Spritz RA, Bailin T, Nicholls RD, et al. Hypopigmentation in the Prader-Willi syndrome correlates with P gene deletion but not with haplotype of the hemizygous P allele. Am J Med Genet 1997;71:57–62.
83. Rebbeck TR, Kanetsky PA, Walker AH, et al. P gene as an inherited biomarker of human eye color. Cancer Epidemiol Biomarkers Prev 2002;11:782–784.
84. Eiberg H, Mohr J. Assignment of genes coding for brown eye colour (BEY2) and brown hair colour (HCL3) on chromosome 15q. Eur J Hum Genet 1996;4:237–241.
85. Oetting WS, Gardner JM, Fryer JP, et al. Mutations of the human P gene associated with Type II oculocutaneous albinism (OCA2). Mutations in brief no. 205. Hum Mutat 1998;12:434(Online).
86. Ito S. Biochemistry and physiology of melanin. In: Levine N, ed. Pigmentation and Pigmentary Disorders. CRC, Boca Raton, FL: 1993, pp. 33–59.
87. Hearing VJ, Tsukamoto K. Enzymatic control of pigmentation in mammals. FASEB J 1991;5:2902–2909.
88. Tripathi RK, Giebel LB, Strunk KM, Spritz RA. A polymorphism of the human tyrosinase gene is associated with temperature-sensitive enzymatic activity. Gene Expr 1991;1:103–110.
89. Camand O, Marchant D, Boutboul S, et al. Mutation analysis of the tyrosinase gene in oculocutaneous albinism. Hum Mutat 2001;17:352.
90. King RA, Pietsch J, Fryer JP, et al. Tyrosinase gene mutations in oculocutaneous albinism 1 (OCA1): definition of the phenotype. Hum Genet 2003;113:502–513.
91. Albinism database. International Albinism Center, University of Minnesota. http://albinismdb.med.umn.edu/. Last modified April 6, 2004.
92. Giebel LB, Spritz RA. RFLP for MboI in the human tyrosinase (TYR) gene detected by PCR. Nucleic Acids Res 1990;18:3103.
93. Zhao H, Eling DJ, Medrano EE, Boissy RE. Retroviral infection with human tyrosinase-related protein-1 (TRP-1) cDNA upregulates tyrosinase activity and melanin synthesis in a TRP-1–deficient melanoma cell line. J Invest Dermatol 1996;106:744–752.
94. Kuzumaki T, Matsuda A, Wakamatsu K, Ito S, Ishikawa K. Eumelanin biosynthesis is regulated by coordinate expression of tyrosinase and tyrosinase-related protein-1 genes. Exper Cell Res 1993;207:33–40.
95. Manga P, Kromberg JG, Box NF, Sturm RA, Jenkins T, Ramsay M. Rufous oculocutaneous albinism in southern African Blacks is caused by mutations in the TYRP1 gene. Am J Hum Genet 1997;61:1095–1101.
96. Boissy RE, Zhao H, Oetting WS, et al. Mutation in and lack of expression of tyrosinase-related protein-1 (TRP-1) in melanocytes from an individual with brown oculocutaneous albinism: a new subtype of albinism classified as "OCA3". Am J Hum Genet 1996;58:1145–1156.
97. Box NF, Wyeth JR, Mayne CJ, O'Gorman LE, Martin NG, Sturm RA. Complete sequence and polymorphism study of the human TYRP1 gene encoding tyrosinase-related protein 1. Mamm Genome 1998;9:50–53.
98. Wildenberg SC, King RA, Oetting WS. Detection of a Tsp509I polymorphism in the 3' UTR of the human tyrosinase related protein-1 (TYRP) gene. Hum Genet 1995;95:247.
99. Sturm RA, O'Sullivan BJ, Box NF, et al. Chromosomal structure of the human TYRP1 and TYRP2 loci and comparison of the tyrosinase-related protein gene family. Genomics 1995;29:24–34.
100. Budd PS, Jackson IJ. Structure of the mouse tyrosinase-related protein-2/dopachrome tautomerase (Tyrp2/Dct) gene and sequence of two novel slaty alleles. Genomics 1995;29:35–43.
101. King RA, Willaert RK, Schmidt RM, et al. MC1R mutations modify the classic phenotype of oculocutaneous albinism type 2 (OCA2). Am J Hum Genet 2003;73:638–645.

20 The Biology of Melanoma Progression

From Melanocyte to Metastatic Seed

A. Neil Crowson, Cynthia Magro, and Martin C. Mihm, Jr.

Summary

The last two decades have seen spectacular advances in our understanding of the biology of melanoma and, in particular, the mechanisms operative in disease initiation and progression. In disease initiation, the genetics of melanoma, and, in particular, the impact of genetic defects on dysregulation of the cell cycle, are key issues in malignant transformation and a major focus of this chapter. Regarding disease progression, consideration is also given herein to the acquisition of growth factor autonomy by neoplastic clones and to the acquisition of capabilities for invasion and metastasis from the standpoint of cell adhesion, motility, and matrix digestion. These events have specific morphological correlates which will be discussed briefly.

Key Words: Melanoma biology; metastasis; clonal autonomy.

From: *From Melanocytes to Melanoma: The Progression to Malignancy*
Edited by: V. J. Hearing and S. P. L. Leong © Humana Press Inc., Totowa, NJ

INTRODUCTION

At current incidence rates, roughly 1 in 74 Americans will develop melanoma in their lifetime *(1)*. It is estimated that in 2005 there will be 55,000 new cases of invasive melanoma and 41,000 new cases of *in situ* melanoma in the United States. Although the most effective preventative measure is avoidance of sunlight, recent surveys suggest that the population at large is not responding as intended to educational programs calling for more effective use of sunscreens, contributing to rising melanoma incidence rates. Clearly, therefore, a better understanding of melanoma biology is needed, along with more effective therapeutic modalities that will flow therefrom. Advances in our understanding of the biology of melanoma have illuminated the nature of disease initiation and progression. In disease initiation the genetics of melanoma, and, in particular, the impact of genetic defects on dysregulation of the cell cycle, are key issues in the malignant transformation of the nevomelanocyte. In disease progression, consideration is given in this chapter to the acquisition of growth factor autonomy by neoplastic clones, and to the acquisition of capabilities for invasion and metastasis from the standpoint of cell adhesion, motility, and matrix digestion. We will also briefly discuss, where appropriate, how these biological determinants of behavior correlate to histomorphology.

THE GENETIC BASIS OF MALIGNANT MELANOMA: CELL CYCLE DYSREGULATION AND THE MALIGNANT PHENOTYPE

The first observation that melanoma might have a hereditary component was made by Norris in 1820, who reported the case of a father and son with the disease *(2)*. The subsequent recognition by Wallace Clark and coworkers of kindreds whose members expressed numerous abnormal nevi and an increased risk of melanoma was a signal event in the history of clinical oncology, because it led to an intense investigative effort that enhanced our comprehension of the biological basis of human neoplasia. Early studies of the dysplastic nevus syndrome suggested a possible linkage to the short arm of chromosome 1 *(3,4)*. Other candidate regions were subsequently reported; in particular, most tumor cell lines manifest deletions that implicate 9p as the possible site for an aberrant tumor suppressor gene. More refined techniques using molecular probes to establish conversion to homozygosity have defined 9p as the location of consistent deletions in early melanomas; one case study demonstrated a reciprocal translocation involving 5p and 9p with the breakpoint near 9p21, implicating 9p as the probable locus of a melanoma susceptibility gene. Roughly 50% of all familial melanoma kindreds have since been shown to manifest a defect within this region *(5–12)*. It has become clear that genetic abnormalities inherent in melanomas consistently impact genes that encode for cell cycle regulatory proteins, a phenomenon that results in unrestricted cell proliferation under growth factor-deprived conditions in vitro *(13)*. In particular, 9p21 is the location of the *CDKN2A* (or *p16*) gene, which is frequently deleted in sporadic melanomas, as well as in those associated with familial clustering *(11,14–20)*. Some 8–12% of all cases of melanoma in North America appear to be a consequence of a defect or a combination of defects inherited in an autosomal dominant fashion, a large subset of these reflecting germline mutations of the *CDKN2A* gene *(21)*. Regarding the incidence of this mutation in sporadic melanoma, 5 of 33 patients in one series of multiple melanoma had *CDKN2A* mutations, 2 of whom were subsequently proved to have previously unknown family histories of melanoma *(22)*. This finding suggests that genetic testing of multiple melanoma patients has a role to play in promoting closer surveillance of family members.

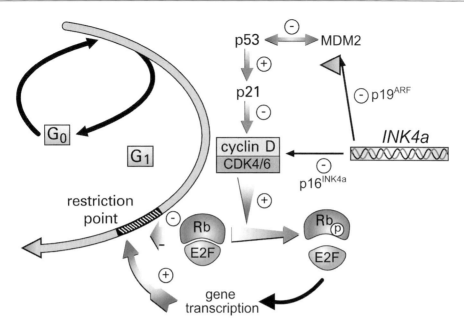

Fig. 1. The cell cycle, a highly ordered series of recurrent events that effect the duplication and transmission of DNA to daughter cells, is regulated at discrete replicative "check points," including the gap 1 (G1) phase and the interval between mitosis and DNA synthesis (the S phase). The external stimuli that affect the progress from the resting, or G0 phase, are communicated through a cascade of intracellular phosphorylation events through upregulated expression of the cyclin-dependent kinases (CDKs). CDK is the catalytic partner that acts by complexing with its regulatory unit, the corresponding cyclin, a process mediated by the synthesis of its substrates and their subsequent proteolytic degradation. The D cyclins complex with and activate CDKs 4 and 6 to effect phosphorylation of the protein product of the *retinoblastoma* gene (pRb), which is the essential checkpoint to prevent progression of the cell cycle in the event of sublethal genotoxic injury. Unphosphorylated or hypophosphorylated pRb complexes with the E2F transcription factor proteins to prevent DNA transcription. After phosphorylation, however, pRb dissociates from E2F, allowing E2F to transcribe the responder genes and, thus, to permit passage past the transcription check-point. The phosphorylation of pRb is controlled through the tumor suppressor gene, *p53*, the level of which is negligible in normal dividing cells. *p53* is regulated in a reciprocal fashion by the murine double-minute 2 (MDM2) protein, which downregulates *p53* expression, binds p53 protein to inactivate it, and mediates its export from the nucleus into the cytosol for ubiquination and proteosomal degradation. p53 controls the cell cycle via transcriptional upregulation of the CDK inhibitor p21; the inhibition of kinase activity prevents phosphorylation of pRb and, in consequence, the cell remains in G1 to allow time for DNA repair. The *INK4a* gene encodes for two discrete protein products, one of which, p16^{INK4a}, specifically inhibits CDK4/6.

The *CDKN2A (p16)* gene (Fig. 1) belongs to a family of genes that encode for proteins termed cyclin-dependent kinase (CDK) inhibitors. These are negative regulators of the cell cycle that operate through their interaction with multiunit complexes comprising CDKs and their activating, homologous protein partners, the cyclins *(23)*. The CDKs constitute a group of serine/threonine kinases that are responsible for driving the orderly progression of the cell cycle through a series of sequential phosphorylation events involving target proteins critical to nuclear transcription that become operative after their activation. Key to this process are the cyclins, proteins that activate the CDKs through other phosphorylation events. The CDK inhibitor, CDKN2A, acts at a critical checkpoint in the cell cycle, preventing progression from G1 to S phase. This effect is mediated through the complexing of p16, cyclin D1/CDK4, and pRB, the protein product of the *retinoblastoma* gene. The hypophosphorylated form of pRB is believed to be the activated form *(24)*. Hypophosphorylated pRB binds to proteins including the transcription factor E2F, which appears to positively induce the transcription of genes whose products are essential for the synthesis of DNA, i.e., progression to S phase. Mutations can occur at several different basepair stations in the *CDKN2* gene *(25)*; the key to oncogenesis is that such mutations must disable the ability of p16 to bind to CDK4/6 and, thus, block the inhibition by p16 of the activation of cyclin D1 *(26)*.

As mentioned, p16 mutations and deletions are seen both in familial dysplastic nevus syndrome and in sporadic cases of melanoma and dysplastic nevi. These findings are confirmed in cell lines derived from sporadic melanomas and may be associated with CC→TT translocations that are the hallmark of ultraviolet light (UVL)-induced mutagenesis *(19)*. Some melanoma cell lines that have metastatic capability lack p16 mutations, implying that cell cycle dysregulation is not an essential feature of the metastatic phenotype *(19)*, or, alternatively, that cell cycle dysregulation is an earlier event that becomes redundant when the metastatic seed is established. Loss of heterozygosity studies on sporadic dysplastic nevi show hemizygous deletions of 9p21–22 (p16) *(27,28)* at one or more loci, and specific point mutations bearing the UVL fingerprint C→T in some cases *(27)*. In contrast, no loss of heterozygosity for p16 was seen in any of 13 benign intradermal nevi studied *(28)*. As regards the role of defects in p16 or other tumor suppressor genes in cases of familial atypical mole–melanoma syndrome, it seems logical that a germline mutation of one allele, inherited as an autosomal dominant trait, might lead to the eruption of dysplastic nevi in the first and second decades of life, and that UVL-induced mutagenesis then transforms an individual dysplastic nevus into melanoma by inducing a defect in the tumor suppressor gene borne by the other allele. This seems to be the probable operative mechanism in at least some cases of heredofamilial melanoma.

There is strong evidence that melanoma manifests genetic heterogeneity even in the setting of familial dysplastic nevus syndrome, because some patients do not manifest abnormalities of 9p21 *(10)* and because cases of childhood melanoma arising in the setting of familial dysplastic nevus syndrome only rarely express p16 mutations *(29)*. One potential culprit would be a mutation or deletion of *CDK4* itself, such that binding of p16 would not occur; however, such mutations are uncommon *(25)*. One study showed that although allelic loss at 9p21 was frequent in sporadic melanoma, being seen in 63% of metastatic cutaneous melanomas and 32% of primary uveal tract melanomas, homozygous deletions of the CDKN2 locus were unusual, implying that genes in the 9p21–p23 region other than p16 may be responsible for inducing melanoma in the setting of a preexisting 9p21 mutation or deletion at one allele *(17)*, or that the complex of p16 abnormalities included a deletion at one allele and a mutation at the other. One study has localized a melanoma tumor suppressor gene to a small (<2 Mb) region on 11q23 *(30)*, whereas another group of familial melanoma patients showed linkage of a susceptibility gene to chromosome 6p in 5 of 16 families *(31)*. Two-locus linkage analysis in another study suggested that a chromosome locus at 1p contributed both to melanoma and to dysplastic nevi, whereas 9p anomalies correlated to melanoma in the absence of familial dysplastic nevus syndrome *(32)*. Germline mutations of CDKN2A were identified in 8% of Swedish familial melanoma kindreds that each included at least two first-degree relatives with melanoma and dysplastic nevus syndrome *(20)*, although the same families had no abnormalities of the closely related genes *CDKN2B* or *CDKN2C*, the latter located at 1p32 and encoding the CDK inhibitor, p18 *(33)*. What is clear is that complex genetic aberrations are involved in the genesis of familial dysplastic nevi and melanoma. It would seem that different populations have different genetic bases for familial melanoma. The early work by Clark and his coworkers *(3,4)* studied, as a matter of geographic selection, particular kindreds whose melanomas were induced, in part, by p18 defects.

It appears that phenotypic penetrance of the melanoma-predisposing gene or genes that link to chromosome 9p is increasing; one study of 18 familial melanoma kindreds in Australia showed a 21-fold increase in melanoma incidence and an earlier age at onset of melanoma (21 vs 45 yr) in those born after 1959 vs those born before 1900 *(34)*. This provides presumptive evidence for an epigenetic factor in inducing a second allelic deletion or mutation to generate homozygous loss of function of the implicated gene or genes. Increasing UVL irradiation because of human habits or perhaps reflecting a depleted ozone layer would seem a logical culprit.

It is possible to measure p16 expression immunohistochemically. In one study, it appeared that lack of immunoreactivity to an antibody to p16 correlated highly with aggressive biological behavior and inversely with survival *(35)*; only 46% of primary melanomas were immunoreactive for p16, implying that a homozygous p16 defect was operative in over half of cases. Using immunohistochemical markers on frozen tissue, one group noted complete loss of the p16 protein in 15% of 39 uncultured primary melanomas, prompting the authors to suggest that inactivation of p16 was perhaps not as common as earlier thought and that primary, uncultured melanomas should be used instead of cell culture lines to examine early events in tumorigenesis *(36)*.

These disparate data prompt several speculations. It is possible that differences in the frequencies of any given mutation or deletion may reflect differences in the ethnicity of the particular population under study, or it may be that tumor cell lines in culture manifest genotypic alterations that are not expressed in vivo. Alternatively, perhaps genotypic aberrancy of melanoma is plastic, evolving constantly because of interactions between tumor, the host soil, and the immune system; and that cell lines with a metastatic capability have a more advanced profile of genetic abnormalities. Recent studies have shown that early melanoma lesions manifest losses of 9p and 10p, whereas melanoma progression is associated with anomalies of chromosomes 6q, 18q, 1p, 11q, and 17q *(18,37–41)*. Loss of heterozygosity studies on lymph node metastases showed abnormalities of 6q, 11q, and 7q not detected in primary lesions, whereas the most common abnormality involved loss of p16 expression, even though no somatic mutations were identified in the primary or metastatic tumors studied *(42)*. The authors held the data to constitute evidence that different subclones lost different alleles of 9p during tumor progression. By immunohistochemical means, they showed that some primary tumors and skin metastases did not express p16, whereas corresponding lymph node metastases did *(42)*, a profile that raises several possibilities, including protein inactivation by epigenetic mechanisms, gene inactivation, repair of genetic abnormalities during tumor progression, and clonal selection.

The RB1/p16INK4a gene products are affected not only by genetic events, but also by epigenetic ones, such as promotor methylation. Promotor methylation causes silencing of RB1/p16INK4a in melanoma and other brain-metastasizing cell lines *(43)*.

It is important to recognize that the p16INK4a/CDK4/pRB/E2F1 mechanism impacts not only cell proliferation but also cell death. Normal senescence of melanocytes requires p16 activity *(44)*; the presence of epidermal-derived cytokines in p16-deficient melanoma cell lines reduces apoptosis, whereas further perturbation of p53 function extends the lifespan of p16-deficient cells dramatically. Another epidermal-derived cytokine, α-melanocyte-stimulating hormone, acts through a cyclic adenosine mono-phosphate (cAMP)-dependent pathway to elicit proliferative arrest and senescence in normal human pigment-bearing melanocytes *(45)*. Under experimental conditions designed to promote melanogenesis, melanocytes derived from light-skinned individuals accumulate less melanin than do melanocytes derived from dark-skinned individuals, and continue to proliferate for several additional division cycles. The delayed senescence associated with UVL-induced melanogenesis in melanocytes from light-skinned persons may, in part, reflect a reduced association of p16 with CDK4 *(45)*. This mechanism might explain the seemingly paradoxical epidemiological evidence that increased UVL exposure in dark-tanning individuals is associated with a reduced risk of melanoma *(46)*. Because biallelic mutation of the *p16 (INK4a)* gene and its alternate reading frame locus confer resistance to cellular senescence induced by the *Ras* gene and its down-stream regulators, Ets1 and Ets2 *(47)*, one can conclude that dysfunction of this gene locus in familial dysplastic nevus syndrome simultaneously promotes upregulated cell proliferation and delayed cell senescence.

P53, BCL-2, FAS, TELOMERASES, AND THE APOPTOTIC PATHWAYS

Although some malignant neoplasms destroy native tissue by virtue of their relatively greater proliferation rates or via enhanced tissue lysis and invasion, others appear to replace native tissue by virtue of enhanced cell longevity. For the most part, this can be achieved through one or both of two mechanisms: reducing the impact of those sequences which lead to preprogrammed cell death or avoiding the replication-limiting effects of cell senescence. The first of these processes appears to be dominantly mediated by the B-cell lymphoma gene, *bcl-2*, and more specifically by the bcl-2/bax homeostatic system, as well as by ligation of Fas (APO/CD95) (Fig. 2). In addition to perturbation of the apoptotic pathway sequences in melanomagenesis, it is necessary to consider the effects of the prohibition of cell senescence by overexpression of telomerase activity.

Enhanced expression of *bcl-2* has been shown in benign, dysplastic, and malignant melanocytic proliferations *(48,49)*. Expression of *bcl-2* appears to decrease with disease progression, with absent or focally absent expression becoming increasingly common in metastatic deposits *(50)*, in which the intensity of immunoreactivity is also reduced *(51)*. We have shown similar findings in human basal cell carcinoma and have advanced the hypothesis that *bcl-2* expression may play a role in initiating events leading to malignant transformation by inhibiting apoptosis and, thus, promoting cellular longevity with attendant enhanced risk of UVL-induced mutagenesis *(52,53)*. The *p53* tumor-suppressor gene is particularly susceptible and has been shown to mutate in some human melanomas. Only 13% of melanomas in one series had loss of heterozygosity at 17p, the site of *p53 (54)*, in contrast to 40% of cases that showed loss of heterozygosity at 9p21;

Fig. 2. (*opposite page*) Apoptosis, the major physiological mechanism for cell removal, affects the death of cells that are irreparably injured or that have reached the end of their lifespan and achieved replicative senescence. The major endogenous mechanism for apoptosis is mediated via p53, which binds directly to DNA to recognize DNA damage, mediate cell cycle arrest (*see* Fig. 1), or to promote apoptosis. In the event that DNA repair is impossible, p53 moves the cell into

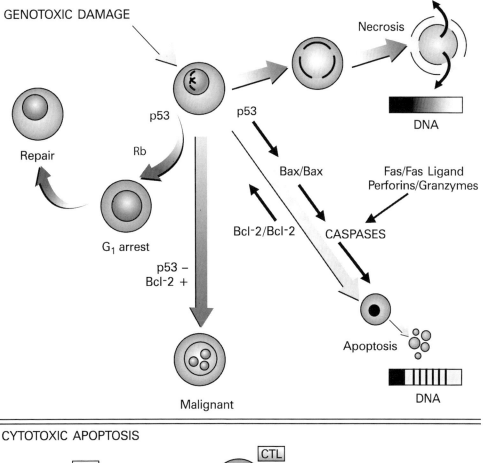

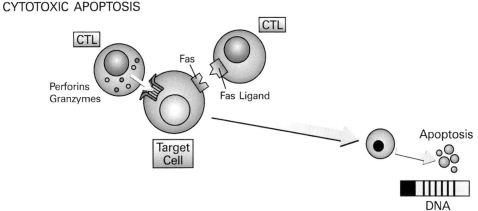

Fig. 2. (*continued from opposite page*) apoptosis through the bcl-2/bax system. High expression of the bcl-2/bcl-X_L group inhibits apoptosis, whereas high expression of the complementary members of this homodimeric protein family, bad and bax, reduce the antiapoptotic function. The final death event, disruption of the cell structure, is mediated through the caspases. In addition to the endogenous mechanisms mediated through p53, external triggers can affect apoptosis; in particular, the Fas/Fas ligand system, a component of the tumor necrosis factor (TNF/TNF ligand) family. The ligands bind to cell membrane receptors that assemble into trimeric proteins that contain specific cytoplasmic death domains that oligomerize and activate procaspase-8 to generate the latter's autocatalytic activation.

thus, a *p53* defect is felt to impact only a minority of cases, but is of particular significance in those tumors which are expressed in sun-exposed skin sites *(55)*.

The *p53* gene encodes a 53-kDa nuclear phosphoprotein that is a member of a group of proteins that regulates the cell cycle. The p53 protein product functions both as a suppressor of cell proliferation and, through regulation of the bcl-2/bax system and via enhanced surface Fas expression, as a regulator of processes that lead to programmed cell death *(56,57)*. Wild-type p53 operates through the CDK inhibitor, p21[waf1/cip1] (p21), to arrest the cell cycle; elevated expression of wild-type p53 correlates with cell cycle arrest via elevated p21, which acts by phosphorylating the pRB through CDK CDC2, and preventing transition from G1 to S phase *(58)*. Mutant-type p53 correlates with low p21 levels and cell proliferation. p53 protein detected in formalin-fixed tissue often reflects posttranslational stabilization of long-lived mutant protein, as opposed to short-lived wild-type protein, which normally does not accumulate to sufficient levels to permit immunohistochemical detection. Nonmutational stabilization of p53 occurs through complexing with cellular or viral oncoproteins, such as mdm-2 or HPV-16 E6 *(59)*. Although correlation between high p53 expression and molecular evidence of mutation is not consistent, it has been postulated that secondary stabilization of wild-type p53 detectable in formalin-fixed tissue may also correlate with a loss of function. Overexpression of wild-type p53 is inducible by UVL *(60)*. Correlation of p53 and p21 expression in paraffin-embedded tissue would provide presumptive evidence of whether expressed p53 protein was mutant or wild type *(53)*. Molecular methods for detection of mutations in p53 have an inherent limitation in that numerous mutations of p53 have been described, and their detection by polymerase chain reaction requires application of a variety of different primer sequences *(58)*. As one might expect from the foregoing, demonstration in melanomas of elevated levels of p21 has been associated with a more favorable prognosis *(61)*. However, high expression of p53 in the quoted study was also associated with high expression of proliferating cell nuclear antigen (PCNA) (*see* page 377), implying that the cell cycle regulatory effects of p21 may be overcome by other mechanisms. Furthermore, it appears that p21, although it expresses an inhibitory effect on the cell cycle at high concentrations, is present at low levels in active cyclin–CDK complexes, as well as CDK–cyclin–PCNA complexes *(62,63)*. It seems that the relationship of p21 expression to the cell cycle is an exquisitely complex one.

The ubiquitinylation of p53 with export into the cytosol leads to its elimination through the proteosomal system. Proteosome function can itself be abrogated by specific inhibitors, thus providing a potential avenue for therapeutic intervention *(64)*.

The Fas/Fas ligand (CD95/CD95L) system represents a parallel control mechanism to that of the bcl-2/bax system for initiation of cell-death sequences through the activation of caspases that are involved in the apoptotic process *(57)*. Fas ligand is a member of the tumor necrosis factor (TNF) family. Fas-mediated keratinocyte apoptosis induced by UVL prevents the accumulation within keratinocytes of p53 mutations by deleting those keratinocytes that bear mutant p53 *(65)*. It would appear that interleukin (IL)-6 downregulates the expression of the Fas receptor and is associated with refractoriness to therapy in melanoma patients, in concert with a decrease in the percentage of HMB-45 positive cells expressing CD95 *(66)*. Melanomas have the capacity to produce IL-6 in an autocrine and paracrine fashion, and could theoretically abrogate their own cell-death activation in this fashion *(66)*. The role of CD95 and its ligand in melanomagenesis is a controversial one. One study showed high expression of CD95, but not of its ligand, in most melanoma lines studied (67). Expression of C95 in those systems was not associated with apoptosis of tumor cells, but induced expression of CD95L resulted in apoptosis through activation of the caspase cascade (67). Interferon-γ enhances CD95 expression in melanoma cell lines and, in combination with anti-Fas antibody, decreases bcl-2 expression in cells destined for apoptosis (68). Melanoma cells have been shown to avoid immune surveillance via high expression of Fas ligand, through which they induce apoptosis in attacking natural-killer T-lymphocytes (69). Elevated levels of soluble Fas and Fas ligand may be associated with poor prognosis in advanced melanoma (70). The expression of Fas appears to be significantly higher in primary than in metastatic melanoma cells, whereas Fas ligand expression appears to be significantly increased in metastases as opposed to primary tumors and also correlates with progressively greater primary tumor thickness (71,72).

Although cell immortality is not a necessary prerequisite in tumorigenesis, it appears to be essential for development of the metastatic phenotype, perhaps enabling an expansion of the number of possible cell divisions needed to acquire the genetic aberrations that characterize malignant tumors (63). Also theoretically capable of conferring a selective survival advantage on melanoma cells over their nontransformed counterparts, through enhanced longevity, would be an increase in the activity of telomerase, a ribonucleoprotein reverse transcriptase complex responsible for telomere reconstitution that, by delay of telomere attrition, has the capacity to immortalize cell lines (73,74). Telomeres enable correct mitotic segregation of sister chromatids during mitosis and facilitate pairing of homologous chromosomes. Typically, cell lines manifest approx 60 to 80 doublings before replicative senescence. Without telomeres, chromosomes rapidly undergo fusion and degradation (63). During division, the length of telomeres, 4- to 15-kb simple DNA repeats (TTAGGG), is successively reduced. Although variable in length in different chromosomes in the same species, telomeres are typically approx 450 nucleotides long in humans. It is believed that progressive shortening of telomeres, which provide a protective DNA cap at ends of chromosomes to prevent genetic instability (73,75), is a key mechanism in cell senescence. Telomerase activity correlates with the malignant phenotype in neoplasms, such as those of ovary (76), cervix (75,77), breast (78), brain (79), and stomach (80). In vitro models indicate that increased telomerase activity, including that from ectopic sources, is associated with resistance of cells to apoptosis (81) and to the prevention of ultimate cell senescence in fibroblast lines transformed by viral oncogenes (82). Immortalized human fibroblasts containing active telomerases continue to proliferate after many generations even if telomeres are ultimately shortened, suggesting alternate protective pathways by which telomerases can allow cell proliferation to occur (82). A clear relationship of telomerase activity to enhanced cell cycle activity is not demonstrated in most systems (76). Senescent cells, which manifest upregulated expression of cyclins D1 and E, cyclin E–CDK2, and cyclin D–CDK4/6 complexes in the absence of phosphorylated pRB, may instead be impacted by an inhibitor of cyclin activity, such as the molecule, statin (62).

Enhanced telomerase activity in human cancers does not necessarily reflect increased transcription of telomerase genes but also may result from decreased function of the catalytic subunit responsible for telomerase degradation (80), or from loss of a putative telomerase suppressor gene on chromosome 5 (83). Suppression of telomerase activity is one function of drug cytotoxicity in human cancer cell lines (74). Increased telomerase activity has been identified in the serum of melanoma patients (84), in metastatic and primary melanoma cell lines, and in dysplastic nevi, with only weak increases in telomerase activity in normal melanocytes compared with adjacent normal skin. *Ab initio*, the relative overexpression of telomerase in *in situ* melanoma in concert with enhanced expression of the apoptotic markers, calcium channel receptors P2X *(1–3)* and P2Y *(2)*, suggests that the role of telomerase initially may be that of overwhelming the apoptotic defense in the early melanoma *(85)*. An association between high telomerase activity and early metastatic spread in melanoma has been demonstrated by others who showed focal marked elevation of telomerase activity in otherwise banal nevi, perhaps a factor promoting malignant progression *(86)*. Overexpression of the heat-shock protein, Hsp90, which is essential to the integrity and stability of the telomerase complex, has been shown on the cell surface of melanoma cells by flow cytometry, and, by immunohistochemistry, at a higher level in melanomas and in their metastases than in benign nevi *(87)*. It is interesting that in the lower-order eukaryotic species studied to date, induced abnormalities of telomeres generates giant, misshapen "monster cells," which are incapable of normal cell division *(88)* and are morphologically akin to the cells seen in so-called senescent atypia. Telomer shortening may represent the biological basis underlying the morphology of senescent atypia. Kerl and coworkers have described a lesion they term the "ancient melanocytic nevus," which has features of senescent atypia mimicking melanoma in large dome-shaped nevi on the head and neck of the elderly *(89)*.

To further complicate the issue, it must be recognized that there are telomerase-independent mechanisms that induce melanoma cell senescence, such as one recently localized to the 1q42.3 region *(90)*. In any event, the telomerase system may afford a novel strategy for melanoma therapy in the future. For example, inducing telomerase expression by transduction of cytotoxic T-lymphocytes with the human telomerase reverse transcriptase gene, presumably by rendering those T-cells resistive to melanoma cell-induced apoptosis, resulted in enhanced antitumor activity in one study *(91)*.

ONCOGENES AND PROTO-ONCOGENES

Most oncogenes and proto-oncogenes expressed in experimental and human cancers act through protein tyrosyl phosphorylation, an essential component of intercellular signaling with impacts on diverse biological functions, including cell proliferation, migration, differentiation, and death *(92)*. Protein tyrosyl phosphorylation is controlled by a balance between the activity of the protein tryosine phosphatases and the protein tyrosine kinases (PTKs). Differentially expressed PTKs are considered candidates for gene products important in the development of melanoma.

Specific PTKs are overexpressed in human melanoma lines, such as basic fibroblast growth factor (bFGF) receptor, FGF-R4. Certain PTKs are expressed constitutively in benign and malignant melanocytes, such as insulin-like growth factor (IGF), FGF-R1, Her2/Neu, and FAK *(92)*. A receptor tyrosine kinase controlling endothelial cell growth, and thus critical for neoangiogenesis in malignant neoplasms, is the receptor for vascular endothelial growth factor (VEGF) *(93)*. Different subtypes of melanoma, perhaps reflecting anatomic distribution, selectively express different oncogenes with different impacts on cell proliferation and death. Oncogenic *ras*, as was demonstrated in acral melanoma, downregulates CD95 (*Fas*) expression, apparently at the transcriptional level, and, thus, contributes to resistance to Fas-mediated cell death *(94)*.

The oncogene profile expressed in a given tumor may impact its histomorphology, as well as its metastatic potential. In a murine melanoma model, epithelioid cell, spindle cell, small round cell, and anaplastic growth patterns are associated respectively with transformation by *H-ras*, *neu*, *E1a*, and *myc* oncogenes *(95)*. Morphological heterogeneity of human melanomas may thus reflect the activation of different oncogenes in different regions of a given neoplasm. Round as opposed to spindled vertical growth phases correlate with the metastatic phenotype in logistic regression models *(96)*; spindled vertical growth phase clinically portends stubborn local persistence and invasion rather than widespread metastasis. Expression levels of oncogenes and their protein products may have prognostic significance because high levels of myc expression in acral lentiginous melanomas studied by flow cytometry appear to correlate with shorter disease-free survival *(97,98)*. The role of myc in melanoma progression is a complex one, because this gene can have proapoptotic or antiapoptotic effects depending on other genetic and epigenetic influences *(99)*. The mechanism by which c-myc induces cell crisis and proliferative arrest appears to depend on cooperative effects between telomerase dysfunction and simultaneous oxidative stress *(100)*. Inhibition of the c-myc proto-oncogene using liposome-mediated antisense oligonucleotides promoted apoptosis and inhibited tumor growth and metastases in one study *(101)*, suggesting a role for specific target liposomal therapy. In contrast, analysis of c-myc transfection in a p53-deficient cell line suggested that c-myc itself appears to sensitize melanoma cells to diverse apoptotic triggers *(102)*. This could reflect the fact that p53 acts via modulation of the bcl-2/bax ratio. High coexpression levels of bcl-2 and c-myc have been shown in metastatic melanoma but not in primary tumors or nevi *(103)*. Enhanced c-myc expression appears to promote cell growth, but antiapoptotic bcl-2, which abrogates the proapoptotic effects of c-myc, appears to confer a huge selective growth and survival advantage on metastatic melanoma *(103)*. Overexpression of c-myc binding protein in melanoma, but not in nevi, has been shown using DNA microarray technology *(104)*.

Comparative Genomic Hybridization

Through comparative genomic hybridization (CGH) of metaphase chromosomes, one can map DNA sequence copy number variation throughout the entire human genome onto a cytogenetic map *(105)*. Through the use of arrays of genomic bacterial artificial chromosomes clones, relative copy number can be measured at loci specified by those clones through the hybridization of fluorochrome-labeled test and reference DNA *(106,107)*. Although the prior resolution limit was 10- to 20-Mb segments, the new technology, termed "array genomic hybridization," has resolution limited only by the extent of genomic spacing and length of target DNA clone segments. Because each cloned segment contains an expressed sequence tag, the location of the clonal DNA segments on the human genome can be precisely identified. Array genomic hybridization permits the accurate quantification of DNA copy number variations across a wide array of genes, detects single copy deletions and duplications, and improves resolution and sensitivity in the analysis of the tumor genome *(108,109)*.

DNA Copy Number Changes in Primary Cutaneous Melanoma

CGH can be performed on formalin fixed, paraffin-embedded primary cutaneous melanomas *(110)*. The most common aberrations in one such study were losses of chromosome 9p, demonstrated in 81% of melanomas, most of which were of the superficial spreading type *(110)*. Other frequently affected chromosomes were 10 (63%), 6q (28%), and 8p (22%). Gains in copy number were seen in chromosomes 7 (50%), 8q (34%), 6p (28%), 1q (25%), 20 (13%), 17 (13%), and 2 (13%) *(110)*. Most acral lentiginous melanomas studied had only one or two amplified genes, as compared with a control set of superficial spreading melanomas of similar thickness, in which only 2 of 15 (13%) had one amplification each *(111)*; at least 15 different genomic regions were amplified in acral lentiginous tumors, attesting to their more complex genomic anomalies. The most commonly amplified regions were at 11q13 (47%), 22q11–13 (40%), and 5p15 (20%) *(110)*. Many of the amplified chromosome segments contain genes implicated in melanoma; for example, 11q13 contains the *cyclin D1* gene that is overexpressed in all cases with the amplification and in approx 20% of melanomas without it *(112)*. In in vitro models, the use of antisense RNA to inhibit cyclin D1 expression in mouse melanoma cell lines that amplify or overexpress the *cyclin D1* gene leads to apoptosis and reduction of tumor size *(111)*. These genomic differences between acral lentiginous and other histological melanoma subtypes appear to be expressed in a site-dependent fashion; that is, superficial spreading or nodular melanomas of non-hair-bearing acral sites seemed to have more genomic similarities with acral lentiginous melanomas than with their nonacral counterparts, whereas lentigo maligna and other melanomas arising on sun-damaged skin show more frequent losses of chromosomes 17p and 13q *(55)*.

Genomic Instability in Spitz and Otherwise Banal Melanocytic Nevi

Unlike melanomas, which tend to have multiple chromosomal aberrations, Spitz nevi typically express a normal chromosomal complement by CGH, with a minority showing an increased copy number of chromosome 11p *(113)*. Employing fluorescence *in situ* hybridization probes, Bastian and coworkers determined that 12 of 102 cases (11.8%) had at least a threefold copy number increase of chromosome 11p, the site of the *HRAS* oncogene *(111)*. The *HRAS* gene in two-thirds of those cases with increased copy numbers had oncogenic mutations, whereas only 5% of studied cases with normal 11p copy numbers had an *HRAS* mutation *(111)*. Those Spitz nevi with 11p copy number increases were larger, more often dominantly intradermal, and had more pronounced stromal desmoplasia with characteristic cytology, but were clearly distinctive from melanoma in terms of their biological behavior *(111)*. A minority of Spitz nevi are aneuploid *(114)*, albeit with lower DNA indices than melanoma; we regard these aneuploid Spitz nevi as biologically unstable neoplasms, in which subsequent mutagenic "hits" have the potential to induce a lesion with invasive and/or metastatic capacity *(115)*, and, in consequence, we advise complete removal of all biopsied Spitz nevi.

Mutations in the *BRAF* oncogene are described in other forms of melanocytic proliferation *(116)*. Operating immediately downstream in the mitogen activated protein kinase (MAPK) pathway, the *BRAF* gene is frequently mutated in melanoma *(117)*, but, by itself, appears insufficient to enable malignant transformation of melanocytes. *BRAF* mutations in primary cutaneous melanoma correlate highly with those tumors that arise in sun-exposed skin *(118)*. Just as RAS genes require activation of other oncogenes or inactivation of p53 or p16 to effect neoplastic transformation of normal cells, cells in Spitz nevi that possess *HRAS* mutations may, for example, undergo senescence caused by degenerating telomeres or have G1 arrest that prevents cell replication. Proliferation rates in most genetically anomalous Spitz nevi are typically low, but those with the 11p gain may have an increased risk of recurrence *(111,119)*. Although most Spitz nevi show enhanced MAPK pathway activation, those with 11p copy number increases also have increased cyclin D1 expression despite low proliferative activity *(120)*. It would appear that the majority of primary melanomas express multiple chromosomal aberrations, whereas the great majority of nevi manifest a normal chromosomal complement. Benign nevi that do manifest chromosomal aberrations most often express a restricted set of abnormalities uncharacteristic of melanoma.

A better understanding of the oncogenes and their molecular mechanisms of action holds the promise of novel therapies for melanoma. For example, the use of a Ras antagonist has been shown to inhibit the growth of N-Ras-transformed human melanoma cells in vitro and also to reverse the transformed phenotype *(121)*. Another example would be the generation of specific peptide vaccines designed to promote the formation of antibodies that block growth factor–receptor interactions. Antibodies to FGF-2 that restrict neoangiogenesis are associated with a reduced incidence of metastatic events in animal models (*see* "Cell–Matrix Interactions") *(122)*.

MARKERS OF CELL-PROLIFERATIVE ACTIVITY

Ki-67/MIB-1 and Proliferating Cell Nuclear Antigen

The biomechanics of cell cycle dysregulation result in higher proliferation rates in melanoma as opposed to benign nevomelanocytes. Several markers of proliferative activity have been used in an attempt to distinguish benign from malignant melanocytic proliferations. MIB-1 is a monoclonal antibody that recognizes a Ki-67 epitope, but, unlike Ki-67 antibody, which requires fresh or frozen tissue, MIB-1 antibody can be used in formalin-fixed, paraffin-embedded material *(123)*; high MIB-1 reactivity (defined as immunoreactivity in >20% of tumor cells) correlates with a reduction in cause-specific survival in thick (>4.0 mm Breslow depth) stage I melanomas. MIB-1 expression is progressively greater from benign nevi through primary to metastatic melanomas, and correlates with Clark level of invasion and Breslow depth *(124)*.

Proliferating cell nuclear antigen (PCNA) is a polymerase accessory protein expressed during the cell cycle from G1 to G2, peaking at the G1/S phase; PCNA can be detected in formalin-fixed, paraffin-embedded tissue by a monoclonal antibody. The PCNA index, as defined by the number of immunoreactive cells per 1000 tumor cells, was 7.2 in nevi and 248.5 in melanoma *(125)*. The PCNA index in one study was more efficacious than the Breslow depth in predicting locoregional recurrence and metastasis *(126)*. Ki-67 expression correlated more closely in one study of uveal melanoma with S phase, shorter survival, histological type, and tumor size than did PCNA expression *(127)*; similar greater predictive power has been reported for Ki-67 over PCNA expression in animal models *(128)*. Ki-67 and PCNA expression correlate with survival *(129)* and/or meta-static behavior *(130)*.

Flow cytometric analysis showing an aneuploid DNA content is associated with a higher risk of metastatic progression in level III and IV melanomas *(131)*. Mitotic indices, which are a morphological reflection of the proliferation status of a melanoma, correlate inversely with survivorship in large series *(132)* and have recently emerged as a powerful prognostic indicator *(133)*. Combinations of data elements and large sample sizes improve prognostic power *(134)*. The correlation of sensitive immunohistochemical markers to historically tested outcome determinates may soon permit prognostication on a personal level and with a previously impossible degree of accuracy, a practice referred to by some authorities as "ultrastaging" *(135)*.

Argyrophilic Nucleolar Organizer Region

Argyrophilic nucleolar organizer regions (AgNORs) are loops of DNA that transcribe ribosomal RNA. Because cells showing prominent transcription are thought to have more AgNORs, the staining of AgNORs is a histological technique that has been used to distinguish benign from malignant tumors. Melanomas have a higher number of black nucleolar and extranucleolar dots than benign nevi, including Spitz nevi, and in one study, melanomas with more than 3.62 AgNORs per cell were more likely to be associated with aggressive disease than melanomas with fewer AgNORs *(136)*. Although dysplastic nevi and Spitz nevi show significantly lower AgNOR expression than melanomas *(137)*, there is no significant difference in some observers' hands between dysplastic nevi and banal common acquired nevi *(138)*. Stepwise increases in AgNORs seem to parallel melanocytic progression from benign nevi through radial growth phase to vertical growth phase melanoma in a fashion that corresponds to Ki-67 immunoreactivity *(139)*.

Metallopanstimulin/S27 Ribosomal Protein

Human metallopanstimulin (MPS)-1 is a 9.4-kDa multifunctional ribosomal S27 nuclear protein expressed at high levels in a wide variety of cultured proliferating cells and neoplasms, including melanoma *(140–142)*, but at only at low levels in nonmalignant neoplasms and cell lines *(140)*. Levels of MPS antigens circulating in the peripheral blood stream, as detected by radioimmunoassay, correlate with more advanced stages of prostatic carcinoma, for example, and are reduced when tumors are in remission *(142)*. Elevated MPS levels identify neoplasia with greater than 90% confidence in a wide array of tumor types *(143)*. MPS-1 protein is weakly expressed in benign nevi, in which expression is usually confined to the more superficial type A nevomelanocytic component; the deeper, more mature components do not manifest expression. A parallel expression gradient is observed in congenital nevi, in which superficially disposed proliferation nodules are often positive. Reactivity of neoplastic melanocytes in melanoma is variable throughout the lesion, unlike the aforementioned gradient expression pattern seen in congenital or common benign acquired nevi *(144)*.

GROWTH FACTOR INTERDEPENDENCE AND REGULATORY PATHWAYS IN MALIGNANT MELANOMA

Normal melanocytes are subject to the cytokine-mediated growth-regulatory effects of keratinocytes and Langerhans' cells. In the human epidermis, a functional symbiosis exists between keratinocytes and melanocytes, whereby the keratinocytes control the dendritic character and growth activities of the melanocytes *(145)*. Keratinocytes produce IL-1 constitutively and can be stimulated to produce IL-6, IL-8, colony-stimulating factors, and TNF-α in vitro. IL-1β inhibits neonatal tyrosinase activity, and, thus, melanin synthesis, but lacks an inhibitory effect on melanocyte proliferation. Neonatal human melanocyte proliferation is inhibited by IL-1α, TNF-α, and IL-6. It has been established through immunohistochemical means and through polymerase chain reaction studies that normal and neoplastic melanocytes synthesize IL-1α and IL-1β in vitro *(146)*.

In contrast to nontransformed melanocytes, melanoma cells do not require exogenous growth factors to promote continuous growth. Melanoma cells instead become refractory to the keratinocyte-mediated regulation of their growth activities. This loss of regulatory dominance by keratinocytes is associated with downregulation of E-cadherin expression *(145)*. Transduction of E-cadherin expression in previously E-cadherin-negative melanoma cell lines results in melanoma cell adhesion to keratinocytes, and downregulates expression of the invasion-associated adhesion receptors, melanoma cell adhesion molecule (MCAM)/MUC-18 (*see* "Cell–Matrix Interactions in Melanoma Progression") and β-3 integrin, and also induces apoptosis *(145)*. It is believed that autonomy from keratinocyte-derived growth factors confers a selective growth advantage on neoplastic melanocytes. In particular, melanocytes harvested from common acquired and dysplastic nevi have similar growth factor requirements, namely, for bFGF and IGF-1. Similarly, radial growth phase melanoma cells, which lack the biological capacity for metastasis in vivo, require bFGF and IGF-1 for sustained growth; the combination of bFGF and IGF-1 has the greatest effect on growth promotion in certain specific melanoma cell lines *(147)*. Cells harvested from vertical growth phase melanoma cells or from metastatic melanoma, however, have an indefinite life-span in culture and do not require exogenous bFGF. It appears that stepwise transformation occurs, in that vertical growth phase melanoma cells still require exogenous IGF-1 for sustenance, whereas metastatic melanoma cells do not. The reason for growth factor autonomy is thought to reflect autocrine elaboration of growth factors by the melanoma cells. By Northern blot analysis or RNA-polymerase chain reaction assays, growth factor transcripts including platelet-derived growth factor (PDGF)-α and PDGF-β, transforming growth factor (TGF)-α and TGF-β, bFGF, IL-1α, IL-6, and IL-8 have been detected in vertical growth phase melanoma cell lines. Most notably, bFGF, PDGF-α and PDGF-β, TGF-α and -β, and IL-1-α have been found to be constitutively enhanced in vertical growth phase melanoma cells. Thus, vertical growth phase melanoma cells appear to acquire the capacity for autocrine and paracrine stimulation, the latter reflecting an ability of vertical growth phase melanoma cells to enhance and to perturb the growth of their neoplastic and nonneoplastic neighbors *(146)*. Similarly, melanomas appear to have the capacity to increase receptor density for growth-promoting cytokines; whereas epidermal growth factor receptor can be demonstrated in tissue sections in both benign and malignant melanocytic proliferations, the expression is greater in malignant than in benign melanocytic proliferations *(148)*.

Certain cytokines, such as IL-6, generate a response from melanocytes that is dependent on the state of disease progression. Thus, whereas bFGF stimulates melanocyte growth at all states of progression, IL-6 inhibits growth of early-stage melanoma cells, and different late-stage melanoma lines are either resistant to or stimulated by Il-6. A similar bidirectional growth regulator in melanoma is TGF-β. Although radial growth phase melanoma cells are sensitive in vitro to growth inhibition by TGF-β, IL-6, IL-1, and TNF-α, vertical growth phase melanoma cells are insensitive. It appears that constitutive enhancement of synthesis of one cytokine in isolation does not, by itself, reflect a metastatic phenotype, implying a "multi-hit" mechanism of neoplastic transformation. Some of these cell culture findings can be confirmed *in situ*. Immunohistochemical studies comparing nevi and thin primary melanomas to thick primary and metastatic tumors seem to indicate that weak TNF-α, TGF-β, and IL-8 expression correlates with benign nevi and early malignancy, whereas marked upregulation of expression of TNF-α, TGF-β, granulocyte macrophage colony-stimulating factor (GM-CSF), stem cell factor, and IL-6, IL-8, and IL-1α correlates with more biologically advanced (i.e., thick) melanomas *(149)*. Increased production of TGF-β, along with resistance to its growth-inhibitory effects, is characteristic of metastatic melanoma cell lines (150); TGF-β appears to be a key cytokine in upregulation of β-integrin expression, and plays a role in downregulation of the immune response to melanoma. Expression of TGF-β appears to be a marker of metastatic dissemination (149). The coexpression of both ligand and receptor for TGF-β, GM-CSF, and IL-6 suggests autocrine production of these growth factors. Although TGF-β2 expression correlates with thick melanoma and is not seen in benign nevi, including Spitz nevi (151), TGF-β1, which stimulates the motility of melanoma cells in culture in the presence of collagen type I, also requires the presence of surface CD44 expression to have effect (see "Cell–Matrix Interactions in Melanoma Progression") (152).

The elaboration of IL-1 by melanoma cells may play a role in tumor invasiveness and the acquisition of metastatic capability. IL-1α is known to enhance melanoma cell motility, whereas blockade of IL-1 receptors has been shown to decrease the size and number of hepatic metastases in mouse models. IL-1 upregulates the expression of mannose receptors in murine endothelia, a phenomenon associated with increased melanoma cell adhesion. Increased IL-1 levels are seen in the setting of inflammation and infection and correlate, in murine models, with greater adhesion of melanoma cells to endothelia.

CELL–MATRIX INTERACTIONS IN MELANOMA PROGRESSION

Cell-Surface Adhesion Molecules and Their Expression in Melanoma

The expression of certain adhesion molecules on the surfaces and in the cytoplasms of melanoma cells correlates with acquisition of the metastatic phenotype. Specific surface glycoproteins that correlate to vertical growth phase and metastatic melanoma include the integrins $\alpha v\beta 3$ (153) and $\alpha 4\beta 1$, the immunoglobulins intercellular adhesion molecule (ICAM)-1 and MCAM (MUC18 or CD146), and specific subtypes of CD44.

The integrins are a family of cell-surface adhesion molecules that coordinate cell–cell and cell–matrix interactions. The integrins exist as transmembrane molecules that comprise a heterodimer of α- and β-subunits, of which there are currently at least 22 distinctly recognized forms (154). The integrin includes a cell-surface ligand and an intracellular component that is in contact with the cytoskeleton. Cell surface interactions impact cell motility, as well as adhesion and, thus, play a role in processes as diverse as wound healing and malignant transformation (155,156). The integrins manifest differential substrate binding in the extracellular matrix. For example, $\alpha 3\beta 1$ integrin binds to collagen types I and IV. Alterations of the integrin profile attend the acquisition of the malignant phenotype in solid tumors. Whereas $\alpha 6\beta 1$ integrin is said to be expressed at significantly higher levels in benign nevomelanocytic lesions (157), $\alpha 3\beta 1$ integrin has been shown to be upregulated in melanoma cells and correlates with increased invasive and metastatic potential (158,159). There is a high expression level of $\alpha 3$ integrin in metastatic deposits (159,160). Localization of $\alpha 3$ integrin in basal lamina around melanoma cells is demonstrable by immunoelectron microscopy (154); tumor cells may elaborate basement membrane material to promote invasion and/or as protection from immunocompetent cells. The $\alpha 3\beta 3$ integrin has emerged as a key mediator of angiogenesis, and its expression on endothelia and melanocytes is a relatively specific and sensitive marker of melanoma (161). Blockage of $\alpha v\beta 3$ integrin, the vitronectin receptor, inhibits tumoral neoangiogenesis in mice (162,163). Treatment of melanoma cells in culture with αv integrin antagonists has been shown to disrupt the actin cytoskeleton, to induce molecular disassembly of cell-to-cell contacts, and to cause melanoma cells to round up and detach from culture plate surfaces *(164)*. By downregulating expression of the vitronectin receptor and the laminin receptor, as well as 72-kDa collagenase activity, retinoic acid therapy has been shown to inhibit the metastatic potential of the B16 melanoma cell line *(165)*.

The intensity of β3 integrin expression is an independent prognostic variable that correlates with tumor thickness, with vertical, as opposed to radial, growth phase melanomas *(153)*, with lung metastases *(166)*, and with death *(167)*. In contrast, β1 integrin expression correlates with lymph node metastases *(168)*. β3 integrin expression is absent in benign nevi but has an expression profile in Spitz nevi that strongly resembles that of vertical growth phase melanoma *(153)* and is upregulated by TGF-β, which is elaborated in an autocrine fashion by melanoma cell lines capable of metastasis *(169)*. The expression of TGF-β also correlates with increased cell proliferation, as measured by Ki67 expression *(169)*. There is a correlation between the expression of β3 integrin and of matrix metalloproteinase (MMP)-9 in one human melanoma cell line *(170)*. Because one of the roles of metalloproteinases is basement membrane lysis, it is of interest that specific NC1 domains of type IV collagen actually may inhibit angiogenesis, providing an additional mechanism by which metalloproteinases, through the digestion of such domains, could negate their antiangiogenic properties and, thus, promote tumor growth and metastasis *(171)*. These NC1 domains also regulate endothelial cell adhesion and tumor migration through αvβ1 integrin-dependent mechanisms *(171)*. Tumor cell chemotaxis induced by type IV collagen appears to be dependent, at least in part, on mechanisms involving CD47/integrin-associated protein and αvβ3 integrin *(172)*. It appears that CD36 expression in melanoma cells may induce the sequestration of specific integrins into membrane microdomains to promote cell migration *(173)*. The distinctive capacity of melanoma subclones to selectively metastasize to different organs *(174)* may in part reflect the integrin profiles on the cell surfaces of those subclones.

As determined by zymography of cell lysates, the expression of integrin αvβ3 has been shown to correlate with the activity levels of membrane-type (MT)-1MMP and MMP-2 in human melanoma cells *(175)*. The import of integrin αvβ3 expression appears to be dependent on the morphological subtype of melanoma analyzed. In particular, integrin αvβ3 expression correlated to tumor thickness and recurrence in lesions of nodular melanoma, superficial spreading melanoma, lentigo maligna melanoma, and mucosal melanoma, but did not correlate with those parameters in lesions of acral lentiginous melanoma *(176)*. Furthermore, although the expression profiles of integrins appear to fluctuate during transition from radial to vertical growth phases in the skin, in particular by virtue of the acquisition of αvβ3 expression, this pattern does not hold true for uveal tract melanoma *(177)*. It may well be that the integrin expression profile also fluctuates during vascular ingress and egress *(177)*.

Components of the stroma also impact cell proliferation and synthetic capacities. Fibrillar collagen has been shown to inhibit melanoma cell proliferation by upregulating p27^{kip1} expression *(178)*. It is plausible that basement membrane material, which is secreted by and surrounds melanoma cells before their expression of MT-1 MMP, serves as a barrier to prevent type I collagen from contacting the cell surface and causing cell-growth arrest. These regulatory effects appear to be mediated by interactions between type I collagen and the collagen-binding integrin, $\alpha2\beta1$ *(179)*. Another way for melanoma cells to escape these downregulating mechanisms would be to digest type I collagen or to alter surface integrin expression. The former activity would require MMP elaboration and/or activation. Epithelioid melanoma cells from vertical growth phase tumors generally have the most aggressive metastatic capability. One study of four uveal tract melanoma cell lines showed that the most aggressive phenotype was associated with an epithelioid cytomorphology that correlated not only with the highest expression of 117-kDa MMP-2, but also with the lowest expression of integrin $\alpha v\beta1$ *(179)*. The investigators attributed the aggressive behavior to the MMP-2 expression, and the epithelioid cytomorphology to the loss of integrin $\alpha v\beta1$ expression *(179)*. With respect to $\beta1$ integrin expression, one study of 38 metastatic melanomas in 27 patients found that those patients whose tumors had higher $\beta1$ integrin expression had significantly longer disease-free (median 38 vs 7 mo) and overall (median 70 vs 23 mo) survival than those patients whose tumors had low levels of $\beta1$ integrin expression *(180)*.

The members of the CD44 family of transmembrane glycoproteins are the binding receptors for hyaluronate, a major component of the extracellular matrix. The CD44 protein exists in standard (CD44s) and variant isomers, of which, at least 10 (CD44v1–10) have been identified to date. When expressed at the cell surface, CD44 can mediate binding to collagens type I and IV and fibronectin, with a potential role in tumor cell motility and invasion *(152)*. In mouse models, melanomas with high levels of CD44s expression have a greater propensity for hematogenous metastases than do cell lines with low levels *(181)*. The expression of CD44s in human melanoma metastases has been said to parallel that of primary neoplasms and to correlate inversely with tumor size, depth, and level of invasion *(182)*, whereas nevi uniformly and strongly express CD44s. In contrast, CD44v6 expression appears to be restricted to malignant tumors. Others have found no reliable correlation between CD44 isomer expression and neoplastic transformation *(183)*. The CD44 molecule appears to be the binding site of the ezrin, radixin, and moesin glycoprotein family members, thought to play a role in attachment to the cell membrane of actin filaments involved in cell locomotion. Moesin expression is progressively reduced in those melanomas showing deeper levels of invasion or metastasis, but is intense in benign melanocytic proliferations and *in situ* melanomas *(184)*. Reduced moesin expression may play a role in reducing contact inhibition of motility.

Osteonectin (BM40 or SPARC—secreted protein, acidic, and rich in cysteine) is a cell matrix protein involved in tissue mineralization, angiogenesis, and cell–stroma interaction. Its overexpression in a group of thin primary melanomas was associated with aggressive biological behavior as compared with a control group of biologically indolent tumors of similar thickness *(185)*, leading the authors to conclude that osteonectin expression correlates highly with the metastatic phenotype.

The cell-surface adhesion molecule, MCAM (MUC18/CD146), the gene for which is located on chromosome 11q *(186)*, appears to play a role in heterophilic interactions between melanoma cells and endothelia and is strongly expressed in melanoma cell lines with metastatic capability *(187,188)*; transfection of non-MCAM-expressing, nonmetastasizing cell lines with MCAM complementary DNA leads to acquisition of metastatic capability *(189)*. Expression of MCAM in melanoma cells lines is downregulated by transfection with mutated transcription factors of the activating transcription factor/cyclic adenosine monophosphate response element-binding (CREB) protein family; the CREB protein transcription factors play a role in cell adhesion and the acquisition of the metastatic phenotype *(190)*. Cells transfected with mutant CREB protein display downregulation of the 72-kDa collagenase type IV (MMP-2), which is involved in the lysis of basement membrane materials in the dermo–epidermal interface and in blood vessels *(190–192)*. Such mutant CREB protein-containing cells also manifest downregulated expression of MCAM/MUC18 *(192)* and increased radiosensitivity, the latter suggesting that CREB factors promote survival in human melanoma cells *(193)*. In addition to enhancing radioresistance, a feature that characterizes metastatic melanoma cell lines, activating transcription factor -2 confers drug resistance to several classes of cytoreductive agents *(194)*.

Cell-to-cell contact appears to influence events that trigger the apoptotic pathways, because, in a canine melanoma cell culture system, cell contact led to the expression of p53 and p21$^{waf1/cip1}$. This expression of p21$^{waf1/cip1}$ did not prevent apoptosis *(195)*, although prolonged growth arrest without restimulation did lead to apoptosis, whereas discontinuance of serum deprivation or release from contact inhibition caused reentry of the growth cycle. Metastatic melanoma cells producing growth factors in an autocrine and paracrine fashion appear to survive insults that provoke apoptosis in healthy cells.

CYTOSKELETAL COMPONENTS, INVASION, AND THE METASTATIC PATHWAY

Cell skeleton intermediate filaments, such as actin, present not only in smooth muscle cells but in keratinocytes *(196)* and in melanocytes as well, play a role in cell motility. Typically below the detection threshold of routine histochemistry, some melanomas, such as desmoplastic melanomas, may express cytosolic actin demonstrable in conventional immunoperoxidase preparations *(197)*. Actin filaments are arranged in configurations including loose and tight bundles and branching arrays. To effect locomotion, the cell must be able to solubilize or disassemble and then reassemble these arrays, a function that is dependent on actin-binding protein and gelsolin, a protein that enables or effects their reassembly *(198)*. Metastatic melanoma and the fibroblasts of the host stromal reaction to metastatic melanoma manifest a qualitative and quantitative difference in actin filament expression. Primary melanoma cells strongly express cytoplasmic actin filaments *(199)*, whereas benign nevi and their stromal cells do not express α-actin. By immunohistochemistry and Western blot analysis, the bulk of α-actin surrounding metastatic melanoma can be shown to derive from myofibroblasts, a cell species perhaps derived from fibroblasts in response to cytokine elaboration by the melanoma cells *(200)*. Transfection of B16 melanoma cell cultures with variant actins reduces metastatic capability *(201)*. Other cytoskeletal filaments also play a role in structural integrity and presumably also in locomotion. Cotransfection of a low metastatic capability, vimentin-expressing melanoma cell line in vitro with keratins 8 and 18 enhanced invasion of basement membrane matrix and migration through gelatin, leading to speculation that coexpression of vimentin and keratins results in cytoskeletal interactions at contact points between tumor and matrix and, thus, contributes to enhanced migratory behavior *(202)*.

Complementary to cytosolic actin filaments are the actin-binding proteins. One such protein, α-actinin, is expressed only in the superficial portions of benign nevi and superficial spreading melanomas but is strongly expressed in a pandermal fashion in nodular melanomas and their metastases *(203)*. Lentiginous and pagetoid intraepidermal melanoma cells do not express actin-binding protein, whereas the nested neoplastic cells of both benign nevi and primary melanomas do *(204)*. Differential expression of this

adhesion protein may play a role in the adhesive character of subpopulations of melanoma with differing metastatic capabilities. α-Actinin is postulated to affect linkage of
actin to β-1 integrins, whose expression relates to malignant potential. Metastatic cell
lines have a high ratio of α-actinin to actin *(205)*.

The degree of actin organization and the presence of vinculin-containing adhesion
plaques correlates inversely with metastatic capability of cultured cell lines in some
systems *(206)*, although there is controversy regarding how the ability of cells to highly
organize their cytoskeleton correlates to metastatic capability. Melanoma cell lines with
high metastatic ability are those that are most effective at acutely increasing their cytosolic levels of F-actin and vimentin in response to agents that reduce cell attachment and
invasion of fibronectin in vitro *(207)*. Using confocal laser microscopy, it has been
shown that melanoma cell shapes are highly plastic during transendothelial migration,
being round and having cortical F-actin expression before migration but manifesting a
pseudopod-like morphology with blebs protruding from contact surfaces during
transendothelial migration *(208)*. These effects are promoted by TNF *(208)*, except in
cell lines deficient in actin-binding protein, in which TNF fails to impact signal transduction in cell *(209)*. Melanoma cell lines deficient in actin-binding proteins are those
with impaired locomotion, suggesting that actin-binding protein is important for the
stabilization of cortical actin in vivo, and, thus, a prerequisite for locomotion *(198)*. The
ability to rapidly and reversibly alter the cytoskeleton is a property of cells capable of
successfully moving through and around stromal barriers and of gaining vascular access.

MATRIX METALLOPROTEINASES

The MMPs are zinc-dependent enzymes capable of lysing components of the extracellular matrix and are classified based on the substrate that they preferentially digest;
therefore, members of this family include collagenases, stromelysins, gelatinases, and
so on. The subclass of gelatinases, including MMP-2 and MMP-9, are capable of digest-
ing type IV collagen, which constitutes a major constituent of basement membrane
material. Although earlier studies showed a high correlation between expression of
MMP-2 by melanoma cells and hematogenous metastasis *(210)*, it is now believed that
the expression of MMPs 1, 2, 3, 9, 14, 15, and 16 correlates with the metastatic phenotype
(211). The MMP system exhibits a dynamic balance with tissue inhibitors of
metalloproteinases (TIMPs). The downregulation of TIMP activity can have the same
effect as upregulation of its corresponding MMP. Some MMPs are elaborated or secreted
in an inactive state and require cofactors for their activation, such as the 72-kDa gelatinase
that is activated by MT-1 MMP and TIMP-2 in cultured melanoma cells *(212)*. Certain
products of some MMP digestion events are capable of acting as cofactors for other
MMPs. Thus, the basement membrane that is elaborated around benign nevus cells and
early melanoma cells, but is absent in late stage melanomas, may act as a semipermeable
barrier for the accumulation of growth-promoting tissue factors, such as bFGF, until
growth factor autonomy is established by a given neoplastic clone. Expression of
MT-1 MMP is upregulated in melanoma and those tumor cells that do express MT-1
MMP manifest enhanced mobility in response to laminin-1, a basement membrane
component *(213)*. Tumor-stromal signaling is a critical, but as yet poorly understood
factor in melanoma progression *(214,215)*. For example, stimulation of MT-1 MMP
activity by the stromal cell-derived factor-1α, has been documented and is dependent on

the expression by melanoma cells of the stromal cell-derived factor-1α receptor, CXCR4 *(156)*. The expression of CXCR4 is augmented by TGF-β, whereas antibodies to TGF-β inhibit CXCR4 expression and melanoma cell invasion *(156)*. Alternatively, TGF-β may inhibit melanoma growth by blocking the plasminogen activation system *(216)*.

The importance of enzyme degradation in acquisition of the metastatic phenotype is underscored by logistic regression models that highlight a relationship between type IV collagenase, as well as cathepsins B and D, and metastatic capability *(96)*. Cathepsin D is expressed in the great majority of primary and metastatic melanomas and dysplastic nevi but only in a minority of common acquired nevi and not in normal melanocytes *(217)*. Further, dermal nevus cells derived from congenital nevi lack the capacity to activate MMP-2 *(218)*.

MMPs may also play a role in angiogenesis. The MMP inhibitor, batimastat, inhibits angiogenesis in hepatic metastases of B16F1 melanoma cell lines *(219)*.

MMPs and their inhibitors are also involved in the initiation of the cell-death cascade. The overexpression of TIMP-2 inhibits tumor cell growth in severe combined immuno-deficient mice, dependent on the presence of fibrillar type I collagen in the matrix of the infiltrated stroma, which induces melanoma cells to undergo a cell cycle arrest at the G1 to S phase transition through a mechanism that involves upregulation of the cell cycle inhibitor, p27^{kip1} *(220)*. The metalloproteinase inhibitor TIMP-3 promotes apoptosis, further suggesting that in some cases the signal for cell death is an extracellular one *(221)*. The induction of TIMP-3 expression by an adenoviral vector results in stabilization of CD95, TNF receptor, and the TNF-related apoptosis-inducing ligand receptor, thereby sensitizing melanoma cell lines to apoptosis induced by TNF-α, Fas antibody, and TNF-related apoptosis-inducing ligand *(222)*. These effects can be blocked by selective and coselective caspase inhibitors, suggesting that the role of TIMP-3 in promoting apoptosis is mediated through stabilization of the aforementioned cell death receptors and the activation of the apoptotic signal cascade through caspase 8 *(222)*.

The MMP system affords a potential therapeutic target. Topical imiquimod, for example, which has been used successfully to treat lentigo maligna *(223)*, has been shown to downregulate MMP-9 activity and, thus, to inhibit angiogenesis *(224)*.

P75 NERVE GROWTH FACTOR RECEPTOR AND BRAIN METASTASES

The p75 nerve growth factor receptor, a cysteine-rich transmembrane glycoprotein receptor for nerve growth factor (neurotrophin), is present on the surface of neural crest-derived cells. Highly expressed in spindle cell melanomas, p75 is thought to mediate perineural spread of desmoplastic melanoma *(225)*. Its stimulation by neurotrophin enhances heparinase activity in melanoma cell lines with high metastatic potential, in a fashion that correlates with the brain-metastasizing melanoma phenotype. Expression of p75 appears to promote the survival of brain-metastasizing cell lines, but not normal melanocytes, under stressed culture conditions *(226)*.

ANGIOGENESIS AND THE METASTATIC PHENOTYPE

Vascular access is a key event in metastatic progression. VEGF, bFGF, IL-8 and platelet-derived endothelial cell growth factor play a synergistic role in promoting neoangiogenesis in human melanoma *(227,228)*; opposed to these angiogenesis promoters in malignant neoplasms are antiangiogenesis agents, such as angiostatin, endostatin, and vasculostatin, derived from the proteolytic cleavage of plasminogen, collagen, and transthyretin *(228–230)*. The vascular supply issue is a vital piece to the puzzle of melanoma metastases and may partly explain, for example, why melanoma micrometastases appear to remain dormant in a given lymph node station, perhaps for years. When compared with clinically apparent and biologically significant macro-metastases, it has been established that micrometastatic deposits have low proliferation rates that correlate to hypovascularity *(231)*. In the future, certain growth factors will likely be proven to be essential prerequisites to the acquisition of the metastasizing melanoma phenotype and, of these, some may emerge as possible therapeutic targets.

VEGF and ICAM-1

VEGF is a homodimeric endothelial cytokine that increases vascular permeability *(232)* and promotes endothelial mitogenesis. The expression of VEGF correlates with thick, as opposed to thin, melanoma and with the absence of regression *(233)*. Transition from radial to vertical growth phase melanoma is associated with the accumulation of VEGF in tumor stroma *(234)*. In concert with the expression of VEGF, all melanoma cell lines tested in one in vitro study also expressed receptors for VEGF, flt-1, and KDR *(235)*. Dysplastic, Spitz, and blue nevi do not express VEGF *(233)*. The *Ha-Ras* gene appears to exercise some regulatory control over VEGF expression *(236)*. Using sensitive radioimmunoassay, elevated levels of soluble VEGF are demonstrable in patients with melanoma vs normal controls, although it is not clear that survival correlates with the level of expression *(237)*. One study showed that 6 of 10 patients with VEGF-expressing primary melanomas developed metastases, whereas all of four VEGF-negative primary tumors remained disease-free at 5-yr follow-up *(238)*. Cofunctional ligands of the VEGF receptor that inhibit VEGF binding inhibit neoangiogenesis and lung metastases in murine melanoma cell lines *(239)*. The morphological hallmark of mela-noma angiogenesis is a glomeruloid pattern of microvascular proliferation typically associated with upregulated expression in tumor endothelia of the VEGF-A receptors KDR, FLT-1, and neuropilin-1, as well as VEGF protein, associated with stromal ex-pression of thrombospondin-1 *(240)*. All isoforms of VEGF-A appear to be operative in vertical growth phase melanoma *(241)*.

Expression of VEGF appears not to be mediated through upregulation of ICAM-1 expression by endothelia *(242)*. The soluble form of ICAM-1 is elaborated by melanoma cells in a fashion that correlates with tumor progression *(242)*; melanoma-secreted interferon-1α upregulates the shedding of ICAM-1 by endothelia and thus affords a mechanism by which melanoma cells can enhance their angio-adhesive properties. There appear to be other independent and distinctive pathways of tumor angiogenesis. One of these is the tyrosine kinase with immunoglobulin-like and epidermal growth factor homology domains, or Tie family *(243)*. Both the Tie pathway and VEGF proved essen-tial to tumor angiogenesis in one in vitro study *(243)*.

Melanomas appear to be capable of producing their own lymphatic supply as well, including in the context of tumor emboli; intratumoral lymphatics as demonstrated with the lymphatic endothelial marker LYVE-1 correlate with poor disease-free survival *(244)*. Through a real-time polymerase chain reaction methodology, expression levels of LYVE-1 were found to correlate with those of VEGF-C messenger RNA in vertical, as opposed to horizontal, growth phase melanoma, as well as with local recurrence and metastatic disease *(245)*. It appears that VEGF-C has high specificity for lymphatic endothelium and is differentially expressed in melanoma cells harvested from lymph node deposits *(246)*.

Basic Fibroblast Growth Factor

bFGF is a heparin-binding polypeptide that has potent angiogenic properties. Although not expressed in normal melanocytes but a requisite for their sustenance in culture, bFGF is expressed early in the acquisition of the invasive melanoma phenotype *(247)*. The transduction of normal melanocytes by bFGF in culture systems results in the acquisition of a transformed phenotype manifesting anchorage-independent growth in agar *(248)*. It appears that bFGF plays a decisive role in the acquisition of the early tumorigenic phenotype, because the growth and migration of radial growth phase melanoma cells in skin reconstructs and tumorigenicity in vivo occurs only after transduction of early radial growth phase melanoma cells with a vector bearing the *bFGF* gene *(249)*. Lentigo maligna, which has a longer *in situ* phase than superficial spreading melanoma, also expresses significantly less bFGF in tumor cells and manifests lower dermal microvessel density *(250)*. Melanoma cell lines in culture express bFGF in proportion to their meta-static capability *(251)*, and, when injected into nude mice, cell lines expressing the highest levels of bFGF have the greatest angiogenic impact *(252)*. Administration of a liposome-based FGF peptide vaccine to mice resulted in the generation of a specific anti-FGF antibody response, blocking neovascularization in an in vitro model and inhibiting experimental metastases by more than 90% *(122)*. Microvessel density is low in common acquired nevi and increases proportionately in dysplastic nevi, primary melanoma, and metastases in a fashion that correlates with FGF2 expression *(253)*. The expression of bFGF in peritumoral mast cells may suggest a role for mast cell-induced angiogenesis; melanomas produce mast cell chemoattractant and degranulating factors *(254,255)*. Mast cell densities and tryptase expression correlate with FGF-2 elaboration and with microvessel density in melanocytic tumor progression *(253)*.

The expression of bFGF in desmoplastic melanoma has been thought to be one potential explanation for the fibroblastic stromal reaction in these tumors. When analyzing the distribution of bFGF by immunohistochemical means, one group found nuclear and/or cytoplasmic expression in 95% of desmoplastic melanomas vs only 31% of nonsclerosing tumors, in which bFGF is expressed only at the advancing edge of the lesions *(255)*. Immunoreactivity of peritumoral and intratumoral endothelia for the same antibody was demonstrated, supporting a role for bFGF in promoting angiogenesis in vivo. Cell culture studies provide support for a potential role for bFGF in tumoral fibrogenesis as a function of cooperation between melanoma cells and fibroblasts in co-culture *(256)*. The expression of bFGF in areas of fibroplasia around dysplastic nevi and in regressed areas of melanoma provides further support for an important role for this cytokine in tumor–stromal interactions *(247)*. The elaboration of bFGF by vertical growth phase melanoma cells in vivo could explain the seeming paradox of the correlation between regression and metastatic events, in concert with both the neoangiogenesis and the fibroplasia at the regressed primary tumor sites. As noted on page 379, clonal autonomy in melanoma is associated with the autocrine stimulation of melanoma cells through their acquisition of the capacity to elaborate bFGF, a growth factor on which intra-epidermal melanocytes are dependent for sustained growth *(146)*.

Laminin Expression and Extravascular Migratory Metastasis

In addition to endovascular hematogenous trafficking of melanoma cells during the establishment of metastatic deposits, melanomas can, in animal models, grow through the extracellular matrix by extending along the abluminal surface of endothelia through an amorphous extracellular laminin-rich matrix *(257)*. The source of laminin appears to derive from endothelia after their interaction with melanoma cells *(258,259)*; β-2 laminin is consistently and selectively expressed in an angiocentric disposition around tumor microvessels *(260)* and may play a role in the promotion of tumor cell migration along the abluminal vascular surface, a phenomenon termed *extravascular migratory metastasis*. This laminin-rich extravascular matrix is observed in both primary and secondary neoplasms *(260)*.

CD40

CD40, a receptor on the surface of lymphocytes, has important functions in the immune response and has been demonstrated in various carcinomas and melanomas, in which it may function as a receptor for mitogenic signals. CD40 manifests variable expression in radial and vertical growth phase components of melanoma, in which patients whose tumors show CD40 expression have a significantly shorter disease-free survival. Patients whose tumors express the CD40 ligand in addition to CD40 also have a shorter disease-free survival time relative to those who do not express CD40 ligand. CD40 expression is seen in benign melanocytic lesions, confined mainly to the superficial components along the dermoepidermal junction and within proliferative nodules of congenital nevi *(261)*.

CONCLUSIONS AND PERSPECTIVES

The stepwise events that lead to the neoplastic degeneration of the melanocyte follow a specific, apparently site-dependent path, which is variable and has different possible outcomes depending on the nature of the host genomic soil, on the microenvironment in which the tumor arises, and on epigenetic factors that modulate the transforming events. Our understanding of melanoma biology will lead to a better comprehension not only of prevention, but also of treatment and of the morphological hallmarks of each step on the path from melanocyte to metastatic seed.

ACKNOWLEDGMENTS

We are indebted to Dr. Esther Israels of Winnipeg, MB and to David Searle of Core Health Services, Concord, ON, for permitting use of figures from *Mechanisms in Hematology*, 3rd Ed. (2002).

REFERENCES

1. Rigel DS, Carucci JA. Malignant melanoma: prevention, early detection, and treatment in the 21st century. CA Cancer J Clin 2000;50:215–236.
2. Hecht F. The annals of cancer genetics. The description by Norris of hereditary malignant melanoma of the skin in 1820. Cancer Genet Cytogenet 1989;42:153–156.
3. Greene MH, Goldin LR, Clark WH Jr, et al. Familial cutaneous malignant melanoma: autosomal trait possibly linked to the Rh locus. Proc Natl Acad Sci USA 1993;80:6071–6075.
4. Bale SJ, Dracopoli NC, Tucker MA, et al. Mapping the gene for hereditary cutaneous malignant melanoma-dysplastic nevus to chromosome 1p. N Engl J Med 1989;320:1367–1372.

5. Cannon-Albright LA, Goldgar ME, Meyer LJ, et al. Assignment of a locus for familial melanoma, MLM, to chromosome 9p13–p22. Science 1992;258:1148–1152.

6. Nancarrow DJ, Mann GJ, Holland EA, et al. Confirmation of chromosome 9p linkage to familial melanoma. Am J Hum Genet 1993;53:936–942.

7. Gruis NA, Sandkuijl LA, Weber JL, et al. Linkage analysis in Dutch familial atypical multiple-mole melanoma (FAMMM) syndrome families. Effect of naevus count. Melanoma Res 1993;3:271–277.

8. Goldstein AM, Dracopoli NC, Engelstein M, Fraser MC, Clark WH Jr, Tucker MA. Linkage of cutaneous malignant melanoma/dysplastic nevi to chromosome 9p, and evidence for genetic heterogeneity. Am J Hum Genet 1994;54:489–496.

9. Hussussian CJ, Struewing JP, Goldstein AM, et al. Germline p16 mutations in familial melanoma. Nat Genet 1994;8:15–21.

10. MacGeoch C, Bishop JA, Bataille V, et al. Genetic heterogeneity in familial malignant melanoma. Hum Mol Genet 1994;3:2195–2200.

11. Holland EA, Beaton SC, Becker TM, et al. Analysis of the p16 gene, CDKN2, in 17 Australian melanoma kindreds. Oncogene 1995;11:2289–2294.

12. Flores J, Pollock PM, Walker GJ, et al. Analysis of the CDK2NA, CDKN2B and CDK4 genes in 48 Australian melanoma kindreds. Oncogene 1997;15:2999–3005.

13. Halaban R, Miglarese MR, Smicun Y, Puig S. Melanomas, from the cell cycle point of view. Int J Mol Med 1998;1:419–425.

14. Isshiki K, Seng BA, Elder DE, Guerry D, Linnenbach AJ. Chromosome 9 deletion in sporadic and familial melanomas in vivo. Oncogene 1994;9:1649–1653.

15. Nobori T, Miura K, Wu DJ, Lois A, Takabayashi K, Carson DA. Deletions of the cyclin-dependent kinase-4 inhibitor gene in multiple human cancers. Nature 1994;268:753–756.

16. Ohta M, Nagai H, Shimizu M, et al. Rarity of somatic and germline mutations of the cyclin-dependent kinase 4 inhibitor gene, CDK4I, in melanoma. Cancer Res 1994;54:5269–5272.

17. Ohta M, Berd D, Shimizu M, et al. Deletion mapping of chromosome region 9p21–p22 surrounding the CDKN2 locus in melanoma. Int J Cancer 1996;65:762–767.

18. Walker GJ, Palmer JM, Walters MK, Hayward NKA. Genetic models of melanoma tumorigenesis based on allelic losses. Genes Chromosomes Cancer 1995;12:134–141.

19. Luca M, Xie S, Gutman M, Huang S, Bar-Eli M. Abnormalities in the CDKN2A (p16INK4/MTS-1) gene in human melanoma cells: relevance to tumor growth and metastasis. Oncogene 1995;11:1399–1402.

20. Platz A, Hansson J, Mansson-Brahms E, et al. Screening of germline mutations in the CDKN2A genes in Swedish families with hereditary utaneous melanoma. J Natl Cancer Inst 1997;89:697–702.

21. Hogg D, Brill H, Liu L, et al. Role of the cyclin-dependent kinase inhibitor CDKN2A in familial melanoma. J Cutan Med Surg 1998;2:172–179.

22. Monzon J, Liu L, Brill H, et al. CDKN2A mutations in multiple primary melanomas. N Engl J Med 1998;338:879–887.

23. Kovar H, Jug G, Ayre DNT, et al. Among genes involved in the RB dependent cell cycle regulatory cascade, the p16 tumor suppressor gene is frequently lost in the Ewing family of tumors. Oncogene 1997;165:2225–2232.

24. Grana X, Reddy EP. Cell cycle control in mammalian cells: role of cyclins, cyclin dependent kinases (CDK's), growth suppressor genes and cyclin-dependent kinase inhibitors (CKI's). Oncogene 1995;11:211–219.

25. Harland M, Meloni R, Gruis N, et al. Germline mutations of the CDKN2 gene in UK melanoma families. Hum Mol Genet 1997;6:2061–2067.

26. Hashemi J, Linder S, Platz A, Hansson J. Melanoma development in relation to non-functional p16/INK4a protein and dysplastic nevus syndrome in Swedish melanoma kindreds. Melanoma Res 1999;9:21–30.

27. Lee JY, Dong SM, Shin MS, et al. Genetic alterations of p16INK4a and p53 genes in sporadic dysplastic nevus. Biochem Biophys Res Commun 1997;237:667–672.

28. Park WS, Vortmeyer AO, Pack S, et al. Allelic deletion at chromosome 9p21 (p16) and 17p13 (p53) in microdissected sporadic dysplastic nevus. Hum Pathol 1998;29:127–130.

29. Whiteman DC, Milligan A, Welch J, Green AC, Hayward NK. Germline CDKN2A mutations in childhood melanoma (letter). J Natl Cancer Inst 1997;89:1460.

30. Robertson GP, Goldberg EK, Lugo TG, Fountain JW. Functional localization of a melanoma tumor suppressor gene to a small (< or = 2 Mb) region on 11q23. Oncogene 1999;18:3173–3180.

31. Walker GJ, Nancarrow DJ, Walters MK, Palmer JM, Weber JL, Hayward NK. Linkage analysis in familial melanoma kindreds to markers on chromosome 6p. Int J Cancer 1994;59:771–775.
32. Goldstein AM, Goldin LR, Dracopoli, NC, Clark WH Jr, Tucker MA. Two-locus linkage analysis of cutaneous malignant melanoma/dysplastic nevi. Am J Hum Genet 1996;58:1050–1056.
33. Platz A, Hansson J, Ringborg U. Screening of germline mutations in the CDK4, CDKN2C and TP53 genes in familial melanoma: a clinic-based population study. Int J Cancer 1998;78:13–15.
34. Battistutta D, Palmer J, Walters M, Walker G, Nancarrow D, Hayward N. Incidence of familial melanoma and MLM2 gene. Lancet 1994;344:1607–1608.
35. Soler-Carrillo J, Puig S, Palou J, Castel T, Lecha M. p16 protein expression as an important prognostic factor in primary cutaneous malignant melanoma (abstract). Am J Dermatopathol 1998;20:603.
36. Fujimoto A, Morita R, Hatta N, Takehara K, Takata M. p16INK4a inactivation is not frequent in uncultured sporadic primary melanoma. Oncogene 1999;18:2527–2532.
37. Hecht F, Hecht BK. Chromosome rearrangements in dysplastic nevus syndrome predisposing to malignant melanoma. Cancer Genet Cytogenet 1998;35:73–78.
38. Puig S, Ruiz A, Lazaro C, et al. Chromosome 9p deletions in cutaneous malignant melanoma tumors: the minimal deleted region involves markers outside the p16 (CDNK2) gene. Am J Hum Genet 1995;57:395–402.
39. Healy E, Rehman I, Angus B, Rees JL. Loss of heterozygosity in sporadic primary melanoma. Genes Chromosomes Cancer 1995;12:152–156.
40. Healy E, Belgaid CE, Takata M, et al. Allelotypes of primary cutaneous melanoma and benign melanocytic nevi. Cancer Res 1996;56:589–593.
41. Dracopoli NC, Fountain JW. CDNK2 mutations in melanoma. Cancer Surv 1995;26:115–132.
42. Morita R, Fujimoto A, Hatta N, Takehara K, Takata M. Comparison of genetic profiles between primary melanomas and their metastases reveals genetic alterations and clonal evolution during progression. J Invest Dermatol 1998;111:919–924.
43. Gonzalez-Gomes P, Bello MJ, Alonso ME, et al. Promotor methylation status of multiple genes in brain metastases of solid tumors. Int J Mol Med 2004;13:93–98.
44. Sviderskaya EV, Gray-Schopfer VC, Hill SP, et al. p16/cyclin-dependent kinase inhibitor 2A deficiency in human melanocyte senescence, apoptosis, and immortalization: possible implications for melanoma progression. J Natl Cancer Inst 2003;95:723–732.
45. Bandyopadhyay D, Medrano EE. Melanin accumulation accelerates melanocyte sensescence by a mechanism involving p16INK4a/CDK4/pRB and E2F1. Ann NY Acad Sci 2000;908:71–84.
46. Moan J, Dahlback A, Setlow RB. Epidemiological support for an hypothesis for melanoma induction indication a role for UVA radiation. Photochem Photobiol 1999;70:243–247.
47. Huot TJ, Rowe J, Harland M, et al. Biallelic mutations in p16(INK4a) confer resistance to Ras- and Ets-induced senescence in human diploid fibroblasts. Mol Cell Biol 2002;22:8135–8143.
48. Cerroni L, Soyer P, Kerl H. bcl-2 protein expression in cutaneous malignant melanoma and benign melanocytic nevi. Am J Dermatopathol 1995;17:7–11.
49. Morales-Ducret CRJ, van de Rijn M, Smoller BR. Bcl-2 expression in melanocytic nevi. Arch Dermatol 1995;131:915–918.
50. Ramsey JA, From L, Kahn HJ. Bcl-2 protein expression in melanocytic neoplasms of the skin. Mod Pathol 1995;8:150–154.
51. Saenz-Santamaria MC, Reed JA, McNutt NS, Shea CR. Immunohistochemical expression of BCL-2 in melanomas and intradermal nevi. J Cutan Pathol 1994;21:393–397.
52. Crowson AN, Magro CM, Kadin M, Stranc M. Differential expression of bcl-2 oncogene in human basal cell carcinoma. Hum Pathol 1996;27:355–359.
53. Crowson AN, Pilavdzic D, Stranc M, Magro CM. Expression of p21[WAF1/CIP1] in aggressive- versus non-aggressive-growth basal cell carcinoma: a comparative study. Lab Invest 1999;79:56A (abstract).
54. Peris K, Keller G, Chimenti S, et al. Microsatellite instability and loss of heterozygosity in melanoma. J Invest Dermatol 1995;105:625–628.
55. Bastian BC, Olshen AB, LeBoit PE, Pinkel D. Classifying melanocytic tumors based on DNA copy number changes. Am J Pathol 2003;163:1765–1770.
56. Oltvai ZN, Korsmeyer SJ. Checkpoints of dueling dimers foil death wishes. Cell 1994;79:189–192.
57. Zhuang L, Wang B, Sauder DN. Molecular mechanisms of ultraviolet-induced keratinocyte apoptosis. J Interferon Cytokine Res 2000;20:445–454.
58. Smith KJ, Barrett TL, Smith WF, Skelton HM. A review of tumor suppressor genes in cutaneous neoplasms with emphasis on cell cycle regulators. Am J Dermatopathol 1998;20:302–313.

59. Rolfe M, Beer-Romero P, Glass S, et al. Reconstitution of p53-ubiquitinylation reactions from purified components: the role of human ubiquitin-conjugating enzyme UBC4 and E6-associated protein (E6AP). Proc Natl Acad Sci USA 1995;92:3264–3269.
60. Campbell C, Quinn AG, Angus B, et al. Wavelength specific patterns of p53 induction in human skin following exposure to UV radiation. Cancer Res 1993;53:2697–2699.
61. Karjalainen JM, Eskelinen MJ, Kellokoski JK, Reinkainen M, Alhava EM, Kosma VM. P21 (WAF1/CIP1) expression in stage I cutaneous malignant melanoma: its relationship with p53, cell proliferation and survival. Br J Cancer 1999;79:895–902.
62. Stein GH, Dulic B. Molecular mechanisms for the senescent cell cycle arrest. J Invest Dermatol Symp Pro 1998;5:14.
63. Smith KJ, Germain M, Skelton HM. Perspectives in dermatopathology: telomeres and telomerase in ageing and cancer; with emphasis on cutaneous disease. J Cutan Pathol 2000;27:2–18.
64. Elliott PJ, Ross JS. The proteosome. A new target for novel drug therapies. Am J Clin Pathol 2001;116:637–646.
65. Wehrli P, Viard I, Bullani R, Tschopp J, French LE. Death receptors in cutaneous biology and disease. J Invest Dermatol 2000;115:141–148.
66. Mouawad R, Antoine EC, Khayat D, Soubrane C. Effect of endogenous interleukin-6 on Fas (APO-1/CD95) receptor expression in advanced melanoma patients. Cytokines Cell Mol Ther 2000;6:135–140.
67. Eberle J, Fecker LF, Hossini AM, et al. CD95/Fas signaling in human melanoma cells: conditional expression of CD95L/FasL overcomes the intrinsic apoptosis resistance of malignant melanoma and inhibits growth and progression of human melanoma xenotransplants. Oncogene 2003;22:9131–9141.
68. Kamei T, Inui M, Nakamura S, Okumura K, Goto A, Tagawa T. Interferon-gamma and anti-Fas antibody-induced apoptosis in human melanoma cell lines and its relationship to bcl-2 cleavage. Melanoma Res 2003;13:153–159.
69. Aragane Y, Maeda A, Cui CY, Tezuka T, Kaneda Y, Schwarz T. Inhibition of growth of melanoma cells by CD95 (Fas/APO-1) gene transfer in vivo. J Invest Dermatol 2000;115:1008–1014.
70. Mouawad R, Khayat D, Soubrane C. Plasma Fas ligand, an inducer of apoptosis, and plasma soluble Fas, an inhibitor of apoptosis, in advanced melanoma. Melanoma Res 2000;10:461–467.
71. Ekmekcioglu S, Okcu MF, Colome-Grimmer MI, Owen-Schaub L, Buzaid AC, Grimm EA. Differential increase of Fas ligand expression on metastatic and thin or thick primary melanoma cells compared with interleukin-10. Melanoma Res 1999;9:261–272.
72. Soubrane C, Mouawad R, Antoine EC, Verola O, Gil-Delgado M, Khayat D. A comparative study of Fas and Fas-ligand expression during melanoma progression. Br J Dermatol 2000;143:307–312.
73. Blackburn EH. Structure and function of telomeres. Nature 1991;350:569–573.
74. Faraoni I, Graziani G, Turriziani M, et al. Suppression of telomerase activity as an indicator of drug-induced cytotoxicity against cancer cells: in vitro studies with fresh human tumor samples. Lab Invest 1999;79:993–1005.
75. Anderson S, Shera K, Ihle J, et al. Telomerase activation in cervical cancer. Am J Pathol 1997;151:25–31.
76. Terasawa K, Sagae S, Takeda T, Ishioka S, Kobayashi K, Kudo R. Telomerase activity in malignant ovarian tumors with deregulation of cell cycle regulatory proteins. Cancer Lett 1999;142:207–217.
77. Nakano K, Watney E, MacDougall JK. Telomerase activity and expression of telomerase RNA component and telomerase catalytic subunit gene in cervical cancer. Am J Pathol 1998;153:857–864.
78. Mokbel K, Parris CN, Ghilchik M, Williams G, Newbold RF. The association between telomerase, histopathological parameters, and Ki-67 expression in breast cancer. Am J Surg Pathol 1999;178:69–72.
79. Poremba C, Willenbring H, Hero B, et al. Telomerase activity distinguishes between neuroblastomas with good and poor prognosis. Ann Oncol 1999;10:715–721.
80. Jong HS, Park YI, Sim S, et al. Up-regulation of human telomerase catalytic subunit during gastric carcinogenesis. Cancer 1999;86:559–565.
81. Holt SE, Glinksy VV, Ivanova AB, Glinsky GV. Resistance to apoptosis in human cells conferred by telomerase function and telomere stability. Mol Carcinog 1999;25:241–248.
82. Zhu J, Wang H, Bishop JM, Blackburn EH. Telomerase extends the lifespan of virus-transformed human cells without net telomere lengthening. Proc Natl Acad Sci USA 1999;96:3723–3728.
83. Kugoh H, Shigenami K, Funaki K, Barrett JC, Oshimura M. Human chromosome 5 carries a putative telomerase repressor gene. Genes Chromosomes Cancer 2003;36:37–47.
84. Novakovic S, Hocevar M, Zgajnar J, Besic N, Stegel V. Detection of telomerase RNA in the plasma of patients with breast cancer, malignant melanoma or thyroid cancer. Oncol Rep 2004;11:245–252.

85. Slater M, Scolyer RA, Gidley-Baird A, Thompson JF, Barend JA. Increased expression of apoptoic markes in melanoma. Melanoma Res 2003;13:137–145.

86. Rudolph P, Schubert C, Tamm S, et al. Telomerase activity in melanocytic lesions: a potential marker of tumor biology. Am J Pathol 2000;156:1425–1432.

87. Becker B, Muthoff G, Farkas B, et al. Induction of Hsp90 protein expression in malignant melanomas and melanoma metastases. Exp Dermatol 2004;13:27–32.

88. Smith CD, Blackburn EH. Uncapping and deregulation of telomeres lead to detrimental consequences in yeast. J Cell Biol 1999;145:203–214.

89. Kerl H, Soyer HP, Cerroni L, Wolf IH, Ackerman AB. Ancient melanocytic nevus. Semin Diagn Pathol 1998;15:210–215.

90. Yawata T, Kamino H, Kugoh H, et al. Identification of a </=600-kb region on human chromosome 1q42.3 inducing cellular senescence. Oncogene 2003;22:281–290.

91. Verra NC, Jorritsma A, Weijer K, et al. Human telomerase reverse transcriptase-transduced human cytotoxic T-cells suppress the growth of human melanoma in immunodeficient mice. Cancer Res 2004;64:2153–2161.

92. Easty DJ, Bennett DC. Protein tyrosine kinases in malignant melanoma. Melanoma Res 2000;10:401-411.

93. McMahon G. VEGF signalling in tumor angiogenesis. Oncologist 2000;5(Suppl 1):3–10.

94. Urquhart JL, Meech SJ, Marr DG, Shellman YG, Duke RC, Norris DA. Regulation of Fas-mediated apoptosis by N-ras in melanomas. J Invest Dermatol 2002;119:556–561.

95. Ramon y Cajal S, Suster S, Halaban R, Filvaroff E, Dotto GP. Induction of different morphological features of malignant melanoma and pigmented lesions after transformation of murine melanocytes with bFGF-cDNA and H-ras, myc, neu and E1a oncogenes. Am J Pathol 1991;138:349–358.

96. Otto FJ, Goldmann T, Biess B, Lippold A, Suter L, Westhoff U. Prognostic classification of malignant melanoma by combining clinical, histological, and immunohistochemical parameters. Oncology 1999;56:208–214.

97. Grover R, Chana J, Grobbelaar AO, et al. Measurement of c-myc oncogene expression provides an accurate prognostic marker for acral lentiginous melanoma. Br J Plast Surg 1999;52:122–126.

98. Grover R, Pacifico MD, Wilson GD, Sanders R. Use of oncogene expression as an independent prognostic marker for primary melanoma. Ann Plast Surg 2003;50:183–187.

99. Hussein MR, Haemel AK, Wood GS. Apoptosis and melanoma: molecular mechansisms. J Pathol 2003;199:275–288.

100. Biroccio A, Amodei S, Antonelli A, Benassi B, Zupi G. Inhibition of c-Myc oncoprotein limits the growth of human melanoma cells by inducing cellular crisis. J Biol Chem 2003;278:35,693–35,701.

101. Pastorino F, Brignole C, Marimpietri D, et al. Targeted liposomal c-myc antisense oligodeoxynucleotides induce apoptosis and inhibit tumor growth and metastases in human melanoma models. Clin Cancer Res 2003;9:4594–4605.

102. Peltenburg LT, de Bruin EC, Meersma D, Wilting S, Jurgensmeier JM, Schrier PI. C-Myc is able to sensitize human melanoma cells to diverse apoptotic triggers. Melanoma Res 2004;14:3–12.

103. Utikal J, Leiter U, Udart M, Kaskal P, Peter RU, Krahn GM. Expression of c-myc and bcl-2 in primary and advanced cutaneous melanoma. Cancer Invest 2002;20:914–921.

104. Seykora JT, Jih D, Elenitsas R, Horng WH, Elder DE. Gene expression profiling of melanocytic tumors. Am J Dermatopathol 2003;25:6–11.

105. Kallioniemi A, Kallioniemi OP, Sudar D, et al. Comparative genomic hybridization for molecular cytogenetic analysis of solid tumors. Science 1992;258:818–821.

106. Pinkel D, Segraves R, Sudar D, et al. High resolution analysis of DNA copy number variation using comparative genomic hybridization to microarrays. Nat Genet 1998;20:207–211.

107. Snijders AM, Nowak N, Segraves R, et al. Assembly of microarrays for genome-wide measurement of DNA copy number. Nat Genet 2001;29:263–264.

108. Albertson DG, Ylstra B, Segraves R, et al. Quantitative mapping of amplicon structure by array CGH identified CYP24 as a candidate oncogene. Nat Genet 2000;25:144–146.

109. Ishkanian AS, Malloff CA, Watson SK, et al. A tiling resolution DNA microarray with complete coverage of the human genome. Nat Genet 2004;36:299–303.

110. Bastian BC, LeBoit PE, Hamm H, Brocker EB, Pinkel D. Chromosomal gains and losses in primary cutaneous melanomas detected by comparative genomic hybridization. Cancer Res 1998;58:2170–2175.

111. Bastian BC, Kashani-Sabet M, Hamm H, et al. Gene amplifications characterize acral melanomas and permit the detection of occult tumor cells in the surrounding skin. Cancer Res 2000;60:1968–1973.

112. Sauter ER, Yeo UC, vonStemm A, et al. Cyclin D1 is a candidate oncogene in cutaneous melanoma. Cancer Res 2002;62:3200–3206.

113. Bastian BC, Wesselmann U, Pinkel D, LeBoit PE. Molecular cytogenetic analysis of Spitz nevi shows clear differences to melanoma. J Invest Dermatol 1999;113:1065–1069.

114. Winokur TS, Palazzo JP, Johnson WC, Duray PH. Evaluation of DNA ploidy in dysplastic and Spitz nevi by flow cytometry. J Cutan Pathol 1990;17:342–347.

115. Crowson AN, Magro CM, Mihm MC Jr. The biology of malignant melanoma. In: The Melanocytic Proliferations: A Comprehensive Textbook of Pigmented Lesions. John Wiley and Sons, New York, NY, 2001: pp. 449–476.

116. Pollock PM, Harper UL, Hansen KS, et al. High frequency of BRAF mutations in nevi. Nat Genet 2003;33:19–20.

117. Davies H, Bignell GR, Cox C, et al. Mutations of the BRAF gene in human cancer. Nature 2002;417:949–954.

118. Maldonado JL, Fridlyand J, Patel H, et al. Determinants of BRAF mutations in primary melanomas. J Natl Cancer Inst 2003;95:1878–1890.

119. Harvell JD, Bastian BC, LeBoit PE. Persistent (recurrent) Spitz nevi: a histopathologic, immunohistochemical, and molecular pathologic study of 22 cases. Am J Surg Pathol 2002;26:654–661.

120. Maldonado JL, Timmerman L, Fridlyand J, Bastian BC. Mechanisms of cell-cycle arrest in Spitz nevi with constitutive activation of the MAP-kinase pathway. Am J Pathol 2004;164:1783–1787.

121. Jansen B, Schlagbauer-Wadl H, Kahr H, et al. Novel Ras antagonist blocks human melanoma growth. Proc Natl Acad Sci USA 1999;96:14,019–14,029.

122. Plum SM, Holaday JW, Ruiz A, Madsen JW, Fogler WE, Fortier AH. Administration of a liposomal FGF-2 peptide vaccine leads to abrogation of FGF-2-mediated angiogenesis and tumor development. Vaccine 2000;19:1294–1303.

123. Ramsay JA, From L, Iscoe NA, Kahn HJ. MIB-1 proliferative activity is a significant prognostic factor in primary thick cutaneous melanomas. J Invest Dermatol 1995;105:22–26.

124. Sparrow LE, English DR, Taran JM, Heenan PJ. Prognostic significance of MIB-1 proliferative activity in thin melanomas and immunohistochemical analysis of MIB-1 proliferative activity in melanocytic tumors. Am J Dermatopathol 1998;20:12–16.

125. Penneys N, Seigfried E, Nahass G, Vogler C. Expression of proliferating cell nuclear antigen in Spitz nevus. J Am Acad Dermatol 1995;32:964–967.

126. Vecchiato A, Rossi CR, Montesco MC, et al. Proliferating cell nuclear antigen (PCNA) and recurrence in patients with cutaneous melanoma. Melanoma Res 1994;4:207–211.

127. Karlsson M, Boeryd B, Carstensen J, et al. Correlation of Ki-67 and PCNA to DNA ploidy, S-phase fraction and survival in uveal melanoma. Eur J Cancer 1996;32A:357–362.

128. Roels S, Tilmant K, Ducatelle R. PCNA and Ki67 proliferation markers as criteria for prediction of clinical behaviour of melanocytic tumours in cats and dogs. J Comp Pathol 1999;121:13–24.

129. Niezabitowski A, Czajecki K, Rys J, et al. Prognostic evaluation of cutaneous malignant melanoma: a clinicopathological and immunohistochemical study. J Surg Oncol 1999;70:150–160.

130. Goldmann T, Ribbert D, Suter L, Brode M, Otto F. Tumor characteristics involved in the metastatic behaviour as an improvement in primary cutaneous melanoma prognostics. J Exp Clin Cancer Res 1998;17:483–489.

131. Reddy VB, Gattuso P, Aranha G, Carson HJ. Cell proliferation markers in predicting metastases in malignant melanoma. J Cutan Pathol 1995;22:248–251.

132. Karjalainen JM, Eskelinen MJ, Nordling S, Lipponen PK, Alhava EM, Kosma VM. Mitotic rate and S-phase fraction as prognostic factors in stage I cutaneous malignant melanoma. Br J Cancer 1998;77:1917–1925.

133. Azzola MF, Shaw HM, Thompson JF, et al. Tumor mitotic rate is a more powerful prognostic indicator than ulceration in patients with primary cutaneous melanoma: an analysis of 3661 patients from a single center. Cancer 2003;97:1488–1498.

134. Balch CM, Buzaid AC, Atkins MB, et al. A new American Joint Committee on Cancer staging system for cutaneous melanoma. Cancer 2000;88:1484–1491.

135. Cochran AJ. Prediction of outcome for patients with cutaneous melanoma. Pigment Cell Res 1997;10:162–167.

136. Rebora A. Prognosing melanomas: the argyrophilic nucleolar organizer region approach. Dermatology 1992;185:166–168.

137. Heinisch G, Barth J. [AgNOR expression in skin tumors. Studies of melanocytic, epidermal and fibrohistiocytic lesions]. Hautarzt 1995;46:177–185.

138. Howat AJ, Wright AL, Cotton DW, Reeve S. AgNORs in benign, dysplastic and malignant melanocytic skin lesions. Am J Dermatopathol 1990;12:156–161.
139. Fogt F, Vortmeyer AO, Tahan SR. Nucleolar organizer regions (AgNOR) and Ki-67 immunostaining in melanocytic skin lesions. Am J Dermatopathol 1995;17:12–17.
140. Fernandez-Pol JA, Klos DJ, Hamilton PD. A growth factor-inducible gene encodes a novel nuclear protein with a zinc finger structure. J Biol Chem 1993;268:21,198–21,204.
141. Ganger DR, Hamilton PD, Fletcher JW, Fernandez-Pol JA. Metallopanstimulin is overexpressed in a patient with colonic carcinoma. Anticancer Res 1997;17:1993–1999.
142. Fernandez-Pol JA, Fletcher FW, Hamilton PD, Klos DJ. Expression of metallopanstimulin and oncogenesis in human prostatic carcinoma. Anticancer Res 1997;17:1519–1530.
143. Fernandez-Pol JA. Metallopanstimulin as a novel tumor marker in sera of patients with various types of common cancers: implications for prevention and therapy. Anticancer Res 1996;16:2177–2185.
144. Santa Cruz DJ, Hamilton PD, Klos DJ, Fernandez-Pol JA. Differential expression of metallopanstimulin/S27 ribosomal protein in melanocytic lesions of the skin. J Cutan Pathol 1997;24:533–542.
145. Hsu MY, Meier FE, Nesbit M, et al. E-cadherin expression in melanoma cells restores keratinocyte-mediated growth control and down-regulates expression of invasion-associated adhesion receptors. Am J Pathol 2000;156:1515–1525.
146. Shih IM, Herlyn M. Role of growth factors and their receptors in the development and progression of melanoma. J Invest Dermatol 1993;100(Suppl 2):196S–203S.
147. Kato J, Wanebo H, Calabresi P, Clark JW. Basic fibroblast growth factor production and growth factor receptors as potential targets for melanoma therapy. Melanoma Res 1992;2:13–23.
148. Sparrow LE, Heenan PJ. Differential expression of epidermal growth factor receptor in melanocytic tumours demonstrated by immunohistochemistry and mRNA in situ hybridization. Australas J Dermatol 1999;40:19–24.
149. Moretti S, Pinzi C, Spallanzani A, et al. Immunohistochemical evidence of cytokine networks during progression of human melanocytic lesions. Int J Cancer 1999;84:160–168.
150. Rodeck U, Nishiyama T, Mauviel A. Independent regulation of growth and SMAD-mediated transcription by transforming growth factor beta in human melanoma cells. Cancer Res 1999;59:547–550.
151. Reed JA, McNutt NS, Prieto VG, Albino AP. Expression of transforming growth factor-beta 2 in malignant melanoma correlates with depth of tumor invasion. Implications for tumor progression. Am J Pathol 1994;145:97–104.
152. Faasen AE, Mooradian DL, Tranquillo RT, et al. Cell surface CD44-related chondroitin sulfate proteoglycan is required for transforming growth factor-stimulated mouse melanoma cell motility and invasive behaviour on type I collagen. J Cell Sci 1993;106:501–511.
153. Van Belle PA, Elenitsas R, Satyamoorthy K, et al. Progression-related expression of β3 integrin in melanomas and nevi. Hum Pathol 1999;33:562–567.
154. Schumacher D, Schaumberg-Lever G. Ultrastructural localization of alpha-3 integrin subunit in malignant melanoma and adjacent epidermis. J Cutan Pathol 1999;26:321–326.
155. Hynes RO. Integrins: versatility, modulation and signalling in cell adhesion. Cell 1992;69:11–25.
156. Bartolome RA, Galvez BG, Longo N, et al. Stromal cell-derived factor-1 alpha promotes melanoma cell invasion across basement membranes involving stimulation of membrane-type 1 matrix metalloproteinase and Rho GTPase activities. Cancer Res 2004;64:2534–2543.
157. Moretti S, Martini L, Berti E, Pinzi C, Gianotti B. Adhesion molecule profile and malignancy of melanocytic lesions. Melanoma Res 1993;3:235–239.
158. Melchiori A, Mortarini R, Carlone S, et al. The alpha 3 beta 1 integrin is involved in melanoma cell migration and invasion. Exp Cell Res 1995;219:233–242.
159. Natali PG, Hamby CV, Felding-Habermann B, et al. Clinical significance of alpha(v)beta3 integrin and intercellular adhesion molecule-1 expression in cutaneous malignant melanoma lesions. Cancer Res 1997;57:1554–1560.
160. Goldbrunner RH, Haugland HK, Klein CE, Kerkau S, Roosen K, Tonn JC. ECM dependent and integrin mediated tumor cell migration of human glioma and melanoma cell lines under serum-free conditions. Anticancer Res 1996;16:3679–3687.
161. Kageshita T, Hamby CV, Hirai S, Kimura T, Ono T, Ferrone S. Differential clinical significance of alpha(v)beta3 expression in primary lesions of acral lentiginous melanoma and of other melanoma histotypes. Int J Cancer 2000;89:153–159.
162. Kang IC, Kim DS, Jang Y, Chung KH. Suppressive mechanism of salmosin, a novel disintegrin in B16 melanoma cell metastasis. Biochem Biophys Res Commun 2000;275:169–173.

163. Mitjans F, Meyer T, Fittschen C, et al. In vivo therapy of malignant melanoma by means of antago-nists of alpha v integrins. Int J Cancer 2000;87:716–723.

164. Castel S, Pagan R, Garcia R, et al. Alpha v integrin antagonists induce the disassembly of focal contacts in melanoma cells. Eur J Cell Biol 2000;79:502–512.

165. Sengupta S, Ray S, Chattopadhyay N, Biswas N, Chatterjee A. Effect of retinoic acid on integrin receptors of B16 F10 melanoma cells. J Exp Clin Cancer Res 2000;19:81–87.

166. Hieken TJ, Ronan SG, Farolan M, Shilkaitis AL, Das Gupta TK. Molecular prognostic markers in intermediate-thickness cutaneous malignant melanoma. Cancer 1999;85:375–382.

167. Hieken TJ, Farolan M, Ronan SG, Shilkaitis A, Wild L, Das Gupta TK. Beta3 integrin expression in melanoma predicts subsequent metastasis. J Surg Res 1996;63:169–173.

168. Hieken TJ, Ronan SG, Farolan M, Shilkaitis AL, Das Gupta TK. Beta 1 integrin expression: a marker of lymphatic metastases in cutaneous malignant melanoma. Anticancer Res 1996;16:2321–2324.

169. Moretti S, Pinzi C, Berti E, et al. In situ expression of transforming growth factor beta is associated with melanoma progression and correlates with Ki67, HLA-DR and beta 3 integrin expression. Melanoma Res 1997;7:313–321.

170. Gouon V, Tucker GC, Kraus-Berthier L, Arassi G, Kieffer N. Up-regulated expression of the beta3 integrin and the 92kDa gelatinase in human HT-144 melanoma cell tumors grown in nude mice. Int J Cancer 1996;68:650–662.

171. Peticlerc E, Boutaud A, Presayko A, et al. New functions for non-collagenous domains of human collagen type IV. Novel integrin ligands inhibiting angiogenesis and tumor growth in vivo. J Biol Chem 2000;275:8051–8061.

172. Shahan TA, Fawzi A, Bellon G, Monboisse JC, Kefalides NA. Regulation of tumor cell chemtoaxis by type IV collagen is mediated by a Ca(2+)-dependent mechanism requiring CD47 and the integrin alpha(v)beta(3). J Biol Chem 2000;275:4796–4802.

173. Thorne RF, Marshall JF, Shafren DR, Gibson PG, Hart IR, Burns GF. The inetgrins alpha 3 beta 1 and alpha 6 beta 1 physically and functionally associate with CD36 in human melanoma cells. J Biol Chem 2000;275:35,264–35,275.

174. Fidler IJ, Schackert G, Zhang RD, Radinsky R, Fujimaki T. The biology of melanoma brain metas-tasis. Cancer Metastasis Rev 1999;18:387–400.

175. Hofmann UB, Westphal JR, van Kraats AA, Ruiter DJ, van Muijen GN. Expression of integrin alpha(v)beta(3) correlates with activation of membrane-type matrix metalloproteinase-1 (MT1-MMP) and matrix metalloproteinase-2 (MMP-2) in human melanoma cells in vitro and in vivo. Int J Cancer 2000;87:12–19.

176. Kageshita T, Hamby CV, Hirai S, Kimura T, Ono T, Ferrone S. Alpha(v)beta3 expression on blood vessels and melanoma cells in primary lesions: differential association with tumor progression and clinical prognosis. Cancer Immunol Immunother 2000;49:314–318.

177. Seftor RE, Seftor EA, Hendrix MJ. Molecular role(s) for integrins in human melanoma invasion. Cancer Metastasis Rev 1999;18:359–375.

178. Henriet P, Zhong ZD, Brooks PC, Weinberg KI, DeClerck YA. Contact with fibrillar collagen inhibits melanoma cell proliferation by up-regulating p27KIP1. Proc Natl Acad Sci USA 2000;97:10,026–10,031.

179. Beliveau A, Berube M, Rousseau A, Pelletier G, Guerin SL. Expression of integrin alpha5beta1 and MMPs associated with epithelioid cytomorphology and malignancy of uveal melanoma. Invest Ophthalmol Vis Sci 2000;41:2363–2372.

180. Vihinen P, Nikkola J, Vlaykova T, et al. Prognostic value of beta1 integrin expression in metastatic melanoma. Melanoma Res 2000;10:243–251.

181. Birch M, Mitchell S, Hart IR. Isolation and characterization of human melanoma cell variants expressing high and low levels of CD44. Cancer Res 1991;51:6660–6667.

182. Leigh CJ, Palechek PL, Knutson JR, McCarthy JB, Cohen MB, Argenyi AB. CD44 expression in benign and malignant nevomelanocytic lesions. Hum Pathol 1996;27:1288–1294.

183. Schaider H, Soyer HP, Heider KH, et al. CD44 and variants in melanocytic skin neoplasms. J Cutan Pathol 1998;25:199–203.

184. Ichikawa T, Matsumoto J, Kaneko M, Saida T, Sagara J, Taniguchi S. Moesin and CD44 expression in cutaneous melanocytic tumours. Br J Dermatol 1998;138:763–768.

185. Massi D, Franchi A, Borgogni L, Reali UM, Santucci M. Osteonectin expression correlates with clinical outcome in thin cutaneous malignant melanomas. Hum Pathol 1999;30:339–344.

186. Kuske MD, Johnson JP. Assignment of the human melanoma cell adhesion molecule gene (MCAM) to chromosome 11 band q23.3 by radiation hybrid mapping. Cytogenet Cell Genet 1999;87:258.

187. Shih IM, Speicher D, Hsu MY, Levine E, Herlyn M. Melanoma cell-cell interactions are mediated through heterophile Mel-CAM/ligand interaction. Cancer Res 1997;57:3835–3840.
188. Mintz-Weber CS, Johnson JP. Identification of the elements regulating the expression of the cell adhesion molecule MCAM/MUC18. J Biol Chem 2000;275:34,672–34,680.
189. Xie S, Luca M, Huang S, et al. Expression of MCAM/MUC 18 by human melanoma cells leads to increased tumor growth and metastasis. Cancer Res 1997;57:2295–2303.
190. Xie S, Price JE, Luca M, Jean D, Ronai Z, Bar-Eli M. Dominant-negative CREB inhibits tumor growth and metastasis of human melanoma cells. Oncogene 1997;15:2069–2075.
191. Shih IM. The role of CD146 (Mel-CAM) in biology and pathology. J Pathol 1999;189:4–11.
192. Jean D, Bar-Eli M. Regulation of tumor growth and metastasis of human melanoma by the CREB transcription factor family. Mol Cell Biochem 2000;212:19–28.
193. Jean D, Harbison M, McConkey DJ, Ronai Z, Bar-Eli M. CREB and its associated proteins act as survival factors for human melanoma cells. J Biol Chem 1998;273:24,884–24,890.
194. Ronai Z, Yang YM, Fuchs SY, Adler V, Sardana M, Herlyn M. ATF2 confers radiation resistance to human melanoma cells. Oncogene 1998;16:523–531.
195. Modiano JF, Ritt MG, Wojcieszyn J, Mith R 3rd. Growth arrest of melanoma cells is differentially regulated by contact inhibition and serum deprivation. DNA Cell Biol 1999;18:357–367.
196. Tada S, Hatoko M, Tanaka A, Kuwahara M, Muramatsu T. Expression of desmoglein I and plakoglobin in skin carcinomas. J Cutan Pathol 2000;27:24–29.
197. Riccioni L, Di Tommaso L, Collina G. Actin-rich desmoplastic malignant melanoma. Am J Dermatopathol 1999;21:537–541.
198. Cunningham CC. Actin-binding protein requirement for cortical stability and efficient locomotion. Science 1992;255:325–327.
199. Puches R, Smolle J, Rieger E, Soyer HP, Kerl H. Expression of cytoskeletal components in melanocytic skin lesions. An immunohistochemical study. Am J Dermatopathol 1991;13:137–144.
200. Tsukamoto H, Mishima Y, Hayashibe K, Sasase A. Alpha-smooth muscle actin expression in tumor and stromal cells of benign and malignant human pigment tumors. J Invest Dermatol 1992;98:116–120.
201. Shimokawa-Kuroki R, Sadano H, Taniguchi S. A variant actin (beta m) reduces metastases of mouse B16 melanoma. Int J Cancer 1994;56:689–697.
202. Chu YW, Sefor EA, Romer LH, Hendrix MJ. Experimental coexpression of vimentin and keratin intermediate filaments in human melanoma cells augments motility. Am J Pathol 1996;148:63–69.
203. Duncan LM, Bouffard D, Howard C, Mihm MC Jr, Byers HR. In situ distribution of integrin alpha 2 beta 1 and alpha-actinin in melanocytic proliferations. Mod Pathol 1996;9:938–943.
204. Bouffard D, Duncan LM, Howard CA, Mihm MC Jr, Byers HR. Actin-binding protein expression in benign and malignant melanocytic proliferations. Hum Pathol 1994;25:709–714.
205. Byers HR, Etoh T, Vink J, Franklin N, Gattoni-Celli S, Mihm MC Jr. Actin organization and cell migration of melanoma cells relate to differential expression of integrins and actin-associated proteins. J Dermatol 1992;19:847–852.
206. Helige C, Zellnig G, Hofman-Wellenhof R, Finkes-Puches R, Smolle J, Tritthart HA. Interrelation of motility, cytoskeletal organization and gap junctional communication with invasiveness of melanocytic cells in vitro. Invasion Metastasis 1997;17:26–41.
207. Dewhurst LO, Rennie IG, MacNeil S. Positive attachment between cytoskeletal changes, melanoma cell attachment and invasion in vitro. Melanoma Res 1998;8:303–311.
208. Voura EB, Sandig M, Kalnins VI, Siu C. Cell shape changes and cytoskelton reorganization during transmigration of human melanoma cells. Cell Tissue Res 1998;293:375–387.
209. Leonardi A, Ellinger-Ziegelbauer H, Franzoso G, Brown K, Siebenlist U. Physical and functional interaction of filamin (actin-binding protein 280) and tumor necrosis factor receptor-associated factor 2. J Biol Chem 2000;2745:271–278.
210. Vaisanen A, Kallioinen M, Taskinen PJ, Turpeenniemi-Hujanen T. Prognostic value of MMP-2 immunoreactive protein (72kD type IV collagenase) in primary skin melanoma. J Pathol 1998;186:51–58.
211. Ntayi C, Hornebeck W, Bernard P. [Involvement of matrix metalloproteinases (MMPs) in cutaneous melanoma progression]. Pathol Biol (Paris) 2004;52:154–159.
212. Airola K, Karonen T, Vaalamo M, et al. Expression of collagenases-1 and -3 and their inhibitors TIMP-1 and -3 correlates with the level of invasion in malignant melanomas. Br J Cancer 1999;80:733–743.
213. Iida J, Wilhelmson KL, Price MA, et al. Membrane type-1 matrix metalloproteinase promotes human melanoma invasion and growth. J Invest Dermatol 2004;122:167–176.

214. Eves P, Katerinaki E, Simpson C, et al. Melanoma invasion in reconstructed human skin is influenced by skin cells—investigation of the role of proteolytic enzymes. Clin Exp Metastasis 2003;20:685–700.

215. Ntayi C, Hornebeck W, Bernard P. Influence of cultured dermal fibroblasts on human melanoma cell proliferation, matrix metalloproteinase-2 (MMP-2) expression and invasion in vitro. Arch Dermatol Res 2003;295:236–241.

216. Ramont L, Pasco S, Hornebeck W, Maquart FX, Monboise JC. Transforming growth factor-beta 1 inhibits tumor growth in a mouse model by down-regulating the plasminogen activation system. Exp Cell Res 2003;291:1–10.

217. Podhajcer OL, Bover L, Bravo AI, et al. Expression of cathepsin D in primary and metastatic melanoma and dysplastic nevi. J Invest Dermatol 1995;104:340–344.

218. Gontier E, Cario-Andre M, Vergnes P, Bizik J, Surleve-Bazeille JE, Taieb A. The 'Abtropfung phenonmenon' revisited: demal nevus cells from congenital nevi cannot activiate matrix metalloproteinase 2 (MMP-2). Pigment Cell Res 2003;16:366–373.

219. Wylie S, MacDonald IC, Varghese HJ, et al. The matrix metalloproteinase inhibitor batimastat inhibits angiogenesis in liver metastases of B16F1 melanoma cells. Clin Exp Metastasis 1999;17:111–117.

220. Henriet P, Blavier L, Declerck YA. Tissue inhibitors of metalloproteinase (TIMP) in invasion and proliferation. APMIS 1999;107:111–119.

221. Baker AH, George SJ, Zaltsman AB, Murphy G, Newby AC. Inhibition of invasion and induction of cell death of cancer cell lines by overexpression of TIMP-3. Br J Cancer 1999;79:1347–1355.

222. Ahonene M, Poukkula M, Baker AH, et al. Tissue inhibitor of metalloproteinase-3 induces apoptosis in melanoma cells by stabilization of death receptors. Oncogene 2003;22:2121–2134.

223. Naylor MF, Crowson N, Kuwahara R, et al. Treatment of lentigo maligna with topical imiquimod. Br J Dermatol 2003;149(suppl 66):66–69.

224. Hesling C, D'Incan M, Mansard S, et al. In vivo and in situ modulation of the expression of genes involved in metastasis and angiogenesis in a patient treated with topical imiquimod for melanoma skin metastases. Br J Dermatol 2004;150:761–767.

225. Iwamoto S, Odland PB, Piepkorn M, Bothwell M. Evidence that the p75 neurotrophin receptor mediates perineural spread of desmoplastic melanoma. J Am Acad Dermatol 1996;35(5 Pt 1):725–731.

226. Marchetti D, Aucoin R, Blust J, Murray B, Greiter-Wilke A. p75 neurotrophin receptor functions as a survival receptor in brain-metastastic melanoma cells. J Cell Biochem 2004;91:206–215.

227. Rofstad EK, Halsor EF. Vascular endothelial growth factor, interleukin 8, platelet-derived endothelial growth factor, and basic fibroblast growth factor promote angiogenesis and metastasis in human melanoma xenografts. Cancer Res 2000;60:4932–4938.

228. Westphal JR, van't Hullenaar R, Peek R, et al. Angiogenic balance in human melanoma: expression of VEGF, bFGF, IL-8, PDGF and angiostatin in relation to vascular density of xenografts in vivo. Int J Cancer 2000;96:768–776.

229. Hanahan D, Folkman J. Patterns and emerging mechanisms of the angiogenic switch during tumorigenesis. Cell 1996;86:353–364.

230. Bergers G, Javaherian K, Lo KM, Folkman J, Hanahan D. Effects of angiogenesis inhibitors on mutistage carcinogenesis in mice. Science 1999;284:808–812.

231. Barnhill RL. The biology of melanoma micrometastases. Recent Results Cancer Res 2001;158:3–13.

232. Reed JA, Albino AP. Update of diagnostic and prognostic markers in cutaneous malignant melanoma. Dermatol Clin 1999;17:631–643.

233. Bayer-Garner IB, Hough AJ Jr, Smoller BR. Vascular endothelial growth factor expression in malignant melanoma: prognostic versus diagnostic usefulness. Mod Pathol 1999;12:770–774.

234. Erhhard H, Rietveld FJR, van Altena MC, Brocker E-B, Ruiter DJ, de Waal RMW. Transition of horizontal to vertical growth phase melanoma is accompanied by induction of vascular endothelial growth factor expression and angiogenesis. Melanoma Res 1997;7(Suppl 2):S19–S26.

235. Graeven U, Fiedler W, Karpinski, et al. Melanoma-associated expression of vascular endothelial growth factor and its receptors FLT-1 and KDR. J Cancer Res Clin Oncol 1999;125:621–629.

236. Chin L, Tam A, Pomerantz J, et al. Essential role for oncogenic Ras in tumour maintenance. Nature 1999;400:468–472.

237. Van Muijen GN, Danzen EH, de Vries TJ, Quax PH, Verheijen JH, Ruiter DJ. Properties of metastasizing and non-metastasizing human melanoma cells. Recent Results Cancer Res 1995;139:105–122.

238. Redondo P, Sanchez-Carpintero I, Bauza A, Idoate M, Solano T, Mihm MC Jr. Immunologic escape and angiogenesis in human malignant melanoma. J Am Acad Dermatol 2003;49:255–263.

239. Sun J, Blaskovich MA, Jain RK, et al. Blocking angiogenesis and tumorigenesis with GFA-116, a synthetic molecule that inhibits binding of vascular endothelial growth factor to its receptor. Cancer Res 2004;64:3586–3592.

240. Straume O, Akslen LA. Increased expression of VEGF-receptors (FLT-1, KDR, NRP-1) and thrombospondin-1 is associated with glomeruloid microvascular prolferation, an aggressive phenotype in malignant melanoma. Angiogenesis 2003;6:295–301.

241. Gorski DH, Leal AD, Goydos JS. Differential expression of vascular endothelial growth factor-A isoforms at different stages of melanoma progression. J Am Coll Surg 2003;197:408–418.

242. Fonsatti E, Lamaj E, Coral S, et al. In vitro analysis of the melanoma/endothelium interaction increasing the release of soluble intercellular adhesion molecule 1 by endothelial cells. Cancer Immunol Immunother 1999;48:132–138.

242. Siemeister G, Schirner M, Weindel K, et al.Two independent mechanisms essential for tumor angiogenesis: inhibition of human melanoma xenograft growth by interfering with either the vascular endothelial growth factor receptor pathway or the Tie-2 pathway. Cancer Res 1999;59:3185–3191.

243. Siemeister G, Schirner M, Weindel, et al. Two independent mechanisms essential for tumor angiogenesis: inhibition of human melanoma xenograft growth by interfering with either the vascular endothelial growth factor receptor pathway or the Tie-2 pathway. Cancer Res 1999;59:3185–3191.

244. Dadras SS, Paul T, Bertoncini J, et al. Tumor lymphangiogenesis: a novel prognostic indicator for cutaneous metastases and survival. Am J Pathol 2003;162:1951–1960.

245. Goydos JS, Gorski DH. Vascular endothelial growth factor C mRNA expression correlates with stage of progression in patients with melanoma. Clin Cancer Res 2003;9:5962–5967.

246. Schietroma C, Cianfarani F, Lacal PM, et al. Vascular endothelial growth factor-C expression correlates with lymph node localization of human melanoma metastases. Cancer 2003;98:789–797.

247. Reed JA, McNutt NS, Albino AP. Differential expression of basic fibroblastic growth factor (bFGF) in melanocytic lesions demonstrated by in situ hybridization. Implications for tumor progression. Am J Pathol 1994;144:329–336.

248. Nesbit M, Nesbit HK, Bennett J, et al. Basic fibroblast growth factor induces a transformed phenotype in normal human melanocytes. Oncogene 1999;18:6469–6476.

249. Meir F, Nesbit M, Hsu MY, et al. Human melanoma progression in skin reconstructs: biological significance of bFGF. Am J Pathol 2000;156:193–200.

250. Auslender S, Barzilai A, Goldberg I, Kopolovic J, Trau H. Lentigo maligna and superficial spreading melanoma are different in their in situ phase: an immunohistochemical study. Hum Pathol 2002;33:1001–1005.

251. Singh RK, Gutman M, Radinsky R. Heterogeneity of cytokine and growth factor gene expression in human melanoma cells with metastatic potentials. J Interferon Cytokine Res 1995;15:81–87.

252. Danielsen T, Fofstad EK. VEGF, bFGF and EGF in the angiogenesis of human melanoma xenografts. Int J Cancer 1998;76:836–841.

253. Ribatti D, Vacca A, Ria R, et al. Neovascularization, expression of fibroblast growth factore-2 and mast cells with tryptase activity increase simultaneously with pathological expression in human malignant melanoma. Eur J Cancer 2003;39:666–674.

254. Reed JA, McNutt NS, Bogdany JK, Albino AP. Expression of the mast cell growth factor interleukin-3 in melanocytic lesions correlates with an increased number of mast cells in the perilesional stroma: implications for melanoma progression. J Cutan Pathol 1996;23:495–505.

255. Al-Alousi S, Carlson JA, Blessing K, Cook M, Karaoli T, Barnhill RL. Expression of basic fibroblast growth factor in desmoplastic melanoma. J Cutan Pathol 1996;23:118–125.

256. Fearns C, Dowdle EB. The desmoplastic response: induction of collagen synthesis by melanoma cells in vitro. Int J Cancer 1992;50:621–627.

257. Lugassy C, Christensen L, Le Charpentier M, Faure E, Escande JP. Ultrastructural observations concerning laminin in B16 melanoma. Is an amorphous form of laminin promoting a non hematogenous migration of tumor cells? J Submicrosc Cytol Pathol 1998;30:137–144.

258. Lugassy C, Christensen L, Le Charpentier M, Faure E, Escande JP. Angio-tumoral laminin in murine tumors derived from human melanoma cell lines. Immunohistochemical and ultrastructural observations. J Submicrosc Cytol Pathol 1998;30:231–237.

259. Lugassy C, Dickersin GR, Christensen L, et al. Ultrastructural and immunohistochemical studies of the periendothelial matrix in human melanoma: evidence for an amorphous matrix containing laminin. J Cutan Pathol 1999;26:78–83.

260. Lugassy C, Shahsafaei A, Bonitz P, Busam KJ, Barnhill RL. Tumor microvessels in melanoma express the beta-2 chain of laminin. Implications for melanoma metastases. J Cutan Pathol 1999;26:222–226.

261. Van den Oord JJ, Maes A, Stas M, et al. CD40 is a prognostic marker in primary cutaneous malignant melanoma. Am J Pathol 1996;149:1953–1961.

21 Optical Imaging Analysis of Atypical Nevi and Melanoma

Amanda Pfaff Smith and Dorothea Becker

CONTENTS

Summary

Optical imaging has become a powerful tool for visualizing and tracking, spatially and in real time, the expression and function of individual genes and proteins, and biological processes at large. In this chapter, we review recent advances in optical imaging techniques, discuss optical imaging-based biological and biomedical studies in live cells and organisms, and present examples for the application of optical imaging in the context of molecular investigations of melanoma and its precursor lesions.

Key Words: Melanoma; optical imaging; applications.

FUNDAMENTALS OF OPTICAL IMAGING

Since the building of the first practical microscopes by Anton Van Leeuwenhoek in the 17th century, optical imaging has undergone steady advances, but in the past two decades, the field has taken major leaps. The development of bioluminescent reporters, new fluorescent probes, and digital imaging workstations that integrate optics, electronics, and software have opened avenues for real-time, functional imaging of mammalian development, the neurosciences, gene therapy, and animal models of human biology and disease.

Fluorescent Probes

Molecular cloning of the jellyfish *Aequorea victoria*-derived green fluorescent protein (GFP) *(1)* and its first use as a marker for gene expression *(2)*, initiated, in a major fashion, the application of optical imaging to biological systems *(3)*. Furthermore, subsequent engineering of mutant GFPs, collectively termed *Aequora* fluorescent proteins (AFPs), has provided the means to visualize and record gene expression and protein

From: *From Melanocytes to Melanoma: The Progression to Malignancy*
Edited by: V. J. Hearing and S. P. L. Leong © Humana Press Inc., Totowa, NJ

localization in complex biological processes, both in vitro and in vivo. Although the development of AFPs is an ongoing process, currently available fluorescent proteins that have different spectral characteristics, and photostable organic dyes, which do not disintegrate on exposure to light, provide the basis for multicolor, multiparameter analyses *(4)*.

A major challenge for optical imaging, particularly when used for in vivo studies, is the scattering of light caused by tissue autofluorescence, and the presence of light-absorbing biological molecules, such as hemoglobin. Performing optical imaging analyses in the near-infrared (NIR) spectrum helps to minimize some of these technical obstacles, and therefore, NIR probes are best suited for imaging live organisms and tissue samples. Water-soluble NIR and far-red emitting cyanine dyes, such as Cy3, Cy5, and Cy7 can easily be conjugated to DNA, RNA, proteins, peptides, and antibodies. Furthermore, semiconductor quantum dots, which are hydrophilic, bioconjugatable zinc sulfide-coated cadmium selenide nanocrystals, have recently been introduced as fluorescent probes *(5,6)*. Compared with organic dyes, quantum dots are brighter, more stable, and more resistant to photobleaching (the irreversible destruction of a fluorophore under illumination), and thus, they will significantly broaden the range of optical imaging applications.

Imaging Systems for Basic Research and Clinical Investigation

Optical imaging techniques exploit different physical parameters of light to allow the capture of images derived from fluorescent or bioluminescent reporters, or from the absorption, emission, and scattering effects of biological structures. In fluorescence microscopy, light from an external source excites a fluorophore, the core portion of a molecule that is responsible for absorbing and re-emitting photons, and thereupon, that energy is nearly instantaneously emitted at a lower magnitude (longer wavelength). The most commonly used fluorescence microscope is an epi-fluorescence microscope in which excitation light, generated from a mercury or xenon lamp, or a laser, illuminates the object, and fluorescence emission is viewed through the same objective lens used for excitation (Fig. 1). The weaker emission light, back-scattering from the object, is separated from the excitation light through a fluorescence filter cube and focused into a charged-coupled device camera that produces images by converting light photons into electrons according to the intensity of incoming energy.

Because a fluorescence-labeled object glows brightly and obscures the captured image above and below the focus plane, standard epi-fluorescence microscopes have limits with respect to the extent of optical resolution. Confocal and multiphoton microscopy *(7)* overcome these problems. Confocal microscopes enhance resolution by blocking out-of-focus light from above or below the imaging plane through spatial filtering, whereas multiphoton microscopes limit excitation to the focal volume, minimizing photobleaching and photodamage. To further minimize phototoxicity, multiphoton microscopes can be adapted for second harmonic imaging. With this technique, highly polarizable, ordered biological structures, such as collagen, produce strong second harmonic signals on illumination with intense laser light *(8)*.

For bioluminescence imaging (BLI), which has become the presently most widely used technique for in vivo imaging *(9)*, cells are tagged in vitro with a reporter gene, such as luciferase, a light-generating enzyme that catalyzes the oxidation of substrate in the presence of adenosine triphosphate. Although BLI produces somewhat diffuse two-

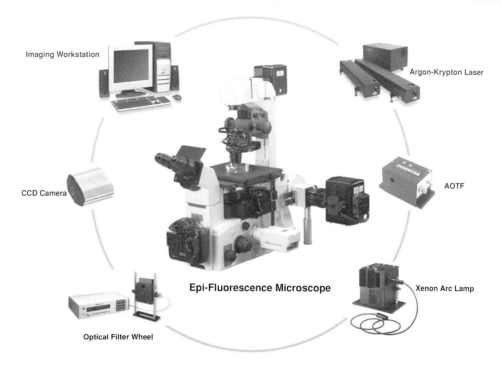

Fig. 1. Inverted epi-fluorescence microscope system. Optical imaging systems, which are versatile, can be equipped with mercury or xenon lamps for standard illumination, mixed gas or pulsed lasers for specialized applications, filter wheels or acousto-optic tunable filters for ultrafast multichannel imaging, and charged-coupled device cameras or photomultiplier tubes for sensitive detection.

dimensional images that are pseudocolored based on intensity, future systems may facilitate the imaging of animals from multiple angles, yielding three-dimensional or even tomographic information.

Fluorescence molecular tomography has the ability to three-dimensionally localize and quantify fluorescent probes in a living animal *(10)*. In this approach, a single light beam is directed into tissue, and both the excitation and emission light are detected at multiple points of the tissue boundary. Measurements are tomographically combined to yield quantitative maps of fluorochrome distributions. A similar approach, diffuse optical tomography (DOT), produces two-dimensional optical slices of tissue after intrinsic and extrinsic absorption and scattering of NIR light. Although images obtained with DOT have less spatial resolution than those acquired with fluorescence molecular tomography, DOT technology is currently assessed in the clinic for early detection of breast cancer *(11)*.

Of the different optical imaging systems reviewed here, optical coherence tomography (OCT) has made the furthest inroads into the clinic, generating *in situ* images for diagnosis of retinal, intravascular, gastrointestinal, and esophageal diseases *(12)*. Similar to ultrasound imaging, but using light rather than sound waves, an optical beam emitted by a low-coherence-length light source is scanned across the tissue, and light reflected or back-scattered from inside the tissue is measured by correlation with light that has traveled a known reference path. Because OCT penetrates tissues to acquire cross-sectional or *en face* images on the micron scale, the resulting data sets yield images with resolutions approaching that of conventional histology.

OPTIMAL IMAGING IN NEUROBIOLOGY, IMMUNOLOGY, AND CANCER

In this section, we present examples of how single molecules, protein interactions, cell motility and migration, and complex pathophysiological events can be characterized in individual cells or in complex live organisms, both spatially and temporally.

Multimodal Imaging of Neuron Development

Although the glycine receptor has been indicated to represent the major inhibitory neurotransmitter receptor in the adult spinal cord, past studies have precluded observation of the receptor's dynamics in the synaptic cleft. Quantum dot labeling of the glycine receptor in the neuronal membrane of live cells has enabled observation of the receptor's lateral dynamics among extrasynaptic and synaptic domains, and silver-intensified quantum dot-based electron microscopy images demonstrated that labeled receptors can access the synaptic core *(13)*. Advances in neural development have also been documented via transgenic mice that express AFPs in motor neurons. During mammalian development, axon branches of several motor neurons coinnervate the same muscle fiber, yet all but one are eliminated in a competitive process with unknown mechanisms. Laser scanning confocal microscopy of two or more fluorescently labeled neurons with multiple neuromuscular junctions suggests that at each coinnervated junction where competition exists the same neuron overpowers its competitor *(14)*. Furthermore, the winning neuronal competitor has a more powerful neurotransmission *(15)*. Thus, fluorescence imaging has established that neuronal identity determines the outcome at each synaptic competition and that this process occurs as a result of differences in relative axonal activity.

Optical Imaging in Immunology and Cancer

Intravital optical imaging combined with two-photon laser microscopy has started to redefine the classical model of lymphocyte trafficking deep inside lymphoid structures. To initiate an immune response, antigen-presenting dendritic cells (DCs) must contact T-cells within the complex lymph node microenvironment, and classical models suggest that T-cells are attracted to DCs by pervasive chemokine gradients. However, unlike the behavior expected of T-cells following graded chemotactic paths, fluorescently labeled naive T-cells in surgically exposed lymph nodes of an anesthetized mouse migrate independently and randomly in all three dimensions *(16)*. Based on the data from these fluorescence imaging studies, it has become evident that the mechanism by which DCs solicit T-cell interaction is not through chemokine gradients but rather by increasing their surface area with numerous fine dendritic processes *(17)*. Furthermore, intravital two-photon and second harmonic imaging have most recently been employed to study tumor dynamics, such as migration, intravasation, and host immune infiltration *(18)*.

Despite the application of intravital imaging in pharmacokinetics studies, it still requires a surgical procedure that yields a window to molecular events in a restricted locality. In vivo BLI, on the other hand, confers the ability to detect tumor stasis and necrosis noninvasively, such that the timing and dosage of immunotherapy, chemotherapy, or gene therapy can be investigated before clinical trials *(19)*. For example, the luciferase gene incorporated into an adenoviral vector containing a therapeutic transgene was used to monitor gene expression after intratumoral injection of brain tumors *(20)*. The sensitivity of BLI also makes it a useful tool for detecting relapse. In addition to monitoring tumor growth and gene transfer, BLI has been used to track the localization of bacterial infection *(21)* and to characterize early events in hematopoietic stem cell reconstitution *(22)*.

The p53–Mdm2 negative feedback loop, wherein p53 transcriptionally activates Mdm-2, and Mdm-2, in turn, targets p53 for degradation, is modulated in response to DNA damage. Past studies suggested that p53 and Mdm-2 undergo dampened oscillations after DNA damage, and the greater the DNA damage, the stronger the amplitude of the average response. By tracking p53 and Mdm2 protein conjugated to AFPs, Lahav et al. demonstrated by way of optical imaging that the number of pulses, but not their amplitude, is dependent on the extent of irradiation-induced damage *(23)*. Similarly, epidermal growth factor-loaded quantum dots and fluorescent-labeled erbB/HER receptors were followed through ligand binding, receptor activation, endocytic uptake, and endosomal trafficking to provide new insights into receptor specificity and endosomal transport patterns in live cells *(24)*.

Increasingly, intramolecular and intermolecular events are investigated by fluorescence resonance energy transfer (FRET), wherein energy is transferred from a fluorescence donor to a fluorescence acceptor, given that the two fluorochromes are in proximity of less than 80 Å. FRET is recorded by determining the ratio of acceptor to donor fluorescence, or by measuring lifetime rather than intensity of a fluorescent signal transfer through fluorescence lifetime microscopy *(25)*. Although FRET is predominantly used to visualize molecular interactions and conformations, it has also been employed in molecular beacons that dynamically trace the movement of messenger RNA in live cells *(26)*.

APPLICATIONS OF OPTICAL IMAGING TO MELANOMA

Because light interacts with molecular probes and subcellular structures in different ways, optical imaging techniques have the potential to detect subtle molecular and structural differences in the composition of tissues. Nowhere are these properties more applicable than in the research and detection of melanoma, in which visualization of tumor composition, growth, and regression is integral in animal models; histological staging and gene expression studies are most often conducted with ex vivo tissue sections; and early diagnosis typically hinges on the identification of suspicious lesions on the surface of the body.

Monitoring Angiogenesis, Growth, and Metastasis in Human Melanoma Xenografts

The first fluorescent melanoma bone and organ metastasis models were developed through establishment of stable GFP expression transductants of the murine B16 melanoma and LOX human melanoma cell lines *(27)*. Lung, pleural membrane, liver, kidney, adrenal gland, lymph node, and skeletal metastases were observed after tail vein or intradermal injection of transduced cells, many of which could not be detected by brightfield microscopy. Furthermore, when red fluorescent protein-expressing tumors were grown in GFP-expressing transgenic mice, host angiogenic and DCs could be distinguished from B16 tumor cells in live tissue *(28)*.

Melanomas and their interspersing vasculature can also be visualized through fluorochrome-conjugated antibodies and fluorescence reflectance imaging *(29)*. Advanced-stage melanomas are very vascular and produce high levels of basic fibroblast growth factor (bFGF) and fibroblast growth factor receptor (FGFR)-1, but when human melanomas grown as subcutaneous tumors in nude mice are exposed to antisense bFGF and FGFR-1 constructs, tumor growth and angiogenesis are blocked *(30)*. To determine whether bFGF/FGFR-1 signaling occurs between melanoma cells, endothelial cells, or bidirectionally, antisense constructs containing the human tyrosinase promoter to specifically inhibit expression of bFGF and FGFR-1 in the melanoma cells were intratumorally injected into human melanoma xenografts, and tumor growth and vasculature were noninvasively imaged with Cy7-S100 and Cy5-CD31 antibodies, respectively *(31)*. Dual-color in vivo fluorescence images obtained over a 2-wk period of antisense treatment (Fig. 2A), and simultaneous imaging of targeted tumors injected with the fluorescent apoptosis marker, acridine orange, indicated that tumors were regressing as a result of a massive onset of apoptosis. Subsequent ex vivo immunofluorescent images of tissue sections, probed for bFGF, FGFR-1, and vascular endothelial growth factor, confirmed that the treated tumors were not expressing bFGF or its receptor, and implied that the tumors failed to upregulate expression of another angiogenic molecule, such as vascular endothelial growth factor, to circumvent bFGF and FGFR-1 antisense treatments.

Optical Imaging of Gene Expression in Nevus and Melanoma Tissue Specimens

Much effort has been focused on characterizing the genes that govern the progression from atypical nevi to metastatic melanoma, but imaging methods are seldom used. Optical imaging analysis of formalin-fixed, paraffin-embedded and snap-frozen nevus and melanoma tissue sections yields several benefits over standard immunohistochemistry or *in situ* hybridization: tissue pigmentation does not interfere with visualization of fluorescent or spectral signals; multiple proteins or cellular structures can be clearly localized and colocalized in the same tissue section with spectrally separated probes; and intensity-based analysis of a fluorescent signal in spatially segmented digital images provides an objective means for comparing gene expression in multiple specimens. Spectral imaging of tissue sections illustrates these properties because it enables the determination of the presence or absence of spectrally distinct signals through the acqui-

---

Fig. 2. (A) *(opposite page)* Noninvasive optical imaging of melanoma xenografts. Human melanoma cells, grown as subcutaneous tumors in nude mice, were injected intratumorally with a pREP7 plasmid (a), or a pREP7 plasmid containing human basic fibroblast growth factor or fibroblast growth factor receptor 1 full-length antisense-oriented complimentary DNA (b). Images, captured by illuminating mice placed under a charged-coupled device camera with appropriate filters, were collected after intratumoral injection of a Cy5-conjugated antibody that binds to the endothelial cell marker CD31 (pseudocolored red) and a Cy7-conjugated antibody that recognizes S100 antigen expressed on melanoma cells (pseudocolored green). **(B)** Quantitative determination of gene expression in melanoma-positive lymph nodes. Two adjacent tissue sections from a metastatic melanoma-positive lymph node were probed with a Cy7-conjugated antibody to the T-cell marker, CD3 (a), pseudocolored yellow; and a Cy5-labeled S100 antibody (b) pseudocolored red; to visualize T-cells and melanoma cells. Average gray-scale values, represented by arbitrary units of fluorescence (c), reflect the relative levels of antibody

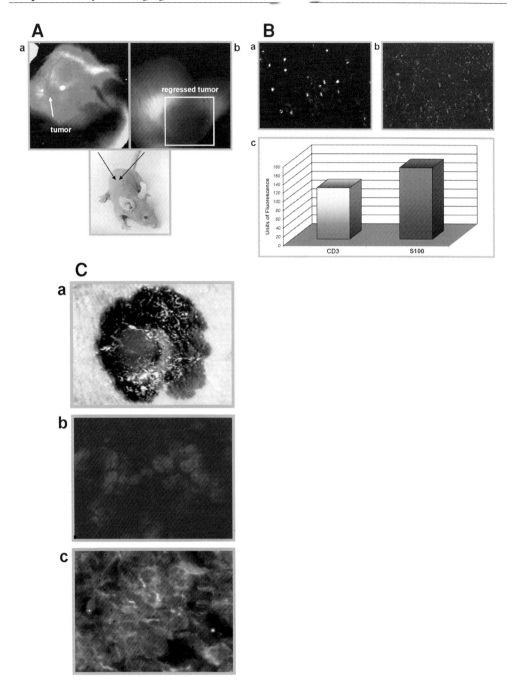

Fig. 2. (A) (*continued from opposite page*) hybridization and fluorescence in the tissue sections. (C) Colocalization of the Hsc70-interacting protein, Hip, and the chemokine receptor, CXCR2, in melanoma tissue sections. A tissue section from a melanoma (a) was counterstained with fluorescent 4',6-diamidino-2-phenylindole (DAPI) (b) pseudocolored blue; and an adjacent tissue section was triple-stained with fluorescent DAPI (pseudocolored blue), a Cy3-conjugated CXCR2 antibody (pseudocolored green), and a Cy5-labeled Hip antibody (pseudocolored red). Images were captured in the respective channels for DAPI, Cy3, and Cy5. Areas of colocalization of Hip and CXCR2 are pseudocolored orange. (Please *see* color insert following p. 430.)

sition of a high-resolution spectrum, intensity as a function of wavelength, at each pixel in an image *(32)*. In a study involving microscopic spectral imaging of atypical nevus sections probed with antibodies to signal transducer and activator of transcription (STAT) proteins, it was found that systemic low-dose interferon-α treatment inactivates the transcription factors STAT1 and STAT3 *(33)*. To further investigate the proteins involved in STAT signal transduction, immunofluorescence images of upstream regulators and downstream targets of STAT3 established gene expression and cellular localization profiles in atypical nevi obtained before and after low-dose interferon-α treatment. Software designed to determine cell boundaries and quantitate the average fluorescent signal on a cell-by-cell basis (Fig. 2B) suggested that STAT inactivation does not occur via upregulation or downregulation of the proteins involved in STAT signaling *(34)*. Similarly, fluorochrome-labeled antibodies and oligonucleotides were used to visualize expression of novel candidate genes in melanoma that were identified by gene expression profiling techniques, such as Serial Analysis of Gene Expression *(35)* and microarrays (Fig. 2C) *(36)*.

In Situ *Spectral Imaging of Atypical Nevi and Melanomas*

Digital photography and standard dermoscopy are the two optical methods that are most often used to monitor clinically suspicious changes in atypical nevi. For patients who have a large number of atypical nevi, Dysplastic Nevus Syndrome, or a clinical history of sporadic or familial melanoma, it would be of great benefit to have an automated, noninvasive means to identify high-risk nevocytic lesions. OCT has been used in ophthalmology to diagnose retinal diseases, such as glaucoma and macular degeneration, but, to date, its feasibility in melanoma detection has not been investigated. In vivo confocal scanning laser microscopy images of pigmented lesions allow recognition of melanocytes, which contain melanin for endogenous contrast, with a resolution approaching histological detail *(37)*.

Unlike optical methods that monitor the histology of lesions, macroscopic spectral imaging has been shown to have the ability to identify melanoma *in situ* present in contiguous association with atypical nevi in patients with a clinical history of melanoma, by spectrally identifying areas of interest based on their interaction with light at various wavelengths *(38)*. Using light that spans the visible to NIR regions of the spectrum, information that may or may not be available to the naked eye is collected from various depths of the lesion present on the skin. If, in the near future, this information can serve as the basis for building spectral signatures for histological stages of melanoma development, spectral imaging may become an invaluable tool in the clinical setting for automated detection of early-stage melanoma.

CONCLUSIONS AND PERSPECTIVES

Examples of recent advances in optical imaging, reviewed in this chapter, illustrate their growing range of applications in biology and medicine. Availability of bioluminescent reporters and the continuous development of new fluorescent probes and digital imaging workstations that integrate optics, electronics, and software have opened avenues for real-time, functional imaging of mammalian development, the neurosciences, gene therapy, and animal models of human biology and disease. In the case of melanoma, optical imaging devices are expected to help detect the disease before it becomes visible to the naked eye, and to provide important insights into the spatiotemporal expression and function of genes regulating melanoma cell proliferation, adhesion, angiogenesis, and metastasis.

REFERENCES

1. Prasher DC, Eckenrode VK, Ward WW, Prendergast FG, Cormier MJ. Primary structure of the Aequorea victoria green-fluorescent protein. Gene 1992;111:229–233.
2. Chalfie M, Tu Y, Euskirchen G, Ward WW, Prasher DC. Green fluorescent protein as a marker for gene expression. Science 1994;263:802–805.
3. Tsien RY. The green fluorescent protein. Annu Rev Biochem 1998;67:509–544.
4. Zhang J, Campbell RE, Ting AY, Tsien RY. Creating new fluorescent probes for cell biology. Nat Rev Mol Cell Biol 2002;3:906–918.
5. Bruchez M Jr, Moronne M, Gin P, Weiss S, Alivisatos AP. Semiconductor nanocrystals as fluorescent biological labels. Science 1998;281:2013–2016.
6. Chan WC, Nie S. Quantum dot bioconjugates for ultrasensitive nonisotopic detection. Science 1998;281:2016–2018.
7. Stephens DJ, Allan VJ. Light microscopy techniques for live cell imaging. Science 2003;300:82–86.
8. Campagnola PJ, Loew LM. Second-harmonic imaging in microscopy for visualizing biomolecular arrays in cells, tissues and organisms. Nat Biotechnol 2003;21:1356–1360.
9. Contag CH, Bachmann MH. Advances in in vivo bioluminescence imaging of gene expression. Annu Rev Biomed Eng 2002;4:235–260.
10. Ntziachristos V, Tung CH, Bremer C, Weissleder R. Fluorescence molecular tomography resolves protease activity in vivo. Nat Med 2002;8:757–760.
11. Ntziachristos V, Yodh AG, Schnall M, Chance B. Concurrent MRI and diffuse optical tomography of breast after indocyanine green enhancement. Proc Natl Acad Sci USA 2000;97:2767–2772.
12. Fujimoto JG. Optical coherence tomography for ultrahigh resolution in vivo imaging. Nat Biotechnol 2003;21:1361–1367.
13. Dahan M, Levi S, Luccardini C, Rostaing P, Riveau B, Triller A. Diffusion dynamics of glycine receptors revealed by single-quantum dot tracking. Science 2003;302:442–445.
14. Kasthuri N, Lichtman JW. The role of neuronal identity in synaptic competition. Nature 2003;424:426–430.
15. Buffelli M, Burgess RW, Feng G, Lobe CG, Lichtman JW, Sanes JR. Genetic evidence that relative synaptic efficacy biases the outcome of synaptic competition. Nature 2003;424:430–434.
16. Miller MJ, Wei SH, Cahalan MD, Parker I. Autonomous T cell trafficking examined in vivo with intravital two-photon microscopy. Proc Natl Acad Sci USA 2003;100:2604–2609.
17. Miller MJ, Hejazi AS, Wei SH, Cahalan MD, Parker I. T cell repertoire scanning is promoted by dynamic dendritic cell behavior and random T cell motility in the lymph node. Proc Natl Acad Sci USA 2004;100:998–1003.
18. Condeelis J, Segall JE. Intravital imaging of cell movement in tumours. Nat Rev Cancer 2003;3:921–930.
19. Edinger M, Cao YA, Hornig YS, et al. Advancing animal models of neoplasia through in vivo bioluminescence imaging. Eur J Cancer 2002;38:2128–2136.
20. Rehemtulla A, Hall DE, Stegman LD, et al. Molecular imaging of gene expression and efficacy following adenoviral-mediated brain tumor gene therapy. Mol Imaging 2002;1:43–55.
21. Hardy J, Francis KP, DeBoer M, Chu P, Gibbs K, Contag CH. Extracellular replication of Listeria Monocytogenes in the murine gall bladder. Science 2004;303:851–853.
22. Cao YA, Wagers AJ, Beilhack A, et al. Shifting foci of hematopoiesis during reconstitution from single stem cells. Proc Natl Acad Sci USA 2004;101:221–226.
23. Lahav G, Rosenfeld N, Sigal A, et al. Dynamics of the p53-Mdm2 feedback loop in individual cells. Nat Genet 2004;36:147–150.
24. Lidke DS, Nagy P, Heintzmann R, et al. Quantum dot ligands provide new insights into erbB/HER receptor-mediated signal transduction. Nat Biotechnol 2004;22:198–203.
25. Jares-Erijman EA, Jovin TM. FRET imaging. Nat Biotechnol 2003;21:1387–1395.
26. Bratu DP, Cha BJ, Mhlanga MM, Kramer FR, Tyagi S. Visualizing the distribution and transport of mRNAs in living cells. Proc Natl Acad Sci USA 2003;100:13,308–13,313.
27. Yang M, Jiang P, An Z, et al. Genetically fluorescent melanoma bone and organ metastasis models. Clin Cancer Res 1999;5:3549–3559.

28. Yang M, Li L, Jiang P, Moossa AR, Penman S, Hoffman RM. Dual-color fluorescence imaging distinguishes tumor cells from induced host angiogenic vessels and stromal cells. Proc Natl Acad Sci USA 2003;100:14,259–14,262.

29. Ballou B, Fisher GW, Deng JS, Hakala TR, Srivastava M, Farkas DL. Cyanine fluorochrome-labeled antibodies in vivo: assessment of tumor imaging using Cy3, Cy5, Cy5.5, and Cy7. Cancer Detect Prev 1998;22:251–257.

30. Wang Y, Becker D. Antisense targeting of basic fibroblast growth factor and fibroblast growth factor receptor 1 in human melanomas blocks intratumoral angiogenesis and tumor growth. Nat Med 1997;3:887–893.

31. Valesky M, Spang AJ, Fisher GW, Farkas DL, Becker D. Noninvasive dynamic fluorescence imaging of human melanomas reveals that targeted inhibition of bFGF or FGFR-1 in melanoma cells blocks tumor growth by apoptosis. Mol Med 2002;8:103–112.

32. Farkas DL, Du C, Fisher GW, et al. Non-invasive image acquisition and advanced processing in optical bioimaging. Comput Med Imaging Graph 1998;22:89–102.

33. Kirkwood JM, Farkas DL, Chakraborty A, et al. Systemic interferon-alpha (IFN-alpha) treatment leads to Stat3 inactivation in melanoma precursor lesions. Mol Med 1999;5:11–20.

34. Smith AP, Kirkwood JM, Edington HD, Jukic DM, Farkas DL, Becker D. Fluorescence imaging analysis of upstream regulators and downstream targets of STAT3 in melanoma precursor lesions obtained from patients before and after systemic low-dose interferon-alpha treatment. Mol Imaging 2003;2:65–73.

35. Smith AP, Weeraratna AT, Spears JR, Meltzer PS, Becker D. SAGE Identification and fluorescence imaging analysis of genes and transcripts in melanomas and precursor lesions. Cancer Biol Ther 2004;3:104–109.

36. McDonald SL, Edington HD, Kirkwood JM, Becker D. Expression analysis of genes identified by molecular profiling of VGP melanomas and MGP melanoma-positive lymph nodes. Cancer Biol Ther 2004;3:110–120.

37. Busam KJ, Charles C, Lohmann CM, Marghoob A, Goldgeier M, Halpern AC. Detection of intraepidermal malignant melanoma in vivo by confocal scanning laser microscopy. Melanoma Res 2002;12:349–355.

38. Farkas DL, Becker D. Applications of spectral imaging: detection and analysis of human melanoma and its precursors. Pigment Cell Res 2001;14:2–8.

22

Proteomics Analysis of Melanoma Cell Lines and Cultured Melanocytes

Katheryn A. Resing and Natalie G. Ahn

Summary

Biochemical, molecular biological, and genetic studies suggest carcinogenesis results in progressive release from growth regulation and apoptosis surveillance, and increasing likelihood of metastasis. In melanoma, this progression is reflected in histopathological stages, including radial growth phase, vertical growth phase, and metastasis. Understanding melanoma progression is complicated by the difficulty of distinguishing these stages at a molecular level. In addition, the complexity of cancer cell behavior involving altered stromal interactions, angiogenesis, resistance to drugs and immune surveillance, and metastasis to various tissues, makes it difficult to directly or quantitatively connect functional responses to mutations or regulatory events. More precise ways are needed to delineate molecular phenotypes in a manner that is quantifiable and directly related to mutation or underlying signaling status. One approach that shows great promise is proteomic profiling, in which new methods for sensitive and reproducible identification and quantification of thousands of different proteins in cells are being applied to analyze molecular changes in melanoma.

Key Words: 2D-PAGE; mass spectrometry; hepatoma-derived growth factor; shotgun proteomics.

INTRODUCTION

The proteomics revolution is driven by the success of genome sequencing endeavors, the development of new methods for ionizing peptides and proteins, and the availability of new mass spectrometers capable of high-throughput protein analysis. Two approaches to protein profiling are "top-down," which analyzes intact proteins in complex mixtures,

From: *From Melanocytes to Melanoma: The Progression to Malignancy*
Edited by: V. J. Hearing and S. P. L. Leong © Humana Press Inc., Totowa, NJ

and "bottom-up," which involves proteolytic digestion of the proteins and reconstruction of protein profiles from analysis of the peptides. Protein identification in either approach depends on fragmentation of the analytes in the mass spectrometer, generating sequencing spectra (MS/MS); the data from the MS/MS spectra are input into protein sequence database search programs that allow identification of peptides or proteins. Although few proteomics studies have been carried out in melanoma, emerging studies suggest that this approach can be useful for understanding disease progression in this cancer type.

A method often used for proteomics profiling is a top-down approach, involving separation of proteins by two-dimensional polyacrylamide gel electrophoresis (2D-PAGE) followed by excision of protein spots for in-gel digestion and protein identification by peptide mass spectrometry (MS). Interest in using 2D-PAGE to profile protein expression was stimulated in 1996 when Matthias Mann's laboratory combined these approaches with a search program that could use MS information to identify proteins from protein databases (1). This application depends on high-sensitivity MS, using various types of ionization methods that "volatilize" peptides (2). Typical methods used for peptides and proteins involve electrospray ionization (ESI) or matrix-assisted laser desorption ionization (MALDI), the importance of which was recognized by the 2002 Nobel Prize in chemistry going to developers John Fenn and Koichi Tanaka. Rapid improvement in analytical methods in recent years now allows analysis of very complex samples containing thousands of proteins. New methodological improvements and studies applying these methods to cancer are appearing almost daily. Here we address some of the major methodologies and their capabilities and limitations, and provide references to recent reviews or studies evaluating the methods.

Analytical MS Methods Underlying the Proteomics Revolution

A confusing array of mass spectrometers is used in proteomics applications (3). The most commonly used MS instruments are based on the following four types of mass analyzers:

1. Time-of-flight (TOF) instruments that accelerate ions then measure the time they take to traverse a field-free flight tube.
2. Quadrupole instruments that analyze a stream of ions in a quadrupole field, scanning through the mass range in small, discrete windows to produce a mass spectrum.
3. Three-dimensional (3D) ion trap instruments that trap ions in a 3D field then scan the masses by sequentially destabilizing small mass ranges of ions.
4. Ion cyclotron resonance (ICR) instruments that use a large magnet to trap ions as with 3D ion traps, but have very high mass accuracy and can fragment proteins.

Often, these analyzers are combined to produce hybrid instruments, such as the QqTOF configuration that combines a quadrupole and a TOF; or tandem instruments, such as the TOF–TOF. These combinations provide unique analytical capabilities or increased mass accuracy of the MS/MS spectra. New linear ion trap mass spectrometers are emerging as popular instruments for high throughput bottom-up proteomics, because of their fast scanning rates, which enable more rapid data collection; and their larger trapping field, enabling a working sensitivity at less than 250 attomoles of peptide when combined with a nanoscale chromatography system.

Two types of MS data are used to identify proteins, peptide masses or peptide sequences, and several analytical methods have been developed to obtain these data (4). In experiments involving recovery of proteins from gel pieces by in-gel digestion, peptide mass "fingerprinting" is often carried out using a MALDI-TOF MS. The low recovery of peptides from in-gel digests (typically 25–40% sequence coverage is obtained) *(5)* and overlap of masses between highly homologous proteins produces ambiguity in some cases. Despite the limits, this approach is able to identify most prokaryotic proteins and up to 80% of higher eukaryotic proteins from in-gel digests if a sequenced genome is available and the protein is homogeneous. Peptide sequencing is a more reliable method for protein identification, and can identify related protein homologs when the protein is not in a database *(6)*. Peptide sequencing can be carried out using MALDI interfaced with TOF–TOF, ion trap, or QqTOF detectors, or by ESI interfaced with several types of MS instruments. High sensitivity in ESI systems is often achieved using low-flow capillary chromatography systems with microionspray or nanospray ionization sources *(7)*. Protein digests of simple composition may be applied via a nanospray tip, delivering sample to the MS by electrically assisted evaporation or analyzed on a reverse-phase column directly coupled to the MS. Sequence information is reported by fragmenting peptides at peptide bonds by introducing energy, either by collisional or resonance activation, producing fragment ions of varying sizes differing by the mass of constituent amino acids *(8)*. The resulting spectra are often referred to as MS/MS data, because, historically, such spectra were produced in tandem MS instruments.

Computer Search Programs for MS/MS Data

Obviously critical to successful protein identification are computer search programs that match peptide mass and/or MS/MS data to protein sequences within databases *(9)*. Five commonly used search programs are website accessible and allow analysis of single peptide fingerprints or MS/MS files; some allow analysis of moderately sized data sets. These include: Mascot (www.matrixscience.com), PeptideSearch (www.mann.embl-heidelberg.de/Services/PeptideSearch/), MSTag (prospector.ucsf.edu/htmlucsf/mstag.htm), Profound (prowl.rockefeller.edu/cgi-bin/Profound), and OMSSA (pubchem.ncbi.nlm.nih.gov/omssa). MSTag and related programs at the University of California at San Francisco are particularly useful, providing a wide range of tools for MS data analysis. Database search engines available from MS vendors include: Sequest (ThermoElectron), ProID (Applied Biosystems), MassLynx (Waters), and SpectrumMill (Agilent). Recent reviews have discussed these and other software applications for proteomics, including those that are open source, free to academic researchers by licensing, or commercially available *(9,10)*.

2D GEL ELECTROPHORESIS

The attractiveness of 2D-PAGE for proteomic profiling is its integrated view of expression levels from staining intensities and posttranslational modifications from pI or size separations *(11,12)*. The use of immobilized pH gradient gels has improved reproducibility and capacity over previously used tube gels *(13)*. Gels are dehydrated onto a plastic backing to produce a "dry strip" that is then rehydrated with the sample for isoelectric focusing (IEF). Spreading the proteins throughout the strip at the beginning reduces much of the aggregation that plagues IEF methods, enabling 0.1 to 1 mg of protein to be loaded without loss of resolution, depending on the sample. The dry strip technology is limited to analysis of proteins that can be absorbed into the gel during rehydration or can remain in the strip during equilibration with sodium dodecyl sulfate

(SDS) before 2D SDS-PAGE. Thus, both large and small proteins, as well as insoluble proteins, are underrepresented. Despite these limitations, a survey of the high to moderate abundance proteins can still be used to monitor the signaling status of cells, e.g., through altered expression and/or posttranslational modifications of proteins that control cell morphology, protein synthesis, and protein stability.

Silver staining allows detection of some proteins at nanogram levels, or approx 50,000 copies/cell for proteins from mammalian cells (approx 0.1 nM cellular concentration). For larger proteins, the sensitivity is lower. However, the highest sensitivity silver staining methods interfere with subsequent MS analysis. Fluorescent dyes are often used instead; a common fluorescent stain is SyproRuby, but newer stains that show lower background staining of low-abundance proteins (e.g., Deep Purple) or less saturation with more abundant proteins (C-16F) provide reasonable alternatives *(14)*. Higher protein loadings can be achieved using IEF strips with narrow overlapping isoelectrc point (pI) ranges. In an example analyzing the proteome of *Escherichia coli (15)*, which has 4288 predicted open reading frames *(16)*, a wide pI range strip revealed 2364 spots representing approx 1691 gene products, whereas multiple narrow range pI strips revealed 4950 spots representing approx 3535 gene products. The detection limit was estimated to be a few copies of protein per *E. coli* cell. In contrast, proteomic profiling of higher eukaryotes is more difficult, because of the greater complexity and larger dynamic range of protein expression. Protein extracts can be prefractionated and concentrated before analysis to enhance sensitivity, although this greatly increases data collection and analysis effort.

Few studies attempt to identify all the proteins observed by 2D-PAGE, and the majority of proteins on 2D gels do not change significantly, even under conditions of large experimental perturbation. Therefore, most experimentalists focus on protein "spots" that change in intensity. Comparison of proteins can be complicated by slight shifts in protein mobility caused by variations between gels that are not reproducible, so that gel images cannot be superimposed directly. Efficient comparison between multiple gels requires computer-aided image analysis *(17,18)*, and several commercial programs are available to "warp" gel images to enable overlay and comparison. These programs are not entirely satisfactory, but image analysis is an area of active development, and steady improvements have been made during past years.

Characterizing Gel Quality and Quantification in 2D-PAGE Studies

In comparative studies, reproducibility is often not addressed adequately. When 2D-PAGE is properly carried out on a cell lysate, the image should have more than 1800 spots that can be distinguished and quantified by the program (as in Fig. 1). To determine significant differences, changes should be observed on at least three gels representing different experimental repeats. It is typical for investigators to report only the intensity differences that are targeted in a study. However, an assessment of the similarity between the replicate gels also should be reported. For example, in Fig. 2, the reproducibility of the spots in corresponding areas of two replicate gels is shown. Even in replicate gels of the same sample, variation between some spots can be extreme in certain regions of the gel because of staining variations, requiring spot changes to be assessed against unchanging "landmark" spots in the surrounding region.

A promising method to deal with nonreproducibility is the use of different fluorescent chromophores to derivatize proteins in different samples to be compared, followed by

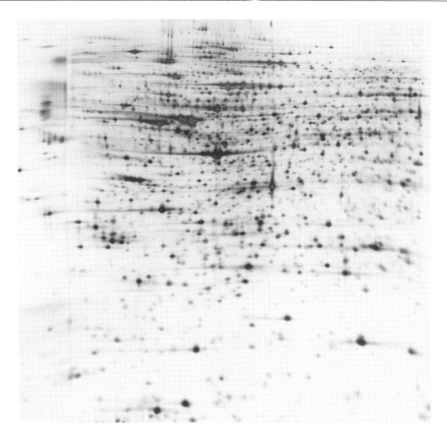

Fig. 1. Analysis of melanoma cell lines by 2D-PAGE. Cell lines, culture methods, and 2D gel analysis details are described in Bernard et al. *(25)*. A pI 4–7 dry strip was rehydrated with 100 µg of cell extract for the first dimension (acidic on the left of the final gel) and 12% SDS-PAGE was used for the second dimension. Gels were silver stained. Analysis of this gel yielded more than 1800 features.

sample mixing and 2D gel separation (DIGE technology) *(19)*. Mobility changes of one sample compared with another are identified by overlapping the images at different emission wavelengths. The use of fluorescent stains requires sensitive fluorescence detectors, sophisticated image analysis, and robotic excision, requiring a significant infrastructure commitment. Furthermore, this approach poses significant problems in sensitivity, because gel-to-gel variation is high, primarily because of background staining (signal-to-noise issue), and log ratio distributions are not normal and are biased *(20)*. More sensitive chromophores with higher signal-to-background ratios would increase the attractiveness of this approach.

Despite methodological limitations, relatively low-abundance signaling proteins have been identified by 2D-PAGE. In an early study of proteins phosphorylated in response to platelet-derived growth factor treatment of fibroblasts, proteins identified included calmodulin kinase; the guanidine nucleotide-binding protein, Gα phospholipase C; tyrosine phosphatase PTP-2; Rac b; ERK1; and AKT *(21)*. Our lab identified several targets of mitogen-activated protein kinase signaling in human cells, including covalently modified proteins and signaling pathway components *(22)*.

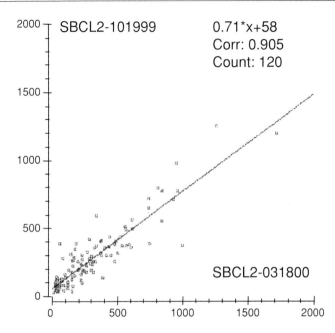

Fig. 2. Correlation of features between two replicate gels of the same cell line (SBCL2) run on different days. Gels were aligned and peak area was determined for 120 features from an area in the upper right hand area of 2D-PAGE gels run as described in Fig. 1. The intensity is given in arbitrary units on the *x* and *y* axes, for the two samples. The parameters for the best-fit line are shown. Note that some features show significant variation; this delineates the range of values that a difference must exceed to be considered significant when comparing gels from different cell lines.

2D Gel Studies of Melanoma

Several studies have been published in the last 2 yr investigating melanoma cell types by proteomics. In studies using gels surveying about 1000 proteins, Sinha and coworkers *(23)* identified several high-abundance proteins that changed when melanoma cell lines were treated with various chemotherapy compounds, including proteins involved in drug detoxification, as well as protein chaperones. Craven and coworkers *(24)* examined protein responses accompanying interferon-α-induced proliferation in two melanoma cell lines (MM418, MeWo), surveying approx 1500 proteins. Induced by interferon-α treatment, were a number of gene products previously identified as type I interferon-responsive (tryptophanyl tRNA synthetase, leucine aminopeptidase, ubiquitin cross-reactive protein, gelsolin, far upstream element-binding protein 2, and human polynucleotide phosphorylase), as well as proteins not previously known to be regulated by this signaling pathway (cathepsin B, proteasomal activator 28a, and a-SNAP). Most of these candidates changed in a similar manner between the two cell lines, although a large difference in basal level of cathepsin B between the two lines suggested a possible role in modulating the response to interferon-α treatment.

Our lab examined 12 melanoma cell lines representing radial growth phase (RGP), vertical growth phase (VGP), and metastatic stages against two primary melanocyte cell lines, in an effort to identify markers for stages of melanoma progression. Eight protein spots (summarized in Table 1) showed consistent increased or decreased intensities in

Table 1

Eight Proteins Identified in 2D-PAGE That Correlate With Progression Stages in Melanoma

Protein	NCBI no.	Comments
Hepatoma-derived growth factor	gi4758516	Low in melanocytes
Nucleophosmin	gi6307090	Low in melanocytes
Cathepsin D/spot a	P07339	High in melanocytes
Cathepsin D/spot b		High in melanocytes; low in Met; variable in RGP and VGP
Quinolinate phosphoribosyl-transferase	Q15274	High in melanocytes and RGP
Trp-tRNA synthetase	P23381	High in melanocytes
Glutathione-*S*-transferase-Ω	P78417	Not seen in melanocytes; high in RGP; variable in VGP and Met
14-3-3-γ	Q9UN99	Increased in VGP

As described in ref. *25*.

NCBI, National Center for Biotechnology Information; RGP, radial growth phase; VGP, vertical growth phase.

a manner correlating with tumorigenicity and metastatic potential of the cell lines *(25)*. Identification of these spots by MS revealed four that had been associated with melanoma or other cancers. When examined by 2D-PAGE followed by Western blotting, three proteins each appeared as multiple spots, of which, one or two varied in intensity but others were constant, indicating that changes in covalent modification, not expression, were correlated with melanoma. It is likely that such changes do not reflect primary control of gene expression, but, rather, represent alterations in the balance between cellular signaling pathways. This type of change is not an ideal candidate for a biomarker, because a significant amount of follow-up work is necessary to identify the altered regulatory processes, which may be quite subtle.

Among the potential markers, hepatoma-derived growth factor (HDGF) showed consistent increased expression in all melanoma lines compared with melanocytes. HDGF is a protein of unknown function, first discovered as a factor from conditioned media of hepatoma cells with mitogenic activity toward endothelial cells. It localizes to nuclei as well as extracellular pools, and its mitogenic activity has been shown to depend on a nuclear translocation signal sequence. In histochemical analysis of human melanoma biopsies, melanocytes and normal nevi showed very low immunoreactivity for HDGF, consistent with the low expression of HDGF in primary melanocyte cell culture. Atypical melanocytes sometimes showed higher reactivity, although expression was variable. However, advanced tumors showed intense immunoreactivity, greater than that of surrounding cells. Furthermore, the percentage of cells expressing high levels of HDGF increased with tumor malignancy, with lower percentages of cells expressing high HDGF in RGP melanomas, and higher percentages in VGP or metastatic tumors. This HDGF expression in cell lines recapitulates the expression pattern in tumors, suggesting that this may be a useful diagnostic marker for early stage melanoma with a potential functional role in cancer progression.

We also examined whether overall expression patterns reflected the progression stages. Most striking was the large range of protein changes between different lines.

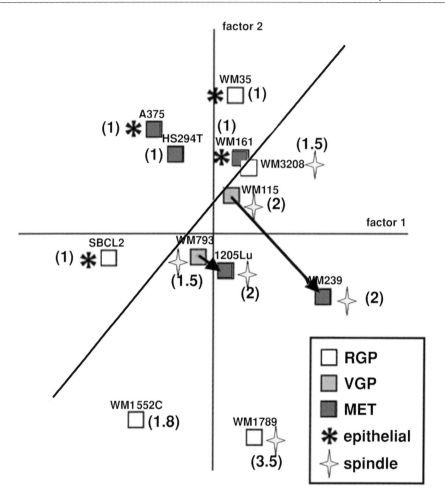

Fig. 3. Principle component analysis of 11 cell lines. Gels were aligned and intensities of features determined. The principle component analysis module of Melanie 2 was used to characterize the variability, and the first two components accounted for 83% of the variability. The number in parentheses by each cell line is the doubling time for that cell line. The symbol represents whether the cell line assumed to be an epithelial or spindle morphology in culture.

Pairwise comparisons between cells showed changes ranging between a handful of spot changes to as many as 200 changes, and, overall, approximately one-third of gel spots showed large variations between cell lines. Similar numbers of genes showed changes in messenger RNA expression between cell lines when monitored with Affymetrix microarrays. In contrast, published proteomics analyses often show very few changes between different cell lines. Surprisingly, there was no correlation between the protein phenotype and classifications of the cell lines into RGP, VGP, and metastatic stages (RGP, no tumors when injected into nude mice; VGP, tumors when injected into nude mice; metastatic, lung tumors when injected into a tail vein). A weak correlation was observed between the protein phenotypes and cell morphology and growth rates of the cell lines (Fig. 3). In fact, a pair of VGP and metastatic cell lines isolated from the same patient showed a shift along the same axis, but inversely to what one might expect, in that the metastatic cells grew more slowly.

Importantly, the observed protein changes were not completely random, in that spots varying between two cell types were more likely to vary in at least one other pairwise comparison involving other cell lines. Highly malignant cells may evolve by successive cycles of molecular diversification as a result of genetic instability, with consequent accumulation of genetic changes; only a few of these may be relevant to disease progression, although they may be relevant to the specific behavior of a given cell line or differences between tumors that may be overlooked. Thus, the wide range of protein differences between the cell lines may reflect genetic instability; however, our data suggest that genetic instability leads to altered expression of a limited subset of proteins. The remaining protein changes may represent events involved in other aspects of cell behavior, for example, survival in cell culture.

In support of the lack of correlation of the 2D-PAGE expression pattern with progression states, the two cell lines that showed the most similar 2D gel patterns were WM793, isolated from a primary melanoma with relatively low metastatic potential when injected in a mouse tail vein, and 1205Lu, isolated from a mouse lung metastasis produced after injection of WM793 cells. 1205Lu was highly metastatic in the tail vein assay, indicating metastatic conversion had occurred in comparison to the parent WM793 line. This result is consistent with other studies on sequential selection of malignant or metastatic variants in animals *(26)*. It has been suggested that an inherent limitation in studying properties of metastatic cells is that it is preceded by a transient and unstable state that limits the ability of cells to colonize a remote site. In this model, a critical event in solid tumor formation involves changes in shed cells that allow colonization of new sites followed by proliferation *(27)*. Thus, the motile "shedding" phenotype may be transient and early metastatic cells may be slow growing. Cells expressing melanocyte markers are observed in circulating blood of melanoma patients, supporting this model. Thus, critical shifts may involve changes in invasive potential and ability to survive the suspended state in the blood or lymph, as well as being capable of extravasation and tissue colonization *(28)*. On the other hand, early metastases often appear in sentinel lymph nodes, suggesting that, initially, shed cells move through the lymph system.

ACTIVITY-BASED PROTEOMIC PROFILING

In addition to determining changes in protein expression, methods for surveying changes in enzymatic activities are also emerging. Of particular interest in cancer biology is extracellular protease activity, which is important in invasion and cell–matrix interactions. A recent study used chemical inhibitors to target classes of serine hydrolase enzymes in human breast and melanoma cell lines *(29)*, separating the proteins by SDS-PAGE and using a fluorescent form of the inhibitor to allow detection of the active enzymes in the original sample. A set of proteases, lipases, and esterases were identified that distinguished breast from melanoma cancer cell lines. The activities of these enzymes were mostly downregulated in the most invasive lines. Activities of secreted enzymes that were upregulated included urokinase, a protease with known involvement in tumor progression, and a previously uncharacterized hydrolase. Although limited in sensitivity by the gel-based method in this study, activity profiling shows promise of improved sensitivity and resolution when using liquid chromatography/MS *(30)*. Other broad-spectrum inhibitor probes are available for other enzyme classes, such as hydroxamate inhibitors of zinc-dependent hydrolases, including metalloproteases and histone deacetylases *(31)*.

SURFACE-ENHANCED LASER DESORPTION IONIZATION
AS A METHOD FOR PROFILING CLINICAL SAMPLES

In search of better clinical assays for cancer, many investigators have turned their attention to proteomic profiling of serum or other body fluids, using methods that are less labor intensive than 2D-PAGE. One approach that has gained much attention is a new top-down profiling technology, using partially selective matrices that bind a subset of the analytes in the sample surface-enhanced laser desorption ionization (SELDI), thus, simplifying the sample to enhance analyte detection *(32)*. Combined with TOF MS detection, SELDI provides profiles of intact proteins in serum primarily in the low mass range (3000–20,000 Dalton). Machine learning algorithms have been used to identify combinations of peaks that may serve as molecular markers of cancer prognosis or responses to therapy. A serious problem with SELDI is that differences in sample handling between controls and patient samples can generate artifactual differences *(33)*, therefore, studies should be carefully designed to control for that possibility, including collection and processing of serum in an identical manner, carrying out analyses on samples that have not been repeatedly frozen and thawed, and interleaving control and experimental samples for the MS analyses (because MALDI ionization methods are highly variable from day to day). Furthermore, although there are now a few studies that indicate that it is possible to distinguish serum from late stage metastatic cancer vs controls, the limited dynamic range of this approach may be inadequate to detect changes in very early stage tumors.

Many groups are exploring this approach in clinical settings with other bodily fluids than serum. For example, a recent SELDI study reported two markers for uveal melanoma (4543 and 6853 Dalton) in 89% of aqueous humoral samples from patient eyes *(34)*. This study demonstrates another problem with SELDI proteomics, in that the analytes were not identified. In general, MS instruments commonly used in these studies are not able to fragment the analytes of interest to identify them. Samples can be analyzed by high-resolution instrumentation with the ability to fragment large analytes, but often the ion of interest is not observed in the second MS instrument. Most investigators resort to purification to homogeneity, which is a difficult undertaking. The small size of the marker candidates suggests that these are likely proteolytic fragments, and, indeed, that has been the case in most cases identified to date. This then begs the question of whether the physiologically relevant change is in the detected protein or in protease or protease inhibitors in serum or at the tumor. For translation of a SELDI assay into the clinic, sample preparation becomes critical to control artifactual proteolysis in samples.

To survey larger proteins in complex mixtures and achieve higher dynamic range, a few researchers are now using top-down methods with high-resolution ICR MS instruments. This technique directly couples multidimensional chromatography, capillary electrophoresis, or free-flow electrophoresis to the ICR, which is capable of fragmenting the very large protein analytes *(35)*. This approach has demonstrated very complex posttranslational patterns on histones *(36)*, providing a method to study combinatorial signaling between different regulatory sites. To date, these studies have focused on proteins that are easily ionized; in general, top-down approaches using MS detection of the intact proteins suffers from the fact that proteins often are hard to ionize. Even when using an MS capable of fragmentation, our understanding of gas-phase fragmentation of large analytes is poor, making identification difficult. Before top-down MS is a routine profiling approach for complex samples, new methods for fractionating and ionizing proteins and new computational and informatics tools for analysis of the complex data sets are needed.

An interesting application of SELDI to analysis of archival samples has recently been published *(37)*. Rapid Romanowsky-stained cytocentrifuged specimens from fine-needle aspirates of metastatic malignant melanoma (with both known cutaneous primary and unknown primary sites), clear cell sarcoma, and renal cell carcinoma each had a unique MS spectrum when examined using the SELDI technology. These preliminary findings suggest a substantial potential for SELDI applications to specific pathological diagnoses. In addition, combination of laser capture microdissection *(34,35)* with SELDI or other proteomics approaches may be particularly powerful in pathology. Another approach similar to SELDI is the direct scanning of a tissue section in a MALDI source *(38,39)*. Both laser capture microdissection and tissue scanning will be important in making the transition from studies with cell lines to understanding tumor biology. However, both of these approaches are subject to the same limitations described for SELDI, and careful experimental design will be required to exploit these methods in analysis of disease.

ARRAY-BASED PROTEOMICS ASSAYS

Protein array technologies are another approach under development for high-through-put proteomic screening. In one type of array, sets of predicted open reading frames are immobilized at high density onto slides, allowing screening for protein interactions, activities, modifications, and regulation *(40)*. Zhu et al. *(41)* constructed a protein array containing more than 5800 individually cloned, overexpressed, and purified yeast proteins. By probing this array with calmodulin or various phosphatidylinositides, 33 new and 6 known calmodulin binding proteins were found, and 150 proteins were identified as phosphatidylinositide-binding proteins, 52 of which were previously uncharacterized. Likewise, substrates for protein kinases were screened *(42)* using a protein array containing nearly all known protein kinases in yeast (119 of 122). Thus, protein microarrays show promise in screens for protein function and association, and for mapping pathways and elucidating biochemical activities of individual components in signaling pathways. Current limitations reflect quality of expressed protein targets and representation of relevant posttranslational modifications and splice variants, as well as the fact that most eukaryotic proteins require unique conditions to ensure proper folding and enzyme activity.

Another array approach under development for protein profiling is analogous to DNA microarrays, using antibody or aptamer probes covalently bound to surfaces, for direct or sandwich binding assays of proteins in complex mixtures *(43)*. Protein array technologies are more difficult than DNA arrays, because of fundamental differences between oligonucleotide and protein chemistries. Oligonucleotide analytes are chemically similar and stable, simplifying sample preparation and providing specific binding of analytes to targets. The oligonucleotide targets are stable on surfaces and can be polymerized on the target using inexpensive technology developed for printers. In contrast, proteins vary in solubility and stability, complicating sample preparation. Antibody arrays are easiest to produce, but antibodies are generally unstable on surfaces. Recent works with hydrogels show promise for providing an appropriate platform *(44)*. Some targeted arrays have been developed for specific proteins, such as antibody arrays for cytokines

(45), but it is not yet clear whether protein chip-based arrays can provide the necessary global information on splicing and posttranslational modifications required for full proteome profiling.

BOTTOM-UP OR "SHOTGUN" PROTEOMICS

A different approach, referred to as bottom-up or shotgun proteomics, or multidimensional protein identification technology (MudPIT), is now under development in many labs. Bottom-up or shotgun proteomics uses solution proteolysis of a complex sample, such as a soluble cell extract or a membrane fraction, followed by multidimensional chromatographic separation of the peptides, which are then sequenced by MS. By coupling the last chromatographic step to a mass spectrometer (LC/MS), thousands of peptide MS/MS spectra can be collected in a few hours. An early paper using this technique identified more than 1400 proteins from *Saccharomyces cerevisiae (46)*, representing 25% of the open reading frames; this and other studies by several labs indicate that this is an extremely powerful method for identifying a large number of proteins from complex mixtures.

The first critical issue in bottom-up proteomic profiling is the magnitude of the analytical problem, especially for mammalian cells. A typical MudPIT analysis identifies 800 to 1700 proteins, similar to the number of proteins typically surveyed using 2D-PAGE, and provides sufficient analytical power to analyze a bacterial proteome. However, a mammalian cell proteome likely has more than 12,000 expressed open reading frames (not counting splice variants or posttranslational modifications) *(47)*. As in 2D-PAGE, the large dynamic range of protein expression in higher eukaryotes interferes with detection of lower abundance proteins by MudPIT. In MudPIT, this interference is caused by resampling of the most abundant peptides and also by sampling of fragments of those peptides produced artifactually during the analysis (this refers to ions produced during the MS scans, not during the MS/MS scans). To minimize repetitive collection of data on the most abundant peptides, the MS instrument is set to ignore sequenced ions for a given time after the initial detection (referred to as dynamic exclusion); nevertheless, resampling rates are still high. Simplification of the sample can be used to reduce complexity down to less than 1000 proteins, at which the MudPIT method provides adequate sampling. For example, using sampling statistics, we estimate that the soluble extract from human K562 erythroleukemia cells has approx 6500 proteins present at a detection range of 50,000 copies/cell or greater (>0.1 μM). When the extract is subfractionated to produce a sample with fewer than 1000 proteins, there is high sampling of the less abundant proteins, and more than 85% of the proteins have two or more peptides identified.

However, the time required for complete mammalian cell profiling becomes prohibitive with fractionation levels needed to achieve sampling rates sufficient to detect low-abundance proteins. Each protein fraction generates many peptide fractions, and each peptide fraction requires several greater than 2-h chromatographic runs for optimal peptide capture. Thus, a MudPIT experiment on a single protein fraction from gel exclusion chromatography required 9 d for data collection using the 3D ion trap MS instrument most commonly used in MudPIT experiments, and detection of more than 5000 proteins in a soluble mammalian cell extract fractionated by gel filtration required 85 d *(48)*. At this rate, we estimate a full cell profile with compartmental subfractionation would require approx 2 yr using 3D ion trap instruments, a formidable undertaking, even with multiplexing. Fortunately, new linear ion trap MS instruments provide significantly increased scan rates, as well as higher sensitivity, reducing times required to adequately sample a mammalian proteome to approx 80 d *(49)*. Although still challenging, this is a reasonable time-scale, and detailed studies of specific cell compartments, such as the plasma membrane, are now very feasible.

Another issue for shotgun proteomics is that low sequence coverage is obtained for all but the most abundant proteins. This is caused by low sampling of less-abundant proteins, as well as limitations in what can be observed by MudPIT protocols. The average mammalian protein is approx 53 kDa and yields approx 50 tryptic peptides, of which approx 33 are experimentally observable because many peptides fail to bind chromatography resins and some peptides fragment poorly or are weakly ionizable. In the analysis of the 5000 proteins from a soluble human cell extract *(48)* described above, the peptides identified represented less than 11% of potentially observable peptides expected from proteins in the sample. These sampling constraints cause low reproducibility in identifying low abundance proteins. In addition, this also lowers the probability of observing covalently modified peptides. This is a serious limitation of proteomics, and much work is currently directed at overcoming it, in particular regarding phosphorylation *(50)*. Many investigators attempt to enrich phosphopeptides or phosphoproteins chromatographically before MS analysis. Alternatively, new mass spectrometers are able to detect specific fragmentations in the gas phase that are diagnostic of a phosphopeptide, thus ensuring that the MS/MS spectrum of that ion is taken during an analysis, despite its low intensity compared with other ions.

Another critical issue in bottom-up proteomics is validation of peptide assignments. Scoring methods of search programs (e.g., Sequest, Mascot) are poor at distinguishing correct from incorrect sequence assignments, leading to high false-positive and false-negative rates *(48,51)*. Typically, less than half of potentially identifiable MS/MS spectra are identified with high confidence. The last 2 yr have seen extensive research in improving the method of scoring the search results. In addition, alternative methods for validating sequence assignments use peptide properties other than the fragmentation pattern, such as exact mass measurements *(52)*, probability of proteolytic cleavages generating the sequence, and consistency of peptide sequence with observed chromatographic properties. Using an information fusion approach, combining several low discrimination methods based on both peptide chemical properties and the scoring of the MS/MS spectra greatly improves sensitivity and accuracy, and provides a significant increase in capture of peptide sequences from a data set *(48)*. In combination with the research on new scoring methods, it is likely that a good method of extracting maximum information from the MS data sets will emerge in the next year.

Comparing Bottom-Up Proteomic Analyses

The most common application of proteomic profiling is to compare different samples, requiring quantitative assessment of the relative or absolute changes in different proteins. Top-down proteomics enables straightforward quantification. In bottom-up proteomics, many peptides are generated for each protein, but because of variable ionization efficiencies, the ion intensities of peptides from a single protein may vary by greater than 1000-fold. When peptide sampling is low, different peptides may be detected in each experiment, increasing the difficulty of absolute quantification of low abundance proteins. One solution is use stable isotopic and/or mass tag labeling of peptides; two samples to be compared are labeled with different isotopic moieties, the samples are mixed and analyzed, and the relative quantification is determined from the ratio of intensities between the differentially labeled peaks (for example, ref. 53). However, the proteins detected by isotope-labeling methods in recent publications are so far within the abundance range observable by 2D-PAGE (54). This is most likely caused by kinetic limitations of the labeling reactions when components are subfemtomole and by the fact that both ions must be sampled to quantify the change reliably. A recent study shows that the error frequency in this approach can be substantial (55). In vivo labeling has also been used, but is not practical in many cases (clinical samples, for example). Another serious limitation of the isotope-labeling methods is that comparisons must be made pairwise, and studies comparing results between many samples or between different labs would be difficult.

Label-free quantification methods would represent a useful solution to these problems, and recently, two label-free methods involving comparison of peptide ion intensities or counting spectra have been proposed. Spectral counting is based on the fact that resampling is proportional to protein concentration (56) and is particularly useful when large changes in protein expression occur. Comparison of ion intensities requires programs that connect the MS/MS data to the ion intensity of the parent. Because the mass spectrometer is collecting information about the ion intensity before it carries out MS/MS, and ion intensity is related to peptide concentration, a peak area can be calculated as a function of elution from the chromatographic column used during the MS analysis. Preliminary experiments from several labs show that both methods are feasible (57,58), although their dynamic range and robustness are not yet clear. In our experience, combining both label-free quantification methods yields results comparable to published studies using stable isotope-labeling methods, thus, equivalent results can be obtained with either 2D gels or the shotgun approach. This should improve as new linear traps provide the increased sampling rates allowing improved sensitivity of label-free approaches.

BIOINFORMATICS IS THE NEXT CHALLENGE TO THIS FIELD

The instrument and computational advances in the last 2 yr now allow high-coverage proteomic profiling. The next big challenge is to integrate the information into higher-order systems views of the samples (10,59). This presents significant challenges. For example, display of proteomics data is complicated by variations in splicing and post-translational modifications. Simple green/red heat maps, such as those used to display microarray data sets, cannot fully represent the complexity of protein variations. Challenges common to proteomics and microarray studies are that analyses of protein or messenger RNA expression changes of gene products must be mapped to higher-order pathways or regulatory networks. More facile methods to achieve this will be needed to shift the focus of the experiment from marker discovery to more fundamental understanding of cell phenotypes. Because of the complexity of signaling, protein expression changes do not automatically convert to an understanding of effects on cellular regulatory networks. Better bioinformatics tools, surveys with pharmacological inhibitors and activators, and responses to varying expression of signaling components and modulators will be required to expand the "alphabet" of signaling rules. Cancer research will shift from an emphasis on linear responses to signaling pathways toward responses that involve measurement and analysis of combinatorial signaling patterns.

CONCLUSIONS AND PERSPECTIVES

Recent MS instrument and methodology improvements have been applied in biomarker discovery and in cell phenotyping; however, these methods have yet to have a significant impact in understanding disease processes. In part, this is because of limited profiling capabilities of the current approaches and naiveté regarding the complexity of the problems. However, the great need for increased analytical power in clinical settings is providing impetus for a large investment in this technology, and promising results are beginning to appear in the literature. The new linear ion traps are expected to greatly enhance the usefulness of proteomics, but many careful and controlled studies, and education of investigators in the complex issues in systems biology will be required for proteomics to become a mature field. However, even at this early stage, proteomics will likely play an important role in providing a better understanding of melanoma tumor biology and a solid biochemical underpinning for targeting signaling pathways in anti-cancer therapy.

REFERENCES

1. Shevchenko A, Jensen ON, Podtelejnikov AV. Linking genome and proteome by mass spectrometry: large scale identification of yeast proteins from 2D gels. Proc Natl Acad Sci USA 1979;93: 14,440–14,445.
2. Cristoni S, Bernardi LR. Development of new methodologies for the mass spectrometry study of bioorganic macromolecules. Mass Spectrom Rev 2003;22:369–406.
3. Sleno L, Volmer DA. Ion activation methods for tandem mass spectrometry. J Mass Spectrom. 2004;39:1091–1112.
4. Gygi SP, Corthals GL, Zhang Y, Rochon Y, Aebersold R. Evaluation of two-dimensional gel electrophoresis-based proteome analysis technology. Proc Natl Acad Sci USA. 2000;97:9390–9395.
5. Resing KA, Ahn NG. Identification of proteins by in-gel digestion and mass spectrometry. In: Speicher DW, ed. Proteome Analysis: Interpreting the Genome. Elsevier Science, Inc. 2003: pp. 163–182.
6. Steen H, Mann M. The ABC's (and XYZ's) of peptide sequencing. Nat Rev Mol Cell Biol 2004;5:699–711.
7. Lion N, Reymond F, Girault HH, Rossier JS. Why the move to microfluidics for protein analysis? Curr Opin Biotechnol 2004;15:31–37.
8. Wysocki VH, Tsaprailis G, Smith LL, Breci LA. Mobile and localized protons: a framework for understanding peptide dissociation. J Mass Spectrom 2000;35:1399–1406.
9. Sadygov RG, Cociorva D, Yates JR 3rd. Large-scale database searching using tandem mass spectra: looking up the answer in the back of the book. Nat Methods 2004;1:195–202.
10. Russell SA, Old W, Resing KA, Hunter L. Proteomic informatics. Int Rev Neurobiol 2004; 6127–6157.
11. O'Farrell PH. High resolution two-dimensional electrophoresis of proteins. J Biol Chem 1975; 250:4007–4021.
12. Gorg A, Weiss W, Dunn MJ. Current two-dimensional electrophoresis technology for proteomics. Proteomics 2004;4:3665–3685.
13. Cargile BJ, Talley DL, Stephenson JL Jr. Immobilized pH gradients as a first dimension in shotgun proteomics and analysis of the accuracy of pI predictability of peptides. Electrophoresis 2004;25: 936–945.
14. Chevalier F, Rofidal V, Vanova P, Bergoin A, Rossignol M. Proteomic capacity of recent fluorescent dyes for protein staining. Phytochemistry 2004;65:1499–1506.
15. Tonella L, Hoogland C, Binz PA, Appel RD, Hochstrasser DF, Sanchez JC. New perspectives in the Escherichia coli proteome investigation. Proteomics 2001;1:409–423.
16. Blattner FR, Plunkett G III, Bloch CA, et al. The complete genome sequence of *Escherichia coli* K-12. Science 1997;277:1453–1462.
17. Rosengren AT, Salmi JM, Aittokallio T, et al. Comparison of PDQuest and Progenesis software packages in the analysis of two-dimensional electrophoresis gels. Proteomics 2003;3:1936–1946.

18. Righetti PG, Castagna A, Antonucci F, et al. Critical survey of quantitative proteomics in two-dimensional electrophoretic approaches. J Chromatogr A 2004;1051:3–17,
19. Tonge R, Shaw J, Middleton B, et al. Validation and development of fluorescence two-dimensional differential gel electrophoresis proteomics technology. Proteomics 2001 1:377–396.
20. Karp NA, Kreil DP, Lilley KS. Determining a significant change in protein expression with DeCyder during a pair-wise comparison using two-dimensional difference gel electrophoresis. Proteomics 2004;4:1421–1432.
21. Soskic V, Gorlach M, Poznanovic S, Boehmer FD, Godovac-Zimmermann J. Functional proteomics analysis of signal transduction pathways of the platelet-derived growth factor beta receptor. Biochemisty 1999;38:1757–1764.
22. Lewis TS, Hunt JB, Aveline LD, et al. Identification of Novel MAP kinase pathway signaling targets by functional proteomics and mass spectrometry. Molecular Cell 2001;6:1–20.
23. Sinha P, Poland J, Kohl S, et al. Study of the development of chemoresistance in melanoma cell lines using proteome analysis. Electrophoresis 2003;24:2386–2404.
24. Craven RA, Stanley AJ, Hanrahan S, et al. Identification of proteins regulated by interferon-α in resistant and sensitive malignant melanoma cell lines. Proteomics 2004;4:3998–4009
25. Bernard K, Litman E, Fitzpatrick JL, et al. Functional proteomic analysis of melanoma progression. Cancer Res 2003;63:6716–6725.
26. Cross M, Dexter TM. Growth factors in development, transformation, and tumorigenesis. Cell 1991;64:271–280.
27. Vander Griend DJ, Rinker-Schaeffer CW. A new look at an old problem: the survival and organ-specific growth of metastases. Sci STKE 2004;2004:pe3.
28. Pepper MS. Lymphangiogenesis and tumor metastasis: myth or reality? Clin Cancer Res 2001; 7:462–468.
29. Jessani N, Liu Y, Humphrey M, Cravatt BF. Enzyme activity profiles of the secreted and membrane proteome that depict cancer cell invasiveness. Proc Natl Acad Sci USA 2002;99:10,335–10,340.
30. Adam GC, Burbaum J, Kozarich JW, Patricelli MP, Cravatt BF. Mapping enzyme active sites in complex proteomes. J Am Chem Soc 2004;126:1363–1368.
31. Marks PA, Richon VM, Breslow R, Rifkind RA. Histone deacetylase inhibitors as new cancer drugs. Curr Opin Oncol 2001;13:477–483.
32. Conrads TP, Hood BL, Issaq HJ, Veenstra TD. Proteomic patterns as a diagnostic tool for early-stage cancer: a review of its progress to a clinically relevant tool. Mol Diagn 2004;8:77–85.
33. Check E. Running before we can walk? Nature 2004;429:496–497.
34. Missotten GS, Beijnen JH, Keunen JE, Bonfrer JM. Proteomics in uveal melanoma. Melanoma Res 2003;13:627–629.
35. Kelleher NL. Top-down proteomics. Anal Chem 2004;76:197A–203A.
36. Pesavento JJ, Kim YB, Taylor GK, Kelleher NL. Shotgun annotation of histone modifications: a new approach for streamlined characterization of proteins by top down mass spectrometry. J Am Chem Soc 2004;126:3386–3387.
37. Emmert-Buck MR, Bonner RF, Smith PD, et al. Laser capture microdissection. Science 1996; 274:998–1001.
38. Ornstein DK, Gillespie JW, Paweletz CP. Proteomic analysis of laser capture microdissection human prostate cancer and in vitro prostate cell. Electrophoresis 2000;21:2235–2240.
39. Chaurand P, Sanders ME, Jensen RA, Caprioli RM. Proteomics in diagnostic pathology: profiling and imaging proteins directly in tissue sections. Am J Pathol 2004;165:1057–1068.
40. Zhu H, Snyder M. Protein chip technology. Curr Opin Chem Biol 2003;7:55–763.
41. Zhu H, Bilgin M, Bangham R, et al. Global analysis of protein activities using proteome chips. Science 2001;293:2101–2105.
42. Zhu H, Klemic JF, Chang S, et al. Analysis of yeast protein kinases using protein chips. Nat Genct 2000;26:283–289.
43. Smith AH, Vrtis JM, Kodadek T. The potential of protein-detecting microarrays for clinical diagnostics. Adv Clin Chem 2004;38:217–238.
44. Yoshimura I, Miyahara Y, Kasagi N, Yamane H, Ojida A, Hamachi I. Molecular recognition in a supramolecular hydrogel to afford a semi-wet sensor chip. J Am Chem Soc 2004;126:12,204–12,205.
45. Li Y, Schutte RJ, Abu-Shakra A, Reichert WM. Protein array method for assessing in vitro biomaterial-induced cytokine expression. Biomaterials 2005;26:1081–1085.
46. Washburn, MP, Wolters D, Yates JR. Large-scale analysis of the yeast proteome by multidimensional protein identification technology. Nat Biotechnol 2001;19:242–247.

47. Harrison PM, Kumar A, Lang N, Snyder M, Gerstein M. A question of size: the eukaryotic proteome and the problem in defining it. Nucleic Acids Res 2002;30:1083–1090.

48. Resing KA, Meyer-Arendt K, Mendoza AM, et al. Improving reproducibility and sensitivity in identifying human proteins by shotgun proteomics. Analytical Chem 2004;76:3556–3568.

49. Resing KA. Current progress in protein profiling of complex samples. Expert Rev Proteomics 2004;1:137–140

50. Kalume DE, Molina H, Pandey A. Tackling the phosphoproteome: tools and strategies. Curr Opin Chem Biol 2003;7:64–69.

51. Keller A, Nesvizhskii AI, Kolker E, Aebersold R. Empirical statistical model to estimate the accuracy of peptide identifications made by MS/MS and database search. Anal Chem 2002;74:5383–5392.

52. Lipton MS, Pasa-Tolic' L, Anderson GA, et al. Global analysis of the Deinococcus radiodurans proteome by using accurate mass tags. Proc Natl Acad Sci USA 2002; 99:11,049–11,054.

53. Gygi SP, Rist B, Griffin TJ, Eng J, Aebersold R. Proteome analysis of low-abundance proteins using multidimensional chromatography and isotope-coded affinity tags. J Proteome Res 2002;1:47–54.

54. Gygi, SP, Corthals GL, Zhang Y, Rochon Y, Aebersold R. Evaluation of two-dimensional gel electrophoresis-based proteome analysis technology. Proc Natl Acad Sci USA 2000;97:9390–9395.

55. Parker KC, Patterson D, Williamson B, et al. Depth of proteome issues: a yeast isotope-coded affinity tag reagent study. Mol Cell Proteomics 2004;3:625–659.

56. Liu H, Sadygov RG, Yates JR 3rd. A model for random sampling and estimation of relative protein abundance in shotgun proteomics. Anal Chem 2004;76:4193–4201.

57. Bondarenko PV, Chelius D, Shaler TA. Identification and relative quantitation of protein mixtures by enzymatic digestion followed by capillary reversed-phase liquid chromatography-tandem mass spectrometry. Anal Chem 2002;74:4741–4749.

58. Wang W, Zhou H, Lin H, et al. Quantification of proteins and metabolites by mass spectrometry without isotopic labeling or spiked standards. Anal Chem 2003;75:4818–4826.

59. Russell SA, Old W, Resing KA, Hunter L. Proteomic Informatics. International Review of Neurobiology 2004;61:129–157.

III

PRIMARY INVASIVE MELANOMA TO METASTATIC MELANOMA

23

Paradigm of Metastasis for Malignant Melanoma

Stanley P. L. Leong

CONTENTS

Summary

Melanomas usually progress from an *in situ* growth to a radial growth phase in which they expand into a vertical growth phase that is associated with an increased risk of metastasis. In general, the process of metastasis occurs in an orderly fashion from the primary site to the regional sentinel lymph nodes before systemic dissemination. Occasionally, early blood-borne metastasis may occur. The role of selective sentinel lymphadenectomy is to provide accurate staging at the initial diagnosis of primary invasive melanoma, 1 mm or greater in depth; because the staging result is often accurate, the morbidity is reduced and the cost is less. Melanoma may spread to almost all organs. Autopsy reports have shown widespread dissemination with predominance to lymph nodes and lungs. The survival is dismal with visceral metastasis. Early diagnosis of melanoma through education and surveillance should be encouraged. Because treatments for metastatic cancer are still limited, it is imperative for oncologists to detect and resect an early cancer as soon as possible. Multifaceted aspects of micrometastasis, including proliferation and differentiation of various clones from the primary tumor, the acquisition of adhesion molecules, the process of angiogenesis, and host interaction with the microscopic tumor may shed new lights on the biology and mechanism of early metastasis. Molecular and genetic tools may be used to dissect the mechanisms of lymphatic and hematogenous routes of metastasis. Understanding such mechanisms may help us to develop therapeutic strategies to prevent the process of micrometastasis.

Key Words: Melanoma; metastasis; lymphovascular system; sentinel nodes.

From: *From Melanocytes to Melanoma: The Progression to Malignancy*
Edited by: V. J. Hearing and S. P. L. Leong © Humana Press Inc., Totowa, NJ

INTRODUCTION

The incidence of malignant melanoma is still increasing rapidly, with 1 of 75 Americans being diagnosed with melanoma annually, but the overall mortality rate has risen only slightly. This trend indicates that most of the melanoma being diagnosed is of the thin level that can be treated effectively by surgical excision *(1)*. Both clinical and histological features have been used to predict the prognosis of primary melanoma *(2)*. In stage I melanoma, the Clark model is about 89% accurate in predicting survival based on tumor progression *(3)*. Melanomas usually progress from an *in situ* growth to a radial growth phase in which they expand into a vertical growth phase that is associated with increased risk of metastasis. Breslow tumor thickness, as measured from the stratum granulosum of the epidermis to the deepest depth of the tumor, is considered the best predictor of clinical outcome *(4)*. The survival rate drops to single digits when metastasis is found beyond the regional lymph nodes, especially in visceral sites *(5)*.

PATTERNS OF MELANOMA METASTASIS IN THE PRE-SENTINEL LYMPH NODE ERA

Nodal status is the most important predictor of clinical outcome in melanoma *(5,6)*. It is known that the number of positive lymph nodes greater than four signifies a poor prognosis *(5)*. These studies of the pre-sentinel lymph node (SLN) era strongly suggest that, in general, tumor progression in a primary site resulted in metastasis to regional nodes at first and then to distant sites. Thus, the premise of treatment for melanoma rested on the eradication of the primary tumor and the nodal disease. Oftentimes, a regional lymph node dissection was performed to make sure that all of the lymph nodes were harvested to stage the patient. Further, such lymph nodes would harbor microscopic disease, thus, their removal could potentially prevent systemic metastasis.

In the pre-SLN era, based on multiple clinical collative retrospective studies, it has been noted that regional nodal basins are the most common sites of metastasis. Patients with primary lesions ranging from 0.76- to 1.5-mm thick may develop nodal recurrence 25% of the time within 3 yr. When the Breslow thickness increases to 1.5–4 mm, the percentage of nodal metastasis increases to 60% within 3 yr. On the other hand, systemic metastases are less common but their incidence is also correlated with the thickness of the primary tumor. Patients with primary lesions from 1.5- to 4-mm thick may develop systemic metastasis 15% of the time within 5 yr of the diagnosis *(7)*. These retrospective studies indicate that, in general, during the early phase of melanoma proliferation, the pattern of metastasis to the regional nodal basin is the predominant pattern, but a minority of the patients will develop systemic disease. Often, the tumor progresses in an orderly fashion from the primary lesion to the regional nodal basin and later to systemic metastasis. This is the reason why most patients who experience recurrence in the nodal basin after lymphadenectomy may result in 5-yr survival rates between 20 and 50% *(7)*. This implies that between 20 and 50% of patients are "cured" by removing the lymph nodes. On the other hand, patients with thin melanoma may develop recurrence, indicating early dissemination of the disease in a minority of patients (approx 4.8%) *(8)*. The phenomenon of dormancy may exist in melanoma, as shown by a very late metastasis of more than 10 yr. However, such late metastasis was relatively rare, in 168 patients (2.8%) from a large series of 7104 patients *(9)*. During dormancy, whether the cancer cells are quiescent or the host exerts a suppressive effect on the cancer cells is not known.

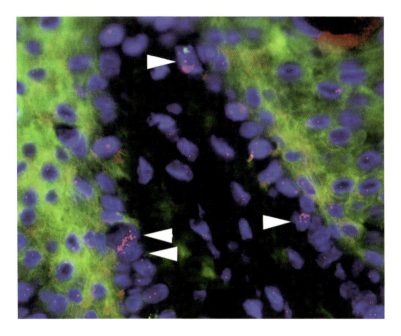

Color Plate 1, Fig. 2. Field cells in acral melanoma detected by fluorescence *in situ* hybridization. Single basal melanocytes with amplifications of cyclin D1 highlighted by arrowheads. (*See* discussion in Chapter 11 on p. 203.)

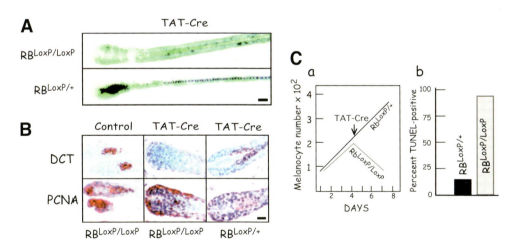

Color Plate 1, Fig. 6. RB is required to suppress apoptosis in normal melanocytes. (**A**) Nonpigmented hair shaft of TAT-Cre-treated RB$^{LoxP/LoxP}$ hair follicles compared with pigmented RB$^{LoxP/+}$ hair shaft. (*See* complete caption in Chapter 13 on p. 234 and discussion on pp. 233–234.)

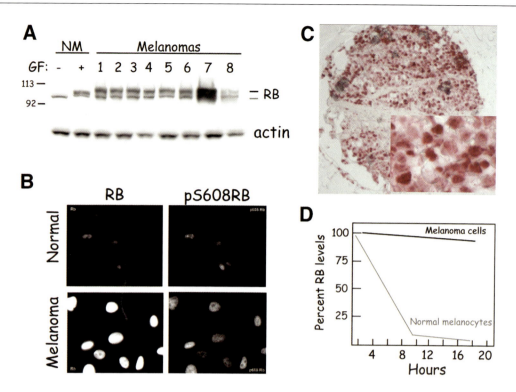

Color Plate 2, Fig. 7. RB is highly abundant in melanoma cells relative to normal melanocytes. **(A)** Western blot showing expression of RB in normal melanocytes (NM) vs melanoma cell strains from different tumors (1–8). (*See* complete caption in Chapter 13 on p. 233 and discussion on pp. 232–233.)

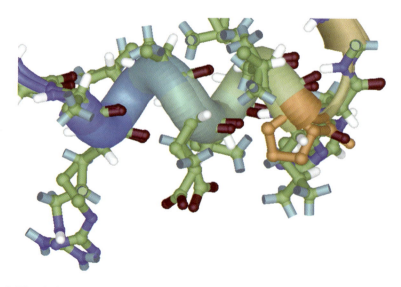

Color Plate 2, Fig. 4. Structural model of the leucine to proline substitution at position 65 of p16 (from ref. *72*). The model shows that the proline amino acid (indicated in orange), differently from the leucine (behind the proline), no longer makes hydrogen atoms available to the surface of the protein, possibly affecting the ability of this protein to complex or bind with its ligand. (*See* discussion in Chapter 18 on p. 336.)

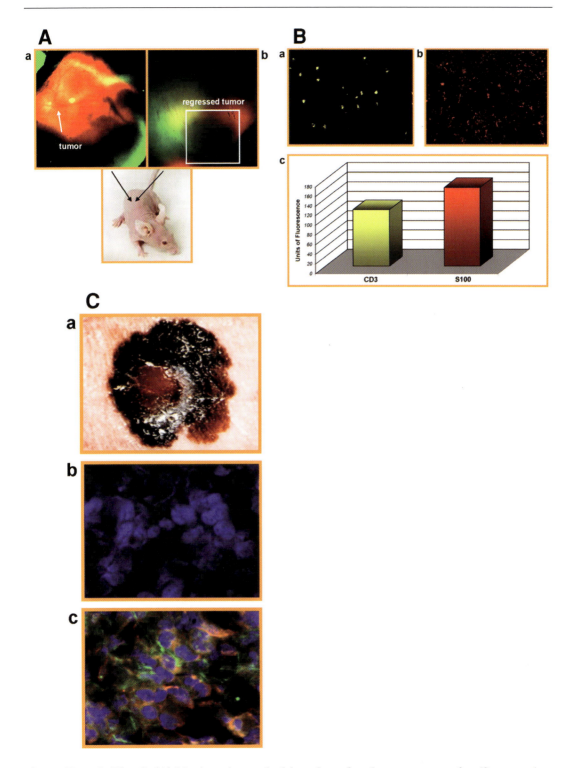

Color Plate 3, Fig. 2. (A) Noninvasive optical imaging of melanoma xenografts. (*See* complete caption in Chapter 21 on pp. 406–407 and discussion on p. 406.)

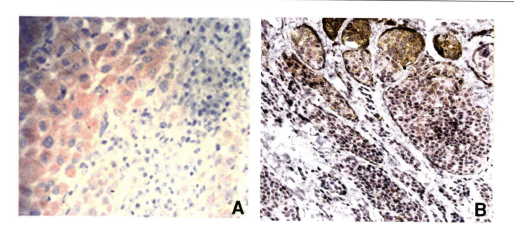

Color Plate 4, Fig. 2. Detection of melanoma inhibitory activity (MIA) by immunohistochemistry. (*See* complete caption in Chapter 26 on p. 479 and discussion on p. 478.)

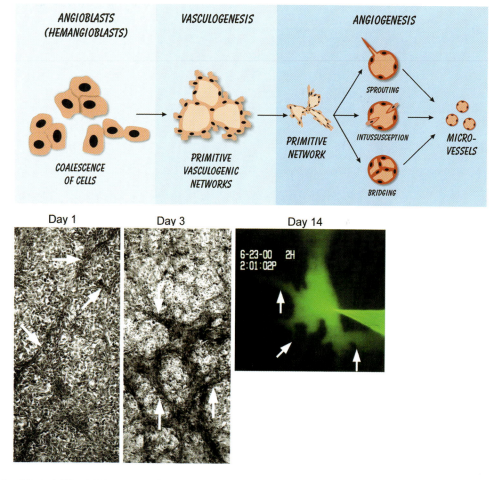

Color Plate 4, Fig. 1. Diagrammatic representation of vasculogenesis, angiogenesis, and photomicroscopy of tumor cell vasculogenic mimicry. (*See* complete caption in Chapter 30 on p. 537 and discussion on p. 536.)

Table 1
Autopsy Reports of 216 Melanoma Patients
Showing That Lymph Nodes and Lungs
Are the Most Frequent Sites of Involvement

Lymph nodes	73.6%
Lung	71.3%
Liver	58.3%
Brain	54.6%
Adrenals	46.8%
Gastrointestinal	43.5%
Skin	10.6%

Adapted from refs. *10* and *12*.

Detailed patterns of metastasis both from clinical studies and autopsy reports have been described *(10)*. Melanoma may metastasize to almost all organs; hence the nickname of "syphilis" of cancer. For patterns of dissemination, autopsy results represent the most accurate distribution of metastasis. In a series of 216 melanoma patients, Patel et al. *(12)* found that the lymph nodes and lungs are the most frequent sites of involvement (Table 1). Further, melanoma may be found in multiple organs (Table 2), indicating that in late stages of the disease, dissemination may be widespread. Based on the autopsy reports *(11,12)*, clinical and histological features do not predict patterns of metastasis. However, when melanoma disseminates widely, the survival is usually short. On the other hand, when dissemination is limited, the survival is longer. Indeed, isolated metastasis may potentially be resected, resulting in a better survival *(13)*. Patients with multiple metastasis usually do quite poorly *(7)*. The unanswered question is whether the melanoma is pluripotential to multiple sites or whether multiple clones are present from the primary site with each clone directed to certain specific organs as in the "seed and soil" hypothesis proposed by Paget *(14,15)*.

PATTERNS OF MELANOMA METASTASIS IN THE SLN ERA

SLNs are the first nodes in the regional nodal basin that cancer cells metastasize to from a primary site. The validation of the SLN concept in human solid cancer is definitely a turning point in the management of human solid cancer and, in particular, for melanoma. The rapid adoption of this technique by surgical oncologists at large has quickly made the debate of whether an elective lymph node dissection should be done vs watchful observation, when the primary invasive melanoma is at least 1 mm or greater in depth, irrelevant. Although the therapeutic role of selective sentinel lymphadenectomy (SSL) to harvest the SLNs in melanoma has not been determined, and the conclusions will come forth after the completion of the Multicenter Sentinel Lymphadenectomy Trial by Morton et al. *(16)*, the practical significance is that it is being applied widely as a staging procedure so that a negative SLN can spare a patient a radical regional lymph node dissection and the associated morbidity of such a procedure *(17)*.

The relationship between Breslow thickness and the sentinel node status is linearly correlated *(18)*. Because of the accuracy of SSL as a staging method, the 6th edition of the American Joint Committee on Cancer for melanoma has been revised with incorporation of the SLN status *(19)*. Melanoma progression can be further defined in terms of

Table 2
Patterns of Metastasis of Melanoma
in Different Organs Based on Autopsy Reports of 216 Cases

Respiratory	Lungs	71.3%
	Upper respiratory tract	7.9%
Gastrointestinal	Liver	58.3%
	Oral cavity/esophagus	9.3%
	Stomach	22.7%
	Peritoneum	42.6%
	Pancreas	37.5%
	Small bowel	35.6%
	Spleen	30.6%
	Colon	28.2%
	Biliary tract	8.8%
Cardiovascular	Heart	47.2%
	Pericardium	24.1%
	Major vessels	6.0%
Endocrine	Adrenal	35.6%
	Thyroid	25.5%
	Parathyroid, pituitary	16.2%
CNS	Brain	49.1%
	Meninges	24.1%
	Medulla, pons	12.9%
Urinary tract	Kidney, left	34.7%
	Kidney, right	31.9%
	Lower urinary tract	13.0%
Bone	Vertebrae	41.2%
	Other bones	33.3%
Genital system	Ovaries or testes	
	Left	13.2%
	Right	10.2%
Lymph nodes	Neck	42.0%
	Thorax	55.5%
	Abdominal	56.0%
	Pelvic	37.0%
	Others	32.4%
Soft tissue, muscle	Skin	68.0%

Adapted from refs. 10 and 12.
CNS, central nervous system.

primary melanoma proliferation, metastasis to the SLNs or distant sites, progression from SLNs to non-SLNs, and progression from SLNs or non-SLNs to systemic sites (20). Thus, based on the literature on the pre-SLN and the SLN era, metastatic melanoma cells are generated as a result of proliferation (Fig. 1). Early metastasis occurs mostly in the regional SLN and metastasis to SLN is a poor prognostic factor with respect to disease-free and overall survival (Fig. 2) (21). In general, the paradigm of metastasis for melanoma is characterized by initial proliferation and metastasis to SLNs then to non-SLNs before systemic metastasis. Occasionally, it is possible for the cancer cells to spread via the systemic circulation to distant sites from the primary site, SLN(s) or non-SLN(s).

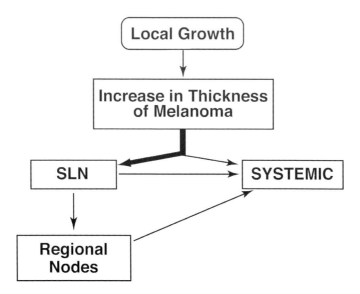

Fig. 1. Paradigm of metastasis for melanoma starts as a local growth, and proliferation results in more aggressive clones to metastasize to sentinel lymph nodes (SLNs) and subsequently to non-SLNs before systemic metastasis. Occasionally, either from the primary site, SLNs, or non-SLNs, tumor cells may spread via systemic circulation to distant sites. Thus, based on the literature on the pre-SLN and the SLN era, melanoma metastatic cells are generated as a result of proliferation. (Reprinted with permission from Leong, ref. *50*.)

Thus, it is important to define the patterns of metastasis of melanoma with respect to the incubator hypothesis vs the marker hypothesis *(22)*. In the SLN era, both retrospective and prospective studies indicate that most likely in most cases, in melanoma, the incubator hypothesis may describe the situation more appropriately than the marker hypothesis *(22)*. Although it has been argued that upstaging by SSL may result in a "lead time" basis, recent studies with longer follow-up suggest that the SLN status is indeed a strong and reliable prognostic indicator *(21)*. Therefore, prospective and long-term follow-up of these patients is essential to further define the biology of nodal micrometastasis. The unresolved issue is when is the critical point of that progression when the cancer can be arrested before metastasis either to the SLNs or to systemic sites. An attempt has been made to define the tumor burden by S-classification to predict the clinical outcome of the disease *(23)*. Even when only the SLNs are involved, can the removal of the positive SLNs render the patient cured? Recent studies by Kretschmer et al. have shown that melanoma patients with lymphatic metastasis may benefit from sentinel lymphadenectomy and early excision of their nodal disease *(24)*.

IMPLICATIONS OF INCUBATOR VS MARKER HYPOTHESIS

The clinical implication is that, with the incubator hypothesis there is a definite window of opportunity during which, when the primary tumor or the metastasis in the locoregional basin is being removed, the patient is rendered free of disease. If indeed the incubator hypothesis is correct, then the removal of the involved SLNs or the regional lymph nodes may result in the cure of patients at the stage when metastatic cells are only captured within the SLNs or regional lymph nodes. Therefore, in patients with positive

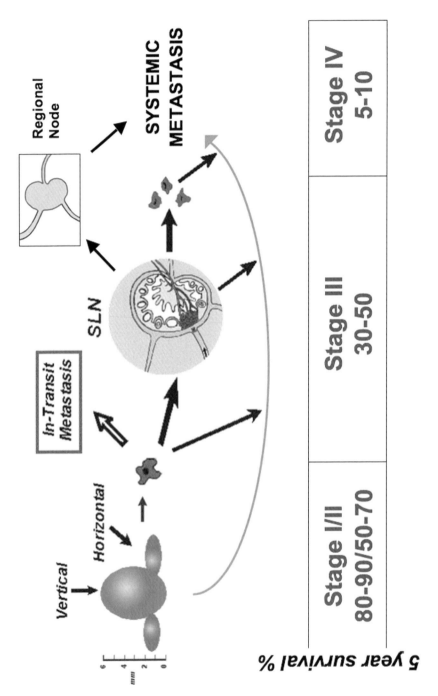

Fig. 2. Specific pattern of metastasis with corresponding survival rates for melanoma. (Reprinted with permission from Leong, ref. *20.*)

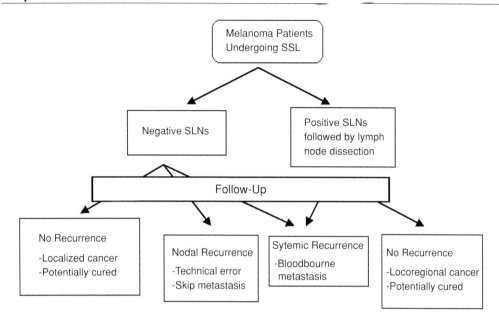

Fig. 3. Importance of follow-up of melanoma patients undergoing selective sentinel lymphadenec-tomy. It is important to establish the patterns of metastasis for primary melanoma. Clinical characteristics and outcome of patients may be correlated with the histological features and molecular markers of the primary tumor and sentinel lymph nodes to define high-risk subgroups to be accrued for adjuvant clinical trials.

SLNs, at least a subgroup of these patients may be cured, provided that melanomas in these patients have not yet initiated the process of blood-borne metastasis. On the other hand, with the marker hypothesis, the removal of the SLNs or regional lymph nodes being positive will not result in a cure of the patients, because the positive SLNs or regional lymph nodes only serve as a marker that the patient has systemic metastasis. Current clinical and histological risk factors are not able to pinpoint such subgroups of patients. Molecular markers are being developed to further define such subgroups. Therefore, in the future, if the molecular markers can segregate the patients whose pattern of metastasis is that of the incubator type vs those patients whose pattern is that of the marker type, then adjuvant therapy, even if it is toxic, will become more appropriate to treat those patients known to have the marker pattern of metastasis.

Thin melanomas are usually curable when treated only with wide local excision *(1)*. To date, surgical resection of early melanoma is of vital importance to control the spread of melanoma and achieve a greater benefit of survival. It is critical for all melanoma surgeons to keep a computerized database so that patients undergoing SSL can be followed in a prospective fashion. Each point of follow-up, as shown in Fig. 3, is a yardstick in its correlation with molecular markers of the tumor. The extensive genetic profiles being obtained by microarray technology may be correlated with the clinical outcome to bring out the genes responsible for such clinical manifestations *(25,26)*. Thus, further prognostic markers and therapeutic innovations may be developed. Early diagnosis of melanoma through education and surveillance should be encouraged *(27)*. The challenge in the future would be to determine the mechanisms of metastasis via the lymphatic system vs the circulatory system on a molecular and genetic level, to subgroup patients according to incubator vs marker hypothesis. Such information will be critical to select high-risk patients for adjuvant therapy.

The crucial question is whether melanoma spreads through the lymphatic system first, then from the lymphatic system to the systemic system, thereby involving the distant organs; vs the other possibility that melanoma at the onset spreads by a vascular route to the bloodstream and thereby distant sites. In general, based on clinical observations, both in carcinomas and in melanoma, the lymph node predicts the outcome of the patients. On the other hand, mesenchymal tumors, such as sarcomas, in general, spread through the blood stream rather than the lymphatic system. In this sense, melanomas and carcinomas behave similarly. Of course, a minority of melanoma patients may manifest locoregional and systemic metastasis simultaneously.

MOLECULAR DETECTION OF MELANOMA METASTASIS

Molecular staging using the polymerase chain reaction (PCR) technique to detect the *tyrosinase* gene messenger (m)RNA has been shown to increase detection of submicroscopic disease in SLNs *(28)*. Obviously, the advantage of PCR determination is that it examines the entire lymph node being processed via mRNA detection, thus, sampling errors may be eliminated. PCR has enhanced our ability to detect even several cells in the SLNs, and accuracy may be increased by using multiple markers. Because usually a few SLNs are involved, the cost would be much reduced, as compared with application of this technique to multiple lymph nodes from elective lymph node dissection.

A major breakthrough has been made in the development of assessing specific mRNA markers in archival paraffin-embedded specimens. Not only can this technique be employed to study gene expression of micrometastasis in SLNs more precisely, with microscopic guidance to the sections containing micrometastasis, but also the patients' clinical outcome is also readily available. Thus, the biological significance of the gene markers can be assessed with respect to the clinical outcome *(29)*. Further, in archival specimens with hemotoxylin and eosin-negative SLNs, subgroups can be differentiated using a multigene reverse transcription (RT)-PCR assay to correlate with the clinical outcome *(22,30)*.

Using paraffin-embedded tissues, the immunohistochemistry (IHC)-negative group can be further subgrouped. Both SLN- and PCR-negative patients enjoy survivals approaching nearly 100%, indicating that melanoma with no metastasis to the SLN(s) can potentially be cured. Patients who are SLN-negative but PCR-positive have a significant recurrence rate compared with the SLN-negative and PCR-negative group. In the report by Morton et al. *(22)*, when paraffin-embedded SLNs from 162 IHC-negative patients were further studied using multimarker RT-PCR, 41 (25%) showed positive signals; 5-yr rates of recurrence were 40, 63, and 78% when SLNs expressed 1, 2, and melanoma markers, respectively, vs only 4% for PCR-negative SLNs (p 0.001). This difference suggests that the IHC method fails to detect 25% of SLN micrometastasis. Thus, PCR is not only more sensitive than IHC in the detection of micrometastasis in SLNs, but is also clinically significant for recurrence. This is consistent with the high cure rate of patients with early invasive primary melanoma. Prospective clinical follow-up of patients will further define the validity of molecular staging.

In view of the recent finding that melanoma patients with PCR positivity in the lymph node have a worse prognosis than PCR-negative patients, it is possible that early dissemination of microscopic cells via the circulatory system may occur *(22)*. Although attempts have been made to detect melanoma cells in the circulation by RT-PCR, the specificity has yet to be optimized *(31–33)*.

EVIDENCE FOR EARLY MELANOMA METASTASIS THROUGH THE LYMPHATIC SYSTEM

Recent advances in the biology of chemokine receptors have shed light on the mechanism of melanoma metastasis through the lymphatic system. Chemokine receptors have been found on dendritic cells, Langerhans' cells, T-cells, and natural-killer cells, which migrate from the skin to the draining lymph node in response to these chemokines *(34–40)*. It has been hypothesized that the role of chemokines is to recruit solid tumor cells to draining lymph nodes *(41)*. One chemokine of interest is cc-ligand-21/secondary lymphoid tissue chemokine (CCL21/SLC), which has been shown to recruit CCR7(+) naive T-cells, natural-killer cells, memory T-cells, and dendritic cells *(34–46)*. CCL21/SLC is constitutively expressed in the high endothelial venules of lymph nodes, Peyer's patches, thymus, spleen, and mucosal tissue *(38,47)*. CCL21/SLC produced by high endothelial venules cells recruits CCR7 cells to draining lymph nodes *(36,40,42,43,46,47)* which, when stimulated by antigen, become activated and express CCL21/SLC. This expression results in the activation of CCR7(+) immune cells *(38,40,45)*. Melanoma cells have been found to express CCR7, which may be selectively recruited to the SLNs. The metastatic cells may downregulate the production of CCL21/SLC in the SLNs, resulting in a decreased recruitment of T-cells into the SLNs as a possible mechanism of immunosuppression *(48)*. Further, CCR7 expression was assessed in primary melanomas by IHC and quantitative real-time RT-PCR and shown to be significantly ($p < 0.02$) correlated to Breslow thickness by quantitative real-time RT-PCR. The studies also demonstrated that SLN produced significant levels of CCL21 when SLN was negative for tumor cells; however, in the presence of tumor metastasis, the levels of CCL21 were significantly reduced. In the assessment of 55 SLNs from melanoma patients by quantitative real-time RT-PCR, Takeuchi et al. *(48)* demonstrated that CCL21 mRNA expression level was significantly ($p = 0.008$) higher in pathologically melanoma-negative SLNs than in melanoma-positive SLNs. This supported the hypothesis that a subset of melanoma cells can use the CCR7–CCL21 axis system to home to SLN. The study also indicated that the reduction of CCL21 may be a significant indicator of immunoregulation in the SLN, affecting not only tumor cells, but also dendritic cell and T-cell recruitment. The chemokine ligand receptor interaction is an important finding to be pursued, to further delineate its role and mechanism in downregulating the immune response in melanoma SLNs.

Recently, a novel molecular marker for cutaneous melanoma metastasis and survival was shown to be related to the ability of the melanoma to spread through the lymphatic system to the regional lymph nodes. Using double immunolabeling for the novel lymphatic endothelial marker, LYVE-1, and for the paravascular marker, CD31, tumor samples were obtained from clinical and histological closely matched cases of primary melanomas with early lymph node metastasis and nonmetastatic melanoma. The incidence of intratumoral lymphatics was significantly higher in metastatic melanomas and correlated with poor disease-free survival. These results reveal tumor lymphangiogenesis as a novel prognosticator for the risk of lymph node metastasis in cutaneous melanoma *(49)*.

CONCLUSIONS AND PERSPECTIVES

Melanomas usually progress from an *in situ* growth to a radial growth phase from which they expand into a vertical growth phase that is associated with an increased risk of metastasis. In general, the process of metastasis occurs in an orderly fashion from the primary site to the regional sentinel lymph nodes before systemic dissemination. The role of SSL is to provide accurate staging at the initial diagnosis of primary invasive melanoma, 1 mm or greater in depth *(50)*, because the staging result is often accurate, the morbidity is reduced, and the cost is less. Because treatments for metastatic cancer are still limited, it is imperative for oncologists to detect and resect cancers as soon as possible.

In the future, molecular markers will further define the subgroups, and thereby pinpoint the subgroups of patients that will require either only SSL or complete lymph node dissection to cure their metastatic disease. Multifaceted aspects of micrometastasis, including proliferation and differentiation of various clones from the primary tumor, the acquisition of adhesion molecules, the process of angiogenesis, and host interaction with the microscopic tumor may shed new light on the biology and mechanism of early metastasis *(15)*. Molecular and genetic tools may be used to dissect the mechanisms of lymphatic and hematogenous routes of metastasis. Understanding such mechanisms may help us to develop therapeutic strategies to prevent the process of micrometastasis.

REFERENCES

1. Reintgen D, Balch CM, Kirkwood J, Ross M. Recent advances in the care of the patient with malignant melanoma. Annal Surg 1997;225(1):1–14.
2. Zettersten E, Shaikh L, Ramirez R, Kashani-Sabet M. Prognostic factors in primary cutaneous melanoma. Surg Clin North Am 2003;83(1):61–75.
3. Clark WH, Elder DE, DuPont G IV, et al. Model predicting survival in Stage I melanoma based on tumor progression. J Natl Cancer Inst 1989;81(24):1893–1904.
4. Liu V, Mihm MC. Pathology of malignant melanoma. Surg Clin North Am 2003;83(1):31–60.
5. Balch CM, Buzaid AC, Soong S, et al. Final version of the American joint committee on cancer staging system for cutaneous melanoma. J Clin Oncol 2001;19(16):3635–3648.
6. Reintgen DS, Cruse CW, Wells K, et al. The orderly progression of melanoma nodal metastases. Ann Surg 1994;220:759–767.
7. Allen PJ, Coit DG. The surgical management of metastatic melanoma. Ann Surg Oncol 2002; 9(8):762–770.
8. Slingluff CL Jr, Seigler HF. "Thin" malignant melanoma: risk factors and clinical management. Ann Plast Surg 1992;28(1):89–94.
9. Crowley NJ, Darrow TL, Quinn-Allen MA, Seigler HF. MHC-restricted recognition of autologous melanoma by tumor-specific cytotoxic T cells. Evidence for restriction by a dominant HLA-A allele. J Immunol 1991;146(5):1692–1699.
10. Debois J. The Anatomy and Clinics of Metastatic Cancer. Kluwer Academic, Norwell, MA: 2002.
11. Akslen LA, Heuch I, Hartveit F. Metastatic patterns in autopsy cases of cutaneous melanoma. Invasion Metastasis. 1988;8(4).193–204.
12. Patel JK, Didolkar MS, Pickren JW, Moore RH. Metastatic pattern of malignant melanoma. A study of 216 autopsy cases. Am J Surg 1978;135(6):807–810.
13. Essner R. Surgical treatment of malignant melanoma. Surg Clin North Am 2003;83(1):109–156.
14. Paget S. The distribution of secondary growths in cancer of the breast. 1889. Cancer Metastasis Rev 1989;8(2):98–101.
15. Fidler IJ. The pathogenesis of cancer metastasis: the "seed and soil" hypothesis revisited. Nat Rev Cancer 2003;3(6):453–458.
16. Morton DL, Thompson JF, Essner R, et al. Validation of the accuracy of intraoperative lymphatic mapping and sentinel lymphadenectomy for early-stage melanoma: a multicenter trial. Multicenter Selective Lymphadenectomy Trial Group. Ann Surg 1999;230(4):453–463; discussion 463–455.

17. Leong SP. Sentinel lymph node mapping and selective lymphadenectomy: the standard of care for melanoma. Curr Treat Options Oncol. 2004;5(3):185–194.
18. Leong SP. Selective sentinel lymphadenectomy for malignant melanoma. Surg Clin North Am 2003;83(1):157–185.
19. AJCC. Cancer Staging Manual. 6th ed. Springer, New York, NY: 2003.
20. Leong SP. Paradigm of metastasis for melanoma and breast cancer based on the sentinel lymph node experience. Ann Surg Oncol 2004;11(suppl 3):192S–197S.
21. Leong SP, Kashani-Sabet M, Desmond R, et al. Clinical significance of occult metastatic melanoma to sentinel lymph nodes and other high risk factors based on long-term follow-up. World J Surg 2005;29:683–689.
22. Morton DL, Hoon DS, Cochran AJ, et al. Lymphatic mapping and sentinel lymphadenectomy for early-stage melanoma: therapeutic utility and implications of nodal microanatomy and molecular staging for improving the accuracy of detection of nodal micrometastases. Ann Surg 2003;238(4):538–549; discussion 549–550.
23. Starz H, Siedlecki K, Balda BR. Sentinel lymphonodectomy and s-classification: a successful strategy for better prediction and improvement of outcome of melanoma. Ann Surg Oncol 2004;11(Suppl 3):162S–168S.
24. Kretschmer L, Hilgers R, Mohrle M, et al. Patients with lymphatic metastasis of cutaneous malignant melanoma benefit from sentinel lymphonodectomy and early excision of their nodal disease. Eur J Cancer 2004;40(2):212–218.
25. Wang E, Miller LD, Ohnmacht GA, et al. Prospective molecular profiling of melanoma metastases suggests classifiers of immune responsiveness. Cancer Res 2002;62(13):3581–3586.
26. Kim CJ, Reintgen DS, Yeatman TJ. The promise of microarray technology in melanoma care. Cancer Control 2002;9(1):49–53.
27. Leong SP. Future perspectives on malignant melanoma. Surg Clin North Am 2003;83(2):453–456.
28. Shivers SC, Li W, Lin J, Stall A, Stafford M, Messina J. The clinical relevance of molecular staging for melanoma. Recent Results Cancer Res 2001;158:187–199.
29. Paik S, Shak S, Tang G, et al. A multigene assay to predict recurrence of tamoxifen-treated, node-negative breast cancer. N Engl J Med 2004;351(27):2817–2826.
30. Takeuchi H, Morton DL, Kuo C, et al. Prognostic significance of molecular upstaging of paraffin-embedded sentinel lymph nodes in melanoma patients. J Clin Oncol 2004;22(13):2671–2680.
31. Muhlbauer M, Langenbach N, Stolz W, et al. Detection of melanoma cells in the blood of melanoma patients by melanoma-inhibitory activity (MIA) reverse transcription-PCR. Clin Cancer Res 1999;5(5):1099–1105.
32. Hoon DS, Wang Y, Dale PS, et al. Detection of occult melanoma cells in blood with a multiple-marker polymerase chain reaction assay. J Clin Oncol 1995;13(8):2109–2116.
33. Samija M, Juretic A, Solaric M, et al. RT-PCR detection of tyrosinase, gp100, MART1/Melan-A, and TRP-2 gene transcripts in peripheral blood of melanoma patients. Croat Med J 2001;42(4):478–483.
34. Murphy PM, Baggiolini M, Charo IF, et al. International union of pharmacology. XXII. Nomenclature for chemokine receptors. Pharmacol Rev 2000;52(1):145–176.
35. Dieu MC, Vanbervliet B, Vicari A, et al. Selective recruitment of immature and mature dendritic cells by distinct chemokines expressed in different anatomic sites. J Exp Med 1998;188(2):373–386.
36. Forster R, Schubel A, Breitfeld D, et al. CCR7 coordinates the primary immune response by establishing functional microenvironments in secondary lymphoid organs. Cell 1999;99(1):23–33.
37. Nakano H, Tamura T, Yoshimoto T, et al. Genetic defect in T lymphocyte-specific homing into peripheral lymph nodes. Eur J Immunol 1997;27(1):215–221.
38. Willimann K, Legler DF, Loetscher M, et al. The chemokine SLC is expressed in T cell areas of lymph nodes and mucosal lymphoid tissues and attracts activated T cells via CCR7. Eur J Immunol 1998;28(6):2025–2034.
39. Zlotnik A, Yoshie O. Chemokines: a new classification system and their role in immunity. Immunity 2000;12(2):121–127.
40. Moretta A. Natural killer cells and dendritic cells: rendezvous in abused tissues. Nat Rev Immunol 2002;2(12):957–964.
41. Rofstad EK, Halsor EF. Vascular endothelial growth factor, interleukin 8, platelet-derived endothelial cell growth factor, and basic fibroblast growth factor promote angiogenesis and metastasis in human melanoma xenografts. Cancer Res 2000;60(17):4932–4938.
42. Yoshida R, Nagira M, Imai T, et al. EBI1-ligand chemokine (ELC) attracts a broad spectrum of lymphocytes: activated T cells strongly up-regulate CCR7 and efficiently migrate toward ELC. Int Immunol 1998;10(7):901–910.

43. Yoshida R, Nagira M, Kitaura M, Imagawa N, Imai T, Yoshie O. Secondary lymphoid-tissue chemokine is a functional ligand for the CC chemokine receptor CCR7. J Biol Chem 1998;273(12): 7118–7122.

44. Geissmann F, Dieu-Nosjean MC, Dezutter C, et al. Accumulation of immature Langerhans cells in human lymph nodes draining chronically inflamed skin. J Exp Med 2002;196(4):417–430.

45. Yanagihara S, Komura E, Nagafune J, Watarai H, Yamaguchi Y. EBI1/CCR7 is a new member of dendritic cell chemokine receptor that is up-regulated upon maturation. J Immunol 1998;161(6): 3096–3102.

46. Gunn MD, Kyuwa S, Tam C, et al. Mice lacking expression of secondary lymphoid organ chemokine have defects in lymphocyte homing and dendritic cell localization. J Exp Med 1999;189(3):451–460.

47. Gunn MD, Tangemann K, Tam C, Cyster JG, Rosen SD, Williams LT. A chemokine expressed in lymphoid high endothelial venules promotes the adhesion and chemotaxis of naive T lymphocytes. Proc Natl Acad Sci USA 1998;95(1):258–263.

48. Takeuchi H, Fujimoto A, Tanaka M, Yamano T, Hsueh E, Hoon DS. CCL21 chemokine regulates chemokine receptor CCR7 bearing malignant melanoma cells. Clin Cancer Res 2004;10(7): 2351–2358.

49. Dadras SS, Paul T, Bertoncini J, et al. Tumor lymphangiogenesis: a novel prognostic indicator for cutaneous melanoma metastasis and survival. Am J Pathol 2003;162(6):1951–1960.

50. Leong SP. Selective sentinel lymphadenectomy for malignant melanoma, merkel cell carcinoma, and squamous cell carcinoma. Cancer Treat Res 2005;127:39–76.

24

Repair of UV-Induced DNA Damage and Melanoma Risk

Qingyi Wei

Summary

Melanoma is relatively uncommon compared with nonmelanoma skin cancers, but it causes a vast majority of skin-cancer deaths. Sunlight exposure, particularly intermittent sun exposure early in life, is a well-established risk factor for melanoma. Because only a fraction of those exposed to sunlight ever developed melanoma, genetic susceptibility has long been suspected to be an etiological factor in sunlight-induced melanoma. For example, people who have a strong family history of dysplastic nevus syndrome have an increased risk of melanoma. The extremely high frequency and early onset of melanomas in patients with xeroderma pigmentosum (XP), a rare autosomal-recessive disease of mutated DNA repair genes that confer hypersensitivity to ultraviolet light, suggest that DNA repair is involved in the etiology of melanoma. Until recently, not enough population-based data were available to support the idea that DNA repair plays a role in the etiology of sporadic melanoma, but recent studies suggest that patients with sporadic melanoma, particularly those with sunlight-sensitive skin, have a low DNA repair capacity (DRC). This theory was also supported by studies showing that patients with melanomas on sun-exposed skin had a lower DRC than did patients with melanomas on unexposed skin. Furthermore, studies found that the risk of melanoma increased as DRC decreased. Taken together, these new data suggest that reduced DRC contributes to genetic susceptibility to sunlight-induced sporadic melanoma in the general population. More studies are needed to validate that DRC is a marker for genetic susceptibility to melanoma. With advances in high-throughput technology, individuals at increased risk for melanoma could be screened for functional variants of DNA repair genes, leading to primary prevention of sunlight-induced melanoma in the general population.

Key Words: Biomarker; DNA repair; genetic susceptibility; genotype; molecular epidemiology; phenotype; skin cancers.

From: *From Melanocytes to Melanoma: The Progression to Malignancy*
Edited by: V. J. Hearing and S. P. L. Leong © Humana Press Inc., Totowa, NJ

EPIDEMIOLOGY OF MELANOMA

Melanoma is relatively uncommon compared with nonmelanoma skin cancers (NMSC), but it is the most lethal cancer of the skin, causing the vast majority of skin cancer-related deaths. Since the 1970s, a melanoma "epidemic" has been occurring in the United States (1,2) and in other parts of the industrialized world, including Australia, New Zealand, and southern Europe (3,4). The incidence rate of melanoma has increased by approx 3 to 7% per year since the 1970s, although it has leveled off lately. In 2004, an estimated 7910 people died of melanoma and 55,000 new melanoma cases were diagnosed in the United States (5). It is predicted that the incidence rate of melanoma will continue to increase as the concentration of stratospheric ozone continues to decrease (6,7) and as people spend more time doing sunlight-related recreational activities, such as sunbathing (8).

SUNLIGHT EXPOSURE AND MELANOMA

Sunlight exposure, particularly intermittent sun exposure early in life, as opposed to cumulative sun exposure, is a well-established risk factor for melanoma development in humans (9–11). Increased sensitivity to the acute effects of sunlight exposure—erythema and sunburns—is also a risk factor for developing melanoma (12,13). For example, children immigrating to Australia, where ambient ultraviolet (UV) light exposure is the highest in the world, have an increased risk of melanoma compared with those who stayed in their original countries, and the risk increases with age and in those with light skin color, who freckle, sunburn easily, and are unable to tan (14,15). These data suggest that sunlight plays a very important role in the etiology of melanoma. Risk of melanoma is also associated with recreational sunlight exposure and exposure to artificial sunlight or UV radiation (UVR) (16,17). Other minor risk factors are related to occupations (18,19), diet (20,21), and hormones (22,23), although reported results have been contradictory (24).

UV light induces melanocytes to proliferate in both exposed and shielded areas of the skin (25). Fibroblasts and lymphocytes from melanoma patients are more sensitive to genetic damage induced by UVR than are cells from the controls (26). Several molecular mechanisms of UV light-induced carcinogenesis have been postulated, including alterations in growth factors, mutations of tumor suppressor genes, and immune suppression (27). However, unlike NMSC, in which the incidence is clearly related to solar radiation exposure, the incidence of melanoma is much less dependent on sunlight exposure (17). Furthermore, some melanomas occur on unexposed body sites and some melanoma patients have a strong family history of melanoma and premalignant lesions, such as inherited cutaneous moles or nevi that are not directly related to sun exposure (28). Therefore, the exact role of UV light in the etiology of melanoma warrants further investigation.

GENETIC FACTORS IN MELANOMA

Epidemiological studies found that a high frequency of common nevi in childhood is also associated with an increased risk of melanoma (29,30). In familial atypical multiple-mole melanoma syndrome, inherited cutaneous moles or nevi appear to be the precursors of malignant lesions (31,32). The relative risk of developing melanoma is greater than

300-fold for people whose relatives have melanoma and greater than 85-fold in those whose relatives have dysplastic nevi *(33)*. Several high-penetrance melanoma susceptibility genes, including *p16/MTS1/CDKN2A/p14ARF* and *CDK4*, have been cloned and mapped to the human chromosomes 9p and 12q respectively, in familial melanoma patients *(34–38)*, but hereditary melanoma cases account for only about 10% of all melanomas *(39)*.

Therefore, some low-penetrance melanoma susceptibility genes exist, whose polymorphisms or variants appear to modify the risk associated with sunlight exposure. However, to date, no published study has been large enough to provide solid evidence for an association between variants of these low-penetrance genes and risk of melanoma. One of these genes is the melanocortin 1 receptor (*MC1R*) gene, whose variants are associated with red hair and fair skin and have been shown to be risk factors for melanoma *(40,41)*. However, later studies have produced mixed results *(42–44)*. Two polymorphisms of *CDKN2A* (C500G and C540T) were found to be associated with an increased risk of developing melanoma *(45,46)*, but a later study did not confirm these findings *(47)*. A newly identified functional epidermal growth factor was found to be associated with an increased risk of risk of developing melanoma *(48)*, but a later study could not replicate these findings, instead observing that this factor play a role in melanoma progression *(49)*. The results from one study on polymorphisms of the *GSTM1*, *GSTT1*, *CYP2D6*, and *VDR* genes were inconclusive *(50)*.

Because benign, atypical, and dysplastic nevi are also independent predictors of sporadic melanomas *(51–53)*, with about 40% of patients with sporadic melanoma having dysplastic nevi compared with 7% of the general population *(52)*, additional host susceptibility factors other than the known susceptibility genes may play a role in the etiology of sporadic melanoma in the general population. The high frequency and early onset of melanoma in patients with xeroderma pigmentosum (XP)—a rare autosomal recessive disease of mutated DNA repair genes that confers hypersensitivity to UV light and has an incidence rate of 1 in 250,000 in the United States *(54)*—suggest that genetically determined DNA repair capacity (DRC) may be involved in the pathogenesis of human melanoma.

UV LIGHT-INDUCED DNA DAMAGE IN MELANOMA ETIOLOGY

UV light induces DNA damage, also called photoproducts, which are usually thought of as bulky lesions involving more than one nucleotide in the skin; UV light also produces free radicals that cause oxidative damage to DNA, resulting in oxidative stress in the cells *(55)*. Several glutathione-*S*-transferase (GST) isoenzymes encoded by the GST supergene family, which includes the *GSTM*, *GSTT*, and *GSTP* gene families, catalyze the conjugation of reduced glutathiones with a wide range of carcinogenic electrophiles and oxidized DNA *(56,57)*. Therefore, it is biologically plausible that a deficiency in these isoenzymes contributes to the risk of UV light-induced melanoma. Studies of polymorphisms in the GST supergene family have shown that individuals who carry the null *GSTM1* or *GSTT1* alleles and who have light skin (and thus are prone to photoproduct formation after exposure to sunlight) have a higher risk of developing multiple basal cell carcinomas (BCCs) than do controls *(58,59)*. Immunohistochemistry showed that the human GSTM1 protein is present in normal skin, nevi, and melanocytes *(60)*, and that individuals who have the *GSTM1*-null genotype tend to have an increased risk of developing melanoma *(61)*. GSTM1 may also be involved in the DNA repair associated with drug resistance *(56,62)*. Therefore, to understand the extent to which the *GSTM1*-null and *GSTT1*-null genotypes contribute to the risk of developing melanoma, studies that evaluate both GST genotypes and DRC are needed to determine the genotypes' individual and combined roles in the etiology of melanoma *(50)*.

NUCLEOTIDE EXCISION REPAIR IN MELANOMA ETIOLOGY

The role of DNA repair in human skin carcinogenesis was first demonstrated in XP patients *(63,64)*, in whom there was a defect in the repair system for UV light-induced DNA damage coupled with a 2000-fold increased frequency of having sunlight-induced skin cancers compared with the general population *(54)*. Malignant skin neoplasms are present in 70% of patients with XP and appear at a median age of 8 yr, which is 50 yr younger than in the general US, non-Hispanic, white population *(65)*. Unrepaired UV light-induced damage in DNA undergoing replication leads to mutation fixation *(66)*, as seen in the mutations frequently found in the *ras* and *p53* genes (often C→T or CC→TT, the so-called UV signature mutations) of skin tumors on sun-exposed body sites of both XP patients *(67,68)* and persons with sporadic skin cancers *(69,70)*.

UV light-induced DNA damage is effectively removed by the nucleotide excision repair (NER) pathway, which involves at least 20 genes *(71)*. XP is genetically heterogeneous, and mutations in seven genes (*XPA* through *XPG*) are known to cause this disease. All seven XP gene products are involved in NER, which removes a wide variety of DNA damages by incision on both sides of the lesion *(71)*. An in vitro NER system for UV light-induced damage can be reconstituted with the proteins XPA, replication protein A, XPC–HR23B complex, transcription factor II H (containing XPD), XPF–ERCC1 complex, XPG, and damage DNA-binding protein *(72)*. A number of NER genes are so-called core factors that participate in NER activities; any functional mutation in these genes will lead to NER abnormalities and therefore susceptibility to cancers, including skin cancer in XP patients.

One study found a nonsignificant difference in DRC between patients with hereditary dysplastic nevi and healthy controls *(73)*. Other studies with fibroblast and lymphoblastoid cell lines derived from patients with and without melanoma and dysplastic nevi suggested that patients with familial melanoma had abnormal sensitivity to sunlight *(74)* and a defect in the repair of UV light-induced DNA damage *(75)*. These relatively small studies suggest that inherited DRC plays a role in the pathogenesis of sporadic melanoma.

DRC Phenotype and Risk of Skin Cancers

XP provides an excellent disease model with which to study the etiology of skin cancers. Kraemer et al. published the first comprehensive estimation of the risk of developing neoplasms in 726 XP patients from 41 countries from 1874 to 1982. Compared with the general population, XP patients younger than 20 yr had an estimated 2000-fold increased risk of having BCCs and squamous cell carcinoma (SCC) of the skin, cutaneous melanoma, and other cancers involving UV light exposure *(76)*. However, until recently, the role of DRC in sunlight-induced skin cancers in the general population was largely unknown.

BASAL CELL CARCINOMAS

Because the incidence of BCC, compared with SCC, is less dependent on exposure to sunlight (17), genetic factors are more likely to play a role in the etiology of BCC than of SCC. Furthermore, an extraordinarily high incidence rate of BCC among XP patients suggests that abnormal DRC plays a role (77). Therefore, BCC serves as an excellent disease model for studying the role of DRC and gene–environment interactions in skin cancer. In the 1990s, investigators began to design laboratory assays that would allow the role of DRC in the etiology of BCC to be studied in the general population.

The first hospital-based, case–control study of skin cancer and DRC was the Baltimore Study, which was conducted between 1987 and 1990 (78). To increase the study's efficiency for testing genetic susceptibility, investigators enrolled subjects between 20 and 60 yr of age because genetically determined cancer risk is characterized by an early onset of cancer, as seen in XP patients. Patients with BCC and selected controls free of known hereditary skin diseases and cancers were frequency matched by age. This kind of study design allowed the investigators to control for confounding by age and other genetic factors. Blood samples were drawn from the subjects, and the lymphocytes were cryopreserved and later assayed in batches. This approach was designed to avoid experimental variation in the assays caused by differences in daily laboratory procedures. The DRC was measured by a newly developed host cell reactivation (HCR) assay (79), with the plasmids harboring the chloramphenicol acetyltransferase reporter gene. The plasmids were damaged by an incident dose of 254 nm of UVR (700 J/m^2; 30 J/m^2 produces one pyrimidine dimer per plasmid) before transfection. Preliminary data from 88 patients with BCC and 135 cancer-free controls suggested that the distribution of DRCs among subjects was approximately normal, with a fivefold variation between individuals; however, the DRC decreased significantly as age increased (78). DRCs below the upper 30th percentile of the controls were associated with a greater than twofold increased risk for BCCs. This risk was even higher in subgroups with lighter skin (>threefold); six or more severe sunburns in a lifetime (>fourfold); and moderate or severe actinic elastosis (>fourfold), who had low DRC but not in those subgroups with high DRC (80). Furthermore, the number of skin tumors among patients with BCCs significantly increased as the DRC decreased, after adjustment for age (81). The inverse relationship between DRC and risk of BCCs is consistent with the notion that the underlying mechanism for sunlight-induced BCC is defective DRC.

The results of the Baltimore Study were not confirmed by a later population-based, case–control study of NMSC (including BCC and SCC) in Western Australia (82). This study used the same HCR–DRC assay as that used in the Baltimore Study, but with a lower dose of UVR (254 nm, 350 J/m^2) to damage the plasmids. The investigators performed the assays on T-lymphocytes isolated from 86 skin cancer cases (76 BCCs and 25 SCCs) and 87 healthy controls between the ages of 44 and 68 yr. They found no evidence for a difference in DRC between the cases and controls.

Differences between the Baltimore Study and the Australian Study, including different BCC patient sample sizes, different age ranges of the subjects, and, more importantly, different degrees of ambient sunlight exposure, may account for the observed discrepancies. For example, the incidence of BCCs was not sunlight dependent but the incidence of SCC was in Maryland fishermen (83); in Australia, both BCC and SCC were sunlight dependent, but the incidence of SCCs was more sunlight-dependent than that of BCCs, and the incidence of melanoma was the least sunlight-dependent (17).

These incidence data suggest that the BCCs in Maryland may be more genetically determined, with a low threshold of sunlight exposure, whereas BCC in Australia may be more sunlight related, because saturated sunlight exposure could have overcome even a proficient DRC. However, this hypothesis needs to be further tested.

In 1999, D'Errico et al. (84) investigated the role of DRC in 49 patients with BCC and 68 cancer-free controls in Italy. This study used the same HCR–DRC assay as that used in the Baltimore and Australian studies. The authors found a statistically significant age-related decline in DRC observed among controls from 20 to 70 yr of age but not among BCC cases. They also found significant differences in DRC between the cases and controls. These findings are similar to those of the Baltimore Study (78,80). More interestingly, the authors of the Italian study also found that tobacco smoking may enhance DRC among older patients, a finding that was later confirmed by a larger study (85).

Using the same HCR assay, Dybdahl et al. (86) studied DRC among patients with psoriasis in Denmark; they were investigating the importance of DRC in chemically induced skin cancer. They observed a significantly lower DRC among 20 psoriasis patients with skin cancer than among 20 psoriasis patients without skin cancer. Individuals who had a low DRC had a greater than sixfold increased risk of skin cancer compared with individuals with high DRC. The lower the level of DRC, the earlier the patients had their first skin tumor. Interestingly, they found no difference in DRC between 20 BCC patients without psoriasis and 20 healthy controls.

More recently, Matta et al. (87) conducted a larger study of 288 NMSC patients (78% had BCC) and 177 cancer-free controls in Puerto Rico. They measured DRC using a modified HCR assay with a luciferase reporter gene instead of a chloramphenicol acetyltransferase reporter gene. The authors found a clear age-related decline in DRC among the controls; the patients had a 42% reduction in DRC compared with the controls, and this difference contributed to a nearly fourfold increased risk of skin cancer. The number of tumors increased as DRC decreased. These findings further confirmed the findings from the Baltimore Study (78,81,88).

MELANOMA

The link between the occurrence of melanoma and defective DRC is supported by analyses of skin cancers in XP patients, but is less obvious in the general population because of a lack of data from population-based studies. Kraemer et al. (76) analyzed published reports of 132 XP patients and found that 22% of these patients had melanoma. The frequency of melanomas was increased greater than 1000-fold in patients with XP who were younger than 20 yr compared with the general population. These findings suggest that sunlight exposure and poor DRC cause melanoma in patients with XP. Until recently, there was a lack of evidence showing that defective DRC leads to an increased risk of developing melanoma in the general population.

An Italian Hospital-Based, Case–Control Study. Landi et al. (89) conducted a molecular epidemiological study on DRC and melanoma in Italy between 1994 and 1999. This study included 183 patients with melanoma and 179 control subjects who were recruited from the Dermatology Unit of the Bufalini Hospital in Cesena, Italy. Approximately 85% of the melanoma patients were from the Northern Marche and Southern Romagna areas, and approx 55% of the control subjects were spouses or close friends of the case patients. The majority of subjects had no occupational sun exposure but did have prolonged recreational (intermittent) sun exposure. The final analysis included 132 patients with melanoma and 145 control subjects whose DRC was tested by the HCR assay *(17)*; the plasmids were damaged by one 254-nm dose of UVR (350 J/m^2).

The investigators found that overall melanoma risk and DRC were not associated in this Italian population. Among cases with dysplastic nevi, DRC was not associated with known risk factors for melanoma (except for recreational lifetime sun exposure) including age; the color of the hair, eyes, and skin; and skin response to sunlight exposure; nor was between DRC associated with melanoma characteristics. DRC decreased with increasing age among control subjects without dysplastic nevi or with few nevi, but increased with increasing age among control subjects with dysplastic nevi or with many nevi. These findings suggest that the effect of dysplastic nevi on risk of melanoma is independent of DRC. In other words, dysplastic nevi and DRC may have different genetic implications and play different roles in the etiology of melanoma. Low DRC was a risk factor only in subjects who had a low tanning ability. Individuals with a low tanning ability and a low DRC had a greater than eightfold increased risk of melanoma compared with subjects with a high or medium tanning ability and a high DRC. This finding suggests low DRC may have played a role in the development of sunlight-induced melanoma in this Italian population.

An American Hospital-Based, Case–Control Study. Between 1994 and 2001, we conducted a molecular epidemiological study on DRC and melanoma in Texas *(90)*, where exposure to ambient sunlight is much higher than in Northern Italy. This study is perhaps the largest case–control study of its kind to date; 312 melanoma patients were recruited at The University of Texas M. D. Anderson Cancer Center in Houston, TX, and 324 cancer-free subjects were selected from genetically unrelated clinic visitors (83%) and spouses (17%). The melanoma patients and cancer-free controls were frequency matched by age (±5 yr) and sex; all subjects were non-Hispanic whites who resided in Texas. DRC was measured by the HCR assay *(17)*, with the plasmids damaged by an incident dose of 800 J/m^2 of UVR. The results revealed that an increased risk for melanoma was associated with having naturally blonde or red hair (>twofold) compared with black or brown hair; blue eye color (>1.5-fold) compared with other eye colors; fair or light brown skin (>3.5-fold) compared with dark skin; poor or low tanning ability (nearly twofold) compared with good or high tanning ability; and more than one sunburn (>twofold) compared with zero or one sunburn throughout life. These findings suggest that sunlight exposure played a role in the etiology of melanomas in this study population.

Overall, the melanoma patients in our study had a significant reduction in mean DRC (by 19%) compared with cancer-free controls. Low DRC was associated with a nearly twofold increased risk of melanoma. Notably, female patients had significantly lower DRC than did male patients, and this sex-related difference was not observed among the controls. This sex difference in patients with cancer was also observed in our previous studies on BCC and lung cancer *(78,85)*. Among the patients only, the subgroups that tended to have low DRC were those with blonde or red hair, blue eyes, fair skin, and poor tanning ability, but the differences were not statistically significant. These data suggest that low DRC is the underlying molecular mechanism for these known risk factors, as well as for the genetic susceptibility that contributes to the risk of UV light-induced melanoma.

When the control subjects' DRC values were divided into tertiles (i.e., efficient, medium, and poor), a dose–response relationship was observed between increased risk and decreased DRC in an unconditional logistic model after adjustment for age, sex, hair color, eye color, skin color, tanning ability after prolonged sun exposure, lifetime sun-burns with blisters, freckling after sun exposure as a child, and presence of moles and dysplastic nevi. These findings provide evidence that low DRC is an independent risk factor for melanoma and may play a role in the etiology of sporadic melanoma. Not only are these results consistent with the results of previous studies of XP patients, in which defective DRC was associated with sunlight-induced skin cancers, including melanoma; but also they are consistent with results of earlier studies of NMSC, in which reduced DRC was shown to be associated with increased risk of BCC in the general population.

Modification of DRC Phenotype by Genotypes of DNA Repair Genes

Phenotypic studies have revealed that DRC varies among individuals up to fivefold and may be modulated by genetic and environmental factors *(81,85,91)*. Because the DRC phenotype assay is labor intensive, costly, and potentially influenced by environmental factors, there is a need to identify genotypes that are correlated with DRC and amenable to high-throughput analysis. The advantage of genotypic assays is that the assays are not affected by environmental factors. In our pilot studies of 102 cancer-free subjects, we performed the chloramphenicol acetyltransferase and luciferase HCR–DRC assays and genotyped for four variants of the *XPC* and *XPD* genes (*XPC* PAT+ in intron 9 and *XPD* 156Arg, 312Asn, and 751Gln) *(91,92)*.

Based on the DRC data generated by the chloramphenicol acetyltransferase assay, we found that individuals with the *XPC* PAT$^{+/+}$ genotype, but not the heterozygotes (PAT$^{-/+}$), had statistically significantly lower DRC than those with wild-type homozygotes (PAT$^{-/-}$). Similarly, *XPD* homozygotes, but not *XPD* heterozygotes, were consistently correlated with lower DRC than were wild-type homozygotes, but none of the differences was statistically significant. These results suggest that these variant alleles have a recessive effect on DRC phenotype. Because relatively few individuals were homozygous for the *XPC* and *XPD* variant alleles compared with other genotypes, we combined individuals with these variant homozygotes into one group. Based on the data generated by the luciferase assays, which appeared to improve precision and reduce variation in the measurements, the group with one or more XP variant homozygous genotypes ($n = 45$) had a significantly lower DRC than did the other genotype group ($n = 57$); more inter-estingly, the DRC measured by the luciferase assay decreased as the number of variant homozygous genotypes increased *(91)*.

These phenotype and genotype correlation data suggest that DRC for NER is modu-lated by genetic polymorphisms of NER genes, such as *XPC* and *XPD*. Furthermore, each variant NER allele or genotype may partially contribute to the NER phenotype and, thus, to genetic susceptibility to cancer. Therefore, a combination of several variant genotypes of the NER genes that determine the DRC phenotype should be identifiable. In molecular epidemiology studies of the association between DRC and genetic suscep-tibility to cancer, a large number of samples need to be evaluated for the DRC phenotype. Further investigations are needed to identify a DNA repair pathway genotype that pre-dicts the DRC phenotype and that can then be used for population-based studies, even-tually leading to mass screening for individuals at risk.

DNA REPAIR GENE POLYMORPHISMS IN MELANOMA ETIOLOGY

Recent completion of the Human Genome Project has provided timely information on sequence variations of known DNA repair genes. In their pioneer work to identify the molecular basis for variations in DRC, Mohrenweiser and colleagues resequenced 37 DNA repair genes in 164 biologically unrelated individuals and identified 127 amino acid-substitution variants resulting from single-nucleotide polymorphisms *(93,94)*. The single-nucleotide polymorphism databases on DNA repair genes will be a huge resource for future molecular epidemiology studies on the DNA repair gene genotype and phenotype correlation and their associations with cancer risk. The findings of Mohrenweiser et al. have stimulated a large number of studies that contribute to our understanding of the role of variants of DNA repair genes in individual susceptibility to cancer *(95)*. However, relatively few studies on melanoma and DNA repair gene polymorphisms have been conducted to date.

The first United Kingdom case–control study on melanoma and DNA repair gene polymorphisms was reported by Winsey et al. *(96)*. They investigated the association between polymorphisms of five DNA repair genes (*XRCC1*, *ERCC1*, *XPD*, *XPF*, and *XRCC3*) and the risk for developing melanoma in 125 patients with melanoma and 211 cancer-free controls. Except for *XRCC3*, none of the variants selected was associated with an increased risk of melanoma. *XRCC3* is involved in double-strand break repair and the variant is a T-allele in exon 7 (position 18067 and codon 241 [Thr241Met]) of *XRCC3*, and was found to be associated with an approximately twofold increased risk of developing melanoma *(96)*. However, this finding was not confirmed in our larger study of 305 patients with melanoma and 319 non-Hispanic white controls in Texas *(97)* or in subsequent studies on NMSC in Denmark *(98)*. A later study investigated the role of polymorphisms in exon 4 of *ERCC1* (G→A) and exons 6 (A→C), 22 (C→T), and 23 (A→C) of *XPD* in 56 patients with melanoma and 66 cancer-free controls *(99)*. Although this study was small, the *XPD* exon 22 (C→T) and 23 (A→C) polymorphisms appeared to be associated with an increased risk of melanoma. In a more recent study, an Italian research group investigated the genetic basis for reduced DRC in melanoma and genotyped the *XPD* Asp312Asn (exon 10) and Lys751Gln (exon 23) polymorphisms *(100)*. Although the Italian researchers did not observe an association between these *XPD* polymorphisms and increased melanoma risk in 176 cases and 177 cancer-free controls, they found an increased risk for melanoma among subgroups of older subjects (>50 yr), subjects without dysplastic nevi, and subjects with low tanning ability. These findings provide further support for a role of inherited low DRC in sunlight-induced, sporadic melanoma in the general population.

CONCLUSIONS AND PERSPECTIVES

Emerging data, both from laboratory and population studies, suggest that variations in NER capacity phenotype and polymorphisms in NER genes are potential risk factors for sporadic melanoma and that polymorphisms in NER genes contribute to variations in DRC phenotype in the general population. A combined NER pathway genotype could be identified that may predict the NER phenotype and risk of melanoma better than any single genotype; therefore, this combined pathway genotype may serve as a better tool for studying interactions between genetic factors and sunlight exposure in the etiology of sporadic melanoma. More studies are needed to further validate DRC as a marker for genetic susceptibility to melanoma and to search for genetic variants that could better predict DRC phenotype and risk of melanoma. With advances in high-throughput technology, individuals at increased risk for melanoma could be screened for several functional variants of DNA repair genes, leading to primary prevention of sunlight-induced melanoma in the general population.

REFERENCES

1. Lamberg L. "Epidemic" of malignant melanoma: true increase or better detection? JAMA 2002;287:2201.
2. Beddingfield FC 3rd. The melanoma epidemic: res ipsa loquitur. Oncologist 2003;8:459–465.
3. Bulliard JL. Site-specific risk of cutaneous malignant melanoma and pattern sun exposure in New Zealand. Int J Cancer 2000;85:627–632.
4. Sides BA. The melanoma epidemic. Figures have risen by over 150% over 10 years. BMJ 1996;312:1363.
5. American Cancer Society, Inc. Cancer Facts & Figures 2004. American Cancer Society. Atlanta, GA: 2004.
6. Mettlin CJ. Skin cancer and ozone depletion: the case for global action. J Surg Oncol 2001;77:76–78.
7. de Gruijl FR, Longstreth J, Norval M, et al. Health effects from stratospheric ozone depletion and interactions with climate change. Photochem Photobiol Sci 2003;2:16–28.
8. Wingo PA, Ries LA, Rosenberg HM, Miller DS, Edwards BK.Cancer incidence and mortality, 1973–1995: a report card for the U.S. Cancer 1998;82:1197–1207.
9. International Agency for Research on Cancer. IARC Monographs on the Evaluation of Carcinogenic Risk to Human. Ultraviolet Radiation. Vol. 55. International Agency for Research on Cancer, Lyon, France: 1992.
10. Armstrong BK. How much melanoma is not caused by sun exposure? Melanoma Res 1993; 3(Suppl):10.
11. Woodhead AD, Setlow RB, Tanaka M. Environmental factors in nonmelanoma and melanoma skin cancer. J Epidemiol 1999;9(Suppl 6):S102–114.
12. Brenner AV, Lubin JH, Calista D, Landi MT. Instrumental measurements of skin color and skin ultraviolet light sensitivity and risk of cutaneous malignant melanoma: a case-control study in an Italian population. Am J Epidemiol 2002;156:353–362.
13. Tabenkin H, Tamir A, Sperber AD, Shapira M, Shvartzman P. A case-control study of malignant melanoma in Israeli Kibbutzin. Isr Med Assoc J 1999;1:154–157.
14. Khlat M, Vail A, Parkin M, Green A. Mortality from melanoma in migrants to Australia: variation by age at arrival and duration of stay. Am J Epidemiol 1992;135:1103–1113.
15. McCredie M, Williams S, Coates M. Cancer mortality in migrants from the British Isles and continental Europe to New South Wales, Australia, 1975–1995. Int J Cancer 1999;83:179–185.
16. Chen YT, Dubrow R, Zheng T, Barnhill RL, Fine J, Berwick M. Sunlamp use and the risk of cutaneous malignant melanoma: a population-based case-control study in Connecticut, USA. Int J Epidemiol 1998;27:758–765.
17. Armstrong BK, Kricker A. The epidemiology of UV induced skin cancer. J Photochem Photobiol B 2001;63:8–18.
18. Nelemans PJ, Verbeek ALM, Rampen FHJ. Nonsolar factors in melanoma risk. Clin Dermatol 1992;10:51–63.
19. Rafnsson V, Hrafnkelsson J, Tulinius H. Incidence of cancer among commercial airline pilots. Occup Environ Med 2000;57:175–179.
20. Moon T. Diet, nutrition in melanoma etiology. Melanoma Res 1993;3(Suppl 1):11.
21. Manson JE, Rexrode KM, Garland FC, Garland CF, Weinstock MA. The case for a comprehensive national campaign to prevent melanoma and associated mortality. Epidemiology 2000;11:728–734.
22. Smith MA, Fine JA, Barnhill RL, Berwick M. Hormonal and reproductive influences and risk of melanoma in women. Int J Epidemiol 1998;27:751–757.
23. Feskanich D, Hunter DJ, Willett WC, et al. Oral contraceptive use and risk of melanoma in premenopausal women. Br Cancer 1999;81:918–923.
24. Veierod MB, Thelle DS, Laake P. Diet and risk of cutaneous malignant melanoma: a prospective study of 50,757 Norwegian men and women. Int J Cancer 1997;71:600–604.
25. Stierner U, Rosdahl I, Augustsson A, et al. UVB irradiation induced melanocyte increase in both exposed and shield human skin. J Invest Dermatol 1989;92:561–564.
26. Roser M, Bohm A, Oldigs M. Ultraviolet-induced formation of micronuclei and sister chromotid exchange in cultured fibroblasts of patients with cutaneous malignant melanoma. Cancer Genet Cytogenet 1989;41:129–137.
27. Halaban R. Molecular correlates in the progression of normal melanocytes to melanoma. Semin Cancer Biol 1993;4:171–181.

28. Weinstock MA. Issues in the epidemiology of melanoma. Hematol Oncol Clin North Am 1998;12:681–698.

29. Gallagher RP, McLean DI, Yang CP, et al. Anatomic distribution of acquired melanocytic nevi in white children. A comparison with melanoma: the Vancouver Mole Study. Arch Dermatol 1990;126:466–471.

30. Masback A, Westerdahl J, Ingvar C, Olsson H, Jonsson N. Clinical and histopathological characteristics in relation to aetiological risk factors in cutaneous melanoma: a population-based study. Melanoma Res 1999;9:189–197.

31. Greene MH, Clark WH Jr, Tucker MA, et al. Acquired precursor of cutaneous malignant melanoma: the familial dysplastic nevus syndrome. N Engl Med Med 1985;312:91–97.

32. Greene MH. The genetics of hereditary melanoma and nevi. 1998 update. Cancer 1999; 86(Suppl 11):2464–2477.

33. Tucker MA, Fraser MC, Goldstein AM, Elder DE, Guerry D 4th, Organic SM. Risk of melanoma and other cancers in melanoma-prone families. J Invest Dermatol 1993;100:350S–355S.

34. Dracopoli NC, Harnett P, Bale SJ, et al. Loss of alleles from the distal short arm of chromosome 1 occurs late in melanoma tumor progression. Proc Natl Acad Sci USA 1989;86:4614–4618.

35. Cannon-Albright LA, Goldgar DE, Meyer LJ, et al. Assignment of a locus for familial melanoma, MLM, to chromosome 9p13-p22. Science 1992;258:1148–1152.

36. Fountain JW, Karayiorgou M, Ernstoff MS, et al. Homozygous deletions within human chromosome band 9p21 in melanoma. Proc Natl Acad Sci USA 1992;89:10,557–10,561.

37. Goldstein AM, Struewing JP, Chidambaram A, Fraser MC, Tucker MA. Genotype-phenotype relationships in US melanoma-prone families with CDKN2A and CDK4 mutations. J Natl Cancer Inst 2000;92:1006–1010.

38. Gillanders E, Juo SH, Holland EA, et al. Lund Melanoma Study Group; Melanoma Genetics Consortium. Localization of a novel melanoma susceptibility locus to 1p22. Am J Hum Genet 2003;73:301–313.

39. Platz A, Ringborg U, Hansson J. Hereditary cutaneous melanoma. Semin Cancer Biol 2000; 10:319–326.

40. Valverde P, Healy E, Jackson I, Rees JL, Thody AJ. Variants of the melanocyte-stimulating hormone receptor gene are associated with red hair and fair skin in humans. Nat Genet 1995;11:328–330.

41. Valverde P, Healy E, Sikkink S, et al. The Asp84Glu variant of the melanocortin 1 receptor (MC1R) is associated with melanoma. Hum Mol Genet 1996;5:1663–1666.

42. Ichii-Jones F, Lear JT, Heagerty AH, et al. Susceptibility to melanoma: influence of skin type and polymorphism in the melanocyte stimulating hormone receptor gene. J Invest Dermatol 1998;111: 218–221.

43. Palmer JS, Duffy DL, Box NF, et al. Melanocortin-1 receptor polymorphisms and risk of melanoma: is the association explained solely by pigmentation phenotype? Am J Hum Genet 2000;66:176–186.

44. Kennedy C, ter Huurne J, Berkhout M, et al. Melanocortin 1 receptor (MC1R) gene variants are associated with an increased risk for cutaneous melanoma which is largely independent of skin type and hair color. J Invest Dermatol 2001;117:294–300.

45. Aitken J, Welch J, Duffy D, et al. CDKN2A variants in a population-based sample of Queensland families with melanoma. J Natl Cancer Inst 1999;91:446–452.

46. Kumar R, Smeds J, Berggren P, et al. A single nucleotide polymorphism in the 3'untranslated region of the CDKN2A gene is common in sporadic primary melanomas but mutations in the CDKN2B, CDKN2C, CDK4 and p53 genes are rare. Int J Cancer 2001;95:388–393.

47. Zheng Y, Shen H, Sturgis EM, et al. Haplotypes of two variants in p16 (CDK2/MTS-1/INK4A) exon 3 and risk of squamous cell carcinoma of the head and neck—a case-control study. Cancer Epidemiol Biomarkers Prev 2002;11:640–645.

48. Shahbazi M, Pravica V, Nasreen N, et al. Association between functional polymorphism in EGF gene and malignant melanoma. Lancet 2002;359:397–401.

49. McCarron SL, Bateman AC, Theaker JM, Howell WM. EGF +61 gene polymorphism and susceptibility to and prognostic markers in cutaneous malignant melanoma. Int J Cancer 2003;107:673–675.

50. Hayward NK. Genetics of melanoma predisposition. Oncogene 2003;22:3053–3062.

51. Roush GC, Nordlund JJ, Forget B, Gruber SB, Kirkwood JM. Independence of dysplastic nevi from total nevi in determining risk for nonfamilial melanoma. Prev Med 1988;17:273–279.

52. Halpern AC, Guerry D 4th, Elder DE, et al. Dysplastic nevi as risk markers of sporadic (nonfamilial) melanoma. Arch Dermatol 1991;127:995–999.

53. Armstrong BK, English DR. Cutaneous malignant melanoma. In: Schottenfeld D and Fraumeni JF Jr, eds. Cancer Epidemiology and Prevention. 2nd ed. Oxford Press, New York, NY: 1996, pp. 1282–1312.

54. Cleaver JE, Kraemer K. Xeroderma pigmentosum. In: Scriver CR, Beauber AL, Sly WS, et al., eds. The Metabolic Basis of Inherited Diseases II. McGraw-Hill, New York, NY: 1989, pp. 2949–2471.

55. Meyskens FL Jr, Farmer P, Fruehauf JP. Redox regulation in human melanocytes and melanoma. Pigment Cell Res 2001;14:148–154.

56. Jernstrom B, Morgenstern R, Moldeus P. Protective role of glutathione, thiols, and analogues in mutagenesis and carcinogenesis. Basic Life Sci 1993;61:137–147.

57. Hayes JD, Strange RC. Potential contribution of the glutathione S-transferase supergene family to resistance to oxidative stress. Free Radical Res 1995;22:193–207.

58. Heagerty A, Smith A, English J, et al. Susceptibility to multiple cutaneous basal cell carcinomas: significant interactions between glutathione S-transferase GSTM1 genotypes, skin type and male gender. Br J Cancer 1996;73:44–48.

59. Lear JT, Heagerty AH, Smith A, et al. Multiple cutaneous basal cell carcinomas: glutathione S-transferase (GSTM1, GSTT1) and cytochrome P450 (CYP2D6, CYP1A1) polymorphisms influence tumour numbers and accrual. Carcinogenesis 1996;17:1891–1896.

60. Moral A, Palou J, Lafuente A, et al. Immunohistochemical study of alpha, mu and pi class glutathione S transferase expression in malignant melanoma. Multidisciplinary Malignant Melanoma Group. Br J Dermatol 1997;136:345–350.

61. Lafuente A, Molina R, Castel T, et al. Phenotype of glutathoine S transferase mu (GSTM1) and susceptibility to malignant melanoma. Br J Cancer 1995;72:324–326.

62. Tew KD. Glutathione-associated enzymes in anticancer drug resistance. Cancer Res 1994;54: 4313–4320.

63. Cleaver JE. Defective replication of DNA in xeroderma pigmen¬ tosum. Nature 1968;218:652–656.

64. Setlow RB, Regan JD, German J, et al. Evidence that xeroderma pigmentosum cells do not perform the first step in the repair of ultraviolet damage to their DNA. Proc Natl Acad Sci USA 1969;64: 1035–1041.

65. Kraemer KH, Lee MM, Andrews AD, Lambert WC. The role of sunlight and DNA repair in melanoma and nonmelanoma skin cancer. The xeroderma pigmentosum paradigm. Arch Dermatol 1994;130:1018–1021.

66. Carty MP, Hauser J, Levien AS, Dixon K. Replication and mutagenesis of UV,Ä'damaged DNA templates in human and monkey cell extracts. Mol Cell Biol 1993;13:533–542.

67. Suarez HG, Daya-Grosjean L, Schlaifer D, et al. Activated oncogenes in human skin tumors from a repair-deficient syndrome, xeroderma pigmentosum. Cancer Res 1989;49:1223–1228.

68. Sato M, Nishigori C, Zghal M, et al. Ultraviolet mutations in p53 genes in skin tumors in xeroderma pigmentosum patients. Cancer Res 1993;53:2944–2946.

69. Ananthaswamy H, Price JE, Goldberg LH, Bales ES. Detection and identification of activated oncogenes in human skin cancer occurring on sun-exposed body sites. Cancer Res 1988;48: 3341–3346.

70. Brash DE, Rudolph JA, Simon JA, et al. A role for sunlight in skin cancer: UV-induced p53 mutations in squamous cell carcinoma. Proc Natl Acad Sci USA 1991;88:10,124–10,128.

71. Sancar A. DNA repair in human. Annu Rev Genet 1995;29:69–105.

72. Wakasugi M, Shimizu M, Morioka H, Linn S, Nikaido O, Matsunaga T. Damaged DNA-binding protein DDB stimulates the excision of cyclobutane pyrimidine dimers in vitro in concert with XPA and replication protein A. J Biol Chem 2001;276:15,434–15,440.

73. Hansson J, Loow H. Normal reactivation of plasmid DNA inactivation by UV irradiation by lymphocytes from individuals with hereditary dysplastic naevus syndrome. Melanoma Res 1994;4:163–167.

74. Howell JN, Greene MH, Corner RC, Maher VM, McCormick JJ. Fibroblasts from patients with hereditary cutaneous malignant melanoma are abnormally sensitive to the mutagenic effect of similated sunlight and 4-nitroquinolibne-1-oxide. Proc Natl Acad Sci USA 1984;81:1179–1183.

75. Moriwasi SI, Tarone RE, Tucker MA, Goldstein AM, Kraemer KH. Hypermutability of UV-treated plasmids in dysplastic nevus/familial melanoma cell lines. Cancer Res 1997;57:4637–4641.

76. Kraemer KH, Lee MM, Scotto J. DNA repair protects against cutaneous and internal neoplasia: evidence from xeroderma pigmentosum. Carcinogenesis 1984;5:511–514.

77. Vitasa BC, Taylor HR, Strickland PT, et al. Association of nonmelanoma skin cancer and actinic keratosis with cumulative solar ultraviolet exposure in Maryland watermen. Cancer 1990;65: 2811–2817.

78. Wei Q, Matanoski GM, Farmer ER, Hedayati MA, Grossman L. DNA repair and aging in basal cell carcinoma: a molecular epidemiology study. Proc Natl Acad Sci USA 1993;90:1614–1618.

79. Athas AF, Hedayati M, Matanoski GM, et al. Development and field-test validation of an assay for DNA repair in circulating human lymphocytes. Cancer Res 1991;51:5786–5793.

80. Wei Q, Matanoski GM, Farmer ER, Hedayati MA, Grossman L. DNA repair related to multiple skin cancers and drug use. Cancer Res 1994;54:437–440.

81. Wei Q, Matanoski GM, Farmer ER, Hedayati MA, Grossman L. DNA repair and susceptibility to basal cell carcinoma: a case-control study. Am J Epidemiol 1994;140:598–607.

82. Hall J, English DR, Artuso M, Armstrong BK, Winter M. DNA repair capacity as a risk factor for non-melanocytic skin cancer—a molecular epidemiological study. Int J Cancer 1994;58:179–84.

83. Strickland PT, Vitasa BC, West SK, Rosenthal FS, Emmett EA, Taylor HR. Quantitative carcinogenesis in man: solar ultraviolet B dose dependence of skin cancer in Maryland watermen. J Natl Cancer Inst 1989;81:1910–1913.

84. D'Errico M, Calcagnile A, Iavarone I, et al. Factors that influence the DNA repair capacity of normal and skin cancer-affected individuals. Cancer Epidemiol Biomarkers Prev 1999;8:553–559.

85. Wei Q, Cheng L, Amos CI, et al. Repair of tobacco carcinogen-induced DNA adducts and lung cancer risk: a molecular epidemiological study. J Natl Cancer Inst 2000;92:1764–1772.

86. Dybdahl M, Frentz G, Vogel U, Wallin H, Nexo BA. Low DNA repair is a risk factor in skin carcinogenesis: a study of basal cell carcinoma in psoriasis patients. Mutat Res 1999;433:15–22.

87. Matta JL, Villa JL, Ramos JM, et al. DNA repair and nonmelanoma skin cancer in Puerto Rican populations. J Am Acad Dermatol 2003;49:433–439.

88. Wei Q, Matanoski GM, Farmer ER, Hedayati MA, Grossman L. DNA repair related to multiple skin cancers and drug use. Cancer Res 1994;54:437–440.

89. Landi MT, Baccarelli A, Tarone RE, et al. DNA repair, dysplastic nevi, and sunlight sensitivity in the development of cutaneous malignant melanoma. J Natl Cancer Inst 2002;94:94–101.

90. Wei Q, Lee JE, Strom SS, et al. Repair of ultraviolet-light induced DNA damage and risk of cutaneous malignant melanoma—a case-control study. J Natl Cancer Inst 2000;92:1764–1772.

91. Qiao Y, Spitz MR, Shen H, et al. Modulation of repair of ultraviolet damage in the host-cell reactivation assay by polymorphic XPC and XPD/ERCC2 genotypes. Carcinogenesis 2002;23:295–299.

92. Qiao Y, Spitz MR, Guo Z, et al. Rapid assessment of repair of ultraviolet DNA damage with a modified host-cell reactivation assay using a luciferase reporter gene and correlation with polymorphisms of DNA repair genes in normal human lymphocytes. Mutat Res 2002;509:165–174.

93. Shen MR, Jones IM, Mohrenweiser H. Nonconservative amino acid substitution variants exist at polymorphic frequency in DNA repair genes in healthy humans. Cancer Res 1998;58:604–608.

94. Mohrenweiser HW, Xi T, Vazquez-Matias J, Jones IM. Identification of 127 amino acid substitution variants in screening 37 DNA repair genes in humans. Cancer Epidemiol Biomarkers Prev 2002;11:1054–1064.

95. Goode EL, Ulrich CM, Potter JD. Polymorphisms in DNA repair genes and associations with cancer risk. Cancer Epidemiol Biomarkers Prev 2002;11:1513–1530.

96. Winsey SL, Haldar NA, Marsh HP, et al. A variant within the DNA repair gene XRCC3 is associated with the development of melanoma skin cancer. Cancer Res 2000;60:5612–5616.

97. Duan Z, Shen H, Lee JE, et al. DNA repair gene XRCC3 241Met variant is not associated with risk of cutaneous malignant melanoma. Cancer Epidemiol Biomarkers Prev 2002;11:1142–1143.

98. Jacobsen NR, Nexo BA, Olsen A, et al. No association between the DNA repair gene XRCC3 T241M polymorphism and risk of skin cancer and breast cancer. Cancer Epidemiol Biomarkers Prev 2003;12:584–585.

99. Tomescu D, Kavanagh G, Ha T, Campbell H, Melton DW. Nucleotide excision repair gene XPD polymorphisms and genetic predisposition to melanoma. Carcinogenesis 2001;22:403–408.

100. Baccarelli A, Calista D, Minghetti P, et al. XPD gene polymorphism and host characteristics in the association with cutaneous malignant melanoma risk. Br J Cancer 2004;90:497–502.

25 High-Risk Factors for Melanoma Metastasis

Neil A. Accortt and Seng-jaw Soong

Summary

Survival from melanoma varies greatly depending on the characteristics of the subject and the tumor. The purpose of this chapter is to summarize the factors associated with melanoma metastasis and poor survival. The risk factors are presented according to the staging system developed by the American Joint Committee on Cancer (AJCC). There are four distinct stages of cutaneous melanoma, with different risk factors for each stage, although the factors for stages I and II are often combined.

Although many risk factors for melanoma have been established for over 30 yr, new risk factors are being identified as larger population-based studies are being conducted and more research is done in the area of biomarkers. The sections on biological markers as predictors of survival are presented as only an introduction into this area. Much research still needs to be done to determine which biomarkers prove to be consistent predictors of melanoma survival. Continued identification of prognostic factors will aid in the improvement of prognosis and subsequent treatment of melanoma.

Key Words: Melanoma; survival; risk factors; staging; biomarkers.

INTRODUCTION

Survival from melanoma is highly variable. Studies have shown that 10-yr survival can range from 95% to less than 30% *(1)*, depending on the characteristics of the subject and the tumor at the time of diagnosis. To better understand the prognosis for survival from primary melanoma, the American Joint Committee on Cancer (AJCC) has developed a staging system for primary melanoma *(2)*. This system has evolved over the last 10 yr as more studies on larger populations are conducted on melanoma patients *(1,3)*.

The current staging system was implemented in 2002 and consists of four stages *(1,4)*. Stages I and II can both be described as localized disease. Stage III consists of disease

From: *From Melanocytes to Melanoma: The Progression to Malignancy*
Edited by: V. J. Hearing and S. P. L. Leong © Humana Press Inc., Totowa, NJ

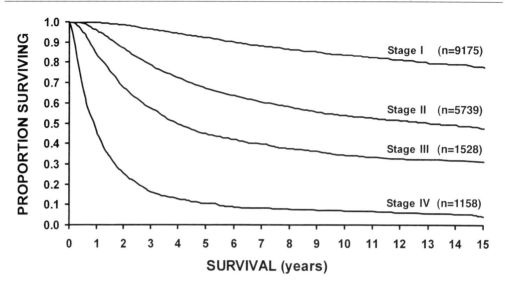

Fig. 1. Survival curve by American Joint Committee on Cancer (AJCC) stage for melanoma patients. (Reprinted with permission from ref. *1*.)

that has spread to regional sites and stage IV consists of tumors that have spread to distant sites. Differences in survival by stage of cancer diagnosis have clearly been established (Fig. 1).

The current staging system also incorporates the advancement of lymphatic mapping and sentinel lymph node biopsy through the definition of a clinical stage and a pathological stage *(1)*. This change is particularly apparent in stage III melanoma in which the clinical staging, based solely on clinical and/or radiological assessment of the regional lymph nodes, has no subgrouping. However, with the technological advancement of lymphatic mapping, patients can be staged using both pathological information on both the primary tumor and the regional lymph nodes. Patients previously determined to be clinically node negative are now subgrouped according to their nodal status. An analysis by Balch et al. showed that there were statistically significant differences in 5 and 10-yr survival rates between clinically and pathologically staged patients for all T stages except for T4b (tissue thickness >4.0 mm, with ulceration) *(1)*. The decreases in 5-yr survival rates for the significant results between clinically and pathologically staged disease ranged from 15 to 30%.

The AJCC staging system for melanoma provides a consistent nomenclature for physicians and researchers. Furthermore, the risk factors for disease-free survival and overall survival differ by stage. For these reasons, the prognostic risk factors in this chapter will be discussed within each melanoma stage.

PROGNOSTIC FACTORS FOR STAGE I AND STAGE II MELANOMA

Stage I and stage II melanoma are characterized as localized disease. The prognosis for disease diagnosed at these stages is generally good. As Fig. 1 shows, the overall survival for subjects diagnosed at either of these two stages is much better than for stages III or IV *(1)*. However, there is definite variation in the prognosis within these stages. Fig. 2 displays the overall survival for subcategories of localized disease. The differ-

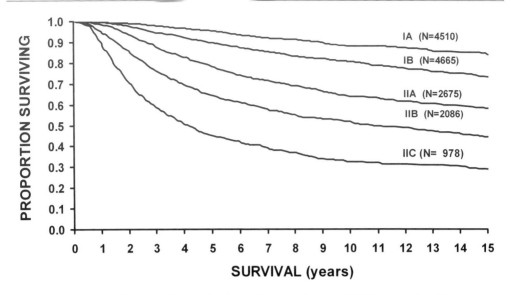

Fig. 2. Survival curve for American Joint Committee on Cancer (AJCC) stage I and II melanoma patients. (Reprinted with permission from ref. *1*.)

ences in survival are multifactorial and include tumor thickness, ulceration, Clark level of invasion, mitotic rate, gender, age, anatomical site of the tumor, and other factors. The following sections discuss these factors in detail in their recognized order of importance.

Tumor Thickness

Tumor thickness is one of three factors used by the AJCC melanoma staging system to stage localized melanoma. Tumor thickness has been identified as the most important prognostic risk factor for localized tumors *(1,4–9)*. A study of 13,581 melanoma patients found tumor thickness to be the more important predictor of melanoma survival *(4)*. This finding has been duplicated in numerous other studies *(5–9)*.

Some discussion does exist over the ideal categorization of tumor thickness. The categories currently used by the AJCC staging system are less than or equal to 1.00 mm, 1.01 to 2.00 mm, 2.01 to 4.00 mm, and greater than 4.00 mm *(1)*. Breslow first identified the differences in survival by tumor thickness proposing a categorization of six categories in 1970 *(5)*. More recent studies have used fewer categories and/or different cutoff points *(1,2,9,10)*. However, all have reached the same conclusion: thinner tumors have better survival than thicker tumors and survival correlates with thickness in a trend-like fashion. This last point is best demonstrated in Fig. 3. Therefore, the current cutoff system is used for its simplicity (even integer categories), its statistical validity, and its compatibility with current thresholds in clinical decision making *(1,4)*. Figure 4 displays the overall survival curve of localized melanoma using the current categorization.

Tumor Ulceration

Ulcerated melanomas have consistently shown worse survival than nonulcerated tumors *(4,6,8,10–15)*. The reason for this worsened prognosis is thought to be that tumors with histological ulceration tend to invade the epidermis rather than displace normal cells *(9)*. Ulceration is more common in men (26%) than women (20%) *(9)*.

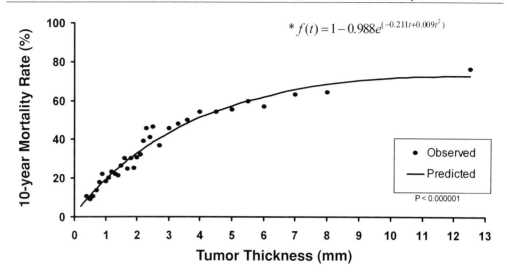

$$* f(t) = 1 - 0.988e^{(-0.211t + 0.009t^2)}$$

Fig. 3. Observed vs predicted 10-yr mortality rates for American Joint Committee on Cancer stage I and II melanoma patients. *T, measured tumor thickness in millimeters; f(t), 10-yr melanoma-specific mortality rates. (Reprinted with permission from ref. *4*.)

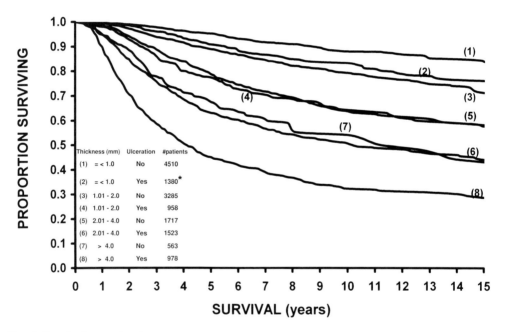

Fig. 4. Survival curve for American Joint Committee on Cancer stage I and II melanoma patients stratified by thickness and ulceration. **Note:** Group (2) includes patients with ulceration or level IV/V (i.e., TNM classification T1b). (Reprinted with permission from ref. *4*.)

Tumor ulceration has been shown to be a significant predictor of poor survival in multifactorial regression models and in one analysis was shown to be the second most important predictor of overall survival, behind tumor thickness (Table 1). However, tumor thickness and ulceration are closely correlated. Balch et al. found that the thinner the tumor the lower the prevalence of ulceration *(4)*. Analysis of the AJCC database

Table 1
Predictors of Survival
for AJCC Stage I and II Melanoma Patients

Variable	χ^2	p value
Thickness	244.3	< 0.0001
Ulceration	189.5	< 0.0001
Age	45.6	< 0.0001
Site	41.0	< 0.0001
Level	32.7	< 0.0001
Sex	15.1	0.001

Reprinted with permission from ref. *4*.

found that 6% of thin tumors (<1 mm) were ulcerated, whereas 63% of thick tumors (>4 mm) were ulcerated.

The most recent staging version of the AJCC system includes tumor ulceration as one of three factors in the staging system *(1)*. Ulcerated tumors are placed in the same category as thicker tumors with no ulceration. For example, a 1.0–2.0-mm tumor with ulceration is categorized the same as a 2.01 to 4.0 mm tumor without ulceration. This result is displayed graphically in Fig. 4, showing the similar survival between thinner tumors with ulceration and thicker tumors with no ulceration. Figure 2 displays the combination of these categories into five substages of stage I and stage II melanoma.

Clark Level of Invasion

Clark level of invasion is the third prognostic factor to be included in the most recent AJCC staging system for melanoma for stage I and II *(1)*. The higher the level of invasion, the worse the prognosis is for melanoma cases. However, this finding has not been as consistent as tumor thickness has been for disease prognosis. In a review by Vollmer, the author found that in 54 studies conducted before 1988, tumor thickness was a more significant factor than level of invasion in 42 of the studies *(16)*. Furthermore, only 8 of 48 studies found level of invasion to be statistically significant.

When looking only at thin tumors (<1.0 mm), level of invasion has been found to be a significant prognostic factor. An analysis of the AJCC melanoma database found that Clark level was a more important prognostic factor for thin melanomas than ulceration *(4)*. In the substaging of stage I melanoma, Clark level is only incorporated into stages IA and IB (Fig. 2). Table 2 shows that level is the most important predictor among thin melanomas but becomes less important as the tumors get thicker, although it does remain significant for tumors of all thickness categories.

Tumor Mitotic Rate

Tumor mitotic rate (TMR) has recently been identified as an independent predictor of survival. A study from the Sydney Melanoma Unit (SMU) of 3661 subjects, defining TMR as the number of mitoses/mm^2 in the dermal area of the tumor in which mitoses were seen, found that mitotic index was second only to tumor thickness when predicting patient survival *(17)*. This finding was limited to a certain categorization of TMR (0, 1–4, 5–10, and >11 mitoses/mm^2). However, when recategorized to three different

Table 2
χ^2 Values (p Values) for Predictors of Survival
for AJCC Stage I and II Melanoma Patients: Stratified by Tumor Thickness Category

Tumor thickness	Ulceration	Level	Age	Site	Sex
1.00 mm	17.239	24.778	12.563	6.940	5.506
($n = 5299$)	(<0.0001)	(<0.0001)	(0.0004)	(0.0084)	(0.0189)
1.01–2.00 mm	57.215	6.656	11.613	24.085	2.668
($n = 3943$)	(<0.0001)	(0.0099)	(0.0007)	(<0.0001)	(0.1024)
2.01–4.00 mm	62.291	4.451	12.529	12.342	3.165
($n = 2959$)	(<0.0001)	(0.0349)	(0.0004)	(0.0004)	(0.0752)
>4.00 mm	47.246	4.065	8.745	2.547	2.875
($n = 1380$)	(<0.0001)	(0.0438)	(0.0031)	(0.1106)	(0.0951)

Reprinted with permission from ref. 4.

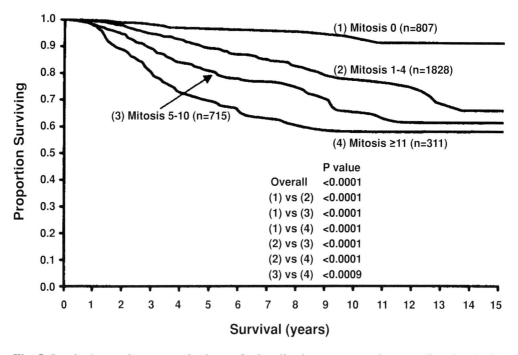

Fig. 5. Survival curve by tumor mitotic rate for localized cutaneous melanoma. (Reprinted with permission from ref. 17.)

categories (0–1, 2–4, >5 mitoses/mm^2), TMR was still a highly significant independent predictor of overall survival. These results support evidence that has shown that a mitotic index of greater than 5 is associated with poorer survival (18). The univariate survival curves for TMR subdivided into four categories are shown in Fig. 5. A recent study by Francken et al. confirmed that TMR is an independent predictor of survival, even after controlling for stage of disease (19).

Age

Older subjects have worse survival than younger subjects *(4,20,21)*. This finding may be expected because older patients tend to present with thicker tumors. However, in multivariate analyses of the University of Alabama at Birmingham (UAB)–SMU database, age has been found to be an independent predictor of survival *(9)*. Age was found to be a significant independent predictor within each of the thickness categories for stage I and II tumors (Table 2). Balch et al. found consistently decreasing 5-yr and 10-yr survival rates for melanoma subjects as they age in 10-yr increments *(4)*. Although age has been found to be an independent predictor, it has also been shown that increasing age is associated with increased tumor thickness, increased prevalence of ulcerated tumors, an increased prevalence of tumors on the head and neck, and a higher proportion of male subjects *(22)*.

Anatomic Site of the Primary Tumor

The anatomic location of the primary tumor has also consistently been found to be a significant predictor of melanoma survival *(4,8,9,20,23,24)*. Although melanoma can occur anywhere, the site is generally categorized into extremities (including the arms, legs, hands, and feet) and nonextremities (usually consisting of the head and neck or trunk area). Analyses of the UAB–SMU database found that extremity tumors had significantly (*p* < 0.0001) better survival than nonextremity tumors *(9)*. Several other studies have duplicated this finding *(4,8,20,23,24)*.

Interestingly, in the UAB–SMU data set, there was no difference in survival between lower extremities and upper extremities, but tumors located on the hands and feet had worse prognosis than tumors on the arms and legs *(9)*. However, this finding is not consistent, because Wells et al. found no difference in survival for tumors on the hands and feet after controlling for tumor thickness *(25)*.

Women are more likely to have tumors located on the extremities, whereas men are more likely to have tumors on their head and neck or trunk area *(9)*. However, when six specific tumor locations (back, chest, arm, leg, foot, and hand) were compared in the UAB–SMU database, women had better survival than men for all locations *(9)*.

Gender

As expected from the differences between men and women for specific sites, women tend to have better overall survival than men *(4,9,20)*. In addition to having more tumors located on the extremities, tumors in female patients are thinner and less likely to be ulcerated *(9)*. In the overall analysis of 13,581 patients in the AJCC melanoma database, gender was a significant predictor of survival in a multifactorial Cox model *(4)*. However, when the analysis was stratified by thickness, gender was only a significant independent predictor for tumors less than 1.0 mm in diameter (Table 2).

Other Pathological Variables

Research on prognostic factors for melanoma outcomes has been rather extensive and includes many variables for which the results are not as consistent as those already discussed. These factors will be mentioned here, in brief. Although some research does exist for each of these factors, no conclusive evidence currently exists in the literature.

Lymphocyte infiltration is one factor with inconsistent findings. Infiltration of the melanoma by lymphocytes is believed to represent a more vigorous host response to the tumor. Analyses of the UAB–SMU database found that tumor thickness and lymphocyte infiltration were inversely correlated, i.e., thinner tumors had more infiltration, thicker tumors had less infiltration (9). However, tumor infiltration was no longer significant once tumor thickness was controlled for in a multivariate model. However, other investigators have found tumor infiltration to be an independent predictor of melanoma survival (26–28).

As with lymphocyte infiltration, the role of tumor vascularity and microvessel density is, as yet, undetermined, and the findings of recent research are inconsistent. Srivastava found that increased vascular density was associated with poor prognosis (29,30). Similarly, Kashani-Sabat et al. found that tumor vascularity (categorized as absent, sparse, moderate, and prominent) was the most important predictor of overall survival in a multivariate analysis (31). However, these findings have not been duplicated in other research (32–34).

Microsatellites have been defined as "discrete nests of melanoma cells, greater than 0.05 mm in diameter, noncontiguous, and clearly separated from the main body of the tumor by normal reticular dermal collagen or subcutaneous fat (35)." Leon et al. and Kelly et al., in separate studies, have shown that microsatellites are associated with clinically worse outcomes (35,36). However, the number of studies on microsatellites is limited, and more research is needed before its importance in melanoma prognosis can be determined.

Although tumor regression has been found to be an independent prognostic factor in a few studies (26,37), other studies found no difference in survival between subjects exhibiting regression and those who do not exhibit regression (9,38,39).

The growth pattern of stage I and II tumors has been studied to some extent. The four growth patterns are superficial spreading melanoma, lentigo maligna melanoma (LMM), nodular melanoma, and acral lentiginous melanoma. Analyses of the UAB–SMU database showed that growth pattern was a significant prognostic indicator in a univariate analysis, but not in the multivariate analysis (9). When grouped according to tumor thickness, superficial spreading melanoma and nodular melanoma had similar 10-yr survival rates, whereas LMM had the best survival rates and acral lentiginous melanoma had the worst survival rates (9). LMM patients tend to have thinner lesions, although Garbe et al. found that even LMM patients with thicker tumors (>3.0 mm) had 80% survival at 10 yr (40).

Desmoplastic neurotropic melanoma is a rare variant of malignant melanoma, accounting for approx 1% of all cases (41,42). These tumors tend to invade locally around the peripheral nerves, especially in the head and neck area. Carlson et al. conducted a literature review and found an overall survival rate of 60%, a local recurrence rate of 50%, and distant metastases at a rate of 25% (41). Among the thickest desmoplastic neurotropic melanoma (>4.0 mm), Carlson et al. found a survival rate of 72%, much higher than found in thicker, conventional melanomas.

Molecular Variables

Much of the current research in melanoma focuses on the molecular markers of melanoma tumors and their use as predictors of survival. The literature on molecular markers is quite extensive, although relatively new. This section serves as only a brief summary of the factors most often mentioned in the literature. A tabular summary of these factors is provided (Table 3).

Table 3
Summary of Literature on Molecular Variables as Predictors of Melanoma Survival

Stage	Variables	Authors
I and II	P53	Gelsleichter et al. *(45)* (1995); Yamamoto et al. *(46)* (1995); Weiss et al. *(54)* (1995); Saenz-Santamaria et al. *(55)* (1995); Kanter-Lewensohn et al. *(43)* (1997); Hieken et al. *(56)* (1999); Kaleem et al. *(44)* (2000)
	P16	Reed et al. *(51)* (1995); Talve et al. *(50)* (1997); Straume et al. *(53)* (1997); Sparrow et al. *(49)* (1998); Funk et al. *(48)* (1998); Grover et al. *(52)* (1998); Piepkorn et al. *(47)* (2000)
	B_1 and B_3 integrins	Hieken et al. *(57)* (1995); Natali et al. *(61)* (1997); Hieken et al. *(56)* (1999); VanBelle et al. *(58)* (1999); Vihinen et al. *(59)* (2000); Kageshita et al. *(60)* (2000)
	CD44	Schaider et al. *(63)* (1998); Karjalainen et al. *(62)* (2000)
	CEACAM1	Thies et al. *(64)* (2002)
	S-100β	Bonfrer et al. *(65)* (1998); Kaskel et al. *(66)* (1999); Garbe et al. *(68)* (2003)
	MIA	Bosserhoff et al. *(67)* (2001); Garbe et al. *(68)* (2003)
	Metallothioneins	Weinlich et al. *(69)* (2003)
	MART-1/Tyrosinase	Mellado et al. *(71)* (1996); Farthmann et al. *(70)* (1998); Garbe et al. *(68)* (2003)
III	S-100β	Kaskel et al. *(66)* (1999); Garbe et al. *(68)* (2003)
	MIA	Garbe et al. *(68)* (2003)
	MART-1/Tyrosinase	Mellado et al. *(71)* (1996); Garbe et al. *(68)* (2003); Palmieri et al. *(76)* (2003)
	B_1 integrins	Vihinen et al. *(59)* (2000)

Several tumor suppressor genes have been studied in relation to melanoma. Expressions of the *p53* gene and the *p16* gene have both been shown to correlate with melanoma progression *(43–53)*. Although one study has shown that overexpression of *p53* in thick tumors (>3 mm) was associated with metastasis and death *(43)*, other reports have not supported this finding *(54–56)*. The data on *p16* is somewhat more consistent. Several studies have shown a correlation between loss of *p16* expression and advanced stages of melanoma progression *(49–53)*.

Integrins are glycoproteins that play a role in the cell–cell and cell–extracellular matrix interactions. B_1 and B_3 integrins have been found to be markers of poor prognosis in primary melanoma *(56–61)*. Both markers have been shown to positively correlate with worse prognoses in primary melanoma for both overall survival and disease-free survival *(56,61)*. The role of integrins as a prognostic factor needs to be studied more extensively before it can be used as a prognostic indicator of melanoma progression.

CD44 is another cell adhesion molecule that has been studied in relation to melanoma. Again, the literature, although limited, is contradictory. Karjalainen et al. found that reduced expression of CD44 led to poorer prognosis on melanoma patients *(62)*, whereas Schaider et al. found no correlation between CD44 expression and melanoma progression *(63)*.

CEACAM1, another cell adhesion molecule, has evidence in one study that it is a significant, independent predictor of metastatic disease. Thies et al., in a multivariate analysis of 40 subjects, found that CEACAM1 was superior to tumor thickness in its predictive value *(64)*.

A series of proteins have also been studied as risk factors for melanoma progression. Melanoma inhibitory activity (MIA) and S-100B are two proteins that have been studied in relation to melanoma. Although both MIA and S-100B levels have been shown to be better predictors for stage IV melanoma *(65–67)*, Garbe et al. did conclude that MIA and S-100B have clinical prognostic significance for stage II cases *(68)*.

Metallothioneins (MTs), proteins with a high affinity for heavy metal ions, have been shown to be associated with melanoma progression and survival. Weinlich et al. found that overexpression of MTs in tumor cells was a significant and independent predictor of disease progression and reduced survival compared with MT-negative tumors *(69)*.

Melanoma antigen recognized by T-cells-1 and tyrosinase are both recognized as markers that occur in circulating melanoma cells. New methods to detect these genes, particularly reverse transcription-polymerase chain reaction (RT-PCR) are allowing researchers to quantify the prognostic abilities of these molecular markers. Although the exact prognostic abilities of these markers is inconclusive at this point *(68,70,71)*, research continues in this area as technology continues to improve.

Summary of Stage I and Stage II Melanomas

In summary, tumor thickness, which was identified as a major risk factor for patient survival more than 30 yr ago *(5)*, remains the most important predictor of disease progression today. Other factors, such as tumor ulceration, level of invasion, site of primary tumor, mitotic rate, and age do still play an important role in assessing the risk for disease progression. The research on other factors is more inconsistent, but may still play an important role in the prognosis of melanoma survival. The newest area of research focuses on the molecular markers and although still inconsistent, offers promising venues for the detection of new prognostic factors that will aid in the improvement of prognosis and subsequent treatment for localized melanoma.

PROGNOSTIC FACTORS FOR STAGE III MELANOMA

Stage III melanoma is considered to be regionalized disease. This category encompasses tumors found in either the regional lymph nodes or intralymphatic metastases manifesting as either satellite or in-transit metastases. Survival rates are worse than those for stage I and II melanomas, with overall 5-yr survival rates approx 50% (Fig. 1). However, within the stage III category, there is a range of 5-yr survival from approx 25 to 70% depending on the subject and tumor characteristics *(1)*. Prognostic factors for stage III tumors are fewer than that for stage I and II tumors and also not as closely associated with the characteristics of the primary tumor. Again, these factors will be discussed in their currently accepted order of importance for prediction of survival.

Number of Nodes

The number of nodes involved has been found to be the most important predictor of survival for stage III melanoma *(4,10,72–74)*. Table 4 displays the results of the multifactorial Cox regression analysis of the AJCC database. Among 1151 subjects with stage III disease, number of metastatic nodes was the most important predictor of overall survival *(4)*. A univariate survival analysis of the AJCC database showed that survival decreases as the number of positive nodes increases ($p < 0.0001$) *(4)*.

Table 4
Predictors of Survival for AJCC Stage III Melanoma Patients

Variable	χ^2	p Value
Number of metastatic nodes	57.616	<0.0001
Tumor burden	40.301	<0.0001
Ulceration	23.282	<0.0001
Site	17.843	0.0001
Age	13.369	0.0003
Thickness	1.964	0.1611
Level	0.219	0.6396
Sex	0.006	0.9407

Reprinted with permission from ref. 4.

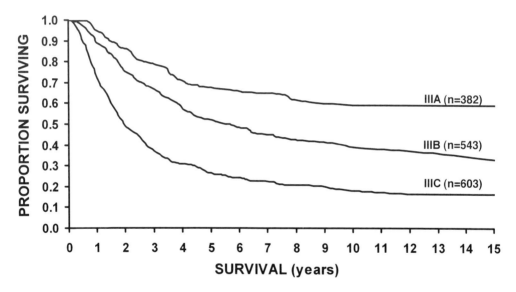

Fig. 6. Survival curve for American Joint Committee on Cancer stage III melanoma patients. (Reprinted with permission from ref. 1.)

Using this same data set, researchers were able to determine that the categorization of the number of nodes that best predicted survival was one node, two or three nodes, and four or more nodes (4). This categorization has been incorporated into a subcategorization of stage III disease: N1, N2, and N3. These separate N categories form the basis for the subdivision of stage III disease into stage IIIA, IIIB, and IIIC. Figure 6 displays the difference in survival for the three subcategories of stage III melanoma (1). Tumor burden and ulceration are the two other factors included in the subcategorization of stage III disease.

Tumor Burden

Tumor burden is the distinction between microscopic (or clinically occult) tumors vs macroscopic (or clinically apparent) tumors. Multivariate analysis has shown that tumor burden is the second most important predictor of tumor survival (Table 4). Table 5

Table 5
Five-Year Survival Rates for AJCC Stage III Patients Stratified by Number of Metastatic Nodes, Ulceration, and Tumor Burden

Melanoma Ulceration	Microscopic						Macroscopic					
	1+ Node		2–3 Nodes		>3 Nodes		1+ Node		2–3 Nodes		>3 Nodes	
	% ± SE	No.	% ± SE	No.	% ± SE	No.	% ± SE	No.	% ± SE	No.	% ± SE	No.
Absent	69 ± 3.72	52	63 ± 5.6	130	27 ± 9.3	57	59 ± 4.7	122	46 ± 5.5	93	27 ± 4.6	109
Present	52 ± 4.1	217	50 ± 5.7	111	37 ± 8.8	46	29 ± 5.0	98	25 ± 4.4	109	13 ± 3.5	104

Reprinted with permission from ref. 4.
SE, standard error.

displays the decreasing 5-yr survival of stage III patients as the number of positive nodes increases. When stratified by tumor burden, Balch et al. found that, for each nodal category, microscopic nodes had improved survival compared with the macroscopic nodes, and this improvement was statistically significant for all but one category *(4)*. Table 5 displays the importance of tumor burden in the prediction of survival and why it is included in the subcategorization of stage III disease.

Ulceration of Primary Tumor

Tumor ulceration is the one factor that is included in the categorization of both stage I and II disease, as well as stage III disease. In the analysis of the AJCC database, ulceration was the only primary tumor characteristic that was a significant predictor of survival in the multivariate model (Table 4). Similar to the stratification done by Balch et al. for tumor burden, the number of nodes was stratified by the presence or absence of ulceration. The results of this analysis showed that those patients with ulcerated primary tumors had significantly worse survival than those without ulceration for all numbers of positive nodes, except when the number of nodes was greater than three and microscopic tumors were involved (Table 5) *(9)*.

As mentioned previously, ulceration is the third factor used in the staging of stage III tumors. Microscopic tumors with one to three nodes and ulceration were found to have worse survival than these same tumors without ulceration. Similarly, macroscopic tumors of 1 to 3 nodes and ulceration have worse survival than similar tumors without ulceration.

Other Factors

Primary tumor site and subject age were also found to be significant prognostic factors in the multivariate analysis of the AJCC database (Table 4). As with the earlier stage disease, stage III tumors on the extremities fared better than those on the head and neck or trunk area *(4)*. This finding was also supported by analysis of the UAB–SMU database *(9)*.

Increasing age was correlated with worse survival in the AJCC database. And although no overall difference was found for gender, Balch et al. found that the age effect was more pronounced in men than women *(4)*. When stratified by gender, the difference in survival by age (50 vs >50) was much more disparate among men ($p = 0.0006$) than among women ($p = 0.02$) *(9)*.

Although tumor thickness is not as important a factor in predicting survival for stage III tumors as it is for stage I and II, it has been found to be a prognostic factor in a univariate analysis. Thinner tumors have been shown to have better overall survival than thicker tumors *(9)*.

Molecular Variables

The research investigating molecular variables as prognostic factors for stage III disease is not as extensive as it is for stage I and II. However, several factors have been investigated as prognostic variables for stage III disease. This section will serve as a brief discussion of those factors (Table 3).

One of the more comprehensive studies of molecular markers was done by Garbe et al. on 296 subjects, 129 of which were stage III (the remaining were stage II) *(68)*. Although the analyses were not stratified for the different stages, the authors did find that the proteins S-100B and MIA were significantly associated with increased risk of developing metastases. The finding of S-100B as a prognostic factor is supported in an earlier study by Kaskel et al. *(75)*.

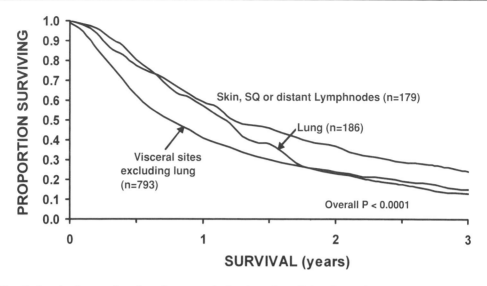

Fig. 7. Survival curve by site of metastasis for American Joint Committee on Cancer stage IV melanoma patients. (Reprinted with permission from ref. *4.*)

In a study from 1996, Mellado et al. found that stage II and III patients who were RT-PCR-positive for tyrosinase did significantly worse than RT-PCR-negative patients for both disease-free survival and death *(71)*. Later research has not supported this finding. Garbe et al. did not find RT-PCR to be a significant predictor of increased recurrence-free survival time *(68)*. Similarly, in a study of stage I to III subjects, Palmieri et al. found that RT-PCR was significant as a univariate predictor but did not remain significant in a multivariate model *(76)*. In contrast to its role for early stage tumors, B1 integrin is positively correlated with longer disease-free and overall survival in patients with metastatic tumors *(59)*.

PROGNOSTIC FACTORS FOR STAGE IV MELANOMA

Stage IV melanoma is considered metastatic disease that has spread to distant sites. The overall survival for late-stage disease is much lower than that for the other stages (Fig. 1), with median survival from time of diagnosis ranging from 6 to 8 mo *(9)* and 5-yr survival rates less than 10% *(9,77–79)*. As with other stages, several factors have been identified that differentiate the prognosis associated with stage IV disease.

Site of Distant Metastasis

The site to which the tumor has metastasized is one of the important predictors of survival for stage IV disease *(9,77–80)*. Using data from the AJCC database, stage IV subjects were subdivided by site using the following categorization: metastasis in the skin, subcutaneous tissue, or distant lymph nodes; metastasis to the lung; and metastasis to visceral sites other than lung. The survival curves for these three groups are shown in Fig. 7. Survival differences were significant between the nonvisceral sites and the lung metastasis (*p* < 0.0003) and the other visceral sites (*p* < 0.0001). The differences between the lung metastasis and the other visceral sites were only significant up to year 1 (*p* < 0.0001) *(4)*.

Number of Metastatic Sites

The number of metastatic sites involved has been found to be a significant predictor of survival. Subjects with only one site involved have a significantly better outcome than those with two or more sites involved ($p < 0.0001$). Similarly, subjects with two sites involved fare better than those with three or more sites involved ($p = 0.03$) *(81)*. The median survival time for the subjects in the UAB–SMU database ranged from 7 mo for those with one site involved, to 4 mo for two sites, and 2 mo for three or more sites.

Serum Lactic Dehydrogenase

Elevated levels of serum lactic dehydrogenase (LDH) have been associated with worse survival among stage IV subjects *(77,81,82)*. Multiple studies have demonstrated elevated LDH as an independent risk factor for decreased survival. Sirott et al. found decreased survival time in patients with elevated LDH levels when compared with patients with normal LDH levels (median survival of 3 mo vs 11 mo) *(82)*, whereas Manola et al., found median survival times of 6.6 mo and 12.4 mo for abnormal vs normal LDH *(79)*.

Other Variables

Gender has had mixed results as a prognostic factor for stage IV disease. A few studies have shown that women had better survival than men *(10,71,80)*, although others did not reach this same result *(9,78)*. Age has not been found to be a prognostic indicator of survival among stage IV patients *(9,77)*. Duration of disease-free survival has been found in at least one study to be predictive of improved survival *(77)*. Barth et al. found that subjects who had experienced at least 72 mo of disease remission fared significantly better than subjects with a remission time of less than 72 mo. However, Balch et al. did not find a correlation between disease-free survival and worse prognosis *(9)*.

Performance status has been found by several researchers to positively correlate with prognosis, i.e., the worse the performance score, the worse the prognosis *(78–80)*. A multivariate analysis by Manola et al. showed that an Eastern Cooperative Oncology Group performance score of 1 or greater was independently associated with worse survival (hazard ratio, 1.49; 95% confidence interval, 1.3–1.7) *(79)*. Using a different performance score, the Southwest Oncology Group also found performance score to be highly predictive of worse survival *(80)*.

CONCLUSIONS AND PERSPECTIVES

This review provides a comprehensive list of those factors that have been well studied as prognostic factors for melanoma survival. It also includes brief descriptions of more recently studied factors and also considers some factors for which the evidence is still controversial. As the data has shown, the overall survival from melanoma is highly variable.

Not only do these factors differentiate survival between different stages, the research has shown that, within stages, subjects can have very different outcomes depending on the combinations of several different factors. As the stage of disease progresses, it becomes apparent that individual factors (such as age and gender) become less important. Also, for the later stages of disease, the characteristics of the primary tumor become less important.

The importance of discussing these factors is twofold. First, it provides a basis for the AJCC staging system that leads to a consistency of diagnosis for physicians. Second, it provides physicians with a way of predicting disease outcome in their subjects and subsequently deciding the proper treatment protocol. Investigation of newer markers as independent prognostic factors, as well as their possible interaction with existing factors, will further enhance the prognostic abilities of physicians, and therefore potentially lead to even more focused treatment regimens that will eventually lead to improved survival among all stages of melanoma subjects.

REFERENCES

1. Balch CM, Buzaid AC, Soong SJ, et al. Final version of the American Joint Committee on Cancer staging system for cutaneous melanoma. J Clin Oncol 2001;19:3635–3648.
2. Beahrs OH, Henson DE, Hutter RVP, Myers MH. Manual for Staging of Cancer. 3rd ed. American Joint Committee on Cancer. JB Lippincott, Philadelphia, PA: 1988, p. 139.
3. Balch CM, Buzaid AC, Atkins MB, et al. A new American Joint Committee on Cancer staging system for cutaneous melanoma. Cancer 2000;88:1484–1491.
4. Balch CM, Soong SJ, Gershenwald JE, et al. Prognostic factors analysis of 17,600 melanoma patients: validation of the American Joint Committee on Cancer melanoma staging system. J Clin Oncol 2001;19:3622–3624.
5. Breslow A. Thickness, cross-sectional areas and depth of invasion in the prognosis of cutaneous melanoma. Ann Surg 1970;172:902–908.
6. Balch CM, Murad TM, Soong SJ, et al. A multifactorial analysis of melanoma: prognostic histopathological features comparing Clark's and Breslow's staging methods. Ann Surg 1978;188:732–742.
7. Eldh J, Boeryd B, Peterson LE. Prognostic factors in cutaneous malignant melanoma in stage I. A clinical, morphological and multivariate analysis. Scand J Plast Reconstr Surg 1978;12:243–255.
8. Clark WH, Elder DE, Guerry D, et al. Model predicting survival in stage I melanoma based on tumor progression. J Natl Cancer Inst 1989;81:1893–1904.
9. Stadelmann WK, Rapaport DP, Soong SJ et al. Prognostic clinical and pathologic features. In: Balch CM, Houghton AN, Sober AJ, Soong SJ, eds. Cutaneous Melanoma. 3rd ed. Quality Medical Publishing, St Louis, MO: 1998, pp. 11–35.
10. Buzaid AC, Ross MI, Balch CM, et al. Critical analysis of the current American Joint Committee on Cancer staging system. Clin Oncol 1997;15:1039–1051.
11. Averbrook BJ, Russo LJ, Mansour EG. A long-term analysis of 620 patients with malignant melanoma at a major referral center. Surgery 1988;124:746–755; discussion 755–756.
12. Shaw HM, Balch CM, Soong SJ, et al. Prognostic histopathological factors in malignant melanoma. Pathology 1985;17:271–274.
13. Balch CM, Wilkerson JA, Murad TM, et al. The prognostic significance of ulceration of cutaneous melanoma. Cancer 1980;45:3012–3017.
14. Balch CM, Soong SJ, Milton GW, et al. A comparison of prognostic factors and surgical results in 1,786 patients with localized (stage I) melanoma treated in Alabama, USA, and New South Wales, Australia. Ann Surg 1982;196:677–684.
15. McGovern VJ, Shaw HM, Milton GW, et al. Ulceration and prognosis in cutaneous malignant melanoma. Histopathology 1982;6:399–407.
16. Vollmer RT, Malignant melanoma. A multivariate analysis of prognostic factors. Pathol Annu 1989;24(Pt 1):383–407.
17. Azzola MF, Shaw HM, Thompson JF, et al. Tumor mitotic rate is a more powerful prognostic indicator than ulceration in patients with primary cutaneous melanoma. Cancer 2003;97:1488–1498.
18. Salman SM, Rogers GS. Prognostic factors in thin cutaneous malignant melanoma. J Dermatol Surg Oncol 1990;16:413–418.
19. Francken AB, Shaw HM, Thompson JF, et al. The prognostic importance of tumor mitotic rate confirmed in 1317 patients with primary cutaneous melanoma and long follow-up. Ann Surg Oncol 2004;11:426–433.
20. Schuchter L, Schultz DJ, Synnestvedt M, et al. A prognostic model for predicting 10-year survival in patients with primary melanoma. The Pigmented Lesion Group. Ann Intern Med 1996;25:369–375.

21. Austin PF, Cruse CW, Lyman G, et al. Age as a prognostic factor in the malignant melanoma population. Ann Surg Oncol 1994;1:487–494.

22. Balch CM, Soong SJ. Melanoma in the elderly: older age as an independent prognostic factor. ASCO, Orlando, FL; 2002(Abstract).

23. Carmichael V, Davidson VV, Wilson KS. Analysis of prognostic factors in clinical stage I cutaneous malignant melanoma (CMM): British Columbia Agency (BCAA) experience. Proc Am Soc Clin Oncol 1992;119.

24. Garbe C, Buttner P, Bertz J, et al. Primary cutaneous melanoma. Prognostic classification of anatomic location. Cancer 1995;75:2492–2498.

25. Wells KE, Reintgen DS, Cruse CW. The current management and prognosis of acral lentiginous melanoma. Ann Plast Surg 1992;28:100–103.

26. Clark WH Jr, Elder DE, Guerry DT, et al. Model predicting survival in stage I melanoma based on tumor progression. J Natl Cancer Inst 1989;81:1893–1904.

27. Mihm MC Jr, Clemente CG, Cascinelli N. Tumor infiltrating lymphocytes in lymph node melanoma metastases: a histopathologic prognostic indicator and an expression of local immune response. Lab Invest 1996;74:43–47.

28. Clemente CG, Mihm MC Jr, Bufalino R, et al. Prognostic value of tumor infiltrating lymphocytes in the vertical growth phase of primary cutaneous melanoma. Cancer 1996;77:1303–1310.

29. Srivastava A. The prognostic significance of tumor vascularity in intermediate-thickness (0.76–4.0 mm thick) skin melanoma. A quantitative histologic study. Am J Pathol 1988;133:419–423.

30. Srivastava A. Vascularity in cutaneous melanoma detected by Doppler sonography and histology: correlation with tumour behaviour. Br J Cancer 1989;59:89–91.

31. Kashani-Sabet M, Sagebiel RW, Ferreira CMM, et al. Tumor vascularity in the prognostic assessment of primary cutaneous melanoma. J Clin Oncol 2002;20:1826–1831.

32. Ilmonen S, Kariniemi AL, Vlaykova T, Muhonen T, Pyrhonen S, Asko-Seljavaara S. Prognostic value of tumour vascularity in primary melanoma. Melanoma Res 1999;9:273–278.

33. Barnhill RL, Fandrey K, Levy MA, Mihm MC Jr, Hyman B. Angiogenesis and tumor progression of melanoma. Quantification of vascularity in melanocytic nevi and cutaneous malignant melanoma. Lab Invest 1992;67:331–337.

34. Busam KJ, Berwick M, Blessing K, et al. Tumor vascularity is not a prognostic factor for malignant melanoma of the skin. Am J Pathol 1995;147:1049–1056.

35. Leon P, Daly JM, Synnestvedt M, et al. The prognostic implications of microscopic satellites in patients with clinical stage I melanoma. Arch Surg 1991;126:1461–1468.

36. Kelly JW, Sagebiel RW, Calderon W. The frequency of local recurrence and microsatellites as a guide to re-excision margins for cutaneous malignant melanoma. Ann Surg 1984;200:759–763.

37. Paladugu RR, Yonemoto RH. Biologic behavior of thin malignant melanomas with regressive changes. Arch Surg 1983;118:41–44.

38. McGovern VJ, Shaw HM, Milton GW. Prognosis in patients with thin malignant melanoma: influence of regression. Histopathology 1983;7:673–680.

39. Wanebo HJ, Cooper PH, Hagar RW. Thin (1 mm) melanomas of the extremities are biologically favorable lesions not influenced by regression. Ann Surg 1985;201:499–504.

40. Garbe C, Büttner P, Bertz J, et al. Primary cutaneous melanoma. Identification of prognostic groups and estimation of individual prognosis for 5,093 patients. Cancer 1995;75:2484–2491.

41. Carlson JA, Dickersin GR, Sober AJ, et al. Desmoplastic neurotropic melanoma. A clinicopathologic analysis of 28 cases. Cancer 1995;75:478–494.

42. Quinn MJ, Crotty KA, Thompson JF, et al. Desmoplastic and desmoplastic neurotropic melanoma: experience with 280 patients. Cancer 1998;83:1128–1135.

43. Kanter-Lewensohn L, Hedblad MA, Wejde J, Larsson O. Immunohistochemical markers for distinguishing Spitz nevi from malignant melanomas. Mod Pathol 1997;10:917–920.

44. Kaleem Z, Lind AC, Humphrey PA, et al. Concurrent Ki-67 and p53 immunolabeling in cutaneous melanocytic neoplasms: an adjunct for recognition of the vertical growth phase in malignant melanomas? Mod Pathol 2000;13:217–222.

45. Gelsleichter L, Gown AM, Zarbo RJ, Wang E, Coltrera MD. P53 and mdm-2 expression in malignant melanoma: an immunocytochemical study of expression of p53, mdm-2, and markers of cell proliferation in primary verses metastatic tumors. Mod Pathol 1995;8:530–535.

46. Yamamoto M, Takahashi H, Saitoh K, Horikoshi T, Takahashi M. Expression of the p53 protein in malignant melanomas as a prognostic indicator. Arch Dermatol Res 1995;287:146–151.

47. Piepkorn M. Melanoma genetics: an update with focus on the CDKN2A (p16)/ARF tumor suppressors. J Am Acad Dermatol 2000;42:705–722 (quiz, 723).

48. Funk JO, Schiller PI, Barrett MT, et al. p16INK4a expression is frequently decreased and associated with 9p21 loss of heterozygosity in sporadic melanoma. J Cutan Pathol 1998;25:291–296.

49. Sparrow LE, Eldon MJ, English DR, Hennan PJ. P16 and p21WAF1 protein expression in melanocytic tumors by immunohistochemistry. Am J Dermatopathol 1998;20:255–261.

50. Talve L, Sauroja I, Collan Y, Punnomen K, Ekfors T. Loss of expression of the p16INK4/CDKN2 gene in cutaneous malignant melanoma correlates with tumor cell proliferation and invasive stage. Int J Cancer 1997;74:255–259.

51. Reed JA, Loganzo F Jr, Shea CR, et al. Loss of expression of the p16/cyclin-dependent kinase inhibitor 2 tumor suppressor gene in melanocytic lesions correlates with invasive stage of tumor progression. Cancer Res 1995;55:2713–2718.

52. Grover R, Chana JS, Wilson GD, et al. An analysis of p16 protein expression in sporadic malignant melanoma. Melanoma Res 1998;8:267–272.

53. Straume O, Akslen LA. Alterations and prognostic significance of p16 and p53 protein expression in subgroups of subcutaneous melanoma. Int J Cancer 1997;74:535–539.

54. Weiss J, Heine M, Korner B, Pilch H, Jung EG. Expression of p53 protein in malignant melanoma: clinicopathological and prognostic implications. Br J Dermatol 1995;133:23–31.

55. Saenz-Santamariz MC, McNutt NS, Bogdany JK, Shea CR. P53 expression is rare in cutaneous melanomas. Am J Dermatopathol 1995;17:344–349.

56. Hieken TJ, Ronan SG, Farolan M, Shilkaitis AL, Das Gupta TK. Molecular prognostic markers in intermediate-thickness cutaneous malignant melanoma. Cancer 1999;85:375–382.

57. Hieken TJ, Ronan SG, Farolan M, et al. Beta 1 integrin expression in malignant melanoma predicts occult lymph node metastasis. Surgery 1995;118:669–673, discussion, 673–675.

58. VanBelle PA, Elenitsas R, Satyamoorthy K, et al. Progression-related expression of beta3 integrin in melanomas and nevi. Hum Pathol 1999;30:562–567.

59. Vihinen P, Nikkola J, Vlaykova T, et al. Prognostic value of beta1 integrin expression in metastatic melanoma. Melanoma Res 2000;10:243–251.

60. Kageshita T, Hamby CV, Hirai S, et al. Differential clinical significance of alpha (v) Beta (3) expression in primary lesions of acral lentiginous melanoma and other melanoma histotypes. Int J Cancer 2000;89:153–159.

61. Natali PG, Hamby CV, Felding-Habermann B, et al. Clinical significance of alpha (v) beta3 integrin and intercellular adhesion molecule-1 expression in cutaneous malignant melanoma lesions. Cancer Res 1997;57:1554–1560.

62. Karjalainen JM, Tammi RH, Tammi MI, et al. Reduced level of CD44 and hyaluronan associated with unfavorable prognosis in clinical stage 1 cutaneous melanoma. Am J Pathol 2000;157:957–965.

63. Schaider H, Soyer HP, Heider KH, et al. CD44 and variants in melanocytic skin neoplasms. J Cutan Pathol 1998;25:199–203.

64. Thies A, Moll I, Berger J, et al. CEACAMI expression in cutaneous malignant melanoma predicts the development of metastatic disease. J Clin Oncol 2002;20:2530–2536.

65. Bonfrer JM, Korse CM, Nieweg OE, Rankin EM. The luminescence immunoassay S-100: a sensitive test to measure circulating S-100B: its prognostic value in malignant melanoma. Br J Cancer 1998;77:2210–2214.

66. Kaskel P, Berking C, Sander S, et al. S-100 protein in peripheral blood: a marker for melanoma metastases: a prospective 2-center study of 570 patients with melanoma. J Am Acad Dermatol 1999;41:962–969.

67. Bosserhoff AK, Dreau D, Hein R, et al. Melanoma inhibitory activity (MIA), a serological marker of malignant melanoma. Recent Results Cancer Res 2001;158:158–168.

68. Garbe C, Leiter U, Ellwanger U, et al. Diagnostic value and prognostic significance of protein S-100β, melanoma-inhibitory activity, and tyrosinase/mart-1 reverse transcription-polymerase chain reaction in the follow-up of high-risk melanoma patients. Cancer 2003;97:1737–1745.

69. Weinlich G, Bitterlich W, Mayr V, Fritsch PO, Zelger B. Metallothionein-overexpression as a prognostic factor for progression and survival in melanoma. A prospective study on 520 patients. Br J Dermatol 2003;149:535–541.

70. Farthmann B, Eberle J, Krasagakis K, et al. RT-PCR for tyrosinase-m-RNA–positive cells in peripheral blood: evaluation strategy and correlation with known prognostic markers in 123 melanoma patients. J Invest Dermatol 1998;110:263–267.

71. Mellado B, Colomer D, Castel T, et al. Detection of circulating neoplastic cells by reverse-transcriptase polymerase chain reaction in malignant melanoma: association with clinical stage and prognosis. J Clin Oncol 1996;14:2091–2097.

72. Buzaid AC, Tinoco LA, Jendiroba D, et al. Prognostic value of size of lymph node metastases in patients with cutaneous melanoma. J Clin Oncol 1995;13:2361–2368.

73. Morton DL, Wanek L, Nizze JA, et al. Improved long-term survival after lymphadenectomy of melanoma metastatic to regional nodes: analysis of prognostic factors in 1134 patients from the John Wayne Cancer Clinic. Ann Surg 1991;214:491–499; discussion 499–501.

74. Balch CM, Soong SJ, Murad TM, et al. A multifactorial analysis of melanoma. III. Prognostic factors in melanoma patients with lymph node metastases (stage II). Ann Surg 1981;193:377–388.

75. Kaskel P, Berking C, Sander S, Volkenandt M, Peter RU, Krahn G. S-100 protein in peripheral blood: a marker for melanoma metastases. A prospective 2-center study of 570 patients with melanoma. J Am Acad Dermatol 1999;41:962–969.

76. Palmieri G, Ascierto PA, Perrone F, et al. Prognostic value of circulating melanoma cells detected by reverse transcriptase-polymerase chain reaction. J Clin Oncol 2003;21:767–773.

77. Barth A, Wanek LA, Morton DL. Prognostic factors in 1,512 melanoma patients with distant metastases. J Am Coll Surg 1995;181:193–201.

78. Unger JM, Flaherty LE, Liu PY, et al. Gender and other survival predictors in patients with metastatic melanoma on Southwest Oncology Group trials. Cancer 2001;91:1148–1155.

79. Manola J, Atkins M, Ibrahim J, et al. Prognostic factors in metastatic melanoma: a pooled analysis of Eastern Cooperative Oncology Group Trials. J Clin Oncol 2000;18:3782–3793.

80. Ryan L, Kramar A, Borden E. Prognostic factors in metastatic melanoma. Cancer 1993;71:2995–3005.

81. Balch CM, Soong SJ, Murad TM, et al. A multifactorial analysis of melanoma. IV. Prognostic factors in 200 melanoma patients with distant metastases (stage III). J Clin Oncol 1983;1:126–134.

82. Sirott MN, Bajorin DF, Wong GY, et al. Prognostic factors in patients with metastatic malignant melanoma. A multivariate analysis. Cancer 1993;72:3091–3098.

26

Role of Melanoma Inhibitory Activity in Early Development of Malignant Melanoma

Anja-Katrin Bosserhoff

CONTENTS

Summary

Despite its ambiguous name, the protein melanoma inhibitory activity (MIA) was identified as a key molecule involved in the progression and metastasis of malignant melanomas. In this review, we update current knowledge on MIA with a focus on its role in early development of malignant melanoma. A search for autocrine growth-regulatory factors secreted by melanoma cells identified MIA, which was purified in 1989 and cloned in 1994. Subsequent analyses of nonneoplastic tissues revealed specific expression of MIA in cartilage. In neoplastic tissues, MIA expression was detected in malignant melanomas and chondrosarcomas. In melanoma cells, the regulation of MIA expression is controlled at the level of messenger RNA transcription by defined transcription factors. Probably, the same transcription factors regulating MIA expression also have an impact on the expression of other melanoma-associated molecules. Evidence obtained from in vitro and in vivo experiments indicated that MIA plays an important functional role in melanoma metastasis and invasion. Determination of the three-dimensional structure in solution identified MIA as the first member of a novel family of secreted extracellular proteins adopting an SH3 domain-like fold. These findings suggest specific protein–protein interactions with components of the extracellular matrix and possibly epitopes on cellular surfaces. The exact mechanisms of these interactions are unknown but certainly attract further investigations. A number of studies from different laboratories evaluated MIA as a highly specific and sensitive prognostic marker, clinically useful for follow-up and therapy monitoring of patients with malignant melanomas.

Key Words: Malignant melanoma; MIA; invasion; metastasis; serum marker; transcriptional regulation.

From: *From Melanocytes to Melanoma: The Progression to Malignancy*
Edited by: V. J. Hearing and S. P. L. Leong © Humana Press Inc., Totowa, NJ

INTRODUCTION

Regulation of tumor progression is influenced by a complex network of inhibiting and stimulating factors produced both by tumor cells and by the local environment. By characterizing autocrine growth-regulatory factors in malignant melanoma, the melanoma inhibitory activity (MIA) protein was identified within a growth-inhibiting activity purified from the tissue culture supernatant of the human melanoma cell line, HTZ-19d *(1,2)*. Initially, MIA was thought to act as a tumor suppressor, because when purified and added to melanoma cells in vitro, MIA caused alterations in cell morphology, cell rounding, detachment from tissue culture plastic, and growth inhibition *(3,4)*. Based on partial peptide sequences obtained by Edman degradation, a complementary (c)DNA fragment was amplified by reverse transcriptase-polymerase chain reaction (RT-PCR) and used as a probe to isolate the fully encoding cDNA *(3)*.

Cloning of MIA

The first human MIA cDNA sequence was obtained by screening a cDNA library of the human melanoma cell line HTZ-19d, and was verified by cDNA and genomic clones obtained from different sources. Until today, no mutations in the MIA sequence have been detected. MIA mRNA was identified independently by a differential display approach comparing differentiated and dedifferentiated chondrocytes in vitro. Because dedifferentiation was accelerated by retinoic acid in this study, MIA was also referred to as CD-RAP (cartilage-derived retinoic acid-sensitive protein) *(5)*. Subsequent studies of murine embryos and murine adult tissues demonstrated cartilage-specific mRNA expression patterns *(6)*.

Both human and murine genomic *MIA* sequences were determined and deposited in the gene bank (X84707, X97965). The *MIA* locus was mapped as a single-copy gene to human chromosome 19q13.32-13.33 *(7)* and murine chromosome 7 *(6,8)*. The gene consists of four exons and the exon–intron structure is highly conserved, because it was also found in all other species that have been analyzed so far, even in pufferfish (Tetraodon).

Expression Pattern of MIA

Analysis of normal skin and skin-derived melanocytic tumors by semiquantitative RT-PCR did not reveal significant MIA mRNA levels in normal skin and melanocytes, but revealed moderate levels in some benign melanocytic nevi and very high levels in all primary and metastatic malignant melanomas (Fig. 1) *(3,9)*. Subsequent studies confirmed specific expression patterns of MIA mRNA and protein in malignant melanomas and the absence of MIA mRNA expression in benign melanocytes cultured from normal skin biopsies *(10–12)*. The expression pattern data obtained by RT-PCR studies were supported by *in situ* hybridization and coincided with protein expression visualized by immunohistochemistry (Fig. 2).

The finding that MIA is already expressed in some nevi led to the hypothesis that upregulation of MIA is an early process in melanoma initiation. However, the regulation of expression in nevi is not strictly regulated because some nevi also present as negative for MIA.

In summary, these results indicate that expression of MIA in nonneoplastic tissues is limited to cartilage. However, under pathological circumstances, high expression levels occur in melanomas and in chondrosarcomas.

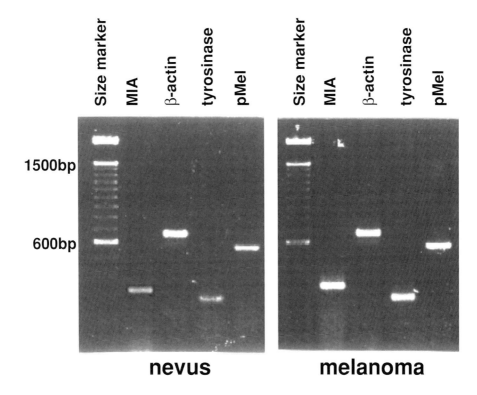

Fig. 1. Melanoma inhibitory activity (MIA) messenger RNA expression in nevi and melanoma. MIA complementary DNA was amplified by reverse transcriptase-polymerase chain reaction (PCR). Strong expression was detected in malignant melanoma, weak expression in some of the nevi. As a control, β-actin (to verify RNA integrity), tyrosinase, and pMel (to verify melanocytic origin) were amplified. The PCR products were separated on 1.5% agarose gels, stained with ethidium bromide, and visualized under ultraviolet light.

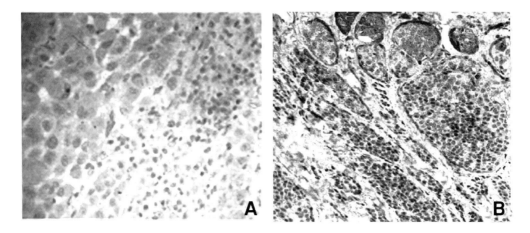

Fig. 2. Detection of melanoma inhibitory activity (MIA) by immunohistochemistry. Primary cutaneous melanoma (**A**) and intradermal nevi (**B**) were immunoreacted with a specific antibody for MIA. A strong signal (AEC staining, red) was found in melanoma (original magnification, ×100), weak staining was found in nevi (original magnification, ×40). Please *see* color insert following p. 430.

MIA PROTEIN

Characterization of MIA Protein

MIA is translated as a 131-amino-acid precursor molecule and is processed during translation into the mature 107-amino-acid protein after cleavage of a hydrophobic peptide *(3)*. These first 24 amino acids of the 11-kDa putative protein correspond to a signaling peptide that results in the release of MIA into the extracellular compartment. The MIA amino acid sequence is highly conserved between species from fish to mammals, suggesting functional conservation (Fig. 3A,B).

MIA Protein Structure

Recently, it has been shown by multidimensional NMR that recombinant human MIA adopts an Src homology 3 (SH3) domain-like fold in solution *(13–15)*, a structure with two perpendicular, antiparallel, three- and five-stranded β-sheets (Fig. 4A). SH3 domains are small (55–70 amino acids) noncatalytic protein modules that are found in many intracellular signaling proteins. Different from previously solved structures of proteins with SH3 domain folds, MIA is a single-domain protein and contains an additional antiparallel β-sheet and two disulfide bonds. These two disulfide bonds are absolutely necessary for correct folding and function, as revealed by mutation analysis *(15)*. Obviously, additional stabilization of the SH3 domain is needed in the extracellular compartment. SH3 domains mediate protein–protein interactions by binding to proline-rich peptide sequences. More than 50 SH3 domains are known, and these SH3 domains are widely distributed. For example, SH3 domains have been identified in kinases, lipases, guanosine triphosphatases, adapter proteins, structural proteins, and viral regulatory proteins, all of which represent intracellular proteins. In contrast, human MIA appears to be the first extracellular protein adopting an SH3 domain-like fold in solution. Nuclear magnetic resonance data were recently confirmed by X-ray crystallography *(16,17)*. Peptides identified as ligands for human MIA in a heptapeptide phage display experiment are strikingly similar to the consensus sequence XPPLPXR for SH3 domains.

Furthermore, it was shown that MIA interacts with fibronectin (FN) and that MIA-interacting peptide ligands identified by phage display screening are similar to the consensus sequence of type III human FN repeats, especially FN14 *(14,18)*. Functional data suggest that FN12–14 is able to promote melanoma cell adhesion activity and is sensitive to antibodies to α4 β1 integrin, suggesting a direct interaction between FN12–14 and α4 β1 integrin *(19)*. Therefore, while bound to the FN14 domain of FN, human MIA might sterically interfere with the binding of FN to α4 β1 integrin (Fig. 4B).

Additionally, intact FN has binding surfaces for several molecules, including collagens, fibrin, integrins, heparin, DNA, and so on. In vivo, it may be occupied at multiple sites by multiple ligands *(20,21)*. This might also be true for the binding of human MIA to FN, because the identified target peptides share sequence similarities with several

---

Fig. 3. (*opposite page*) Human melanoma inhibitory activity (MIA) protein sequence. **(A)** The signal sequence responsible for translocation into the endoplasmic reticulum and subsequent secretion is in *italics*. MIA is translated as a 131-amino-acid precursor molecule and processed into a mature 107-amino-acid protein after cleavage of the N-terminal secretion signal *(3)*. The consensus sequence displays the high homology comparing the species. **(B)** The phylogenetic tree further supports the high homology of MIA between the species (generated using the program DNAMAN, Lynnon Biosoft, Quebec, Canada).

A

```
HUMAN              MARSLVCLGVIILLSAFSGPGVRGGPMPKLADRKLCADQE        40
BOVINE             MAwSLVfLG.vvLLSAFpGPsagGrPMPKLADRKmCADeE         39
RAT                MvcSpVlLG.IviLSvFSGlsradraMPKLADRKLCADeE         39
MOUSE              MvwSpVlLG.IvvLSvFSGPsradraMPKLADwKLCADeE         39
SALMON             MsarrVCLwgvvfLcvvS.vcqaGrqMPKLsnkKmCADaE         39
ZEBRAFISH                  lviigvcfvcdsathtalMdKLADtKiCADrd         32
TETRAODON_(PARTIAL)                                                 0
Consensus                  SIGNAL SEQUENCE   mpklad k cad e


HUMAN              CSHPISMAVALQDYMAPDCRFLTIHRGQVVYVFS.KLK.G        78
BOVINE             CSHPISvAVALQDYvAPDCRFLTIHqGQVVYiFS.KLK.G        77
RAT                CSHPISMAVALQDYvAPDCRFLTIyRGQVVYVFS.KLK.G        77
MOUSE              CSHPISMAVALQDYvAPDCRFLTIyRGQVVYVFS.KLK.G        77
SALMON             CSHPIliArALeDYypgDCRFislrqGQVVYVya.lLK.d        77
ZEBRAFISH          CSyvISvAsALeDYvAPDCRFinlrRGQkiYVFfsKLrpa        72
TETRAODON_(PARTIAL)   nPImiArALQDYypaDCxFipIrqGQliYVya.mLK.G       36
Consensus          cshpis avalqdyvapdcrflti rgqvvyvfs klk g


HUMAN              RGR.LFWGGSVQGDYYGDLAARLGYFPSSIVREDQTLKPG       117
BOVINE             RGR.LFWGGSVQGDYYGDgAARLGYFPSSIVREDQTLKPa       116
RAT                RGR.LFWGGSVQGDYYGDLAAhLGYFPSSIVREDlTLKPG       116
MOUSE              RGR.LFWGGSVQGgYYGDLAARLGYFPSSIVREDlTLKPG       116
SALMON             RGn.mFWaGSVQGsYYGeqeARLGhFPSSvVeEthaLmPa       116
ZEBRAFISH          eGagvFWsGSVyGerYvDqmgiiGYFPSnyinEtQvfqkn       112
TETRAODON(PARTIAL) RGs.qFWaGSVQdsYYGqqeARiGhFPSSIVeEthpLmaa        75
Consensus          rgr lfwggsvqg yygd aarlgyfpssivred tlkp


HUMAN              KVDVKTDKWDFYCQ                                 131
BOVINE             KtDVKTDiWDFYCQ                                 130
RAT                KVDmKTDeWDFYCQ                                 130
MOUSE              KiDmKTDqWDFYCQ                                 130
SALMON             tneVmTDnWDFYCQ                                 129
ZEBRAFISH          tVeipTtdmDFlCQ                                 125
TETRAODON_(PARTIAL) qteVKTsnWDFYCx                                 89
Consensus          k dvktd wdfycq
```

B

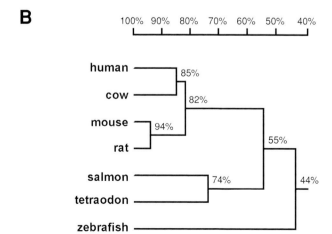

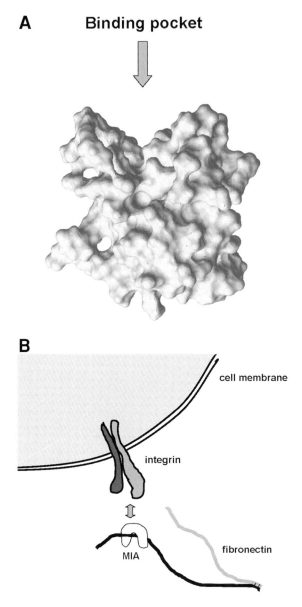

A   **Binding pocket**

B

cell membrane

integrin

MIA

fibronectin

Fig. 4. Three-dimensional structure of melanoma inhibitory activity (MIA) protein in solution. **(A)** Multidimensional nuclear magnetic resonance studies revealed that MIA adopts an Src homology 3 domain-like fold. The model shows the three-dimensional structure of MIA. The binding pocket is indicated *(13–15)*. **(B)** MIA binding to fibronectin was verified by several studies. This leads to masking of the integrin binding sites and subsequently causes the detachment of the cells.

domains in FN. The matching sequence of all human type III FN repeats suggests the intriguing possibility of a multiple binding of human MIA to several FN repeats, but at least to FN6, FN10, and FN14. Experiments suggest that four MIA proteins bind to one FN molecule, inhibit the binding of integrins to FN, and thereby cause the detachment of cells from the extracellular matrix (ECM) *(14)*.

These findings may provide a mechanistic explanation for the role of MIA in metastasis in vivo (*see* following subheading) and support a model in which the binding of human MIA to type III repeats of FN competes with integrin binding, thus, detaching cells from the ECM.

Interestingly, inhibitory antibodies against α4 or α5 integrin recognize recombinant MIA *(18)*. By sequence comparison of MIA and α4 or α5 integrin, weak homology in amino acid identity (18% or 15.6%) and homology in predicted secondary structure by hydrophobicity blots is detectable. Homology was found in the region of the W6 and W7 β-propeller structure in α4 and α5 integrin, a region known to be involved in ligand binding. Because denatured human MIA does not crossreact with anti-α4 and -α5 integrin, these antibodies obviously recognize a three-dimensional epitope in human MIA. However, a detailed analysis on the molecular level awaits the structure elucidation of α4 and/or α5 integrin. This will allow one to address the question of which regions of human MIA are structurally similar to α4 and α5 integrin.

MIA Function

Based on monitoring biological activity during purification of the protein from tissue culture supernatants, MIA was initially believed to elicit antitumor activity by inhibiting melanoma cell proliferation in vitro *(2,3)*. However, further analysis revealed an expression pattern inconsistent with that of a tumor suppressor. Expression of MIA was not detected in normal skin and melanocytes, but was associated with progression of melanocytic tumors (*see* "MIA Protein Structure") *(10,11)*. More recently, it was observed that MIA specifically inhibits attachment of melanoma cells to FN and laminin by masking the binding site of integrins to these ECM components and, thereby, promoting invasion and metastasis in vivo (Fig. 4B) *(13–15,18)*. Thus, the growth-inhibitory activity in vitro may reflect the ability of the protein to interfere with the attachment of cell lines to culture dishes in vitro. In conclusion, there is evidence for the potential molecular mechanism by which MIA promotes invasion and metastasis: MIA binds to human FN type III repeats, thus, inhibiting the attachment of melanoma cells. In general, the structure of human MIA suggests a new mechanism of metastasis: binding of the extracellular SH3-like domain to type III repeats of FN competes with integrin binding and leads to detachment of the melanoma cells from the ECM.

Further experiments in hamsters and mice were performed to analyze the in vivo role of MIA during melanoma metastasis *(22,23)*. In a study of Guba et al., A-mel 3 hamster melanoma cells were transfected with sense or antisense MIA cDNA and analyzed for changes in their tumorigenic and metastatic potential. The metastatic potential of A-mel 3 cells with enforced expression of MIA was significantly increased compared with control- or antisense-transfected cells, but did not affect the growth rate of the primary tumor, cell proliferation, or apoptosis. In addition, MIA overexpressing cell clones showed a higher rate, both of tumor cell invasion and of extravasation, as analyzed by intravital microscopy. Consistently, cell clones transfected with an antisense MIA cDNA expression plasmid revealed significantly reduced metastatic potential. The changes in metastatic behavior in correlation to the expression level of MIA provide evidence that upregulation of MIA during malignant transformation of melanocytic cells is causally involved in acquisition of the malignant cancer cell phenotype.

This hypothesis was further confirmed by a second study analyzing B16 mouse melanoma cells secreting different amounts of MIA generated by stable transfection

(23). The capacity of these cell clones to form lung metastases in syngeneic C57Bl6 mice was strictly correlated to the level of MIA expression. B16 melanoma cells over-expressing MIA showed increased metastatic progression compared with untreated controls, whereas the antisense MIA-transfected B16 cells displayed a strongly reduced metastatic potential. Again, no effects on cell proliferation were observed.

These positive effects on migration can be explained by the MIA protein structure containing an SH3-like domain that binds to type III repeats of FN (*see* "MIA Protein Structure"). This results in a decrease in the ability of α4 β1 integrin on the cell surface to bind to FN, promoting cell detachment from the ECM *(14)*.

Based on these findings, it could be speculated that MIA enables melanoma cells to detach from some of their ECM contacts. In accordance with that, adhesion of melanoma cells to FN, laminin, and tenascin was shown to be reduced by 30–50% *(18)*. Taken together, these data identify active detachment through secretion of MIA as a molecular mechanism by which neoplastic melanocytes specifically change their attachment to components of the ECM and basement membranes to enhance their metastatic capability.

Interactions between cell-surface molecules and matrix components do not only mediate physical adhesion but also provide other important signals for melanocytic cells. Detachment of melanoma cells by MIA may also be implicated in regulating migration, apoptosis, secretion of proteases, or matrix proteins and cell growth (*see* section entitled 3.4.). It is known that such interactions between melanocytic cells and ECM involve foremost the binding of integrins to specific epitopes within FN and depend to a significant extent on activation of α4 β1 and α5 β1 integrins *(24)*. Detachment from ECM molecules within the local milieu is a key prerequisite for melanoma cells to migrate, invade, and finally metastasize. A previous study has demonstrated that overexpression of functionally active α4 β1 integrin in B16 cells strongly reduced matrigel invasion and pulmonary metastasis *(25)*. These findings indicate that MIA particularly affects interactions between ECM molecules and integrins, which play critical roles in controlling melanoma cell metastasis at the invasive stage. Active detachment promoted by MIA secretion appears to be a highly regulated and cell-type specific mechanism because other cell types known to actively migrate, including macrophages or lymphocytes, do not express MIA *(3)*.

Downstream Effects of MIA Expression

Because MIA expression seems to be an early event in melanoma development, it was speculated that further molecules involved in melanoma development and progression could be regulated by MIA. To follow up on this question, MIA expression was omitted by an antisense approach in a human melanoma cell line *(25a)*. Changes in the expression profile were analyzed by cDNA and protein arrays. Interestingly, several genes associated with melanoma progression, such as MT1-MMP or β3 integrin, were markedly downregulated in the melanoma cell clone without functional MIA. These findings lead to the hypothesis that MIA is not only involved in melanoma migration and invasion but also in regulating gene expression.

TRANSCRIPTIONAL REGULATION OF MIA IN MALIGNANT MELANOMA

Because MIA is highly specifically expressed in melanomas but not in benign melanocytes, the mechanism of transcriptional regulation is of particular interest. As discussed in "MIA Protein Structure," the upregulation or induction of MIA expression seems to be an early event in melanoma development. This is supported by the finding that MIA expression is already found in some nevi and in all melanomas *in situ*.

Changes in the activity of the *MIA* promoter could provide insights into gene regulatory mechanisms prototypic for malignant transformation of melanomas. A fragment of approx 1.4 kb in the 5' flanking DNA of the human gene conferred strong reporter gene expression in melanoma cells but not in melanocytes *(9)*. Regulation of promoter activity usually results from the binding of transcription factors that specifically activate or repress the rate of transcription. To search for transcription factors involved in regulating MIA expression, reporter constructs with a series of different truncated *MIA* promoter fragments were analyzed. This study identified important active *cis*-regulatory elements on the MIA promoter between nucleic acids –230 and –130, relative to the translation start site *(26)*. Promoter constructs with that particular region revealed melanoma-specific expression of the reporter gene, but no activity in melanocytes or nonmelanocytic cells. Gel mobility shift assays and Southwestern blots led to the identification of further specific DNA–protein complexes in melanoma cells. Fine mutational analysis of the *cis*-regulatory promoter elements revealed that two critical nucleic acid residues are essential for transcriptional activity, because mutagenesis of both base pairs abolished the entire promoter activity. Using an affinity purification approach, a protein of approx 32 kDa was isolated from melanoma cells and referred to as MATF (melanoma-associated transcription factor) *(26)*. After protein sequencing, MATF was revealed to be a high-mobility group (HMG)-1 protein. HMG proteins are known as abundant and ubiquitous nonhistone proteins. They can be classified into three families: HMG1/2/4, HMG14/17, and HMG-I. The family of HMG1/2/4 was recently renamed to HMGB (with HMG1 as HMGB1, HMG2 as HMGB2, and HMG4 as HMGB3). The structure of the three family members is highly conserved. They are composed of three different domains and two DNA-binding domains, called HMG boxes *(27)*. Until this finding, HMG-1 was commonly described as a DNA-bending molecule without specific DNA-binding and transcriptional activating activity. In the study of Poser et al. *(28)*, it was shown that HMG-1 expression is strongly upregulated in malignant melanoma in comparison with melanocytes. Furthermore, the experiments revealed that HMG-1 in concert with p65, a member of the nuclear factor-κB family, positively regulates the *MIA* promoter. This study revealed HMG-1 and p65 as important factors in MIA regulation and melanoma progression, and further defined HMG-1 as a gene-specific transregulatory protein (Fig. 5).

In addition to the positive regulation of MIA expression by HMG-1, C-terminal binding protein (CtBP), a negative regulator of the T-cell factor (TCF)/lymphoid enhancer factor family of transcription factors, was shown to be an inhibitor of MIA expression in primary melanocytes *(29)*. Testing mutated constructs of the *MIA* promoter gave additional evidence for a negative *cis*-regulatory element located 5' adjacent to the HMG-1-binding region, and it was shown that this element is critically important in melanoma-specific expression. Defects in this promoter element lead to loss of its specific expression and to unscheduled activity of the promoter in MIA negative cells, such as HeLa cells or primary melanocytes. Further analysis revealed that TCF4 binds to this region. Interestingly, β-catenin does not seem to function as a co-regulator of this TCF-dependent element. Therefore, the TCF co-repressor, CtBP1, was analyzed. CtBP1 was first identified as a cytoplasmic protein binding to the C-terminal region of the adenoviral protein, E1A, and attenuating its ability to activate transcription. CtBP recognizes PXDLS motifs in DNA-binding proteins and functions as a transcriptional co-repressor in *Drosophila*, *Xenopus*, and mammals. As previously shown for the tran-

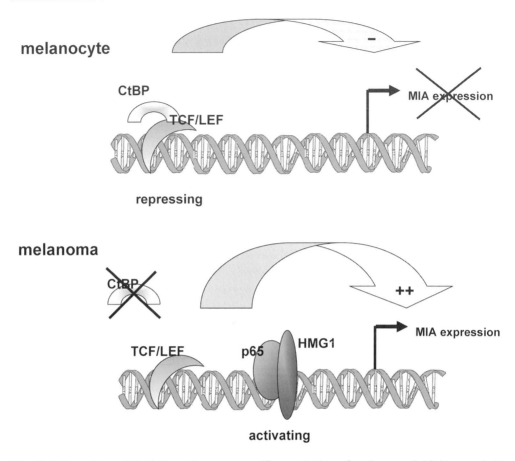

Fig. 5. Schematic model of the melanoma-specific regulation of melanoma inhibitory activity (MIA) expression. In melanocytes, the transcriptional repressor C-terminal binding protein (CtBP) is expressed and suppresses MIA expression. Further, positive regulators, such as p65 and high-mobility group (HMG)-1 are missing. The lower figure represents the situation in melanoma cells. The repressor CtBP is lost and HMG-1, as a positive regulator of MIA expression, is strongly upregulated. This results in induction of MIA expression.

scriptional regulator, Sox6, the study by Poser et al. implies that TCF4 can act as a transcriptional repressor depending on the context of co-regulatory factors. In vitro reporter gene assays revealed that CtBP1 functions as a strong repressor of *MIA* promoter activity and that this repressor function requires the TCF-binding element within the MIA promoter. Expression studies further indicate that the loss of TCF/CtBP1 binding and, consequently, the loss of suppression of MIA expression, may be important for melanoma progression. In the context of the MIA promoter, TCF is obviously used as a negative regulator in combination with CtBP1. This could be proven by simultaneous transfections of TCF4 and CtBP1 expression plasmids into melanoma cells. Here, TCF4 negatively regulates CtBP1-induced repression of MIA promoter activity by interacting with CtBP1 (Fig. 5).

Further analysis revealed CtBP1 to be strongly expressed in primary melanocytes. In contrast, melanoma cells in vitro and in vivo were shown to have strongly downregulated or lost wild-type CtBP1 expression.

CtBP has been speculated to be involved in normal cell growth control. Furthermore, invasion assays pointed to a role of CtBP1 in cell migration because re-expression of CtBP1 in melanoma cells induced a reduction of the invasive potential.

MIA AS A SERUM MARKER IN PATIENTS WITH MALIGNANT MELANOMAS

Proteins strongly expressed by and released from tumor cells can be used as markers to monitor the development and systemic spread of the tumor disease. Because studies of melanocytic tumors in vitro and in vivo indicated that MIA mRNA expression correlates with tumor progression, it was investigated whether MIA provides a clinically useful parameter in patients with primary or metastatic melanoma. Therefore, a quantitative enzyme-linked immunosorbent assay was designed and MIA serum levels were correlated with clinically determined melanoma stages *(30–35)*.

In the first study *(30)*, the cut-off for positive values (97th percentile) was set at 6.5 ng/mL, based on measuring sera from a control group of healthy blood donors. Of sera obtained from patients with metastatic malignant melanomas in stage IV, 97% revealed enhanced MIA values and 81% of the sera from patients in stage III revealed enhanced MIA values. After surgery, MIA serum levels dropped significantly. Interestingly, patients responding to chemotherapy also showed decreasing MIA serum levels, whereas patients with progressive disease during or after chemotherapy had increasing MIA serum levels. Furthermore, slightly enhanced MIA serum levels in 13 and 23% of patients with stage I and II disease, respectively, were reported. In repeated measurements of the sera of 350 patients with a history of stage I or II melanoma during follow-up, 32 patients developed positive MIA values. At the time of serum analysis, 15 of the patients had recurrent metastatic disease and 1 further patient presented with metastatic disease 6 mo later. In contrast, none of the patients with normal MIA serum levels developed metastases during the follow-up period of 6–12 mo. Therefore, it was concluded that MIA represents a clinically useful, novel serum marker for systemic malignant melanomas, revealing a very high sensitivity and specificity. Potential clinical applications included detection of occult metastases, detection of progression from localized to metastatic disease during follow-up, and monitoring therapy of advanced melanomas *(30)*. Several follow-up studies confirmed these results with minor differences in sensitivity and specificity *(31,33–35)*.

CONCLUSIONS AND PERSPECTIVES

In summary, the protein MIA was characterized as a secreted molecule playing a role in invasion and metastasis of malignant melanoma. The solution of the three-dimensional structure identified MIA as the first extracellular protein adopting an SH3 domain-like fold, and will have great future impact on basic research addressing protein interactions within the ECM. It was clearly shown that MIA has the ability to bind to specific matrix proteins, such as FN, a process which leads to controlled detachment of the cells from the surrounding matrix and supports migration. In addition, by analyzing the regulation of MIA expression on the promoter level, several transcriptional regulators, such as HMG-1 and CtBP, were identified. Future studies should reveal whether these factors are also involved in the regulation of expression of other proteins that are upregulated early in melanoma development or progression.

Clinically, MIA has already been established as a serum marker for patients with cutaneous and uveal melanomas.

ACKNOWLEDGMENTS

The following people supported the work on the protein MIA: R. Buettner, U. Bogdahn, I. Poser, M. Golob, M. Guba, M. Steinbauer, B. Echtenacher, F. Hofstädter, R. Hein, M. Landthaler, T. Holak, R. Stoll, B. Kaluza, M. Hergersberger, M. Kaufmann, and Reinhard Fässler.

REFERENCES

1. Apfel R, Lottspeich F, Hoppe J, Behl C, Durr G, Bogdahn U. Purification and analysis of growth regulating proteins secreted by a human melanoma cell line. Melanoma Res 1992; 2(5–6):327–336.
2. Bogdahn U, Apfel R, Hahn M, et al. Autocrine tumor cell growth-inhibiting activities from human malignant melanoma. Cancer Res 1989;49(19):5358–5363.
3. Blesch A, Bosserhoff AK, Apfel R, et al. Cloning of a novel malignant melanoma-derived growth-regulatory protein, MIA. Cancer Res 1994;54(21):5695–5701.
4. Weilbach FX, Bogdahn U, Poot M, et al. Melanoma-inhibiting activity inhibits cell proliferation by prolongation of the S-phase and arrest of cells in the G2 compartment. Cancer Res 1990;50(21): 6981–6986.
5. Dietz UH, Sandell LJ. Cloning of a retinoic acid-sensitive mRNA expressed in cartilage and during chondrogenesis. J Biol Chem 1996;271(6):3311–3316.
6. Bosserhoff AK, Kondo S, Moser M, et al. Mouse CD-RAP/MIA gene: structure, chromosomal localization, and expression in cartilage and chondrosarcoma. Dev Dyn 1997;208(4):516–525.
7. Koehler MR, Bosserhoff A, von Beust G, et al. Assignment of the human melanoma inhibitory activity gene (MIA) to 19q13.32-q13.33 by fluorescence in situ hybridization (FISH). Genomics 1996;35(1):265–267.
8. Koehler MR, Bosserhoff A, von Beust G, et al. Assignment of the human melanoma inhibitory activity gene (MIA) to 19q13.32-q13.33 by fluorescence in situ hybridization (FISH). Genomics 1996;35(1):265–267.
9. Bosserhoff AK, Hein R, Bogdahn U, Buettner R. Structure and promoter analysis of the gene encoding the human melanoma-inhibiting protein MIA. J Biol Chem 1996;271(1):490–495.
10. van Groningen JJ, Bloemers HP, Swart GW. Identification of melanoma inhibitory activity and other differentially expressed messenger RNAs in human melanoma cell lines with different metastatic capacity by messenger RNA differential display. Cancer Res 1995;55(24):6237–6243.
11. Bosserhoff AK, Moser M, Hein R, Landthaler M, Buettner R. In situ expression patterns of melanoma-inhibiting activity (MIA) in melanomas and breast cancers. J Pathol 1999;187(4):446–454.
12. Perez RP, Zhang P, Bosserhoff AK, Buettner R, Abu-Hadid M. Expression of melanoma inhibitory activity in melanoma and nonmelanoma tissue specimens. Hum Pathol 2000;31(11):1381–1388.
13. Stoll R, Renner C, Ambrosius D, et al. Sequence-specific 1H, 13C, and 15N assignment of the human melanoma inhibitory activity (MIA) protein. J Biomol NMR 2000;17(1):87–88.
14. Stoll R, Renner C, Zweckstetter M, et al. The extracellular human melanoma inhibitory activity (MIA) protein adopts an SH3 domain-like fold. EMBO J 2001;20(3):340–349.
15. Stoll R, Renner C, Buettner R, Voelter W, Bosserhoff AK, Holak TA. Backbone dynamics of the human MIA protein studied by (15)N NMR relaxation: implications for extended interactions of SH3 domains. Protein Sci 2003;12(3):510–519.
16. Lougheed JC, Holton JM, Alber T, Bazan JF, Handel TM. Structure of melanoma inhibitory activity protein, a member of a recently identified family of secreted proteins. Proc Natl Acad Sci U S A 2001;98(10):5515–5520.
17. Lougheed JC, Domaille PJ, Handel TM. Solution structure and dynamics of melanoma inhibitory activity protein. J Biomol NMR 2002;22(3):211–223.
18. Bosserhoff AK, Stoll R, Sleeman JP, Bataille F, Buettner R, Holak TA. Active detachment involves inhibition of cell-matrix contacts of malignant melanoma cells by secretion of melanoma inhibitory activity. Lab Invest 2003;83(11):1583–1594.

19. Mould AP, Humphries MJ. Identification of a novel recognition sequence for the integrin alpha 4 beta 1 in the COOH-terminal heparin-binding domain of fibronectin. EMBO J 1991;10(13):4089–4095.

20. Potts JR, Campbell ID. Fibronectin structure and assembly. Curr Opin Cell Biol 1994;6(5):648–655.

21. Grant RP, Spitzfaden C, Altroff H, Campbell ID, Mardon HJ. Structural requirements for biological activity of the ninth and tenth FIII domains of human fibronectin. J Biol Chem 1997;272(10): 6159–6166.

22. Guba M, Steinbauer M, Ruhland V, et al. Elevated MIA serum levels are predictors of poor prognosis after surgical resection of metastatic malignant melanoma. Oncol Rep 2002;9(5):981–984.

23. Bosserhoff AK, Echtenacher B, Hein R, Buettner R. Functional role of melanoma inhibitory activity in regulating invasion and metastasis of malignant melanoma cells in vivo. Melanoma Res 2001;11(4):417–421.

24. Scott G, Ryan DH, McCarthy JB. Molecular mechanisms of human melanocyte attachment to fibronectin. J Invest Dermatol 1992;99(6):787–794.

25. Qian F, Vaux DL, Weissman IL. Expression of the integrin alpha 4 beta 1 on melanoma cells can inhibit the invasive stage of metastasis formation. Cell 1994;77(3):335–347.

25a. Poser I, Tatzel J, Kuphal S, Bosserhoff AK. Functional role of MIA in melanocytes and early development of melanoma. Oncogene 2004;23:6115–6124.

26. Golob M, Buettner R, Bosserhoff AK. Characterization of a transcription factor binding site, specifically activating MIA transcription in melanoma. J Invest Dermatol 2000;115(1):42–47.

27. Travers A. Recognition of distorted DNA structures by HMG domains. Curr Opin Struct Biol 2000;10(1):102–109.

28. Poser I, Golob M, Buettner R, Bosserhoff AK. Upregulation of HMG1 leads to melanoma inhibitory activity expression in malignant melanoma cells and contributes to their malignancy phenotype. Mol Cell Biol 2003;23(8):2991–2998.

29. Poser I, Golob M, Weidner M, Buettner R, Bosserhoff AK. Down-regulation of COOH-terminal binding protein expression in malignant melanomas leads to induction of MIA expression. Cancer Res 2002;62(20):5962–5966.

30. Bosserhoff AK, Kaufmann M, Kaluza B, et al. Melanoma-inhibiting activity, a novel serum marker for progression of malignant melanoma. Cancer Res 1997;57(15):3149–3153.

31. Dreau D, Bosserhoff AK, White RL, Buettner R, Holder WD. Melanoma-inhibitory activity protein concentrations in blood of melanoma patients treated with immunotherapy. Oncol Res 1999; 11(1):55–61.

32. Deichmann M, Benner A, Kuner N, Wacker J, Waldmann V, Naher H. Are responses to therapy of metastasized malignant melanoma reflected by decreasing serum values of S100beta or melanoma inhibitory activity (MIA)? Melanoma Res 2001;11(3):291–296.

33. Stahlecker J, Gauger A, Bosserhoff A, Buttner R, Ring J, Hein R. MIA as a reliable tumor marker in the serum of patients with malignant melanoma. Anticancer Res 2000;20(6D):5041–5044.

34. Schmitz C, Brenner W, Henze E, Christophers E, Hauschild A. Comparative study on the clinical use of protein S-100B and MIA (melanoma inhibitory activity) in melanoma patients. Anticancer Res 2000;20(6D):5059–5063.

35. Bosserhoff AK, Hauschild A, Hein R, et al. Elevated MIA serum levels are of relevance for management of metastasized malignant melanomas: results of a German multicenter study. J Invest Dermatol 2000;114(2):395–396.

27 Role and Regulation of PAR-1 in Melanoma Progression

Carmen Tellez and Menashe Bar-Eli

Contents

Summary

To determine treatment strategies and predict the clinical outcome of patients with melanoma it is important to understand the etiology of this disease. Recently, there has been some insight into the molecular basis of melanoma, including identification of a few of the regulatory factors and genes involved in this disease. For instance, the transcription factor, activator protein (AP)-2α, plays a tumor suppressor-like role in melanoma progression by regulating genes involved in tumor growth and metastasis. Previously, we have shown that the progression of human melanoma to the metastatic phenotype is associated with loss of AP-2 expression and deregulation of target genes, such as *MUC18/MCAM*, *c-KIT*, and *MMP-2*. This chapter focuses on the expression of the thrombin receptor (protease-activated receptor [PAR]-1) in human melanoma and its regulation by AP-2 and specificity protein (Sp)-1. We demonstrate that the metastatic potential of human melanoma cells correlates with overexpression of PAR-1. We also provide evidence that an inverse correlation exists between the expression of AP-2 and the expression of PAR-1 in human melanoma cells. The regulatory region of the *PAR-1* gene contains multiple AP-2 consensus elements overlapping multiple Sp1 consensus elements. Our analysis of the highly overlapping AP-2 and Sp1 binding elements (complex 1, bp −365 to −329) within the regulatory region demonstrates that AP-2 and Sp1 bind to this region in a mutually exclusive manner to promote repression or activation, respectively. We propose that loss of AP-2 results in increased expression of the thrombin receptor, which subsequently contributes to the metastatic phenotype of melanoma by upregulating the expression of adhesion molecules, proteases, and angiogenic molecules.

Key Words: Melanoma; gene regulation; transcription factor; gene expression; AP-2; angiogenesis; metastasis; thrombin receptor.

From: *From Melanocytes to Melanoma: The Progression to Malignancy*
Edited by: V. J. Hearing and S. P. L. Leong © Humana Press Inc., Totowa, NJ

INTRODUCTION

Melanoma develops and progresses through a multistep process. In humans, it progresses from melanocytes to nevi with structurally normal melanocytes, to dysplastic nevus with structural and architectural atypia, to early radial growth phase primary melanoma, to advanced vertical growth phase primary melanoma with competence for metastasis, and finally to metastatic melanoma *(1)*. The transition of normal melanocytes to clinical melanoma is associated with genetic and molecular changes. The mechanisms that mediate the differential expression of genes that contribute to the process remain largely unknown, however, and are under investigation. Nevertheless, there has been some progress in our understanding of the molecular and genetic changes associated with the development of this disease. Of particular relevance are recent results concerning aberrant expression of transcription factors, which modulate gene expression through activation or repression of a multitude of genes that can enhance tumor development and metastasis of melanoma. Recent investigations have demonstrated the contributions of abnormalities in expression of transcription factors, which, in turn, modulate the expression of several genes involved in malignant progression, including activating transcription factor-1 *(2,3)*; cyclic adenosine monophosphate response element-binding protein *(4–6)*; microphthalmia transcription factor *(7,8)*; nuclear factor-κB *(9)*; transcriptional repressor, Snail *(10)*; and activator protein (AP)-2α *(11–13)*.

In this chapter, we focus on the expression of the transcription factor AP-2α, a 52-kDa protein first purified from HeLa cells. Partial peptide sequences led to the isolation of the complementary (c)DNA from a HeLa cell library *(14)*, and the gene was mapped to a region on the short arm of chromosome 6 near the HLA locus *(15)*. The AP-2α protein binds to a consensus palindromic sequence, 5'-GCCNNNGGC-3', as a homodimer *(14,16)*, although a number of sites that are specifically footprinted by AP-2α have been shown to differ from this consensus sequence *(17)*. The DNA-binding domain is located within the C-terminal half of the 52-kDa protein and consists of two putative amphipathic α-helices separated by a 92-amino acid sequence that is both necessary and sufficient for homodimer formation *(18)*. Buettner's group *(19)* cloned an alternatively spliced AP-2α protein, AP-2αB, which differs in its C-terminus and acts as a dominant-negative to AP-2α.

Transcriptional activity of AP-2α as a positive or negative transcriptional regulator can be seen in its response to different signal-transducing agents. For example, phorbol esters and signals that enhance cyclic adenosine monophosphate levels induce AP-2α activity independently of protein synthesis, whereas retinoic acid treatment of teratocarcinoma cell lines transiently induces increase in AP-2α transcription *(17,20,21)*. Other signals demonstrated to stimulate AP-2α expression and activate transcription of target genes include ultraviolet-A radiation and singlet oxygen *(22–24)*.

AP-2α mediates programmed gene expression during both embryonic morphogenesis and adult cell differentiation. *In situ* hybridization has demonstrated a restricted spatial and temporal expression pattern during murine embryogenesis. In particular, regulated AP-2α expression appeared in neural crest-derived cell lineages (from which melanocytes are derived) and in facial and limb bud mesenchyme *(25)*. Two studies of AP-2α-null mutant mice demonstrated that AP-2α is important for development of the cranial region and for midline fusions; the AP-2α-null mice have multiple congenital defects and die at birth *(26,27)*. The identification of AP-2α target genes involved in development and differentiation remain under investigation. Numerous studies have identified AP-2α target genes that contain functional AP-2α-binding elements in the enhancer regions; these include viral genes, such as simian virus 40 (*SV40*) *(28,29)*; the human T-cell leukemia virus type I *(30)*; and such cellular genes as those for the murine major histocompatibility complex, *H-2Kb (31)*; human metallothionein-IIa, *huMTIIa (32)*; human proenkephalin *(33)*; and human keratin, *K14 (34)*.

AP-2α is a cell type-specific transcription factor expressed in neural crest- and ecto-derm-derived tissues, including craniofacial, skin, and urogenital tissues *(25–27)*. It has been implicated as a critical regulator of gene expression during mammalian develop-ment, differentiation, and carcinogenesis *(26,27,34,35)*. Loss of AP-2α has been impli-cated in the development and progression of many different types of cancers, including human melanoma, prostate, breast, and colorectal carcinomas. For example, immuno-fluorescent staining of malignant human prostate tissues indicated that loss of AP-2α expression occurs early in the development of prostate adenocarcinomas *(36)*. In clinical specimens of invasive breast cancer, a correlation between low AP-2α expression and disease progression was demonstrated, suggesting a tumor suppressor-like role for AP-2α *(37)*. In colorectal carcinoma, AP-2α expression correlates with p21/WAF1 expression and recurrence-free survival *(38)*. These observations indicate that AP-2α plays mul-tiple roles in both normal development and the development and progression of cancer.

ROLE OF AP-2α IN MELANOMA PROGRESSION

We have previously demonstrated that loss of AP-2 is an important molecular event in melanoma progression. The transition of melanoma cells from radial growth phase to vertical growth phase is associated with a loss of expression of AP-2α, which results in deregulation of AP-2 target genes involved in tumor growth and metastasis *(39)*. For example, loss of AP-2 expression in metastatic melanoma cells resulted in overexpression of the melanoma cell adhesion molecule (MCAM/MUC18) *(13)* and lack of expression of the tyrosine kinase receptor, c-KIT *(12)*. Increased expression of MUC18 allowed the metastatic cells to adhere to the endothelial cells in blood vessels and supported their migration to the metastatic site *(40)*, whereas low c-KIT expression rendered the cells resistant to apoptosis *(41)*. In addition, inactivation of AP-2 in AP-2-positive primary cutaneous melanoma cells by means of transfection with a dominant-negative *AP-2* gene (*AP-2B*) led to deregulation of the *matrix metalloproteinase-2* (*MMP-2*) gene *(11)*. Functional AP-2-binding elements have been identified in other genes involved in the progression of human melanoma, including *p21/WAF1 (42)*, intercellular adhesion molecule *(23)*, c-erbB-2/HER-2/neu *(43–45)*, plasminogen activator inhibitor type I *(46)*, insulin-like growth factor binding protein-5 *(47)*, transforming growth factor-α *(48)*, vascular endothelial growth factor *(22,49)*, E-cadherin *(50)*, and hepatocyte growth factor *(51)*.

Loss of AP-2α was also observed in clinical specimens of advanced primary and metastatic melanoma and was associated with malignant transformation and elevated risk of tumor progression; the loss of AP-2 expression correlated with low p21/WAF1, E-cadherin, and c-KIT expression and poor prognosis *(52,53)*, thus, supporting the hypothesis that loss of AP-2α is a crucial event in the progression and metastasis of melanoma. In this chapter, we summarize our recent data demonstrating an inverse correlation between the expression of AP-2α and the thrombin receptor (PAR-1), which correlates with the malignant phenotype of human melanoma.

ROLE AND REGULATION OF THE THROMBIN RECEPTOR (PAR-1) IN HUMAN MELANOMA

Seven-transmembrane G protein-coupled receptors compose the largest group of receptors in mammalian systems. A recently described novel subset of this group, the PARs, has been shown to have a unique mechanism of activation. PAR-1, the first PAR to be cloned *(54)*, is activated when the N-terminus is proteolytically cleaved by the serine protease, thrombin, irreversibly activating the receptor, thus, leading to downstream cell-signaling events that evoke a variety of cellular responses *(54,55)*. The pathway of cellular activation and induction of mitogenesis by thrombin is well characterized for fibroblasts and other cell types. PAR-1 can couple to members of the G12/13, Gq, and Gi families and, hence, to a host of intracellular effectors *(56)*. The interaction of PAR-1 with multiple G protein subunits allows for signaling via several transduction pathways, including increases in Ca^{2+} and activation of protein kinase C via second messengers, inositol 1,4,5-triphosphate, and diacylglycerol *(57)*; activation of mitogen-activated protein kinases *(55)*; activation of phosphoinositide-3 kinase *(58,59)*; and activation of Rho kinases *(60,61)*.

The thrombin receptor has recently been assigned a central role in tumorigenesis and metastasis *(62–64)*. Overexpression of PAR-1 has been detected in human carcinoma cell lines, including colon adenocarcinoma *(65)*, and laryngeal *(66)*, breast *(62,63)*, pancreatic *(67)*, and oral squamous cell carcinoma *(68)*. We have recently demonstrated that metastatic melanoma cells have increased expression of PAR-1 *(69)*. In human melanoma cells, thrombin acts as a growth factor, suggesting that signaling by PAR-1 is involved in the biological response of these cells, which likely involves downstream regulation of gene products contributing to their metastatic phenotype *(64,70,71)*. To that end, PAR-1 was reported to be a rate-limiting factor in thrombin-enhanced experimental pulmonary metastasis in a murine melanoma cell line, demonstrating a potential role of PAR-1 in the metastatic process of melanoma *(64)*. Activation of PAR-1 induces intracellular signaling molecules, such as Rho kinase, phosphoinositide-3 kinase, and mitogen-activated protein kinases, which have been shown to be involved in cell growth, tumor promotion, and carcinogenesis *(55,72)*. These signaling effector molecules can elicit a range of cellular responses and expression of thrombin-responsive genes. For example, some of these gene products are precisely those that would be required for angiogenesis and tumor invasion of melanoma, such as interleukin-8 *(73)*, vascular endothelial growth factor *(74)*, basic fibroblast growth factor *(75)*, platelet-derived growth factor *(76)*, MMP-2 *(77)*, and αvβ3 integrins *(78)*. Therefore, PAR-1 activation may facilitate angiogenesis, tumor invasion, and metastasis through the induction and stimulation of secreted angiogenic factors, matrix-degrading proteases, and expression of cell adhesion molecules.

Despite the extensive data regarding the cellular signaling pathways mediated by PAR-1, little is known about the regulatory mechanism of this receptor. The regulatory region of the *PAR-1* gene has been cloned, and DNA sequence analysis indicates the presence of binding sites for Ets, TEF-1, NF-E1, Octamer, AP-2-like elements, and multiple putative AP-2 and specificity protein (Sp)-1 regulatory elements (Fig. 1) *(79,80)*. Transcription factor sequence analysis indicates the presence of two complexes that contain highly overlapping binding motifs for the transcription factors AP-2 and Sp1 at the proximal 3' region of the PAR-1 promoter *(79)*. Overall, these complexes contain

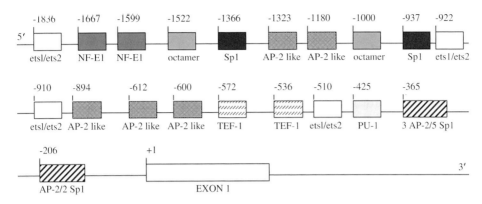

Fig. 1. Schematic summarizing the putative regulatory sequences within the protease-activated receptor (PAR)-1 promoter, including the 5' flanking sequence of the *PAR-1* gene and potential regulatory motifs. Overlapping activator protein-2 and specificity protein-1 binding motifs are noted with dashes. Translation start codon position is defined as +1, and the first base upstream of +1 is defined as −1.

four putative AP-2-binding elements and seven Sp1-binding elements, suggesting that these transcription factors likely mediate PAR-1 promoter activity. Furthermore, we found that the regulatory region of the thrombin receptor shares remarkable similarities with other AP-2 target genes, such as a G+C-rich sequence, lack of conventional TATA and CAAT sequences, and multiple AP-2-binding elements, which makes the PAR-1 gene a likely candidate for regulation by the transcription factor AP-2.

The cell lines in our investigation included primary and metastatic human melanoma cells with different tumorigenic and metastatic potentials in nude mice. Because the regulatory region of the *PAR-1* gene contains several putative AP-2 binding sites, a panel of AP-2-negative metastatic, and AP-2-positive nonmetastatic melanoma cell lines was surveyed for differential expression of PAR-1 (Fig. 2). To further investigate the contribution of AP-2 in human melanoma, we re-expressed AP-2 in the human metastatic melanoma cell line, WM266-4 (AP-2 C8, AP-2 C12A). We observed that the expression of PAR-1 was significantly lower in AP-2-positive than in AP-2-negative melanoma cell lines. The expression of the PAR-1 was significantly lower in cells transfected with the full-length *AP-2* gene construct, WM266-4-AP-2, than in the WM266-4 parental and control transfected cell line. These data demonstrate an inverse correlation between the expression of AP-2 and the expression of PAR-1 in human melanoma, and a correlation between the level of PAR-1 expression and the metastatic potential of human melanoma cell lines *(69)*. Our results suggest that loss of AP-2 results in an increase in the expression of the thrombin receptor in metastatic melanoma cells.

Although AP-2 generally serves as an activator of target gene expression, it has been shown to negatively regulate the transcription of several genes, including K3 keratin *(81)*, acetylcholinesterase *(82)*, C/EBPα *(83)*, and manganese superoxide dismutase *(84,85)*. In all of these studies, it was proposed that AP-2 functions as a repressor by inhibiting or competing with a transcriptional activator that has a binding motif that overlaps or is adjacent to the AP-2-binding site. Several lines of evidence indicate that AP-2 represses Sp1-dependent promoters through transcriptional steric interference with the general transcription machinery *(81)*. Sp1 was the first mammalian transcrip-

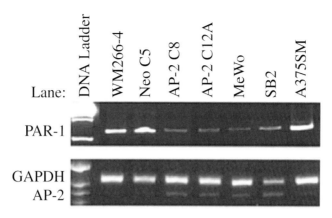

Fig. 2. Expression of activator protein (AP)-2 and protease-activated receptor (PAR)-1 in human melanoma cell lines. Reverse transcriptase-polymerase chain reaction analysis for the expression of PAR-1 and AP-2 in human melanoma cell lines. High levels of PAR-1 expression were observed in WM266-4, neotransfected (Neo C5), and A375SM cell lines, which expressed negligible levels of AP-2. AP-2-transfected C8 and C12A, MeWo, and SB2 melanoma cell lines expressed high levels of AP-2 and low levels of PAR-1.

tion factor to be cloned *(86)*. It binds to GC-rich elements, such as GC (GGGGGCGGGG) and GT (GGTGTGGGG) boxes *(87)*. Early studies indicated that Sp1 was responsible for recruiting TATA-binding protein and fixing the transcriptional start site at TATAA-less promoters *(88)*. These findings, together with the fact that GC/GT-rich sequences are found in promoters of many housekeeping genes, led to the widely held notions that Sp1 acts as a basal transcription factor and that these GC/GT-rich elements represent constitutive promoter elements that support basal transcription *(88)*. However, Sp1 was also shown to undergo extensive posttranslational modification by both glycosylation and phosphorylation, indicating that its activity was likely to be regulated *(89)*. Other mechanisms that mediate Sp1 transcriptional activity act in part through complex interactions with Sp-related proteins, other transcriptional activators, and members of the basal transcriptional complex *(90,91)*.

To further investigate the role of AP-2 and Sp1 in regulating the expression of PAR-1, we investigated whether these nuclear proteins were associated with the PAR-1 promoter in vivo, using the chromatin immunoprecipitation assay (Fig. 3). Chromatin fragments from cultured cells were immunoprecipitated with an antibody to either AP-2 or Sp1, and DNA from the immunoprecipitates was isolated. From this DNA, a 276-bp fragment of the PAR-1 promoter region was amplified by polymerase chain reaction. This region of the promoter contains two AP-2/Sp1 complexes with overlapping binding motifs for these transcription factors *(79)*. In AP-2-negative cell line (WM266-4), Sp1 was predominantly bound to the PAR-1 promoter. In contrast, in AP-2-positive cell line (WM266-4-AP-2 C8), 9- to 10-fold more AP-2 was bound to the same region of the promoter *(69)*. These data demonstrate that both AP-2 and Sp1 bind to the 3' regulatory region of the PAR-1 promoter in a mutually exclusive manner.

To determine which nuclear proteins were bound to the regulatory region, we performed electrophoretic mobility shift assays using wild-type and mutant oligonucleotide probes that corresponded to bp −365 to −329 (complex 1) and bp −206 to −180 (complex 2) of the 5' flanking sequence of the *PAR-1* gene *(79)*. Incubation of the

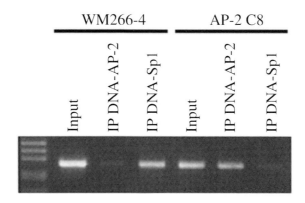

Fig. 3. ChIP assay to determine transcription factors binding to the protease-activated receptor (PAR)-1 promoter in vivo. Chromatin fragments from cultured cells were immunoprecipitated with an antibody to either activator protein (AP)-2 or specificity protein (Sp)-1, and a 276-bp fragment of the PAR-1 promoter region was amplified by polymerase chain reaction. This region containing complex 1 and complex 2 of the PAR-1 promoter demonstrated that in the AP-2-negative cell line, WM266-4, Sp1 was predominantly bound to the PAR-1 promoter. In contrast, in the AP-2–positive cell line, WM266-4-AP-2 C8, AP-2 was bound to the same region of the promoter.

radiolabeled complex 1 probe with nuclear extracts from AP-2-transfected melanoma cells (WM266-4-AP-2) cells demonstrated functional binding of AP-2, Sp1, and an Sp1 family member, Sp3, bound to overlapping motifs within complex 1 of the human PAR-1 promoter in a mutually exclusive manner *(69)*. In contrast, the formation of DNA–protein complexes with the sequence corresponding to complex 2 of the promoter did not involve AP-2 binding; however, Sp1 and Sp3 demonstrated functional binding to this region *(69)*.

To define the functional elements responsible for *PAR-1* gene regulation, we constructed a series of luciferase reporter plasmids containing serial 5' deletions. These plasmid constructs were transfected into a panel of melanoma cell lines that differentially express PAR-1 (Table 1). We observed that the promoter activity driven by the full-length promoter (–1400 bp to +1 bp, –1400/PAR1-Luc) reporter construct was increased in AP-2-negative cell lines and decreased in AP-2-positive cell lines *(69)*. Deletion of bp –1400 to –889, to create the –890 bp reporter construct (–890/PAR1-Luc) did not produce any marked differences in PAR-1 promoter activity, which implied that the elements in this region were not required for basal activity of the PAR-1 promoter. Further deletions of sequences from bp –890 to –499, which left intact the remaining 500-bp region of the promoter (–500/PAR1-Luc), doubled PAR-1 promoter activity in AP-2-negative cell lines, whereas only a minimal effect was observed in AP-2-positive cell lines. This indicated that this –500 bp to +1 bp segment of the promoter is driven by a strong transcriptional activator. Furthermore, this 500-bp region of the promoter contains both complex 1 (bp –365 to –329) and complex 2 (bp –206 to –180), implicating these regulatory motifs in the regulation of this gene. To further determine the effects of AP-2 and Sp1 on PAR-1 promoter activity, expression constructs containing cDNA encoding for AP-2 and Sp1 or an empty vector (pcDNA3.1-Neo) were transiently cotransfected with –500 bp to +1 bp reporter construct in WM266-4 and WM266-4-AP-2 cell lines. In comparison with the reporter construct cotransfected with pcDNA3.1-

Table 1
Deletion Analysis of PAR-1 Promoter in Human Melanoma Cell Lines

Plasmids	Cell lines (relative luciferase activity)				
	A375SM	WM266-4	AP-2 C8	SB2	MeWo
−1400/PAR1-Luc	0.580 ± 0.143	0.507 ± 0.186	0.189 ± 0.041	0.211 ± 0.075	0.222 ± 0.037
−890/PAR1-Luc	0.730 ± 0.090	0.764 ± 0.125	0.257 ± 0.083	0.264 ± 0.047	0.209 ± 0.067
−500/PAR1-Luc	1.334 ± 0.193	0.957 ± 0.078	0.517 ± 0.163	0.294 ± 0.120	0.207 ± 0.035

5' deletion of PAR-1 promoter luciferase reporter construct were transfected in A375SM, WM266-4, WM266-4-AP-2 C8, SB2, and MeWo cell lines. Constructs were cotransfected with pRL–β-actin to correct for transfection efficiency. Luciferase activity is expressed as relative luciferase units. Data shown are cumulative of three independent experiments performed in triplicate (means ± SEM).

Neo, transfection with the reporter construct and AP-2 markedly decreased reporter gene activity in WM266-4 cells and further decreased activity in WM266-4-AP-2 cells. In contrast, cotransfection of the reporter construct with Sp1 markedly increased promoter activity, by 2- to 2.5-fold. These results demonstrate that AP-2 functioned as a transcription repressor of PAR-1, whereas Sp1 was a strong transcriptional activator of PAR-1.

To ascertain the functional role of complex 1 in *PAR-1* gene regulation, we performed site-directed mutagenesis within the Sp1 and AP-2 sites. Mutant reporter constructs were transiently transfected into the WM266-4 and WM266-4-AP-2 melanoma cell lines, and their activity was compared with that of the −500 bp to +1 bp reporter construct, which contained the native PAR-1 promoter sequences. Disruption of complex 1 with 2-bp mutations at the distal and middle regions increased promoter activity in the WM266-4-AP-2 cells by 1.4-fold, but no changes in luciferase activity were observed in WM266-4 cells compared with the native reporter construct. Cotransfection of mutant reporter construct with AP-2 in WM266-4 and WM266-4-AP-2 cell lines had no effect on promoter activity. Transfection with Sp1 resulted in a twofold increase in luciferase activity. Similarly, 2-bp mutations in the middle and proximal regions of complex 1 decreased promoter activity by 0.5- to 2-fold in WM266-4 and WM266-4-AP-2 cell lines. Introduction of AP-2 had no effect on promoter activity, whereas Sp1 had a minimal increase in the promoter activity of luciferase. When 2-bp mutations were introduced in the distal and proximal region of complex 1, we observed a onefold to twofold increase in promoter activity in WM266-4 and WM266-4-AP-2 cell lines compared with native reporter construct. Transfection with AP-2 had little effect on promoter activity, whereas Sp1 transactivated the promoter construct. To our surprise, when 2-bp mutations were introduced simultaneously at the distal, middle, and proximal region of complex 1, promoter activity was abolished in WM266-4 and WM266-4-AP-2 cell lines, thus inhibiting the positive effect of Sp1 transactivation on complex 1.

The results of this targeted mutation analysis of the PAR-1 promoter, in conjunction with the deletion analysis and cotransfection with AP-2 and Sp1 expression plasmids, demonstrated that complex 1 was necessary for activation by Sp1 and repression by AP-2. Furthermore, when this region was significantly mutated, the promoter activity was lost, which suggests that complex 2 may have a minimal role in promoter activation.

Table 2
AP-2 and Sp1 DNA-Binding Activity in Human Melanoma Cell Lines

Plasmids	Cell lines				
	A375SM	WM266-4	AP-2 C8	SB2	MeWo
3xAP-2-Luc	0.605 ± 0.295	0.546 ± 0.176	1.489 ± 0.013	2.737 ± 0.176	3.359 ± 0.322
3xSp1-Luc	2.604 ± 0.355	2.424 ± 0.085	2.184 ± 0.120	1.876 ± 0.477	1.068 ± 0.141
AP-2:Sp1 ratio	0.232	0.225	0.681	1.458	3.145

Luciferase activity of 3xAP-2 and 3xSp1 reporter plasmids in A375SM, WM266-4, WM266-4-AP-2 C8, SB2, and MeWo cell lines. Constructs were cotransfected with pRL–β-actin to correct for transfection efficiency. Luciferase activity is expressed as relative luciferase units. The ratio of AP-2:Sp1 DNA-binding activity was determined from the relative luciferase activity of 3xAP-2 and 3xSp1. Data shown are cumulative of three independent experiments performed in triplicate (means ± SEM).

Our promoter analysis of the overlapping AP-2- and Sp1-binding motifs within the PAR-1 promoter suggests that AP-2 likely repressed expression of this gene by interfering with activated or basal transcription. Therefore, the levels of AP-2- and Sp1-DNA binding activity and expression in relation to the level of PAR-1 expression were examined by reporter assay and Western blot analysis (69). To determine the DNA-binding activity of AP-2 and Sp1, we performed luciferase reporter assays using either a reporter construct that contained three AP-2-binding sites (3xAP-2-Luc) or a vector that contained three Sp1-binding motifs (3xSp1-Luc) in a panel of human melanoma cell lines (Table 2). We demonstrated that AP-2-negative melanoma cell lines had significantly lower AP-2 binding activity than AP-2-positive melanoma cell lines. The AP-2-binding activity was 2.7-fold higher in WM266-4-AP-2 cell line than in the parental WM266-4 cell line.

Sp1 DNA-binding activity was similar in the AP-2-positive cell lines. The Sp1 activity was only slightly lower in SB2 cell line than in the A375SM and WM266-4 cell lines. However, we observed a marked decrease in Sp1 DNA-binding activity in the MeWo cell line. To calculate the ratio of AP-2 to Sp1 DNA-binding activity we used their relative luciferase activities. We determined that the AP-2-negative melanoma cell lines had a low AP-2:Sp1 ratio and the AP-2-positive melanoma cell lines had significantly higher ratios, of 3.1 and 1.4, respectively. The WM266-4-AP-2 cells, in which AP-2 activity has been restored, had a low AP-2:Sp1 ratio, which suggests that the balance of the transcriptional regulators determines the level of PAR-1 expression in melanoma cells.

Similarly, the AP-2:Sp1 ratio was determined by Western blot and densitometry analyses. The AP-2-negative melanoma cell lines had a low ratio. In contrast, the AP-2-positive melanoma cell lines had a high AP-2:Sp1 ratio and expressed minimal levels of PAR-1. The WM266-4-AP-2 cells displayed an increase in the ratio of AP-2:Sp1, which coincided with decreased PAR-1 expression. We conclude that the loss of AP-2 in melanoma cells resulted in a noticeable decrease in the ratio of AP-2:Sp1 and correlated with high expression levels of PAR-1. Furthermore, re-expression of AP-2 restored the ratio of AP-2 expression to Sp1 expression in melanoma cells and resulted in downregulation of PAR-1.

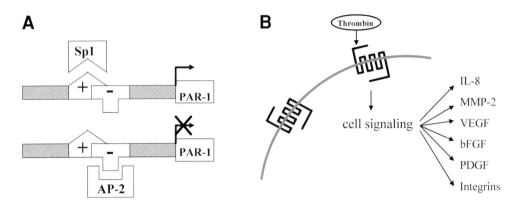

Fig. 4. Scheme showing how activation of protease-activated receptor-1 contributes to the acquisition of the metastatic phenotype in human melanoma.

CONCLUSIONS AND PERSPECTIVES

In our continued investigation of AP-2α, we identified *PAR-1* as an additional AP-2 target gene that can play an active role in melanoma progression *(92)*. Previously, we determined that *c-KIT (12)*, *MCAM/MUC18 (13)*, and *MMP-2 (11)* genes, all of which contribute to the malignant phenotype of human melanoma, are regulated by AP-2. The investigation described here offers evidence that loss of AP-2 increases expression of PAR-1 in metastatic human melanoma cells. We noted with special interest the presence of multiple AP-2 consensus sequences in the PAR-1 promoter. Analysis of the PAR-1 promoter region revealed putative binding sites for many sequence-specific transcription factors, including Sp1, which is ubiquitously expressed, and AP-2, which is a cell type-specific transcriptional regulator. Taken together, these observations point to a strong link between thrombin, its receptor, PAR-1, and the invasive properties of malignant melanoma. Figure 4 summarizes our view of how activation of PAR-1 contributes to the acquisition of the metastatic phenotype in human melanoma. Inhibitors of PAR-1-signaling cascade are now under investigation as potential modalities to inhibit tumor growth and metastasis of melanoma.

REFERENCES

1. Meier F, Satyamoorthy K, Nesbit M, et al. Molecular events in melanoma development and progression. Front Biosci 1998;3:D1005–D1010.
2. Jean D, Tellez C, Huang S, et al. Inhibition of tumor growth and metastasis of human melanoma by intracellular anti-ATF-1 single chain Fv fragment. Oncogene 2000;19(22):2721–2730.
3. Bohm M, Moellmann G, Cheng E, et al. Identification of p90RSK as the probable CREB-Ser133 kinase in human melanocytes. Cell Growth Differ 1995;6(3):291–302.
4. Xie S, Price JE, Luca M, Jean D, Ronai Z, Bar-Eli M. Dominant-negative CREB inhibits tumor growth and metastasis of human melanoma cells. Oncogene 1997;15(17):2069–2075.
5. Rutberg SE, Goldstein IM, Yang YM, Stackpole CW, Ronai Z. Expression and transcriptional activity of AP-1, CRE, and URE binding proteins in B16 mouse melanoma subclones. Mol Carcinog 1994;10(2):82–87.
6. Jean D, Harbison M, McConkey DJ, Ronai Z, Bar-Eli M. CREB and its associated proteins act as survival factors for human melanoma cells. J Biol Chem 1998;273(38):24,884–24,890.
7. Goding CR. Mitf from neural crest to melanoma: signal transduction and transcription in the melanocyte lineage. Genes Dev 2000;14(14):1712–1728.

8. King R, Weilbaecher KN, McGill G, Cooley E, Mihm M, Fisher DE. Microphthalmia transcription factor. A sensitive and specific melanocyte marker for melanoma diagnosis. Am J Pathol 1999;155(3):731–738.

9. Huang S, DeGuzman A, Bucana CD, Fidler IJ. Nuclear factor-kappaB activity correlates with growth, angiogenesis, and metastasis of human melanoma cells in nude mice. Clin Cancer Res 2000;6(6): 2573–2581.

10. Poser I, Dominguez D, de Herreros AG, Varnai A, Buettner R, Bosserhoff AK. Loss of E-cadherin expression in melanoma cells involves up-regulation of the transcriptional repressor Snail. J Biol Chem 2001;276(27):24,661–24,666.

11. Gershenwald JE, Sumner W, Calderone T, Wang Z, Huang S, Bar-Eli M. Dominant-negative transcription factor AP-2 augments SB-2 melanoma tumor growth in vivo. Oncogene 2001; 20(26):3363–3375.

12. Huang S, Jean D, Luca M, Tainsky MA, Bar-Eli M. Loss of AP-2 results in downregulation of c-KIT and enhancement of melanoma tumorigenicity and metastasis. EMBO J 1998;17(15):4358–4369.

13. Jean D, Gershenwald JE, Huang S, et al. Loss of AP-2 results in up-regulation of MCAM/MUC18 and an increase in tumor growth and metastasis of human melanoma cells. J Biol Chem 1998; 273(26):16,501–16,508.

14. Williams T, Admon A, Luscher B, Tjian R. Cloning and expression of AP-2, a cell-type-specific transcription factor that activates inducible enhancer elements. Genes Dev 1988;2(12A):1557–1569.

15. Gaynor RB, Muchardt C, Xia YR, et al. Localization of the gene for the DNA-binding protein AP-2 to human chromosome 6p22.3-pter. Genomics 1991;10(4):1100–1102.

16. Bauer R, Imhof A, Pscherer A, et al. The genomic structure of the human AP-2 transcription factor. Nucleic Acids Res 1994;22(8):1413–1420.

17. Imagawa M, Chiu R, Karin M. Transcription factor AP-2 mediates induction by two different signal-transduction pathways: protein kinase C and cAMP. Cell 1987;51(2):251–260.

18. Williams T, Tjian R. Characterization of a dimerization motif in AP-2 and its function in heterologous DNA-binding proteins. Science 1991;251(4997):1067–1071.

19. Buettner R, Kannan P, Imhof A, et al. An alternatively spliced mRNA from the AP-2 gene encodes a negative regulator of transcriptional activation by AP-2. Mol Cell Biol 1993;13(7):4174–4185.

20. Buettner R, Bauer R, Imhof A, Tainsky MA, Hofstaedter F. [AP-2: a nuclear effector of malignant transformation by ras oncogene]. Verh Dtsch Ges Pathol 1993;77:271–275.

21. Luscher B, Mitchell PJ, Williams T, Tjian R. Regulation of transcription factor AP-2 by the morphogen retinoic acid and by second messengers. Genes Dev 1989;3(10):1507–1517.

22. Gille J, Reisinger K, Asbe-Vollkopf A, Hardt-Weinelt K, Kaufmann R. Ultraviolet-A-induced transactivation of the vascular endothelial growth factor gene in HaCaT keratinocytes is conveyed by activator protein-2 transcription factor. J Invest Dermatol 2000;115(1):30–36.

23. Grether-Beck S, Olaizola-Horn S, Schmitt H, et al. Activation of transcription factor AP-2 mediates UVA radiation- and singlet oxygen-induced expression of the human intercellular adhesion molecule 1 gene. Proc Natl Acad Sci USA 1996;93(25):14,586–14,591.

24. Huang Y, Domann FE. Redox modulation of AP-2 DNA binding activity in vitro. Biochem Biophys Res Commun 1998;249(2):307–312.

25. Mitchell PJ, Timmons PM, Hebert JM, Rigby PW, Tjian R. Transcription factor AP-2 is expressed in neural crest cell lineages during mouse embryogenesis. Genes Dev 1991;5(1):105–119.

26. Schorle H, Meier P, Buchert M, Jaenisch R, Mitchell PJ. Transcription factor AP-2 essential for cranial closure and craniofacial development. Nature 1996;381(6579):235–238.

27. Zhang J, Hagopian-Donaldson S, Serbedzija G, et al. Neural tube, skeletal and body wall defects in mice lacking transcription factor AP-2. Nature 1996;381(6579):238–41.

28. Lee W, Haslinger A, Karin M, Tjian R. Activation of transcription by two factors that bind promoter and enhancer sequences of the human metallothionein gene and SV40. Nature 1987;325(6102): 368–372.

29. Mitchell PJ, Wang C, Tjian R. Positive and negative regulation of transcription in vitro: enhancer-binding protein AP-2 is inhibited by SV40 T antigen. Cell 1987;50(6):847–861.

30. Nyborg JK, Dynan WS. Interaction of cellular proteins with the human T-cell leukemia virus type I transcriptional control region. Purification of cellular proteins that bind the 21-base pair repeat elements. J Biol Chem 1990;265(14):8230–8236.

31. Kanno M, Fromental C, Staub A, Ruffenach F, Davidson I, Chambon P. The SV40 TC-II(kappa B) and the related H-2Kb enhansons exhibit different cell type specific and inducible proto-enhancer

activities, but the SV40 core sequence and the AP-2 binding site have no enhanson properties. EMBO J 1989;8(13):4205–4214.

32. Haslinger A, Karin M. Upstream promoter element of the human metallothionein-IIA gene can act like an enhancer element. Proc Natl Acad Sci USA 1985;82(24):8572–8576.

33. Hyman SE, Comb M, Pearlberg J, Goodman HM. An AP-2 element acts synergistically with the cyclic AMP- and phorbol ester-inducible enhancer of the human proenkephalin gene. Mol Cell Biol 1989;9(1):321–324.

34. Leask A, Byrne C, Fuchs E. Transcription factor AP2 and its role in epidermal-specific gene expression. Proc Natl Acad Sci USA 1991;88(18):7948–7952.

35. Nottoli T, Hagopian-Donaldson S, Zhang J, Perkins A, Williams T. AP-2-null cells disrupt morphogenesis of the eye, face, and limbs in chimeric mice. Proc Natl Acad Sci USA 1998;95(23): 13,714–13,719.

36. Ruiz M, Troncoso P, Bruns C, Bar-Eli M. Activator protein 2alpha transcription factor expression is associated with luminal differentiation and is lost in prostate cancer. Clin Cancer Res 2001;7(12): 4086–4095.

37. Gee JM, Robertson JF, Ellis IO, Nicholson RI, Hurst HC. Immunohistochemical analysis reveals a tumour suppressor-like role for the transcription factor AP-2 in invasive breast cancer. J Pathol 1999;189(4):514–520.

38. Ropponen KM, Kellokoski JK, Lipponen PK, et al. p22/WAF1 expression in human colorectal carcinoma: association with p53, transcription factor AP-2 and prognosis. Br J Cancer 1999; 81(1):133–140.

39. Bar-Eli M. Gene regulation in melanoma progression by the AP-2 transcription factor. Pigment Cell Res 2001;14(2):78–85.

40. Johnson JP, Bar-Eli M, Jansen B, Markhof E. Melanoma progression-associated glycoprotein MUC18/MCAM mediates homotypic cell adhesion through interaction with a heterophilic ligand. Int J Cancer 1997;73(5):769–774.

41. Huang S, Luca M, Gutman M, et al. Enforced c-KIT expression renders highly metastatic human melanoma cells susceptible to stem cell factor-induced apoptosis and inhibits their tumorigenic and metastatic potential. Oncogene 1996;13(11):2339–2347.

42. Zeng YX, Somasundaram K, El-Deiry WS. AP2 inhibits cancer cell growth and activates p21WAF1/CIP1 expression. Nat Genet 1997;15(1):78–82.

43. Bosher JM, Williams T, Hurst HC. The developmentally regulated transcription factor AP-2 is involved in c-erbB-2 overexpression in human mammary carcinoma. Proc Natl Acad Sci USA 1995;92(3):744–747.

44. Hollywood DP, Hurst HC. A novel transcription factor, OB2-1, is required for overexpression of the proto-oncogene c-erbB-2 in mammary tumour lines. EMBO J 1993;12(6):2369–2375.

45. Turner BC, Zhang J, Gumbs AA, et al. Expression of AP-2 transcription factors in human breast cancer correlates with the regulation of multiple growth factor signalling pathways. Cancer Res 1998;58(23): 5466–5472.

46. Descheemaeker KA, Wyns S, Nelles L, Auwerx J, Ny T, Collen D. Interaction of AP-1-, AP-2-, and Sp1-like proteins with two distinct sites in the upstream regulatory region of the plasminogen activator inhibitor-1 gene mediates the phorbol 12-myristate 13-acetate response. J Biol Chem 1992;267(21): 15,086–15,091.

47. Duan C, Clemmons DR. Transcription factor AP-2 regulates human insulin-like growth factor binding protein-5 gene expression. J Biol Chem 1995;270(42):24,844–24,851.

48. Wang D, Shin TH, Kudlow JE. Transcription factor AP-2 controls transcription of the human transforming growth factor-alpha gene. J Biol Chem 1997;272(22):14,244–14,250.

49. Gille J, Swerlick RA, Caughman SW. Transforming growth factor-alpha-induced transcriptional activation of the vascular permeability factor (VPF/VEGF) gene requires AP-2-dependent DNA binding and transactivation. EMBO J 1997;16(4):750–759.

50. Batsche E, Muchardt C, Behrens J, Hurst HC, Cremisi C. RB and c-Myc activate expression of the E-cadherin gene in epithelial cells through interaction with transcription factor AP-2. Mol Cell Biol 1998;18(7):3647–3658.

51. Jiang JG, DeFrances MC, Machen J, Johnson C, Zarnegar R. The repressive function of AP2 transcription factor on the hepatocyte growth factor gene promoter. Biochem Biophys Res Commun 2000;272(3):882–886.

52. Karjalainen JM, Kellokoski JK, Eskelinen MJ, Alhava EM, Kosma VM. Downregulation of transcription factor AP-2 predicts poor survival in stage I cutaneous malignant melanoma. J Clin Oncol 1998;16(11):3584–3591.

53. Baldi A, Santini D, Battista T, et al. Expression of AP-2 transcription factor and of its downstream target genes c-kit, E-cadherin and p21 in human cutaneous melanoma. J Cell Biochem 2001; 83(3):364–372.

54. Vu TK, Hung DT, Wheaton VI, Coughlin SR. Molecular cloning of a functional thrombin receptor reveals a novel proteolytic mechanism of receptor activation. Cell 1991;64(6):1057–1068.

55. Grand RJ, Turnell AS, Grabham PW. Cellular consequences of thrombin-receptor activation. Biochem J 1996;313(Pt 2):353–368.

56. Coughlin SR. Thrombin signalling and protease-activated receptors. Nature 2000;407(6801): 258–264.

57. Vouret-Craviari V, Van Obberghen-Schilling E, Rasmussen UB, Pavirani A, Lecocq JP, Pouyssegur J. Synthetic alpha-thrombin receptor peptides activate G protein-coupled signaling pathways but are unable to induce mitogenesis. Mol Biol Cell 1992;3(1):95–102.

58. Mitchell CA, Jefferson AB, Bejeck BE, Brugge JS, Deuel TF, Majerus PW. Thrombin-stimulated immunoprecipitation of phosphatidylinositol 3-kinase from human platelets. Proc Natl Acad Sci USA 1990;87(23):9396–9400.

59. Walker TR, Moore SM, Lawson MF, Panettieri RA Jr, Chilvers ER. Platelet-derived growth factor-BB and thrombin activate phosphoinositide 3-kinase and protein kinase B: role in mediating airway smooth muscle proliferation. Mol Pharmacol 1998;54(6):1007–1015.

60. Seasholtz TM, Majumdar M, Kaplan DD, Brown JH. Rho and Rho kinase mediate thrombin-stimulated vascular smooth muscle cell DNA synthesis and migration. Circ Res 1999;84(10):1186–1193.

61. Carbajal JM, Gratrix ML, Yu CH, Schaeffer RC Jr. ROCK mediates thrombin's endothelial barrier dysfunction. Am J Physiol Cell Physiol 2000;279(1):C195–204.

62. Even-Ram S, Uziely B, Cohen P, et al. Thrombin receptor overexpression in malignant and physiological invasion processes. Nat Med 1998;4(8):909–914.

63. Henrikson KP, Salazar SL, Fenton JW 2nd, Pentecost BT. Role of thrombin receptor in breast cancer invasiveness. Br J Cancer 1999;79(3-4):401–406.

64. Nierodzik ML, Chen K, Takeshita K, et al. Protease-activated receptor 1 (PAR-1) is required and rate-limiting for thrombin-enhanced experimental pulmonary metastasis. Blood 1998;92(10):3694–3700.

65. Wojtukiewicz MZ, Tang DG, Ben-Josef E, Renaud C, Walz DA, Honn KV. Solid tumor cells express functional "tethered ligand" thrombin receptor. Cancer Res 1995;55(3):698–704.

66. Kaufmann R, Schafberg H, Rudroff C, Nowak G. Thrombin receptor activation results in calcium signaling and protein kinase C-dependent stimulation of DNA synthesis in HEp-2g laryngeal carcinoma cells. Cancer 1997;80(11):2068–2074.

67. Rudroff C, Schafberg H, Nowak G, Weinel R, Scheele J, Kaufmann R. Characterization of functional thrombin receptors in human pancreatic tumor cells (MIA PACA-2). Pancreas 1998;16(2):189–194.

68. Liu Y, Gilcrease MZ, Henderson Y, Yuan XH, Clayman GL, Chen Z. Expression of protease-activated receptor 1 in oral squamous cell carcinoma. Cancer Lett 2001;169(2):173–180.

69. Tellez C, McCarty M, Ruiz M, Bar-Eli M. Loss of activator protein-2alpha results in overexpression of protease-activated receptor-1 and correlates with the malignant phenotype of human melanoma. J Biol Chem 2003;278(47):46,632–46,642.

70. Fischer EG, Ruf W, Mueller BM. Tissue factor-initiated thrombin generation activates the signaling thrombin receptor on malignant melanoma cells. Cancer Res 1995;55(8):1629–1632.

71. Wojtukiewicz MZ, Tang DG, Nelson KK, Walz DA, Diglio CA, Honn KV. Thrombin enhances tumor cell adhesive and metastatic properties via increased alpha IIb beta 3 expression on the cell surface. Thromb Res 1992;68(3):233–245.

72. Macfarlane SR, Seatter MJ, Kanke T, Hunter GD, Plevin R. Proteinase-activated receptors. Pharmacol Rev 2001;53(2):245–282.

73. Ueno A, Murakami K, Yamanouchi K, Watanabe M, Kondo T. Thrombin stimulates production of interleukin-8 in human umbilical vein endothelial cells. Immunology 1996;88(1):76–81.

74. Huang YQ, Li JJ, Hu L, Lee M, Karpatkin S. Thrombin induces increased expression and secretion of VEGF from human FS4 fibroblasts, DU145 prostate cells and CHRF megakaryocytes. Thromb Haemost 2001;86(4):1094–1098.

75. Cucina A, Borrelli V, Di Carlo A, et al. Thrombin induces production of growth factors from aortic smooth muscle cells. J Surg Res 1999;82(1):61–66.

76. Shimizu S, Gabazza EC, Hayashi T, Ido M, Adachi Y, Suzuki K. Thrombin stimulates the expression of PDGF in lung epithelial cells. Am J Physiol Lung Cell Mol Physiol 2000;279(3):L503–L510.
77. Zucker S, Conner C, DiMassmo BI, et al. Thrombin induces the activation of progelatinase A in vascular endothelial cells. Physiologic regulation of angiogenesis. J Biol Chem 1995;270(40): 23,730–23,738.
78. Even-Ram SC, Maoz M, Pokroy E, et al. Tumor cell invasion is promoted by activation of protease activated receptor-1 in cooperation with the alpha vbeta 5 integrin. J Biol Chem 2001;276(14): 10,952–10,962.
79. Li F, Baykal D, Horaist C, et al. Cloning and identification of regulatory sequences of the human thrombin receptor gene. J Biol Chem 1996;271(42):26,320–26,328.
80. Schmidt VA, Vitale E, Bahou WF. Genomic cloning and characterization of the human thrombin receptor gene. Structural similarity to the proteinase activated receptor-2 gene. J Biol Chem 1996;271(16):9307–9312.
81. Chen TT, Wu RL, Castro-Munozledo F, Sun TT. Regulation of K3 keratin gene transcription by Sp1 and AP-2 in differentiating rabbit corneal epithelial cells. Mol Cell Biol 1997;17(6):3056–3064.
82. Getman DK, Mutero A, Inoue K, Taylor P. Transcription factor repression and activation of the human acetylcholinesterase gene. J Biol Chem 1995;270(40):23,511–23,519.
83. Jiang MS, Lane MD. Sequential repression and activation of the CCAAT enhancer-binding protein-alpha (C/EBPalpha) gene during adipogenesis. Proc Natl Acad Sci USA 2000;97(23):12,519–12,523.
84. Yeh CC, Wan XS, St Clair DK. Transcriptional regulation of the 5' proximal promoter of the human manganese superoxide dismutase gene. DNA Cell Biol 1998;17(11):921–930.
85. Zhu CH, Huang Y, Oberley LW, Domann FE. A family of AP-2 proteins down-regulate manganese superoxide dismutase expression. J Biol Chem 2001;276(17):14,407–14,413.
86. Kadonaga JT, Carner KR, Masiarz FR, Tjian R. Isolation of cDNA encoding transcription factor Sp1 and functional analysis of the DNA binding domain. Cell 1987;51(6):1079–1090.
87. Philipsen S, Suske G. A tale of three fingers: the family of mammalian Sp/XKLF transcription factors. Nucleic Acids Res 1999;27(15):2991–3000.
88. Black AR, Black JD, Azizkhan-Clifford J. Sp1 and kruppel-like factor family of transcription factors in cell growth regulation and cancer. J Cell Physiol 2001;188(2):143–160.
89. Suske G. The Sp-family of transcription factors. Gene 1999;238(2):291–300.
90. Pascal E, Tjian R. Different activation domains of Sp1 govern formation of multimers and mediate transcriptional synergism. Genes Dev 1991;5(9):1646–1656.
91. Su W, Jackson S, Tjian R, Echols H. DNA looping between sites for transcriptional activation: self-association of DNA-bound Sp1. Genes Dev 1991;5(5):820–826.
92. Tellez C, Bar-Eli M. Role and regulation of the thrombin receptor (PAR-1) in human melanoma. Oncogene 2003;22(20):3130–3137.

28 Molecular Mechanisms of Melanoma Metastasis

Mohammed Kashani-Sabet

Contents

Summary

The recent development of powerful and efficient systemic gene delivery techniques has allowed the identification of a number of genes and pathways critical to the progression of melanoma in murine models. Using this approach, the nuclear factor-κB (NF-κB)-signaling pathway has been identified as playing an important role in the metastatic progression of melanoma. Moreover, recent prognostic analyses using a large cohort of patients from the University of California at San Francisco Melanoma Center database have identified interactions between tumor cells and the tumor vasculature that play a dominant role in the survival associated with melanoma. Translational studies using tissue microarrays have identified expression of the p65 subunit of NF-κB to be tightly correlated with the development of tumor vascularity and vascular invasion. Finally, recent studies on tumor lymphangiogenesis have clarified the nature of the relevant vasculature in the progression of cutaneous melanoma. This chapter will discuss the recent understanding of the molecular mechanisms and pathways underlying the development of traditional and novel histological prognostic markers in melanoma.

Key Words: Melanoma; metastasis; ribozymes; vascularity.

INTRODUCTION

Malignant melanoma is a disease with an unpredictable clinical behavior. Although patients with thin tumors have an excellent 5-yr survival based on the most recent analysis performed by the American Joint Committee on Cancer (AJCC) staging system for melanoma *(1)*, a small but clinically important subset of these patients with thin

From: *From Melanocytes to Melanoma: The Progression to Malignancy*
Edited by: V. J. Hearing and S. P. L. Leong © Humana Press Inc., Totowa, NJ

tumors relapse and die as a result of their melanoma. Conversely, a substantial proportion of patients with thick tumors are free of metastasis. Thus, the development of prognostic markers that provide important prognostic information regarding the risk of relapse and death independent of the tumor thickness represents an important area of melanoma research. In addition, understanding the molecular basis of these pathological prognostic factors is crucial to the identification of molecular markers of melanoma outcome that may represent important targets for novel therapies for advanced melanoma.

BIOLOGY OF TUMOR METASTASIS

Based on recent prognostic analyses of melanoma, lymph node metastasis is well-recognized as one of the most important prognostic factors for predicting survival in patients with cutaneous melanoma *(1,2)*. The identification of the pathological events and underlying molecular factors that are crucial for the development of both lymph node and distant metastasis would improve our risk assessment of melanoma patients, resulting in potentially different algorithms for identifying patients who may benefit from sentinel lymph node dissection or systemic adjuvant therapies.

Recent studies in murine models have shed light on the biology of tumor metastasis. Metastasis is a highly complicated biological process that has been broken down into a number of different steps: detachment from the primary tumor, migration, invasion into lymphatic or blood vessels (intravasation), survival in the lymphatic or blood circulation, egress from the lymphatic or blood vessels (extravasation), angiogenesis, and cell proliferation *(3)*. Many of these steps require the interaction of the tumor cell with the extracellular matrix or with vascular endothelial cells. As a result, the identification of molecular factors that play a role in these interactions would greatly improve our understanding of steps crucial to the metastatic cascade. Intriguingly, recent studies have revealed that distal steps in the cascade (i.e., those following extravasation) are crucial to the development of clinically apparent metastases *(4)*. Thus, the important factors that result in the success or failure of tumor metastasis appear to occur at the level of metastatic progression. Although much of cancer research has been devoted to the identification of genes involved in tumor initiation (such as activating mutations in oncogenes and losses in tumor suppressor genes), until recently, little attention has been paid to the identification of genes that drive metastatic progression and the onset of lethal tumor metastasis. Understanding genes and pathways that promote the distal steps of the metastatic cascade may be important in the identification of novel targeted therapies for lethal melanoma metastasis.

SYSTEMIC GENE DELIVERY IN THE IDENTIFICATION
OF MELANOMA PROGRESSION GENES

Recent advances in gene delivery have demonstrated the utility of cationic liposome–DNA complexes (CLDCs) in the identification of genes and pathways crucial to the metastatic progression of melanoma. An extensive discussion of gene delivery is beyond the scope of this chapter; however, a brief review of systemic gene transfer techniques will be undertaken. For systemic gene therapy to be successful, the genetic construct of interest (comprising the complementary [c]DNA of a gene with tumor suppressor activity, or an anti-gene, such as antisense, ribozyme, or small interfering RNA [siRNA], targeting a tumor-promoting gene) must be delivered systemically and expressed effi-

results suggested that NF κB mediates its prometastatic effects in melanoma primarily through effects on tumor invasion, rather than through apoptosis, mitosis, or angiogenesis.

Additional studies have used CLDC-based delivery to identify the genes regulated by NF-κB that could mediate its effects on tumor invasion. Initial studies focused on integrin β3 and platelet endothelial cell-adhesion molecule-1, which form a ligand–receptor pair linked to cell adhesion and invasion (17), and are known to be regulated by NF-κB. Systemic administration of ribozymes targeting integrin β3 and platelet endothelial cell-adhesion molecule-1 also significantly suppressed the metastatic progression of B16 cells (15), suggesting that this ligand–receptor pair may help mediate the effects of NF-κB on tumor invasion and metastasis in tumor cells and/or vascular endothelial cells.

Subsequently, gene expression profiling was used to identify additional genes involved in NF-κB-mediated effects on tumor invasion. cDNA microarray analysis of the B16 clone stably expressing the anti-p65 ribozyme compared with the control transformant clone demonstrated the upregulation of FKBPr38, a previously uncharacterized member of the FK-506 binding protein (FKBP) gene family, in ribozyme-expressing cells. We then used systemic gene transfer to assign novel anti-invasive and antimetastatic functions to FKBPr38, and subsequently to FKBP12 (18). cDNA microarray analysis was then combined with FKBP gene transfer to show that FKBP gene expression coordinately induced the anti-invasive *syndecan-1* gene and suppressed the proinvasive *MMP-9* gene. Conversely, suppression of FKBP12 expression by anti-FKBP12 siRNA treatment significantly reduced cellular levels of syndecan-1 protein, whereas it increased matrix metalloproteinase (MMP)-9 levels and tumor invasiveness. Taken together, these studies have identified a network of adhesion- and matrix-remodeling genes that appear to be responsible for the ability of the NF-κB pathway to control tumor invasion and metastasis.

VASCULAR FACTORS IN THE PROGRESSION OF CUTANEOUS MELANOMA

Recent prognostic analyses from the University of California at San Francisco Melanoma Center database have identified novel histological prognostic factors that appear to play an important role in the progression of cutaneous melanoma. Our initial study (19) examined the role of vascular invasion as a prognostic marker. Vascular invasion is a known marker of poor outcome in a number of different malignancies, but has not been traditionally recognized as an independent marker of survival in melanoma. As a result, presence or absence of vascular invasion is not routinely recorded in most melanoma pathology reports. We examined the role of vascular invasion in a database of 526 patients with primary cutaneous melanoma who had 2 yr of follow-up or documented first relapse. In this data set, 78 patients were identified with two patterns of vascular involvement: definite vascular invasion, with melanoma cells identified within vascular spaces, and incipient vascular invasion, with tumor cells abutting the tumor vasculature, without evidence of definite invasion. The presence of either type of vascular involvement significantly increased the risk of relapse and death, and reduced the survival associated with melanoma. Intriguingly, vascular involvement increased the risk of both regional and distant metastasis. The impact of vascular involvement on these outcomes was similar to that of ulceration. Furthermore, the risk of metastasis and death from tumors exhibiting incipient invasion was as high as those exhibiting definite vascular invasion, suggesting the poor prognosis associated with this finding. By multivariate analysis, vascular involvement was an independent predictor of relapse-free and overall survival. There was no difference between the two patterns of vascular involvement with respect to overall relapse or death rate, and rate of regional nodal or distant metastasis. However, the relapse-free survival of cases with uncertain vascular invasion was significantly lower than those with definite invasion. This observation suggested that the group with incipient vascular invasion occupies an important earlier step in tumor progression.

In addition, we evaluated the impact of morphological patterns of tumor vascularity in the outcome associated with melanoma *(20)*. Four patterns of tumor vascularity were recorded: absent, sparse, moderate, and prominent. By univariate analysis, increasing tumor vascularity was associated with a significantly increased risk of relapse (consisting of both regional and distant metastasis) and death associated with melanoma. In addition, increased vascularity correlated with significantly reduced relapse-free and overall survival. By multivariate analysis, tumor vascularity was an independent predictor of relapse-free and overall survival. Intriguingly, the prevalence of ulceration increased with increased vascularity, such that ulceration was present in almost 50% of cases with the prominent pattern of tumor vascularity.

Finally, we analyzed the interactions between these vascular factors in the progression of cutaneous melanoma *(21)*. To begin with, Cox regression analysis of factors evaluated by the AJCC melanoma staging committee reproduced the powerful impact of tumor thickness and ulceration in the University of California at San Francisco data set, thereby establishing comparability between the two databases and analyses. Thus, when the six factors used by the AJCC were incorporated into the model, tumor thickness and ulceration emerged as the most powerful prognostic factors, with risk ratios strikingly similar to those demonstrated by the AJCC analysis. Intriguingly, when vascular involvement and tumor vascularity were added to the model, they emerged as the most powerful predictors of melanoma survival by multivariate analysis *(21)*. With the inclusion of these two factors in the model, ulceration was no longer an independent predictor of overall survival. Finally, increasing tumor vascularity was shown to predispose to the development of vascular invasion, and the presence of both of these factors increased the prevalence of ulceration. These results suggested that melanomas invade more commonly into newly formed vessels than pre-existing ones, and that ulceration may reflect the interactions between the tumor and the tumor vasculature, as evidenced by tumor vascularity and vascular involvement.

Based on these observations, we have developed a model of melanoma progression that takes into account the dominant role played by these vascular factors in the progression of cutaneous melanoma and in the development of ulceration, which has now been incorporated into the AJCC staging classification for melanoma *(1)*. In this model, tumor vascularity represents the initial vascular factor that is necessary for the development of melanoma metastases. The presence of increased vascularity increases the likelihood (and potentially enables the development) of both vascular invasion and ulceration. Although tumors can metastasize with the presence of increased tumor vascularity alone, the presence of either vascular invasion or ulceration (or both) greatly increases the likelihood of metastatic spread.

MOLECULAR ANALYSIS OF THE TUMOR VASCULATURE IN PRIMARY MELANOMA

Given the powerful role played by these vascular pathways in melanoma progression, determining the molecular events that underlie the development of these factors would potentially result in the identification of novel molecular prognostic factors for melanoma. It is intriguing to note that melanoma cell invasiveness was the dominant mechanism identified by our gene targeting studies in mice, as well as the dominant prognostic factor in patients with cutaneous melanoma. Thus, we hypothesized that the NF-κB pathway, which drove tumor metastasis in murine models by virtue of effects on tumor invasion, could also be involved in mediating the development of tumor invasiveness in human melanoma specimens. To examine this possible association further, we performed a matched-pair analysis of human primary melanomas using tissue microarray technology. We identified 24 cases with documented vascular involvement and increased tumor vascularity and 24 controls with no vascular involvement and limited tumor vascularity but matched for a number of other known melanoma prognostic factors, including tumor thickness, gender, age, anatomical location, histogenetic subtype, and Clark level. The pairs were not matched for ulceration, given that the presence of vascular factors would automatically create an imbalance in the presence of ulceration. Immunohistochemical assay of the tissue array with an antibody targeting NF-κB/p65 showed higher levels of p65 protein in 17 cases with vascular factors present. In addition, the cases more commonly expressed higher levels of p65 expression than the controls *(21)*. These results suggested a correlation between elevated expression of NF-κB/p65 and the presence of increased tumor vascularity and vascular involvement in human melanoma tissues. Given the powerful impact of these histological prognostic factors on melanoma survival, these studies also suggest that NF-κB may serve as a molecular marker of melanoma outcome.

With the important role of NF-κB in melanoma progression, the identification of downstream genes that may mediate the development of tumor vascularity would be of great interest. In this regard, recent studies examining the role of lymphangiogenesis in melanoma progression have yielded significant insights into the nature of the relevant tumor vasculature in melanoma. These studies have identified vascular endothelial growth factor (VEGF)-C and VEGF-D as potent lymphangiogenic agents, and lymphatic endothelial hyaluronan receptor-1 as a specific marker for lymphatic vessels *(22)*. Dadras et al. *(23)* used lymphatic endothelial hyaluronan receptor-1 immunohistochemistry on primary melanoma specimens to examine the correlation of lymphatic vessel density and melanoma metastasis to the regional lymph nodes. In a matched-pair study of 18 melanoma patients with lymph node metastasis and 19 patients without metastasis, a significantly higher number of intratumoral lymphatic vessels and a significant increase in peritumoral lymphatic vascular area was observed in metastatic vs nonmetastatic primary melanomas. In contrast, there was no difference in the blood vessel density (as determined by CD31 immunohistochemistry) between the matched pairs. By multivariate analysis, only peritumoral lymphatic vascular area was found to be an independent predictor of lymph node metastasis. Increasing lymphatic density was also associated with significantly reduced disease-free and overall survival. These results suggest lymphangiogenesis as a novel molecular prognostic marker for melanoma. The further identification of relevant lymphangiogenic factors in melanoma would be of great interest. In this regard, it is intriguing to note that one candidate lymphangiogenic factor, VEGF-C, has been shown to be regulated by NF-κB *(24)*, thereby further implicating the NF-κB pathway in the development of increased tumor vascularity by virtue of promoting lymphangiogenesis in primary cutaneous melanoma.

CONCLUSIONS AND PERSPECTIVES

In conclusion, recent studies have demonstrated the dominant impact of interactions between melanoma cells and the tumor vasculature in the progression of melanoma. As a result, tumor vascularity, vascular involvement, and tumor lymphangiogenesis have emerged as powerful prognostic factors for melanoma. These studies have clarified the contribution of lymphatic vs blood vessels in the metastatic cascade of primary melanoma. These studies have also shown that coordinate regulation of the NF-κB-signaling pathway plays an important role in mediating these effects, resulting in the lethal metastasis of melanoma.

REFERENCES

1. Balch CM, Buzaid AC, Soong SJ, et al. Final version of the American Joint Committee on Cancer staging system for cutaneous melanoma. J Clin Oncol 2001;19:3635–3648.
2. Gershenwald JE, Thompson W, Mansfield PF, et al. Multi-institutional melanoma lymphatic mapping experience: the prognostic value of sentinel lymph node status in 612 stage I or II melanoma patients. J Clin Oncol 1999;17:976–983.
3. Pantel K, Brakenhoff RH. Dissecting the metastatic cascade. Nat Rev Cancer 2004;4:448–456.
4. Chambers AF, Groom AC, MacDonald IC. Dissemination and growth of cancer cells in metastatic sites. Nature Rev Cancer 2002;2:563–572.
5. Sandrin V, Russell SJ, Cossett FL. Targeting retroviral and lentiviral vectors. Curr Top Microbiol Immunol 2003;281:137–178.
6. Imperiale MJ, Kochaneck S. Adenovirus vectors: biology, design, and production. Curr Top Microbiol Immunol 2004;273:335–357.
7. Liu Y, Fong S, Debs RJ. Cationic liposome-mediated gene delivery in vivo. Methods Enzymol 2003;373:536–550.
8. Tu G, Kirchmaier AL, Liggitt D, et al. Non-replicating Epstein-Barr virus-based plasmids extend gene expression and can improve gene therapy in vivo. J Biol Chem 2000;275:30,408–30,416.
9. Liu Y, Thor A, Shtivelman E, et al. Systemic gene delivery expands the repertoire of effective anti-angiogenic agents. J Biol Chem 1999;274:13,338–13,344.
10. Bagheri S, Kashani-Sabet M. Ribozymes in the age of molecular therapeutics. Current Molecular Med 2004;4:489–506.
11. Scherer LJ, Rossi JJ. Approaches for the sequence-specific knockdown of mRNA. Nat Biotech 2003;21:1457–1465.
12. Kashani-Sabet M. Ribozyme therapeutics. J Invest Dermatol Symp Proc 2002;7:76–78.
13. Nosrati M, Li S, Bageri S, et al. Anti-tumor activity of systemically delivered ribozymes targeting murine telomerase RNA. Clin Cancer Res 2004;10:4983–4990.
14. Aggarwal BB. Nuclear factor-kappaB: the enemy within. Cancer Cell 2004;6:203–208.
15. Kashani-Sabet M, Liu Y, Fong S, et al. Identification of gene function and functional pathways by systemic plasmid-based ribozyme targeting in adult mice. Proc Natl Acad Sci USA 2002;99: 3878–3883.
16. Liu Y, Mounkes LC, Liggitt HD, et al. Factors influencing the efficiency of cationic liposome-mediated intravenous gene delivery. Nature Biotechnol 1997;15:167–173.
17. Piali L, Hammel P, Uherek C, et al. CD31/PECAM-1 is a ligand for alpha v beta 3 integrin involved in adhesion of leukocytes to endothelium. J Cell Biol 1995;130:451–460.
18. Fong S, Mounkes L, Liu Y, et al. Functional identification of distinct sets of anti-tumor activities mediated by the FKBP gene family. Proc Natl Acad Sci USA 2003;100:14,253–14,258.

19. Kashani-Sabet M, Sagebiel RW, Ferreira CM, Nosrati M, Miller JR 3rd. Vascular involvement in the prognosis of primary cutaneous melanoma. Arch Dermatol 2001;137:1169–1173.20. Kashani-Sabet M, Sagebiel RW, Ferreira CM, et al. Tumor vascularity in the prognostic assessment of primary cutaneous melanoma. J Clin Oncol 2002;20:1826–1831.

21. Kashani-Sabet M, Shaikh L, Miller JR 3rd, et al. NF-kappa B in the vascular progression of melanoma. J Clin Oncol 2004;22:617–623.

22. Banerji S, Ni J, Wang SX, et al. LYVE-1, a new homologue of the CD44 glycoprotein, is a lymph-specific receptor for hyaluronan. J Cell Biol 1999;144:789–801.

23. Dadras SS, Paul T, Bertoncini J, et al. Tumor lymphangiogenesis: a novel prognostic indicator for cutaneous melanoma metastasis and survival. Am J Pathol 2003;162:1951–1960.

24. Tsai PW, Shiah SG, Lin MT, et al. Up-regulation of vascular endothelial growth factor C in breast cancer cells by heregulin-beta 1. A critical role of p38/nuclear factor-kappa B signaling pathway. J Biol Chem 2003;278:5750–5759.

29 Overview of Tumor Progression in Melanoma

David E. Elder

Summary

radial

Primary melanomas may arise in precursor nevi, and may evolve through two stages, the ~~rapid~~ growth phase (RGP) and the vertical growth phase (VGP). The RGP may be *in situ* or microinvasive but is nontumorigenic, whereas the VGP is tumorigenic and/or mitogenic. The prognosis in RGP is excellent regardless of thickness or other variables, whereas the prognosis in VGP depends on multiple attributes, including thickness and ulceration, which are the major variables used in the currently standard American Joint Committee on Cancer prognostic model and staging system for melanoma. In addition, the mitotic rate and the presence of lymphocytic infiltrates within the VGP are powerful predictors of survival. In thin (i.e., good prognosis) melanomas, three simple variables—the presence of any dermal mitoses, the presence or absence of tumorigenicity, and the patient gender—can divide patients into groups at very low or quite high risk of metastatic disease. These clinical findings based on tumor progression can be used to generate biological hypotheses suitable for testing in basic science laboratories and in clinical trials.

Key Words: Tumor progression; melanoma; radial growth phase; vertical growth phase; melanocytic nevus; dysplastic nevus; tumorigenic; mitogenic; prognosis; diagnosis; histopathology.

INTRODUCTION

In this chapter, aspects of tumor progression in melanoma are reviewed, primarily from a historical perspective while also indicating areas of new discovery and potential for future research. Much of the new genetic progression information is covered in other chapters of this book. Topics to be considered here include the nature and significance of melanocytic nevi, of nontumorigenic and tumorigenic melanomas, and of metastatic melanoma. The term *tumor progression* was attributed by Leslie Foulds to Rous, who in 1935 described it as "the process whereby tumors go from bad to worse" *(1)*. Tumors do not, however, merely expand in space and time, but rather progress by a stepwise

From: *From Melanocytes to Melanoma: The Progression to Malignancy*
Edited by: V. J. Hearing and S. P. L. Leong © Humana Press Inc., Totowa, NJ

process. This stepwise progression is now believed to correlate with a sequential acquisition of genetic changes. These genetic changes are only recently beginning to be understood in melanoma. However, the morphology of the tumor progression stages has long been well described, although useful markers for the specific diagnosis of melanoma are few and nonspecific, as is also true in other tumors. These progression stages include common nevi, dysplastic nevi, *in situ* and microinvasive radial growth phase (RGP) melanoma, tumorigenic vertical growth phase (VGP) melanoma, and metastatic melanoma. Clark described the stages of tumor progression, which, according to him, include class I lesions, which are stable after a period of growth; class II lesions, which appear to proliferate inexorably yet lack competence for metastasis; and class III primary lesions, which are tumorigenic and have competence for metastasis *(2,3)*. The class I melanocytic lesions include common and congenital nevi, and dysplastic nevi. These have importance as markers of increased risk, and as simulants of melanoma. Although melanomas may arise in these nevi, which are therefore potential precursors, the risk of progression of individual nevi is low. The class II lesions represent the so-called RGP, or nontumorigenic phase of melanoma development. Melanomas in this stage are quite likely to progress to the next stage, VGP (a class III lesion), which is a lesion that is both tumorigenic and has competence for metastasis. Metastatic or secondary melanomas are also tumorigenic and have the capacity to give rise to tertiary metastases.

MELANOCYTIC NEVI
Nature and Significance of Melanocytic Nevi

Melanocytic nevi are benign neoplasms of melanocytes. Melanocytes are so-called "labile" cells, which normally reside in the epidermis just above the basement membrane, and are capable of cell division in response to appropriate stimuli, such as ultraviolet (UV) light or wound healing *(4–6)*. Melanocytes synthesize melanin pigment and transfer it to adjacent keratinocytes, a process that is modulated by UV irradiation *(7)*. Melanin pigment synthesis is under the control of several genes, including the melanocortin receptor (*MC1R*) and the Agouti-signaling protein (*ASP*) *(8)*. Melanocytes in a normal epidermis are not themselves conspicuously pigmented in light-skinned individuals.

In response to stimuli that are perhaps related to UV light exposure, nevi may arise from melanocytes. Nevi are localized proliferations of abnormal melanocytes, termed nevus cells, which are defined under "Common Acquired Melanocytic Nevi as Simulants of Melanoma." Epidemiologically, nevi share risk factors with melanoma, including a relationship with UV light exposure, especially in childhood, and a relationship with UV susceptibility *(9–13)*. There is also a familial tendency and other evidence consistent with a genetic background to susceptibility *(11,14)*.

Although the term *nevus* historically refers to a hamartomatous malformation in dermatology, melanocytic nevi are considered to be neoplasms. The unqualified term nevus in current usage typically refers to a melanocytic nevus. Clonality studies have generally, although not in every study, demonstrated that the lesions are clonal *(15–17)*. The so-called "common acquired nevi" first appear in childhood, usually beginning in the second year, and becoming most numerous in the second and third decades *(12,18)*. Thereafter, their numbers decline, either because the lesions senesce and disappear, and/ or, perhaps in part, because of cohort effects, with younger generations having a rising incidence of the lesions. However, new acquired nevi continue to appear, albeit at a reduced rate, in adulthood.

With some exceptions in the case of so-called "giant" congenital nevi, which have major cosmetic significance and may be precursors of melanomas, but are, fortunately, rare, melanocytic nevi are of importance only in relation to melanoma. Their significance may be discussed in terms of three main topics: as simulants of melanomas, as markers of individuals at increased risk for melanoma, and as potential precursors of melanomas. First, the morphology of the major types of nevi—common acquired melanocytic nevi and dysplastic nevi—will be discussed. This morphology is the basis of distinguishing nevi from melanomas, which is a daily problem in dermatology clinics and in dermatology and dermatopathology laboratories, because melanocytic nevi represent the major potential simulants from which melanomas need to be distinguished.

Common Acquired Melanocytic Nevi as Simulants of Melanoma

A newly evolving acquired melanocytic nevus, in a child or an adult, arises as a patch of hyperpigmentation in the skin, corresponding histologically to a junctional nevus, in which nests of nevus cells are present in the epidermis. Nevus cells, also often called nevomelanocytes, were defined by Whimster in terms of three essential differences from ordinary melanocytes (19). First, the cells tend to have rounded cell bodies rather than the more dendritic processes typical of melanocytes. Second, the nevus cells tend to retain pigment rather than transfer it to keratinocytes. Third, the nevus cells tend to lose the inhibition that appears to separate melanocytes from one another, forming rounded balls or "nests." These nests are perhaps the most uniformly observed feature that allows for recognition of a melanocytic nevus in histological sections. The formation of nests appears to correlate with changes in adhesion and communication between cells, although the molecular determinants of nevogenesis remain to be fully elucidated (20,21). As the lesions evolve, the junctional nests appear to descend into the dermis, although, in all likelihood, this appearance of dermal descent is actually caused by elevation of the epidermis as additional nests accrete onto the initial ones, to build up the lesion, much as a brick wall is constructed. A melanocytic nevus with lesional cells in the epidermis and in the dermis is termed a *compound nevus*. As time progresses, the junctional nests are lost, and the lesion is now a *dermal nevus*. With loss of nests in the epidermis, pigmentation, which is initially confined to the junctional nests and superficial dermal nests, gradually disappears. The lesions in adults therefore become flesh-colored or pink, rather than the tan or brown pigmented lesions more usual in children. Typical acquired melanocytic nevi are relatively small, usually less than 4–5 mm in diameter and rarely greater than 1 cm. They are symmetrical, uniformly colored, and have sharp discrete borders which are raised above the level of the skin in compound and dermal nevi.

Common acquired melanocytic nevi with the above features are usually readily distinguished from melanomas. However, there is a subset of melanomas that share morphological features with nevi, termed *nevoid melanomas (22–24)*. These melanomas may be relatively symmetrical, and they may be comprised of small nevoid melanocytes, rather than the larger more epithelioid or spindle-shaped melanocytes that comprise most melanomas. Clues to diagnosis include the presence of cytological atypia, albeit subtle, and the failure of the normal maturation that is seen from superficial to deep in nevi. In addition, at least a few mitotic figures are observed. This latter finding is only occasionally seen in benign nevi, including dysplastic nevi.

Dysplastic Melanocytic Nevi

Dysplastic nevi were recognized initially by Clark and Green in hereditary melanoma kindreds, and were presented in a national meeting in 1976 (25). They were initially named BK moles after the initial letters of the names of the first two kindreds. Another kindred was published by Lynch and colleagues, under the term familial atypical multiple mole melanoma syndrome (26,27). The Clark group later referred to these lesions as dysplastic nevi, recognizing the architectural and cytological abnormalities that characterize these lesions, and the analogy with other tumor systems mentioned in the next paragraph (28,29). The association of dysplastic nevi with hereditary melanoma was referred to as the dysplastic nevus syndrome. Initial observations suggested that the dysplastic nevi might be transmitted in an autosomal dominant fashion, but, later, more detailed studies ruled out this simple genetic model, so that it is best not to refer to this condition as if it were a simple genetic syndrome (30). There is, however, a characteristic constellation of findings in patients and their families affected by these lesions.

Dysplastic nevi are benign nevi in which there is architectural and cytological disorder by comparison with common acquired nevi and congenital nevi. The term *dysplasia* refers, as in other systems, to architectural, as well as to cytological features (28,29). For example, dysplasia in the cervix of the uterus is characterized by cytological atypia and occurs in metaplastic (architecturally abnormal) squamous epithelium, not in the native squamous or glandular epithelium. Similarly, dysplasia in Barrett's esophagus occurs in relation to metaplastic intestinal epithelium. Melanocytic dysplasia may develop *de novo*, or in association with a pre-existing nevus. *De novo* dysplasia represents a strictly junctional proliferation and is a variant of the junctional nevus. Melanocytic dysplasia may also be associated with dermal nevus cells, which typically are seen in the center of the lesion, creating a lesion with a papular "head" and adjacent flat "shoulders." The shoulder region is the junctional component of the nevus at the periphery of the dermal component and is the region in which the dysplasia is typically best seen. As in other tumor systems, the dysplasia apparently represents a relative failure of maturation, in this case of the junctional component, which fails to undergo the typical progression from junctional to compound nevus throughout the entire extent of the lesion. However, as with more banal nevi, the lesion retains a general tendency to symmetry, to limitation in size, and to growth stability after an initial period of growth in which the lesion is formed.

Dysplastic nevi are the most important potential simulants of melanoma, both clinically and histologically (29,31). Clinically, the lesions are characterized by slight to moderate enlargement compared with common nevi (5 mm or greater by definition, although not often much greater than 1 cm). They are entirely macular, or have a macular or flat periphery, which is ill-defined, "fuzzy," and nonpalpable. If there is a dermal component, this may be papular and is located in the center of the macular component, to produce a characteristic "fried egg" or "target" appearance. This may represent a phenomenon of tumor progression in which dysplasia develops at the periphery of a pre-existing dermal nevus, or, alternatively, the dermal nevus component may be comprised of dermal dysplastic nevus cells.

The advent of epiluminescence microscopy has provided additional criteria to assist with the distinction between dysplastic nevi and melanomas. Nevertheless, histology remains the gold standard for this distinction (32). Dysplastic nevi are characterized histologically by architectural and cytological features (25,29,33–37) (Fig. 1).

The architectural features include the presence of nested and single melanocytes along the dermal–epidermal junction. These are located mainly along the tips and sides of elongated rete ridges, with some nests bridging between adjacent rete. In the dermis, there are stromal reactions, including concentric and sometimes lamellar fibroplasia. The latter appears to represent desmoplastic collagen produced by spindle-shaped lesional nevomelanocytes. In addition, there is a lymphocytic response characterized by

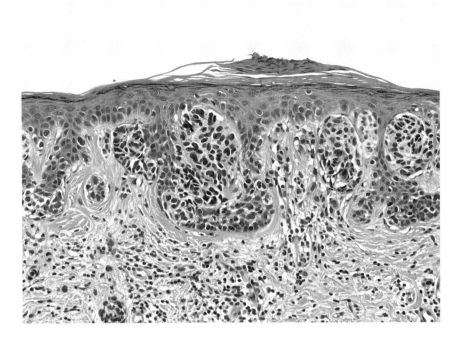

Fig. 1. Compound dysplastic nevus. There is an increased number of nevoid melanocytes arranged near the dermal–epidermal junction, predominantly in nests, predominantly near the tips and sides of the elongated rete ridges, with bridging of nests between adjacent the elongated rete ridges, and without continuous proliferation between the rete, or pagetoid extension of lesional cells into the epidermis. Cytologically, there is moderate to severe atypia characterized by enlargement, irregularity, and hyperchromatism of randomly scattered lesional cell nuclei—random cytological atypia.

patchy perivascular lymphocytes. Cytologically, there is nuclear atypia in the form of enlargement, slight irregularity, and sometimes nucleolation, of randomly scattered lesional cell nuclei. This is termed *random nuclear atypia*, to distinguish it from the more uniform atypia seen in melanomas (Fig. 1).

Significance of Nevi as Precursors of Melanoma

In most tumor systems, as reviewed by Foulds, the initial lesions of tumor progression are benign and self-limited *(1)*. Only a few of these lesions undertake the next step of a stepwise progression sequence that may ultimately lead to a fully developed cancer. In the melanocytic system, most nevi are symmetrical, well-circumscribed, or "well-made" benign lesions. The majority of these are stable, and, with time, many of them senesce and disappear. Only a few lesions undertake the next step *(38)*. In some cases, this represents the development of melanocytic dysplasia at the periphery of the nevus, whereas, in other cases, there may be direct progression to melanoma without an intervening step of dysplasia. In addition, melanoma may develop *de novo* without an antecedent nevus.

The evidence that nevi and the dysplastic nevi are potential precursors of melanoma is primarily histological and usually inferential, because the rarity of progression in nevi usually precludes direct observation. However, in pigmented lesion clinics, occasional examples of direct progression of a previously photographed nevus have anecdotally been observed. The usual finding is the appearance of a focal area of darker pigmentation developing within a pre-existing nevus. Although this finding is suspicious for melanoma, most nevi with small focal dark areas are not melanomas *(39)*. Because it is quite rare for a nevus to progress to melanoma, these lesion should be regarded as potential precursors rather than precursors of melanomas.

Paradoxically, because nevi are vastly more common than melanomas, it is quite rare for any given nevus to progress to melanoma, although it is common for a putative precursor nevus to be found in association with any given melanoma. Although this association provides putative evidence of a precursor relationship, it is also possible that this relationship could occur by chance. Recently, molecular studies have provided more direct evidence of a precursor relationship. Mutations in the mitogen-activated protein kinase pathway, either in the *BRAF* or *RAS* oncogenes, have been detected in melanomas, and the same mutation has also been found in a contiguous putative precursor nevus, indicating that the two parts of the lesion share a common biological genesis *(40,41)*.

Estimates of the frequency of melanoma in association with nevi have been derived from histological evidence of nevi in contiguity with melanomas. Large studies of the relationship between nevi and melanomas have been published *(42–48)*. In these studies, between 5 and 39% (median, 22%) of melanomas exhibited a contiguous dysplastic nevus and banal (dermal) nevic cells are present in an additional 10–21% (median, 15%) of cases. The incidence of a putative precursor nevus appears to be higher in relation to melanomas in high-risk populations, and to melanomas that are diagnosed in surveillance programs *(49,50)*. Gruber et al. *(47)* found that a precursor nevus was 22 times more frequent in relation to melanomas of superficial-spreading type compared with those of the lentigo maligna type. This supports the concept of the nevocytic and melanocytic pathways of melanoma pathogenesis proposed by Mishima *(51)*, and the histogenetic classification of melanoma proposed by Clark *(2,52,53)*. Molecular evidence for this distinction has been recently provided by Bastian *(54)*.

Based on these histological observations, it seems that dysplastic nevi are overrepresented as precursor lesions, and it is also possible that many lesions associated with a remnant dermal nevus component represent lesions whose junctional dysplastic component was overrun by the melanoma. In many instances, the dermal nevic component demonstrates so-called "congenital pattern features," namely descent of nevus cells into the reticular dermis and around or within skin appendages. This finding has led to considerations that small congenital nevi, like dysplastic nevi, may be overrepresented as precursors *(55,56)*. Nevertheless, simple calculations demonstrate that there are thousands of nevi or dysplastic nevi for every one of these lesions that progresses to a melanoma *(38)*. The low frequency of progression of these lesions suggests that they should not be managed as high-risk precursors. For example, population-based screening programs are not indicated to identify and excise dysplastic and small congenital nevi.

Significance of Clinically Dysplastic Nevi as Markers of Risk for Melanoma

The greatest significance of melanocytic nevi is as markers of individuals at increased risk for melanoma. Although nevi appear to be ubiquitous in human populations, the number and type of nevi correlate with melanoma risk. This has been demonstrated in multiple case control studies. These studies have shown that clinically dysplastic nevi are relatively common in the community, their incidence ranging in various studies from

Table 1
Relative Risk Estimates for Common and Dysplastic (Atypical) Nevi

	Study adjusted relative risks	
	Common Nevi	*Dysplastic Nevi*
Nordlund et al., 1985		
Australia *(62)*		7.7 (any atypical nevi)
Holly et al., 1987	4.4 (26–50 nevi)	3.8 (1–5 dysplastic nevi)
California *(60)*	6.2 (51–100 nevi)	6.3 (6+ dysplastic nevi)
Garbe et al., 1989	7.3 (41–60 nevi)	11.4 (1–2 atypical nevi)
Germany *(59)*	14.7 (>60 nevi)	6.0 (>2 atypical nevi)
Swerdlow et al., 1989	6.7 (>20 nevi)	2.1 (1–2 atypical nevi)
Glasgow *(61)*		4.4 (3+ atypical nevi)
Halpern et al., 1990	6.5 (>25 nevi)	6.8 (any dysplastic nevi)
Pennsylvania *(58)*		
Augustsson et al., 1991	1.4 (75–149 nevi)	2.5 (1–2 atypical nevi)
Stockholm *(57)*	3.9 (>149 nevi)	15.6 (>2 atypical nevi)
	4.6 (histological dysplasia)	
Tucker et al., 1997	1.8 (25–49 nevi)	2.3 (1 dysplastic nevus)
Pennsylvania,	3.0 (50–99 nevi)	7.3 (2–4 dysplastic nevi)
California *(31)*	3.4 (100+ nevi)	4.9 (5–9 dysplastic nevi)
	7.3 (10+ dysplastic nevi)	

5 to 20% (median, 13%) *(31,57–62)*. Other risk markers identified in case–control studies have included total number of nevi *(58,63,64)*; the presence and number of freckles *(65)*; the number of large nevi; a derivative of nevus number and size called total nevus density *(66,67)*; the quantitative history of sunburn *(68)*; and sometimes other markers of sun exposure or susceptibility.

In these studies, estimates of the frequency of nevi and dysplastic nevi in populations vary considerably according to geographic and genetic factors, as well as according to criteria for diagnosis, especially in the case of dysplastic nevi. Estimates of the frequency of common acquired nevi are also dependent on criteria. In some studies, lesions less than 2 mm in diameter were not counted, because of the difficulty of distinguishing among small junctional nevi, lentigines, and ephelids or freckles. In studies that included these lesions, the nevus counts are much higher. Therefore, comparability among different studies from different geographic regions and time periods is difficult. Similarly, with dysplastic nevi, criteria for diagnosis vary among studies. For example, some studies required a 4-mm size, whereas others required a 5-mm size cut off. Others required all of the diagnostic features mentioned on page 518. Yet other studies required only a subset of the diagnostic features. In a case–control format, these differences among studies are corrected for because the same criteria are applied to cases and controls. Table 1 provides relative risk estimates for common and dysplastic nevi, derived from several large case–control studies.

It is worth noting in Table 1 that the number of dysplastic nevi required to create a given relative risk is much smaller than the number of common nevi; however, common nevi are also risk factors for melanoma. The relative risk estimates are quite consistent among different geographic areas, and, unlike incidence rates, are not dependent on criteria. Several of the studies demonstrate a dose–response relationship between increasing numbers of nevi and increasing relative risk. The relative risks for dysplastic nevi tend to be higher, and associated with smaller numbers of lesions, i.e., dysplastic nevi are stronger than nondysplastic nevi as melanoma risk factors. The estimates in these studies are, in general, adjusted for most of the other important risk factors for melanoma—age, family history of melanoma, personal history of melanoma, evidence of chronic sun exposure in the form of freckles, skin sun-susceptibility type, and the history of acute (sunburn) and chronic exposure to the sun. The history of sun exposure appears to be most significant in childhood, but the significance of sun exposure persists into adult life. None of these studies has been well correlated, as yet, with genotype (e.g., *CDKN2A* or *MC1R* polymorphisms).

Significance of Histologically Dysplastic Nevi as Risk Markers for Melanoma

The risk estimates provided above are based on clinical diagnosis of nevi and dysplastic nevi. Case–control studies involving histological dysplasia are difficult to accomplish for two reasons. First, it is difficult to achieve compliance from controls in donation of nevus biopsies for research studies. Second, it is not reasonable to examine histologically all of the nevi on any one person's skin, so that a single nevus has to serve for the entire nevus phenotype. Therefore, only a few studies have attempted to correlate histological atypia with epidemiological risk. In one of these studies, slides were circulated among six observers from different institutions, from a unique set of nevi for melanoma cases, their relatives, and random population controls, collected by Larry Meyer of the University of Utah *(69)*. The six observers had no knowledge of case status or clinical diagnosis and made no attempt to adopt unified criteria. Although intraobserver reproducibility was substantial, interobserver reproducibility was fair as judged by κ-statistics, indicating that criteria differed among the observers but that they were applied consistently. Nevertheless, histological dysplasia, as defined variously by the observers, was associated with the clinical phenotype of total nevus number for all six observers, and with clinical atypia of the individual nevus for four of the observers. Except for one "outlier" observation of 32%, five of the six observers determined prevalence rates between 7 and 19%, similar to clinical estimates reviewed in "Significance of Clinically Dysplastic Nevi as Markers of Risk for Melanoma." The relative incidence of histological dysplasia in cases vs controls (an approximation of relative risk) was 1.3 to 3.6 for four of the six observers. The study therefore provides suggestive evidence that histological dysplasia is associated with melanoma risk.

In a formal case–control study from Sweden, Augustsson et al. *(57)* reported a relative risk estimate of 4.6 for histological dysplasia as a risk marker for melanoma, using pattern criteria in which cytological atypia was not an explicit criterion and was considered to be rarely seen. This relative risk is in the same range as in the clinical studies reviewed above that have established clinically atypical nevi as generally accepted risk markers for melanoma. It is of considerable interest that pattern histological features (judged by observers who do not consider cytological atypia to be a criterion) appear to be associated with risk in the Scandinavian data *(57)*, as well as in the Utah data *(69)* (not shown in Table 1).

In an important recent study, McNutt and colleagues have addressed the relationship of histological dysplasia and melanoma, using criteria that include both architectural and cytological features, nevi with architectural disorder and cytological atypia (NAD). From a total of 20,275 nevi retrospectively reviewed, 6275 were diagnosed as NAD (also known as dysplastic nevi), which were present in 4481 patients. These patients were divided into those whose worst NAD was mild (2504), moderate (1657), or severe (320). A personal history of melanoma was present in 5.7% of patients with mild, 8.1% with moderate, and 19.7% with severe atypia. The odds ratio for the association of NAD and a history of melanoma was 4.08 for NAD-severe vs NAD-mild, 2.81 for NAD-severe vs NAD-moderate, and 1.45 for NAD-moderate vs NAD-mild. Because of the study design, the relative risk for nevi with no atypia vs nevi with atypia could not be determined. These data were interpreted by the authors to show that the probability of a personal history of melanoma correlates with the architectural and cytological grade in a nevus biopsy submitted for clinical purposes, and that the risk of melanoma is greater for individuals who tend to make nevi with high-grade histological atypia *(70)*.

Taken together, these studies suggest that histological dysplasia appears to be quite strongly associated with melanoma risk status, but it is not yet known whether this effect is independent of clinical atypia. The recent studies of Arumia-Uria have resolved an important question by demonstrating that risk is associated with increasing degrees of cytological and architectural atypia of nevi *(70)*. The relative contribution of architectural and cytological features remains to be dissected. The clinical cohort and case–control studies reviewed beginning on page 520 confirm the predictive value of clinical morphology originally described in the context of dysplastic nevi in hereditary kindreds. These considerations suggest that the clinical morphology should at present be considered the gold standard for assessment of risk based on analysis of nevi. Future studies will determine with more precision whether the association of histological dysplasia with melanoma risk is independent of clinical atypia, and whether this association can be strengthened by paying more attention to cytological atypia.

TUMOR PROGRESSION IN MALIGNANT MELANOMA

Salient Diagnostic Features of Melanomas

Whether it arises in a pre-existing nevus or not, melanoma arises in most instances by a process of stepwise tumor progression. In their earliest stage, most melanomas arise in the epidermis as a proliferation of neoplastic melanocytes. Some exceptions occur, but these are outside the mainstream of tumor progression in melanoma. This intra-epidermal proliferation in melanoma differs from that of junctional nevi in terms of architecture and cytology. Architecturally, melanomas are characterized primarily by a greater cell density compared with nevi. This is expressed in the diagnostic descriptions of contiguous or confluent proliferation. In addition, melanoma cells compared with nevus cells tend to lose their tendency to form nests, being present along the dermal–epidermal junction as single cells in what is termed a *lentiginous pattern*, and they lose their tendency to be anchored to the basement membrane, leading to extension up into the epidermis in what is termed a *pagetoid pattern* (Fig. 2).

The terms *contiguous proliferation*, *lentiginous proliferation*, and *pagetoid proliferation* describe the salient architectural features of most melanomas in the epidermis.

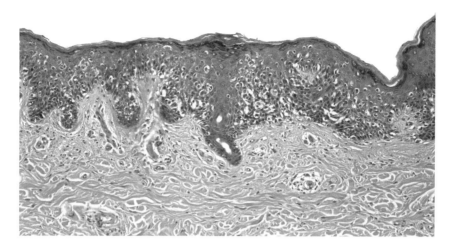

Fig. 2. Melanoma *in situ*, pagetoid pattern (superficial spreading melanoma). There is "buckshot scatter" of uniformly to moderately atypical epithelioid melanocytes in the epidermis. These have abundant cytoplasm with retraction artifact that readily distinguishes them from the surrounding keratinocytes. The basement membrane is intact in this example, with no evidence of invasion of the dermis.

Cytologically, melanomas in the epidermis or in the dermis are characterized by uniform cytological atypia, which is atypia that is observable in a majority of the lesional cells, rather than a minority of them, as in dysplastic nevi. Melanomas in the dermis are uniformly atypical and may be present in the form of single cells or small groups (nontumorigenic melanomas), or may form a focal mass lesion (tumorigenic melanoma).

In Situ *and Microinvasive Radial Growth Phase Melanoma*

A melanoma that is confined to the epidermis is known as "melanoma *in situ*" (MIS). In such a lesion, the proliferation is entirely above the basement membrane, and lesional cells do not enter into contact with dermal stroma, vasculature, or lymphocytes. As in nevi, however, the cells of MIS appear to have an innate tendency to migrate downward into the dermis. Whether this is termed invasion or not, depends on one's perspective. The same phenomenon in a junctional nevus is usually termed *migration*. As in nevi, the lesional cells may not travel very far in space as they move from the epidermis to the dermis. Indeed, the epidermis may become raised above the lesional cells that have just separated from it, forming a plaque-like, slightly raised lesion clinically, although histologically the dermal melanoma cells remain close to the region of the former basement membrane. This has been demonstrated by the finding of type VII collagen, a basement membrane-associated protein, in relation to invasive cells that appear to lie in the deep papillary dermis *(71)*.

Melanomas that have entered the dermis are traditionally called "invasive," whatever the biology of this process. However, this invasion, taken alone, does not appear to be the key step establishing competence for metastasis. One or both of two properties appears to be necessary for competence for metastasis to be established. These are tumorigenicity, and mitotic activity or "mitogenicity." The prognosis of melanomas that lack these two properties does not differ from that of MIS *(72,73)*. Although MIS is often considered to be associated with a 100% probability of survival, anecdotal observations and a few small cohort studies suggest that there is an approx 1% risk of metastasis in association with these lesions *(74)*, probably because a small invasive component was missed either because of sampling error or regression. The same is true for invasive melanomas that lack tumorigenicity and mitotic activity *(72,73)*. Taken together, nontumorigenic and nonmitotic melanomas (either *in situ* or invasive) have been termed radial growth phase (RGP) melanomas. This is a clinical term that was originally proposed by the late Scott Blois *(2)*. The term is intended to describe the clinical evolution of lesions along the radii of a more or less imperfect circle in the skin. Histologically, translated into the two dimensions of a microscopic slide, the RGP appears linear and has often been termed, in consequence, the horizontal growth phase by pathologists. Alternatively, these lesions can be more specifically described as either *in situ*, or microinvasive, a term that, by definition, implies lack of tumorigenicity and lack of mitogenicity.

Tumorigenic and Mitogenic Vertical Growth Phase Melanoma

The next step of progression, in a melanoma that has entered the dermis, is from the RGP to the vertical growth phase (VGP). In a recent study, point mutations in the *n-Ras* oncogene were present in both the RGP and the VGP of the same lesion, indicative of clonal progression between the two growth phases *(41)*. The critical biological feature that distinguishes VGP from RGP is the capacity for proliferation of melanoma cells in the dermis to form an expansile mass. In contrast, RGP melanoma cells have the capacity to proliferate more or less inexorably in the epidermal compartment, but not in the dermis. This concept of VGP is based on the concept that cell proliferation in a matrix of a distant site is essential to the development of a clinical metastasis, and that a tumor that lacks the capacity to proliferate in the matrix at its local site of origin is not likely to have this capacity in a distant site either.

Definition of VGP

The definition of VGP depends on the presence of either or both of the properties of tumorigenicity and mitogenicity, either of which is an expression of the capacity of the lesional cells to proliferate in the matrix at the local site, as follows *(75,76)*:

> Tumorigenic: A mass of melanoma cells is present in the dermis that contains at least one cluster (nest) that is larger than the largest intra-epidermal cluster (indicative of a tumor with capacity for expansile growth in the dermis) (Fig. 3).
>
> Mitogenic: the presence of any mitoses in the dermal component of the melanoma is indicative of a tumor with capacity for expansile growth in the dermis, even if this expansile growth has not yet occurred, and defines typical VGP even in the absence of the criterion of tumorigenicity.
>
> The definition of RGP or microinvasive melanoma is the converse of the above. That is, no mass of melanoma cells is present in the dermis and there are no mitoses in the dermal component of the melanoma (Fig. 4).

Other attributes tend to differ between RGP and VGP, in addition to the properties of tumorigenicity and mitogenicity. For example, the cells in the dermis tend to resemble those in the epidermis in RGP melanomas, whereas in the VGP they tend to be larger and more atypical than the cells of the adjacent RGP component. RGP melanomas are usually level I or II, whereas VGP melanomas may be level II but are more commonly level

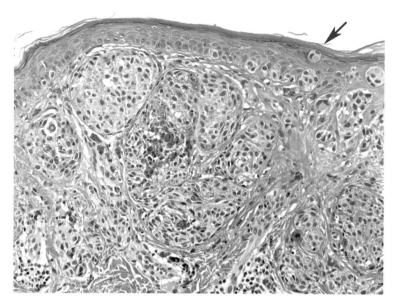

Fig. 3. Vertical growth phase melanoma. In the dermis, there are clusters of uniformly atypical epithelioid melanocytes, considerably larger than the largest clusters in the overlying epidermis, where there is focal pagetoid proliferation (arrow).

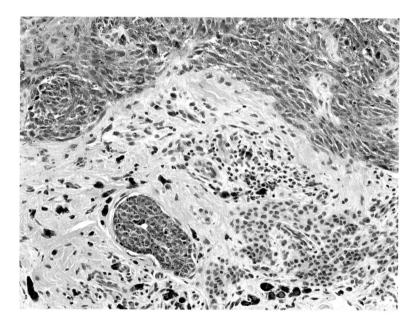

Fig. 4. Invasive radial growth phase (RGP) melanoma and an associated dermal nevus. In the epidermis, there is confluence of nests, comprised of uniformly atypical epithelioid to somewhat spindle-shaped melanocytes, consistent with melanoma *in situ* with a partly lentiginous pattern. Elsewhere in the lesion, pagetoid proliferation was observed. In the dermis on the left, there is a cluster of nested melanocytes that are morphologically similar to those in the epidermis. This cluster is not larger than the largest clusters in the epidermis, consistent with invasive RGP or microinvasive melanoma. To the right of the image in the dermis, there are clusters of orderly nevus cells, distinguished from the melanoma cells by lacking cytological atypia.

Table 2
Summary of Tumor Progression Biology in Melanoma

	RGP	*VGP*	*Metastases*
Growth in culture	Slow	Rapid	Rapid
Permanent lines	Few	Yes	Yes
Tumorigenicity in mice	No	Yes	Yes
Cytogenetic abnormalities	Few, random	More, some nonrandom	Many, some nonrandom
Growth factor production	No	Yes	Yes
Growth factor independence	No	Infrequent	Often
Progression antigens	Low	High	High

Adapted from refs. *83,111,112*. RGP, radial growth phase; VGP, vertical growth phase.

III or greater, and greater than 0.76 mm in Breslow thickness. The tumor-infiltrating lymphocytes (TIL) response is usually less in the VGP than in the RGP, and the clusters of cells in the VGP tend to compress or distort surrounding tissue, as if they have growth preference over the stromal cells. Finally, ulceration, vascular invasion, and satellites are all rare in RGP melanomas.

The reproducibility of diagnosis of VGP in thin melanomas (<1 mm in greatest thickness according to the criteria of Breslow) has been studied by two groups, and found to be acceptable for clinical use *(77,78)*.

Biology of RGP vs VGP Melanoma

The biology of tumor progression in melanoma has been reviewed *(79–82)*. Several lines of evidence are consistent with the hypothesis that the cells of RGP and VGP lesions differ in several important properties that relate to the malignant phenotype. First, despite considerable effort, only a few permanent cell lines have been established from RGP cells *(83)*. Such cells have tended to proliferate slowly for a time, but never reach confluence, and ultimately senesce, taking on a spindled fibroblast-like morphology. In contrast, cell lines are readily established from VGP primary tumors and from metastases. Furthermore, cells from short-term culture of RGP lesions are not tumorigenic in immunodeficient mice, in contrast to VGP and metastatic melanoma cells, which often readily form tumors in these animals. In human skin reconstruct models, cells from RGP melanoma remain confined to the epidermis and undergo apoptosis if they enter the artificial dermis. These cells can be protected from apoptosis by transfection with the β3 integrin gene, which, when ligated with collagen fragments or other matrix molecules, activates a cell death protection pathway *(84)*. β3 integrin expression also serves as a strong marker for VGP, compared with RGP *(85)*. Another strong marker that can distinguish VGP from RGP in tissue sections is Ki-67, a marker of cells in the G1-S phase of the cell cycle. However, neither of these markers is diagnostic of melanoma; for example, each of them may be expressed in Spitz nevi, which are diagnostically troublesome simulants of melanoma.

In terms of biological, as well as clinical, attributes, the cells of VGP melanoma tend to resemble those of metastatic melanoma more closely than those of the RGP within which they may arise. Some of these differences and similarities are summarized in Table 2.

Prognosis in VGP Melanoma

These considerations have important clinical significance. In early studies from the University of Pennsylvania's Pigmented Lesion Clinic, it was demonstrated that invasive RGP melanomas, lacking the properties of tumorigenicity and mitogenicity, were not associated with competence for metastasis *(72,73)*. Indeed, in these early studies, the survival of a cohort of patients followed for more than 10 yr was literally 100%, with a statistical confidence interval of 1%. In the latest follow-up studies from this same, but now greatly expanded, database, an incidence of metastasis of approx 1% has now been observed. As already mentioned, this metastatic rate does not appear to differ significantly from that associated with MIS. Studies that have observed metastasis in thin melanomas have also noted the presence of partial regression in the lesion *(74,75)*. Thus, it is possible that a portion of the tumor that was thicker may have metastasized, then regressed, leaving a "footprint" of regressive histology and clinical morphology behind.

The prognosis in "pure" RGP melanoma—a melanoma that lacks both the properties of tumorigenicity and mitogenicity—is close to 100%, irrespective of other attributes *(72,73)*. This simple model is good enough for clinical use for these lesions. In VGP, on the other hand, there is a wide range of prognosis, from close to 100%, to a very low probability of survival at the other extreme.

Prognostic models for melanoma have described phenotypic attributes of the lesions that are associated with survival, and therefore are likely associated with mechanisms of metastasis. The prognostic model in widest use at this time is that of the American Joint Committee for Cancer (AJCC) *(86)*. This model uses the property of tumor thickness described by Breslow in 1970, modified by the presence or absence of ulceration and, in thin melanomas, by level IV invasion, as described by Clark in 1967 *(2,52)*. Ulceration has been identified as an important prognostic attribute in many studies *(87–91)*; however, the effect of ulceration seems to be diminished or absent in some studies that have included additional variables, such as the tumor mitotic rate or vascular invasion *(75,90–92)*. The AJCC model provides good stratification of risk of metastasis and death from melanoma. However, in thin melanomas, there is an approx 12% risk of death at 10 yr. Thus, this is not an especially low-risk category.

Studies from the University of Pennsylvania's Pigmented Lesion Clinic database have demonstrated that additional prognostic attributes have significance in thin (and also in thicker) VGP melanomas *(75)*. The two most important attributes are TIL and mitotic rate:

TIL: The prognosis for patients with "brisk" lymphocytes in their VGP is approx 12 times better than that for patients with no infiltrating lymphocytes *(75,93)*. This finding of a beneficial effect of TIL, defined as lymphocytes that are in contact with melanoma cells, is also true for metastatic disease *(94)*, and is encouraging for investigators who are attempting to define immunogenic antigens suitable for therapeutic use in melanoma patients.

Mitotic rate: The prognosis for patients with no mitoses is approx 11 times better than that for patients with greater than 6 mitoses/mm^2. This finding doubtless represents a loss of the normal control of proliferation pathways, such as mitogen-activated protein kinase (MAP-kinase) *(95)*, and suppressor pathways, such as p16/RB *(96)*.

In addition to these major attributes, other attributes have been found to have weaker associations with prognosis, in studies based on tumor progression and in numerous other studies *(75,88–90,93,97–104)*. These include the following: patient gender—in

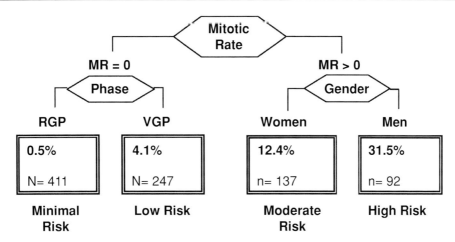

Fig. 5. Metastasis-free survival in thin melanomas (*n* = 887) *(110)*. Cartesian regression analysis of 887 cases of thin primary melanoma (American Joint Committee on Cancer stage 1, <1 mm Breslow thickness), all followed 10 yr or more (Gimotty et al., Penn Pigmented Lesion Clinic, ref. *110*). MR, mitotic rate; RGP, radial growth phase; VGP, vertical growth phase.

the Clark model, the prognosis for women is approximately three times better than for men *(75)*; lesional location—the prognosis for melanomas on the extremities is approximately four times better than for melanomas on the trunk; RGP regression—the prognosis is approximately twofold worse when regression is present in an area of the RGP, possibly because this conceals an area of early VGP that had been at risk of metastasizing before it regressed. The prognostic significance of attributes related to vascularity and vascular involvement has been controversial *(92,99,105–109)*; however, recent studies from the University of California at San Francisco database have produced strong evidence for the significance of these attributes *(92,108,109)*.

In recent studies using Cartesian regression tree analysis, Gimotty and colleagues demonstrated interesting interactions among several of the variables discussed in this section *(110)*. For example, in an analysis of 887 thin melanomas (i.e., <1 mm in Breslow thickness), the Cartesian model divided the cases first on mitogenicity, a mitotic rate of zero vs greater than zero. Mitotic rate zero groups were divided on the basis of tumorigenicity, RGP vs VGP. Melanomas with mitotic rates of greater than zero were divided on the basis of gender. This process identified a group of 411 minimal-risk patients, with 0.5% probability of metastasis; and another group of 92 high-risk patients, with a 31.5% probability of metastasis; with two other groups at intermediate risk. These relationships are illustrated in Fig. 5.

CONCLUSIONS AND PERSPECTIVES

Principles of tumor progression have been reviewed here, mainly from an historical perspective. Clinical, histological, cellular, and molecular evidence are all consistent with a model of progression evolving from clinically and histologically characteristic precursor lesions. These lesions are better described as potential precursors of melanoma, because the majority of potential precursors do not progress (and not all melanomas arise in a precursor). Common acquired nevi and dysplastic nevi are potential precursors of melanoma, and they are also important as simulants of melanoma and as markers of individuals at increased risk of developing melanoma. Melanomas themselves evolve through stages of tumor progression, from an initial plaque-like phase of progression called the RGP, to a more advanced tumorigenic phase, called the VGP. Melanomas lacking VGP do not metastasize, with vanishingly rare exceptions. Melanomas with VGP are recognized histologically by the properties of tumorigenicity and mitogenicity, and may have competence for metastasis. The likelihood of metastasis can be predicted with increasing accuracy by the use of prognostic models. The AJCC staging system, which is in wide use, uses attributes that are commonly available in pathology reports, including Breslow's thickness, Clark's level, and the presence or absence of ulceration. More sophisticated models have added the use of various additional attributes. TIL as a favorable attribute and mitotic rate as an unfavorable attribute have entered into several of these models. Although not yet in common use, future models of this sort will doubtless include biological markers with the capacity not only to predict survival with greater precision (prognostic attributes), but also to identify those tumors that are most likely to respond to particular therapeutic modalities (predictive attributes). Thus, principles derived from clinical studies of tumor progression will continue to have diagnostic and therapeutic relevance.

REFERENCES

1. Foulds L. Neoplastic development. Academic, London and New York, NY: 1969, pp. 41–86.
2. Clark WH Jr, From L, Bernardino EA, Mihm MC Jr. The histogenesis and biologic behavior of primary human malignant melanomas of the skin. Cancer Res 1969;29:705–727.
3. Clark WH Jr, Tucker MA. Problems with lesions related to the development of malignant melanoma: common nevi, dysplastic nevi, malignant melanoma in situ, and radial growth phase malignant melanoma. Hum Pathol 1998;29:8–14.
4. An HT, Yoo JY, Lee MK, et al. Single dose radiation is more effective for the UV-induced activation and proliferation of melanocytes than fractionated dose radiation. Photodermatol Photoimmunol Photomed 2001;17:266–271.
5. Gilchrest BA, Blog FB, Szabo G. Effects of aging and chronic sun exposure on melanocytes in human skin. J Invest Dermatol 1979;73:141–143.
6. Cox PM, Dhillon AP, Howe S, Pittilo RM, Rode J. Repopulation of guinea-pig skin by melanocytes during wound healing: a morphometric study. Br J Exp Pathol 1989;70:679–689.
7. Boissy RE. Melanosome transfer to and translocation in the keratinocyte. Exp Dermatol 2003; 12(Suppl 2):5–12.
8. Abdel-Malek Z, Scott MC, Suzuki I, et al. The melanocortin-1 receptor is a key regulator of human cutaneous pigmentation. Pigment Cell Res 2000;13(Suppl 8):156–162.
9. Autier P, Severi G, Pedeux R, et al. Number and size of nevi are influenced by different sun exposure components: implications for the etiology of cutaneous melanoma (Belgium, Germany, France, Italy). Cancer Causes Control 2003;14:453–459.
10. MacLennan R, Kelly JW, Rivers JK, Harrison SL. The Eastern Australian Childhood Nevus Study: site differences in density and size of melanocytic nevi in relation to latitude and phenotype. J Am Acad Dermatol 2003;48:367–375.
11. Wiecker TS, Luther H, Buettner P, Bauer J, Garbe C. Moderate sun exposure and nevus counts in parents are associated with development of melanocytic nevi in childhood: a risk factor study in 1812 kindergarten children. Cancer 2003;97:628–638.
12. Darlington S, Siskind V, Green L, Green A. Longitudinal study of melanocytic nevi in adolescents. J Am Acad Dermatol 2002;46:715–722.
13. Dulon M, Weichenthal M, Blettner M, et al. Sun exposure and number of nevi in 5- to 6-year-old European children. J Clin Epidemiol 2002;55:1075–1081.
14. Bishop JA, Wachsmuth RC, Harland M, et al. Genotype/phenotype and penetrance studies in melanoma families with germline CDKN2A mutations. J Invest Dermatol 2000;114:28–33.

15. Harada M, Suzuki M, Ikeda T, Kaneko T, Harada S, Fukayama M. Clonality in nevocellular nevus and melanoma: an expression-based clonality analysis at the X-linked genes by polymerase chain reaction. J Invest Dermatol 1997;109:656–660.

16. Hui P, Perkins AS, Glusac EJ. Assessment of clonality in melanocytic nevi. J Cutan Pathol 2001;28:140–144.

17. Robinson WA, Lemon M, Elefanty A, Harrison-Smith M, Markham N, Norris D. Human acquired naevi are clonal. Melanoma Res 1998;8:499–503.

18. MacKie RM, English J, Aitchison TC, Fitzsimmons CP, Wilson P. The number and distribution of benign pigmented moles (melanocytic nevi) in a healthy British population. Brit J Dermatol 1985;113:167–174.

19. Whimster IW. Recurrent pigment cell naevi and their significance in the problem of endogenous carcinogenesis. Ann Ital Dermatol Clin Sper 1965;19:168–191.

20. Silye R, Karayiannakis AJ, Syrigos KN, et al. E-cadherin/catenin complex in benign and malignant melanocytic lesions. J Pathol 1998;186:350–355.

21. Li G, Satyamoorthy K, Herlyn M. Dynamics of cell interactions and communications during melanoma development. Crit Rev Oral Biol Med 2002;13:62–70.

22. Zembowicz A, McCusker M, Chiarelli C, et al. Morphological analysis of nevoid melanoma: a study of 20 cases with a review of the literature. Am J Dermatopathol 2001;23:167–175.

23. Schmoeckel C, Castro CE, Braun-Falco O. Nevoid malignant melanoma. Arch Dermatol Res 1985;277:362–369.

24. Levene A. On the histological diagnosis and prognosis of malignant melanoma. J Clin Pathol 1980;33:101–124.

25. Clark WH Jr, Reimer RR, Greene MH, Ainsworth AA, Mastrangelo MJ. Origin of familial melanomas from heritable melanocytic lesions. "The B-K mole syndrome". Arch Dermatol 1978;114:732–738.

26. Frichot BC, Lynch HT, Guirgis HA, Harris RE, Lynch JF. New cutaneous phenotype in cutaneous malignant melanoma. Lancet 1977;1:864–865.

27. Lynch HT, Fusaro RM, Danes BS, Kimberling WJ, Lynch JF. A review of hereditary malignant melanoma including biomarkers in familial atypical multiple mole melanoma syndrome. Cancer Genet Cytogenet 1983;8:325–358.

28. Elder DE, Goldman LI, Goldman SC, Greene MH, Clark WH Jr. Dysplastic nevus syndrome: a phenotypic association of sporadic cutaneous melanoma. Cancer 1980;46:1787–1794.

29. Elder DE, Green MH, Guerry DIV, Kraemer KH, Clark WH Jr. The dysplastic nevus syndrome: our definition. Am J Dermatopathol 1982;4:455–460.

30. Greene MH. The genetics of hereditary melanoma and nevi: 1998 update. Cancer 1999;86: 2464–2477.

31. Tucker MA, Halpern A, Holly EA, et al. Clinically recognized dysplastic nevi. A central risk factor for cutaneous melanoma. JAMA 1997;277:1439–1444.

32. Robinson JK, Nickoloff BJ. Digital epiluminescence microscopy monitoring of high-risk patients. Arch Dermatol 2004;140:49–56.

33. Barnhill RL, Roush GC, Duray PH. Correlation of histologic architectural and cytoplasmic features with nuclear atypia in atypical (dysplastic) nevomelanocytic nevi. Hum Pathol 1990;21:51–58.

34. Clemente C, Cochran A, Elder DE, et al. Histopathologic diagnosis of dysplastic nevi. Concordance among pathologists convened by the WHO melanoma programme. Hum Pathol 1991;22:313–319.

35. De Wit PEJ, Van't Hof-Grootenboer B, Ruiter DJ, et al. Validity of the histopathological criteria used for diagnosing dysplastic naevi. An interobserver study by the pathology subgroup of the EORTC Malignant Melanoma Cooperative Group. Eur J Cancer [A] 1993;29A:831–839.

36. Duncan LM, Berwick M, Bruijn JA, Byers HR, Mihm MC, Barnhill RL. Histopathologic recognition and grading of dysplastic melanocytic nevi: an interobserver agreement study. J Invest Dermatol 1993;100:318S–321S.

37. National Institutes of Health. National Institutes of Health Consensus Development Conference statement on diagnosis and treatment of early melanoma, January 27–29, 1992. Am J Dermatopathol 1993;15:34–43.

38. Tsao H, Bevona C, Goggins W, Quinn T. The transformation rate of moles (melanocytic nevi) into cutaneous melanoma: a population-based estimate. Arch Dermatol 2003;139:282–288.

39. Bolognia JL, Lin A, Shapiro PE. The significance of eccentric foci of hyperpigmentation ('small dark dots') within melanocytic nevi: analysis of 59 cases. Arch Dermatol 1994;130:1013–1017.

40. Yazdi AS, Palmedo G, Flaig MJ, et al. Mutations of the BRAF gene in benign and malignant melanocytic lesions. J Invest Dermatol 2003;121:1160–1162.

41. Demunter A, Stas M, Degreef H, Wolf-Peeters C, Van den Oord JJ. Analysis of N- and k-ras mutations in the distinctive tumor progression phases of melanoma. J Invest Dermatol 2001;117: 1483–1489.

42. Rhodes AR, Harrist TJ, Day CL, Mihm MC Jr, Fitzpatrick TB, Sober AJ. Dysplastic melanocytic nevi in histologic association with 234 primary cutaneous melanomas. J Am Acad Dermatol 1983;9: 563–574.

43. Clark WH Jr, Elder DE, Guerry DIV, Epstein MN, Greene MH, Van Horn M. A study of tumor progression: the precursor lesions of superficial spreading and nodular melanoma. Hum Pathol 1984;15:1147–1165.

44. Cook MG, Roberston I. Melanocytic dysplasia and melanoma. Histopathology 1985;9:647–658.

45. English DR, Menz J, Heenan PJ, Elder DE, Watt JD, Armstrong BK. The dysplastic naevus syndrome in patients with cutaneous malignant melanoma in Western Australia. Med J Aust 1986;145:194–198.

46. Black WC. Residual dysplastic and other nevi in superficial spreading melanoma. Clinical correlations and association with sun damage. Cancer 1988;62:163–173.

47. Gruber SB, Barnhill RL, Stenn KS, Roush GC. Nevomelanocytic proliferations in association with cutaneous malignant melanoma: a multivariate analysis. J Am Acad Dermatol 1989;21:773–780.

48. Bevona C, Goggins W, Quinn T, Fullerton J, Tsao H. Cutaneous melanomas associated with nevi. Arch Dermatol 2003;139:1620–1624.

49. Greene M, Clark WH Jr, Tucker MA, Kraemer KH, Elder DE, Fraser MC. High risk of malignant melanoma in melanoma-prone families with dysplastic nevi. Ann Intern Med 1985;102:458–465.

50. Masri GD, Clark WH Jr, Guerry DIV, Halpern A, Thompson CJ, Elder DE. Screening and surveillance of patients at high risk for malignant melanoma result in detection of earlier disease. J Am Acad Dermatol 1990;22:1042–1048.

51. Mishima Y. Melanocytic and nevocytic malignant melanomas. Cellular and subcellular differentiation. Cancer 1967;20:632–649.

52. Clark WH Jr. A classification of malignant melanoma in man correlated with histogenesis and biologic behavior. In: Montagna W, Hu F, eds. Advances in the Biology of the Skin Volume VIII. Pergamon, New York, NY: 1967, pp. 621–647.

53. Clark WH Jr, Mihm MC Jr. Lentigo maligna and lentigo-maligna melanoma. Am J Pathol 1969; 55:39–67.

54. Bastian BC, Olshen AB, LeBoit PE, Pinkel D. Classifying melanocytic tumors based on DNA copy number changes. Am J Pathol 2003;163:1765–1770.

55. Rhodes AR, Sober AJ, Day CL, et al. The malignant potential of small congenital nevocellular nevi. An estimate of association based on a histologic study of 234 primary cutaneous melanomas. J Am Acad Dermatol 1982;6:230–241.

56. Illig L, Weidner F, Hundeiker M, et al. Congenital nevi less than or equal to 10 cm as precursors to melanoma. 52 cases, a review, and a new conception. Arch Dermatol 1985;121:1274–1281.

57. Augustsson A, Stierner U, Rosdahl I, Suurküla M. Common and dysplastic naevi as risk factors for cutaneous malignant melanoma in a Swedish population. Acta Derm Venereol (Stockh) 1991; 71:518–524.

58. Halpern AC, Guerry DIV, Elder DE, et al. Dysplastic nevi as risk markers of sporadic (non-familial) melanoma: a case–control study. Arch Dermatol 1991;127:995–999.

59. Garbe C, Kruger S, Stadler R, Guggenmoos-Holzmann I, Orfanos CE. Markers and relative risk in a German population for developing malignant melanoma. Int J Dermatol 1989;28:517–523.

60. Holly EA, Kelly JW, Shpall SN, Chiu S-H. Number of melanocytic nevi as a major risk factor for malignant melanoma. J Am Acad Dermatol 1987;17:459–468.

61. Swerdlow AJ, English J, MacKie RM, et al. Benign melanocytic naevi as a risk factor for malignant melanoma. Brit Med J 1986;292:1555–1559.

62. Nordlund JJ, Kirkwood J, Forget BM, et al. Demographic study of clinically atypical (dysplastic) nevi in patients with melanoma and comparison subjects. Cancer Res 1985;45:1855–1861.

63. Holly EA, Kelly JW, Shpall SN, Chiu S-H. Number of melanocytic nevi as a risk factor for malignant melanoma. J Am Acad Dermatol 1987;17:459–468.

64. Grob JJ, Gouvernet J, Aymar D, et al. Count of benign melanocytic nevi as a major risk factor for nonfamilial nodular and superficial spreading melanoma. Cancer 1990;66:387–395.

65. MacKie RM, Freudenberger T, Aitchison TC. Personal risk-factor chart for cutaneous melanoma. Lancet 1989;2:487–490.

66. Meyer LJ, Goldgar DE, Cannon-Albright LA, et al. Number, size, and histopathology of nevi in Utah kindreds. Cytogenet Cell Genet 1992;59:167–169.

67. Goldgar DE, Cannon-Albright LA, Meyer LJ, Piepkorn MW, Zone JJ, Skolnick MH. Inheritance of nevus number and size in melanoma/DNS kindreds. Cytogenet Cell Genet 1992;59:200–202.

68. Green A, Siskind V, Bain C, Alexander J. Sunburn and malignant melanoma. Br J Cancer 1985;51:393–397.

69. Piepkorn MW, Barnhill RL, Cannon-Albright LA, et al. A multiobserver, population-based analysis of histologic dysplasia in melanocytic nevi. J Am Acad Dermatol 1994;30:707–714.

70. Arumi-Uria M, McNutt NS, Finnerty B. Grading of atypia in nevi: correlation with melanoma risk. Mod Pathol 2003;16:764–771.

71. Kirkham N, Price ML, Gibson B, Leigh IM, Coburn P, Darley CR. Type VII collagen antibody LH 7.2 identifies basement membrane characteristics of thin malignant melanomas. J Pathol 1989;157:243–247.

72. Elder DE, Guerry DIV, Epstein MN, et al. Invasive malignant melanomas lacking competence for metastasis. Am J Dermatopathol 1984;6:55–62.

73. Guerry DIV, Synnestvedt M, Elder DE, Schultz D. Lessons from tumor progression: the invasive radial growth phase of melanoma is common, incapable of metastasis, and indolent. J Invest Dermatol 1993;100:342S–345S.

74. Guitart J, Lowe L, Piepkorn M, et al. Histological characteristics of metastasizing thin melanomas: a case-control study of 43 cases. Arch Dermatol 2002;138:603–608.

75. Clark WH Jr, Elder DE, Guerry DIV, et al. Model predicting survival in stage I melanoma based on tumor progression. JNCI 1989;81:1893–1904.

76. Elder DE, Murphy GF. Melanocytic tumors of the skin. Washington, D.C. Armed Forces Institute of Pathology, 1991.

77. Cook MG, Clarke TJ, Humphreys S, et al. A nationwide survey of observer variation in the diagnosis of thin cutaneous malignant melanoma including the MIN terminology. J Clin Pathol 1997;50:202–205.

78. McDermott NC, Hayes DP, al-Sader MH, et al. Identification of vertical growth phase in malignant melanoma. A study of interobserver agreement. Am J Clin Pathol 1998;110:753–757.

79. Herlyn M. Molecular and cellular biology of melanoma. R. G. Landes, Austin, TX: 1993.

80. Kath R, Rodeck U, Menssen HD, et al. Tumor progression in the human melanocytic system. Anticancer Res 1989;9:865–872.

81. Herlyn M. Human melanoma: development and progression. Cancer Metastasis Rev 1990;9:101–112.

82. Herlyn M. Structure and function of molecules produced by melanoma cells. In: Herlyn M, ed. Molecular and Cellular Biology of Melanoma. R. G. Landes, Austin, TX: 1993, pp. 44–92.

83. Hsu M-Y, Elder DE, Herlyn M. The Wistar (WM) melanoma cell lines. In: Masters JRW, Palsson B, eds. Human Cell Culture. Vol. 2, Cancer Cell Lines, Part 2 (Human Cell Culture) Springer, 1989.

84. Hsu M-Y, Shih D-T, Meier F, et al. Adenoviral gene transfer of β3 integrin subunit induces conversion from radial to vertical growth phase in primary human melanoma. Am J Pathol 1998;153:1347–1351.

85. Van Belle PA, Elenitsas R, Satyamoorthy K, et al. Progression-related expression of beta3 integrin in melanomas and nevi. Hum Pathol 1999;30:562–567.

86. Balch CM, Sober AJ, Soong SJ, Gershenwald JE. The new melanoma staging system. Semin Cutan Med Surg 2003;22:42–54.

87. MacKie RM, Aitchison T, Sirel JM, McLaren K, Watt DC. Prognostic models for subgroups of melanoma patients from the Scottish Melanoma Group database 1979–86, and their subsequent validation. Br J Cancer 1995;71:173–176.

88. Cochran AJ, Elashoff D, Morton DL, Elashoff R. Individualized prognosis for melanoma patients. Hum Pathol 2000;31:327–331.

89. Balch CM, Soong SJ, Gershenwald JE, et al. Prognostic factors analysis of 17,600 melanoma patients: validation of the american joint committee on cancer melanoma staging system. J Clin Oncol 2001;19:3622–3634.

90. Tuthill RJ, Unger JM, Liu PY, Flaherty LE, Sondak VK. Risk assessment in localized primary cutaneous melanoma: a Southwest Oncology Group study evaluating nine factors and a test of the Clark logistic regression prediction model. Am J Clin Pathol 2002;118:504–511.

91. Azzola MF, Shaw HM, Thompson JF, et al. Tumor mitotic rate is a more powerful prognostic indicator than ulceration in patients with primary cutaneous melanoma: an analysis of 3661 patients from a single center. Cancer 2003;97:1488–1498.

92. Kashani-Sabet M, Shaikh L, Miller JR III, et al. NF-kappa B in the vascular progression of melanoma. J Clin Oncol 2004;22:617–623.

93. Clemente CG, Mihm MG, Bufalino R, Zurrida S, Collini P, Cascinelli N. Prognostic value of tumor infiltrating lymphocytes in the vertical growth phase of primary cutaneous melanoma. Cancer 1996;77:1303–1310.

94. Mihm MC Jr, Clemente CG, Cascinelli N. Tumor infiltrating lymphocytes in lymph node melanoma metastases: a histopathologic prognostic indicator and an expression of local immune response. Lab Invest 1996;74:43–47.

95. Satyamoorthy K, Li G, Gerrero MR, et al. Constitutive mitogen-activated protein kinase activation in melanoma is mediated by both BRAF mutations and autocrine growth factor stimulation. Cancer Res 2003;63:756–759.

96. Straume O, Akslen LA. Alterations and prognostic significance of p16 and p53 protein expression in subgroups of cutaneous melanoma. Int J Cancer 1997;74:535–539.

97. Averbook BJ, Fu P, Rao JS, Mansour EG. A long-term analysis of 1018 patients with melanoma by classic Cox regression and tree-structured survival analysis at a major referral center: implications on the future of cancer staging. Surgery 2002;132:589–604.

98. Gimotty PA, Guerry D, Elder DE. Validation of prognostic models for melanoma. Am J Clin Pathol 2002;118:489–491.

99. Barnhill RL, Fine JA, Roush GC, Berwick M. Predicting five-year outcome for patients with cutaneous melanoma in a population-based study. Cancer 1996;78:427–432.

100. MacKie RM, Aitchison T, Sirel JM, McLaren K, Watt DC. Prognostic models for subgroups of melanoma patients from the Scottish Melanoma Group database 1979–86, and their subsequent validation. Br J Cancer 1996;71:173–176.

101. Garbe C, Büttner P, Bertz J, et al. Primary cutaneous melanoma: identification of prognostic groups and estimation of individual prognosis for 5093 patients. Cancer 1995;75:2484–2491.

102. Soong SJ. A computerized mathematical model and scoring system for predicting outcome in melanoma patients. In: Balch CM, Milton GW, eds. Cutaneous Melanoma. Lippincot, Philadelphia, PA: 1985, pp. 353–367.

103. Day CL Jr, Lew RA, Mihm MC Jr, et al. A multivariate analysis of prognostic factors for melanoma patients with lesions greater than or equal to 3.65 mm in thickness. The importance of revealing alternative Cox models. Ann Surg 1982;195:44–49.

104. Day CL Jr, Mihm MC Jr, Lew RA, et al. Prognostic factors for patients with clinical stage I melanoma of intermediate thickness (1.51–3.39 mm). A conceptual model for tumor growth and metastasis. Ann Surg 1982;195:35–43.

105. Ilmonen S, Kariniemi AL, Vlaykova T, Muhonen T, Pyrhonen S, Asko-Seljavaara S. Prognostic value of tumour vascularity in primary melanoma. Melanoma Res 1999;9:273–278.

106. Straume O, Salvesen HB, Akslen LA. Angiogenesis is prognostically important in vertical growth phase melanomas. Int J Oncol 1999;15:595–599.

107. Massi D, Borgognoni L, Franchi A, Martini L, Reali UM, Santucci M. Thick cutaneous malignant melanoma: a reappraisal of prognostic factors. Melanoma Res 2000;10:153–164.

108. Kashani-Sabet M, Sagebiel RW, Ferreira CM, Nosrati M, Miller JR III. Vascular involvement in the prognosis of primary cutaneous melanoma. Arch Dermatol 2001;137:1169–1173.

109. Kashani-Sabet M, Sagebiel RW, Ferreira CM, Nosrati M, Miller JR III. Tumor vascularity in the prognostic assessment of primary cutaneous melanoma. J Clin Oncol 2002;20:1826–1831.

110. Gimotty PA, Guerry DIV, Ming ME, et al. Thin primary cutaneous malignant melanoma: a prognostic tree for ten-year metastasis is more accurate than AJCC staging. Am J Clin Oncol 2004; 22:3668–3676.

111. Herlyn M, Balaban G, Bennicelli J, et al. Primary melanoma cells of the vertical growth phase: similarities to metastatic cells. J Natl Cancer Inst 1985;74:283–289.

112. Rodeck U, Herlyn M. Characteristics of cultured human melanocytes from different stages of tumor progression. Cancer Treat Res 1988;43:3–16.

30 The Plasticity of Melanoma Cells and Associated Clinical Implications

Mary J. C. Hendrix, Elisabeth A. Seftor, Angela R. Hess, and Richard E. B. Seftor

CONTENTS

Summary

The molecular signature of aggressive cutaneous and uveal melanoma cells is consistent with an undifferentiated cell with a genetic profile similar to that of embryonic cells. The associated plastic phenotype may explain how aggressive melanoma cells can mimic endothelial cells, participate in neovascularization of tissues, and form a fluid-conducting meshwork through a process called *vasculogenic mimicry*. Although elucidation of the biological steps of melanoma vasculogenic mimicry should lead to improved diagnostic and therapeutic strategies, the clinical management of cutaneous and uveal melanoma (as well as many other types of cancers), would benefit from the identification of valid predictors of disease progression and metastatic potential. In this regard, recent studies aimed at characterizing the molecular signature of melanoma tumor cells has resulted in a classification scheme for malignant cutaneous melanoma, as well as a molecular profile for uveal melanoma, which may contribute to improving the diagnosis and treatment of this and possibly other cancers.

Key Words: Melanoma; vasculogenic mimicry; plasticity; angiogenesis.

DIFFERENTIAL GENE EXPRESSION OF HIGHLY AGGRESSIVE VS POORLY AGGRESSIVE HUMAN CUTANEOUS AND UVEAL MELANOMA CELL LINES

Microarray analyses of differential gene expression of highly aggressive compared with poorly aggressive human cutaneous and uveal melanoma cell lines revealed the

From: *From Melanocytes to Melanoma: The Progression to Malignancy*
Edited by: V. J. Hearing and S. P. L. Leong © Humana Press Inc., Totowa, NJ

co-expression of multiple phenotype-specific genes by aggressive tumor cells. These cell types include: endothelia, epithelia, pericytes, fibroblasts, hematopoietic lineage, kidney, neuronal lineage, muscle, and several other precursor cell types *(1–3)*, which suggests that aggressive melanoma cells may undergo a genetic reversion to a undifferentiated, embryonic-like phenotype indicative of a deregulated cell. Although the biological significance of these unexpected findings remains enigmatic, these observations have prompted further investigation into the relevance of a "plastic" tumor cell phenotype and they challenge our current thinking concerning the identification and subsequent therapeutic targeting of tumor cells that may masquerade as other cell types.

VASCULOGENIC MIMICRY AS A MODEL FOR MELANOMA CELL PLASTICITY

Many of the biological properties relevant to embryogenesis are also important in tumor growth. As an example, the formation of primary vascular networks during embryonic development occurs by the process called *vasculogenesis*, the *in situ* differentiation of mesodermal progenitor cells (angioblasts and hemangioblasts) to endothelial cells that organize into a primitive network (for reviews, *see* refs. *4–6*) (Fig. 1). The remodeling of this initial vasculogenic network subsequently into a more refined microvasculature occurs through the process of angiogenesis, the sprouting of new capillaries from pre-existing networks. In this regard, it is widely accepted that, during cancer progression, tumors not only require a blood supply for growth, but also use this vehicle for metastatic dissemination (for review, *see* refs. *7–14*).

The molecular profile of aggressive melanoma cells, along with novel in vitro observations (using three-dimensional [3D] matrices) and appropriate correlative histopathological findings, led our laboratory and collaborators to introduce the concept of vasculogenic mimicry (VM) in 1999 *(15)*. Initially, VM described the unique characteristic of aggressive melanoma tumor cells to express endothelial-associated genes and form extracellular matrix (ECM)-rich (highlighted by periodic acid-Schiff [PAS] staining) vasculogenic-like networks in 3D culture that recapitulate embryonic vasculogenic networks (Fig. 1). These in vitro networks appear to correlate with the distinctive patterned, ECM-rich networks observed in patients' aggressive tumors *(2,15–23)*. Additional studies have reported intriguing observations regarding VM in various tumors and have resulted in an evolution in thinking with respect to the concept of VM we presently use.

In both xenograft models and human melanomas representative of aggressive disease, the patterned networks appear in the form of loops (and arcs) that tightly encircle spheroidal nests of melanoma that are lined by tumor cells. These networks are rich in laminin (and presumably by other, as yet undetermined, ECM components), and appear in tissue sections to have either small channel-like spaces between them or to be partially or totally occluded ECM sheets surrounding nests of tumor cells. Some of the channel-like spaces were originally called vascular channels because they appear to contain red blood cells (RBC) and plasma and were thought to possibly provide a perfusion mechanism and dissemination route within the tumor compartment. These channels were thought to function either independently of, or simultaneously with, angiogenesis, or possibly with other sources of vascularization, such as vessel co-option. Although patients with melanomas that exhibit VM have a poor prognosis *(17–23)*, little is known concerning the

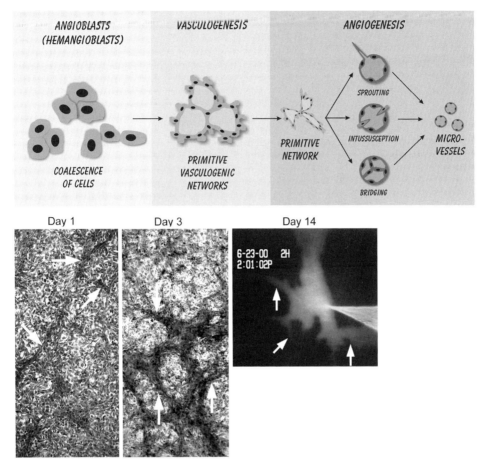

Fig. 1. Diagrammatic representation of vasculogenesis, angiogenesis, and photomicroscopy of tumor cell vasculogenic mimicry. The upper panel provides a diagrammatic overview of vasculogenesis and angiogenesis and shows how endothelial precursors (angioblasts and hemangioblasts) coalesce, differentiate into endothelial cells, and form primitive vasculogenic networks (vasculogenesis). The remodeling of these networks occurs via angiogenesis and results in the formation of microvessels. (Diagram adapted from Carmeliet review of angiogenesis and arteriogenesis, ref. 5, and created by Dr. Dawn A. Kirschmann.) The lower panel contains photomicroscopic images showing the unique characteristic of aggressive melanoma cells forming *de novo* vasculogenic-like networks (arrows) in three-dimensional collagen I gels (in vitro), which are capable of conducting a green fluorescent dye when microinjected after 14 d. Please *see* color insert following p. 430.

biological relevance of this phenomenon. Other studies have reported VM in several other tumor types, including breast, lung, prostatic, and ovarian carcinoma, and have attempted to address some key molecular mechanisms underlying this unique process, including the demonstration of a viable connection of blood flow between tumor cell-lined vascular spaces and endothelial-lined and/or mature vasculature *(24)*.

The significance of these findings relate to the etiology of VM and are particularly important with respect to the ongoing investigations aimed at identifying key regulators of this dynamic process. Specifically, these regulators appear to involve dysregulation

Table 1
Angiogenesis/Vasculogenesis-Related Genes in Melanoma

Gene name	Biological function	Ratio
Melan-A (*MLANA*)	Melanoma surface antigen	0.044 (22)
Microphthalmia-associated transcription factor (*MITF*)	Melanocyte development TF	0.029 (34)
Tyrosinase (*TYR*)	Catalyzes the conversion of tyrosine to melanin	0.027 (37)
Tyrosinase-related protein I (*TYRP1*)	Catalyzes the conversion of tyrosine to melanin	0.004 (>100)
Melanoma cell-adhesion molecule (*MCAM*)	Cell-surface glycoprotein	27
TIE-1 (*TIE*)	Endothelial tyrosine kinase	25
Epithelial cell kinase (*EphA2*)	Receptor tyrosine kinase, ECK	13
VEGF-C (*VEGFC*)	flt-4 ligand	6.5
Neuropilin (*NRP1*)	VEGF receptor	5.3
VE–Cadherin, cadherin-5 (*CDH5*)	Cell–cell adhesion molecule	11
Selectin E (*SELE*)	Adhesion molecule	6.6
Endoglin (*ENG*)	TGF-β1 receptor	4.3
CD34	Stem cell marker, sialomucin	2.5
Hypoxia inducible factor 1α (*HIF1A*)	bHLH transcription factor	3.1
Tissue factor pathway inhibitor (*TFPI*)	Coagulation inhibitor	4.0
Tissue factor pathway inhibitor-2 (*TFPI2*)	Coagulation inhibitor	8.5
Laminin 5γ2 (*LAMC2*)	Extracellular matrix (ECM)	50
Fibronectin (*FN1*)	ECM	27
Collagen IV,α2 (*COL4A2*)	ECM	3.6
Fibrillin-1 (*FBN1*)	ECM	5.0
Endothelial differentiation receptor (*EDG1*)	G coupled receptor	3.7
Endothelial cell specific molecule (*ESM1*)	Endothelial-specific signaling molecule	41
Endothelial differentiation-related factor-1 (*EDF1*)	Endothelial cell differentiation regulator	4.8
Plasminogen activator inhibitor-1 (*PAI1*)	Serine protease inhibitor	31

TF, transcription factor; ECK, epithelial cell kinase; VEGF, vascular endothelial growth factor; TGF, transforming growth factor; bHLH, basic helix–loop–helix.

of the tumor-specific phenotype and a concomitant transdifferentiation of aggressive tumor cells into other cell types, such as endothelial cells, which may be detected using multiple phenotype-specific markers. These observations are significant because results from current angiogenesis inhibitor trials *(25)* suggest that new information regarding effective mechanisms to destroy tumor-associated vasculature in human models is needed in light of recent in vivo and in vitro studies that show that tumor cell VM is relatively unaffected by endostatin *(26)*.

Table 2
Hematopoietic-Associated Markers in Melanoma

Gene name	Biological function	Ratio
Neutral endopeptidase (*CALLA*)	Cell adhesion molecule, CD10	4.7
Hematopoietic-lineage cell-specific protein (*HCLS1*)	LYN tyrosine kinase substrate	5.7
Activated leukocyte cell adhesion molecule (*ALCAM*)	CD6 ligand	17.5
Lymphocyte-specific protein 1 (*LSP1*)	Signal transduction	2.9
Trophoblast-lymphocyte cross-reactive antigen (*MCP*)	Membrane cofactor protein, CD46	3.9
5' nucleotidase (*NT5*)	Lymphocyte differentiation, CD73	36
Macrophage maturation-associated protein (*MMA*)	Differentiation molecule	4.5

LYN, *lck/yes*-related novel tyrosine kinase.

MELANOMA VASCULOGENIC PHENOTYPE

Previous clinical studies in melanoma have shown a strong correlation between the appearance of ECM-rich (PAS positive), patterned, looping networks (resembling vasculogenic patterned networks) in aggressive tumors and poor disease outcome *(17–23)*. These looping networks were originally thought to provide a unique microcirculation to a growing tumor mass within certain areas of aggressive melanoma tumors that contained little vasculature and no necrosis. However, because the biological basis for VM was unclear at the time it was introduced in 1999 *(15)*, interpretation of these findings *(27)* was highly controversial (discussed further under "Biological Implications of VM"). Additional studies focused on the unique differences between highly aggressive and poorly aggressive melanomas in relation to VM, and revealed a number of interesting findings. Aggressive melanoma cells seeded on collagen I 3D matrices form *de novo* ECM-rich patterned networks that surround nests of tumor cells (Fig. 1), similar to the patterned, looping networks observed in histological sections of tumors from patients *(15,28)*. Furthermore, these in vitro networks were shown to be perfusable, by microinjecting a fluorescent dye into these structures (Fig. 1). However, unlike the aggressive melanoma cells, poorly aggressive melanoma cells did not form patterned networks under the same culture conditions *(2,15,28)*.

Molecular analyses of more than 45 human cutaneous and uveal melanoma cell lines revealed unusual and unexpected findings regarding the phenotype of aggressive tumors' cells *(1–3)* (highlights of selected differentially expressed genes from the molecular analyses are shown in Tables 1 and 2). Highly aggressive vs poorly aggressive melanoma cells, including genetically matched highly and poorly aggressive cell lines from melanoma patients, were hybridized to complementary cDNA microarrays, which allowed the simultaneous expression analysis of 6000 genes *(1)*. The spectrum of upregulated genes reflects multiple molecular phenotypes and includes those associated with progenitor cells, endothelia, epithelia, fibroblasts, hematopoietic lineage, kidney, neuronal lineage, muscle, pericytes, and placental cell types. This unusual expression of diverse phenotypes was also accompanied by the downregulation of many melanoma-specific proteins, except for melanoma cell-adhesion molecule, shown in Table 1.

The molecular profile suggests that aggressive melanoma cells exhibit a deregulated genotype with a genetic footprint reminiscent of an embryonic-like cell with an undifferentiated phenotype and leads to a major question under investigation at this time, which focuses on the regulation of melanocyte-associated genes. As such, it is interesting to note that microphthalmia-associated transcription factor is downregulated 34-fold in aggressive melanoma cells compared with poorly aggressive tumor cells (Table 1; ref. *1*). Microphthalmia-associated transcription factor activates expression of the gene that encodes tyrosinase, which is an enzyme involved in melanocyte differentiation *(29)*. The *tyrosinase* and *tyrosinase-related protein-1* genes are also downregulated by 37-fold and greater than 100-fold in the same tumor cells, respectively (Table 1), compared with poorly aggressive tumor cells, which indicates that several of the melanocyte-specific genes are diminished in aggressive melanoma. These results appear to suggest that aggressive melanoma cells have dedifferentiated *in situ* and may be more difficult to identify with routine histopathology methods.

Many of the genes upregulated by the aggressive cancer cells include those involved in angiogenesis and vasculogenesis, including vascular endothelial (VE)-cadherin (CD144 or cadherin 5); erythropoietin-producing hepatocellular carcinoma-A2 (EphA2); and laminin 5 γ2 chain (Table 1; refs. *28,30,31*). These molecules (and their binding partners) are required for the formation and maintenance of blood vessels *(4–6,32)*. VE-cadherin is an adhesive protein, which was previously considered to be endothelial cell specific, that belongs to the cadherin family of transmembrane proteins promoting homotypic cell-to-cell interaction *(33–36)*. EphA2 is a receptor protein tyrosine kinase that is part of a large family of ephrin receptors *(37)*, and when EphA2 binds to its ligand, ephrin-A1, EphA2 becomes phosphorylated on tyrosine. There is also evidence that EphA2 can be constitutively phosphorylated in unstimulated cells *(38)*. The high expression levels of EphA2 and ephrin-A1 have been associated with increased melanoma thickness and decreased survival, and the EphA2/ephrin-A1 pathway has been linked to tumor cell proliferation *(39,40)*.

Laminins are major components of basement membranes and are involved in neurite outgrowth, tumor metastasis, cell attachment and migration, and angiogenesis *(39,41,42)*. Proteolytic cleavage of laminin, particularly the laminin 5 γ2 chain, can alter and regulate the integrin-mediated migratory behavior of certain cells *(39,43–45)*, which suggests its potential importance as a molecular trigger in the microenvironment.

VE-cadherin, EphA2, and laminin 5 γ2 chain proteins are expressed only by aggressive tumor cells and not by nonaggressive or poorly aggressive melanoma cells *(28,30,31)*. The biological relevance of these molecules in VM was demonstrated by downregulating their expression independently and measuring the consequences on the formation of vasculogenic-like networks in vitro. These studies demonstrated that downregulation of VE-cadherin, EphA2, or laminin 5 γ2 chain results in the complete inability of aggressive melanoma cells to engage in the formation of vasculogenic-like networks in 3D culture *(28,30,31)*.

Additional experiments focused more closely on the aggressive tumor cell-associated ECM rather than the cells themselves. These studies revealed that a microenvironment preconditioned or remodeled by aggressive melanoma cells (and subsequent to their removal) can induce poorly aggressive melanoma cells to assume a vasculogenic and more migratory phenotype *(31)*. Furthermore, cooperative interactions between laminin 5 γ2 chain, matrix metalloproteinase (MMP-2), and membrane type-1 MMP (MT1-MMP) were shown to be required for melanoma VM, and laminin was observed to colocalize with PAS-positive VM networks in vitro and in vivo. These findings contributed to our present conceptual model: that highly aggressive melanoma cells deposit molecular messages or signals in their microenvironment (such as laminin 5 γ2' and γ2x promigratory fragments generated by proteolytic cleavage of laminin 5 γ2 chain by MT1-MMP and MMP-2) that may induce a vasculogenic phenotype in poorly aggressive cells, which results in the formation of vasculogenic-like networks and the concomitant expression of vascular-associated genes (VE-cadherin, EphA2, and laminin 5 γ2 chain; Fig. 2). In support of this model, the inductive potential of the tumor cell microenvironment can be abrogated using a potent inhibitor of MMP activity, COL-3 *(46)*, a chemically modified tetracycline.

VM SIGNALING CASCADE

The signal transduction pathways that regulate blood vessel formation and stabilization during vasculogenesis and angiogenesis are beginning to emerge *(5,47,48)* and an examination of the signaling events that regulate melanoma VM is in progress *(49)*. Microarray analysis led to the identification of EphA2 as an important receptor tyrosine kinase in melanoma VM *(28)*. Other key signal-transduction molecules in this process include VE-cadherin, focal adhesion kinase, and phosphoinositide 3-kinase (PI3K) *(50)*. Various experimental approaches are being used to provide a clearer understanding of the signaling cascade that facilitates melanoma VM, and a model highlighting some of the molecules involved is presented in Fig. 2. As shown in this model, phosphorylated EphA2 can colocalize with VE-cadherin on the membrane of highly aggressive melanoma cells. Furthermore, phosphorylated EphA2 can also associate with focal adhesion kinase. Because both VE-cadherin and EphA2 have been shown to activate PI3K in other systems, this would support placing the PI3K-signaling pathway downstream of EphA2 and VE-cadherin signaling. This is significant because recent studies have shown that inhibition of PI3K activity also inhibits VM *(49)*. Furthermore, inhibition of PI3K activity appears to directly affect the regulation of MT1-MMP expression and activity and the subsequent activation of MMP-2, which are required for VM *(31)*. This model suggests key molecular pathways involved in regulating melanoma cell VM and, with additional studies, could provide a basis for designing new therapeutic strategies for targeting the aggressive melanoma phenotype.

BIOLOGICAL IMPLICATIONS OF VM

As with many studies that introduce new concepts, several interpretations of VM have evolved based on various analyses of the original findings. These published studies have reported several scenarios related to VM. Although initial studies focused on a description of PAS-stained patterned networks in tumors, others referred to tumor cells that line spaces or channels containing RBCs or blood lakes. Although subsequent studies equated VM to tumor cells that express endothelial-specific genes, it is also possible that a combination of any of the above scenarios is associated with VM in aggressive cancers. To confuse the point further, the term "vascular mimicry" has been used synonymously with VM, which carries broader implications because it could apply to other vascular-

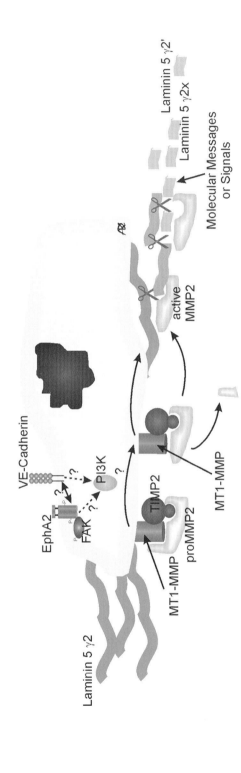

Fig. 2. Vasculogenic mimicry (VM) signaling cascade. The diagram represents a model of the signal-transduction events underlying melanoma tumor cell VM. In this model, phosphorylated epithelial cell kinase (EphA2) and vascular endothelial (VE)-cadherin are colocalized at the cell membrane. Phosphorylated EphA2 subsequently interacts with focal adhesion kinase (FAK), which results in its phosphorylation on key tyrosine residues. The signal-transduction pathways activated by both EphA2 and VE-cadherin may converge to activate phosphoinositide-3 kinase (PI3K). Downstream, PI3K regulates membrane type-1 matrix-metalloproteinase (MT1-MMP) activity, which subsequently activates MMP-2 as an MT1-MMP/tissue inhibitor of metalloproteinase-2 (TIMP-2) pro-MMP-2 ternary complex. Both MT1-MMP and MMP-2 may then promote the cleavage of laminin 5 γ2 chain into promigratory γ2′ and γ2x fragments. The formation of these fragments (molecular messages or signals) into the tumor microenvironment may increase migration, invasion, and, ultimately, VM by aggressive melanoma tumor cells. (Illustration by Dr. Dawn A. Kirschmann.)

associated cell types, such as lymphocytes and macrophages, which represent other molecular phenotypes that could also be expressed by aggressive tumor cells (shown in Table 2).

Subsequent studies that have attempted to address the functional significance of VM in human melanoma and in xenograft models are far more complex than the in vitro cellular and molecular investigations and have generated more questions than answers about the relevance of the in vivo studies. At present, there are two major questions regarding melanoma VM that have been formulated. First, is there a morphological and functional connection between melanoma tumor cell-lined networks and endothelial-lined vasculature? Second, based on their vascular phenotype, is it possible for aggressive melanoma cells to provide a vascular function when challenged to an ischemic, nontumor microenvironment?

The first question addresses a potential biological and functional connection between tumor cell-lined PAS and laminin-positive matrix networks within aggressive melanoma tumors and endothelial-lined vasculature. Several studies in aggressive melanomas (and other tumors, before the introduction of VM) reported that tumor cells could line channels, lakes, and sinuses, and have direct contact with RBCs *(51–53)*. It was unclear, however, whether this was relevant to the functional provision of a blood supply to a growing tumor mass. The prevailing hypothesis at this time was that any blood (RBCs) found in extravascular spaces was probably caused by leaky vessels *(54)*. Additional work showed that PAS-positive patterned networks found in aggressive melanoma tumors and associated with poor clinical outcome *(17–23)* appeared to morphologically converge with blood vessels *(15,16)*. These observations suggested that a putative anastomosis occurred between the tumor cell-lined networks and the endothelial-lined vasculature and contributed to the source of occasional RBCs observed within the network infrastructure *(15)*. This assumption led to the speculation that the tumor cell-lined networks may provide a unique paracirculation that might occur independently of or simultaneously with angiogenesis and/or vessel co-option. Although this is a very complex phenomenon requiring rigorous scientific scrutiny, an orthotopic model for human uveal melanoma in severe combined immunodeficient mice, which might provide important new insights, has been developed to study the generation of the unique network patterning that is characteristic of genetically deregulated aggressive melanoma cells *(55)*.

Significant new findings pertinent to addressing the first question have revealed the presence of a fluid-conducting meshwork (depicted in Fig. 3) in xenografts of human cutaneous and uveal melanoma that corresponds to the PAS- and laminin-positive patterned networks that consist of matrix networks of arcs and back-to-back loops *(56–57)*. Using a combination of intravenous tracers, together with routine, confocal, and immunoelectron microscopy, these studies showed that tracers are found inside traditional, endothelial-lined vasculature and extravascularly along channel-like spaces created by PAS- and laminin-positive patterned loops and networks encasing nests of tumor cells *(56–58)*. This "fluid-conducting meshwork" also contained plasma around the tumor cell-lined nests *(57)*. The plasma, as well as RBCs that were observed in some of the tumors formed PAS- and laminin-positive loops and networks, is likely to be derived from local tumor vessels that are leaky and undergoing remodeling. Although the functional relevance of this finding is still unclear, several theoretical possibilities may exist. The fluid-conducting meshwork may:

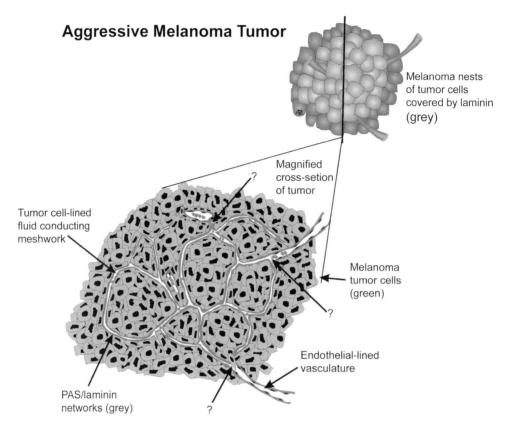

Fig. 3. Model of a melanoma tumor. The biological implications of melanoma vasculogenic mimicry have evolved to a tumor cell-lined fluid-conducting meshwork corresponding to the previously described periodic acid-Schiff-positive and laminin-positive patterned networks. This artistic diagram represents the current interpretation of data generated from several studies *(56–58,61)* involving the use of tracers and perfusion analyses of mice containing aggressive melanoma cells (green) during tumor development. Although the endothelial-lined vasculature is closely apposed to the tumor cell-formed fluid-conducting meshwork, it is presumed, hypothetically, that as the tumor remodels the vasculature, it may become leaky and result in the extravascular conduction of plasma and some red blood cells. However, the biological implication(s) and relationship of the laminin-rich fluid-conducting meshwork to endothelial-lined vasculature is still under investigation. (Illustration by Dr. Dawn A. Kirschmann.)

1. Provide a nutritional exchange for aggressive tumors that might prevent early necrosis.
2. Be analogous to an edematous inflammatory response, in which increased pressure leads to the escape of fluid along connective tissue pathways within intratissue spaces.
3. Act as a suppressive shield against immune surveillance as a result of the complex geometry of the laminin ECM covering that encases the nests of tumor cells.

At present, the consensus is that the microcirculation of aggressive tumors is very complex and, depending on the window of observation, may consist of mosaic vessels *(59)*, co-opted vessels *(60)*, and angiogenic vessels *(7–14)*. There is also strong evidence for intratumoral, tumor cell-lined, ECM-rich patterned networks capable of providing an extravascular fluid pathway, called a fluid-conducting meshwork *(56,57)*. The entire microcirculation in aggressive tumors, therefore, appears to be a combination of these elements and results from destructive tumor growth and remodeling.

Recent studies have used a nude mouse model injected subcutaneously with fluorescent-tagged aggressive human cutaneous melanoma cells to study the blood supply to primary tumors *(61)*. Perfusion of the mouse vasculature with a fluorescent tag and microbeads during tumor development was imaged using confocal microscopy and revealed the close approximation of tumor cell-lined networks with angiogenic mouse vessels at the human–mouse interface. The delivery of microbeads from the endothelial-lined mouse vasculature to the tumor cell-lined networks may indicate a physiological connection between the two compartments. As summarized in Fig. 3, further destructive growth of melanoma into the vasculature led to the observation of RBCs and plasma (presumably caused by leakage) into the tumor cell-lined fluid-conducting meshwork. However, the question of whether a direct morphological and physiological anastomosis exists between endothelial-lined vasculature and tumor cell-lined fluid-conducting meshwork still remains enigmatic.

Attempts are underway to assess physiological blood flow using color Doppler imaging of human melanoma xenografts. Initial work has demonstrated pulsatile turbulent flow at the mouse–human tissue interface (with mouse endothelial-lined neovasculature) and the central region of the tumor, containing melanoma cell-lined networks *(62)*. This functional exchange of blood through a tumor cell-lined meshwork (rich in laminin) could be caused by the overexpression of anticoagulant factors tissue factor pathway inhibitors -1 and -2 by aggressive melanoma cells (Table 1). These tumor cells appear to exhibit similar anticoagulant mechanisms as endothelial cells, which may contribute to the perfusability of the fluid-conducting meshwork. Although these findings are intriguing, more detailed analyses are required to understand the precise sequence of events associated with the establishment of vascularization during tumor growth and remodeling in highly aggressive vs poorly aggressive tumors vs normal tissues.

Another possible fate for the PAS/laminin-rich fluid-conducting meshwork is that it represents an early survival mechanism for nutrient exchange and fluid pressure release. It is also possible that this infrastructure might be subsequently replaced by endothelial cells from either nearby angiogenic vessels or from the bone marrow *(63)*. This intriguing possibility may provide a different perspective on the vasculogenic phenotype of melanoma cells that line these matrix meshworks and appear to disseminate through them, and will require a higher standard of discrimination to unequivocally identify melanoma cells from endothelial cells.

An additional enigmatic finding is the unexpected overexpression by aggressive melanoma cells of VE growth factor *(VEGF)-C*, a lymphangiogenesis-associated gene and growth factor for lymphatic vessels (Table 1). It is interesting that despite the fact that uveal melanomas lack traditional lymphatic vessels, overexpression of VEGF-C has been found by Clarijs and coworkers *(64)*. Although lymphangiogenesis often accompanies angiogenesis, this field has been understudied but is now gaining momentum with new research tools *(65–67)*. Research by Ruoslahti and colleagues have shown localization of the lymphatic vessel marker, LYVE-1, within aggressive cutaneous melanoma *(68)*. These results raise an intriguing possibility that the fluid-conducting meshwork could mimic a lymphatic-like network, with circulating fluid and proteins that might leak out of the blood vasculature.

The second question under investigation concerning the biological implications of VM focuses on the plasticity of aggressive melanoma cells. Experiments have been conducted to challenge melanoma cells to an ischemic, nontumor environment and then assess whether they would participate in neovascularization and/or form a tumor mass. In this study *(69)*, fluorescently tagged human cutaneous metastatic melanoma cells were injected into ischemic hindlimbs of nude mice. After 5 d, the limb vasculature was reperfused. Histological cross-sections of newly formed vasculature of reperfused limbs showed human melanoma cells adjacent to and overlapping with mouse endothelial cells in a linear arrangement and forming chimeric vessels. This evidence demonstrated the powerful influence of the microenvironment on the transendothelial differentiation of malignant melanoma cells involved in neovascularization and reperfusion.

In our investigation of ischemic limb reperfusion, we examined selected Notch proteins that promote the differentiation of endothelial cells into vascular networks *(70,71)*. Notch 4 was highly expressed by malignant melanoma cells as they participated in neovascularization. Activated Notch 4 expression has also been detected in patients' invasive melanomas (personal communication, B. Nickoloff), and interruption of Notch signaling triggers apoptosis of malignant melanoma *(72)*. Notch signaling molecules are integrally involved in cell fate determination of stem cells, particularly angioblasts, and nonterminally differentiated cell types *(70,71)*. Alterations in Notch expression and signaling have also been implicated in human T-cell leukemia *(73)*, cervical carcinoma *(74)*, murine mammary carcinoma *(75)*, prostatic tumor progression *(76)*, and human *Ras*-transformed cells *(77)*. Notch signaling molecules may offer new clues into the regulation of cell fate decision-making pathways that are triggered in the undifferentiated tumor cell phenotype characteristic of aggressive melanoma cells.

These observations advance our understanding of the remarkable inductive nature of the microenvironment on aggressive tumor cells that express vasculogenic/angiogenic/lymphatic molecules, together with cell-fate determination proteins, associated with a transendothelial phenotype. These findings present new possibilities for therapeutic strategies and novel perspectives on tumor cell plasticity, and emphasize the importance of early differentiation pathways, such as those involved in Notch signaling (for review, *see* ref. *78*).

CONCLUSIONS AND PERSPECTIVES

The scientific tools currently available to examine the molecular signature of cancer cells and tissues have contributed significantly to our understanding of the molecular basis of tumor progression (for review, *see* ref. *79*). The molecular analyses of various cancers, particularly melanoma, have generated more questions than answers concerning the biological relevance of the multiple molecular phenotypes expressed by aggressive tumor cells. The implications of these findings pose a significant clinical challenge for the detection and targeting of aggressive cancer cells that could look like endothelia, angioblasts, leukocytes, macrophages, or other cell types. Nonetheless, great hope has been placed in the promise of microarray technology in the classification and clinical management of melanoma *(1,80)*. Without question, the "plastic" phenotype of aggressive melanoma (and other tumor types) confounds the fields of pathology and cancer biology, with respect to properly evaluating both tumor blood supply and microvascular density *(81)*, in particular.

Because aggressive cancer cells can phenotypically mimic other cell types, it is important to improve the detection methodology that is currently applied to identify or discriminate these cells from normal endothelial cells. This could involve the use of two phenotype-specific detection markers, which is highly recommended when studying aggressive melanoma *in situ*—one marker should be tumor specific and the second marker could be endothelial cell specific.

Adding to the clinical challenge is the emerging concept of cancer stem cells *(82)*. Recent studies have challenged previously held dogma with respect to tissue-restricted differentiation of postnatal stem cells, with evidence that demonstrates pluripotency for mesenchymal, neural, and hematopoietic cells *(83–86)*. Transdifferentiation is also emerging as an important phenomenon that adds a new level of complexity to developing rational therapeutic strategies *(87–90)*. In Kaposi's sarcoma, it is interesting to note that endothelial cells transdifferentiate into tumor cells *(91)*, whereas, in aggressive melanoma, these tumor cells transdifferentiate into an endothelial cell phenotype. These observations raise the intriguing possibility that these two cell types may share a common origin or lineage, as well as cell fate determination pathways. Although we have focused on melanoma VM with respect to providing a possible perfusion pathway and dissemination route in aggressive tumors, the mimicry of other cell phenotypes could also provide an evasion mechanism from immune surveillance, based on the expression of genes that are associated with normal cell phenotypes. This is a daunting speculation and will require rigorous scientific investigation.

Although VM is just one example of tumor cell plasticity *(92)*, relatively little is known concerning the molecular switch regulating this event. Our observations indicate that VE-cadherin, EphA2, laminin 5 γ2 chain, MMPs, and Notch proteins are major components of the vasculogenic switch, and current strategies are under assessment to mediate or inhibit their activity. For example, although monoclonal antibodies to VE-cadherin have been shown to inhibit endothelial cell-driven angiogenesis in Lewis lung and epidermoid tumors *(93)*, it remains to be seen whether this therapeutic approach will have widespread use in other tumors. Also, blocking Notch 4 activation triggers rapid apoptosis in melanoma cells, and interference of Notch signaling in melanoma results in the downregulation of the vasculogenic phenotype *(72)*. This novel approach capitalizes on targeting an early angioblast determination gene (*Notch*), and may have significant therapeutic potential not only in melanoma, but also in several other aggressive cancers in which Notch proteins are overexpressed.

A great deal of thought and effort has been devoted to targeting angiogenesis and lymphangiogenesis in cancer patients *(7–10,14,32,65–68,94–101)*. The heterogeneity of the tumor vasculature presents not only an opportunity, but also a significant clinical challenge, which includes issues of drug resistance *(94,99,102,103)*. One approach that appears successful is to target unique molecules on the tumor cell surface that could be expressed concomitantly by both tumor and endothelial cells. Another approach is examining the potential differential effect(s) of angiogenesis inhibitors on tumor cells compared with endothelial cells. Recent studies have demonstrated that although endostatin inhibits endothelial cell-driven angiogenesis, it does not inhibit melanoma cell VM, as shown in Fig. 4 *(26)*. Similar observations have been achieved in vivo by Sausville and colleagues *(104)*. A molecular analysis of endothelial associated genes, including *VE-cadherin* and *EphA2*, revealed that expression of these genes is reduced in the endostatin-treated endothelial cells but remain unaffected in the melanoma cells

Endothelial cells treated
with endostatin

Melanoma cells treated
with endostatin

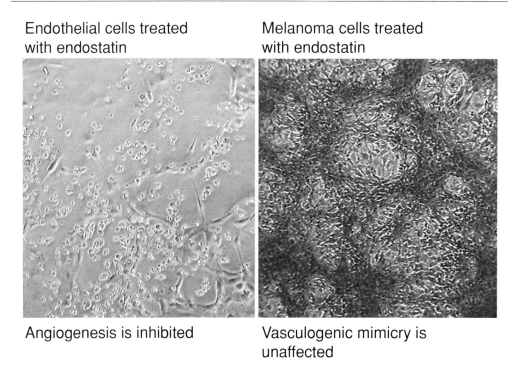

Angiogenesis is inhibited

Vasculogenic mimicry is
unaffected

Fig. 4. The differential effects of endostatin (an angiogenesis inhibitor) on endothelial cells vs melanoma cells in three-dimensional collagen I gels in vitro. Phase contrast microscopy of human microvascular endothelial cells treated with endostatin (left panel) showing inhibition of angiogenesis vs human aggressive melanoma cells treated similarly (right panel), where vasculogenic mimicry network formation is unaffected.

(26). This may indicate a differential response from two different vascular cell phenotypes and suggest key areas to target for the development of more effective antivascular therapies.

Last, although matrix metalloproteinase-inhibitor trials have experienced some challenges, recent observations suggest that this class of proteinases and other matrix-remodeling proteinases are worth further consideration in targeting the tumor microenvironment *(46,105–107)*. As we learn more about the promigratory inductive potential of specific proteolytically cleaved fragments of the ECM, we find that these partially degraded molecules may be prime targets for therapeutic intervention—potentially for use in a combinatorial manner with other therapies that specifically target tumor cells and/or endothelia.

Successful management of malignant melanoma and other aggressive cancers may result in targeting one or more sites in the VM cascade. Furthermore, identification of essential regulatory pathways targeting the undifferentiated, "plastic" tumor cell phenotype, that do not interfere with normal biological processes, holds promise for the generation of new therapeutic strategies. The field of angiogenesis and antivascular targeting contains both challenges and hope as we continue to explore these intriguing scientific questions.

REFERENCES

1. Bittner M, Meltzer P, Chen Y, et al. Molecular classification of cutaneous malignant melanoma by gene expression profiling. Nature 2000;406:536–540.
2. Seftor EA, Seftor, Meltzer PS, et al. Molecular determinants of human uveal melanoma invasion and metastasis. Clin Exp Metastas 2002;19:233–246.
3. Seftor EA, Meltzer PS, Schatteman GC, et al. Expression of multiple molecular phenotypes by aggressive melanoma tumor cells: role in vasculogenic mimicry. Crit Rev Oncol Hematol 2002;44:17–27.
4. Risau W. Mechanisms of angiogenesis. Nature 1997;386:671–674.
5. Carmeliet P. Mechanisms of angiogenesis and arteriogenesis. Nat Med 2000;6:389–395.
6. Tomanek RJ, ed. Assembly of the Vasculature and Its Regulation. Birkhauser, Boston, MA: 2002.
7. Folkman J. Seminars in Medicine of the Beth Israel Hospital, Boston. Clinical applications of research on angiogenesis. New Eng J Med 1995;333:1757–1763.
8. Rak J, Kerbel RS. Treating cancer by inhibiting angiogenesis: new hopes and potential pitfalls. Cancer Metastas Rev 1996;15:231–236.
9. Kumar R, Fidler IJ. Angiogenic molecules and cancer metastasis. In Vivo 1998;12:27–34.
10. Carmeliet P, Jain RK. Angiogenesis in cancer and other diseases. Nature 2000;407:249–257.
11. Gullino PM. Angiogenesis and oncogenesis. J Natl Cancer Inst 1978;61:639–643.
12. Hanahan D, Weinberg RA. The hallmarks of cancer. Cell 2000;100:57–70.
13. Bouck N, Stellmach V, Hsu SC. How tumors become angiogenic. Adv Cancer Res 1996;69:135–174.
14. Kerbel RS. Tumor angiogenesis: past, present and the near future. Carcinogenesis 2000;21:505–515.
15. Maniotis AJ, Folberg R, Hess A, et al. Vascular channel formation by human melanoma cells in vivo and in vitro: vasculogenic mimicry. Am J Pathol 1999;155:739–752.
16. Folberg R, Hendrix MJC, Maniotis AJ. Vasculogenic mimicry and tumor angiogenesis. Am J Pathol 2000;156:361–381.
17. Folberg R, Rummelt V, Parys-Van Ginderdeuren R, et al. Prognostic value of tumor blood vessel morphology in primary uveal melanoma. Ophthalmology 1993;100:1389–1398.
18. Makitie T, Summanen P, Tarkkanen A, Kivela T. Microvascular loops and neworks as prognostic indicators in choroidal and ciliary body melanomas. J Natl Cancer Inst 1999;91:359–367.
19. Sakamoto T, Sakamoto M, Yoshikawa H, et al. Histologic findings and prognosis of uveal malignant melanoma in Japanese patients. Am J Ophthalmol 1996;121:276–283.
20. Seregard S, Spangberg B, Juul C, Oskarsson M. Prognostic accuracy of the mean of the largest nucleoli, vascular patterns, and PC-10 in posterior uveal melanoma. Ophthalmology 1998; 105:485–491.
21. Thies A, Mangold U, Moll I, Schumacher U. PAS-positive loops and networks as a prognostic indicator in cutaneous malignant melanoma. J Pathol 2001;195:537–542.
22. Warso MA, Maniotis AJ, Chen X, et al. Prognostic significance of periodic acid-Schiff-positive patterns in primary cutaneous melanoma. Clin Cancer Res 2001;7:473–477.
23. Rummelt V, Mehaffey MG, Campbell RF, et al. Microcirculation architecture of metastases from primary ciliary body and choroidal melanomas. Am J Ophthalmol 1998;126:303–305.
24. Shirakawa K, Kobayashi H, Heike Y, et al. Hemodynamics in vasculogenic mimicry and angiogenesis of inflammatory breast cancer xenograft. Cancer Res 2002;62:560–566.
25. Garber K. Angiogenesis inhibitors suffer new setback. Nat Biotech 2002;20:1067–1068.
26. van der Schaft DWJ, Seftor, EA, Hess AR, et al. The differential effects of angiogenesis inhibitors on vascular network formation by endothelial cells versus aggressive melanoma tumor cells. Proc AACR 2003;44:696.
27. McDonald DM, Munn L, Jain RK. Vasculogenic mimicry: how convincing, how novel, and how significant? Am J Pathol 2000;156:383–388.
28. Hess AR, Seftor EA, Gardner LMG, et al. Molecular regulation of tumor cell vasculogenic mimicry by tyrosine phosphorylation: role of epithelial cell kinase (Eck/EphA2). Cancer Res 2001;61: 3250–3255.
29. Tachibana M, Takeda K, Nobukuni Y, et al. Ectopic expression of MITF, a gene for Waardenburg syndrome type 2, converts fibroblasts to cells with melanocytes characteristics. Nat Genet 1996; 14:50–54.
30. Hendrix MJC, Seftor EA, Meltzer PS, et al. Expression and functional significance of VE-cadherin in aggressive human melanoma cells: role in vasculogenic mimicry. Proc Natl Acad Sci USA 2001;98:8018–8023.

31. Seftor REB, Seftor EA, Koshikawa N, et al. Cooperative interactions of laminin 5 γ2 chain, matrix metalloproteinase-2, and membrane type-1-matrix/metalloproteinase are required for mimicry of embryonic vasculogenesis by aggressive melanoma. Cancer Res 2001;61:6322–6327.
32. Hynes RO, Bader BL, Hodivala-Diik K. Integrins in vascular development. Braz J Med Biol Res 1999;32:501–510.
33. Hynes RO. Specificity of cell adhesion in development: the cadherin superfamily. Curr Opin Genet Dev 1992;2:621–624.
34. Kemler R. Classical cadherins. Semin Cell Biol 1992;3:149–155.
35. Lampugnani MG. A novel endothelial-specific membrane protein is a marker of cell–cell contacts. J Cell Biol 1992;118:1511–1522.
36. Gumbiner BM. Cell adhesion: the molecular basis of tissue architecture and morphogenesis. Cell 1996;4:345–357.
37. Pasquale EB. The Eph family of receptors. Curr Opin Cell Biol 1997;9:608–615.
38. Rosenburg IM, Goke M, Kana, M, Reinecker HC, Podolsky DK. Epithelial cell kinase-B-61: an autocrine loop modulating intestinal epithelial migration and barrier function. Am J Physiol 1997; 273(4 part 1):G824–G832.
39. Straume O, Akslen LA. Importance of vascular phenotype by basic fibrolast growth factor, and influence of the angiogenic factors basic fibroblast growth factor/fibroblast growth factor receptor-1 and Ephrin-A1/EphA2 on melanoma progression. Am J Pathol 2001;160:1009–1019.
40. Easty DJ, Hill SP, Hsu MY, et al. Up-regulation of ephrin-A1 during melanoma progression. Int J Cancer 1999;84:494–501.
41. Malinda KM, Kleinman HK. The laminins. Int J Biochem Cell Biol 1996;28:957–995.
42. Colognato H, Yurchenco PD. Form and function: the laminin family of heterotrimers. Dev Dynamics 2000;218:213–234.
43. Malinda KM, Nomizu M, Chung M, et al. Identification of laminin α1 and β1 chain peptides active for endothelial cell adhesion, tube formation, and aortic sprouting. FASEB J 1999;13:53–62.
44. Koshikawa N, Giannelli G, Cirulli V, Miyazaki K, Quaranta V. Role of cell surface metalloprotease MT1-MMP in epithelial cell migration over laminin-5. J Cell Biol 2000;148:615–624.
45. Giannelli G, Falk-Marzillier J, Schiraldi O, Stetler-Stevenson WG, Quaranta V. Induction of cell migration by matrix metalloprotease-2 cleavage of laminin-5. Science 1997;277:225–228.
46. Seftor REB, Seftor EA, Kirschmann DA, Hendrix MJC. Targeting the tumor microenvironment with chemically modified tetracyclines: inhibition of laminin 5 γ2 chain promigratory fragments and vasculogenic mimicry. Mol Cancer Therapeut 2002;1:1173–1179.
47. Korpelainen EI, Alitalo K. Signaling angiogenesis and lymphangiogenesis. Curr Opin Cell Biol 1998;10:159–164.
48. Yancopoulos DG, Davis S, Gale NW, Rudge JS, Wiegand SJ, Holash J. Vascular-specific growth factors and blood vessel formation. Nature 2000;407:242–248.
49. Hess AR, Seftor EA, Seftor REB, Hendrix MJC. Phosphoinositide 3-kinase acts downstream of EphA2 to regulate the membrane-type 1 matrix metalloproteinase (MT1-MMP) and matrix metalloproteinase-2 (MMP-2) promoting vasculogenic mimicry in vitro. Mol Biol Cell 2002; 13:210A.
50. Hess AR. Molecular dissection of melanoma tumor cell vasculogenic mimicry. Doctoral Dissertation, The University of Iowa: 2002.
51. Shubik P, Warren BA. Additional literature on "vasculogenic mimicry" not cited. Am J Pathol 2000;156:736.
52. Warren BA, Shubik P. The growth of the blood supply to melanoma transplants in the hamster cheek pouch. Lab Invest 1966;15:464–478.
53. Tímár J, Tóth J. Tumor sinuses-vascular channels. Pathol Oncol Res 2000;6(2):83–86.
54. Hashizume H, Baluk P, Morikawa S, et al. Openings between defective endothelial cells explain tumor vessel leakiness. Am J Pathol 2000;156:1363–1380.
55. Mueller AJ, Maniotis AJ, Freeman WR, et al. An orthotopic model for human uveal melanoma in SCID mice. Microvasc Res 2002;64:207–213.
56. Clarijs R, Otte-Holler I, Ruiter DJ, de Waal RMW. Presence of a fluid-conducting meshwork in xenografted cutaneous and primary human uveal melanoma. Invest Ophthalmol Vis Sci 2002; 43:912–918.
57. Maniotis AJ, Chen X, Garcia C, et al. Control of melanoma morphogenesis, endothelial survival, and perfusion by extracellular matrix. Lab Invest 2002;82:1031–1043.

58. Potgens AJG, van Altena MC, Lubsen NH, Ruiter DJ, de Waal RMW. Analysis of the tumor vasculature and metastatic behavior of xenografts of human melanoma cell lines transfected with vascular permeability factor. Am J Pathol 1996;148:1203–1217.

59. Chang YS, di Tomaso E, McDonald DM, Jones R, Jain RK, Munn LL. Mosaic blood vessels in tumors: frequency of cancer cells in contact with flowing blood. Proc Natl Acad Sci USA 2000;97: 14,608–14,613.

60. Döme B, Paku S, Somlai B, Tímár J. Vascularization of cutaneous melanoma involves vessel co-option and has clinical significance. J Pathol 2002;197:355–362.

61. Hendrix MJC, Seftor EA, Meltzer PS, et al. The plasticity of aggressive melanoma tumor cells: recapitulation of an embryonic stem cell program. Rec Adv Res Updates 2002;3:191–200.

62. Ruf W, Seftor EA, Petrovan R, et al. Differential role of tissue factor pathway inhibitor-1 and 2 (TFPI-1 and 2) in melanoma vasculogenic mimicry. Cancer Res 2003;63:5381–5389.

63. Hattori K, Heissig B, Wu Y, et al. Placental growth factor reconstitutes hematopoiesis by recruiting VEGFR1+ stem cells from bone-marrow microenvironment. Nat Med 2002;8:841–849.

64. Clarijs R, Schalkwijk L, Ruiter DJ, de Waal RMW. Lack of lymphangiogenesis despite coexpression of VEGF-C and its receptor Flt-4 in uveal melanoma. Invest Ophthalmol Vis Sci 2001;42:1422–1428.

65. Witte MH, Bernas MJ, Martin CP, Witte CL. Lymphangiogenesis and lymphangiodysplasia: from molecular to clinical lymphology. Microscopy Res Tech 2001;55:122–145.

66. Alitalo K, Carmeliet P. Molecular mechanisms of lymphangiogenesis in health and disease. Cancer Cell 2002;1:219–227.

67. Padera TP, Kadambi A, Di Tomaso E, et al. Lymphatic metastasis in the absence of functional intratumor lymphatics. Science 2002;296:1883–1886.

68. Laakkonen P, Porkka K, Hoffman JA, Ruoslahti E. A tumor-homing peptide with a targeting specificity related to lymphatic vessels. Nat Med 2002;8:751–755.

69. Hendrix MJC, Seftor REB, Seftor EA, et al. Transendothelial function of human metastatic melanoma cells: role of the microenvironment in cell-fate determination. Cancer Res 2002;62:665–668.

70. Uyttendaele H, Ho J, Rossant J, Kitajewski J. Vascular patterning defects associated with expression of activated Notch4 in embryonic endothelium. Proc Natl Acad Sci USA 2001;98:5643–5648.

71. Gridley T. Notch signaling during vascular development. Proc Natl Acad Sci USA 2001;98: 10,733–10,738.

72. Qin J-Z, Chaturvedi V, Hendrix MJC, et al. Interrupting activated Notch signaling triggers apoptosis in melanoma cells. Soc Intern Invest Derm 2003;0185.

73. Ellisen LW, Bird J, West DC, et al. TAN-1, the human homolog of the Drosophila notch gene, is broken by chromosomal translocations in T lymphoblastic neoplasms. Cell 1991;66:649–661.

74. Robbins J, Blonel BJ, Gallahan D, Callahan R. Mouse mammary tumor gene Int-3: a member of the Notch gene family transforms mammary epithelial cells. J Virol 1992;66:2594–2599.

75. Zagouras P, Stifani S, Blaumueller CM, Carcangiu ML, Artavanis-Tsakonas S. Alterations in Notch signaling in neoplastic lesions of the human cervix. Proc Natl Acad Sci USA 1995;92:6414–6418.

76. Shou J, Ross S, Koeppen H, de Sauvage FJ, Gao W-Q. Dynamics of Notch expression during murine prostate development and tumorigenesis. Cancer Res 2001;61:7291–7297.

77. Weijzen S, Rizzo P, Braid M, et al. Activation of Notch-1 signaling maintains the neoplastic phenotype in human Ras-transformed cells. Nature Med 2002;8:979–986.

78. Allenspach EJ, Maillard I, Aster JC, Pear WS. Notch signaling in cancer. Cancer Biol Therapy 2002;1:466–476.

79. Klausner RD. The fabric of cancer cell biology—weaving together the strands. Cancer Cell 2002;1:3–10.

80. Kim CJ, Reintgen DS, Yeatman TJ. The promise of microarray technology in melanoma care. Cancer Control 2002;9:49–53.

81. Chen X, Maniotis AJ, Majumdar D, Pe'er J, Folberg R. Uveal melanoma cells staining for CD34 and assessment of tumor vascularity. Invest Ophthalmol Vis Sci 2002;43:2533–2539.

82. Reya T, Morrison SJ, Clarke MF, Weissman IL. Stem cells, cancer, and cancer stem cells. Nature 2001;414:105–111.

83. Anderson DJ, Gage FH, Weissman L. Can stem cells cross lineage boundaries? Nature Med 2001;7:393–395.

84. Weissman IL. Stem cells: units of development, units of regeneration, and units in evolution. Cell 2000;100:157–168.

85. Ivanova NB, Dimos JT, Schaniel C, Hackney JA, Moore KA, Lemischka IR. A stem cell molecular signature. Science 2002;298:601–604.
86. Ramalho-Santos M, Yoon S, Matsuzaki Y, Mulligan RC, Melton DA. "Stemness": transcriptional profiling of embryonic and adult stem cells. Science 2002;298:597–600.
87. Stocum DL. A tail of transdifferentiation. Science 2002;298:1901–1903.
88. LaBarge MA, Blau HM. Biological progression from adult bone marrow to mononucleate muscle stem cell to multinucleate muscle fiber in response to injury. Cell 2002;111:589–601.
89. Kon K, Fujiwara T. Transformation of fibroblasts into endothelial cells during angiogenesis. Cell Tissue Res 1994;278:625–628.
90. Condorelli G, Borello U, De Angelis L, et al. Cardiomyocytes induce endothelial cells to transdifferentiate into cardiac muscle: implications for myocardium regeneration. Proc Natl Acad Sci USA 2001;98:10,733–10,738.
91. Nickoloff BJ, Foreman KE. Etiology and pathogenesis of Kaposi's sarcoma. Recent Results Cancer Res 2002;160:332–342.
92. Bissell MJ, Radisky D. Putting tumors in context. Nat Rev Cancer 2001;1:46–54.
93. Liao F, Li Y, O'Connor W, et al. Monoclonal antibody to vascular endothelial-cadherin is a potent inhibitor of angiogenesis, tumor growth, and metastasis. Cancer Res 2000;60:6805–6810.
94. Pasqualini R, Arap W, McDonald DM. Probing the structural and molecular diversity of tumor vasculature. Trends Mol Med 2002;8:563–571.
95. Jain RK. Normalizing tumor vasculature with anti-angiogenic therapy: a new paradigm for combination therapy. Nat Med 2001;7:987–989.
96. O'Reilly MS. Vessel maneuvers: vaccine targets tumor vasculature. Nat Med 2002;8:1352–1354.
97. Miller KD, Sweeney CJ, Sledge GW Jr. The snark is a boojum: the continuing problem of drug resistance in the antiangiogenic era. Ann Oncol 2003;14:20–28.
98. Scappaticci FA. Mechanisms and future directions for angiogenesis-based cancer therapies. J Clin Oncol 2002;20:3906–3927.
99. Gee MS, Procopio WM, Makonnen S, Feldman MD, Yeilding NM, Lee WM. Tumor vessel development and maturation impose limits on th effectiveness of anti-vascular therapy. Am J Pathol 2003;162:183–193.
100. Goetz DE, Yu JL, Kerbel RS, Burns PN, Foster FS. High-frequency Doppler ultrasound monitors the effects of antivascular therapy on tumor blood flow. Cancer Res 2002;62:6371–6375.
101. Hood JD, Bednarski M, Frausto R, et al. Tumor regression by targeted gene delivery to the neovasculature. Science 2002;296:2404–2407.
102. Grossman D, Altieri DC. Drug resistance in melanoma: mechanisms, apoptosis, and new potential therapeutic targets. Cancer Metast Rev 2001;20:3–11.
103. Eberhard A, Kahlert S, Goede V, Hemerlein B, Plate KH, Augustin HG. Heterogeneity of angiogenesis and blood vessel maturation in human tumors: implications for antiangiogenic tumor therapies. Cancer Res 2000;60:1388–1393.
104. Ryback SM, Sanovich E, Hollingshead MG, et al. "Vasocrine" formation of tumor cell-lined vascular spaces: implications for rationale design of antiangiogenic therapies. Cancer Res 2003;63:2812–2819.
105. Coussens LM, Fingleton B, Matrisian LM. Matrix metalloproteinase inhibitors and cancer: trials and tribulations. Science 2002;295:2387–2392.
106. Egeblad M, Werb Z. New functions for the matrix metalloproteinases in cancer progression. Nat Rev Cancer 2002;2:161–174.   107.   Liotta LA, Kohn EC. The microenvironment of the tumor-host interface. Nature 2001;411:375–379.

31

The Clinical Use of Molecular Markers as Predictors of Disease Outcome and Response to Therapy in Malignant Melanoma

Steve R. Martinez, Hiroya Takeuchi, and Dave S. B. Hoon

Summary

Advances in surgical technique, diagnostic imaging, and adjuvant therapy have changed the management of melanoma patients during the last 20 yr. Despite this, several challenges remain. Attempts at using radiographic and nuclear medicine imaging to diagnose disease progression and metastatic disease at a stage early enough to affect survival have not been successful. Similarly, a reliable method of predicting or monitoring response to adjuvant therapy is currently unavailable. The last decade has seen the development of multiple RNA and DNA markers that have been applied toward the diagnosis/ detection of occult disease, prediction of survival, disease surveillance, or as indicators of response to adjuvant therapy. Molecular markers may represent tumor-associated antigens, tumor suppressor genes, oncogenes, cell physiological and transcription factors, or cellular apoptotic mediators. Genomic DNA and RNA molecular markers have been applied to melanoma primary tumors, regional and visceral metastases, serum, cerebral spinal fluid, and bone marrow. The ability to use molecular markers as prognostic indicators will be invaluable as clinicians seek to stratify patients for clinical trials, adjuvant treatments, and clinical follow-up regimens.

Key Words: RNA; DNA; molecular markers; RT-PCR; prognosis; survival.

From: *From Melanocytes to Melanoma: The Progression to Malignancy*
Edited by: V. J. Hearing and S. P. L. Leong © Humana Press Inc., Totowa, NJ

INTRODUCTION

Melanoma is a growing problem in the United States. Approximately 59,580 Americans are diagnosed with melanoma annually and, of these, 7770 patients will die of their disease *(1)*. The prognosis for patients with localized (stage I/II) melanoma is quite good, with an average 10-yr survival rate of 85%. With the diagnosis of regional nodal (stage III) or distant metastatic (stage IV) disease, however, the 10-yr survival rates drop to 35% and 10%, respectively *(2)*.

Improved imaging modalities, such as computed tomography (CT), magnetic resonance imaging (MRI), and positron emission tomography (PET) have facilitated earlier detection of distant metastases *(3–5)*. Such imaging modalities rely on the detection of gross disease, however, and are limited by their ability to reliably detect tumors less than 1 cm in diameter. The early detection of metastatic disease via CT, MRI, or PET has not been shown to confer a survival advantage, but it is plausible that the early detection of occult disease may contribute to an overall survival advantage by identifying subgroups amenable to more aggressive clinical and radiographic follow-up and adjuvant therapy.

Occult regional metastases are routinely identified in stage III melanoma patients because of the widespread adoption of lymphatic mapping and selective lymphadenectomy. Because the sentinel lymph node (SLN) accurately predicts the metastatic status of the draining regional lymph node basin, and lymph node metastasis is the most important determinant of overall survival, then the SLN status likely predicts survival as well. The detection of metastases in the SLN is limited by the accuracy of lymphatic mapping, surgical technique, and sampling error in pathological analysis. Even in cases in which the SLN is deemed free of metastasis, a small but significant percentage of patients will recur *(6,7)*. It is possible that such patients recur because of the presence of undetected subclinical or occult disease.

Despite these advances, the management of metastatic melanoma remains a significant challenge. The last decade has seen the development of multiple RNA and DNA markers that have been applied toward the diagnosis/detection of occult disease, prediction of survival, disease surveillance, or as indicators of response to adjuvant therapy. A list of markers discussed is provided in Table 1.

There is currently no accurate, validated molecular marker for melanoma. When developing new markers, attention must be paid to the degree with which candidate molecular markers address issues relating to the sensitivity and specificity for the disease being detected, as well as technical and logistical considerations. To be clinically relevant, a molecular marker should occur frequently in the disease population being tested. The marker should be detectable only in malignant tissues and, if possible, be specific for a particular tumor histology. Candidate molecular markers may be developed as indicators of tumorigenesis, disease progression, recurrence, response to therapy, or predictors of survival. Logistically, markers should be applied to fluids or tissues that may be easily sampled with little or no associated morbidity and detected using a reproducible, cost-effective, and high-throughput assay.

Molecular markers may represent tumor-associated antigens, tumor suppressor genes, oncogenes, cell physiological factors, transcription factors, or cellular apoptotic mediators that vary in their specificity for melanoma tumor cells. Genomic DNA and RNA molecular markers have been applied to melanoma primary tumors, regional and visceral metastases, serum, cerebral spinal fluid, and bone marrow *(8,9)*.

Table 1
Molecular Markers in Malignant Melanoma Quoted in This Review

Melanoma marker	Nucleic acid	Description
Tyrosinase	RNA	Enzyme in the melanin synthesis pathway
Melanoma antigen recognized by T-cells-1 (*MART-1*)	RNA	Protein recognized by T-cells and antibodies in melanoma patients
Melanoma antigen gene 3 (*MAGE-3*)	RNA	Tumor antigen recognized by cytolytic T-lymphocytes and antibodies
Tyrosinase-related protein-1 (*Trp-1*)	RNA	Melanosomal membrane glycoproteins recognized by antibodies and T-cells
Tyrosinase-related protein-2 (*Trp-2*)	RNA	Melanosomal membrane glycoproteins recognized by antibodies and T-cells
Melanotransferrin (*p97*)	RNA	Membrane glycosylated protein that reversibly binds iron
Melanoma cell adhesion molecule (*MCAM*)/ *MUC18/CD146*	RNA	Membrane glycoprotein and adhesion molecule
Universal MAGE-A (*uMAG-A*)	RNA	Assay detecting expression of multiple major MAGE-A gene family members
β→4-N-acetylgalactos-aminyl-transferase (*GalNac-T*)	RNA	Key glycosyltransferase enzyme in the biosynthetic pathway for the synthesis of the cell-surface gangliosides, GM2 and GD2
Paired-box homeotic gene transcription factor 3 (*Pax3*)	RNA	Regulator of melanin synthesis, cell migration and antiapoptosis
Retinoic acid receptor-β (*RAR-β2*)	DNA	Mediates the growth inhibitory and apoptotic effects of retinoic acid
RAS association domain family protein 1A (*RASSF1A*)	DNA	Potential tumor suppressor gene
O^6-methylguanine DNA methyltransferase (*MGMT*)	DNA	DNA repair enzyme
Death-associated protein kinase (*DAPK*)	DNA	Ca^{2+}/calmodulin-dependent serine/threonine kinase
Glutathione-*S*-transferase P1 (*GSTP1*)	DNA	Member of a superfamily of glutathione transferases that catalyze the conjugation of reduced glutathione
		Inhibitor of the matrix metalloproteinases
Tissue inhibitor of metallo-proteinase-3 (*TIMP3*)	DNA	Tumor suppressor gene on chromosome 9p21; negative regulator of the cell cycle
p16 (*CDKN2, MTS1*)	DNA	
Apoptotic protease-activating factor 1 (*APAF-1*)	DNA	Coordinator of the mitochondrial apoptotic pathway downstream from *p53*
B-type Raf kinase (*BRAF*)	DNA	Serine/threonine kinase important in cellular proliferation and apoptosis

This review seeks to address the role of DNA and RNA molecular markers in melanoma diagnosis, prognosis, disease surveillance, and monitoring response to adjuvant therapy. Our emphasis will be on the sensitivity and specificity rates, and the advantages and disadvantages of these assays toward a goal of clinical applicability. In so doing, we aim not to enumerate each study published on the use of molecular markers in melanoma. Rather, it is our goal to summarize critical discoveries made by our laboratory and others with respect to the use of DNA and RNA molecular markers as diagnostic, prognostic, and predictive tools in the management of melanoma patients. Our approach will be to review the role of molecular markers in parallel with disease progression from analysis of the primary tumor to the lymph node basin, blood, distant sites, and, finally, to other body fluids. Each section has been further subdivided to discuss our laboratory's RNA and DNA molecular marker experience.

PRIMARY TUMOR

The majority of melanomas are diagnosed by punch or excisional biopsies performed by primary care physicians or dermatologists. By the time patients have been referred to a surgical oncologist for definitive management, it is not uncommon for there to be no clinical trace of melanoma. Furthermore, the pathologist frequently deems the re-excision specimen free of melanoma. The analysis of primary melanoma tumors is limited, therefore, by the availability of intact samples at tertiary referral centers. As most investigators work with fresh or fresh-frozen tissue samples, rather than paraffin-embedded (PE) archival tissues, the ability to coordinate an efficient and timely tissue procurement method is also a limiting factor for the study of primary melanoma. When primary melanoma tissue is obtained, the tumor is often quite small, making the isolation of DNA and RNA extremely challenging. For these reasons, most genetic analyses of melanoma have, unfortunately, focused on cell lines, and regional and distant metastases. In contrast, molecular markers have been extensively studied with respect to primary breast, colorectal, prostate, and lung cancers, among others.

Because the Breslow depth of the primary tumor is an important prognostic indicator, it is informative to identify genetic abnormalities in primary melanomas and correlate them with the vertical growth phase of the lesion *(10)*. Comparisons of the genetic and epigenetic alterations in primary tumors relative to those of benign nevi, dysplastic nevi, regional metastases, circulating tumor cells, and distant metastases may provide a more complete understanding of the genetic aberrations and alterations characteristic of oncogenesis, tumor progression, and metastasis. Such information may facilitate the discovery of novel methods of disease prevention, diagnosis, treatment, and outcome prediction.

DNA Markers

Melanoma is characterized by increasing levels of genetic instability with advancing stage *(11)*. Capitalizing on this, numerous approaches have been employed to detect melanoma-associated genetic aberrations, such as allelic imbalances (AI) *(12–16)*, somatic mutations *(17)*, or epigenetic changes in the form of promoter region CpG island hypermethylation (Table 2) *(18,19)*.

ALLELIC IMBALANCES

Various malignancies have demonstrated AI. Because loss of heterozygosity (LOH) is not typical in nontumor tissues, its presence in tumors suggests the alteration of genomic regions that may affect cellular regulatory genes, tumor suppressor genes, or oncogenes that can regulate oncogenesis or tumor progression. Using a combination of

Table 2
DNA Molecular Marker Studies of Primary Melanoma Tumors

Study (yr)	Patients (No.)	AJCC stage	Markers	Positive patients (%)	Recurrence	Difference in overall survival
Fujiwara et al., *(12)* 1999	40	I–IV	D1S214, D1S228, D3S1293, D6S264, IGFIIR, D9S157, D9S161, D10S212, D10S216, D11S925	85%	NR	NR
Fujimoto et al., *(14)* 2004	18	I	*APAF-1* 6%	NR	No	
	21	II	*APAF-1*	33%	NR	No
	16	III	*APAF-1*	9%	NR	No
	2	IV	*APAF-1*	0%	NR	No
Shinozaki et al., *(17)* 2004	18	I	*BRAF*	33%	No	NR
	16	II	*BRAF*	31%	No	NR
	19	III	*BRAF*	26%	No	NR
	2	IV	*BRAF*	100%	No	NR
Hoon et al., *(19)* 2004	130	NR	*RAR-β2, RASSF1A, MGMT, DAPK, GSTP1, TIMP3, p16*	NR	NR	NR

NR, not reported; AJCC, American Joint Committee on Cancer; APAF-1, apoptotic protease activating factor-1; BRAF, B-type Raf Kinase; RAR-β2, retinoic acid receptor-β2; RASSF1A, RAS association domain family protein 1A; MGMT, O^6 methylguanine DNA methyltransferase; PAPR, death-associated protein kinase; GSTP1, glutathione-*S*-transferase P1; TIMP3, tissue inhibitor of metalloproteinase-3.

genetic linkage and LOH analysis in patients with familial melanoma and dysplastic nevi syndrome, many informative loci were discovered *(20–22)*. With the exception of the *B-type Raf kinase* oncogene *(BRAF)*, mutations of tumor suppressor genes or oncogenes occur rarely in melanoma *(23–25)*. LOH of microsatellites, highly repetitive, polymorphic dimeric to hexameric sequences of base pairs, represents one of the most common genetic alterations found in melanoma and may occur on multiple chromosomes *(10)*. Investigators have correlated increasing levels of AI with a significantly worse prognosis in various cancers, particularly colon cancer *(26)*.

Our laboratory sought to find a correlation between genetic instability in primary melanoma tumors and overall survival. Toward this goal, we examined a total of 60 primary melanomas of Breslow thickness 1–4 mm for LOH. A total of eight microsatellite markers (D9S157, D9S161, D10S212, D11S925, D6S264, D1S214, D1S228, and D3S1293) on six chromosomes were used. To correlate findings with a known clinical prognostic factor, tumors were categorized according to Breslow thickness (Table 3). Overall, 27% of melanomas demonstrated no LOH for any marker, 43% for one marker, and 30% for two to four markers. Patients with LOH of two to four microsatellite markers had significantly worse overall survival rates than those with zero or one positive marker(s) ($p = 0.011$; Cox proportional hazard relative risk = 2.58).

Fujimoto et al. examined the primary tumors of 62 stage I to IV melanoma patients for LOH in the vicinity of the *apoptotic protease activating factor-1* (*APAF-1*) locus on chromosome 12q22-23 *(14)*. *APAF-1* is a potential tumor suppressor gene and coordinator of the mitochondrial apoptotic pathway downstream from *p53*. AI of this gene may lead to oncogenic transformation, tumor growth and disease progression. Four

Table 3
Number of Markers Positive for LOH in 60 Primary Melanomas According to Breslow Thickness

Breslow thickness	LOH 0	LOH 1	LOH 2–4	Total
1–2 mm	8	10	8	26
2–4 mm	5	9	5	19
>4 mm	3	7	5	15

LOH, loss of heterozygosity.

microsatellite markers (D12S1657, D12S393, D12S1706, and D12S346) were used to assess the 12q22-23 chromosomal region for LOH. LOH was found more commonly in metastatic than primary tumors (70 vs 20%, respectively). The predominance of LOH in metastatic relative to primary tumors indicates a role for *APAF-1* in later stages of disease progression. Despite this, no correlation between *APAF-1* LOH in primary melanoma tumors and survival was noted after a short 39-mo follow-up period.

EPIGENETIC ALTERATIONS: HYPERMETHYLATION

Hypermethylation of gene promoter region CpG islands and the role this plays in the development of cancer has recently become an important area of investigation. Genes can be transcriptionally silenced when their promoter region CpG islands contain methylated cytosines 5' to an adjacent guanine. Promoter region hypermethylation of cancer-related genes can be as functionally significant as genetic mutations or deletions in permitting neoplasia and facilitating tumor progression *(27)*.

In the first report of tumor suppressor gene hypermethylation in primary human melanoma tissues, Hoon et al. evaluated the methylation profile of 4 candidate tumor suppressor genes in 20 primary PE melanoma tumors using methylation-specific polymerase chain reaction (MSP) *(19)*. The markers used were O^6-methylguanine DNA methyltransferase *(MGMT)*, retinoic acid receptor *(RAR)β-2*, RAS association domain family protein 1A *(RASSF1A)*, and death-associated protein kinase *(DAPK)*. The authors reported tumor suppressor gene promoter methylation rates as follows: MGMT, 10%; *RARβ-2*, 70%; *RASSF1A*, 15%; and *DAPK*, 0%. Overall, 25% of specimens had no tumor suppressor gene methylation. At least one, two, or three tumor suppressor genes were methylated in 75, 20, and 0% of specimens, respectively. This was the first major report of *RARβ-2* hypermethylation in a large series of melanoma patient tumors. To date, no epigenetic alteration has been reported to occur with such a high frequency in primary melanoma, suggesting a possible role of *RARβ-2* hypermethylation in melanoma development. The authors also examined a series of metastatic tumors and demonstrated higher rates of tumor-related gene hypermethylation compared with primary tumors, leading the authors to suggest that tumor-related gene methylation may play a significant role in melanoma progression. Furthermore, this study demonstrated that the methylation of tumor-related genes may occur early in melanoma development, before regional or distant metastasis. Further validation studies incorporating newly discovered tumor suppressor and tumor-related genes are currently being assessed.

MUTATIONS

Oncogene and tumor suppressor gene mutations are rare in melanoma. Deletions and mutations of known tumor suppressor genes, such as *P53* and *CDKN2*, have been reported, but occur at a low frequency and may play a limited role in nonfamilial melanoma *(20–25)*. An exception to this rule is *BRAF*, one of three Raf proteins in vertebrates. It encodes a key serine/threonine kinase important in the mitogen-activated protein kinase pathway for the transduction of signals from the oncogene *Ras. BRAF* mutations can significantly increase kinase activity, resulting in continuous transcription-mediated proliferation and neoplastic growth. A nucleotide 1796 T→A transversion accounts for 92% of *BRAF* mutations in melanoma and results in a mutant V600E amino acid. Somatic missense mutations of *BRAF* were reported in six of nine (66%) primary melanomas *(28)*. A subsequent study, however, demonstrated essentially identical rates of *BRAF* mutations in nevi of various histologies, primary melanoma, and metastatic melanoma *(29)*. Hence, although *BRAF* mutation may facilitate the neoplastic transformation of melanocytes, its role in tumorigenesis remains somewhat unclear. When compared with nevi that remained unchanged during a 12-mo period, initially benign nevi undergoing structural changes were more likely to be diagnosed as melanoma and harbor a *BRAF* mutation *(30)*. This raises the question of whether *BRAF* mutations in benign nevi are predictive of malignant progression.

In the largest series of primary melanomas, Shinozaki et al. examined 59 stage I to IV primary melanomas for mutations by direct sequencing *(17)*. The highest rates of *BRAF* mutation were seen in stage IV primary tumors (100%), followed by stage I tumors (33%), stage II tumors (31%), and stage III tumors (26%). There was no correlation between mutation status and stage of disease, or with overall survival. Age was the only prognostic factor that correlated with *BRAF* mutation in primary melanoma, with a significantly higher mutation rate seen in patients less than 60 yr old. Debate is ongoing regarding whether *BRAF* mutations correlate with melanoma development or are merely a bystander genetic event.

LYMPH NODE/SENTINEL LYMPH NODE

The presence of lymph node metastasis is the most important prognostic factor for predicting 10-yr survival. Wide local excision is the treatment of choice for localized melanoma and metastectomy has been shown to improve survival in patients with distant disease *(31,32)*. Lymph node dissection is indicated for clinically evident lymph nodes. In the past, melanomas with clinical or histopathological risk factors for lymph node metastasis were relegated either to observation until such time as metastasis became clinically evident or elective lymph node dissection. Because only approx 20% of patients undergoing elective lymph node dissection were subsequently diagnosed with lymph node metastases, a majority of patients did not obtain any therapeutic benefit from this procedure.

Lymphatic mapping and the SLN technique pioneered by Morton et al. has facilitated the detection of sub-clinical nodal metastases within the regional nodal basin without the morbidity associated with a complete lymph node dissection *(33)*. A negative SLN does not eliminate the risk of regional or distant recurrence in all patients, however, as up to 13% of patients with histopathologically negative SLNs will develop regional or distant disease recurrence at 5 yr *(6,7)*, presumably because of the presence of disease undetectable by either hematoxylin and eosin (H&E) staining or immunohistochemistry (IHC). Thus, although the SLN technique can accurately identify subclinical nodal metastases, it remains difficult to predict who will develop regional or distant metastases, particularly among SLN-negative patients.

Because regional nodal involvement often occurs before more widespread distant metastasis, identification of occult disease in the SLN frequently represents the earliest stage of metastatic disease. Depending on the status of the SLN, patients may be offered adjuvant therapy, which may be more effective in the setting of relatively low tumor burden.

Although it is true that the tumor status of the SLN represents the status of the regional draining lymphatic basin, if the pathological analysis of the SLN is inaccurate, then all benefit of the procedure is lost. Standard SLN analysis incorporates both H&E staining and IHC, usually for S100, HMB45, or melanoma antigen recognized by T-cells (MART)-1. Routine pathological analysis is prone to sampling error, however, because even with judicious step-sectioning, less than 5% of the SLN is sampled *(34)*.

Messenger RNA Markers

Messenger (m)RNA markers have been quite successful in detecting micrometastatic disease in SLNs. Our studies and others have demonstrated that molecular upstaging of H&E- and IHC-negative SLNs can predict disease-free status and overall survival. The upstaging of SLN using reverse transcriptase-polymerase chain reaction (RT-PCR) is an approach that has been in use for over a decade and may incorporate single or multiple mRNA markers. The predominant single marker used has been tyrosinase, a rate-limiting enzyme of the melanin synthesis pathway. Other, more reliable, approaches use multiple mRNA markers. Over the last decade, PCR assays have improved dramatically and have become more reliable.

SINGLE MARKERS: TYROSINASE

Several investigators have used a single molecular marker approach to detect submicroscopic disease in the SLN. Boi et al., in an analysis of 74 stage I melanoma patients, detected tyrosinase by RT-PCR in 45% of SLNs but did not perform an analysis of either recurrence or overall survival *(35)*.

Shivers et al. compared tyrosinase RT-PCR on the SLN with standard H&E plus IHC in 114 stage I/II melanoma patients *(36)*. Of 91 patients with no metastases in their SLN by standard techniques, 52% were positive using the RT-PCR assay. With a clinical follow-up period of 28 mo, recurrence rates were highest (61%) for those who were SLN positive by both standard techniques and RT-PCR, whereas lowest recurrence rates (2%) were found in those who were SLN negative using both techniques. Patients who were pathologically negative but RT-PCR positive had an intermediate rate of recurrence (13%). Differences among these groups with respect to survival were significantly different.

A series by Kammula et al. examined the SLN of 112 stage I/II melanoma patients using tyrosinase RT-PCR compared with standard pathological analysis *(37)*. Recurrence rates were calculated at two time periods, 42 mo and 67 mo. Initially, recurrence rates were statistically different among patients who were histologically positive and RT-PCR positive (53%), histologically negative but RT-PCR positive (14%), and histologically negative and RT-PCR negative (0%). At 67 mo, however, the recurrence rate differences between the histologically negative but RT-PCR positive (24%) and histologically negative and RT-PCR negative (15%) were no longer statistically significant. These results support the hypothesis that patients exhibit recurrent or progressive disease proportional to their tumor burden.

MULTIMARKER RT-PCR

A number of reports have documented alarmingly high false-positive rates using tyrosinase as a single marker, questioning the assays reliability for diagnostic or predic-

Table 4
mRNA RT-PCR Multimarker Studies of Melanoma Lymph Node Metastases

Study (yr)	Patients (No.)	AJCC stage	Markers	Correlated with recurrence	Correlated with overall survival
Bostick et al., *(38)* 1999	72	I–III	*Tyrosinase, MAGE-A3,* MART-1	Yes	NR
Palmieri et al., *(39)* 2001	75	I–III	*Tyrosinase, MART-1*	Yes	Yes
Kuo et al., *(40)* 2003	37	SLN +	*Tyrosinase, MART-1, TRP-1, TRP-2*	Yes	Yes
Takeuchi, et al. *(13)* 2004	53	SLN +	*MART-1, MAGE-A3, β1→GalNac-T, Pax3*	Yes	Yes
	162	SLN –	*MART-1, MAGE-A3, β1→GalNac-T, Pax3*	Yes	Yes

NR, not reported; SLN, sentinel lymph node; AJCC, American Joint Committee on Cancer; MAGE-3, melanoma antigen gene-3; MART-1, melanoma antigen recognized by T-cells-1; TRP-1, tyrosinase-related protein-1; TRP-2 tyrosinase-related protein-2; B1→GalNac-T, B1→4-*N*-acetyl galactosaminyl-transferase; Pax3, paired-box homeotic gene transcription factor 3.

tive purposes. Investigators sought to increase the specificity of the RT-PCR assay and address some of its inherent weaknesses by using a multimarker panel for the SLN analysis (Table 4). Multimarker advocates site variable detection rates using tyrosinase alone as the primary reason to abandon the single-marker approach. Using multiple molecular markers improves the sensitivity and specificity of the assay by addressing tumor cell heterogeneity, mRNA half-life and variations in mRNA quantity and quality among specimens. Not all cells within a tumor will necessarily express an individual marker. This is a binary event: either expression is present or absent as measured by the assay. The chance that a tumor cell expresses one out of four markers, however, greatly increases the likelihood of detection.

Although these single-marker studies were performed using frozen SLN tissues cut by the surgeon or pathologist arbitrarily, we developed a more reliable method of sampling the SLN, whereby the SLN is frozen, bivalved, and sequentially sectioned parallel to histopathology sections. This provides a more uniform molecular assessment of the SLN in accordance with the portion of the node submitted for histopathological diagnosis. Arbitrary sampling of a fresh SLN, in contrast, is prone to significant sampling bias and error in analysis.

Bostick et al. combined *tyrosinase*, melanoma antigen gene *(MAGE)-3* and *MART-1* to detect micrometastases in the SLN of 72 stage I to III melanoma patients and compared this with standard H&E plus IHC *(38)*. *MAGE-3* is part of the *MAGE* gene family and is expressed in male germline cells and in tumors of various histologies. *MAGE-3* codes for a tumor-associated antigen that can be recognized by T-lymphocytes. *MART-1* is a melanoma-associated antigen recognized by human leukocyte antigen-A2-restricted tumor-infiltrating lymphocytes. A RT-PCR assay positive for two or more markers was considered positive. RT-PCR markers were positive in 94% of histologically positive SLN metastases and in 36% of histologically negative SLN. After a mean follow-up of

12 mo, RT-PCR-positive patients had a significantly higher rate of disease recurrence. The multimarker RT-PCR assay was able to upstage a significant proportion of patients thought to be without SLN metastases by standard histopathology. Furthermore, the ability to upstage patients using molecular techniques was clinically verified by demonstrating a survival disadvantage in patients with RT-PCR-positive SLNs. Overall, multimarker RT-PCR was a better predictor of recurrence-free survival than H&E plus IHC.

Palmieri et al., using a multimarker panel of *tyrosinase* and *MART-1* in an analysis of SLNs from 75 stage I to III melanoma patients, found that the presence of both markers was associated with a significant risk of recurrence and decrease in overall survival *(39)*.

Kuo et al. performed a semiquantitative RT-PCR and electrochemiluminescence analysis on 37 SLN-positive and 40 SLN-negative patients confirmed by standard H&E plus IHC, but used tyrosinase-related protein *(TRP)-1* and *TRP-2* in addition to *tyrosinase* and *MART-1* as molecular markers *(40)*. TRP-1 and -2 are melanosomal membrane glycoproteins recognized by T-cells of patients with melanoma. Rather than frozen sections, this study analyzed PE archival tissues. The assay sensitivity was good, with at least one RT-PCR marker positive in 95% of cases with histologically confirmed metastases. A significant correlation was found between the number of positive markers and mean Breslow thickness. After a median follow-up of 55 mo, the presence of two or more markers positive by RT-PCR significantly correlated with both disease recurrence and overall survival in histopathologically negative SLN.

The ability to reliably perform RT-PCR using PE specimens is a significant advance. Reliance on frozen tissues may sacrifice tissue necessary for an adequate pathological diagnosis. Additionally, the acquisition and storage of frozen tissues may be prohibitively expensive and labor-intensive. PE tissues are readily available after a pathological diagnosis has been made and have the added advantage of resisting mRNA degradation enough to allow for retrospective studies.

Using another multi-marker panel of *MART-1*, *MAGE-3*, β1→4-*N*-acetylgalacto-saminyl-transferase *(GalNac-T)*, and paired-box homeotic gene transcription factor 3 *(Pax3)*, Takeuchi et al. performed a quantitative RT-PCR (qRT) assay on 53 histologically confirmed positive and 162 negative PE SLNs *(13)*. GalNac-T is a key enzyme in the synthesis of cell-surface gangliosides GM2 and GD2 that are abundant in melanoma cells. Pax3 is a transcription factor that participates in melanocyte development. The qRT assay is a significant improvement over standard RT-PCR assays, providing a means of quantifying individual marker positivity as opposed to relying on subjective gel electrophoresis or Southern blot assays, and may better elucidate differential tumor marker expression among tumors. Study end points were disease-free and overall survival. At a median follow-up of 60 mo, patients with at least one positive marker had statistically higher rates of disease recurrence. Furthermore, patients with one, two, and three positive qRT markers had proportional and statistically significant decreases in disease-free survival (Fig. 1A). The authors correlated qRT marker expression with overall survival. Patients with at least one positive marker had significantly worse over-

Fig. 1. (A) *(opposite page)* Kaplan-Meier curve analysis of disease-free survival according to the number of qRT markers positive in 162 patients with histopathologically negative sentinal lymph node (SLN). **(B)** Kaplan-Meier curve analysis of overall survival according to the number of molecular markers positive in 162 patients with histopathologically negative SLN. **(C)** Kaplan-Meier curve analysis of overall survival according to the qRT multimarker and histopathology status of SLNs in 215 melanoma patients. H+E, hematoxylin and eosin; IHC, immunohistochemistry. (Reprinted with permission from ref. *13*.)

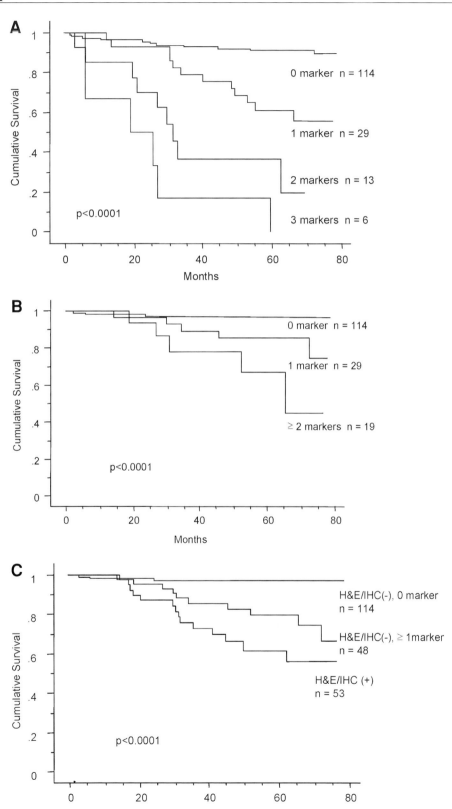

all survival. An increasing number of positive markers correlated with a decrease in disease-free and overall survival (Fig. 1B).

The ability to detect molecular marker expression in SLNs has tremendous translational significance. Identification of these markers effectively stratifies patients into categories of risk for both disease recurrence and overall survival. Those with positive SLNs by conventional and qRT techniques experience the worst outcomes, whereas those with negative SLN using these combined techniques will have the best prognosis (Fig. 1C). Patients with histologically negative but qRT-positive SLN cannot be considered at low risk. Furthermore, Takeuchi et al. have demonstrated that, even among patients with histologically negative but qRT-positive SLNs there are different categories of risk, dependent on the number of molecular markers detected *(13)*. These findings have the potential to serve as a basis for stratifying patients to different treatment pathways based on risk of recurrence and likely survival. Hence, patients at highest risk may undergo more rigorous clinical follow-up, radiographic surveillance, and adjuvant treatment, although those at lowest risk may be followed less aggressively and are perhaps less likely to benefit from adjuvant treatment.

Validation of the prognostic role of multimarker qRT will come from the second Multicenter Selective Lymphadenectomy Trial (MSLT)-II. Patients with negative SLNs by H&E and IHC will undergo multimarker qRT at John Wayne Cancer Institute. Those patients that are SLN negative by qRT will undergo routine follow-up, whereas SLN-positive patients by qRT will be randomized to an observation arm or a completion lymph node dissection arm. If qRT-positive lymph nodes truly represent clinically significant occult disease, then it is expected that patients receiving completion lymph node dissections will receive a survival benefit compared with those undergoing clinical follow-up only. Hence, molecular upstaging of PE SLN will either be validated or refuted. MSLT-II is the first major melanoma clinical trial to randomize patients according to qRT assessment of their SLN. The study is currently underway, with plans to accrue 3500 patients from over 30 countries world wide.

DNA Markers

The analysis of DNA for somatic mutations, LOH, or tumor suppressor gene methylation addresses several of the problems inherent to mRNA RT-PCR assays in melanoma. DNA is significantly more stable than RNA, making these assays technically easier to perform. Furthermore, mRNA expression may be variable and difficult to quantify objectively in standard RT-PCR assays. DNA markers take advantage of detecting a wide variety of genetic anomalies. Furthermore, analysis of DNA markers for somatic alterations of tumor-related genes and oncogenes are tumor-specific and therefore not as vulnerable to false-positive results as are mRNA assays. Investigators have used DNA molecular markers as predictors of disease outcome successfully with respect to lymph node metastases (Table 5). The use of DNA markers for the detection of occult melanoma in the SLN is difficult, because aberrations, such as mutations, may be reliably detected only when they are consistently elevated at a defined site.

Allelic Imbalances

Fujimoto et al. employed a panel of four microsatellite markers surrounding the *APAF-1* locus on chromosomal region 12q22-23 to detect LOH in 44 stage III patients with regional nodal metastases and 39 with in-transit metastases *(14)*. Primary stage III tumors expressed LOH for at least one marker in 9%, but regional nodal metastases

Table 5
DNA Molecular Marker Studies of Melanoma Lymph Node Metastases

Study (yr)	Patients (No.)	AJCC stage	Tissue	Markers	Positive Recurrence patients (%)	Difference in overall survival
Fujimoto et al., *(14)* 2004	83	III	LN metastasis	*APAF-1* 36%	NR	Yes
Shinozaki et al., *(17)* 2004	68	III/IV	LN metastasis, distant metastasis	*BRAF* 57%	No	NR
Spugnardi et al., *(18)* 2003	9	III	LN metastasis	*RASSF1A* 33%, promoter 1 *RASSF1A* promoter 2 22%	NR	NR

LN, lymph node; NR, not reported; AJCC, American Joint Committee on Cancer; APAF, apoptotic protease activating factor 1; BRAF, B-type Raf kinase; RASSF1A, RAS association domain family protein 1A.

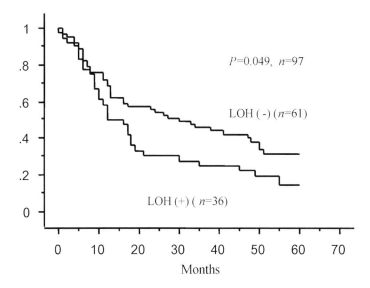

Fig. 2. Kaplan-Meier curve analysis demonstrating the correlation between loss of heterozygosity (LOH) of *APAF-1* and overall survival in American Joint Committee on Cancer stage III/IV metastatic melanoma tumors. (Reprinted with permission from ref. *14.*)

expressed LOH in 28% of cases, supporting the role of *APAF-1* in melanoma progression. In a combined analysis of distant and regional nodal metastases, LOH was correlated with decreased overall survival after 27 mo of follow-up (Fig. 2).

MUTATIONS

Shinozaki et al. examined 68 metastatic tumors, 20 of which were to regional lymph nodes, for mutations of *BRAF* using PCR and automated capillary array electrophoresis *(17)*. The *BRAF* mutation rate was significantly higher in regional nodal metastases (50%) compared with primary tumors (31%). Because *BRAF* mutations have been found in a significant proportion of benign nevi, however, it is unlikely that *BRAF* plays a significant role in regional metastatic melanoma development.

EPIGENETIC ALTERATIONS: HYPERMETHYLATION

Spugnardi et al. detected hypermethylation of *RASSF1A* in nine regional metastases by MSP *(18)*. *RASSF1A* hypermethylation was noted in 33% of lymph node metastases. *RASSF1A* and *RAR-β* promoter region hypermethylation was quantified in 37 stage III melanoma patients with clinically positive lymph nodes by Yao et al. *(41)*. Hypermethylation was detected for *RASSF1A* alone in 16%, *RAR-β* alone in 28%, and both in 14%. By multivariate analysis, *RAR-β* hypermethylation correlated with decreased disease-free and overall survival, confirming that epigenetic inactivation of tumor suppressor genes can be used as predictive markers of disease outcome.

As candidate tumor-related and tumor suppressor genes are identified, MSP will play a prominent role in determining whether hypermethylation influences the neoplastic process from oncogenesis to primary tumor progression and metastasis in melanoma. At this time, it is clear that hypermethylation of promoter regions of tumor-related genes in melanoma play a prominent role, perhaps more so than other genetic aberrations known to date. The hypermethylation of gene promoter regions is a powerful mechanism of silencing gene expression.

BLOOD

Because most tumors, including melanoma, often metastasize and disseminate hematogenously, the detection of tumor-associated molecular markers in the blood is a logical, accessible, and convenient alternative to the examination of primary tumors or metastatic sites. The relative noninvasiveness of routine blood draws makes it possible to monitor disease progression or response to therapeutic interventions at multiple points in time with little or no morbidity.

mRNA Markers

Smith et al. first identified tyrosinase mRNA in the blood of stage III/IV melanoma patients in 1991 *(42)*. The rate of tyrosinase RT-PCR positivity varies widely in published reports, from 0 to 100% *(35–37,42–55)*. Subsequent authors have questioned the specificity of tyrosinase for melanoma, detecting tyrosinase mRNA in up to 11% of normal tissues *(56)*. Possible reasons for these false-positives include detection of illegitimate transcription, benign nevi cells, or PCR contamination. Nevertheless, tyrosinase remains the most common molecular marker assayed in melanoma used either alone or as part of a multimarker panel. The clinical usefulness of detecting circulating blood tyrosinase mRNA was studied extensively in the 1990s, often with conflicting results. The major disadvantage of using a single-marker approach is an unacceptable false-positive rate. Furthermore, these early studies frequently used gel electrophoresis to confirm expression. Such assays are inherently subjective and may fail to detect markers that are expressed in low copy numbers.

SINGLE MARKERS: TYROSINASE

Battayani et al. detected tyrosinase mRNA in 93 stage I to IV melanoma patients rendered disease-free surgically and found that a positive PCR assay predicted recurrence and rapid disease progression *(44)*. Mellado et al. showed that *tyrosinase* RT-PCR positivity correlated with disease stage in 91 stage I to IV melanoma patients *(48)*.

Additionally, blood tyrosinase positivity was associated with lower rates of disease-free survival, although significance was only achieved in stage II/III patients. A later study performed by the same authors failed to correlate tyrosinase positivity with disease stage, but did confirm that RT-PCR-positive patients experienced significantly higher rates of disease recurrence and lower overall survival compared with RT-PCR-negative patients (55). Similarly, Ghossein et al. identified a statistically significant correlation between blood RT-PCR positivity and decreased overall survival in an analysis of 73 patients with stage II to IV melanoma (53).

Conversely, several authors have sought to prove that the detection of the circulating melanoma mRNA marker, tyrosinase, has no clinical use. Because disease stage incorporates several clinical factors that contribute to the risk of disease recurrence, progression, and overall survival, the ability of a molecular marker to correlate with disease stage is not trivial. In stage III and IV disease, when tumor burden and, therefore, the number of circulating tumor cells are presumably greatest, the detection of tyrosinase mRNA has been highly variable, ranging from 0 to 100% (43,44). For this reason, several authors have concluded that blood tyrosinase is of no benefit as a marker of metastatic disease (45,49,51,52,54).

Variation among laboratories in methods of RNA purification and extraction, PCR set-up and cycling, as well as differences in data interpretation, may be partly responsible for these disparate findings. Factors inherent to the biology of each tumor may influence results as well. Tumor cells may be shed in the bloodstream only intermittently, and tumor heterogeneity may lead to clones of cells that do not express the marker being assayed. Additionally, the presence of normal cellular transcripts detected by PCR may dilute the tumor-related mRNA. Similarly, as we would expect fluctuations of tumor cell shedding within each patient from day to day, so should we expect variation in the detection of tyrosinase mRNA between patients, particularly patients in vastly different categories, such as preoperative vs postoperative, and those receiving adjuvant therapy vs those receiving none. Finally, the use of *tyrosinase* as a single marker of melanoma progression or disease recurrence and predictor of overall survival may simply be an inadequate one-dimensional assay for a process that is decidedly complex and multidimensional. As with lymph node analysis, investigators have sought to improve the sensitivity and specificity of the RT-PCR assay by employing multimarker panels (Table 6) (13,34,38,40,57–61).

Multimarker mRNA Panels

The original panel used by Hoon et al. incorporated tyrosinase and the tumor-associated antigens, melanotransferrin (p97) and MAGE-3, and an adhesion-related glycoprotein, melanoma cell-adhesion molecule (*MCAM/MUC18/CD146*) (57). A four-marker PCR assay performed significantly better than *tyrosinase* alone and correlated with both disease stage and progression. An identical multimarker panel was used by the same group to predict overall survival in a cohort of 46 stage II to IV melanoma patients followed-up for 4 yr or longer. The number of positive RT-PCR markers significantly correlated with both disease stage and tumor recurrence, but only approached significance as a predictor of overall survival ($p = 0.068$) (59). Both *MUC18* and *p97* need to be further defined and validated in other tissue and cell types.

Wascher et al. further refined this multimarker panel to incorporate *MART-1* and *universal melanoma antigen gene-A* with *tyrosinase (60)*. The primer set for *universal melanoma antigen gene-A* was designed to detect at least six members of the *MAGE-A*

Table 6
Blood mRNA RT-PCR Multimarker Studies in Melanoma Patients

Study (yr)	Patients (No.)	AJCC stage	Tissue	Markers	Correlated with recurrence?	Correlated with overall survival?
Hoon et al., (57) 1995	119	I–IV	Blood	Tyrosinase, p97, (MCAM/MUC18/ CD146), MAGE-3	NR	NR
Curry et al., (58) 1998	123	I–III	Blood	Tyrosinase, MART-1	Yes	NR
Hoon et al., (59) 2000	46	I–IV	Blood	Tyrosinase, p97, MUC18, MAGE-3	Yes	NR
Palmieri et al. (39) 2001	75	I–III	Blood SLN	Tyrosinase, MART-1	Yes	Yes
Wascher et al., (60) 2003	30	III	Blood	Tyrosinase, MART-1, uMAG-A	Yes	Yes
Mocellin et al., (61) 2004	40	IIBC, IIIAB	Blood	Tyrosinase, MART-1	Yes	NR

NR, not reported; SLN, sentinel lymph node; AJCC, American Joint Committee on Cancer; p97, melanotransferin; MCAM/MUC18/CD146, melanoma cell adhesion molecule; MAGE-3, melanoma antigen gene 3; MART-1, melanoma antigen recognized by T-cells-1; uMAG-A, universal MAG-A.

family. A semiquantitative electrochemiluminescence assay was used to confirm all RT-PCR products. The population assayed in this retrospective study was a select group of 30 stage III patients matched for known clinical prognostic factors and rendered disease-free by surgical resection before treatment with a melanoma vaccine. Peripheral blood specimens were obtained before the first vaccination, and before vaccinations at weeks 8 and 16. Because no validated blood markers for melanoma can reliably predict response to adjuvant therapy, this study sought to use the multimarker RT-PCR assay to detect occult circulating tumor cells early in the course of adjuvant therapy. If circulating tumor cells detected by RT-PCR correlated with either disease recurrence or decreased overall survival, then the assay would have significant clinical applications. Furthermore, because blood samples were obtained during the course of adjuvant therapy, tumor cells detected by RT-PCR could be correlated with disease recurrence and overall survival at these time points as well. Patients were followed-up for a median of 74 mo. Of those who experienced recurrent disease, 53% had at least one RT-PCR marker positive in serial peripheral blood specimens. The presence of at least one RT-PCR marker was associated with a significantly increased risk of disease recurrence in multivariate analysis. Similarly, of those patients dying during the follow-up period, 53% had at least one RT-PCR marker positive in serial peripheral blood specimens. The presence of at least one positive RT-PCR marker was significantly associated with a decreased overall survival (Fig. 3). This study confirmed the usefulness of blood-based multimarker RT-PCR assays in predicting disease recurrence, overall survival, and response to adjuvant therapy.

Using a panel including MART-1 and tyrosinase, Curry examined patterns of recurrence in 123 stage I to III melanoma patients who had blood drawn preoperatively and postoperatively and were followed-up for 18 mo (58). Of note, 65% of patients with a

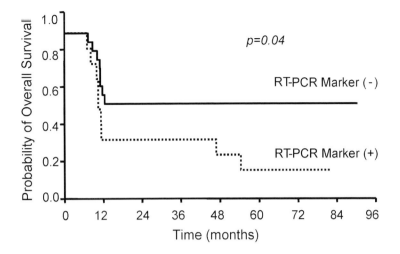

Fig. 3. Kaplan-Meier curve analysis demonstrates a significant correlation between at least one reverse transcriptase-polymerase chain reacion (RT-PCR) marker detected in peripheral blood and overall survival in American Joint Committee on Cancer stage III melanoma patients. All patients had been rendered disease-free surgically and received a melanoma vaccine. (Reprinted with permission from ref. *60.*)

positive result preoperatively converted to a negative result postoperatively, indicating the importance of the temporal relationship between surgery and blood collection and the ability of surgery, unlike adjuvant therapies, to rapidly convert patients to a disease-free status. Up to 34% of recurrences occurring over 18 mo were not predicted by the RT-PCR multimarker panel. Using the same multimarker panel, Palmieri et al. were unable to demonstrate a relationship between the number of positive markers and risk of disease recurrence or improvement in overall survival in 75 stage I to III patients *(39)*.

Multimarker RT-PCR allows tumor-specific mRNA detection with a higher sensitivity than single marker panels. There is abundant variation in results obtained from different laboratories, caused primarily by nonstandardized laboratory techniques and methods of analysis. Our laboratory has pursued the use of blood-based RT-PCR to monitor disease progression and response to therapy. We have recently reported on a blood-based qRT assay incorporating markers initially used to upstage SLN *(13)*. Serial blood draws assessed by multimarker qRT successfully detected tumor cells in the blood of stage III melanoma patients receiving neoadjuvant biochemotherapy (BC) (Koyanagi K, personal communication, 2005). Those patients demonstrating a decrease in circulating tumor cells during therapy tumor had significantly lower rates of disease recurrence compared with patients who showed no change in the number of circulating tumor cells. Thus, multimarker qRT can predict treatment outcome and monitor the effectiveness of different modes of treatment.

Circulating DNA Markers

Free, circulating, tumor-related DNA has been described in various cancers. Levels of circulating total DNA are higher in cancer patients compared with normal healthy volunteers *(62)*. Circulating tumor-related DNA may originate from necrotic, apoptotic, or physically disrupted tumor cells. Circulating tumor-related DNA may represent viable tumor cells shed by the primary or metastatic tumor that lack the ability to metastasize,

Table 7
Circulating DNA Molecular Marker Studies in Melanoma Patients

Study (yr)	Patients (No.)	AJCC stage	Markers	Positive patients (%)	Recurrence	Difference in overall survival?
Fujiwara et al., (12) 1999	76	I–IV	D1S214, D1S228, D3S1293, D6S264, IGFIIR, D9S157, D9S161, D10S212, D10S216, D11S925	58%	NR	NR
Taback et al., (8) 2001	57	I–IV	D1S214, D1S228, D3S1293, D6S264, D9S157, D9S161, D10S216, D11S925	29%	NR	Yes
Fujimoto et al., (15) 2004	49	IV	APAF-1	pre-BC, 36%; post-BC, 36%	NR	Yes
Taback et al., (16) 2004	41	IV	D1S228, D3S1293, D6S264,D9S157, D9S161, D10S212, D11S2000, D14S62, D11S925	29%	NR	Yes
Hoon et al., (19) 2004	130	NR	RAR-β2, RASSF1A, MGMT, DAPK, GSTP1, TIMP3, p16	NR	NR	NR

NR, not reported; BC, biochemotherapy; AJCC, American Joint Committee on Cancer; APAF-1, apoptotic protease activating factor-1; RARβ2, retinoic acid receptor β2; RASSF1A, RAS association domain family protein 1A; MGMT, O^6 methylguanine DNA methyltransferase; DAPK, death-associated protein kinase; GSTP1, glutathione-S-transferase P1; TIMP3, tissue inhibitor of metalloproteinase-3 .

viable tumor cells with metastatic potential, or nonviable tumor cells. Regardless of the scenario, free, circulating, tumor-related nucleic acids have demonstrated diagnostic and prognostic importance and predictive relevance in multiple types of cancer, including melanoma (Table 7) (63).

Free circulating nucleic acids in peripheral blood demonstrate genetic aberrations similar to those found in the primary tumor (12,63). Therefore, circulating DNA may have clinical use as a marker of disease recurrence after surgery. Similarly, the detection of circulating tumor DNA during the administration of adjuvant therapy may be used as a predictor of therapeutic response. Free, circulating, tumor-related DNA may be detected as LOH of DNA microsatellites, methylated DNA, or mutations. The detection of circulating DNA has broadened the role of molecular biomarkers in the diagnosis and prognosis of melanoma and further expanded their use in monitoring patient responses to adjuvant therapy.

ALLELIC IMBALANCES

Fujiwara et al. examined the plasma of 76 stage I to IV melanoma patients for microsatellite loss using 10 markers (D1S214, D1S228, D3S1293, D6S264, IGFIIR, D9S157, D9S161, D10S212, D10S216, and D11S925) on 6 chromosomes (12). LOH of at least one marker was demonstrated in 50% of patients and correlated with disease stage. This was the first major study to show a correlation between circulating DNA and disease progression in melanoma.

Using a different panel of eight microsatellite markers (D1S214, D1S228, D3S1293, D6S264, D9S157, D9S161, D10S216, and D11S925) on six chromosomes, Taback et al. analyzed preoperative and postoperative bloods for LOH in 57 stage I to IV melanoma patients surgically rendered disease free *(13)*. Overall, LOH of at least one marker occurred in 56% of patients and correlated with disease stage. With a median follow-up of 21 mo, a significant risk of death was reported in stage III/IV patients with at least one marker positive for LOH. Because no deaths occurred in the stage I/II cohort during follow-up, survival could not be evaluated in this group.

Because genetic instability increases in melanoma with each advancing American Joint Committee on Cancer stage, patients with regional and distant metastases represent the ideal population on whom to identify AI. Investigators have attempted to use LOH as a predictor of response to therapy in stage IV melanoma patients.

Fujimoto et al. employed a panel of four microsatellite markers surrounding the 12q22-23 locus to detect LOH in the sera of 49 stage IV patients treated with biochemotherapy (BC) *(15)*. Patients were categorized as BC responders or nonresponders. Nonresponders had significantly more LOH than did responders and overall, those with LOH of 12q had significantly worse overall survival.

Similarly, Taback et al. examined the blood of 41 stage IV melanoma patents receiving BC for LOH of nine markers on seven chromosomes *(16)*. Patients were then categorized as BC responders or nonresponders. Responders demonstrated clinical and radiographic complete or partial responses, although nonresponders showed either stable or progressive disease. At the start of BC, LOH of at least one marker was noted in only 9% of responders, but in 56% of responders, a significant difference. Those with LOH of at least one marker had significantly decreased median progression-free and overall survival compared with patients without LOH. This was the first study documenting the association between circulating DNA markers and a patient's response to adjuvant therapy for melanoma.

The usefulness of circulating tumor-related DNA detection lies in the ability to serially assay tumor markers without sampling either the primary or metastatic tumor, each of which may be unavailable or inaccessible. Serial determinations of biomarker status have the most significant implications in the context of adjuvant therapy administration.

The benefit of using molecular techniques as predictors of therapeutic response is clear. Adjuvant therapies, including immune therapy, chemotherapy, and BC, are toxic and associated with significant morbidity and protocol noncompliance. If clinicians could accurately predict, based on molecular marker analysis, the patients most likely to respond, then adjuvant therapy could be offered to this group with significant benefit. More importantly, however, patients who are not likely to respond can avoid potentially toxic therapy that is unlikely to benefit them.

DISTANT METASTASES

It is simplistic to think that information gleaned from a primary melanoma tumor, peripheral blood, or lymph node is identical to that from a distant metastatic site. Tumors from distant metastatic sites often are more undifferentiated than their primary counterparts. Indeed, more advanced stages of malignancy are likely to harbor increasing numbers of genetic and epigenetic aberrations, as has been described in melanoma. Tumor cells at distant metastatic sites are exposed to a vastly different intercellular milieu than their primary tumor cell counterparts, with factors, such as chemokines, cytokines, growth factors, and adhesion molecules, dramatically influencing cellular properties. Metastatic melanomas may even be less pigmented than primary tumors. Hence, it is not unreasonable to seek prognostic data via the molecular analysis of these distant metastases.

mRNA Markers

Just as was performed with primary tumors, Takeuchi et al. used a panel of three mRNA markers consisting of *tyrosinase*, *TRP-2*, and *MART-1* to detect the levels of expression of these melanoma-associated antigens (MAA) in 35 stage IV metastatic tumors *(13)*. Because MAA have been shown to induce T-cell and antibody responses in melanoma patients, the authors hypothesized that their detection in metastatic tumors would correlate with improved overall survival. qRT of mRNA marker expression was as follows: *tyrosinase* was detected in 83% of patients, *TRP-2* in 89%, and *MART-1* in 71%. After follow-up of 60 mo, elevated MAA levels of *tyrosinase* and *TRP-2* significantly correlated with improved overall survival. The authors concluded that detection of MAA mRNA from distant metastases may be a useful predictive factor of disease outcome. Furthermore, the loss of MAA in advanced tumors carries a poor prognosis, whereas those patients carrying immunogenic MAA on their tumors may be more responsive to active, specific immunotherapies. This study demonstrated that disease outcome in stage IV melanoma patients can vary according to both host immunity and antigen expression of the tumor.

DNA Markers

LOSS OF HETEROZYGOSITY

Fujimoto et al. examined microsatellite loss around the *APAF-1* locus at chromosomal region 12q22-23 to determine whether AI of this potential tumor suppressor gene contributes to apoptosis inhibition and resistance to adjuvant therapy *(14)*. A total of 29 distantly metastatic tumors were analyzed using 6 microsatellite markers. LOH of *APAF-1* was found in 38% of specimens and significantly correlated with decreased overall survival. The loss of *APAF-1* may contribute to the resistance of melanoma and other cancers to various therapies.

MUTATIONS

The *BRAF* gene mutation was examined in 13 visceral metastases for sequence mutations *(17)*. Overall, *BRAF* mutations were noted in 62% of distant metastases, a rate significantly higher than that found in primary tumors. Although other studies have reported nearly equivalent rates of *BRAF* mutation occurring in nevi, primary tumors, and metastatic tumors, thereby minimizing any role it may have in tumor progression, our data indicate that *BRAF* mutations may play a part in melanoma progression, particularly in later stages.

EPIGENETIC ALTERATIONS: HYPERMETHYLATION

Spugnardi et al. detected hypermethylation of the *RASSF1A* in 32 distant melanoma metastases by MSP *(18)*. *RASSF1A* hypermethylation was noted in 56% of samples. The potential role of tumor suppressor gene hypermethylation in disease progression was further examined by Hoon et al. *RAR-β*, *RASSF1A*, *MGMT*, and *DAPK* promoter region methylation was determined by MSP in 33 PE metastatic tumors *(19)*. The gene methylation frequencies were as follows: *MGMT*, 27%; *RAR-β2*, 67%; *RASSF1A*, 55%; and *DAPK*, 9%. Although tumor suppressor gene methylation was more common in metastatic than primary tumors, indicating a possible role in tumor progression, no correlation between methylation status and disease-free or overall survival could be made in this patient group studied. Both a larger sample size and additional genes need to be analyzed to more adequately assess the role of epigenetic changes as prognostic factors in advanced metastatic melanoma.

OTHER SITES OF METASTASIS

Central Nervous System Metastasis

Treatment of stage IV melanoma is problematic. Surgical resection has been shown to improve survival in select cases, and is the therapy of choice, when possible *(31,32)*. Chemotherapy alone has not been shown to improve overall survival, and response rates have been disappointingly low *(64)*. Chemotherapy in combination with biological agents and immune adjuvants, or BC, has produced some of the most dramatic response rates to date, although results of its impact on overall survival has not been demonstrated to date *(65)*. This may be partially explained by the fact that the majority of patients responding to BC subsequently succumb to central nervous system (CNS) metastasis *(66)*. Melanoma commonly metastasizes to the CNS, with up to 54% of patients with advanced-stage disease having brain metastases on postmortem examination *(67)*. The early identification of patients with CNS metastasis is difficult using standard clinical and radiographic means of detection. Typically, brain lesions are greater than 1 cm in diameter before they become symptomatic or evident radiographically. Investigators have detected tumor cells in cerebrospinal fluid (CSF) using standard histopathology methods, but with inefficient results *(68)*.

As with the identification of occult tumor cells in circulating blood, Hoon et al. examined the CSF of 37 patients with stage-IV melanoma using a multimarker RT-PCR panel consisting of *tyrosinase*, *MART-1*, and *MAGE-3 (9)*. Patients were also evaluated by routine CSF cytology with IHC and brain MRI. Only 3% of patients were diagnosed with occult CSF metastases using routine histopathology and IHC. MRI identified 11% of patients with CNS metastases. By contrast, multimarker PCR identified occult CNS metastasis in 32% of patients. The combination of *MART-1* and *MAGE-3* positivity was the most sensitive predictor of disease recurrence ($p = 0.04$), but no combination of markers correlated significantly with overall survival. After 4 yr of follow-up, 62% of patients studied developed clinically apparent CNS metastases. Of these, RT-PCR detected approx 50% in a single time-point analysis. It is possible that the sensitivity and specificity of the assay could be improved if CSF was sampled at sequential time points during disease surveillance. However, the clinical applicability of an assay requiring sequential lumbar punctures remains of questionable benefit.

The discovery of sensitive and specific predictive markers of subsequent CNS metastasis may be beneficial for stratifying patients into appropriate surveillance and treatment subgroups. For example, those patients with positive mRNA markers in CSF may be candidates for more aggressive brain MRI imaging to help detect metastases at the earliest stage of clinically evident disease. Furthermore, patients without CSF mRNA markers may be the best cohort of patients to whom adjuvant therapies, such as BC, can be offered, because their survival will likely not be limited by CNS disease.

Bone Marrow Metastasis

Compared with the harsh environment tumor cells encounter in the circulating blood-stream, the bone marrow (BM) provides a relatively hospitable environment. Several investigators have attempted to detect occult melanoma metastases in BM using RT-PCR with the aim of using these results to predict adverse outcome, as has been done in breast cancer *(69)*. To date the results have been conflicting.

Ghossein et al. examined *tyrosinase* expression in the BM of 123 stage II to IV melanoma patients by RT-PCR compared with the level of expression noted in peripheral blood *(53)*. *Tyrosinase* mRNA was detected in 12% of blood samples and 16.5% of BM aspirates. Despite this, blood *tyrosinase* positivity was significantly correlated with overall survival ($p = 0.03$), but BM *tyrosinase* positivity was not.

In contrast, Waldmann et al. concluded that BM is unlikely to be a significant reservoir for melanoma tumor cells *(70)*. *Tyrosinase* expression in blood and BM was examined in 20 stage IV melanoma patients. *Tyrosinase* was detected in the BM of 7 of 20 (35%) patients and the blood of 7 of 20 (35%) patients. Although this is a higher BM *tyrosinase* detection rate than Ghossein reported, the authors did not pursue an outcomes analysis with respect to recurrence-free or overall survival. In a later publication, however, the same authors reported no significant survival difference between patients with and without *tyrosinase* detected in their BM *(71)*.

A multimarker panel consisting of *tyrosinase, TRP-1, Pmel 17/gp100*, and *MCAM/ MUC18/CD146* was used to detect occult melanoma metastases in metastatic tumors, BM, and blood from 26 patients undergoing metastectomy for isolated pulmonary or abdominal metastases *(8)*. Rather than undergoing BM aspiration from the iliac crest, however, these patients had segments of rib excised for analysis as part of routine thoracotomy procedure at the John Wayne Cancer Institute. Tyrosinase was detected in 58% of samples, significantly higher than reported in previous series. The frequency of mRNA expression for the additional markers was as follows: *TRP-1*, 27%; *Pmel 17/ gp100*, 54%; and *MCAM/MUC18/CD146*, 38%. Additionally, 66% of BM samples expressed at least one marker and 65% expressed at least two markers. The highest rates of marker expression were seen in metastatic tumor specimens. For all markers except *Pmel 17/gp100*, marker expression was higher in BM than blood. As with peripheral blood and lymph node studies, the multimarker assay increased the detection of BM metastases compared with single-marker assays using tyrosinase alone.

It could be argued, however, that determining survival differences among patients with and without detectable BM mRNA markers is least important in stage IV patients. This population of patients, with few exceptions, has a uniformly dismal prognosis and, therefore, any difference in BM mRNA marker expression would likely not translate into a survival difference. Rather, the most information on the prognostic value of detecting occult BM metastasis may be obtained from early stage patients without clinical or radiographic evidence of regional or distant metastatic disease. Additionally, patients with minimal metastatic disease may benefit most from adjuvant therapy. Because of cellular heterogeneity within and between tumors, a multimarker panel may provide the most information when seeking to definitively answer the following questions in future studies: do mRNA marker-positive BM aspirates represent true occult metastatic disease, or merely the detection of cells in transit that are incapable of establishing a true metastatic colony? What is the long-term significance of BM mRNA marker positivity with respect to predicting disease recurrence and overall survival? Are these occult metastases more predictive in early-stage or late-stage melanoma patients? What mRNA marker panel detects occult metastases with optimal sensitivity and specificity? These and other questions can only be conclusively answered in the setting of a multicenter, randomized, controlled trial using standardized laboratory techniques.

CONCLUSIONS AND PERSPECTIVES

Improving surgical techniques, diagnostic imaging, and adjuvant therapies for the diagnosis and treatment of melanoma must be matched by a corresponding improvement in methods of molecular diagnosis, outcome prediction, disease surveillance, and monitoring of response to therapy.

The molecular ultrastaging of melanoma tissues, particularly SLN, holds great promise for identifying patients with occult metastatic disease early enough to positively effect their disease outcome. Patients are currently being enrolled in the MSLT-II trial that will hopefully answer this question with respect to the benefit of multimarker qRT. Similarly, we are validating the multi-marker qRT assay in the assessment of circulating tumor cells in stage III and IV melanoma patients in the phase III multicenter Malignant Melanoma Active Immunotherapy Trial. Circulating DNA assays are further being validated in the setting of phase II BC trials, as well as in the Malignant Melanoma Active Immunotherapy Trial. The ability to use molecular markers as prognostic indicators will be invaluable as clinicians seek to stratify patients for clinical trials, adjuvant treatment regimens, and clinical follow-up regimens. The use of molecular markers to investigate clinical melanoma specimens, be they primary tumors or distant metastases, lymph nodes or blood, will lead to new and more sensitive diagnostic evaluations and, potentially, much-needed treatments. Because metastatic melanoma is a disease with few, and very toxic, adjuvant treatment options, the use of molecular markers to monitor a patient's response to therapy will be crucial for determining who will and who will not benefit from that therapy. At the same time, this approach may identify patients unlikely to respond to adjuvant treatments, thereby reducing the number of patients receiving ineffective and unnecessary therapy.

The advent of microarray technology promises the identification of potential molecular markers and candidate tumor-related genes in the future. An emphasis on quantitative rather than subjective or qualitative assays will be important to compare data between and among laboratories. The role of molecular markers in the future of melanoma diagnosis, prognosis, and treatment can only be solidified if data on their usefulness can be confirmed in large, multicenter, randomized, controlled clinical trials.

ACKNOWLEDGMENTS

Supported by funding in part from NIH/NCI grants P01 CA29605, P01 CA12582, and R33 CA100314-02, and the Martin H. Weil Research Laboratories.

The authors would like to thank all past and present members of the Department of Molecular Oncology at John Wayne Cancer Institute for their contributions, and especially Christine Kuo for her assistance with the preparation of this manuscript.

REFERENCES

1. Jemal A, Murray T, Ward E, et al. Cancer statistics, 2005. CA Cancer J Clin 2005;55:10–30.
2. Balch CM, Soong SJ, Atkins MB, et al. An evidence-based staging system for cutaneous melanoma. CA Cancer J Clin 2004;54:131–149; quiz 182–134.

3. Fuster D, Chiang S, Johnson G, Schuchter LM, Zhuang H, Alavi A. Is 18F-FDG PET more accurate than standard diagnostic procedures in the detection of suspected recurrent melanoma? J Nucl Med 2004;45:1323–1327.

4. Kim SY, Kim JS, Park HS, et al. Screening of brain metastasis with limited magnetic resonance imaging (MRI): clinical implications of using limited brain MRI during initial staging for non-small cell lung cancer patients. J Korean Med Sci 2005;20:121–126.

5. Swetter SM, Carroll LA, Johnson DL, Segall GM. Positron emission tomography is superior to computed tomography for metastatic detection in melanoma patients. Ann Surg Oncol 2002;9:646–653.

6. Shivers SC, Li W, Lin J, et al. The clinical relevance of molecular staging for melanoma. Recent Results Cancer Res 2001;158:187–199.

7. Gershenwald JE, Colome MI, Lee JE, et al. Patterns of recurrence following a negative sentinel lymph node biopsy in 243 patients with stage I or II melanoma. J Clin Oncol 1998;16:2253–2260.

8. Taback B, Morton DL, O'Day SJ, Nguyen DH, Nakayama T, Hoon DS. The clinical utility of multimarker RT-PCR in the detection of occult metastasis in patients with melanoma. Recent Results Cancer Res 2001;158:78–92.

9. Hoon DS, Kuo CT, Wascher RA, Fournier P, Wang HJ, O'Day SJ. Molecular detection of metastatic melanoma cells in cerebrospinal fluid in melanoma patients. J Invest Dermatol 2001;117:375–378.

10. Healy E, Rehman I, Angus B, Rees JL. Loss of heterozygosity in sporadic primary cutaneous melanoma. Genes Chromosomes Cancer 1995;12:152–156.

11. Albino AP, Fountain JW. Molecular genetics of human malignant melanoma. Cancer Treat Res 1993;65:201–255.

12. Fujiwara Y, Chi DD, Wang H, et al. Plasma DNA microsatellites as tumor-specific markers and indicators of tumor progression in melanoma patients. Cancer Res 1999;59:1567–1571.

13. Takeuchi H, Morton DL, Kuo C, et al. Prognostic significance of molecular upstaging of paraffin-embedded sentinel lymph nodes in melanoma patients. J Clin Oncol 2004;22:2671–2680.

14. Fujimoto A, Takeuchi H, Taback B, et al. Allelic imbalance of 12q22-23 associated with APAF-1 locus correlates with poor disease outcome in cutaneous melanoma. Cancer Res 2004;64:2245–2250.

15. Fujimoto A, O'Day SJ, Taback B, Elashoff D, Hoon DS. Allelic imbalance on 12q22-23 in serum circulating DNA of melanoma patients predicts disease outcome. Cancer Res 2004;64:4085–4088.

16. Taback B, O'Day SJ, Boasberg PD, et al. Circulating DNA microsatellites: molecular determinants of response to biochemotherapy in patients with metastatic melanoma. J Natl Cancer Inst 2004; 96:152–156.

17. Shinozaki M, Fujimoto A, Morton DL, Hoon DS. Incidence of BRAF oncogene mutation and clinical relevance for primary cutaneous melanomas. Clin Cancer Res 2004;10:1753–1757.

18. Spugnardi M, Tommasi S, Dammann R, Pfeifer GP, Hoon DS. Epigenetic inactivation of RAS association domain family protein 1 (RASSF1A) in malignant cutaneous melanoma. Cancer Res 2003;63:1639–1643.

19. Hoon DS, Spugnardi M, Kuo C, Huang SK, Morton DL, Taback B. Profiling epigenetic inactivation of tumor suppressor genes in tumors and plasma from cutaneous melanoma patients. Oncogene 2004;23:4014–4022.

20. Isshiki K, Seng BA, Elder DE, Guerry D, Linnenbach AJ. Chromosome 9 deletion in sporadic and familial melanomas in vivo. Oncogene 1994;9:1649–1653.

21. Celebi JT, Shendrik I, Silvers DN, Peacocke M. Identification of PTEN mutations in metastatic melanoma specimens. J Med Genet 2000;37:653–657.

22. Florenes VA, Oyjord T, Holm R, et al. TP53 allele loss, mutations and expression in malignant melanoma. Br J Cancer 1994;69:253–259.

23. Essner R, Kuo CT, Wang H, et al. Prognostic implications of p53 overexpression in cutaneous melanoma from sun-exposed and nonexposed sites. Cancer 1998;82:309–316.

24. Holland EA, Beaton SC, Edwards BG, Kefford RF, Mann GJ. Loss of heterozygosity and homozygous deletions on 9p21-22 in melanoma. Oncogene 1994;9:1361–1365.

25. Hussussian CJ, Struewing JP, Goldstein AM, et al. Germline p16 mutations in familial melanoma. Nat Genet 1994;8:15–21.

26. Mao L, Lee DJ, Tockman MS, Erozan YS, Askin F, Sidransky D. Microsatellite alterations as clonal markers for the detection of human cancer. Proc Natl Acad Sci USA 1994;91:9871–9875.

27. Jones PA, Baylin SB. The fundamental role of epigenetic events in cancer. Nat Rev Genet 2002;3:415–428.

28. Davies H, Bignell GR, Cox C, et al. Mutations of the BRAF gene in human cancer. Nature 2002;417:949–954.

29. Pollock PM, Harper UL, Hansen KS, et al. High frequency of BRAF mutations in nevi. Nat Genet 2003;33:19–20.

30. Loewe R, Kittler H, Fischer G, Fae I, Wolff K, Petzelbauer P. BRAF kinase gene V599E mutation in growing melanocytic lesions. J Invest Dermatol 2004;123:733–736.

31. Ollila DW, Hsueh EC, Stern SL, Morton DL. Metastasectomy for recurrent stage IV melanoma. J Surg Oncol 1999;71:209–213.

32. Hsueh EC, Essner R, Foshag LJ, et al. Prolonged survival after complete resection of disseminated melanoma and active immunotherapy with a therapeutic cancer vaccine. J Clin Oncol 2002; 20:4549–4554.

33. Morton DL, Wen DR, Wong JH, et al. Technical details of intraoperative lymphatic mapping for early stage melanoma. Arch Surg 1992;127:392–399.

34. Yu LL, Flotte TJ, Tanabe KK, et al. Detection of microscopic melanoma metastases in sentinel lymph nodes. Cancer 1999;86:617–627.

35. Boi S, Cristofolini P, Togni R, et al. Detection of nodal micrometastases using immunohistochemistry and PCR in melanoma of the arm and trunk. Melanoma Res 2002;12:147–153.

36. Shivers SC, Wang X, Li W, et al. Molecular staging of malignant melanoma: correlation with clinical outcome. Jama 1998;280:1410–1415.

37. Kammula US, Ghossein R, Bhattacharya S, Coit DG. Serial follow-up and the prognostic significance of reverse transcriptase-polymerase chain reaction-staged sentinel lymph nodes from melanoma patients. J Clin Oncol 2004;22:3989–3996.

38. Bostick PJ, Morton DL, Turner RR, et al. Prognostic significance of occult metastases detected by sentinel lymphadenectomy and reverse transcriptase-polymerase chain reaction in early-stage melanoma patients. J Clin Oncol 1999;17:3238–3244.

39. Palmieri G, Ascierto PA, Cossu A, et al. Detection of occult melanoma cells in paraffin-embedded histologically negative sentinel lymph nodes using a reverse transcriptase polymerase chain reaction assay. J Clin Oncol 2001;19:1437–1443.

40. Kuo CT, Hoon DS, Takeuchi H, et al. Prediction of disease outcome in melanoma patients by molecular analysis of paraffin-embedded sentinel lymph nodes. J Clin Oncol 2003;21:3566–3572.

41. Yao K, Kuo C, Wang H, Lai R, Morton D, Hoon D. Prognostic significance of hypermethylated tumor suppressor genes in metastatic melanomas. Ann Surg Oncol 2004;11:S85.

42. Smith B, Selby P, Southgate J, Pittman K, Bradley C, Blair GE. Detection of melanoma cells in peripheral blood by means of reverse transcriptase and polymerase chain reaction. Lancet 1991;338:1227–1229.

43. Brossart P, Keilholz U, Willhauck M, Scheibenbogen C, Mohler T, Hunstein W. Hematogenous spread of malignant melanoma cells in different stages of disease. J Invest Dermatol 1993;101:887–889.

44. Battayani Z, Grob JJ, Xerri L, et al. Polymerase chain reaction detection of circulating melanocytes as a prognostic marker in patients with melanoma. Arch Dermatol 1995;131:443–447.

45. Foss AJ, Guille MJ, Occleston NL, Hykin PG, Hungerford JL, Lightman S. The detection of melanoma cells in peripheral blood by reverse transcription-polymerase chain reaction. Br J Cancer 1995; 72:155–159.

46. Kunter U, Buer J, Probst M, et al. Peripheral blood tyrosinase messenger RNA detection and survival in malignant melanoma. J Natl Cancer Inst 1996;88:590–594.

47. Pittman K, Burchill S, Smith B, et al. Reverse transcriptase-polymerase chain reaction for expression of tyrosinase to identify malignant melanoma cells in peripheral blood. Ann Oncol 1996;7:297–301.

48. Mellado B, Colomer D, Castel T, et al. Detection of circulating neoplastic cells by reverse-transcriptase polymerase chain reaction in malignant melanoma: association with clinical stage and prognosis. J Clin Oncol 1996;14:2091–2097.

49. Glaser R, Rass K, Seiter S, Hauschild A, Christophers E, Tilgen W. Detection of circulating melanoma cells by specific amplification of tyrosinase complementary DNA is not a reliable tumor marker in melanoma patients: a clinical two-center study. J Clin Oncol 1997;15:2818–2825.

50. Jung FA, Buzaid AC, Ross MI, et al. Evaluation of tyrosinase mRNA as a tumor marker in the blood of melanoma patients. J Clin Oncol 1997;15:2826–2831.

51. Reinhold U, Ludtke-Handjery HC, Schnautz S, Kreysel HW, Abken H. The analysis of tyrosinase-specific mRNA in blood samples of melanoma patients by RT-PCR is not a useful test for metastatic tumor progression. J Invest Dermatol 1997;108:166–169.

52. Farthmann B, Eberle J, Krasagakis K, et al. RT-PCR for tyrosinase-mRNA-positive cells in peripheral blood: evaluation strategy and correlation with known prognostic markers in 123 melanoma patients. J Invest Dermatol 1998;110:263–267.

53. Ghossein RA, Coit D, Brennan M, et al. Prognostic significance of peripheral blood and bone marrow tyrosinase messenger RNA in malignant melanoma. Clin Cancer Res 1998;4:419–428.

54. O'Connell CD, Juhasz A, Kuo C, Reeder DJ, Hoon DS. Detection of tyrosinase mRNA in melanoma by reverse transcription-PCR and electrochemiluminescence. Clin Chem 1998;44:1161–1169.

55. Mellado B, Gutierrez L, Castel T, et al. Prognostic significance of the detection of circulating malignant cells by reverse transcriptase-polymerase chain reaction in long-term clinically disease-free melanoma patients. Clin Cancer Res 1999;5:1843–1848.

56. Bieligk SC, Ghossein R, Bhattacharya S, Coit DG. Detection of tyrosinase mRNA by reverse transcription-polymerase chain reaction in melanoma sentinel nodes. Ann Surg Oncol 1999;6:232–240.

57. Hoon DS, Wang Y, Dale PS, et al. Detection of occult melanoma cells in blood with a multiple-marker polymerase chain reaction assay. J Clin Oncol 1995;13:2109–2116.

58. Curry BJ, Myers K, Hersey P. Polymerase chain reaction detection of melanoma cells in the circulation: relation to clinical stage, surgical treatment, and recurrence from melanoma. J Clin Oncol 1998;16:1760–1769.

59. Hoon DS, Bostick P, Kuo C, et al. Molecular markers in blood as surrogate prognostic indicators of melanoma recurrence. Cancer Res 2000;60:2253–2257.

60. Wascher RA, Morton DL, Kuo C, et al. Molecular tumor markers in the blood: early prediction of disease outcome in melanoma patients treated with a melanoma vaccine. J Clin Oncol 2003;21:2558–2563.

61. Mocellin S, Del Fiore P, Guarnieri L, et al. Molecular detection of circulating tumor cells is an independent prognostic factor in patients with high-risk cutaneous melanoma. Int J Cancer 2004;111:741–745.

62. Taback B, Hoon DS. Circulating nucleic acids in plasma and serum: past, present and future. Curr Opin Mol Ther 2004;6:273–278.

63. Nakayama T, Taback B, Nguyen DH, et al. Clinical significance of circulating DNA microsatellite markers in plasma of melanoma patients. Ann NY Acad Sci 2000;906:87–98.

64. Legha SS. Current therapy for malignant melanoma. Semin Oncol 1989;16:34–44.

65. Eton O, Legha SS, Bedikian AY, et al. Sequential biochemotherapy versus chemotherapy for metastatic melanoma: results from a phase III randomized trial. J Clin Oncol 2002;20:2045–2052.

66. Atkins MB, Gollob JA, Sosman JA, et al. A phase II pilot trial of concurrent biochemotherapy with cisplatin, vinblastine, temozolomide, interleukin 2, and IFN-alpha 2B in patients with metastatic melanoma. Clin Cancer Res 2002;8:3075–3081.

67. Fife KM, Colman MH, Stevens GN, et al. Determinants of outcome in melanoma patients with cerebral metastases. J Clin Oncol 2004;22:1293–1300.

68. Fouladi M, Gajjar A, Boyett JM, et al. Comparison of CSF cytology and spinal magnetic resonance imaging in the detection of leptomeningeal disease in pediatric medulloblastoma or primitive neuro-ectodermal tumor. J Clin Oncol 1999;17:3234–3237.

69. Naume B, Wiedswang G, Borgen E, et al. The prognostic value of isolated tumor cells in bone marrow in breast cancer patients: evaluation of morphological categories and the number of clinically significant cells. Clin Cancer Res 2004;10:3091–3097.

70. Waldmann V, Deichmann M, Bock M, Jackel A, Naher H. The detection of tyrosinase-specific mRNA in bone marrow is not more sensitive than in blood for the demonstration of micrometastatic melanoma. Br J Dermatol 1999;140:1060–1064.

71. Waldmann V, Wacker J, Deichmann M, Naher H. No correlation of tyrosinase mRNA in bone marrow with prognosis of metastatic melanoma. Dermatology 2000;201:6–9.

The Role of DCT/TYRP2 in Resistance of Melanoma Cells to Drugs and Radiation

Brian J. Pak and Yaacov Ben-David

Contents

Summary

Intrinsic resistance to both chemotherapy and radiotherapy remains a major obstacle in the clinical treatment of malignant melanoma. Recent advances in cancer research have provided new insights into the molecular mechanisms governing their intrinsic resistance. We have recently demonstrated that DOPAchrome tautomerase (DCT), an enzyme that is well characterized for its function in melanin synthesis, is highly expressed in human melanoma cells that are resistant to both drug and radiation treatments. Conversely, melanoma cells expressing very low levels of DCT are highly susceptible to either type of treatment. Overexpression of DCT in melanoma cells by transfection could confer both radioresistance and chemoresistance. This review will summarize our findings, as well as discuss the possible mechanisms by which DCT overexpression contributes to intrinsic resistance of human malignant melanoma.

Key Words: Radioresistance; chemoresistance; malignant melanoma; DOPAchrome tautomerase (DCT).

From: *From Melanocytes to Melanoma: The Progression to Malignancy*
Edited by: V. J. Hearing and S. P. L. Leong © Humana Press Inc., Totowa, NJ

INTRODUCTION

Conventional cancer therapies involve the selective targeting of actively dividing cells by either the systemic administration of antineoplastic agents or localized treatment with ionizing radiation. There are several different classes of chemotherapeutic drugs that exert their anticancer effects by distinct mechanisms. For example, drugs such as *cis*-diamminedichloroplatinum(II) (CDDP), cyclophosphamide, and dacarbazine generate various forms of DNA damage *(1)*. Other agents, such as paclitaxel and vinblastine bind tubulin, thereby inhibiting the formation of microtubules *(2)*, whereas drugs such as methotrexate and 5-fluorouracil prevent nucleic acid synthesis *(3)*. All of these agents act by blocking specific events during the mitotic cycle, thereby inducing cells to undergo apoptosis. Ionizing radiation, on the other hand, induces DNA strand breaks and dimerization, which, in turn, triggers the apoptotic cascade *(4)*.

Although radiation and chemotherapy remain first-line treatments for cancer, one of the major limitations of these approaches is that many malignancies either acquire resistance to these therapies during the course of treatment or are intrinsically resistant at the time of diagnosis. Several resistance pathways employed by malignant cells have been described in the literature. Drug efflux pumps consisting of groups of integral membrane proteins, such as P-glycoprotein *(5)*, multidrug resistance protein *(6)*, lung resistance protein *(7)*, and breast cancer resistance protein, are expressed in a wide variety of different malignancies *(8)*. Resistance to DNA damage by elevated expression of various DNA repair enzymes, including the nucleotide excision repair enzymes, ERCC1 and XPF, O^6-alkylguanine-DNA alkyltransferase, and O^6-methylguanine-DNA methyltransferase all have been widely described in resistant tumors *(9,10)*. Resistance mechanisms employed by cancer cells are complex and multifactorial, and are likely heterogeneous within a tumor because of random mutations and differences in the tumor microenvironment. As such, a thorough understanding of these resistance pathways are of utmost importance in the effective clinical management of cancer using existing therapies, as well as in the development of novel therapeutic agents.

The treatment of patients with melanoma can vary greatly depending on the stage at which melanoma is diagnosed. In its early stages, melanomas grow superficially on the epidermis and can be treated by surgical excision. However, once the primary tumor disseminates, melanomas become extremely difficult to treat. This is because most late-staged melanoma tumors display intrinsic resistance to chemotherapy and radiation therapy. Indeed, melanoma is virtually unresponsive to most chemotherapeutic drugs administered as a monotherapy *(11,12)*. Combinations of such drugs, however, have been shown to improve tumor response, but rarely lead to complete remission or cures. Currently, the mechanisms underlying intrinsic resistance in melanomas remain poorly understood. Mutations in the tumor suppressor protein, p53, have been shown to enhance drug resistance in many cancer models. However, because most melanomas express wild-type p53, it is widely believed that this resistance phenotype is independent of a p53 mutation *(13–19)*. It has been reported that more than 90% of melanomas express the antiapoptotic protein Bcl-2 *(20–24)* raising the possibility that Bcl-2 expression may contribute to their intrinsic resistance. Studies by Jansen and colleagues *(25)* have shown that the downregulation of Bcl-2 expression in xenograft models using antisense oligonucleotide therapy targeting Bcl-2, improved sensitivity of human melanoma cells to both dacarbazine and CDDP. Such results have also been obtained by treating melanoma

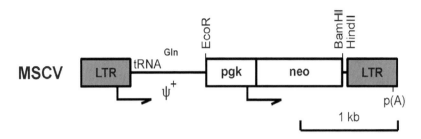

Fig. 1. Restriction map of murine stem cell virus retrovirus.

cells with small interfering RNA *(26,27)*. Other antiapoptotic factors, such as Bcl-xL, Mcl-1, and Survivin have also been reported to be highly expressed in melanoma cells and, therefore, may also contribute to the intrinsic resistance to therapies *(28–31)*.

RETROVIRAL INSERTIONAL MUTAGENESIS AS A METHOD OF GENERATING RESISTANT CELL LINES

In 1994, we described the use of retroviral insertional mutagenesis as a means of rapidly generating resistant variants of drug-sensitive melanoma cell lines *(32)*. This method involves the infection of comparatively drug-sensitive melanoma cells with replication-defective amphotrophic retroviruses to generate mutants of the parental cell line. The integration of proviruses into the host cell genome generates random mutations that can lead to the activation or inactivation of cellular genes depending on the site of integration. For example, if the provirus integrates within a gene, the expression of the gene may be disrupted. Conversely, if the provirus integrates between genes, the transactivating property of the viral long terminal repeats may activate the transcription of adjacent genes. Therefore, mutant cells that harbor a dominantly selectable phenotype can be isolated and characterized. This approach has been used by our group, as well as others, and has yielded several important genes associated with cancer initiation, progression, and resistance, including *Fli-1*, *Spi-1*, *p53*, *NF-E2/p45*, and *CRL-1 (33–38)*.

In an attempt to identify genes that may be associated with drug and radiation resistance in melanoma cells, retroviral insertional mutagenesis was used to create mutants of an early-staged, drug- and radiation-sensitive human melanoma cell line. The retrovirus used was a replication-defective, *neo*-containing murine stem cell virus with an amphotrophic host range *(39)*. Murine stem cell virus is devoid of *env* sequences, and includes an extended packaging region (P$^+$) for high viral titer and a modified 5'-untranslated region with a primer-binding site for tRNA^{Gln} instead of the usual tRNA^{Pro}. Long terminal repeats and *pgk* promoters are used for the expression of viral and *neo* RNA transcripts, respectively (Fig. 1).

Melanoma mutants generated by retroviral insertional mutagenesis were subjected to treatments of lethal doses of CDDP. The rationale was that among the wild-type population of cells, some cells would have acquired a mutation that would confer CDDP resistance. These cells can then be isolated, expanded in culture, and characterized to determine which genes may be associated with CDDP resistance. By this approach, several independently derived CDDP-resistant clones were established. Quite interestingly, more than half of these clones showed the integration of a single provirus at an identical site, which was designated "CDDP resistance locus 1" (*CRL-1*). *CRL-1* was mapped to human chromosome 3p21 (B. J. Pak et al., unpublished data). An analysis of approx 20 kb of genomic DNA flanking *CRL-1* failed to identify exonic sequences. These results were not unexpected because proviruses often alter the expression of target genes located as much as 80 kb from the site of integration *(40)*. Attempts to determine the gene(s) that are directly regulated by proviral integration have, thus far, been unsuccessful.

IDENTIFICATION OF DOPACHROME TAUTOMERASE AS A MEDIATOR OF DRUG RESISTANCE

To screen for genes that are differentially expressed in the CDDP-resistant mutants, subtractive hybridization was employed. Messenger RNA from wild-type cells and from one of the virally derived mutant cells were compared and yielded a single transcript, DCT, also termed tyrosinase-related protein (TYRP)-2, which was upregulated in the CDDP-resistant clone *(41)*. Subsequent Northern blot analysis showed that DOPAchrome tautomerase (DCT) was upregulated in each of the CDDP-resistant clones generated by retroviral insertional mutagenesis. A screen of several other human melanoma cell lines, which had been characterized as CDDP-sensitive or -resistant, showed a consistent correlation between the relative levels of DCT expression and their resistance to CDDP *(41)*. That is, cell lines that express high levels of DCT were characteristically resistant to CDDP, whereas cell lines that express little to no DCT were highly sensitive to CDDP treatment. We further showed that the expression of DCT appeared to be restricted to cells of melanocytic lineage and its expression was not detected in a panel of nonmelanoma human cancer cell lines *(42)*.

Perhaps the best evidence that DCT may play a role in CDDP resistance in melanoma was generated from transfection studies. Wild-type cells were transfected with either a DCT plasmid vector or empty vector. Characterization of the resulting transfectants showed that the wild-type and empty vector cells were equally sensitive to CDDP treatment, whereas each of the isolated DCT transfectants was significantly more resistant. Increased resistance of DCT-overexpressing cells was shown to be associated with a significant decrease in CDDP-induced apoptosis *(41)*. We further observed that DCT-overexpressing melanoma cells not only displayed resistance to CDDP, but were cross-resistant to carboplatin and methotrexate *(41)*. Both of these compounds exert their antineoplastic effects by distinct mechanisms but, similar to CDDP, ultimately interfere with DNA replication. Interestingly, DCT overexpression in these cells did not increase resistance to paclitaxel, a drug that is not directly associated with DNA replication but targets microtubule formation *(2)*. Thus, these results suggest that DCT overexpression confers resistance specifically to agents that interfere with DNA replication.

The association between DCT expression and resistance to DNA-damaging agents was not restricted to cell lines and appeared to be applicable in vivo. In preliminary studies, two human melanoma cell lines, one that expresses high levels of DCT and one that expresses very low levels, were used to generate tumor xenografts in immunodeficient nude mice. After allowing tumors to grow until they were readily palpable, these mice were subjected to treatment with CDDP. After several days of treatment, tumors generated from the low DCT-expressing cell line showed a significant response to CDDP treatment, with a cessation in tumor growth in most animals, and, in a few cases, a complete disappearance of the tumor. Tumor-bearing mice generated by the high DCT-expressing cell line exhibited no evidence of tumor shrinkage during similar treatment (B. J. Pak et al., unpublished data).

MELANOGENESIS AND TYROSINASE-RELATED PROTEINS

The pigment melanin comprises a heterogeneous mixture of indoles and polymers derived from the oxidation of L-tyrosine. Melanin biosynthesis occurs in specialized organelles called melanosomes in cells of the retinal pigment epithelium and dermal melanocytes, and is distributed in the skin, hair bulbs, and the eyes. Two types of melanins, pheomelanin (yellow, red) and eumelanin (black, brown), are synthesized and their relative proportions in pigment cells determine color. In mammals, melanin serves several important protective functions, including photoprotection from solar ultraviolet (UV) radiation, and thermoregulation because of its ability to absorb energy from various forms of radiation. In addition, melanin is a cation chelator and, as such, has been postulated to serve as a free-radical sink *(43)*. The conversion of L-tyrosine to melanin is mediated by the enzymatic activities of the tyrosinase family of proteins, which include tyrosinase, TYRP1, and DCT (Fig. 2), and both quantity and quality of melanin synthesis is dependent on the relative activities of these enzymes.

Tyrosinase (EC 1.14.18.1) is the rate-limiting enzyme in melanogenesis. Tyrosinase mediates the hydroxylation of L-tyrosine to L-dopaquinone *(44,45)* and the oxidation of 5,6-dihydroxyindole (DHI) to indole-5,6-quinone *(46)*. The conversion of L-dopaquinone from L-tyrosine was thought to involve the intermediate formation of DOPA, which subsequently oxidizes to form L-dopaquinone. Recent research, however, has shown that the formation of DOPA from L-tyrosine occurs largely from an indirect, nonenzymatic pathway, independent of tyrosinase *(45)*.

The *tyrosinase* gene maps to the *c (albino/Tyr)* locus on chromosome 7 in mouse and chromosome 11 in human and is comprised of five exons and four introns spanning approx 60–70 kb *(47)*. It encodes a 2.4 kb transcript that translates into a 55-kDa protein, which is glycosylated to a mature size of 65 to 75 kDa.

TYRP1, mapped to the *brown (b/Tyrp)* locus, resides on mouse chromosome 4 and on human chromosome 9p23 *(48)*. The gene is composed of eight exons and seven introns, and encodes a transcript that yields a 537-amino-acid protein with a mature mass of approx 75 kDa. TYRP1 has been suggested to function as a 5,6-dihydroxyindole-2-carboxylic acid (DHICA) oxidase in murine melanocytes, although this remains a subject of dispute *(49,50)*. Recently, it has been suggested that human TYRP1 does not use DHICA as a substrate *(51)*.

DCT (EC 5.3.3.12) mediates the tautomerization of the red melanin precursor, L-DOPAchrome to the colorless DHICA *(52,53)*. In the absence of DCT, l-DOPAchrome is spontaneously converted to the toxic melanin precursor, DHI *(52,54)*. It has been suggested that DCT may function to protect melanocytes against cytotoxicity caused by DHI accumulation by limiting its formation. The *DCT* gene is composed of eight exons and seven introns, and has been mapped to the *slaty (Tyrp2)* locus on chromosome 14 in mouse and chromosome 13 in human. The gene encodes a transcript that contains a 1.6-kb open-reading frame that translates into a mature protein of approx 75 kDa after posttranslational processing *(48)*.

Mutations at the *DCT* locus have been found in mice, all of which leads in pigmentation phenotypes *(55)*. Each of these mutations is a point mutation, designated as Dct[slt], Dct[slt-J], and Dct[slt-Lt], which still express the mutant form. Recently, mice deficient in

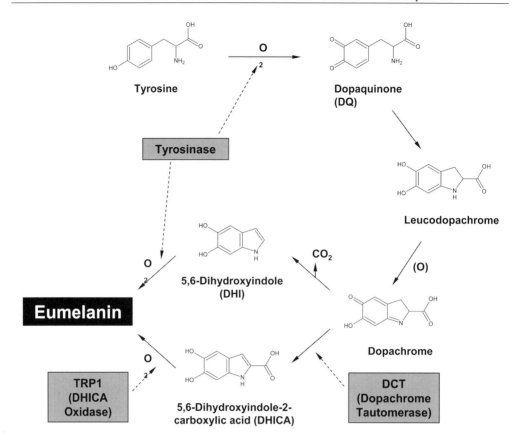

Fig. 2. Schematic of eumelanin synthesis.

DCT have been generated, revealing a diluted coat-color phenotype, which is caused by reduced melanin content in hair *(56)*. Interestingly, this group demonstrated that, in contrast to the knockout mice, the *slaty* mutation (Dct^{slt}/Dct^{slt}) has less melanin and severely effects growth of primary melanocytes *(56)*. This data may suggest involvement of DCT in cell proliferation, in addition to its role in melanin synthesis.

EXPRESSION OF DCT

Although the primary function of DCT is in the synthesis of melanin, its expression is not restricted to melanocytes. DCT expression has been reported in various normal and neoplastic cell types of the neural ectodermal lineage. These include the retinal pigment epithelium *(57)*, retinoblastomas *(58)*, gliomas *(59)*, and glioblastomas *(60)*. However, to our knowledge, DCT expression has not been reported in cells outside of the neural ectodermal lineage. As such, resistance mediated by DCT represents a unique mechanism that is both lineage- and tissue-specific, unlike all other known mechanisms of drug resistance.

In melanomas, DCT is reportedly highly expressed in most primary tumors and cell lines. Orlow and colleagues *(61)* showed that among the tyrosinases, TYRP1 and DCT, only DCT was consistently expressed in all melanoma tumor samples examined. Among the 10 independently derived human melanoma cell lines that are routinely cultured in our laboratory, 7 have been shown to express high levels of DCT. Indeed, reverse transcriptase-polymerase chain reaction (RT-PCR) detection of the *gp100* and *DCT* gene transcripts were identified in metastatic cells collected from the peripheral blood of melanoma patients and was correlated with recurrent and/or metastatic disease *(62)*.

DCT AND RADIATION RESISTANCE

The observation that DCT overexpression appeared to specifically confer resistance to chemotherapeutic agents that later interfere with DNA replication prompted the investigation into whether DCT is associated with resistance to DNA damage induced by ionizing radiation. In a recent study, we employed retroviral insertional mutagenesis, using the same original human melanoma cell line as in our drug resistance study, to generate mutants that display resistance to X-ray irradiation. Characterization of these X-ray resistant mutants showed that each independently derived clone expressed significantly higher levels of DCT compared with the parental cell line, at both the messenger RNA and protein levels *(63)*. X-ray irradiation is known to induce cytotoxicity by generating DNA strand breaks and, as such, these results support the notion that DCT may be associated with resistance to DNA damage.

Exposure to UVB irradiation also induces cytotoxicity. Unlike X-ray radiation, UVB does not induce DNA strand breaks, but causes the formation of pyrimidine dimers, which disrupt the mitotic pathway. An analysis of the X-ray-resistant mutant lines showed that each one of them displayed cross-resistance to UVB radiation *(63)*. Quite interestingly, all of the CDDP-resistant clones showed cross-resistance to UVB irradiation, whereas each of the radiation-resistant clones also showed resistance to CDDP. Moreover, the parental cells that had been transfected with DCT, which had previously been shown to be CDDP resistant, also showed increased resistance to UVB irradiation. Taken together, these results strongly suggest a role for DCT in conferring resistance to DNA damaging effectors.

Recently, Nishioka and colleagues *(64)* reported that DCT overexpression in melanoma cells by transfection abrogates UVB-induced apoptosis. These results provide further evidence of the importance of DCT in drug and radiation resistance. These results also exclude the possibility that DCT may confer resistance by modulating intracellular drug accumulation (i.e., regulating drug efflux pumps, such as P-glycoprotein and multidrug resistance transporter-1), or by enhancing drug detoxification pathways (e.g., increased glutathione or glutathione-*S*-transferase activity). Nishioka et al. also suggest that DCT overexpression may confer resistance by regulating specific apoptotic pathways and/or DNA repair mechanisms.

DCT AND IMMUNOTHERAPY OF HUMAN MELANOMA

Previous studies have demonstrated that various active-specific immunotherapy protocols have the potential to affect melanoma growth and progression. As such, induction of cellular immune responses to melanocyte-specific enzymes, such as tyrosinase, is a goal of clinical studies in melanoma immunotherapy. DCT is an attractive model antigen for melanoma vaccine therapy because it has been shown to be highly immunogenic and is expressed at high levels in melanocytes and melanomas at different stages of tumor progression *(65–67)*. Moreover, upregulation of DCT is also present in the serum of patients with malignant gliomas *(59)*. Several studies over the past decade have demonstrated that immunization with a DCT antigen suppressed tumor progression and significantly enhanced survival of melanoma-bearing mice. Similarly, vaccination with DCT-transfected dendritic cells also significantly increased antimelanoma immunity *(68–70)*. DNA vaccines used against DCT have also been shown to induce T-cell-mediated protection against mouse glioblastoma *(68)*. Taken together, these results suggest that vaccine-induced immune responses against DCT-expressing melanoma cells, as well as malignant gliomas, may leave behind cancer cells that are less intrinsically resistant to conventional cytotoxic agents. If so, a combination of DCT vaccination followed by chemotherapy may improve efficacy of such a treatment.

POSSIBLE MECHANISMS OF DCT-MEDIATED RESISTANCE

Because of the restricted localization of DCT to the melanosomal compartment of pigment-producing cells and its only reported function in melanin synthesis, our initial investigation into its mechanism of action in conferring resistance focused on the process of melanin synthesis. Specifically, the possibility that resistance was associated with an overall increase in melanogenic activity, and not solely DCT, was examined. The levels of tyrosinase, TYRP1, and DCT expression were profiled in a variety of human melanoma cell lines and compared with their relative levels of CDDP resistance. In each cell line examined, the extent of CDDP resistance correlated specifically with DCT expressions and did not bear any relationship to the expressions of tyrosinase or TYRP1 *(42)*. Moreover, the extent of CDDP resistance in these cells was not associated with total cellular melanin content. These results suggest a specific role for DCT in conferring resistance that is independent of overall melanogenic activity.

Given that DCT overexpression appears to be involved specifically with increased resistance to anticancer treatments specifically targeting the DNA, and that this resistance is associated with a decrease in treatment-induced apoptosis, it remains possible that DCT may modulate components of the apoptotic cascade that are triggered in response to DNA damage. A recent study showed DCT localization primarily in the perinuclear/Golgi area and occasionally on the plasma membrane. Very low quantities of DCT were detected in late melanosomes *(71)*. These observations suggest that DCT possibly has a second regulatory function within these cells. There has been increasing evidence in the literature that suggests melanin-related metabolites not only serve as pigment precursors, but also function as regulators of various cellular processes. Indeed, these molecules are highly diffusible and can readily exit the melanosomes and enter other cellular compartments. DHICA, the product of the DCT-mediated isomerization of L-DOPAchrome, is a stable, highly diffusible antioxidant molecule that has been previously shown to exhibit marked reactivity to nitrogen oxides produced by autoxidation of nitric oxide (NO) *(72)*, stimulate NO production by lipopolysaccharide-induced NO synthase *(73)*, and function as a potent inhibitor of lipid peroxidation *(74)*. It remains to be determined whether drug and radiation resistance in DCT-overexpressing melanoma cells is mediated through these melanin precursors. The biological potential of melanin precursors as regulators of cellular processes, independent of their function in the formation of pigmentation, warrants further investigation.

STRESS-DEPENDENT MECHANISMS OF RESISTANCE IN MELANOMAS

Cytotoxicity induced by treatment with either CDDP or UVB has been shown to be mediated, at least in part, by the activation of various cellular stress response pathways *(75,76)*. Thus, the manner in which cancer cells respond to stress may influence the level of resistance to anticancer treatments. Several well-characterized signal transduction pathways involved in the stress response, including p38/ATF, tumor necrosis factor-associated receptor factor 2, tumor necrosis factor-α, and nuclear factor-κB have been shown to play a role in modulating resistance in cancer cells *(75,77–81)*. We have previously noted that DCT-overexpressing melanoma cells, in addition to displaying increased resistance to drug and radiation treatment, also showed resistance to heat shock at 41°C (B. J. Pak et al., unpublished observation). This finding suggests a possible association between DCT expression and stress–response pathways. It is plausible that the differential accumulation of melanin precursors caused by DCT overexpression in these cells may lead to the activation of the stress response, which facilitates survival during subsequent exposure to stress. There are numerous studies that show that pre-exposure to sublethal doses of heat stress and the resulting increase in heat-shock protein expression protects cells from subsequent exposure to heat stress *(82,83)*. To test this hypothesis, melanoma cells were treated with the reducing compound, L-cysteine, which has been shown to enhance the DCT-catalyzed conversion of L-DOPAchrome to DHICA *(84)*. The treatment of melanoma cells with L-cysteine resulted in a dramatic increase in the levels of phospho-extracellular signal-related kinase (ERK), suggesting that increased DCT function may lead to an activation of the ERK/mitogen-activated protein kinase (MAPK) pathway *(63)*. This was supported by the observation that the levels of phospho-ERK were elevated in the DCT-transfected cell lines. Thus, these results suggest that DCT overexpression, possibly through the accumulation of DHICA, activates the ERK/MAPK pathway, and that this activation leads to downstream pathways that result in increased resistance. To test this, melanoma cells were transfected with MEKEE, a constitutively active mutant of MEK/MAPK *(63)*. This leads to an increase in the levels of phospho-ERK expression and conferred increased resistance to UVB treatment in these cells. These results are consistent with a recent report that showed that inhibitors of the ERK/MAPK pathway can sensitize melanoma cells to the toxic effects of chemotherapeutic drugs *(85)*. Therefore, taken together, we propose, based on these findings, that DCT overexpression in melanoma cells results in the activation of the ERK/MAPK pathway, likely through the melanin precursor, DHICA, and that the activation of this pathway results in increased resistance to chemotherapy and radiation therapy that targets DNA damage. Delineation of these pathways is currently ongoing.

CONCLUSIONS AND PERSPECTIVES

The observation that the overexpression of the melanogenic enzyme, DCT, can confer chemoresistance and radioresistance to melanoma cells offers an intriguing therapeutic potential in the treatment of malignant melanoma. The restricted expression of DCT to cells of the neural ectodermal lineage makes it a uniquely tissue-specific therapeutic target. Possible treatment strategies may involve the downregulation of DCT concurrently with chemotherapy or radiation therapy as a means of improving the efficacy of these treatments. Another possible application of these observations is that intratumor levels of DCT can be assayed in melanoma patients as a means to determine whether

these patients will be responsive to DNA-targeting chemotherapeutic agents or radiotherapy. Presently, there is no method of determining which melanoma patients will
respond to conventional therapies, and often patients are subjected to courses of chemotherapy that they are not responsive to and suffer from the adverse side effects of these
drugs. Predicting which patients will be more likely to respond to DNA-targeting
agents or other classes of drugs, such as the tubulin inhibitors, by assaying their serum
levels of DCT may assist in determining the clinical strategy to be considered for the
treatment of melanoma. Studies are currently in progress to identify a therapeutically
effective means of downregulating DCT, as well as to evaluate the validity of DCT as
an indicator of tumor responsiveness to chemotherapy and radiotherapy in melanoma.

REFERENCES

1. Fink D, Aebi S, Howell SB. The role of DNA mismatch repair in drug resistance. Clin Cancer Res
   1998;4(1):1–6.
2. Dumontet C, Sikic BI. Mechanisms of action of and resistance to antitubulin agents: microtubule
   dynamics, drug transport, and cell death. J Clin Oncol 1999;17(3):1061–1070.
3. Kinsella AR, Smith D. Tumor resistance to antimetabolites. Gen Pharmacol 1998;30(5):623–626.
4. Khanna KK, Jackson SP. DNA double-strand breaks: signaling, repair and the cancer connection. Nat
   Genet 2001;27(3):247–254.
5. Kavallaris M. The role of multidrug resistance-associated protein (MRP) expression in multidrug
   resistance. Anticancer Drugs 1997;8(1):17–25.
6. Kruh GD, Belinsky MG. The MRP family of drug efflux pumps. Oncogene 2003;22(47):7537–7552.
7. Izquierdo MA, Scheffer GL, Flens MJ, Shoemaker RH, Rome LH, Scheper RJ. Relationship of LRP-
   human major vault protein to in vitro and clinical resistance to anticancer drugs. Cytotechnology
   1996;19(3):191–197.
8. Doyle LA, Ross DD. Multidrug resistance mediated by the breast cancer resistance protein BCRP
   (ABCG2). Oncogene 2003;22(47):7340–7358.
9. Barret JM, Hill BT. DNA repair mechanisms associated with cellular resistance to antitumor drugs:
   potential novel targets. Anticancer Drugs 1998;9(2):105–123.
10. Cline SD, Hanawalt PC. Who's on first in the cellular response to DNA damage? Nat Rev Mol Cell
    Biol 2003;4(5):361–372.
11. Soengas MS, Lowe SW. Apoptosis and melanoma chemoresistance. Oncogene 2003;22(20):
    3138–3151.
12. Serrone L, Hersey P. The chemoresistance of human malignant melanoma: an update. Melanoma Res
    1999;9(1):51–58.
13. Volkenandt M, Schlegel U, Nanus DM, Albino AP. Mutational analysis of the human p53 gene in
    malignant melanoma. Pigment Cell Res 1991;4:35–40.
14. Weiss J, Schwechheimer K, Cavanee WK, Herlyn M, Arden KC. Mutation and expression of the p53
    gene in malignant melanoma cell lines. Int J Cancer 1993;54:693–699.
15. Weiss J, Heine M, Korner B, Pilch H, Jung EG. Expression of p53 protein in malignant melanoma:
    clinicopathological and prognostic implications. Br J Dermatol 1995;133(1):23–31.
16. Albino AP, Vidal MJ, McNutt NS, et al. Mutation and expression of the p53 gene in human malignant
    melanoma. Melanoma Res 1994;4(1):35–45.
17. Florenes VA, Oyjord T, Holm R, et al. TP53 allele loss, mutations and expression in malignant
    melanoma. Br J Cancer 1994;69(2):253–259.
18. Lubbe J, Reichel M, Burg G, Kleihues P. Absence of p53 gene mutations in cutaneous melanoma.
    J Invest Dermatol 1994;102(5):819–821.
19. Montano X, Shamsher M, Whitehead P, Dawson K, Newton J. Analysis of p53 in human cutaneous
    melanoma cell lines. Oncogene 1994;9(5):1455–1459.
20. Plettenberg A, Ballaun C, Pammer J, et al. Human melanocytes and melanoma cells constitutively
    express the Bcl-2 proto-oncogene in situ and in cell culture. Am J Pathol 1995;146(3):651–659.
21. Cerroni L, Soyer HP, Kerl H. bcl-2 protein expression in cutaneous malignant melanoma and benign
    melanocytic nevi. Am J Dermatopathol 1995;17(1):7–11.

22. Morales-Ducret CR, van de RM, LeBrun DP, Smoller DR. bcl-2 expression in primary malignancies of the skin. Arch Dermatol 1995;131(8):909–912.
23. Tron VA, Krajewski S, Klein-Parker H, Li G, Ho VC, Reed JC. Immunohistochemical analysis of Bcl-2 protein regulation in cutaneous melanoma. Am J Pathol 1995;146(3):643–650.
24. Grover R, Wilson GD. Bcl-2 expression in malignant melanoma and its prognostic significance. Eur J Surg Oncol 1996;22(4):347–349.
25. Jansen B, Schlagbauer-Wadl H, Brown BD, et al. bcl-2 antisense therapy chemosensitizes human melanoma in SCID mice. Nat Med 1998;4(2):232–234.
26. Wacheck V, Losert D, Gunsberg P, et al. Small interfering RNA targeting bcl-2 sensitizes malignant melanoma. Oligonucleotides 2003;13(5):393–400.
27. Yin JQ, Gao J, Shao R, Tian WN, Wang J, Wan Y. siRNA agents inhibit oncogene expression and attenuate human tumor cell growth. J Exp Ther Oncol 2003;3(4):194–204.
28. Thallinger C, Wolschek MF, Wacheck V, et al. Mcl-1 antisense therapy chemosensitizes human melanoma in a SCID mouse xenotransplantation model. J Invest Dermatol 2003;120(6):1081–1086.
29. Gautschi O, Tschopp S, Olie RA, et al. Activity of a novel bcl-2/bcl-xL-bispecific antisense oligo-nucleotide against tumors of diverse histologic origins. J Natl Cancer Inst 2001;93(6):463–471.
30. Olie RA, Hafner C, Kuttel R, et al. Bcl-2 and bcl-xL antisense oligonucleotides induce apoptosis in melanoma cells of different clinical stages. J Invest Dermatol 2002;118(3):505–512.
31. Strasberg RM, Zangemeister-Wittke U, Rieber M. p53-Independent induction of apoptosis in human melanoma cells by a bcl-2/bcl-xL bispecific antisense oligonucleotide. Clin Cancer Res 2001;7(5):1446–1451.
32. Lu S, Man S, Bani MR, et al. Retroviral insertional mutagenesis as a strategy for the identification of genes associated with cis-diamminedichloroplatinum (II) resistance. Cancer Res 1995;55:1139–1145.
33. Ben-David Y, Giddens EB, Bernstein A. Identification and mapping of a common proviral integration site Fli-1 in erythroleukemia cells induced by Friend murine leukemia virus. Proc Natl Acad Sci USA 1990;87:1332–1336.
34. Ben-David Y, Giddens EG, Letwin K, Bernstein A. Erythroleukemia induction by Friend murine leukemia virus: Insertional activation of a new member of the ets gene family, Fli-1, closely linked to c-ets-1. Genes Dev 1991;5:908–918.
35. Moreau-Gachelin F, Tavitian A, Tambourin P. Spi-1 is a putative oncogene in virally induced murine erythroleukaemias. Nature 1988;331:277–280.
36. Ben-David Y, Prideaux VR, Chow V, Benchimol S, Bernstein A. Inactivation of the p53 oncogene by internal deletion or retroviral integration in erythroleukemic cell lines induced by Friend leukemia virus. Oncogene 1988;3:179–185.
37. Lu SJ, Rowan S, Bani MR, Ben-David Y. Retroviral integration within the *FLi-2* locus results in inactivation of the erythroid transcription factor NF-E2 in Friend erythroleukemias: evidence that NF-E2 is essential for globin expression. Proc Natl Acad Sci USA 1994;91:8398–8402.
38. Lu S, Man S, Bani MR, et al. Retroviral insertional mutagenesis as a strategy for the identification of genes associated with cis-diamminedichloroplatinum (II) resistance. Cancer Res 1995;55:1139–1145.
39. Markowitz D, Goff S, Bank A. A safe packaging line for gene transfer: separating viral genes on two different plasmids. J Virol 1988;62:1120–1124.
40. Sola B, Simon D, Mattei MG, et al. Fim-1, Fim-2/c-fms, and Fim-3, three common integration sites of Friend murine leukemia virus in myeloblastic leukemias, map to mouse chromosomes 13, 18, and 3, respectively. J Virol 1988;62(11):3973–3978.
41. Chu W, Pak BJ, Bani MR, et al. Tyrosinase-related protein 2 as a mediator of melanoma specific resistance to cis-diamminedichloroplatinum(II): therapeutic implications. Oncogene 2000;19(3):395–402.
42. Pak BJ, Li Q, Kerbel RS, Ben-David Y. TYRP2-mediated resistance to cis-diamminedichloroplatinum (II) in human melanoma cells is independent of tyrosinase and TYRP1 expression and melanin content. Melanoma Res 2000;10(5):499–505.
43. Riley PA. Melanin. Int J Biochem Cell Biol 1997;29(11):1235–1239.
44. Hearing VJ, Tsukamoto K. Enzymatic control of pigmentation in mammals. FASEB J 1991;5(14):2902–2909.
45. Land EJ, Ramsden CA, Riley PA. Tyrosinase autoactivation and the chemistry of ortho-quinone amines. Acc Chem Res 2003;36(5):300–308.
46. Tripathi RK, Hearing VJ, Urabe K, Aroca P, Spritz RA. Mutational mapping of the catalytic activities of human tyrosinase. J Biol Chem 1992;267(33):23,707–23,712.

47. Barton DE, Kwon BS, Francke U. Human tyrosinase gene, mapped to chromosome 11 (q14----q21), defines second region of homology with mouse chromosome 7. Genomics 1988;3(1):17–24.

48. Sturm RA, O'Sullivan BJ, Box NF, et al. Chromosomal structure of the human TYRP1 and TYRP2 loci and comparison of the tyrosinase-related protein gene family. Genomics 1995;29(1):24–34.

49. Jimenez M, Kameyama K, Maloy WL, Tomita Y, Hearing VJ. Mammalian tyrosinase: biosynthesis, processing, and modulation by melanocyte-stimulating hormone. Proc Natl Acad Sci USA 1988;85(11):3830–3834.

50. Kobayashi T, Urabe K, Winder A, et al. Tyrosinase related protein 1 (TRP1) functions as a DHICA oxidase in melanin biosynthesis. EMBO J 1994;13(24):5818–5825.

51. Boissy RE, Sakai C, Zhao H, Kobayashi T, Hearing VJ. Human tyrosinase related protein-1 (TRP-1) does not function as a DHICA oxidase activity in contrast to murine TRP-1. Exp Dermatol 1998;7(4):198–204.

52. Tsukamoto K, Jackson IJ, Urabe K, Montague PM, Hearing VJ. A second tyrosinase-related protein, TRP-2, is a melanogenic enzyme termed DOPAchrome tautomerase. EMBO J 1992;11(2):519–526.

53. Leonard LJ, Townsend D, King RA. Function of dopachrome oxidoreductase and metal ions in dopachrome conversion in the eumelanin pathway. Biochemistry 1988;27(16):6156–6159.

54. Kroumpouzos G, Urabe K, Kobayashi T, Sakai C, Hearing VJ. Functional analysis of the slaty gene product (TRP2) as dopachrome tautomerase and the effect of a point mutation on its catalytic function. Biochem Biophys Res Commun 1994;202(2):1060–1068.

55. Budd PS, Jackson IJ. Structure of the mouse tyrosinase-related protein-2/dopachrome tautomerase (Tyrp2/Dct) gene and sequence of two novel slaty alleles. Genomics 1995;29(1):35–43.

56. Guyonneau L, Murisier F, Rossier A, Moulin A, Beermann F. Melanocytes and pigmentation are affected in dopachrome tautomerase knockout mice. Mol Cell Biol 2004;24(8):3396–3403.

57. Takeda K, Yokoyama S, Yasumoto K, et al. OTX2 regulates expression of DOPAchrome tautomerase in human retinal pigment epithelium. Biochem Biophys Res Commun 2003;300(4):908–914.

58. Udono T, Takahashi K, Yasumoto K, et al. Expression of tyrosinase-related protein 2/DOPAchrome tautomerase in the retinoblastoma. Exp Eye Res 2001;72(3):225–234.

59. Chi DD, Merchant RE, Rand R, et al. Molecular detection of tumor-associated antigens shared by human cutaneous melanomas and gliomas. Am J Pathol 1997;150(6):2143–2152.

60. Suzuki H, Takahashi K, Yasumoto K, et al. Role of neurofibromin in modulation of expression of the tyrosinase-related protein 2 gene. J Biochem (Tokyo) 1998;124(5):992–998.

61. Orlow SJ, Hearing VJ, Sakai C, et al. Changes in expression of putative antigens encoded by pigment genes in mouse melanomas at different stages of malignant progression. Proc Natl Acad Sci USA 1995;92(22):10,152–10,156.

62. Quaglino P, Savoia P, Fierro MT, Osella-Abate S, Bernengo MG. Clinical significance of sequential tyrosinase expression in the peripheral blood of disease-free melanoma patients: a review of literature data. Melanoma Res 2004;14(2):S17–S19.

63. Pak BJ, Lee J, Thai BL, et al. Radiation resistance of human melanoma analysed by retroviral insertional mutagenesis reveals a possible role for dopachrome tautomerase. Oncogene 2004;23(1):30–38.

64. Nishioka E, Funasaka Y, Kondoh H, Chakraborty AK, Mishima Y, Ichihashi M. Expression of tyrosinase, TRP-1 and TRP-2 in ultraviolet-irradiated human melanomas and melanocytes: TRP-2 protects melanoma cells from ultraviolet B induced apoptosis. Melanoma Res 1999;9(5):433–443.

65. Steitz J, Bruck J, Steinbrink K, Enk A, Knop J, Tuting T. Genetic immunization of mice with human tyrosinase-related protein 2: implications for the immunotherapy of melanoma. Int J Cancer 2000;86(1):89–94.

66. Steitz J, Bruck J, Gambotto A, Knop J, Tuting T. Genetic immunization with a melanocytic self-antigen linked to foreign helper sequences breaks tolerance and induces autoimmunity and tumor immunity. Gene Ther 2002;9(3):208–213.

67. Tanaka M, Kaneda Y, Fujii S, et al. Induction of a systemic immune response by a polyvalent melanoma-associated antigen DNA vaccine for prevention and treatment of malignant melanoma. Mol Ther 2002;5(3):291–299.

68. O I, Blaszczyk-Thurin M, Shen CT, Ertl HC. A DNA vaccine expressing tyrosinase-related protein-2 induces T-cell-mediated protection against mouse glioblastoma. Cancer Gene Ther 2003;10(9):678–688.

69. Prins RM, Odesa SK, Liau LM. Immunotherapeutic targeting of shared melanoma-associated antigens in a murine glioma model. Cancer Res 2003;63(23):8487–8491.

70. Liu G, Khong HT, Wheeler CJ, Yu JS, Black KL, Ying H. Molecular and functional analysis of tyrosinase-related protein (TRP)-2 as a cytotoxic T lymphocyte target in patients with malignant glioma. J Immunother 2003;26(4):301–312.

71. Negroiu G, Dwek RA, Petrescu SM. The inhibition of early N-glycan processing targets TRP-2 to degradation in B16 melanoma cells. J Biol Chem 2003;278(29):27,035–27,042.

72. Novellino L, d'Ischia M, Prota G. Nitric oxide-induced oxidation of 5,6-dihydroxyindole and 5,6-dihydroxyindole-2-carboxylic acid under aerobic conditions: non-enzymatic route to melanin pigments of potential relevance to skin (photo)protection. Biochim Biophys Acta 1998;1425(1):27–35.

73. D'Acquisto F, Carnuccio R, d'Ischia M, Misuraca G. 5,6-Dihydroxyindole-2-carboxylic acid, a diffusible melanin precursor, is a potent stimulator of lipopolysaccharide-induced production of nitric oxide by J774 macrophages. Life Sci 1995;57(26):L401–L406.

74. Memoli S, Napolitano A, d'Ischia M, Misuraca G, Palumbo A, Prota G. Diffusible melanin-related metabolites are potent inhibitors of lipid peroxidation. Biochim Biophys Acta 1997;1346(1):61–68.

75. Dent P, Yacoub A, Contessa J, et al. Stress and radiation-induced activation of multiple intracellular signaling pathways. Radiat Res 2003;159(3):283–300.

76. Zanke BW, Boudreau K, Rubie E, et al. The stress-activated protein kinase pathway mediates cell death following injury induced by cis-platinum, UV irradiation or heat. Curr Biol 1996;6(5):606–613.

77. Storz P, Toker A. NF-kappaB signaling—an alternate pathway for oxidative stress responses. Cell Cycle 2003;2(1):9–10.

78. Raingeaud J, Gupta S, Rogers JS, et al. Pro-inflammatory cytokines and environmental stress cause p38 mitogen-activated protein kinase activation by dual phosphorylation on tyrosine and threonine. J Biol Chem 1995;270(13):7420–7426.

79. Zhang Y, Chen F. Reactive oxygen species (ROS), troublemakers between nuclear factor-kappaB (NF-kappaB) and c-Jun NH(2)-terminal kinase (JNK). Cancer Res 2004;64(6):1902–1905.

80. Legrand-Poels S, Bours V, Piret B, et al. Transcription factor NF-kappa B is activated by photosensitization generating oxidative DNA damages. J Biol Chem 1995;270(12):6925–6934.

81. Natoli G, Costanzo A, Ianni A, et al. Activation of SAPK/JNK by TNF receptor 1 through a noncytotoxic TRAF2-dependent pathway. Science 1997;275(5297):200–203.

82. Subjeck JR, Sciandra JJ, Johnson RJ. Heat shock proteins and thermotolerance; a comparison of induction kinetics. Br J Radiol 1982;55(656):579–584.

83. Li GC, Werb Z. Correlation between synthesis of heat shock proteins and development of thermotolerance in Chinese hamster fibroblasts. Proc Natl Acad Sci USA 1982;79(10):3218–3222.

84. Rosengren E, Rorsman H. Reducing compounds initiate the TRP2-catalyzed conversion of L-dopachrome to DHICA. Melanoma Res 1998;8(5):469–470.

85. Mandic A, Viktorsson K, Heiden T, Hansson J, Shoshan MC. The MEK1 inhibitor PD98059 sensitizes C8161 melanoma cells to cisplatin-induced apoptosis. Melanoma Res 2001;11(1):11–19.

33 How Melanoma Cells Evade Chemotherapy

Role of Transporter-Dependent and -Independent Resistance Mechanisms

Kevin G. Chen and Michael M. Gottesman

CONTENTS

Summary

Melanomas are intrinsically resistant to both radiotherapy and chemotherapy. Chemotherapy is not a very effective way to treat metastatic melanomas. For this reason, therapy of metastatic melanoma has focused on biological approaches, with some significant recent success in immunotherapy. Still, more effective use of chemotherapy in metastatic melanoma would be a vast improvement in treatment of this disease. The design of chemotherapy to treat melanoma has been a challenging task, because the precise mechanisms of drug resistance in melanoma cells are largely unknown. Moreover, in addition to intrinsic resistance of melanoma to chemotherapy, acquired resistance could be achieved by induction or selection of heterogeneous melanoma cells with a selective growth advantage. The most common cause of multidrug resistance (MDR) in human cancers is the expression of one or more energy-dependent multidrug transporters that efflux anticancer drugs out of cells. Melanoma cells express a cluster of such transporters, which include adenosine triphosphate-binding cassette (ABC)-A9, ABCB1 (MDR1, P-glycoprotein), ABCB5, ABCC1 (multidrug resistance-associated protein-1), and ABCC2 (MRP2/canalicular multispecific organic anion transporter). These transporters may be associated with resistance to a broad range of anticancer drugs in melanomas. In addition, other mechanisms of resistance are also important, including overexpression of inhibitors of apoptosis, altered expression of either oncogenes or tumor suppressors, and drug-detoxifying properties of melanosomes. Defining and circumventing these resistance mechanisms would be a major step toward the ultimate goal of improved treatment of melanomas.

Key Words: Melanoma; multidrug resistance; ATP-binding cassette; membrane transporter.

From: *From Melanocytes to Melanoma: The Progression to Malignancy*
Edited by: V. J. Hearing and S. P. L. Leong © Humana Press Inc., Totowa, NJ

INTRODUCTION

Chemotherapy is one of the most effective approaches to the treatment of many types of malignant tumors, especially disseminated cancers, but metastatic melanomas respond poorly to such treatment. Unfortunately, the effectiveness of chemotherapy is limited in cancer cells by various mechanisms that confer multidrug resistance (MDR) (reviewed in refs. *1–4*), but which of these mechanisms are responsible for the intrinsic resistance of melanomas is not known. In many cases, drug resistance appears to be a primitive defense mechanism that both prokaryotic and eukaryotic cells acquired during the evolutionary process to defend against toxins in the environment. Thus, it is not surprising that cancer cells can escape the cytotoxicity of structurally distinct chemotherapeutic agents through either their inherited protective machinery or by acquired MDR during malignant transformation or after exposure to cytotoxic agents. Indeed, the mechanisms that give rise to MDR in cancer cells are extremely complicated, and mainly include:

1. Membrane transporter systems that control drug entry, distribution, and export *(1–4)*.
2. Enzymatic machineries that are able to metabolize cytotoxic drugs *(2,5)*.
3. Antiapoptotic pathways that alter cell death programs *(6–8)*.
4. Tumor physiology and its associated microenvironment *(9,10)*.

Figure 1 hypothesizes several potential drug resistance mechanisms that might account for MDR in melanomas. Understanding the precise mechanisms that control the origin of MDR cells would allow us to design rational approaches to circumventing MDR in cancers such as melanomas.

MDR IN HUMAN CANCER AND IN MELANOMAS

Melanomas, derived from pigment-producing melanocytes, are one of the most aggressive forms of cancer. The incidence of melanomas has increased rapidly and they now rank sixth among the most common cancers in the United States. The drugs (listed sequentially in descending order, according to their response rates as single agents from 20 to 12%) used in current systemic therapy include dacarbazine, nitrosoureas (e.g., carmustine), interleukin-2, cisplatin, interferon-α, carboplatin, taxanes (e.g., paclitaxel), and *Vinca* alkaloids (vinblastine and vincristine). The 5-yr survival rates in advanced stage patients with local node involvement and distant metastases are approx 50% and 10 to 20%, respectively, which account for approx 14% of cancer deaths annually (reviewed in refs. *11–13*). The poor prognosis of melanomas mainly results from intrinsic and/or acquired MDR to conventional chemotherapy or biochemotherapy.

Malignant tumors may be intrinsically resistant to chemotherapy when they originate from tissues that constitutively express molecules with the ability to confer MDR or as a result of events related to malignant transformation (such as mutations in tumor suppressor genes or activation of oncogenes) *(6,7)*. One of the best-characterized intrinsic MDR mechanisms is P-glycoprotein (P-gp)-mediated drug efflux. P-gp is constitutively expressed in the epithelia of the kidney, liver, and intestines; in the endothelial cells of the brain, ovary, testis, the adrenal cortex, and placenta; and in hematopoietic stem cells and other circulating blood cells *(2,14–17)*. These P-gp localizations are consistent with its physiological roles in uptake and excretion of endogenous and exogenous substrates, and in safeguarding blood–brain, blood–testis, blood–ovary, and blood–fetus barriers from cytotoxic drugs. Thus, tumors arising from these tissues consistently show intrinsic

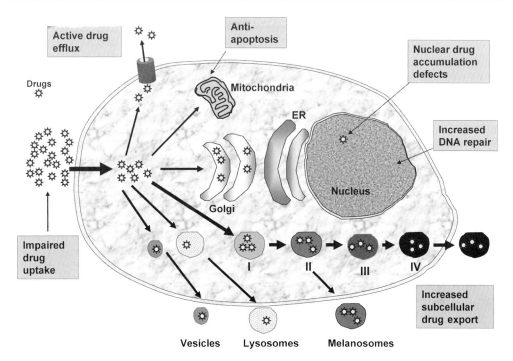

Fig. 1. A schema of potential drug resistance mechanisms in melanomas. Melanoma cells might become resistant to anticancer drugs by several sequentially occurring mechanisms. Initially, drug resistance could occur as a result of reduced drug influx (e.g., reduced endocytosis). Once drugs enter cells, they may be pumped out of cells by energy-dependent drug efflux pumps that are mediated by adenosine triphosphate-dependent transporters (e.g., ABC transporters). Alternatively, drugs could be trapped into subcellular organelles (such as the Golgi apparatus, lysosomes, melanosomes, and other vesicles) and exported out of cells. In cases in which drug accumulation is unchanged, increased DNA repair and overexpression of antiapoptotic factors (e.g., Bcl-2) can promote drug resistance. ER, endoplasmic reticulum; Golgi, the Golgi apparatus; I to IV, stage I to IV melanosomes, respectively.

MDR. It appears that melanomas are also intrinsically resistant to many anticancer drugs that act by producing DNA damage, inhibiting microtubule function, or inhibiting topoisomerases. For example, although platinum-containing drugs have been widely used in current multiagent regimens, fewer than 20% of melanoma patients have benefited from this treatment *(12)*. Hence, intrinsic MDR is obviously a major obstacle that is responsible for an unfavorable chemotherapeutic outcome in melanomas. The mechanisms for intrinsic MDR in melanomas are largely unknown, and could be multifactorial, as discussed in the following sections.

Alternatively, cancer cells may acquire MDR via genetic or epigenetic (e.g., the induction of gene expression) mechanisms, usually by selection or induction of a dominant factor or a specific pathway. Thus, a drug-resistant variant may arise spontaneously from sensitive cells, consistent with certain mutation rates *(18–20)*. Distinguishing whether drug resistant cells originate from spontaneous mutations or by induction has important therapeutic implications. Luria-Delbrück fluctuation analysis provides a powerful genetic tool to differentiate a spontaneous mutational event from an epigenetic alteration *(18–21)*. Drug-resistant variants may also emerge as the result of sublethal selection of a heterogeneous population of cancer cells (i.e., pre-existing variants) with a selective growth advantage developed as an adaptation to stress (e.g., heat shock, serum starvation, and hypoxia). Moreover, P-gp-mediated MDR can be acquired *de novo* from P-gp-negative cells by selection of cells that overexpress this protein, and expression of P-gp in these cells may serve as an adverse prognostic factor *(22)*. Thus, ABCB1/P-gp and its associated family member-mediated adenosine triphosphate-binding cassette (ABC) transporters represent prototypical models to elucidate the mechanisms of MDR in human cancers, including melanomas.

THE ROLE OF TRANSPORTER-DEPENDENT MECHANISMS

P-gp belongs to the ABC superfamily of integral membrane transporters, which typically contain multiple transmembrane domains and one or two nucleotide binding domains. These membrane proteins participate in ATP-dependent membrane transport of structurally diverse molecules ranging from small ions, sugars, and peptides, to more complex organic molecules *(1–4,23)*. At present, there are 48 human ABC transporter proteins that have been identified and classified into seven subfamilies from A to G (http://nutrigene.4t.com/humanabc.htm). It has been clearly shown that several ABC transporters (ABCB1, ABCC1, and ABCG2) have the capacity to confer MDR in vitro and in vivo to many types of cancers.

In the case of melanomas, the contribution of ABC transporters to either their intrinsic or acquired MDR is unclear. Despite frequent reports that link ABC transporters with MDR in melanoma, some studies have questioned the role of ABC transporter-mediated resistance mechanisms in this form of cancer (reviewed in refs. *24* and *25*). One possible reason to doubt their involvement is the lack of clinical data. In these studies, a few melanoma cell lines or samples are usually included and mixed with other types of cancers in both laboratory studies and clinical trials. Second, there are no well-designed intracellular trafficking studies on the relationship between ABC transporter expression/ localization and drug distribution among subcellular organelles in melanoma cells. Third, there is very limited or only preliminary data linking ABC transporters to the melanogenic pathway, which has retarded our understanding of MDR in melanomas. Nevertheless, there is increasing evidence showing that several ABCB and ABCC subfamily members are directly involved in contributing to the development of MDR in melanomas. We have recently shown that the melanoma cell lines included in the NCI-60 cancer cell panel express a specific cluster of ABC transporters (*ABCA9*, *ABCB5*, *ABCC2*, and *ABCD1*) messenger (m)RNAs *(26,27)*, suggesting that a panel of ABC transporters might be associated with both the intrinsic and acquired MDR in melanomas.

Role of ABCB (MDR-TAP) Subfamily Members

There are 11 documented members of the ABCB subfamily. The functions of several transporters included in this subfamily (i.e., ABCB5, ABCB8, ABCB9, and ABCB10) are not well elucidated. However, some ABC transporters (ABCB1/P-gp, ABCB2/TAP1, ABCB3/TAP2, and ABCB5) that have been found to be expressed by melanoma cells may have an effect on the outcome of therapy.

ABCB1/P-GP EXPRESSION IN MELANOMAS

The ability of P-gp to confer MDR in melanoma cells was demonstrated by increased expression of *ABCB1* mRNAs in melanoma cells after drug selection and by enforced expression of *ABCB1* cDNA after transfection *(28,29).* Although P-gp is constitutively expressed in a broad spectrum of normal tissues, it is not found in melanocytes (K. G. Chen and M. M. Gottesman, unpublished data). In the case of melanomas, Goldstein et al. initially reported that they contained undetectable levels of *ABCB1/MDR1* mRNA *(30).* Subsequently, Fuchs et al. examined P-gp expression by the monoclonal antibody, C219, in primary and metastatic human melanomas and found that it was only expressed in 1 of 37 (3%) of primary melanomas and in 1 of 27 (4%) of melanoma metastases *(31).* Miracco et al. studied five melanoma cell lines (Me665/2/21, Me665/2/60, HT-144, SK-MEL-28, and SK-MEL-5) and found only one cell line (SK-MEL-28) with detectable *ABCB1* mRNA *(32).* With quantitative real-time polymerase chain reaction assays, we have recently shown that only two (M14) out of eight melanoma cell lines (M14, MALME-3M LOX-IMVI, SK-MEL-2, SK-MEL-5, SK-MEL-28, UACC-62, and UACC-257) included in the NCI-60 cell panel expressed *ABCB1* mRNA *(26).* In contrast, Molinari et al. *(33)* reported that four untreated human melanoma cell lines (one from a primary culture of metastatic melanoma) did not express P-gp on the plasma membrane, but mislocalized P-gp in the Golgi apparatus. They found that P-gp modulators (verapamil and cyclosporin A) could redistribute the intracellular accumulation of drugs, such as doxorubicin *(33).* Induction and function of P-gp on the plasma membrane was also observed in M14 cells after drug treatment *(34).*

In contrast to the above-mentioned studies, P-gp expression has been detected at higher frequency in certain types of melanomas. For example, McNamara et al. reported that *ABCB1* expression was present in 5 of 12 (42%) ocular melanomas *(35).* Upregulation of P-gp was also found in four cell lines established in short-term culture from ocular melanoma explants. A recurrent tumor was shown to overexpress *ABCB1* mRNA after local excision and radiation. Dunne et al. assessed P-gp expression by immunohistochemistry in 108 cases of melanoma of the uveal tract, and found ABCB1 expression in 80% of cases, apparently associated with poor prognosis of this disease *(36).* Using immunohistochemistry with the JSB-1 antibody, Satherley et al. revealed that P-gp was expressed in 11 of 17 (65%) choroidal melanomas *(37).* Taken together, these studies suggest that ABCB1 is not an intrinsic resistance factor in the majority of common melanomas, but may be involved in intrinsic MDR and tumor propagation in some specific types of melanomas, subject to the usual problems associated with accurately measuring P-gp in clinical samples. In addition, the report of Molinari et al. *(33)* is very interesting, because the mislocalized P-gp may sequester P-gp substrates in subcellular organelles, thereby inactivating the drugs. This represents a possible mechanism for MDR in melanomas. However, the prevalence of this mechanism, or the accuracy of the localization, could not be substantiated because of the small number of samples analyzed in the study and the limited number of antibodies used for localization. Further studies are needed to clarify this issue.

The role of ABCB1 in clinical MDR of melanomas remains elusive. Sequential studies revealed no significant increase in P-gp expression in melanoma cells during and after chemotherapy. It is also conceivable that some types of melanomas do not usually acquire a P-gp-mediated efflux system. Other ABCB subfamily members may be responsible for either MDR or drug sensitivity in this human malignancy.

ABCB2/ABCB3 (TAP1/TAP2) EXPRESSION IN MELANOMAS

Both TAP1 and TAP2 are half-ABC transporters that are associated with antigen processing by loading antigen peptides (derived from endogenous protein degradation) onto major histocompatibility complex class I molecules. The loaded major histocompatibility complex class I then leaves the endoplasmic reticulum and presents its antigenic cargo on the cell surface to cytotoxic T-lymphocytes, by which cancer cells could be eliminated (reviewed in ref. *38*). Impairment of the transporter associated with the antigen processing function can be attributed to a single amino acid alteration of TAP1 *(39)*. Spontaneous tumor regression via destruction of melanoma cells could be achieved by the cytotoxic T-cell recognition of melanoma-associated antigen-derived peptides. An association of TAP1 downregulation in human primary melanoma lesions with a lack of spontaneous regression has been reported *(40)*. It has been shown that several enzymatic and structural proteins of melanosomes (such as tyrosinase, tyrosine-related protein [TRP]1/gp75, silver/gp100, melanoma antigen recognized by T-cells 1 /melan-A, and TRP2/DOPAchrome tautomerase) have been used as molecular targets for inducing cellular and humoral responses to normal melanocytes and to melanomas *(41,42)*. Whether TAP1/2 plays a role in presenting specific peptides as melanoma-associated antigens is unknown, and this could be a fruitful area of further research. Nevertheless, TAP1/2 may represent a prognostic factor for therapy of melanomas.

ABCB5 EXPRESSION IN MELANOMAS

The human ABCB5 gene locus (on the chromosome 7 short arm) encodes a full-length ABC transporter (12 transmembrane domains and 2 ABCs), but is usually expressed as multiple alternatively spliced transcripts, none of which encode the entire predicted ABCB5 protein. We have recently identified two mRNA isoforms, termed *ABCB5α* and *ABCB5β*, representing various parts of the transporter. *ABCB5α* mRNA predicts a 15-kDa protein that lacks the intact domain for a half-transporter protein *(27)*. Whether *ABCB5α* has a role in regulating ABCB5 transporter activity has not been determined, but this isoform is abundant in melanocytes and in melanomas. In contrast, for ABCB5β, the protein topology predicts a half-transporter or more than a half-transporter, with approx 70% similarity to ABCB1/P-gp *(27,43)*. Both *ABCB5α* and *ABCB5β* are usually expressed in pigmented cells (melanocytes and pigmented retinal epithelial cells) and melanomas. However, *ABCB5 α/β* expression was undetectable in two amelanotic melanomas (M14 and LOX-IMVI) included in the NCI-60 cancer cell panel *(27)*. Neither *ABCB5α* nor *ABCB5β* expression was found in a panel of normal tissues *(27)*. Another study indicated that *ABCB5α* was expressed in the testes and uterus *(44)*. Thus, the physiological role of *ABCB5α/β* might be associated with a detoxification process mainly in pigmented cells, such as melanocytes. The other physiological role of *ABCB5* (the *ABCB5β* isoform) may be associated with the regulation of progenitor cell fusion *(43)*.

The pharmacological role of ABCB5 in mediating MDR in melanoma remains to be established. We have recently shown that *ABCB5α/β* expression increases after drug treatment with several different cytotoxic drugs, compared with *ABCB1/P-gp*. Moreover, *ABCB5α* and *ABCB5β* are not coactivated in typical MDR cell lines (such as KB-V1 and MES-SA/Dx5), suggesting that *ABCB5β* might have a distinct transport function (compared with that of P-gp) that has not yet been determined *(27)*. At present, a small interfering RNA directed at *ABCB5* mRNA provides preliminary evidence that *ABCB5* mRNA levels are associated with multidrug sensitivity to several drugs, including camptothecin 10-OH, 5-FU, and mitoxantrone, implying that elevated *ABCB5* mRNA expression may confer drug resistance to these agents *(45)*. However, these results need to be confirmed by transfecting *ABCB5* cDNA into drug-sensitive cells to produce the

MDR phenotype. Nonetheless, melanoma-specific expression of *ABCB5α/β* might allow development of *ABCB5α/β* gene products as additional molecular markers and targets for the differential diagnosis and therapy of melanomas.

The ABCC (CFTR-MRP) Subfamily

The role of the ABCC subfamily in mediating the MDR phenotype has been widely reported. Several ABCC subfamily members (ABCC1/multidrug resistance-associated protein [MRP]1, ABCC2/MRP2/canalicular multispecific organic anion transporter, and ABCC3/MRP3) have been implicated in MDR in human cancers. These ABCC transporters can extrude many natural product drugs out of cancer cells through a cotransport mechanism with glutathione. MRP1 is also an active membrane transporter for organic anions conjugated to glutathione (e.g., leukotriene C4 and glucuronate). MRP2 can export conjugated organic anions and glutathione out of cells, whereas MRP3 fails to export glutathione and, thus, shows a narrow spectrum of MDR *(3,4)*.

ABCC1/MRP1 is widely expressed in many normal tissues and cancers. The contribution of MRP1 expression to melanoma MDR is also unclear. Thus far, only a few studies have been documented in the literature. Depeille et al. reported that MRP1 synergized with glutathione-*S*-transferase M1 to protect melanoma cells from the effects of vincristine *(46)*, consistent with the effect of MRP1 in other nonmelanoma cancers. Another interesting finding of Molinari et al. *(33)* is the absence of plasma membrane expression of MRP1 in all examined melanoma cells. In this case, MRP1 was also mislocalized in a Golgi-like localization in the cytoplasm. The Golgi apparatus appears to be a compartment for trapping certain types (e.g., anthracyclines) of anticancer drugs in some melanoma cells *(33)*. This phenomenon is similar to KB-3-1-derived cisplatin-resistant cells (KB-CP), in which MRP1 was present on the plasma membranes of the parental KB-3-1 cells, but was mislocalized in the cytoplasm of KB-CP cells *(47)*. We have demonstrated that MRP1, located in a lighter and lower-density fraction in KB-CP.5 cells, was co-localized with both a specific marker for the Golgi apparatus and, to some extent, with an endoplasmic reticulum marker, suggesting that the *trans*-Golgi network was involved in MRP1 mislocalization *(47)*. It appears that MRP1 mislocalization might be the hallmark of the MDR phenotype, especially of cisplatin resistance in human cancers, including melanomas. However, in the case of melanomas, the mislocalization of MRP1 is intrinsic. It is conceivable that the mislocalized transporters in the cytoplasm may function as intracellular pumps that sequester anticancer drugs into defined subcellular organelles, such as the Golgi apparatus, lysosomes, melanosomes, or other vesicles. Whether MRP1 is directly involved in sequestering anticancer drugs in subcellular organelles has not been established.

ABCC2/MRP2 has also been reported to be associated with cisplatin resistance. Both increased and decreased expression of MRP2 have been observed in nonmelanoma cell lines *(48,49)*, making its role as a cisplatin efflux pump uncertain. A recent study has shown that elevated expression of MRP2 in melanoma cells causes resistance to cisplatin by reducing the formation of platinum-induced intrastrand crosslinks in the nuclear DNA, concomitant with decreased G2-arrest via an accelerated re-entry into the cell cycle in cisplatin-resistant melanoma cells (MeWo CIS1) *(50)*. Thus, MRP2 could be an attractive molecular target for the reversal of cisplatin resistance in melanomas. When anti-MRP2 hammerhead ribozymes were introduced into A2780RCIS cells, they showed gene-silencing activities and reversed the drug-resistant phenotype *(51)*. No doubt, with pharmacogenomic and molecular biological approaches available in the postgenome era, we will be able to verify all of the contributions of ABC transporters to drug resistance/sensitivity. However, other nontransporter-mediated mechanisms also have been shown to play an important role in determining drug resistance/sensitivity in melanomas.

TRANSPORTER-INDEPENDENT RESISTANCE MECHANISMS

Transporter-independent drug resistance is mainly attributed to insensitivity to chemotherapy-induced apoptosis, which is determined by a broad spectrum of resistance mechanisms that have been extensively reviewed elsewhere *(6–10,24,25)*. Briefly, these mechanisms include:

1. Increased DNA repair to respond to DNA-damaging agents.
2. Methylation-mediated silencing of the *APAF-1* gene.
3. Overexpressed antiapoptotic proteins (e.g., Bcl-2) that impair the ability to undergo programmed cell death.
4. Alterations of G proteins and protein kinases (Ras, B-Raf).
5. Transcription factor effectors (c-Jun, ATF2, Stat3, and NF-κB) that affect tumor necrosis factor, Fas, and tumor necrosis factor-related apoptosis-inducing ligand treatment receptors.

Resistance to chemotherapy-induced apoptosis in melanoma cells is p53-dependent *(52)*, suggesting that the p53 system is also involved in the development of drug resistance.

One unique feature of melanotic melanomas is the presence of the melanosome, an evolutionarily modified lysosomal compartment, and its contents of melanin. Melanin is thought to be able to bind a variety of cytotoxic materials *(53,54)*, and, therefore, the melanosome could act as a receptacle for cytotoxic anticancer drugs, preventing trafficking to their normal intracellular targets, such as the nucleus. How cytotoxic drugs accumulate within melanosomes and whether these melanosomes are retained in the cells or extruded remains to be determined.

Finally, metal-binding proteins have an important role in regulating the homeostasis of trace metals, such as zinc and copper, in melanocytes. Metallothioneins (MTs) are cysteine-rich, have low molecular weights and high affinity for heavy metal ions, e.g. zinc, copper, and cadmium *(55)*. Weinlich et al. recently analyzed MT expression on a large scale (760 cases) in patients with cutaneous melanoma using the monoclonal antibody E5 on routinely fixed and paraffin-embedded tissues. They found that MT overexpression in primary melanoma is associated with an increased risk for disease progression *(56)*. It also has been shown that MT expression was associated with resistance to cisplatin in mouse B16 melanoma cells *(57)*. Indeed, overexpression of MT confers cancer-cell resistance to certain types of drugs, such as cisplatin, via unknown mechanisms *(58,59)*. It has been postulated that the binding of cisplatin to MTs may prevent its further nuclear localization and, thus, reduce cytotoxicity.

CHEMOTHERAPY AND BIOCHEMOTHERAPY OF MELANOMAS

Currently, the mainstream therapy of metastatic melanomas consists of combined drug regimens with the addition of biological modifiers *(12–13,60)*. New clinical trials combining dacarbazine or cisplatin with other cytotoxic agents, such as tamoxifen, or interferon-α have showed promise in clinical phase II/III trials. For example, Rosenberg et al. compared the cisplatin, dacarbazine, and tamoxifen (CDT) regimen with CDT-II (CDT plus both high-dose interleukin-2 and interferon-α) in treatment of stage IV melanoma and found 27 and 44% response rates, respectively *(60)*. Eton et al. compared the cisplatin, dacarbazine, and vinblastine with the cisplatin, dacarbazine, and vinblastine-II regimen and found 25% and 44% response rates, respectively *(60)*. However, there are also reports that phase III trials failed to yield significant results compared with chemotherapy or immunotherapy alone *(13)*. Thus, a proper randomized and well-controlled trial is needed to resolve this controversy.

CONCLUSIONS AND PERSPECTIVES ON MODULATION OF MDR IN MELANOMAS

General Considerations

Over the past decade, tremendous efforts have been made to achieve modulation of clinical MDR through inhibition of the drug efflux pump P-gp in human cancer patients. Although current clinical trials with several generations of P-gp inhibitors have yielded unsatisfactory results, modulation of P-gp-mediated MDR represents a paradigm of translational medicine. We have learned invaluable things from this process, i.e., from identification of molecular targets to clinical phase III trials. It is clear now that the MDR phenotype is a complicated genetic trait, usually mediated by multiple machineries. Thus, simply inhibiting one transporter (e.g., P-gp) would not yield the desired outcome, because of the redundancy of related ABC transporters in the human genome. Moreover, an alternative mechanism of resistance would likely emerge, given that the predominant resistance mechanism is inhibited and the tumor cell population is large. This is determined and programmed by the genomic instability of cancer *(61,62)*. Thus, simultaneous cataloging of all of the major mechanisms of resistance in a specific type of cancer would have great therapeutic implications. Sequential inhibition of these mechanisms at the proper time would enable us to eliminate residual cancer cells with acquired alternative resistance mechanisms. A systematic screening method, such as array-based technologies, would facilitate the identification of molecular targets for melanomas. The unique ABC transporter cluster (ABCA9, ABCC2, ABCB5, and ABCD1) found in melanomas could be a potential molecular target for therapy of melanomas. However, further studies are needed to prove their potential clinical application.

Modulation of MDR in Melanomas: An Extension of Collateral Sensitivity

Using a pharmacogenomic approach, our laboratory has recently identified a compound termed NSC 73306 via analysis of the positive correlation between drug activity and *ABCB1* mRNA expression. This chemical preferentially inhibits growth of *ABCB1*-overexpressing cancer cells *(26)*. The mode of action of NSC 73306 is reminiscent of a classical phenomenon called collateral sensitivity in drug-selected cancer cell lines, which usually show hypersensitivity to some nonselecting agents. However, this phenomenon has not been given much attention. Indeed, some melanoma MDR variants have been shown to have collateral sensitivity to the polyamine analog (N1, N11-diethylnorspermine) *(63)*. Thus, discovery of such "magic bullets" that specifically kill MDR cells would lead to the development of novel anticancer agents to treat resistant melanomas.

Targeting Inhibitors of Apoptosis and Cell Growth Factors

Identification of molecules involved in apoptosis of cancer cells has provided new insights into the molecular basis for melanoma MDR. Thus, targeting of apoptotic regulators may increase the sensitivity of melanoma cells to cytotoxic drugs and provide a promising new therapeutic approach. For example, survivin, an inhibitor of apoptosis, is expressed in melanomas and is required for maintenance of melanoma cell viability. Downregulation of survivin expression by ribozymes could lead to human melanoma cells sensitive to cisplatin-induced apoptosis *(64)*. Currently, more promising new clinical trials combining chemotherapy with demethylating agents, such as 5-aza-2'-deoxycytidine, antisense Bcl-2 oligonucleotides, and RAF inhibitors are ongoing *(13)*. Despite the enthusiasm concerning novel strategies that target antiapoptotic pathways, some of the effective inhibitors that have recently been developed may actually be the substrates of ABC transporters. One example is imatinib mesylate (STI571), a potent tyrosine kinase inhibitor that is a substrate of both multidrug transporters (ABCB1 and ABCG2). Thus, oral administration of STI571 caused cellular resistance and subsequent treatment failure *(65)*. With the knowledge of ABC transporters in mind, the challenge now is to design potent inhibitors that could bypass transporter-mediated resistance mechanisms. Each potential new drug should be routinely screened before clinical trials to determine whether it is a substrate of the transporters.

In summary, both intrinsic and acquired MDR are major obstacles to chemotherapy. Several ABC transporters, including ABCB1 (MDR1), ABCB5, ABCC1 (MRP1), and ABCC2 (MRP2/cMOAT) are implicated in melanoma MDR. ABC transporter-independent resistance mechanisms (including antiapoptosis) are also important determinants of drug resistance. Inhibition or prevention of MDR is the ultimate frontier in current molecular therapeutics of cancer. Even with the best inhibitors of cancer cells, molecular therapy of melanomas is destined to fail given that the cytotoxic molecules could not reach their molecular targets. As more precise primary and secondary resistance mechanisms are revealed, an effective therapeutic regimen could be developed, which could lead to specific inhibition of melanomas.

ACKNOWLEDGMENTS

This work was supported by the Intramural Research Program of the NIH, National Cancer Institute. We thank our colleagues Drs. V. J. Hearing, J. C. Valencia, D. W. Shen, X. J. Liang, F. Rouzaud, J. Paterson, G. Szakacs, and S. V. Ambudkar for critical discussion. We thank Mr. George Leiman for his assistance in preparing this manuscript. We apologize to our colleagues whose original contributions have not been cited or are cited indirectly because of the space limitation of this chapter.

REFERENCES

1. Ling V. Multidrug resistance: molecular mechanisms and clinical relevance. Cancer Chemother Pharmacol 1997;40(Suppl):S3–S8.
2. Gottesman MM, Fojo T, Bates SE. Multidrug resistance in cancer: role of ATP-dependent transporters. Nat Rev Cancer 2002;2:48–58.
3. Borst P, Elferink RO. Mammalian ABC transporters in health and disease. Annu Rev Biochem 2002;71:537–592.
4. Haimeur A, Conseil G, Deeley RG, Cole SP. The MRP-related and BCRP/ABCG2 multidrug resistance proteins: biology, substrate specificity and regulation. Curr Drug Metab 2004;5:21–53.

5. Schuetz EG, Beck WT, Schuetz JD, Modulators and substrates of P glycoprotein and cytochrome P4503A coordinately up-regulate these proteins in human colon carcinoma cells. Mol Pharmacol 1996;49:311–318.

6. El-Deiry WS. The role of p53 in chemosensitivity and radiosensitivity. Oncogene 2003;22: 7486–7495.

7. Soengas MS, Lowe SW. Apoptosis and melanoma chemoresistance. Oncogene 2003;22:3138–3151.

8. Pommier Y, Sordet O, Antony S, Hayward RL, Kohn KW. Apoptosis defects and chemotherapy resistance: molecular interaction maps and networks. Oncogene 2004;23:2934–2949.

9. Jain RK. Therapeutic implications of tumor physiology. Curr Opin Oncol 1991;3:1105–1108.

10. Brown JM, Wilson WR. Exploiting tumour hypoxia in cancer treatment. Nat Rev Cancer 2004; 4:437–447.

11. Kamb A, Herlyn M. Malignant melanoma. In: Vogelstein B, Kinzler KW, eds. The Genetic Basis of Human Cancer. McGraw-Hill: New York, 1998, pp. 507–518.

12. Quan WDY. Melanoma and other skin malignancies. In: Skeel RT, ed. Handbook of Cancer Chemotherapy. 6th ed. Lippincott Williams & Wilkins, Philadephia, PA: 2003, pp. 360–377.

13. Tsao H, Atkins MB, Sober AJ. Management of cutaneous melanoma. N Engl J Med 2004; 351:998–1012.

14. Fojo AT, Ueda K, Slamon DJ, Poplack DG, Gottesman MM, Pastan I. Expression of a multidrug-resistance gene in human tumors and tissues. Proc Natl Acad Sci USA 1987;84:265–269.

15. Thiebaut F, Tsuruo T, Hamada H, Gottesman MM, Pastan I, Willingham MC. Cellular localization of the multidrug-resistance gene product P-glycoprotein in normal human tissues. Proc Natl Acad Sci USA 1987;84:7735–7738.

16. Cordon-Cardo C, O'Brien JP, Boccia J, Casals D, Bertino JR, Melamed MR. Expression of the multidrug resistance gene product (P-glycoprotein) in human normal and tumor tissues. J Histochem Cytochem 1990;38:1277–1287.

17. Chaudhary PM, Roninson IB. Expression and activity of P-glycoprotein, a multidrug efflux pump, in human hematopoietic stem cells. Cell 1991;66:85–94.

18. Chen G, Jaffrezou JP, Fleming WH, Duran GE, Sikic BI. Prevalence of multidrug resistance related to activation of the mdr1 gene in human sarcoma mutants derived by single-step doxorubicin selection. Cancer Res 1994;54:4980–4987.

19. Jaffrezou JP, Chen G, Duran GE, Kuhl JS, Sikic BI. Mutation rates and mechanisms of resistance to etoposide determined from fluctuation analysis. J Natl Cancer Inst 1994;86:1152–1158.

20. Chen GK, Duran GE, Mangili A, Beketic-Oreskovic L, Sikic BI. MDR1 activation is the predominant resistance mechanism selected by vinblastine in MES-SA cells. Br J Cancer 2000;83:892–898.

21. Luria SE, Delbrück M. Mutations of bacteria from virus sensitive to virus resistance. Genetics 1943;28:491–511.

22. Arceci RJ. Clinical significance of P-glycoprotein in multidrug resistance malignancies. Blood 1993;81:2215–2222.

23. Dean M, Allikmets R. Complete characterization of the human ABC gene family. J Bioenerg Biomembr 2001;33:475–479.

24. Grossman D, Altieri DC. Drug resistance in melanoma: mechanisms, apoptosis, and new potential therapeutic targets. Cancer Metastasis 2001;20:3–11.

25. Helmbach H, Rossmann E, Kern MA, Schadendorf D. Human melanoma: drug resistance. Recent Results Cancer Res 2003;161:93–110.

26. Szakacs G, Annereau JP, Lababidi S, et al. Predicting drug sensitivity and resistance: profiling ABC transporter genes in cancer cells. Cancer Cell 2004;6:129–137.

27. Chen KG, Szakacs G, Annereau JP, et al. Principal expression of two mRNA isoforms (ABCB 5alpha and ABCB 5beta) of the ATP-binding cassette transporter gene ABCB5 in melanoma cells and melanocytes. Pigment Cell Res 2005;18:102–112.

28. Lemontt JF, Azzaria M, Gros P. Increased mdr gene expression and decreased drug accumulation in multidrug-resistant human melanoma cells. Cancer Res 1988;48:6348–6353.

29. Lincke CR, van der Bliek AM, Schuurhuis GJ, van der Velde-Koerts T, Smit JJ, Borst P. Multidrug resistance phenotype of human BRO melanoma cells transfected with a wild-type human mdr1 complementary DNA. Cancer Res 1990;50:1779–1785.

30. Goldstein LJ, Galski H, Fojo A, et al. Expression of a multidrug resistance gene in human cancers. J Natl Cancer Inst 1989;81:116–124.

31. Fuchs B, Ostmeier H, Suter L. P-glycoprotein expression in malignant melanoma. J Cancer Res Clin Oncol 1991;117:168–171.

32. Miracco C, Maellaro E, Pacenti L, et al. Evaluation of MDR1, LRP, MRP, and topoisomerase IIalpha gene mRNA transcripts before and after interferon-alpha, and correlation with the mRNA expression level of the telomerase subunits hTERT and TEP1 in five unselected human melanoma cell lines. Int J Oncol 2003;23:213–220.

33. Molinari A, Calcabrini A, Meschini S, et al. Detection of P-glycoprotein in the Golgi apparatus of drug-untreated human melanoma cells. Int J Cancer 1998;75:885–893.

34. Molinari A, Toccacieli L, Calcabrini A, Diociaiuti M, Cianfriglia M, Arancia G. Induction of P-glycoprotein expression on the plasma membrane of human melanoma cells. Anticancer Res 2000;20:2691–2696.

35. McNamara M, Clynes M, Dunne B, et al. Multidrug resistance in ocular melanoma. Br J Ophthalmol 1996;80:1009–1012.

36. Dunne BM, McNamara M, Clynes M, et al. MDR1 expression is associated with adverse survival in melanoma of the uveal tract. Hum Pathol 1998;29:594–598.

37. Satherley K, de Souza L, Neale MH, et al. Relationship between expression of topoisomerase II isoforms and chemosensitivity in choroidal melanoma. J Pathol 2000;192:174–181.

38. Abele R, Tampe R. The ABCs of immunology: structure and function of TAP, the transporter associated with antigen processing. Physiology 2004;19:216–224.

39. Ritz U, Drexler I, Sutter D, Abele R, Huber C, Seliger B. Impaired transporter associated with antigen processing (TAP) function attributable to a single amino acid alteration in the peptide TAP subunit TAP1. J Immunol 2003;170:941–946.

40. Dissemond J, Gotte P, Mors J, et al. Association of TAP1 downregulation in human primary melanoma lesions with lack of spontaneous regression. Melanoma Res 2003;13:253–258.

41. Sakai C, Kawakami Y, Law LW, Furumura M, Hearing VJ. Melanosomal proteins as melanoma-specific immune targets. Melanoma Res 1997;7:8395.

42. Virador V, Matsunaga N, Matsunaga J, et al. Production of melanocyte-specific antibodies to human melanosomal proteins: expression patterns in normal human skin and in cutaneous pigmented lesions. Pigment Cell Res 2001;14:289297.

43. Frank NY, Pendse SS, Lapchak PH, et al. (2003). Regulation of progenitor cell fusion by ABCB5 P-glycoprotein, a novel human ATP-binding cassette transporter. J Biol Chem 2003;278:47,15647,165.

44. Langmann T, Mauerer R, Zahn A, et al. Real-time reverse transcription-PCR expression profiling of the complete human ATP-binding cassette transporter superfamily in various tissues. Clin Chem 2003;49:230238.

45. Huang Y, Anderle P, Bussey KJ, et al. Membrane transporters and channels: role of the transportome in cancer chemosensitivity and chemoresistance. Cancer Res 2004;64:42944301.

46. Depeille P, Cuq P, Mary S, et al. Glutathione S-transferase M1 and multidrug resistance protein 1 act in synergy to protect melanoma cells from vincristine effects. Mol Pharmacol 2004;65:897–905.

47. Liang XJ, Shen DW, Garfield S, Gottesman MM. Mislocalization of membrane proteins associated with multidrug resistance in cisplatin-resistant cancer cell lines. Cancer Res 2003;63:5909–5916.

48. Shen DW, Goldenberg S, Pastan I, Gottesman MM. Decreased accumulation of [^{14}C]carboplatin in human cisplatin-resistant cells results from reduced energy-dependent uptake. J Cell Physiol 2000;183:108–116.

49. Kool M, de Haas M, Scheffer GL, et al. Analysis of expression of cMOAT (MRP2), MRP3, MRP4, and MRP5, homologues of the multidrug resistance-associated protein gene (MRP1), in human cancer cell lines. Cancer Res 1997;57:3537–3547.

50. Liedert B, Materna V, Schadendorf D, Thomale J, Lage H. Overexpression of cMOAT (MRP2/ ABCC2) is associated with decreased formation of platinum-DNA adducts and decreased G2-arrest in melanoma cells resistant to cisplatin. J Invest Dermatol 2003;121:172–176.

51. Materna V, Liedert B, Thomale J, Lage H. Protection of platinum-DNA adduct formation and reversal of cisplatin resistance by anti-MRP2 hammerhead ribozymes in human cancer cells. Int J Cancer 2005;115:393–402.

52. Li G, Tang L, Zhou X, Tron V, Ho V. Chemotherapy-induced apoptosis in melanoma cells is p53 dependent. Melanoma Res 1998;8:17–23.

53. Larsson BS. Interaction between chemicals and melanin. Pigment Cell Res 1993;6:127–133.

54. Mars U, Larsson BS. Pheomelanin as a binding site for drugs and chemicals. Pigment Cell Res 1999;12:266–274.

55. Cherian MG, Howell SB, Imura N, et al. Role of metallothionein in carcinogenesis. Toxicol Appl Pharmacol 1994;126:1–5.

56. Weinlich G, Bitterlich W, Mayr V, Fritsch PO, Zelger B. Metallothionein-overexpression as a prognostic factor for progression and survival in melanoma. A prospective study on 520 patients. Br J Dermatol 2003;149:535–541.

57. Koropatnick J, Pearson J. Zinc treatment, metallothionein expression, and resistance to cisplatin in mouse melanoma cells. Somat Cell Mol Genet 1990;16:529–537.

58. Kondo Y, Woo ES, Michalska AE, Choo KH, Lazo JS. Metallothionein null cells have increased sensitivity to anticancer drugs. Cancer Res 1995;55:2021–2023.

59. Kondo Y, Kuo SM, Watkins SC, Lazo JS. Metallothionein localization and cisplatin resistance in human hormone-independent prostatic tumor cell lines. Cancer Res 1995;55:474–477.

60. Atkins MB. Buzaid AC, Houghton AN Jr. Chemotherapy and biochemotherapy. In: Balch C, Houghton A, Sober A, Soong S, eds. Cutaneous Melanoma. 4th ed. Quality Medical, St. Louis, MO: 2003, pp. 589–604.

61. Campain JA, Padmanabhan R, Hwang J, Gottesman MM, Pastan I. Characterization of an unusual mutant of human melanoma cells resistant to anticancer drugs that inhibit topoisomerase II. J Cell Physiol 1993;155:414–425.

62. Beketic-Oreskovic L, Duran GE, Chen G, Dumontet C, Sikic BI. Decreased mutation rate for cellular resistance to doxorubicin and suppression of *mdr*1 gene activation by the cyclosporin PSC 833. J Natl Cancer Inst 1995;87:1593–1602.

63. Porter CW, Ganis B, Rustum Y, Wrzosek C, Kramer DL, Bergeron RJ. Collateral sensitivity of human melanoma multidrug-resistant variants to the polyamine analogue, N1,N11-diethylnorspermine. Cancer Res 1994;54:5917–5924.

64. Pennati M, Colella G, Folini M, Citti L, Daidone MG, Zaffaroni N. Ribozyme-mediated attenuation of survivin expression sensitizes human melanoma cells to cisplatin-induced apoptosis. J Clin Invest 2002;109:285–286.

65. Burger H, van Tol H, Boersma AW, et al. Imatinib mesylate (STI571) is a substrate for the breast cancer resistance protein (BCRP)/ABCG2 drug pump. Blood 2004;104:2940–2942.

34 Apoptosis in Melanoma

Approaches to Therapy

Heike Röckmann and Dirk Schadendorf

CONTENTS

INTRODUCTION
PROGRAMMED CELL-DEATH PATHWAYS
APOPTOSIS DEFICIENCY AND MELANOMA
REFERENCES

Summary

Apoptosis deficiency seems to be involved in the high resistance of melanoma to therapeutic treatment. This has come into focus because the cytotoxic effects of chemotherapeutic agents via apoptosis are known. Extensive investigations have been made analyzing the role of alterations in the apoptotic pathway in melanoma. The molecular changes affect antiapoptotic, as well as proapoptotic, processes and survival signals and involve various molecules. These mechanisms are also discussed in light of their use in further therapeutical strategies. Actually, a number of these findings have already been employed to test their therapeutical applicability in melanoma treatment. Furthermore, two concepts have been translated from the cell system via animal models into clinical trials.

Key Words: Melanoma; apoptosis; apoptosis deficiency; death receptors; caspases; Bcl-2-family; p53.

INTRODUCTION

Most chemotherapeutic drugs act through induction of apoptosis (programmed cell death). In 1972, Kerr et al. described an experimentally induced killing of tumor cells that involved a coordinated cell disintegration following typical morphological changes, coining the term *apoptosis (1)*. The cytotoxic effect of chemotherapeutic agents appears mainly contributed by apoptosis *(2,3)*. The weak response of metastatic melanoma to anticancer agents gives rise to the hypothesis that the chemoresistance of this malignancy is caused by raising its apoptotic threshold *(2)*. Inactivation of apoptosis is a "hallmark of cancer," an obligate ritual in the malignant transformation of benign cells *(4)*. As a result, these cells enhance their chances of survival and increase their resistance to chemotherapy *(3)*. Indeed, Staunton et al. *(5)* demonstrated a constitutive low level of spontaneous apoptosis in melanoma cells compared with other malignant cell types. An intensive search for cell death factors altered in melanoma has been made. It has been

From: *From Melanocytes to Melanoma: The Progression to Malignancy*
Edited by: V. J. Hearing and S. P. L. Leong © Humana Press Inc., Totowa, NJ

shown that, indeed, various molecular changes in cell-death control in melanoma are present, and three types can be distinguished: activation of antiapoptotic processes, inactivation of proapoptotic effectors, and reinforcement of survival signals.

PROGRAMMED CELL-DEATH PATHWAYS

Apoptosis (programmed cell death) represents a complex genetic program consisting of several pathways that are summarized in Fig. 1. Tremendous efforts have been made to discover and describe the molecular mechanisms of apoptosis, which are discussed elsewhere in detail (6). Briefly, depending on cell type and stimulus, a complex net of sensor and regulator proteins is activated and balanced and there is no unique linear or defined pathway. However, to simplify, two main well-characterized caspase-activating cascades that regulate apoptosis are currently known.

One cascade is triggered from the cell surface by death receptors and the other is initiated by changes of mitochondrial membrane integrity (7). Oligomerization of surface receptors is followed by recruitment of adapter molecules, such as Fas-associated protein with death domain (FADD) and the initiator caspases-8 and -10 (8) into the death-inducing signaling complex (DISC). The subsequent autocatalytic cleavage of procaspase-8 or -10 is followed by activation of effector caspases (e.g., caspase-3) (9) and induction of specific endonucleases, resulting in DNA fragmentation (10,11). These two pathways converge with the activation of effector caspases and induction of specific endonucleases, resulting in DNA fragmentation and cleavage of nuclear proteins essential for nuclear and cellular structure, DNA-repair, and DNA-replication (12,13).

The family of death receptors include CD95 (Fas/APO-1), tumor necrosis factor (TNF)-R1, TNF-receptor apoptosis-inducing ligand receptor (TRAIL-R)1 and TRAIL-R2, DR3 (death receptor 3), and DR6 (reviewed in Locksley et al., ref. 14). Among them, the CD95 receptor, TRAIL-R1 and TRAIL-R2 are the most efficient mediators of apoptosis. Several studies suggest that death receptor–ligand interaction is involved in tumor sensitivity toward chemotherapeutic drugs (15–17). The extrinsic pathway is regulated on multiple levels, whereas the death-inducing signaling complex can also recruit negative and positive regulators of caspase-8 (18,19). Furthermore, in type II cells, the initial activation of caspase-8 is not sufficient. Here, caspase-8 cleaves the Bcl-2 family member, BID, which translocates to the mitochondrial membrane and activates the intrinsic pathway (20). By this mechanism, the death receptor and the mitochondrial pathway is connected.

The intrinsic pathway involves mitochondrial release of cytochrome-c, which binds apoptotic protease activating factor (Apaf)-1, and, in the presence of adenosine triphosphate (ATP), coordinates a series of conformational changes that allow the oligomerization of Apaf-1 into a ring-like complex, referred to as the "apoptosome" (21). The apoptosome binds and activates caspase-9 into the complex (9,22,23), which, in turn, recruits and activates effector caspases (e.g., caspase-3). These are considered as executors of apoptosis.

There are various additional points of control that can modulate apoptosis after cytochrome-c release. The family of inhibitors of apoptosis (IAP), containing X-chromosome-linked IAP (XIAP), neuronal IAP (NIAP), melanoma (ML)-IAP, and survivin, can interfere with the formation of the apoptosome and activation of the downstream caspases (Figs. 1 and 2). IAPs are inhibited by other proapoptotic factors released by the

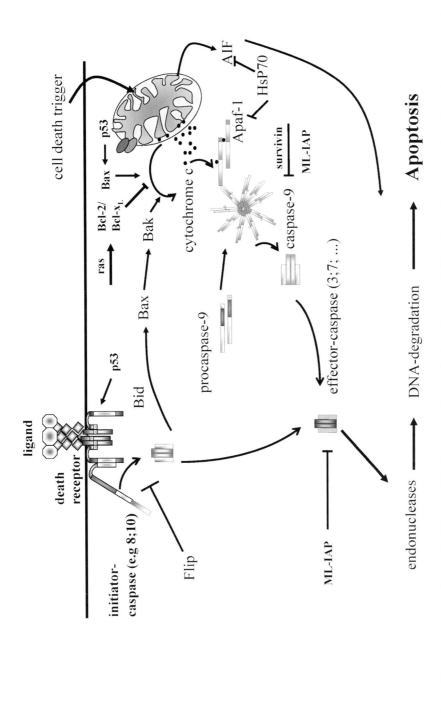

Fig. 1. The apoptotic pathway. In this simplified scheme, the extrinsic pathway is initiated by oligomerization of death receptors after binding ligand and recruitment of initiator caspases (caspase-8 and caspase-10). The intrinsic pathway involves the translocation of proapoptotic Bcl-2 members to mitochondria and release of cytochrome-*c* into the cytosol, oligomerization of apoptotic protease activating factor-1 (Apaf-1) in a co with caspase-9, and the subsequent activation of caspase-3. Receptor-initiated signals can be transduced through the mitochondrial pathwa example, through cleavage of Bid (for details *see* page 608).

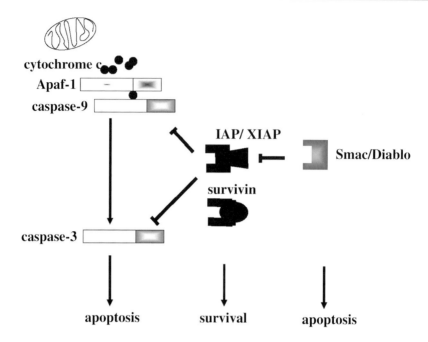

Fig. 2. Caspase regulatory proteins. The inhibitor of apoptosis (IAP) gene family encodes a group of structurally related proteins (e.g., IAP-1, IAP-2, X-chromosome-linked IAP, survivin, and melanoma IAP) that are able to suppress caspase function. They are thought to directly inhibit certain caspases and are controlled by further inhibitory proteins of IAP, Smac (second mitochondrial activator of caspases)/Diablo (direct IAP-binding protein with low pI).

mitochondria, the second mitochondrial activator of caspases (Smac)/Diablo and Omi/ OtrA *(24)*. Furthermore, p53 can modulate the expression of apoptotic effectors, and heat-shock proteins can also regulate the formation of the apoptosome.

APOPTOSIS DEFICIENCY AND MELANOMA

Wild-type p53 promotes cell cycle arrest and apoptosis in response to DNA-damaging drugs most likely by controlling transcriptional regulation of target genes, such as *Bcl-2* and *Bax (25,26)* (Fig. 1), and acts, therefore, as a tumor suppressor. *p53* mutations are common genetic alterations in human cancer. Melanoma cell lines expressing wild-type p53 exhibit a higher response to anticancer agents than melanoma with mutant p53 *(27)*. Mutation of *p53* was associated with metastatic potential *(28)*. Abnormal phosphorylation of *p53* by Ck2 kinase was associated with melanoma resistance to radiotherapy *(29)*. A phase I dose-escalation study of single intratumoral injection of a replication-defective adenoviral expression vector containing *p53* was performed by Dummer et al. in patients with metastatic melanoma. In this study, the therapeutic approach was proven safe, feasible, and biologically effective *(30)*.

Another very common specific gene defect in human melanoma is mutation of activated *ras (31)*. Ras proteins are regulators of multiple signal pathways that control cell growth, differentiation, and apoptosis. The assumed mechanism by which the activated *ras* oncogene is involved in drug resistance is an upregulation of Bcl-2 expression *(32)*. A decreased CD95 surface expression in ras transfectants was demonstrated in melanoma cell lines (33). Indeed, overexpression of activated mutants of N-ras increase cisplatin resistance in melanoma cells and in a SCID (severe combined immunodeficient) mouse model (34). Improved understanding of the molecular mechanisms of Ras processing and membrane targeting provided important tools for the development of molecules that inhibit the association of Ras with the inner cell membrane. Such molecules include inhibitors of farnesyltransferase, prenyl-CAAX protease, methyl-transferase, and inhibitors, such as trans-farnesyl thiosalicylic acid (Fig. 3). Farnesyl thiosalicylic acid, a Ras antagonist, suppresses melanoma growth in vitro and in vivo through a combination of cytostatic and proapoptotic effects (35). Furthermore, a recent study evaluated the effect of farnesyl thiosalicylic acid treatment in combination with dacarbazine on established human melanoma xenografts grown in mice. A significant tumor growth paralleled by an acceptable toxicity profile was shown in a mouse system (36) (Fig. 3).

B-Raf, a Ras effector molecule, was found to be mutated in 66% of human melanomas (37). Previous studies indicated that wild-type B-Raf may inhibit apoptosis downstream of cytochrome-c release by activating nuclear factor (NF)-κB (38).

Extensive efforts have been made in analyzing the involvement of death receptors in melanoma cell death. Downregulation, loss, and mutation of CD95/Fas receptor in melanoma have been described, resulting in triggering resistance to CD95L/Fas ligand (39,40). A respective correlation to clinical response was demonstrated by Mouawad et al. (41). They reported that melanoma patients with low clinical response to various drugs (cisplatin, recombinant interleukin-2, and interferon-α) exhibited a significant increase of soluble sCD95 and sCD95L in the plasma after drug treatment, whereas in the plasma of responders, no changes in sCD95 or sCD95L levels were observed.

Various studies demonstrated that, in contrast to the CD95 receptor, TRAIL-R2 is widely expressed in melanoma. Furthermore, melanoma cell lines were shown to undergo apoptosis after exposure with recombinant TRAIL very readily, whereas melanocytes did not demonstrate such a high TRAIL sensitivity (42). This study also showed that TRAIL-R expression is not predictive of sensitivity. There are some known agents available to upregulate TRAIL-R expression, such as cisplatin, betulinic acid, CD437 retinoid, and TNF-α (overviewed in Hersey et al., ref. 43). Furthermore, Griffith et al. demonstrated increased apoptosis in melanoma cells after TRAIL-expressing adenoviral infection as a possible therapeutic approach (44). Sensitivity toward death-receptor signaling in melanoma cells was also increased using a soluble NF-κB inhibitor (45).

Bcl-2 appears to influence response to chemotherapy by inhibiting apoptosis induction by many cytostatic drugs, including alkylating agents, topoisomerase inhibitors, antimetabolites, and others. The high expression of Bcl-2 in human melanoma and other tumors has been correlated with resistance to chemotherapy and decreased survival (46). Furthermore, Raisova et al. showed that a low Bax:Bcl-2 ratio might be characteristic for drug-resistant melanoma cells (47). Additionally, the oncogenic potential of Bcl-2 seems to be involved in melanoma angiogenesis through vascular endothelial growth factor (VEGF) mRNA stabilization and hypoxia-inducible factor (HIF)-mediated transcriptional activity (48). C-Myc low-expressing compared with high-expressing melanoma lines demonstrated an increased cisplatin sensitivity (49). In a human melanoma xenograft in SCID mouse models, the improvement of chemosensitivity of dacarbazine in combination with bcl-2 oligo–antisense (Augmerosen, Gentasense, G-3139) could be demonstrated (50). Furthermore, Heere-Ress et al. demonstrated recently how antisense

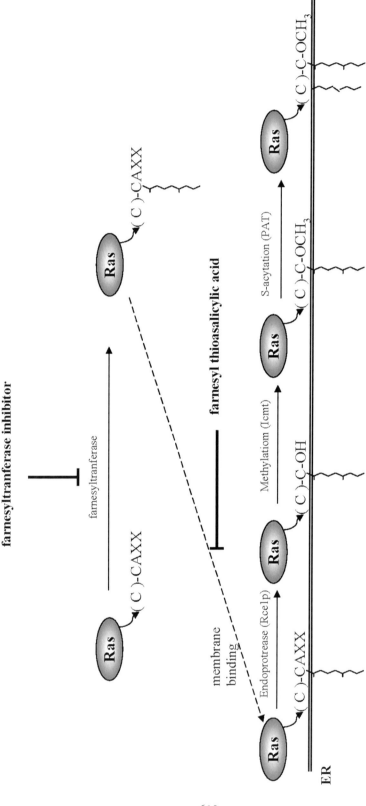

Fig. 3. Ras proteins carry C-terminal lipid modifications, through which they associate with cellular membranes and which are essential for their transforming activity. After initial cytosolic farnesylation, Ras proteins translocate to intercellular membranes. Here they undergo successive removal of the terminal –AXX residues, methylation, and further modification by *S*-acetylation. (Reproduced with permission from ref. 86.)

oligonucleotides reduced Bcl-X$_L$ expression and enhanced the chemosensitivity of melanoma cell lines to cisplatin *(51)*. A recent study showed that the simultaneous downregulation of Bcl-2 and Bcl-X$_L$ expression and induction of apoptosis by antisense oligonucleotides in melanoma cells of different clinical stage may provide an additional clinical benefit *(52)*.

Antisense oligonucleotides are short, single-stranded nucleotides that bind complementary to their respective target mRNA, thus, inhibiting translation and initiating degradation of the targeted mRNA. Antisense oligonucleotides directed against specific genes, such as Bcl-2, associated with neoplastic progression are currently being evaluated in several clinical trials. Therefore, mouse systems *(50)* have been translated into clinical phase I/IIa studies, in which 6 of 14 treated patients showed an antitumor response associated with low Bcl-2 levels and increased apoptosis in melanoma biopsies *(82)*. Recently, a worldwide phase III study recruited 770 patients with metastatic melanoma to compare the efficiency of the standard chemotherapy dacarbazine alone and dacarbazine plus Bcl-2 antisense. The final analysis is currently being performed. Antisense molecules for Bcl-X$_L$ and c-Myc are available, and clinical application can be expected.

Caspase proteases are initially synthesized as precursor proteins with little or no enzymatic activity. The cleaved proteins are the primary apoptotic executers, which act in a cascade ultimately leading to the cleavage of substrates that produce the characteristic features of apoptosis. Caspase proteases are cleaved by upstream molecules (such as caspases, FADD ([Fas-associated protein with death domain], or Apaf-1) and are further controlled by a variety of proteins that directly interact with proteases: IAPs and FLICE (FADD-like interleukin-1-β-converting enzyme inhibitory proteins (FLIPs). Caspase inhibition is achieved by proteins of the IAP family (Fig. 2), which are structurally related by their baculovirus IAP repeat domain. In melanoma, two members of the IAP family (survivin and ML-IAP/Livin) and FLIP have been associated with tumor progression. One of the best-characterized members in melanoma is survivin, which exerts its effect by directly inhibiting caspases and was found in melanoma only (cell lines, metastatic lesions, and invasive melanoma) compared with melanocytes *(54)*. In contrast to other apoptotic inhibitors, survivin expression is cell-cycle dependent. In early mitosis, survivin, linked to the microtubules of the mitotic spindle, inhibits the activation of caspase 3 *(55)*. A recent study by Gradilone et al. showed a significant correlation between survivin expression and outcome of sentinel lymph node-positive melanoma patients *(56)*. Antisense oligonucleotides directed against this molecule were shown to induce spontaneous apoptosis in melanoma in vitro *(54)*. This was proven by the same group by a phosphorylation-defective Thr34 baculoviral IAP repeat (BIR) mutant (the relevant domain in IAPs), which prevented tumor formation and slowed the growth of established tumors in a melanoma xenograft model *(57)*, suggesting that therapeutic targeting of survivin might also be beneficial in patients with recurrent or metastatic melanoma. An additional IAP molecule has been discovered in melanoma by two other groups. ML-IAP/livin is expressed in developed tissues, including melanocytes, but is predominantly overexpressed in melanoma *(58,59)*. ML-IAP acts directly on the mitochondrial pathway by directly inhibiting caspase-9, caspase-3, and the proapoptotic factor, Smac/Diablo *(60)*. Furthermore, this molecule was identified as a possible target for immune-mediated tumor destruction in melanoma *(58,61)*. Further studies found that transfection of an antisense construct against livin could trigger apoptosis specifically in melanoma cell lines expressing *livin* mRNA. This was associated with an increase in DNA fragmentation and in DEVD-like caspase activity *(58)*.

A mitochondria-derived activator of caspase (Smac/Diablo) construct was shown in vitro to sensitize melanoma to TRAIL-induced apoptosis as a very selective tool inhibiting IAP *(62)*. There are strong reasons why caspase inhibitors can be considered characteristic of the drug-resistant phenotype in melanoma cells; caspase inhibitors enhance the ability of the melanoma cells to resist apoptosis and present a rewarding therapeutic target.

FLIP was shown to inhibit caspase-8 and, therefore, to inhibit apoptosis induced by receptor-associated cytokines (e.g., TNF-α, CD95L/Fas ligand, TRAIL). FLIP was shown to be overexpressed in melanoma and associated with resistance *(63)*. Nevertheless, endogenous levels of FLIP do not necessarily correlate with drug response in melanoma patients *(40,64)*.

Apaf-1 represents an essential downstream molecule to induce apoptosis. Soengas et al. reported cases of drug-resistant malignant melanomas in which Apaf-1 expression was impaired *(65)*. Here, cytostatic drugs induced cytochrome-*c* release, but failed to induce caspase-9 activation. This could be reversed by reactivating Apaf-1 with the demethylating agent, 5-aza-2-deoxycytidine, in vitro.

Various studies suggest that increased antiapoptotic, heat-shock protein (HsP) expression, such as HsP70 and HsP90, may be related to drug resistance *(66,67)*. HsP70 antagonizes the caspase-independent apoptotic-inducing factor (AIF) *(68)*. Hsp70 may also interfere with Apaf-1, by inhibiting the oligomerization and/or by blocking the recruitment of caspase-9 to the apoptosome *(69)*. HsP70 was shown to be upregulated in primary melanoma and cell lines *(70,71)*, and an association with resistance to ultraviolet radiation was seen *(72)*. Clinical trials using 17-AAG for Hsp90 inhibition in advanced cancer are currently ongoing *(73)*.

Neef et al. identified the human pleckstin-homology-like domain family A, member 1 (*PHLDA1*)/*TDAG51* gene, which was shown to be downregulated in metastatic melanoma and associated with apoptosis resistance *(74)*. *PHLDA1* expression was associated with reduced cell growth, cloning efficiency, and colony formation, and increased basal apoptosis. Chemosensitivity to doxorubicin and camptothecin was enhanced. Moreover, recently, a group of human melanoma cell populations that are heterogeneously susceptible to C2-ceramide-mediated apoptosis was identified *(75)*. Studies with these melanoma cells revealed a correlation between ceramide-mediated apoptosis and D-NMAPPD, a ceramide analog, confirming the effect of this inhibitor on ceramide signaling in human melanoma cells. These findings suggest ceramidase inhibitors as a potential new therapeutical class of antiproliferative and cytostatic drugs.

NF-κB is a transcription factor linked at the crossroads of life and death (Fig. 4). It functions as a modulator of inflammation, angiogenesis, differentiation, cell cycle, adhesion, migration, and survival *(76)*. NF-κB has been recognized as an possible potential target in cancer treatment *(77)*. In melanoma cells, NF κB can be affected by upregulation of the NF-κB subunit, p50 or Rel A, or downregulation of the NF-κB inhibitor, IκB *(78)*. Subsequently, all target molecules downstream of NF-κB regulation are affected. Therefore antiapoptotic factors, such as c-myc and TNF receptor-associated factor (TRAF)-2, are frequently upregulated in melanoma. In melanoma, gene-transfer approaches targeting NF-κB disruption have been used, inactivating the NF-κB subunit, Rel A *(79)*,and overexpressing IκB *(80)*.

Table 1
Summary of Therapeutic Approaches in Melanoma From In Vitro Studies to Clinical Trials[a]

Target and experimental setting		Reference
Clinical trials		
bcl-2	Antisense oligonucleotides combined (plus dacarbazine)	Jansen et al., 2000 (82)
p53	Intratumoral injection	Dummer et al., 2000 (30)
Mouse systems		
H-ras	Overexpression in SCID-mouse model	Jansen et al., 1997 (34)
ras	Farnesyl thiosalicylic acid combined with dacarbazine in an human melanoma xenograft mouse model	Halaschek-Wiener et al., 2003 (36)
bcl-2	Antisense oligonucleotides	Smalley et al., 2002 (35)
		Jansen et al., 1998 (50)
p53	Adenoviral vector	Cirielli et al., 1995 (83)
survivin	Transient transfection of C85A mutant	Grossman et al., 2001 (57)
p53	Adenoviral vector (plus cyclin D)	Sauter et al., 2002 (84)
In vitro melanoma cell systems		
bcl-X_L	Antisense oligonucleotides	Heere-Ress et al., 2002 (51)
bcl-2/bcl-X_L	Simultaneous downregulation by antisense oligonucleotides	Olie et al., 2002 (52)
survivin	Antisense oligonucleotides	Grossman et al., 1999 (54)
	Conditional expression $T^{34}A$ mutant (plus cisplatin)	Olie et al., 2002 (52)
p53	Adenoviral vector	Cirielli et al., 1995 (83)
H-ras	Ribozyme	Ohta et al., 1996 (85)
	Antisense	Jansen et al., 1997 (34)
apaf-1	Retrovirus, 5aza2dc (plus adriamycin)	Soengas et al., 2001 (65)
ML-lap	Antisense oligonucleotide	Kasof et al., 2001 (58)
relA	Antisense oligonucleotide	McNulty et al., 2001 (79)

[a]Many studies observed single tumor cell lines or limited tissue samples.
SCID, severe combined immunodeficient.

613

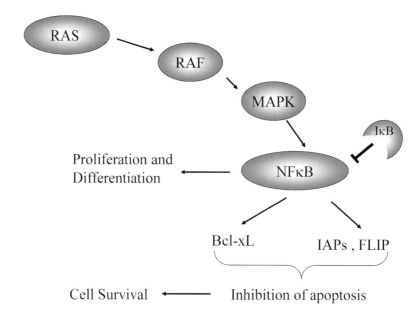

Fig. 4. The nuclear factor (NF)-κB pathway. In the context of cell death control, NF-κB modulates the expression of survival factors.

Apoptosis deficiency appears to be strongly associated with the specific drug-resistant phenotype *(81)*. In this study, cisplatin resistance has been associated with reduced caspase-9 activity and cytochrome-*c* release paralleled by normal DNA fragmentation, whereas no apoptotic events could be induced in etoposide-resistant melanoma cells *(81)*.

Recently, tremendous efforts have been made in identifying new strategies and drug targets inhibiting apoptosis to support melanoma treatment (Table 1). Various investigations in mouse systems could prove the benefit of strategies interfering with apoptotic mechanisms in melanoma. Nevertheless, until now, these strategies could only be transferred in a few clinical trails.

REFERENCES

1. Kerr JF, Wyllie AH, Currie AR. Apoptosis: a basic biological phenomenon with wide-ranging implications in tissue kinetics. Br J Cancer 1972;26:239–257.
2. Kaufmann SH, Earnshaw WC. Induction of apoptosis by cancer chemotherapy. Exp Cell Res 2000:25,642–25,649.
3. Johnstone RW, Ruefli AA, Lowe SW. Apoptosis: a link between cancer genetics and chemotherapy. Cell 2002;108:153–164.
4. Hanahan D, Weinberg RA. The hallmarks of cancer. Cell 2000;100:57–70.
5. Staunton MJ, Gaffney EF. Tumor type is a determinant of susceptibility to apoptosis. Am J Clin Pathol 1995;103:300–307.
6. Leist M, Jaattela M. Triggering of apoptosis by cathepsins. Cell Death Differ 2001;8:324–326.
7. Scaffidi C, et al. Two CD95 (APO-1/Fas) signaling pathways. EMBO J 1998;17:1675–1687.
8. Sprick MR, et al. Caspase-10 is recruited to and activated at the native TRAIL and CD95 death-inducing signalling complex in a FADD-dependent manner but can not functionally substitute caspase-8. EMBO J 2002;21:4520–4530.
9. Zou H, Li Y, Liu X, Wang X. An APAF-1 cytochrome c multimeric complex is a functional apoptosome that activates procaspase-9. J Biol Chem 1999;274:11,549–11,556.
10. Tewari M, et al. Yama/CPP32 beta, a mammalian homolog of CED-3, is a CrmA-inhibitable protease that cleaves the death substrate poly(ADP-ribose) polymerase. Cell 1995;81:801–809.

11. Lazebnik YA, Kaufmann SH, Desnoyers S, Poirier GG, Earnshaw WC. Cleavage of poly(ADP-ribose) polymerase by a proteinase with properties like ICE. Nature 1994;371:346–347.

12. Liu X, Zou H, Slaughter C, Wang X. DFF, a heterodimeric protein that functions downstream of caspase-3 to trigger DNA fragmentation during apoptosis. Cell 1997;89:175–184.

13. Thornberry NA. Caspases: key mediators of apoptosis. Chem Biol 1998;5:1074–5521.

14. Locksley RM, Killeen N, Lenardo MJ. The TNF and TNF receptor superfamilies: integrating mammalian biology. Cell 2001;104:487–501.

15. Fulda S, et al. Cell type specific involvement of death receptor and mitochondrial pathways in drug-induced apoptosis. Oncogene 2001;20:1063–1075.

16. Los M, et al. Cross-resistance of CD95- and drug-induced apoptosis as a consequence of deficient activation of caspases (ICE/Ced-3 proteases). Blood 1997;90:3118–3129.

17. Muller M, et al. Drug-induced apoptosis in hepatoma cells is mediated by the CD95 (APO-1/Fas) receptor/ligand system and involves activation of wild-type p53. J Clin Invest 1997;99:403–413.

18. Tschopp J, Martinon F, Hofmann K. Apoptosis: silencing the death receptors. Curr Biol 1999;9: R389–R384.

19. Wajant H. The Fas signaling pathway: more than a paradigm. Science 2002;296:1635–1636.

20. Strasser A, O'Connor L, Dixit VM. Apoptosis signaling. Annu Rev Biochem 2000;69:217–245.

21. Acehan D, et al. Three-dimensional structure of the apoptosome: implications for assembly, procaspase-9 binding, and activation. Mol Cell 2002;9:423–432.

22. Zou H, Henzel WJ, Liu X, Lutschg A, Wang X. Apaf-1, a human protein homologous to C. elegans CED-4, participates in cytochrome c-dependent activation of caspase-3 [see comments]. Cell 1997;90:405–413.

23. Li P, et al. Cytochrome c and dATP-dependent formation of Apaf-1/caspase-9 complex initiates an apoptotic protease cascade. Cell 1997;91:479–489.

24. Chai JJ, et al. Structural and biochemical basis of apoptotic activation by Smac/DIABLO. Nature 2000;406:855–862.

25. Petty R, Evans A, Duncan I, Kurbacher C, Cree I. Drug resistance in ovarian cancer—the role of p53. Pathol Oncol Res 1998;4:97–102.

26. Miyake H, et al. Enhancement of chemosensitivity in human bladder cancer cells by adenoviral-mediated p53 gene transfer. Anticancer Res 1998;18:3087–3092.

27. Li G, Bush JA, Ho VC. p53-dependent apoptosis in melanoma cells after treatment with camptothecin. J Invest Dermatol 2000;114:514–519.

28. Hartmann A, et al. Overexpression and mutations of p53 in metastatic malignant melanomas. Int J Cancer 1996;67:313–317.

29. Satyamoorthy K, et al. Aberrant regulation and function of wild-type p53 in radioresistant melanoma cells. Cell Growth Differ 2000;11:467–474.

30. Dummer R, et al. Biological activity and safety of adenoviral vector-expressed wild-type p53 after intratumoral injection in melanoma and breast cancer patients with p53-overexpressing tumors. Cancer Gene Ther 2000;7:1069–1076.

31. Serrone L, Hersey P. The chemoresistance of human malignant melanoma: an update. Melanoma Res 1999;9:51–58.

32. Borner C, et al. Mutated N-ras upregulates Bcl-2 in human melanoma in vitro and in SCID mice. Melanoma Res 1999;9:347–350.

33. Urquhart JL, et al. Regulation of Fas-mediated apoptosis by N-ras in melanoma. J Invest Dermatol 2002;119:556–561.

34. Jansen B, et al. Activated N-ras contributes to the chemoresistance of human melanoma in severe combined immunodeficiency (SCID) mice by blocking apoptosis. Cancer Res 1997;57:362–365.

35. Smalley KS, Eisen TG. Farnesyl thiosalicylic acid inhibits the growth of melanoma cells through a combination of cytostatic and pro-apoptotic effects. Int J Cancer 2002;98:514–522.

36. Halaschek-Wiener J, Kloog Y, Wacheck V, Jansen B. Farnesyl thiosalicylic acid chemosensitizes human melanoma in vivo. J Invest Dermatol 2003;120:109–115.

37. Davies H, et al. Mutations of the BRAF gene in human cancer. Nature 2002;417:949–954.

38. Erhardt P, Schremser EJ, Cooper GM. B-Raf inhibits programmed cell death downstream of cytochrome c release from mitochondria by activating the MEK/Erk pathway. Mol Cell Biol 1999;19: 5308–5315.

39. Shin MS, et al. Alterations of Fas (Apo-1/CD95) gene in cutaneous malignant melanoma. Am J Pathol 1999;154:1785–1791.

40. Ugurel S, et al. Heterogenous susceptibility to CD95-induced apoptosis in melanoma cells correlates with bcl-2 and bcl-x expression and is sensitive to modulation by interferon-gamma. Int J Cancer 1999;82:727–736.

41. Mouawad R, Khayat D, Soubrane C. Plasma Fas ligand, an inducer of apoptosis, and plasma soluble Fas, an inhibitor of apoptosis, in advanced melanoma. Melanoma Research 2000;10:461–467.

42. Griffith TS, Chin WA, Jackson GC, Lynch DH, Kubin MZ. Intracellular regulation of TRAIL-induced apoptosis in human melanoma cells. J Immunol 1998;161:2833–2840.

43. Hersey P, Zhang XD. How melanoma cells evade trail-induced apoptosis. Nat Rev Cancer 2001;1:142–150.

44. Griffith TS, Anderson RD, Davidson BL, Williams RD, Ratliff TL. Adenoviral-mediated transfer of the TNF-related apoptosis-inducing ligand/apo-2 ligand gene induces tumor cell apoptosis. J Immunol 2000;165:2886–2894.

45. Franco AV, et al. The role of nf-kappab in tnf-related apoptosis-inducing ligand (trail)-induced apoptosis of melanoma cells. J Immunol 2001;166:5337–5345.

46. Reed JC, Paternostro G. Postmitochondrial regulation of apoptosis during heart failure [comment]. Proc Natl Acad Sci USA 1999;96:7614–7616.

47. Raisova M, et al. The Bax/Bcl-2 ratio determines the susceptibility of human melanoma cells to CD95/Fas-mediated apoptosis. J Invest Dermatol 2001;117:333–340.

48. Iervolino A, et al. Bcl-2 overexpression in human melanoma cells increases angiogenesis through VEGF mRNA stabilization and HIF-1–mediated transcriptional activity. FASEB J 2002;16:1453–1455.

49. Biroccio A, et al. c-Myc down-regulation increases susceptibility to cisplatin through reactive oxygen species-mediated apoptosis in M14 human melanoma cells. Mol Pharmacol 2001;60:174–182.

50. Jansen B, et al. bcl-2 antisense therapy chemosensitizes human melanoma in Scid mice. Nat Med 1998;4:232–234.

51. Heere-Ress E, et al. Bcl-X(L) is a chemoresistance factor in human melanoma cells that can be inhibited by antisense therapy. Int J Cancer 2002;99:29–34.

52. Olie RA, et al. Bcl-2 and bcl-xL antisense oligonucleotides induce apoptosis in melanoma cells of different clinical stages. J Invest Dermatol 2002;118:505–512.

53. Jansen B, et al. Bcl-2 antisense plus dacarbacine therapy for malignan melanoma. Proc Am Assoc Cancer Res Conf Programmed Cell Death Regul 2000;A95.

54. Grossman D, McNiff JM, Li F, Altieri DC. Expression and targeting of the apoptosis inhibitor, survivin, in human melanoma. J Invest Dermatol 1999;113:1076–1081.

55. Li F, et al. Control of apoptosis and mitotic spindle checkpoint by survivin. Nature 1998;396:580–584.

56. Gradilone A, et al. Survivin, bcl-2, bax, and bcl-X gene expression in sentinel lymph nodes from melanoma patients. J Clin Oncol 2003;21:306–312.

57. Grossman D, Kim PJ, Schechner JS, Altieri DC. Inhibition of melanoma tumor growth in vivo by survivin targeting. Proc Natl Acad Sci USA 2001;98:635–640.

58. Kasof GM, Gomes BC. Livin, a novel inhibitor of apoptosis protein family member. J Biol Chem 2001;276:3238–3246.

59. Vucic D, Stennicke HR, Pisabarro MT, Salvesen GS, Dixit VM. ML-IAP, a novel inhibitor of apoptosis that is preferentially expressed in human melanomas. Curr Biol 2000;10:1359–1366.

60. Vucic D, et al. SMAC negatively regulates the anti-apoptotic activity of melanoma inhibitor of apoptosis (ML-IAP). J Biol Chem 2002;277:12,275–12,279.

61. Schmollinger JC, et al. Melanoma inhibitor of apoptosis protein (ML-IAP) is a target for immune-mediated tumor destruction. Proc Natl Acad Sci USA 2003;100:3398–3403.

62. Srinivasula SM, et al. Molecular determinants of the caspase-promoting activity of Smac/DIABLO and its role in the death receptor pathway. J Biol Chem 2000;275:36,152–36,157.

63. Bullani RR, et al. Selective expression of FLIP in malignant melanocytic skin lesions. J Invest Dermatol 2001;117:360–364.

64. Zhang XD, et al. Relation of TNF-related apoptosis-inducing ligand (TRAIL) receptor and FLICE-inhibitory protein expression to TRAIL-induced apoptosis of melanoma. Cancer Res 1999;59:2747–2753.

65. Soengas MS, et al. Inactivation of the apoptosis effector Apaf-1 in malignant melanoma. Nature 2001;409:207–211.

66. Han W, et al. Effects of C(2)-ceramide on the Malme-3M melanoma cell line. J Dermatol Sci 2002;30:10.

67. Sinha P, et al. Identification of novel proteins associated with the development of chemoresistance in malignant melanoma using two-dimensional electrophoresis. Electrophoresis 2000;21:3048–3057.

68. Ravagnan L, et al. Heat-shock protein 70 antagonizes apoptosis-inducing factor. Nat Cell Biol 2001;3:839–843.

69. Saleh A, Srinivasula SM, Balkir L, Robbins PD, Alnemri ES. Negative regulation of the Apaf-1 apoptosome by Hsp70. Nat Cell Biol 2000;2:476–483.

70. Dressel R, Johnson JP, Gunther E. Heterogeneous patterns of constitutive and heat shock induced expression of HLA-linked HSP70-1 and HSP70-2 heat shock genes in human melanoma cell lines. Melanoma Res 1998;8:482–492.

71. Ricaniadis N, Kataki A, Agnantis N, Androulakis G, Karakousis CP. Long-term prognostic significance of HSP-70, c-myc and HLA-DR expression in patients with malignant melanoma. Eur J Surg Oncol 2001;27:88–93.

72. Park KC, et al. Overexpression of HSP70 prevents ultraviolet B-induced apoptosis of a human melanoma cell line. Arch Dermatol Res 2000;292:482–487.

73. Solit DB, Scher HI, Rosen N. Hsp90 as a therapeutic target in prostate cancer. Semin Oncol 2003;30:709–716.

74. Neef R, Kuske MA, Prols E, Johnson JP. Identification of the Human PHLDA1/TDAG51 Gene: downregulation in metastatic melanoma contributes to apoptosis resistance and growth deregulation. Cancer Res 2002;62:5920–5929.

75. Raisova M, et al. Bcl-2 overexpression prevents apoptosis induced by ceramidase inhibitors in malignant melanoma and HaCaT keratinocytes. FEBS Lett 2002;516:47–52.

76. Karin M, Lin A. NF-kappaB at the crossroads of life and death. Nat Immunol 2002;3:221–227.

77. Lin A, Karin M. NF-kappaB in cancer: a marked target Semin Cancer Biol 2003;13:107–114.

78. Yang J, Richmond A. Constitutive IkappaB kinase activity correlates with nuclear factor-kappaB activation in human melanoma cells. Cancer Res 2001;61:4901–4909.

79. McNulty SE, Tohidian NB, Meyskens FL Jr. RelA, p50 and inhibitor of kappa B alpha are elevated in human metastatic melanoma cells and respond aberrantly to ultraviolet light B. Pigment Cell Res 2001;14:456–465.

80. Bakker TR, Reed D, Renno T, Jongeneel CV. Efficient adenoviral transfer of NF-kappaB inhibitor sensitizes melanoma to tumor necrosis factor-mediated apoptosis. Int J Cancer 1999;80:320–323.

81. Helmbach H, et al. Drug-resistance towards etoposide and cisplatin in human melanoma cells is associated with drug-dependent apoptosis deficiency. J Invest Dermatol 2002;118:923–932.

82. Jansen B, et al. Chemosensitisation of malignant melanoma by BCL2 antisense therapy. Lancet 2000;356:1728–1733.

83. Cirielli C, et al. Adenovirus-mediated gene transfer of wild-type p53 results in melanoma cell apoptosis in vitro and in vivo. Int J Cancer 1995;63:673–679.

84. Sauter ER, Takemoto R, Litwin S, Herlyn M. p53 alone or in combination with antisense cyclin D1 induces apoptosis and reduces tumor size in human melanoma. Cancer Gene Ther 2002;9:807–812.

85. Ohta Y, Kijima H, Kashani-Sabet M, Scanlon KJ. Suppression of the malignant phenotype of melanoma cells by anti-oncogene ribozymes. J Invest Dermatol 1996;106:275–280.

86. Silvius JR. Mechanisms of Ras protein targeting in mammilian cells. J Membr Bio 2002; 90:83–92.

35 Role of Melanoma-Associated Antigens

Rishab K. Gupta, Ana M. McElrath-Garza, and Donald L. Morton

Summary

The dynamic interaction between malignant melanoma cells and the host's immune system has a profound influence on the development and progression of disease. Numerous studies have documented the therapeutic potential of immunological manipulation in patients with melanoma, and many tumor-associated antigens have been studied as possible targets of melanoma-specific immunotherapy. This chapter outlines the most significant melanoma-associated antigens, highlighting those with the greatest potential for influencing future treatment modalities. Specific antigens defined by T- and B-cells are discussed, and how these antigens are recognized, processed, and manipulated by the host's immune system is explained. The role of gangliosides in distinguishing different stages of melanocyte differentiation is described, and a 90-kDa tumor-associated glycoprotein antigen which has considerable promise as a marker of melanoma tumor burden is introduced. Finally, this chapter reviews technological advances in assays used to detect various melanoma-associated antigens.

Key Words: Melanoma; melanoma-associated antigens; tumor-associated antigens; immunotherapy; TA90.

INTRODUCTION

The malignant transformation of melanocytes to melanoma can be characterized by changes in cytology, morphology, proliferative index, biochemistry, and gene expression. Activation of genes in transformed cells leads to overexpression and/or unique expression of molecules, such as tumor-associated antigens. Some of these molecules may be present in normal cells but sequestered from the immune system. In transformed

From: *From Melanocytes to Melanoma: The Progression to Malignancy*
Edited by: V. J. Hearing and S. P. L. Leong © Humana Press Inc., Totowa, NJ

cells, the antigens are expressed on nonsequestered sites. Tumor-associated antigens are considered immunogenic when the host recognizes them as nonself and generates an immune response. This chapter reviews the different melanoma-associated antigens (MAA) (e.g., melanoma antigen gene [MAGE]-1, NY-ESO-1, and TA90) and their roles in immune surveillance and the development/progression of melanoma.

More than 40 yr ago, anecdotal reports of an increased incidence of melanoma regression in immunosuppressed patients, such as those with congenital immunodeficiency disorders, suggested an important immune component in the development and control of disease (1–6). The more recent discovery of tissue-specific and common tumor-associated melanoma antigens further supports the key role for the immune system in the development and progression of melanoma. Additional evidence for immune modulation by MAA includes the prognostic significance of lymphocytes and other tumor-cell infiltrates (7–9), the delayed recurrence of rapidly progressive disease after successful treatment of the primary tumor (10–12), the presence of tumor cells in lymphatics, peripheral blood, and operative wounds without subsequent development of metastases (13–20), and the elimination of circulating tumor cells before the establishment of metastatic colonies (21). Ongoing investigations to identify clinically relevant target antigens and enhance the production of corresponding autoantibodies should lead to improvements in immunotherapy for melanoma.

EVIDENCE FOR IMMUNITY TO HUMAN MELANOMA

Spontaneous regression of primary and metastatic melanoma, although rare, has been well documented (1–6). Published reports have correlated regression with minor viral and bacterial infections, fever of unknown origin, changes in hormonal balance, and congenital immunodeficiency disorders. Development of metastases that are histologically and functionally identical to the primary tumor has been reported 10 to 20 yr after successful treatment of the primary tumor. Delayed recurrence suggests a clinically effective antitumor response during the disease-free interval. Although biological, physiological, and endocrine factors could contribute to spontaneous regression and long-term remission, clinical evidence implicates humoral and cellular immunological mechanisms (22,23).

HOST IMMUNE RESPONSE AND DEVELOPMENT
OF MALIGNANT MELANOMA

Because malignant melanoma is one of the most immunogenic solid tumors, it has served as a prototype for investigations of active immunotherapy against cancer (24–27). Determining the mechanisms of tumor escape from immunosurveillance is necessary to formulate effective immunotherapy against tumor cells (28). Despite the highly immunogenic nature of melanoma cells, as evidenced by the infiltration of tumor antigen-specific T-cells, most tumors are not completely destroyed by the host and can lead to progression of disease. An effective immune response against the host's melanoma cells requires immune recognition of target peptides in the context of major histocompatibility complex (MHC) molecules (29–31). This is particularly true for T-cell mediated responses. In addition, co-stimulatory signals are necessary for cell-mediated immunity (32,33). The absence of proper MHC or co-stimulatory molecule expression can prevent an effective antitumor immune response (34). Thus, a melanoma cell that expresses immunogenic MAA may not induce a T-cell mediated antimelanoma response without proper co-stimulation, even if the MAA are recognized by the T-cells. Furthermore, many responses defined as antitumor effector mechanisms can become ineffective or protumorigenic under certain conditions. For example, immune selection pressure could result in outgrowth of resistant tumor variants.

RECOGNITION OF MAA EXPRESSED BY HUMAN MELANOMA CELLS

MAA have been detected by in vitro and in vivo cellular reactions and by in vitro serological tests. T- and B-cells that recognize and reject autologous cells have been widely used to identify MAA *(35)*. In serological approaches, both sera from cancer patients and antisera produced in xenogeneic hosts were used as the source of antibody.

Antigens Defined by T-Cells

Genetic *(36)*, biochemical *(37)*, and immunological *(38)* approaches have been used to identify MAA recognized by cytolytic T-lymphocytes. MAGE-1 *(39)* was the first tumor-associated antigen to be identified by a genetic approach. This antigen belongs to a family of at least 12 closely related genes *(40)* expressed in variable proportions by melanoma cells *(41)*. Expression levels of MAGE antigens, as assessed by polymerase chain reaction technology, vary considerably among tissue samples and cell lines. MAGE-2 and MAGE-3 are the most common. MAGE-1 has been detected by specific monoclonal antibodies (MAbs) in clinical tumor specimens. The pattern of reactivity observed was heterogeneous within individual specimens *(42)*. When MAGE-1 is expressed, MAGE-2 or MAGE-3 is also expressed, making it feasible to use MAGE-1 and MAGE-3 for therapeutic purposes and reduce the risk of tumor escape caused by emergence of antigen-loss variants *(41)*. Benign and dysplastic nevi, as well as *in situ* melanomas, do not express *MAGE* genes *(43–45)*. *MAGE-1, -2, -3* and *-4* are more often expressed by metastatic melanoma than by primary tumors. This difference illustrates the selective activation of certain genes during malignant transformation and progression. Immune responses to the products of these genes may serve as markers of disease status as well as components of a therapeutic antimelanoma response.

Melanoblasts, which are precursors of melanocytes, are presumed to have a phenotypic pattern similar to that of early melanoma cells. MAA such as Melan-A/melanoma antigen recognized by T-cells (MART)-1 *(46–48)*, tyrosinase *(49,50)*, Pme117/gp100 *(37,51)*, gp75/tyrosine-related protein (TRP)-1 *(52)*, and AIM-2 *(53)* are expressed by normally differentiated melanocytes and by melanoma cells. These antigens are melanoma-specific; they are not expressed by other tumor cells. Houghton et al. *(54)* reported that melanoma cells in early stages of differentiation do not express antigens that are present during the later stages (such as tyrosinase). Using a real-time polymerase chain reaction method, Johansson et al. *(55)* found that tyrosinase, TRP-1, TRP-2, and MART-1/ Melan-A expression varied from undetectable to highly detectable levels in the different cell lines at different time intervals.

Peptides derived from these MAA have been used as targets for immunotherapy in several clinical trials. Although a significant proportion of patients with disease limited to the dermis, subcutaneous tissue, and/or lymphatics developed an immune response, only a minority of patients with metastatic disease had regression of the tumor. Studies by Slingluff et al. *(56)* suggest that, if a tumor does not express melanocytic differentiation proteins, immunotherapy should be directed against unique tumor antigens, as well as more frequently encountered melanocytic antigens.

Antigens Defined by B-Cell Factors

Some MAA have been localized on the cell surface, whereas others are found in the cell cytoplasm (57,58). The presence of antinucleolar antibodies in the sera of melanoma patients has also been reported (59). Before the advent of MAbs, numerous studies used patient sera to demonstrate the existence of tumor antigens in melanoma. Use of serological techniques, such as antibody-mediated cytotoxicity, immune adherence, immunofluorescence, mixed hemadsorption, complement fixation, radioimmunoassay, and enzyme immunoassay demonstrated the immunological reactivity between these antigens and sera from melanoma patients. Based on the humoral crossreactivity and absorption studies, MAA can be grouped into four categories: fetal antigens, common MAA, group-specific antigens with variable expression, and individually specific antigens.

Membrane-rich fractions prepared from melanoma tumors showed wide crossreactivity against sera from patients with malignancies of various histological types. However, absorption of the sera with fetal tissue homogenates revealed that the crossreactivity was caused by fetal antigens. Similar wide crossreactivity was observed with the partially purified spent culture medium of a melanoma cell line, suggesting the expression of these antigens by fetal cells and melanoma cells.

Within the last decade, serological expression cloning has been used to identify tumor antigens that elicit a strong antibody response in cancer patients (60). The genes SSX2 (61), NY-ESO-1 (62), and SYCP-1 (63) were identified during serological expression cloning analyses of human cancer. These genes, as well as others such as MAGE, BAGE, and GAGE, have been named "cancer/testis (CT) antigens" (60) because they are expressed predominantly in normal testis and in cancer cells.

CT genes are considered ideal target antigens for a cancer vaccine because of their immunogenicity and lack of expression in normal tissues. Of the various CT antigens, NY-ESO-1 has been the most extensively studied as a potential component of cancer vaccines (64).

There is a clear distinction between CT genes identified by messenger RNA expression analysis and those identified through immunological methods. The former genes have immunogenic potential, whereas the latter are immunogenic in cancer patients (63). Forty-four CT antigen families have been reported. With the exception of a few genes, such as those of the MAGE family, there is no general evolutionary linkage between CT genes. In addition, protein products of only 19 CT gene families have been demonstrated to elicit an immune response in cancer. The responses were strickly humoral in 13 cases, strictly cellular in 3 cases, and cellular plus humoral in 3 cases (63). Some of the antigenic diversity of human malignant melanoma cells could reflect differences in serological assay techniques, antibody sources (patient sera), and target antigen purity. Conditions for in vitro culture are not the same as those for in vivo tumor growth; the selective pressure of culture conditions may change antigenic expression on or in the cultured melanoma cells. In our experience, the expression level of human MAA fluctuates markedly with passage from one generation to another. Incorporation of exogenous components from growth medium into the membrane of cultured cells is well documented (65), and may influence the results of serological assays. This artifact has been minimized by preparing the target antigen from cells cultured in fetal calf serum-free medium or other medium that is free of potentially immunogenic supplements (66).

Hybridoma technology has allowed development of MAbs that recognize tumor-associated antigens expressed in variable levels on autologous cells, melanoma cells, and tumor cells of other histological types. Consistent identification of these antigens—despite varied serological techniques and nonstandardized reagents—confirms existence of the four groups of tumor-associated antigens on melanoma cells. These immunogenic antigens are recognized by allogeneic antibodies and their expression significantly influences the development and progression of melanoma *(67)*.

Gangliosides as Melanoma Antigens

Gangliosides are carbohydrates that have been used to distinguish different stages of melanocyte/melanoma differentiation *(68)*. These acidic glycolipids contain a hydrophobic ceramide moiety and are expressed by both normal melanocytes and melanoma cells. GM_3, GD_3, GM_2, GD_2, and O-acetyl GD_3 are found on the cell membrane of melanocytic cells. Expression of some gangliosides is significantly (>1000-fold, in the case of GD_3) upregulated after malignant transformation of melanocytes *(69)*. Regulation of ganglioside expression could trigger neoplastic transformation of melanocytes and progression of transformed cells. The diversity of ganglioside expression in neoplastically transformed cells is governed by individual genotypic differences. Changes in ganglioside profile of neoplastically transformed melanocytes correlate with changes in the proliferation, migration, and metastasis of malignant cells *(70)*.

Although this chapter is limited to the immunogenic antigens of melanoma, both immunogenic and nonimmunogenic gangliosides play a role in transformation of melanocytes and progression of the transformed cells. The presence of autoantibodies to gangliosides has been correlated with an improved prognosis in melanoma patients *(71–73)*. Sialyl Lewis(a) is not immunogenic in melanoma, but its expression has been correlated with melanoma progression *(74)*.

Antigens Defined by Antibody Phage Display Library Method

A phage-Fab library derived from the B-cells of a melanoma patient in remission after immunotherapy has been used to identify and isolate a 23-kDa glycoprotein *(75)*. The p23 antigen is on the surface and in the cytoplasm of melanoma cells, and it is expressed at high levels by cultured melanoma cell lines, vertical growth-phase primary melanoma, and metastatic melanoma. The antigen is not expressed in radial growth-phase primary melanoma, nevi, and normal skin. By identifying potentially stage-specific MAA and determining the mechanisms involved in neoplastic progression of transformed melanocytes, the antibody phage display library method *(76,77)* may have therapeutic and diagnostic potential *(78)*.

ROLE OF IMMUNOGENIC MAA IN MELANOMA PROGRESSION OR INHIBITION

Reactions observed in vitro between sera and autologous melanoma cells might also occur in vivo. These reactions, which involve both tumor and host functions, could promote or prevent tumor growth and progression *(79)*. Efforts are underway to increase the quality and magnitude of MAA-specific immune responses to a clinically effective level *(80)*. However, the possibility of antigen loss from tumor cells resulting from immunoselection could result in immune escape and subsequent tumor progression *(81–84)*.

Several regulatory pathways and molecules may be involved in melanoma antigen silencing, tumor cell differentiation, and the outcome of antitumor immune responses *(85–87)*. Certain melanoma antigens may be modulated by cytokines. In addition, cell and matrix adhesion molecules, growth factors, proteases, gangliosides, and MHC class I and II molecules contribute to the course of malignant melanoma. Antigens expressed on melanoma cells but not on mature melanocytes may be used as markers for the degree of cell differentiation; dedifferentiation of melanoma cells decreases their antigenic similarity to normal melanocytes *(88)*. Different genes responsible for expression of melanoma antigens have been identified in various stages of the disease and may be used as tumor markers for recurrence or progression.

Modulation of melanoma antigens has been suggested as a mechanism for tumor progression in the presence of cytolytic T-lymphocytes. This might explain the common finding of Melan-A/MART-1-specific tumor-infiltrating lymphocytes in clinically progressing melanomas, and it might represent a possible pathway for therapeutic intervention *(89)*. The antigen-derived T-cell response evoked by early melanoma becomes attenuated with disease progression. A variety of cell adhesion molecules on the surface of melanoma cells may regulate cellular cytotoxicity.

The use of MAA, antiantigen autoantibody levels, and immune complexes (IC) has shown promise for detecting disease and for planning and monitoring treatment. Many reports indicate that appearance of antibodies to MAA is associated with improved prognosis. These circulating antimelanoma antibodies can bind to their corresponding antigens and form IC. A clinically interesting example is the hypopigmentation associated with binding of antimelanoma antibodies to normal melanocytes. Serum from patients with vitiligo contains a high titer of naturally occurring antimelanoma antibodies and reportedly induced regression of melanoma metastases in mice. Although the association with prognosis is not clear, the appearance of hypopigmentation in patients with melanoma serves as evidence for the activity of antimelanoma antibodies *(90)*.

Prognostic Role of Anti-TA90 Immunity in Melanoma

Initial studies used allogeneic antibodies to identify a high molecular weight complex in the urine of patients with metastatic melanoma *(91,92)*. This complex comprises multiple subunits, including an immunogenic 90-kDa glycoprotein called TA90 *(93)*. TA90 is a heat-stable antigen with an isoelectric point of 6.1. It is expressed by about 75% of human solid tumors. Immunochemical analysis, including antibody-blocking studies, revealed that TA90 is distinct from known tumor markers such as carcinoembryonic antigen, prostate-specific antigen, CA15-3, α-fetoprotein, and other oncofetal antigens *(94)*.

Most cancer patients whose tumors express TA90 have endogenous anti-TA90 antibodies of immunoglobulin (Ig)-M and IgG isotypes. In patients with early- or intermediate-stage melanoma, the immune response to TA90 has been correlated with occult nodal disease and survival *(95)*. In addition, evidence suggests that the endogenous immune response to TA90 might determine the postoperative outcome of patients undergoing surgical therapy for metastatic melanoma *(96)*. Despite the fact that tumor cells have been detected in the blood of patients with metastatic melanoma, many of these patients have enjoyed prolonged survival or cure after surgical resection. This suggests that enhancement of a specific antitumor immune response might prolong survival. In fact, melanoma patients receiving a polyvalent specific active immunotherapeutic (Canvaxin, CancerVax Corp, Carlsbad, CA) that contains TA90 exhibit increased humoral (IgM and IgG) and delayed-type hypersensitivity responses *(97,98)*. In a series of investigations in which patients received Canvaxin after surgical resection of melanoma, elevated humoral and delayed-type hypersensitivity responses to Canvaxin were associated with prolonged survival *(99–101)*. These observations were the basis for an immunological model to predict the survival of patients who received Canvaxin for regional metastatic melanoma *(98)*.

In general, the incidence and level of antibodies to TA90 or other MAA are higher when melanoma is localized than when it is disseminated *(102)*. Surgery and immunotherapy with autologous or allogeneic vaccines will affect levels of circulating antibody in melanoma patients.

Prognostic Role of TA90-Specific Immune Complex in Melanoma

When the original high molecular weight glycoprotein complex was purified and used to develop a murine MAb (AD1-40F4) of IgM isotype *(103)*, Western blot analysis revealed that AD1-40F4 recognized a 90-kDa band in urine and serum of cancer patients *(93)*. This epitope is different from the epitope recognized by the autoantibody in the serum of melanoma patients *(104)*. AD1-40F4 was used to develop a TA90-IC assay that discriminated between normal and melanoma sera *(105)*. This assay has a sensitivity of 83% in detecting nodal metastases in melanoma patients undergoing lymphadenectomy *(94)*.

To test the hypothesis that the postoperative serum level of TA90-IC could have a significant correlation with recurrence and survival in patients with thick primary melanomas, postoperative TA90-IC status was correlated with disease-free survival (DFS) and overall survival (OS). Standard prognostic factors for melanoma were then compared with TA90-IC. The sensitivity and specificity of TA90-IC for predicting recurrence were 70% and 85%, respectively. Five-year DFS and OS rates were significantly higher when TA90-IC was negative. At a median follow-up of 25 mo, multivariate analysis identified postoperative TA90-IC status as the only independent predictor of DFS *(106)*. Therefore, a positive postoperative TA90-IC level suggests the presence of micrometastases that may become clinically significant.

Because standard prognostic factors, including precise staging of the regional lymph nodes, cannot accurately determine which early-stage melanomas will metastasize, and because TA90-IC status in thick primary melanoma showed a correlation with survival, TA90-IC was also investigated as a prognostic marker for patients with thin primary melanoma. Patients with 1.01- to 2.00-mm primary melanomas and tumor-negative regional lymph nodes were divided into two groups *(95)*. Group 1 comprised 50 patients who died of metastases within 7 yr after complete surgical treatment; group 2 comprised 50 patients who were matched with group 1 by six standard prognostic factors (including tumor thickness, Clark's level, and presence of ulceration), but who lived at least 10 yr without recurrence. Excluded from study were patients whose stage I melanoma had spread to the regional nodes (stage III disease), either at the time of lymphadenectomy or at any time before the development of distant metastases. This eliminated the possibility of studying patients with occult lymph node metastases or locoregional relapse. In addition, this study excluded any patient who received any form of postoperative adjuvant therapy; this eliminated the possible influence of adjuvant therapy on clinical outcomes. All patients in both groups underwent staging of the regional lymph nodes by complete lymph node dissection or, more recently, by lymphatic mapping and selective dissection of the sentinel lymph node. Postoperative sera from these patients were analyzed for TA90-IC. Standard microscopic examination determined the status of all excised lymph nodes. The incidence of TA90-IC positivity was 82% in group 1 and 18% in group 2 ($p < 0.001$). Thus, positive TA90-IC level correlated with distant metastasis when melanoma was low- or intermediate risk by standard prognostic factors. TA90-IC has been identified in the sera of numerous melanoma patients. The correlation between TA90-IC and overall survival suggests that subclinical metastasis can be detected before surgical treatment of early-stage melanoma.

A subsequent study used postoperative sera to determine TA90-IC levels in patients with melanoma and evaluate their relationship to recurrence and survival *(107)*. Multiple archived serum samples were prospectively collected during postoperative surveillance of 166 patients with American Joint Committee on Cancer stage I, II, or III melanoma. TA90-IC results were correlated with disease recurrence and survival data. The TA90-IC status in the early postoperative period was highly predictive of survival. Five-year OS was 64% for TA90-IC-negative patients and 36% for TA90-IC-positive patients ($p = 0.0001$). Median OS was 40 mo for TA90-IC-positive groups and 160 mo for the negative groups. TA90-IC-positive patients had a 5-yr DFS of only 24%, compared with 74% for TA90-IC-negative patients ($p = 0.0001$). Median DFS was 18 mo and 160 mo in TA90-IC-positive and TA90-IC-negative groups, respectively. In a study of 125 stage IV melanoma patients undergoing complete resection of distant metastases, postoperative TA90-IC positivity was again the most important prognostic variable for DFS *(108)*. Thus, there is ample evidence to suggest that a positive TA90-IC assay strongly correlates with recurrence after surgical resection of American Joint Committee on Cancer stage II, III, and IV melanoma.

CONCLUSIONS AND PERSPECTIVES

Tumor immunology represents a complex interplay of many different factors that affect tumor cell growth. Results of various investigations of immune responses against melanoma antigens indicate that both cellular and humoral immune responses to MAA are critical to the development and control of progressive disease *(109)*. Clinical reports of spontaneous regression of melanoma and the improved outcomes seen in patients receiving experimental vaccines are promising indications of the significant impact that immunotherapy may have on the future treatment of melanoma. However, development of recurrence and the progression of treated disease suggest that melanoma cells may escape immune destruction by losing or downregulating expression of MAA targets. Continued studies of MAA-based interactions may allow the development of antigen-targeted immunotherapy that prevents the malignant transformation of melanocytes to melanoma.

REFERENCES

1. Barnetson RS, Halliday GM. Regression in skin tumours: a common phenomenon. Australas J Dermatol 1997;38:S63–S65.
2. Printz C. Spontaneous regression of melanoma may offer insight into cancer immunology. J Natl Cancer Inst 2001;93:1047–1048.
3. Cochran AJ, Diehl V, Stjernsward J. Regression of primary malignant melanoma associated with a good prognosis despite metastasis to lymph nodes. Rev Eur Etud Clin Biol 1970;15:969–972.

4. Morton DL, Eilber FR, Malmgren RA, et al. Immunological factors which influence response to immunotherapy in malignant melanoma. Surgery 1970;68:158–164.

5. Morton DL, Malmgren RA, Holmes EC, et al. Demonstration of antibodies against human malignant melanoma by immunofluorescence. Surgery 1968;64:233–240.

6. Summer WC, Foraker AG. Spontaneous regression of human melanoma: clinical and experimental studies. Cancer 1960;13:79–81.

7. Movassagh M, Spatz A, Davoust J, et al. Selective accumulation of mature DC-Lamp+ dendritic cells in tumor sites is associated with efficient T-cell–mediated antitumor response and control of metastatic dissemination in melanoma. Cancer Res 2004;64:2192–2198.

8. Mihm MC Jr, Clemente CG, Cascinelli N. Tumor infiltrating lymphocytes in lymph node melanoma metastases: a histopathologic prognostic indicator and an expression of local immune response. Lab Invest 1996;74:43–47.

9. Hersey P, Murray E, Grace J, McCarthy WH. Current research on immunopathology of melanoma: analysis of lymphocyte populations in relation to antigen expression and histological features of melanoma. Pathology 1985;17:385–391.

10. Steiner A, Wolf C, Pehamberger H, Wolff K. Late metastases of cutaneous malignant melanoma. Br J Dermatol 1986;114:737–740.

11. Koh HK, Sober AJ, Fitzpatrick TB. Late recurrence (beyond ten years) of cutaneous malignant melanoma. Report of two cases and a review of the literature. JAMA 1984;251:1859–1862.

12. Lejeune FJ. The impact of surgery on the course of melanoma. Recent Results Cancer Res 2002;160:151–157.

13. Shields JD, Borsetti M, Rigby H, et al. Lymphatic density and metastatic spread in human malignant melanoma. Br J Cancer 2004;90:693–700.

14. Nathanson SD. Insights into the mechanisms of lymph node metastasis. Cancer 2003;98:413–423.

15. Fallowfield ME, Cook MG. Lymphatics in primary cutaneous melanoma. Am J Surg Pathol 1990;14:370–374.

16. Griffiths JD. Circulating cancer cells in surgery. Lond Clin Med J 1966;7:65–71.

17. Roberts SS, Cole WH. Cancer cells in the circulating blood. Semin Int 1961;10:2–10.

18. Keilholz U, Goldin-Lang P, Bechrakis NE, et al. Quantitative detection of circulating tumor cells in cutaneous and ocular melanoma and quality assessment by real-time reverse transcriptase-polymerase chain reaction. Clin Cancer Res 2004;10:1605–1612.

19. Mocellin S, Del Fiore P, Guarnieri L, et al. Molecular detection of circulating tumor cells is an independent prognostic factor in patients with high-risk cutaneous melanoma. Int J Cancer 2004;111:741–745.

20. Palmieri G, Ascierto PA, Perrone F, et al. Prognostic value of circulating melanoma cells detected by reverse transcriptase-polymerase chain reaction. J Clin Oncol 2003;21:767–773.

21. Tsubura E, Yamashita T, Sone S. Inhibition of the arrest of hematogenously disseminated tumor cells. Cancer Metastasis Rev 1983;2:223–237.

22. Morton DL, Sparks FC, Haskell CM. Oncology. In: Swartz SI, Shire CT, Spencer FC, Storer EH, eds. Principles of Surgery, 3rd ed. McGraw Hill, New York, NY: 1979.

23. Vile RG, Chong H, Dorudi S. The immunosurveillance of cancer. In: Tumor Immunology: Immunotherapy and Cancer Vaccines. Dalgleish AG, Browning M, eds. Cambridge University Press, Cambridge, UK: 1996.

24. Wang RF. Human tumor antigens: implications for cancer vaccine development. J Mol Med 1999;77:640–655.

25. Faries MB, Morton DL. Melanoma: is immunotherapy of benefit? Adv Surg 2003;37:139–169.

26. Morton DL, Ollila DW, Hsueh EC, Essner R, Gupta RK. Cytoreductive surgery and adjuvant immunotherapy: a new management paradigm for metastatic melanoma. CA Cancer J Clin 1999;49:101–116.

27. Bitton RJ. Cancer vaccines: a critical review on clinical impact. Curr Opin Mol Ther 2004;6:17–26.

28. Pawelec G. Tumor escape: anti-tumor effectors too much of a good thing? Cancer Immunol Immunother 2004;53:262–274.

29. Parkhurst MR, Riley JP, Robbins PF, Rosenberg SA. Induction of CD4+ Th1 lymphocytes that recognize known and novel class II MHC restricted epitopes from the melanoma antigen gp100 by stimulation with recombinant protein. J Immunother 2004;27:79–91.

30. Mandic M, Almunia C, Vicel S, et al. The alternative open reading frame of LAGE-1 gives rise to multiple promiscuous HLA-DR-restricted epitopes recognized by T-helper 1-type tumor-reactive CD4+ T cells. Cancer Res 2003;63:6506–6515.

31. Maeurer MJ, Storkus WJ, Kirkwood JM, Lotze MT. New treatment options for patients with mela-noma: review of melanoma-derived T-cell epitope-based peptide vaccines. Melanoma Res 1996;6:11–24.
32. Schwartz RH. Acquisition of immunologic self-tolerance. Cell 1989;57:1073–1081.
33. Janeway CA Jr. Approaching the asymptote? Evolution and revolution in immunology. Cold Spring Harb Symp Quant Biol 1989;54 Pt 1:1–13.
34. Chen L, Ashe S, Brady WA, et al. Costimulation of antitumor immunity by the B7 counterreceptor for the T lymphocyte molecules CD28 and CTLA-4. Cell 1992;71:1093–1102.
35. Ramirez-Montagut T, Turk MJ, Wolchok JD, Guevara-Patino JA, Houghton AN. Immunity to mela-noma: unraveling the relation of tumor immunity and autoimmunity. Oncogene 2003;22:3180–3187.
36. Coulie PG, Lehmann F, Lethe B, et al. A mutated intron sequence codes for an antigenic peptide recognized by cytolytic T lymphocytes on a human melanoma. Proc Natl Acad Sci USA 1995;92:7976–7980.
37. Cox AL, Skipper J, Chen Y, et al. Identification of a peptide recognized by five melanoma-specific human cytotoxic T cell lines. Science 1994;264:716–719.
38. Mukherji B, MacAlister TJ. Clonal analysis of cytotoxic T cell response against human melanoma. J Exp Med 1983;158:240–245.
39. van der Bruggen P, Traversari C, Chomez P, et al. A gene encoding an antigen recognized by cytolytic T lymphocytes on a human melanoma. Science 1991;254:1643–1647.
40. De Plaen E, Arden K, Traversari C, et al. Structure, chromosomal localization, and expression of 12 genes of the MAGE family. Immunogenetics 1994;40:360–369.
41. Coulie PG. Human tumor antigens recognized by cytolytic T lymphocytes. In: Tumor Immunology: Immunotherapy and Cancer Vaccines. Cambridge University Press, New York, NY: 1996, pp. 95–125.
42. Zuber M, Spagnoli GC, Kocher T, et al. Heterogeneity of melanoma antigen-1 (MAGE-1) gene and protein expression in malignant melanoma. Eur Surg Res 1997;29:403–410.
43. Van den Eynde B, Peeters O, De Backer O, Gaugler B, Lucas S, Boon T. A new family of genes coding for an antigen recognized by autologous cytolytic T lymphocytes on a human melanoma. J Exp Med 1995;182:689–698.
44. Brasseur F, Rimoldi D, Lienard D, et al. Expression of MAGE genes in primary and metastatic cutaneous melanoma. Int J Cancer 1995;63:375–80.
45. Dalerba P, Ricci A, Russo V, et al. High homogeneity of MAGE, BAGE, GAGE, tyrosinase and Melan-A/MART-1 gene expression in clusters of multiple simultaneous metastases of human mela-noma: implications for protocol design of therapeutic antigen-specific vaccination strategies. Int J Cancer 1998;77:200–204.
46. Kawakami Y, Rosenberg SA. Human tumor antigens recognized by T-cells. Immunol Res 1997;16:313–339.
47. Murer K, Urosevic M, Willers J, et al. Expression of Melan-A/MART-1 in primary melanoma cell cultures has prognostic implication in metastatic melanoma patients. Melanoma Res 2004; 14:257–262.
48. Lee PP, Yee C, Savage PA, et al. Characterization of circulating T cells specific for tumor-associated antigens in melanoma patients. Nat Med 1999;5:677–685.
49. Lotz C, Ferreira EA, Drexler I, et al. Partial tyrosinase-specific self tolerance by HLA-A*0201-restricted cytotoxic T lymphocytes in mice and man. Int J Cancer 2004;108:571–579.
50. Wang RF, Appella E, Kawakami Y, Kang X, Rosenberg SA. Identification of TRP-2 as a human tumor antigen recognized by cytotoxic T lymphocytes. J Exp Med 1996;184:2207–2216.
51. Bakker AB, Schreurs MW, de Boer AJ, et al. Melanocyte lineage-specific antigen gp100 is recog-nized by melanoma-derived tumor-infiltrating lymphocytes. J Exp Med 1994;179:1005–1009.
52. Vijayasaradhi S, Bouchard B, Houghton AN. The melanoma antigen gp75 is the human homologue of the mouse b (brown) locus gene product. Exp Med 1990;171:1375–1380.
53. Harada M, Li YF, El-Gamil M, Rosenberg SA, Robbins PF. Use of an in vitro immunoselected tumor line to identify shared melanoma antigens recognized by HLA-A*0201-restricted T cells. Cancer Res 2001;61:1089–1094.
54. Houghton AN, Vijayasardhi S, Bouchard B, Nazftzger C, Hara I, Chapman PB. Recognition of autoantigens by patients with melanoma. Ann NY Acad Sci 1993;690:59–68.
55. Johansson M, Takasaki A, Lenner L, Arstrand K, Kagedal B. Quantitative relationships between pigment-related mRNA and biochemical melanoma markers in melanoma cell lines. Melanoma Res 2002;12:193–200.

56. Slingluff CL Jr, Colella TA, Thompson L, et al. Melanomas with concordant loss of multiple melanocytic differentiation proteins: immune escape that may be overcome by targeting unique or undefined antigens. Cancer Immunol Immunother 2000;48:661–672.

57. Wolchok JD, Weber JS, Houghton AN, Livingston PO. Melanoma vaccines. In: Balch CM, Houghton AN, Sober AJ, Soong SJ, eds. Cutaneous Melanoma, 4th ed. Quality Medical Publishing, St Louis, MO: 2003.

58. Bar-Dayan Y, Barshack I, Blank M, et al. Antibodies to the cytoplasm, cell membrane and nuclear membrane of malignant neoplasms in pooled normal human polyspecific immunoglobulin G. Int J Oncol 1999;15:1091–1096.

59. Thomas PJ, Kaur JS, Aitcheson CT, Robinson WA, Tan EM. Antinuclear, antinucleolar, and anticytoplasmic antibodies in patients with malignant melanoma. Cancer Res 1983;43:1372–1380.

60. Sahin U, Tureci O, Schmitt H, et al. Human neoplasms elicit multiple specific immune responses in the autologous host. Proc Natl Acad Sci USA 1995;92:11,810–11,813.

61. Chen YT, Scanlan MJ, Sahin U, et al. A testicular antigen aberrantly expressed in human cancers detected by autologous antibody screening. Proc Natl Acad Sci USA 1997;94:1914–1918.

62. Tureci O, Sahin U, Zwick C, Koslowski M, Seitz G, Pfreundschuh M. Identification of a meiosis-specific protein as a member of the class of cancer/testis antigens. Proc Natl Acad Sci USA 1998;95:5211–5216.

63. Scanlon MJ, Simpson AJG, Old LJ. The cancer/testis genes: review, standardization, and commentary. Cancer Immunity 2004;4:1–15.

64. Old LJ. Cancer Vaccine Collaborative 2002: opening address. Cancer Immun 2003;3:1.

65. Natali PG, Wilson BS, Imai K, Bigotti A, Ferrone S. Tissue distribution, molecular profile, and shedding of a cytoplasmic antigen identified by the monoclonal antibody 465.12S to human melanoma cells. Cancer Res 1982;42:583–589.

66. Euhus DM, Gupta RK, Morton DL. Induction of antibodies to a tumor-associated antigen by immunization with a whole melanoma cell vaccine. Cancer Immunol Immunother 1989;29:247–254.

67. Gupta RK, Morton DL. Clinical significance of tumor-associated antigens and antitumor antibodies in human malignant melanoma. In: Reisfeld RA, Ferrone S, eds. Melanoma Antigens and Antibodies. Plenum, New York, NY: 1982, pp. 139–172.

68. Houghton AN, Wolchok JD. Immunology. In: Balch CH, Sober AJ, Soon SJ, eds. Cutaneous Melanoma. Quality Medical Publishing, St. Louis, MO. 2003 pp. 659–668.

69. Albino AP, Sozzi G, Nanus DM, Jhanwar SC, Houghton AN. Malignant transformation of human melanocytes: induction of a complete melanoma phenotype and genotype. Oncogene 1992;7:2315–2321.

70. Ravindranath MH, Tuchida T, Irie RF. Diversity of ganglioside expression in human melanoma: In: Oettgen HF, ed. Gangliosides and Cancer. VCH Publishers, New York, NY: 1989, pp 80–91.

71. Ravindranath MH, Gonzales AM, Nishimoto K, Tam WY, Soh D, Morton DL. Immunology of gangliosides. Indian J Exp Biol 2000;38:301–312.

72. Livingston PO, Wong GY, Adluri S, et al. Improved survival in stage III melanoma patients with GM2 antibodies: a randomized trial of adjuvant vaccination with GM2 ganglioside. J Clin Oncol 1994;12:1036–1044.

73. Ravindranath MH, Morton DL. Immunogenicity of membrane-bound gangliosides in viable whole-cell vaccines. Cancer Invest 1997;15:491–499.

74. Kageshita T, Hirai S, Kimura T, Hanai N, Ohta S, Ono T. Association between sialyl Lewis(a) expression and tumor progression in melanoma. Cancer Res 1995;55:1748–1751.

75. Li J, Pereira S, Van Belle P, et al. Isolation of the melanoma-associated antigen p23 using antibody phage display. J Immunol 2001;166:432–438.

76. Cai X, Garen A. Anti-melanoma antibodies from melanoma patients immunized with genetically modified autologous tumor cells: selection of specific antibodies from single-chain Fv fusion phage libraries. Proc Natl Acad Sci USA 1995;92:6537–6541.

77. Kupsch JM, Tidman NH, Kang NV, et al. Isolation of human tumor-specific antibodies by selection of an antibody phage library on melanoma cells. Clin Cancer Res 1999;5:925–931.

78. Desai SA, Wang X, Noronha EJ, Kageshita T, Ferrone S. Characterization of human anti-high molecular weight-melanoma-associated antigen single-chain Fv fragments isolated from a phage display antibody library. Cancer Res 1998;58:2417–2425.

79. Hanahan D, Lanzavecchia A, Mihich E. Fourteenth Annual Pezcoller Symposium: the novel dichotomy of immune interactions with tumors. Cancer Res 2003;63:3005–3008.

80. Belardelli F, Ferrantini M, Parmiani G, Schlom J, Garaci E. International meeting on cancer vaccines: how can we enhance efficacy of therapeutic vaccines? Cancer Res 2004;64:6827–6830.

81. Cormier JN, Hijazi YM, Abati A, et al. Heterogeneous expression of melanoma-associated antigens and HLA-A2 in metastatic melanoma in vivo. Int J Cancer 1998;75:517–524.

82. Khong HT, Wang QJ, Rosenberg SA. Identification of multiple antigens recognized by tumor-infiltrating lymphocytes from a single patient: tumor escape by antigen loss and loss of MHC expression. J Immunother 2004;27:184–190.

83. Radford KJ, Mallesch J, Hersey P. Suppression of human melanoma cell growth and metastasis by the melanoma-associated antigen CD63 (ME491). Int J Cancer 1995;62:631–635.

84. Kondoh M, Ueda M, Ichihashi M, Mishima Y. Decreased expression of human melanoma-associated antigen ME491 along the progression of melanoma pre-canceroses to invasive and metastatic melanomas. Melanoma Res 1993;3:241–245.

85. Hoek K, Rimm DL, Williams KR, et al. Expression profiling reveals novel pathways in the transformation of melanocytes to melanomas. Cancer Res 2004;64:5270–5282.

86. Du J, Miller AJ, Widlund HR, Horstmann MA, Ramaswamy S, Fisher DE. MLANA/MART1 and SILV/PMEL17/GP100 are transcriptionally regulated by MITF in melanocytes and melanoma. Am J Pathol 2003;163:333–343.

87. Durda PJ, Dunn IS, Rose LB, et al. Induction of "antigen silencing" in melanomas by oncostatin M: down-modulation of melanocyte antigen expression. Mol Cancer Res 2003;1:411–419.

88. Merimsky O, Shoenfeld Y, Chaitchik S, Yecheskel G, Fishman P. Antigens and antibodies in malignant melanoma. Tumour Biol 1994;15:188–202.

89. Ramirez-Montagut T, Andrews DM, Ihara A, et al. Melanoma antigen recognition by tumour-infiltrating T lymphocytes (TIL): effect of differential expression of melan-A/MART-1. Clin Exp Immunol 2000;119:11–18.

90. Merimsky O, Shoenfeld Y, Yecheskel G, Chaitchik S, Azizi E, Fishman P. Vitiligo- and melanoma-associated hypopigmentation: a similar appearance but a different mechanism. Cancer Immunol Immunother 1994;38:411–416.

91. Rote NS, Gupta RK, Morton DL. Tumor-associated antigens detected by autologous sera in urine of patients with solid neoplasms. J Surg Res 1980;29:18–22.

92. Rote NS, Gupta RK, Morton DL. Determination of incidence and partial characterization of tumor-associated antigens found in the urine of patients bearing solid tumors. Int J Cancer 1980;26:203–210.

93. Euhus DM, Gupta RK, Morton DL. Characterization of a 90-100 kDa tumor-associated antigen in the sera of melanoma patients. Int J Cancer 1990;45:1065–1070.

94. Kelley MC, Jones RC, Gupta RK, et al. Tumor-associated antigen TA-90 immune complex assay predicts subclinical metastasis and survival for patients with early stage melanoma. Cancer 1998;83:1355–1361.

95. Litvak DA, Gupta RK, Yee R, Wanek LA, Ye W, Morton DL. Endogenous immune response to early- and intermediate-stage melanoma is correlated with outcomes and is independent of locoregional relapse and standard prognostic factors. J Am Coll Surg 2004;198:227–235.

96. Hsueh EC, Gupta RK, Yee R, Leopoldo ZC, Qi K, Morton DL. Does endogenous immune response determine the outcome of surgical therapy for metastatic melanoma? Ann Surg Oncol 2000; 7:232–238.

97. Euhus DM, Gupta RK, Morton DL. Induction of antibodies to a tumor-associated antigen by immunization with a whole melanoma cell vaccine. Cancer Immunol Immunother 1989;29:247–254.

98. Jones RC, Kelley MC, Gupta RK, et al. Immune response to polyvalent melanoma cell vaccine in AJCC stage III melanoma: an immunologic survival model. Ann Surg Oncol 1996;3:437–445.

99. Chung MH, Gupta RK, Hsueh E, et al. Humoral immune response to a therapeutic polyvalent cancer vaccine after complete resection of thick primary melanoma and sentinel lymphadenectomy. J Clin Oncol 2003;21:313–319.

100. DiFronzo LA, Gupta RK, Essner R, et al. Enhanced humoral immune response correlates with improved disease-free and overall survival in American Joint Committee on Cancer stage II melanoma patients receiving adjuvant polyvalent vaccine. J Clin Oncol 2002;20:3242–3248.

101. Hsueh EC, Gupta RK, Qi K, Morton DL. Correlation of specific immune responses with survival in melanoma patients with distant metastases receiving polyvalent melanoma cell vaccine. J Clin Oncol 1998;16:2913–2920.

102. Wong JH, Gupta RK, Morton DL. Serial determinations of melanoma tumor-associated antigen and antibody in patients with stage I melanoma. Arch Surg 1986;121:1342–1345.

103. Euhus DM, Gupta RK, Morton DL. Detection of a tumor-associated glycoprotein antigen in serum and urine of melanoma patients by murine monoclonal antibody (AD1-40F4) in enzyme immunoassay. J Clin Lab Anal 1989;3:184–190.

104. Euhus DM, Gupta RK, Morton DL. Association between allo-immunoreactive and xeno-immunoreactive subunits of a glycoprotein tumor-associated antigen. Cancer Immunol Immunother 1990;32:214–220.

105. Gupta RK, Morton DL. Monoclonal antibody-based ELISA to detect glycoprotein tumor-associated-antigen specific immune complexes in cancer patients. J Clin Lab Anal 1992;6:329–336.

106. Chung MH, Gupta RK, Essner R, Ye W, Yee R, Morton DL. Serum TA90 immune complex assay can predict outcome after resection of thick (> or =4 mm) primary melanoma and sentinel lymphadenectomy. Ann Surg Oncol 2002;9:120–126.

107. Kelley MC, Gupta RK, Hsueh EC, Yee R, Stern S, Morton DL. Tumor-associated antigen TA90 immune complex assay predicts recurrence and survival after surgical treatment of stage I-III melanoma. J Clin Oncol 2001;19:1176–1182.

108. Hsueh EC, Gupta RK, Qi K, Yee R, Leopoldo ZC, Morton DL. TA90 immune complex predicts survival following surgery and adjuvant vaccine immunotherapy for stage IV melanoma. Cancer J Sci Am 1997;3:364–370.

109. Halliday GM. Skin immunity and melanoma development. In: Thompson JF, Morton DL, Kroon BR, eds. Textbook of Melanoma. Martin Dunitz, Taylor and Francis Group, New York, NY: 2004, pp. 25–42.

36 Host Responses to Melanoma

Implications for Immunotherapy

Julian A. Kim and Ernest Borden

CONTENTS

Summary

Development of immunotherapeutic strategies for the treatment of patients with melanoma have far exceeded that of any other solid malignancy, with the possible exception of renal cell carcinoma. The rationale for use of melanoma as a model for development of immunotherapies is derived from the following observations:

1. Melanoma metastases and primary cutaneous melanomas are among the most common solid tumors to exhibit spontaneous regression.
2. Local intratumoral injections of bacillus-camillus-guerin can lead to regression of not only the injected lesions but also distant lesions, suggesting the successful induction of a systemic immune response.
3. The ability to culture tumor-infiltrating lymphocytes, which recognize melanoma cell lines that share specific major histocompatibility complex alleles could be used to identify shared melanoma-associated rejection antigens.

Key Words: Melanoma; regression; interferon; interleukin; tumor necrosis factor.

INTRODUCTION

The purpose of this chapter will be to highlight observations that demonstrate a natural host immune response to melanoma, which make melanoma particularly suitable to attempts at immunotherapeutic control. Major strategies of immunotherapy will be presented, along with how these strategies have been tested in human clinical trials. The basic categories that will be discussed include "active" forms of immunotherapy, which require a host immune response to exert their activity; and "passive" forms of immunotherapy, which directly target the tumor and can theoretically generate an antitumor

From: *From Melanocytes to Melanoma: The Progression to Malignancy*
Edited by: V. J. Hearing and S. P. L. Leong © Humana Press Inc., Totowa, NJ

effect without a host immune response. Active nonspecific immunotherapies, in the form of systemic administration of cytokines, and active specific immunotherapies, such as cancer vaccines, will be discussed and compared with passive immunotherapies, which consist primarily of monoclonal antibodies and adoptive transfer of T-cells into the tumor-bearing host. Emphasis will be placed on the proposed mechanism of action, antigen(s) that are being targeted, and results of phase II and phase III human clinical trials. Although a detailed analysis of promising therapies that are in preclinical and early clinical development is beyond the scope of this chapter, particularly novel strategies for next-generation immunotherapies will be presented to provide a sense of the future direction of the field.

OBSERVATIONS OF NATURAL IMMUNE RESPONSES TO MELANOMA

Spontaneous Regression of Melanoma

Melanoma is arguably one of the most unpredictable solid tumors in terms of biological behavior, in which there is a documented incidence of spontaneous regression of both the primary cutaneous tumor as well as distant metastases. The percentage of patients who present with partial or complete histological regression of the primary tumor is estimated to be as high as 25 to 40%, although the reports of sustained long-term partial regression are rare *(1–3)*. Interestingly, up to 15% of patients with stage IV metastatic melanoma will live 5 yr, independent of whether they are receiving therapy *(4)*. Many investigators have attributed the regression of primary and metastatic melanomas to the adaptive immune response, although others have shown evidence of alternative mechanisms of tumor growth control, such as apoptosis *(5,6)*.

Several lines of evidence support a central role of immune mediators in spontaneous melanoma regression. Biopsies of regressing lesions have demonstrated overexpression of T-helper (Th)-1 cytokines, such as interferon (IFN)-γ, interleukin (IL)-2, and tumor-necrosis factor-α, when compared with nonregressing lesions *(7)*. In addition, although the reports in the literature are sparse, isolated reports of spontaneous regression of metastatic melanoma have been associated with evidence of increased immune parameters, such as delayed-type hypersensitivity response to skin testing *(8)*. Indirect evidence supporting immune surveillance of primary cutaneous melanoma has been reported in renal transplant patients who not only have a higher risk because of immunosuppression, but also develop cutaneous melanoma from precursor dysplastic nevi, which demonstrated a marked absence of lymphocytic and macrophage infiltrates *(9,10)*. Finally, the presence of a brisk lymphocytic infiltrate in primary cutaneous melanomas has been correlated with improved survival *(11)*. A retrospective analysis of 259 patients with localized primary cutaneous melanoma with median follow-up of 12.3 yr confirmed that the degree of tumor infiltration by lymphocytes was an independent predictor of melanoma-specific mortality *(12)*.

Immune-Cell Infiltrate of Melanoma

Elegant studies directed toward characterizing the immune-cell infiltrate of primary and metastatic malignant melanoma lesions have provided ample evidence of host–tumor immune interaction. Immunohistochemical analysis of immune-cell infiltration have confirmed a preponderance of T-cells, which can range from memory CD4 cells in early (<0.75 mm) superficial spreading melanomas to CD8 cells of cutaneous origin that express HECA 452 *(13)*. Dermal dendritic cells that express human leukocyte antigen-D related (HLA-DR) also appear to infiltrate both vertical growth-phase and radial growth-phase melanomas but not benign compound nevi, and the expression of HLA-DR correlates with the degree of T-cell infiltrate, consistent with the idea that melanoma-associated antigens are being presented to infiltrating T-cells *(14)*. Isolation of tumor-infiltrating lymphocytes (TILs) and long-term culture have resulted in the generation of T-cell clones that recognize melanoma-associated antigens in the context of major histocompatibility complex (MHC) *(15)*.

A variety of cytokines has been identified within the host–melanoma microenvironment that may play a role in either recruitment of T-cells, generation of T-cell effector responses, or both. As has been identified in other solid malignancies, melanoma cells are known to secrete proinflammatory cytokines, such as granulocyte macrophage colony-stimulating factor (GM-CSF) and IL-1 and IL-6, and growth factors, such as vascular endothelial growth factor and basic fibroblast growth factor, which may serve not only as autocrine growth factors but also regulate local cell-mediated immune responses *(16–18)*. Interestingly, melanoma cells have been shown to express a functional IL-4 receptor, which, after ligation, results in decreased cell proliferation and increased MHC II molecule expression *(19)*. Finally, gene-profiling studies of fine-needle aspirations from primary and metastatic subcutaneous melanoma define a subgroup of approx 30 genes, such as chemokines and immune response transcription factors, which were predictive of clinical response to immunotherapy *(20)*. Approximately one-half of the 30 genes with predictive value had function related to T-cell regulation, suggesting that the molecular events which underlie melanoma regression confirm T-cell-mediated mechanisms *(21,22)*.

Tumor-Induced Mechanism of Immune Suppression

Immune-mediated tumor regression can be influenced not only by the efficiency of the host immune response but also counterbalanced by tumor-induced mechanisms of immune evasion. Several observations support the concept that melanoma can either directly or indirectly induce mechanisms of immune evasion. Plasmacytoid dendritic cells that express the tryptophan-degrading enzyme, indoleamine 2,3-dioxygenase, have been found to induce T-cell anergy and direct toward Th2 responses. These cells have been identified in melanoma draining regional lymph nodes in higher numbers as compared with control lymph nodes, suggesting the induction of immunoregulatory antigen-presenting cells (APC) as a mechanism of immune evasion *(23)*. CD4 T-cell clones derived from human melanoma metastases have been shown to decrease cytotoxic T-cell activity in vitro in an antigen-dependent fashion, suggesting the possibility of a subset of T-cells with a suppressor phenotype *(24)*. Melanoma secretion of immunosuppressive cytokines, such as transforming growth factor (TGF)-β and IL-10, and secretion of soluble Fas ligand may also contribute to suppression of local immune responses and deletion of effector T-cells *(25–27)*. Gene-profiling studies have identified suppression of interferon-stimulated genes within primary and metastatic melanomas, and downregulation of MHC class I expression by melanoma cells in vivo has also been observed and is postulated as a mechanism of evasion from antigen-specific CD8 cells *(28,29)*.

Two observations that underscore the importance of melanoma-induced immune evasion are the presence of T-cells in melanoma patients with defective signal transduction pathways and the apparent lack of correlation of the presence of T-cell clonal expansion and melanoma regression. Several studies in patients with both renal cell carcinoma and melanoma have demonstrated T-cells with defective T-cell receptor tyrosine kinase activity, which involves the Src family kinases, lck/fyn, and the ζ-chain of the T-cell receptor *(30–33)*. The putative mechanism of tumor-induced T-cell dysfunction appears to be via soluble factors, and the signaling defects are reversible by administration of certain cytokines, such as IL-2. Melanoma-induced T-cell dysfunction may also explain why recent studies have failed to show a correlation between T-cell clonal expansion within TIL populations and tumor regression *(34)*. Thus, although natural immune responses to melanoma-associated antigens do appear to exist, limitations of the innate and adaptive immune responses may be caused by the inability to overcome melanoma-induced immunosuppressive mechanisms within the tumor–host microenvironment.

IMMUNOTHERAPY OF MELANOMA

Systemic Cytokine Therapy

Immunotherapeutic strategies using systemic administration of recombinant human cytokines represent the most widely studied approach to the treatment of patients with melanoma. The concept of enhancing pre-existing natural immune responses to melanoma-associated antigens by the systemic administration of cytokines has been tested both in the settings of patients with refractory metastatic disease and as adjuvant therapy in patients with high-risk surgically resected disease. Although the efficacy of systemic cytokine administration in generating specific immune responses may be limited by dose-limiting toxicity and a narrow therapeutic window, systemic cytokine administration remains the only Food and Drug Administration (FDA)-approved biological therapy for patients with either metastatic (IL-2) or surgically resected, high-risk (IFN-α-2b) melanoma.

INTERFERON α-2B

Human IFNs are pleiotropic cytokines that exert a broad range of biological effects, including antiviral, antiproliferative, antiangiogenic, apoptosis induction, and immune cell modulation. Preclinical studies in more than 40 freshly derived melanoma tumor cells have confirmed that IFNs exert direct antiproliferative effects and induce apoptosis in vitro via the IFN-stimulated gene, Apo2L ligand (TRAIL) *(35)*. IFNs appear to exert their effects in part via phosphorylation of the intracellular-signaling protein, STAT-1, because the antitumor effects of interferon are abrogated when administered to STAT-1-deficient mice *(36)*. Interestingly, the antitumor efficacy of IFN is preserved in vivo against STAT-1-deficient melanoma tumors growing in syngeneic immunocompetent mice, which demonstrates that stimulation of the host immune response remains an important mechanism of activity *(37)*. Indeed, IFNs have been known to be central regulators of cell-mediated immune responses that involve Th and cytolytic T-cells, as well as professional APCs, such as dendritic cells *(38)*. Finally, IFNs mediate significant antiangiogenic effects in preclinical tumor models via downmodulation of vascular endothelial growth factor gene expression *(39,40)*. These preclinical data provided the rationale for human clinical trials of IFN-α-2b in patients with advanced melanoma.

Human Clinical Trials Using IFN-α-2b. Recombinant IFN-α-2b administered in patients with metastatic disease resulted in an approx 20% clinical response rate. Of note, was that nearly one-third of the responders exhibited complete radiographic responses, with duration of response extending from 1 to 3 yr, suggesting that IFN had significant activity as a single agent *(41)*. Initial early phase studies of combinations of IFN-α-2b with dacarbazine demonstrated clinical response rates approaching 40 to 50%. However, a randomized phase III study comparing combinations of dacarbazine with IFN-α-2b and tamoxifen showed no improvement in time to treatment failure and survival over dacarbazine alone *(42)*. However, because of the significant activity of IFN-α-2b as a single agent, phase III studies in patients with melanoma at high-risk for relapse soon followed.

Numerous clinical trials of adjuvant IFN-α-2b have been conducted in patients with primary cutaneous melanoma greater than 4 mm in thickness or in patients with stage III disease after confirmation of regional lymph node metastasis. The first Eastern Cooperative Oncology Group (ECOG) 1684 study consisted of 287 patients with deep primary (>4 mm thick) or regional lymph node metastatic (N1) disease, which were completely resected and patients were subsequently randomized to treatment with either 20 million U/m^2/d of IFN-α-2b administered intravenously for 4 wk, followed by 10 million U/m^2 of IFN-α-2b three times weekly administered subcutaneously for 48 wk, vs observation. The study demonstrated a significant improvement in relapse-free survival ($p < 0.002$) and overall survival ($p < 0.02$) with a median follow-up of 6.9 yr, and based on this data, IFN-α-2b was later approved by the FDA for adjuvant treatment of patients with resected high-risk melanoma *(43)*. In an attempt to determine whether a low-dose regimen of IFN could retain the same antitumor activity while reducing treatment-related toxicity, an Intergroup study E1690 compared the previously tested high-dose IFN (HDI) regimen for 1 yr with a low-dose regimen for a total of 2 yr *(44)*. At 52 mo median follow-up, the relapse free-survival for the HDI was significantly improved as compared with the low-dose regimen and control observation groups ($p < 0.03$, two-sided) in both node-positive and node-negative patients. Laboratory correlative studies demonstrated increases in tumor cell MHC class II expression and adhesion molecule expression that were dose-dependent but did not predict prolonged disease-free survival *(45)*. Importantly, no improvement in overall survival was demonstrated between the three groups, although this was confounded by the fact that the overall survival in the observation group in E1684 was significantly higher than the same group of patients in E1690 (6 yr vs 2.8 yr). Despite several attempts to reconcile the discrepancy between overall survival in the observation arms of E1690 and E1684, a third study E1694 was initiated that compared 1 yr of adjuvant therapy with either HDI or a ganglioside vaccine, GMK, consisting of the GM2 ganglioside and the adjuvant QS-21 *(46)*. Patients with resected stage IIb or III were randomized to either one of the two treatment arms, because there was no observation control group. The 880 patients were randomized and the trial was closed prematurely, after interim analysis, when it was determined that there was a statistically significant improvement in relapse-free and overall survival in the HDI group as compared with the GMK group ($p < 0.0015$ and $p < 0.009$, respectively). Interestingly, in those patients treated with GMK, antibody titers to GM2 in treated patients' serum were detected and did appear to correlate with improved relapse-free and overall survival. In addition, although patients treated with HDI demonstrated improved survival overall, the largest increase in survival appeared to be in those patients with thick primary tumors that were node negative.

Despite data from these three randomized studies that demonstrated significant improvements in relapse-free and, in two instances, overall survival in patients treated with adjuvant HDI, treatment-related toxicity, such as depression, fatigue, and hepatotoxicity emerged as substantial concerns. A quality-of-life adjusted survival analysis was performed in patients from E1684 that suggested that patients who received HDI experienced severe treatment-related toxicity for an average of 5.8 mo while gaining a mean of 8.9 mo without relapse and 7.0 mo of overall survival. When stratified for tumor burden, it was determined that the greatest quality-of-life adjusted benefit was in the patients who were node positive *(47)*. A recent pooled analysis of the data from the three ECOG and Intergroup trials evaluating over 2000 randomized patients with long-term follow-up (April 2001) confirmed that patients with high-risk, resected melanoma stage IIb or III demonstrated improved relapse-free but not overall survival as compared with observation *(48)*. Although the meta-analysis confirms that IFN-α-2b has significant activity as a single agent in the adjuvant therapy of these patients, there is still considerable need to improve IFN-based adjuvant therapy regarding the overall survival benefit and quality of life *(49)*.

INTERLEUKIN-2

IL-2, first described as T-cell growth factor, was initially isolated from the supernatants of human peripheral blood mononuclear cells after stimulation with lectins, such as phytohemagglutinin *(50,51)*. In vitro studies of recombinant human IL-2 have demonstrated that, after binding of the high affinity IL-2 receptor on the surface of T-cells, activation of signaling molecules within the Janus kinase/signal transducers of and activators of transcription pathways leads to increased transcriptional activity that favors cell proliferation. Because T-cell activation and proliferation is a central component of most strategies of immunotherapy, IL-2 has been one of the most widely studied cytokines in terms of its ability to modulate a therapeutic antitumor immune response.

Early preclinical animal models demonstrated that IL-2 was effective in maintaining long-term T-cell lines and tumor-reactive T-cell clones in culture and represented a significant improvement over lectins and phorbol esters *(52)*. Culture of human peripheral blood lymphocytes with high concentrations of IL-2 (1000–6000 U/mL) resulted in morphological changes that included blast formation and cytoplasmic granules *(53)*. The ability of the resulting cells to lyse a variety of tumor cell targets in vitro led to their classification as lymphokine-activated killer cells (LAK). The hallmark of the LAK phenomenon was that the effector cells lysed a number of tumor cell targets with no apparent MHC restriction but did not lyse normal autologous peripheral blood cells. The theory that emerged from these observations was that tumors of different histological origins shared common or shared antigens that were recognized by LAK cells. The fact that LAK cells did not lyse normal cells provided a significant therapeutic window and the rationale for translation into human clinical trials.

Human Clinical Trials of Systemic IL-2 in Patients With Metastatic Melanoma. Based on the observation of MHC-unrestricted lysis of a variety of tumor cells by lymphocytes in cultures with high concentrations of IL-2, systemic administration of recombinant human IL-2 was initiated in patients with metastatic disease of various histologies *(54)*. Rosenberg et al. reported the experience of the Surgery Branch of the National Cancer Institute, in which over 1039 courses of high-dose IL-2 (720,000 IU/ kg of IL-2, every 8 h for 5-d cycles) were administered in 652 patients, 596 of whom had metastatic cancer. Patients treated with either IL-2 alone ($n = 155$) or IL-2 in combination with ex vivo-generated autologous LAK cells ($n = 214$) demonstrated a 20 to 35% objective response rate in the setting of metastatic melanoma, renal carcinoma, colorectal cancer, and non-Hodgkin's lymphoma. Although the majority of the objective responses were partial regression, of the 18 patients who demonstrated complete radiographic response, 10 demonstrated a duration of complete response from 18 to 52 mo.

Despite the limitations of this reported series of patients with mixed histologies and treatment regimens, two major themes emerged. The first was that systemic administration of a biological agent that had no direct antiproliferative or cytotoxic effect against tumor cells could result in tumor regression in a minority of patients. Thus, in contrast to the interferons, which have been shown to exert some direct effects on tumor cells in vitro, IL-2 therapy demonstrated "proof of principal" that immune mechanisms alone could mediate tumor regression. The second important observation from this study was that subsets of patients with melanoma and renal carcinoma appeared to have the highest chance of tumor regression, which was an important finding because effective conventional cytotoxic chemotherapy was lacking in those particular tumor types. Thus, the initial experience with systemic IL-2 administration led to further randomized studies to define the therapeutic efficacy and mechanism of action in patients with these histologies.

Subsequent studies included a phase II single-armed protocol of high-dose IL-2 therapy in patients with metastatic melanoma and renal cell carcinoma *(55)*. Between September 1985 and December 1992, 283 consecutive patients were treated, and a total of 447 courses were administered. Objective response rates were achieved in 17% of patients with melanoma (7% complete response [CR], 10% partial response [PR]) and 20% of patients with renal carcinoma (7% CR, 13% PR). Based on these and subsequent studies, recombinant human IL-2 was approved for the treatment of patients with metastatic melanoma in 1998. A comparison study of LAK plus IL-2 vs IL-2 alone in 157 patients demonstrated a higher objective response rate in the patients treated with cells plus IL-2, but the difference in patients achieving complete response as well as the development of activated T-cells with MHC-restricted tumor antigen reactivity lead to a gradual decline in the study of LAK adoptive immunotherapy *(56)*.

FUTURE DIRECTIONS

Despite the inherent toxicities of high-dose cytokine therapy, IFN-α-2B and IL-2 remain the only FDA-approved therapies for patients either in the high-risk adjuvant or metastatic melanoma groups. Studies that examined regimens combining IFNs and IL-2 with each other or cytotoxic chemotherapy have yielded only modest increases in objective response rate, but are generally limited by poor tolerability. Methods of delivering cytokines by chemical modification (pegylation of interferon) or the use of carrier proteins, such as monoclonal antibody fragments, has resulted in diminished treatment-related toxicity with apparent maintenance of therapeutic efficacy *(57)*. Preclinical studies identifying novel IFN-stimulated gene pathways to enhance therapeutic efficacy, as well as decrease resistance to IFN therapy, represent an active area of ongoing investigation that may result in targeted therapies for patients with melanoma *(35,58,59)*.

Active Specific Immunotherapy Using Vaccines

Development of therapeutic cancer vaccines for melanoma has been an area of intense investigation in both preclinical animal models and human clinical trials. Although the component structure of vaccines may vary from whole tumor cell preparations, tumor cell lysates, and subcellular fractions, whole proteins and defined peptides administered alone or with professional APCs or gene-modified tumor cells or APCs, the goal of the vaccination is the same. Vaccines are classified as active specific immunotherapy because they require active participation of the host immune system to develop T-cell responses to tumor-associated antigens. Although some vaccines have been demonstrated to result in generation of Th responses that result in antibody production that specifically recognizes and binds the immunogen, most vaccine approaches have focused on the generation of antigen-specific CD8+ cytolytic T-cells. A comprehensive review of the many vaccine strategies is beyond the scope of this chapter. However, examples of several types of vaccines that differ in their composition, as well as resultant immune response, will be highlighted.

WHOLE TUMOR CELL VACCINES

Morton and colleagues pioneered the modern era of the use of irradiated tumor cells as the source of antigen for active specific immunotherapy of melanoma. Initial attempts were focused on the use of autologous melanoma cells irradiated and admixed with bacillus-camillus-guerin (BCG) administered intradermally. However, technical issues surrounding the isolation and expansion of suitable numbers of melanoma cells made the use of autologous tumor cells problematic. Culture of hundreds of melanoma explants resulted in the outgrowth of several melanoma cell lines that could be maintained in vitro and stored using cryopreservation methods. An allogeneic polyvalent melanoma tumor cell vaccine was constructed by combining several cell lines that are now known to express several known melanoma antigens, such as gangliosides, tyrosinase, gp100, and the melanoma antigen recognized by T-cells/melanoma antigen gene proteins. The initial results of a clinical trial using the polyvalent melanoma cell vaccine (MCV) in 136 stage IIIA and IV patients demonstrated significantly increased survival in both groups of patients as compared with historical controls, with no change in the natural history of melanoma in a database of over 1400 patients during that time period (60). Importantly, improved survival correlated significantly with the presence of a delayed-type hypersensitivity reaction and antibody responses to the MCV, suggesting that both cell-mediated and humoral immune responses might be contributing to the survival benefit. Although some of the patients with stage IV disease underwent surgical resection before administration of the vaccine, 9 of 40 patients (23%) who had measurable disease demonstrated evidence of tumor regression, 3 of which were complete responses. These initial observations were followed by three separate reports of prolonged survival as compared with historical controls in patients undergoing vaccination with an allogeneic whole melanoma cell vaccine in patients with stage II, III, and IV disease after complete surgical resection (61–63). These data are the basis for ongoing randomized phase III studies comparing disease-free and overall survival in patients undergoing treatment with either BCG alone or BCG in combination with an allogeneic MCV (Canvaxin™) in patients with either stage III or stage IV melanoma after complete surgical resection. The accrual goal to the trial in stage III patients was met in Fall, 2004, at which time the study was closed to further accrual. The results of the randomized trial in stage III patients may provide an alternative adjuvant therapy for patients who do not wish to be treated with adjuvant IFN-α-2b, although without data comparing Canvaxin and IFN-α-2b there will be continued debate regarding the standard adjuvant therapy for this patient population.

The correlative laboratory studies that accompanied the MCV trials have provided several intriguing results, which may provide insight into potential contributing factors to the mechanism of action. For example, HLA typing of a subset of 69 patients who underwent therapy with MCV demonstrated a significant correlation between the overall survival of the patient and the degree of HLA class I phenotype match with the MCV component cell lines *(64)*. Specific HLA subtypes were also correlated with a better (HLA-A25) or poorer (HLA-B35) outcome. Interestingly, a subset analysis performed in stage III patients treated with an allogeneic melanoma cell-lysate vaccine, as part of a randomized Intergroup study, demonstrated significant correlations with improved overall survival and patients with HLA-A2 or HLA-C3 phenotype *(65)*. Finally, patients treated with Canvaxin that develop immune complexes against the tumor-associated glycoprotein, TA90, have prolonged survival compared with patients that had the TA90 immune complexes before initiation of therapy *(66)*.

TUMOR LYSATE VACCINES

An alternative method to the use of whole tumor cells is the development of tumor lysate vaccines. These preparations have the theoretical advantage over whole tumor cell vaccines of eliminating immunosuppressive factors released by tumor cells (such as IL-10 and TGF-β) but retaining tumor-associated antigens that can be processed and presented by professional APCs. Two examples of melanoma lysate vaccines that have been tested in randomized clinical trials are the Vaccinia Melanoma Oncolysate (VMO) vaccine and Melacine. Interestingly, both vaccines were shown to be ineffective in improving survival in the intent-to-treat analysis, but *post hoc* subset analyses identified subgroups that had improved survival.

The VMO was developed using a live vaccinia virus-augmented allogeneic melanoma lysate. A phase Ib study conducted in patients with American Joint Committee on Cancer (AJCC) stage III melanoma demonstrated a statistically significant increase in disease-free survival as compared with a matched historical control cohort *(67)*. Laboratory studies confirmed a positive correlation between serum titers of antimelanoma immunoglobulin (Ig)G antibodies and disease-free survival. Based on the data, which suggested that VMO may have a protective effect against recurrence in high-risk, surgically resected melanoma patients, a phase III randomized double-blind study was conducted in patients with AJCC stage III, node-positive melanoma. Patients were randomized to receive either adjuvant VMO or vaccinia and followed for disease-free and overall survival. The interim analysis of 217 patients demonstrated no benefit in disease-free survival in patients treated with either agent *(68)*. However, a post-hoc subset analysis suggested that male patients between the ages of 44 and 57 yr with one to five positive nodes appeared to have a survival benefit from VMO therapy. Two subsequent follow-up reports confirmed this observation, with 18.9, 26.8, and 21.3% improvements in survival at 2, 3, and 5 yr, respectively, in the specific male subset who were treated with VMO as compared with vaccinia alone *(69,70)*. In an attempt to determine whether VMO demonstrated therapeutic efficacy as compared with other adjuvant therapy trials in patients with AJCC stage III melanoma, a statistical analysis was performed comparing patients treated with VMO with the survival of patients in the treatment arms of several cooperative group trials of adjuvant IFN-α-2a *(71)*. The results suggested that the survival of patients treated with VMO was comparable to patients treated with adjuvant IFN-α-2a in the ECOG EST 1684, which the authors propose as evidence of therapeutic effect related to treatment with VMO.

A similar sequence of events surrounded a phase III randomized study comparing an allogeneic melanoma lysate (Melacine) to observation in patients with surgically resected, AJCC stage III melanoma *(65)*. Despite a lack of therapeutic efficacy in the intent-to-treat analysis, a subset analysis of patient survival based on HLA type demonstrated that patients who were either HLA-A2 or HLA-C3 had an improved survival when treated with Melacine as compared with observation, with 5-yr, relapse-free survival of 77 vs 64% ($p = 0.004$). These particular HLA serotypes were associated with response to Melacine therapy in patients with stage IV melanoma, suggesting that the allogeneic lysate may contain processed tumor antigens that are presented by professional APCs in the context of these HLA (72). Although the therapeutic efficacy of Melacine was not established by the prospective randomized trial, the subset analysis supports the idea that tumor antigens processed and presented as peptides may represent a valid strategy for vaccine development.

VACCINES USING DEFINED ANTIGENS

The discovery of melanoma-associated antigens, such as those in melanoma antigen gene and melanoma antigen recognized by T-cells families, as well as gp100 and tyrosinase, ushered a new era in active specific immunotherapy using defined peptides that would bind particular MHC motifs (73,74). Preclinical as well as clinical trials of immunotherapy of melanoma over the past 5 yr have been dominated by vaccine strategies using defined antigens. Whole protein antigens or peptides that bind to specific MHC molecules have been used alone, in combination with adjuvants, or, most commonly, after pulsing with autologous dendritic cells (75). Route of administration of antigen-pulsed dendritic cells has ranged from intradermal, subcutaneous, intravenous, and even intranodal.

Although no phase III randomized studies have been reported using defined-antigen melanoma vaccines, a recent review of vaccine trials for patients with melanoma summarizes the current state of the field (76). A review of cancer vaccine clinical trials performed at the Surgery Branch of the National Cancer Institute in 440 patients with metastatic melanoma yielded an objective response rate of only 2.6%. Unfortunately, this response rate was similar to other trials performed in patients with metastatic disease using defined melanoma antigen vaccines. Interestingly, in several of these patients, there was measurable evidence of immunization against the defined antigen, as measured by an increase in the frequency of antigen-specific T-cells in the peripheral blood after vaccine administration (77,78). One hypothesis that the authors present for the presence of antigen-specific T-cells in the face of a lack of melanoma regression is that the cells are not becoming activated at the tumor site to perform their effector function. Evidence of immune selection within melanomas after antigen-specific vaccine therapy has been reported in 532 melanoma lesions in 204 patients in which the tumor expression of the target antigen was reduced, particularly when the vaccine was administered with systemic IL-2 (79). Thus, although there appears to be clear evidence that antigen-specific T-cells can be generated with defined antigen vaccines, with a subsequent elimination of antigen-expressing melanoma cells, clinical tumor regression has been difficult to achieve.

FUTURE DIRECTIONS

Active specific immunotherapy for melanoma appears to be at a crossroads with respect to the management of patients with melanoma. Whole cell vaccination with allogeneic melanoma cell lines that express a variety of melanoma antigens are currently being tested in the adjuvant setting in patients with surgically resected stage III melanoma, the results of which may significantly impact treatment options for patients with melanoma. Newer generations of whole cell vaccines using melanoma cells fused to autologous dendritic cells may provide some improvement over allogeneic vaccines because the melanoma antigens will be presented in the proper MHC context for optimal host T-cell response *(80,81)*. Based on studies that have demonstrated clinical responses in patients with metastatic melanoma after administration of intralesional granulocyte macrophage colony-stimulating factor (GM-CSF) or in combination with a melanoma vaccine *(82,83)*, gene-modified whole cell melanoma vaccines that secrete cytokines, such as GM-CSF or IL-4, are currently under investigation in human clinical trials *(84,85)*. Defined melanoma vaccines have demonstrated the ability to stimulate antigen-specific T-cells in patients with melanoma. However, the observation that the immune response may be too restricted, leading to immune selection and outgrowth of low antigen-expressing melanoma cells, suggests that multiepitope vaccines may provide a better potential for success in future trials.

Adoptive Immunotherapy Using Activated T-Cells

The passive transfer of immunity to the tumor-bearing host by virtue of the administration of activated immune cells is a method that was initially established in preclinical animal models. The translation of this technique into humans has required technological improvements in the culturing and expansion of cells ex vivo, and has evolved into a process that, although cumbersome, can result in the generation of billions of activated, antigen-specific T-cells. Despite the technical hurdles of cell processing, continued testing in human clinical trials is fueled by the occasional observation of striking regression of metastatic melanoma at visceral sites.

TUMOR-INFILTRATING LYMPHOCYTES

The observation that melanoma lesions undergoing regression were infiltrated by immune cells stimulated interest in isolating these cells to determine their antitumor reactivity. Intense research in this area confirmed that long-term culture of TIL from melanoma lesions in both experimental murine models and humans resulted in the outgrowth of T-cells with high avidity for melanoma-associated antigens *(86–88)*. Generation of high numbers of TIL in culture lead to clinical trials of adoptive transfer of these activated cells in combination with systemic IL-2 in patients with metastatic melanoma. Occasional dramatic clinical responses with regression of bulky metastatic tumor provided proof-of-concept that passive transfer of immunity was achievable in select patients. However, the practical limitations of long-term T-cell culture appeared to outweigh the benefit to a small percentage of patients.

Recent studies have shed some insight into potential methods of improving adoptive immunotherapy using TIL. A phase I study of nonmyeloablative chemotherapy in combination with adoptive transfer of autologous melanoma-specific T-cells was devised to induce lymphodepletion before transfer of activated cells. The theoretical premise for this approach was to try to repopulate the tumor-bearing host immune system with the activated transferred cells as the dominant population, as well as to eradicate suppressor T-cells, which might limit the effectiveness of the transferred cells *(89,90)*. Using this treatment strategy, 18 of 35 patients with metastatic melanoma demonstrated an objective clinical response (>50% tumor reduction) *(91)*. Interestingly, the activated transferred cells had high avidity for melanoma antigens but were reactive against several different antigens. This is in stark comparison to adoptive therapy using T-cell clones that were peptide-specific and derived from peripheral blood of patients who were undergoing defined-antigen vaccine therapy, which showed a marked lack of clinical effectiveness (92).

FUTURE DIRECTIONS: TUMOR-DRAINING LYMPH NODE CELLS

Extensive study in preclinical animal models as well as human clinical trials have demonstrated that lymph nodes draining a progressive subcutaneous tumor contain antigen-sensitized T-cells, which, after activation and expansion in culture with anti-CD3/IL-2, mediate effector function in vivo after adoptive transfer (93). One of the most interesting findings within this body of work was that the subpopulation of T-cells that downregulate L-selectin (CD62L) expression contain the subset of antigen-primed cells that mediate therapeutic antitumor effects after culture activation and adoptive transfer (94). Recent studies in mice suggest that restricted V β T-cell receptor usage within the cells that downregulate L-selectin may correspond to antigen-specific T-cells that are clonally derived (95). Human studies looking at lymph nodes draining a melanoma vaccine site demonstrate that T-cells with L-selectin downregulation are skewed toward a type 1 cytokine secretion pattern predictive of clinical response after adoptive transfer (96). These studies provide the rationale for the use of tumor-draining lymph node cells as a source of T-cells for adoptive immunotherapy protocols of the future.

CONCLUSIONS AND PERSPECTIVES

The observations of natural host immune responses to melanoma-associated antigens has resulted in intense research efforts to develop immunotherapy as a treatment option in these patients. The lessons learned from these studies appear to suggest that generation of broad immune responses, such as that seen with systemic cytokine administration, whole cell vaccine therapy, or adoptive transfer of T-cells with broad reactivity, may be beneficial, in that immune selectivity of antigen-expressing tumor cells is less likely. Also, vaccine strategies can result in generation of T-cells with antigen-specificity, but the lack of activation of these T-cells at the tumor site may limit the efficacy in settings of bulky metastatic disease. Further understanding of the mechanism of action of immunotherapy in vivo should provide investigators with a method of balancing the nature of the immune response generated by the treatment to the immune status and the bulk of metastatic disease of the patient. Lessons learned from human clinical trials will undoubtedly extend the use of immunotherapy of patients with melanoma in the future.

REFERENCES

1. Fontaine D, Parkhill W, Greer W, Walsh N. Partial regression of primary cutaneous melanoma: is there an association with sub-clinical sentinel lymph node metastasis? Am J Dermatopathol 2003;25: 371–376.
2. Blessing K, McLaren KM. Histological regression in primary cutaneous melanoma: recognition, prevalence and significance. Histopathology 1992;20:315–322.
3. Baldo M, Schiavon M, Cicogna PA, Boccato P, Mazzoleni F. Spontaneous regression of subcutaneous metastasis of cutaneous melanoma. Plast Reconstr Surg 1992;90:1073–1076.
4. Balch CM, Soong SJ, Gershenwald JE, et al. Prognostic factors analysis of 17,600 melanoma patients: validation of the American Joint Committee on Cancer melanoma staging system. J Clin Oncol 2001;19(16):3622–3634.
5. Papac RJ. Spontaneous regression of cancer: possible mechanisms. In Vivo 1998;12(6):571–578.

6. Printz C. Spontaneous regression of melanoma may offer insight into cancer immunology. J Natl Cancer Inst 2001;93(14):1047–1048.

7. Mocellin S, Ohnmacht GA, Wang E, Marincola FM. Kinetics of cytokine expression in melanoma metastases classifies immune responsiveness. Int J Cancer 2001;93(2):236–242.

8. Bulkley GB, Cohen MH, Banks PM, Char DH, Ketcham AS. Long-term spontaneous regression of malignant melanoma with visceral metastases. Report of a case with immunologic profile. Cancer 1975;36(2):485–494.

9. Greene MH, Young TI, Clark WH Jr. Malignant melanoma in renal-transplant recipients. Lancet 1981;1(8231):1196–1199.

10. Bordea C, Wojnarowska F, Millard PR, Doll H, Welsh K, Morris PJ. Skin cancers in renal-transplant recipients occur more frequently than previously recognized in a temperate climate. Transplantation 2004;77(4):574–579.

11. Elder D. Tumor progression, early diagnosis and prognosis of melanoma. Acta Oncol 1999; 38(5):535–547.

12. Tuthill RJ, Unger JM, Liu PY, Flaherty LE, Sondak VK. Risk assessment in localized primary cutaneous melanoma: a Southwest Oncology Group study evaluating nine factors and a test of the Clark logistic regression prediction model. Am J Clin Pathol 2002;118(4):504–511.

13. Strohal R, Marberger K, Pehamberger H, Stingl G. Immunohistological analysis of anti-melanoma host responses. Arch Dermatol Res 1994;287(1):28–35.

14. Fullen DR, Headington JT. Factor XIIIa-positive dermal dendritic cells and HLA-DR expression in radial versus vertical growth-phase melanomas. J Cutan Pathol 1998;25(10):553–558.

15. Wang RF, Zeng G, Johnston SF, Voo K, Ying H. T cell-mediated immune responses in melanoma: implications for immunotherapy. Crit Rev Oncol Hematol 2002;43(1):1–11.

16. Armstrong CA, Tara DC, Hart CE, Kock A, Luger TA, Ansel JC. Heterogeneity of cytokine production by human malignant melanoma cells. Exp Dermatol 1992;1(1):37–45.

17. Shih IM, Herlyn M. Role of growth factors and their receptors in the development and progression of melanoma. J Invest Dermatol 1993;100(suppl 2):196S–203S.

18. Kruger-Krasagakes S, Krasagakis K, Garbe C, Diamantstein T. Production of cytokines by human melanoma cells and melanocytes. Recent Results Cancer Res 1995;139:155–168.

19. Obiri NI, Siegel JP, Varricchio F, Puri RK. Expression of high-affinity IL-4 receptors on human melanoma, ovarian and breast carcinoma cells. Clin Exp Immunol 1994;95(1):148–155.

20. Wang E, Miller LD, Ohnmacht GA, et al. Prospective molecular profiling of melanoma metastases suggests classifiers of immune responsiveness. Cancer Res 2002;62(13):3581–3586.

21. Wang E, Marincola FM. cDNA arrays and the enigma of melanoma immune responsiveness. Cancer J 2001;7(1):16–24.

22. Wang E, Marincola FM. A natural history of melanoma: serial gene expression analysis. Immunol Today 2000;21(12):619–623.

23. Lee JR, Dalton RR, Messina JL, et al. Pattern of recruitment of immunoregulatory antigen-presenting cells in malignant melanoma. Lab Invest 2003;83(10):1457–1466.

24. Chakraborty NG, Twardzik DR, Sivanandham M, Ergin MT, Hellstrom KE, Mukherji B. Autologous melanoma-induced activation of regulatory T cells that suppress cytotoxic response. J Immunol 1990;145(7):2359–2364.

25. Lazar-Molnar E, Hegyesi H, Toth S, Falus A. Autocrine and paracrine regulation by cytokines and growth factors in melanoma. Cytokine 2000;12(6):547–554.

26. Conrad CT, Ernst NR, Dummer W, Brocker EB, Becker JC. Differential expression of transforming growth factor beta 1 and interleukin 10 in progressing and regressing areas of primary melanoma. J Exp Clin Cancer Res. 1999;18(2):225–232.

27. Real LM, Jimenez P, Kirkin A, et al. Multiple mechanisms of immune evasion can coexist in melanoma tumor cell lines derived from the same patient. Cancer Immunol Immunother 2001;49(11):621–628.

28. Marincola FM, Shamamian P, Simonis TB, et al. Locus-specific analysis of human leukocyte antigen class I expression in melanoma cell lines. J Immunother Emphasis Tumor Immunol 1994; 16(1):13–23.

29. Hoek K, Rimm DL, Williams KR, et al. Expression profiling reveals novel pathways in the transformation of melanocytes to melanomas. Cancer Res 2004;64(15):5270–5282.

30. Finke JH, Zea AH, Stanley J, et al. Loss of T-cell receptor zeta chain and p56lck in T-cells infiltrating human renal cell carcinoma. Cancer Res 1993;53(23):5613–5616.

31. Bukowski RM, Rayman P, Uzzo R, et al. Signal transduction abnormalities in T lymphocytes from patients with advanced renal carcinoma: clinical relevance and effects of cytokine therapy. Clin Cancer Res 1998;4(10):2337–2347.

32. Kolenko V, Wang Q, Riedy MC, et al. Tumor-induced suppression of T lymphocyte proliferation coincides with inhibition of Jak3 expression and IL-2 receptor signaling: role of soluble products from human renal cell carcinomas. J Immunol 1997;159(6):3057–3067.

33. Becker JC, Terheyden P, Brocker EB. Molecular basis of T-cell dysfunction in melanoma. Melanoma Res 1997;7(suppl 2):S51–S57.

34. Bernsen MR, Diepstra JH, van Mil P, et al. Presence and localization of T-cell subsets in relation to melanocyte differentiation antigen expression and tumour regression as assessed by immunohistochemistry and molecular analysis of microdissected T cells. J Pathol 2004;202(1):70–79.

35. Chawla-Sarkar M, Lindner DJ, Liu YF, et al. Apoptosis and interferons: role of interferon-stimulated genes as mediators of apoptosis. Apoptosis 2003;8(3):237–249.

36. Lesinski GB, Anghelina M, Zimmerer J, et al. The antitumor effects of IFN-alpha are abrogated in a STAT1-deficient mouse. J Clin Invest 2003;112(2):170–180.

37. Badgwell B, Lesinski GB, Magro C, Abood G, Skaf A, Carson W 3rd. The antitumor effects of interferon-alpha are maintained in mice challenged with a STAT1-deficient murine melanoma cell line. J Surg Res 2004;116(1):129–136.

38. Kayagaki N, Yamaguchi N, Nakayama M, Eto H, Okumura K, Yagita H. Type I interferons (IFNs) regulate tumor necrosis factor-related apoptosis-inducing ligand (TRAIL) expression on human T cells: a novel mechanism for the antitumor effects of type I IFNs. J Exp Med 1999;189(9):1451–1460.

39. Wang L, Wu WZ, Sun HC, et al. Mechanism of interferon alpha on inhibition of metastasis and angiogenesis of hepatocellular carcinoma after curative resection in nude mice. J Gastrointest Surg 2003;7(5):587–594.

40. von Marschall Z, Scholz A, Cramer T, et al. Effects of interferon alpha on vascular endothelial growth factor gene transcription and tumor angiogenesis. J Natl Cancer Inst 2003;95(6):437–448.

41. Kirkwood JM, Ernstoff M. Melanoma: therapeutic options with recombinant interferons. Semin Oncol 1985;12(4 suppl 5):7–12.

42. Falkson CI, Ibrahim J, Kirkwood JM, Coates AS, Atkins MB, Blum RH. Phase III trial of dacarbazine versus dacarbazine with interferon alpha-2b versus dacarbazine with tamoxifen versus dacarbazine with interferon alpha-2b and tamoxifen in patients with metastatic malignant melanoma: an Eastern Cooperative Oncology Group study. J Clin Oncol 1998;16(5):1743–1751.

43. Kirkwood JM, Strawderman MH, Ernstoff MS, Smith TJ, Borden EC, Blum RH. Interferon alfa-2b adjuvant therapy of high-risk resected cutaneous melanoma: the Eastern Cooperative Oncology Group Trial EST 1684. J Clin Oncol 1996;14(1):7–17.

44. Kirkwood JM, Ibrahim JG, Sondak VK, et al. High- and low-dose interferon alfa-2b in high-risk melanoma: first analysis of intergroup trial E1690/S9111/C9190. J Clin Oncol 2000;18(12):2444–2458.

45. Kirkwood JM, Richards T, Zarour HM, et al. Immunomodulatory effects of high-dose and low-dose interferon alpha2b in patients with high-risk resected melanoma: the E2690 laboratory corollary of intergroup adjuvant trial E1690. Cancer 2002;95(5):1101–1112.

46. Kirkwood JM, Ibrahim JG, Sosman JA, et al. High-dose interferon alfa-2b significantly prolongs relapse-free and overall survival compared with the GM2-KLH/QS-21 vaccine in patients with resected stage IIB-III melanoma: results of intergroup trial E1694/S9512/C509801. J Clin Oncol 2001;19(9):2370–2380.

47. Cole BF, Gelber RD, Kirkwood JM, Goldhirsch A, Barylak E, Borden E. Quality-of-life-adjusted survival analysis of interferon alfa-2b adjuvant treatment of high-risk resected cutaneous melanoma: an Eastern Cooperative Oncology Group study. J Clin Oncol 1996;14(10):2666–2673.

48. Kirkwood JM, Manola J, Ibrahim J, Sondak V, Ernstoff MS, Rao U. A pooled analysis of eastern cooperative oncology group and intergroup trials of adjuvant high-dose interferon for melanoma. Clin Cancer Res 2004;10(5):1670–1677.

49. Schuchter LM. Adjuvant interferon therapy for melanoma: high-dose, low-dose, no dose, which dose? J Clin Oncol 2004;22(1):7–10.

50. Grimm EA, Mazumder A, Zhang HZ, Rosenberg SA. Lymphokine-activated killer cell phenomenon. Lysis of natural killer-resistant fresh solid tumor cells by interleukin 2-activated autologous human peripheral blood lymphocytes. J Exp Med 1982;155(6):1823–1841.

51. Rosenberg SA, Grimm EA, McGrogan M, et al. Biological activity of recombinant human interleukin-2 produced in Escherichia coli. Science 1984;223(4643):1412–1414.

52. Rosenberg SA, Eberlein TJ, Grimm EA, Lotze MT, Mazumder A, Rosenstein M. Development of long-term cell lines and lymphoid clones reactive against murine and human tumors: a new approach to the adoptive immunotherapy of cancer. Surgery 1982;92(2):328–336.

53. Rayner AA, Grimm EA, Lotze MT, Wilson DJ, Rosenberg SA. Lymphokine-activated killer (LAK) cell phenomenon. IV. Lysis by LAK cell clones of fresh human tumor cells from autologous and multiple allogeneic tumors. J Natl Cancer Inst 1985;75(1):67–75.

54. Rosenberg SA, Lotze MT, Yang JC, et al. Experience with the use of high-dose interleukin-2 in the treatment of 652 cancer patients. Ann Surg 1989;210(4):474–484; discussion 484–485.

55. Rosenberg SA, Yang JC, Topalian SL, et al. Treatment of 283 consecutive patients with metastatic melanoma or renal cell cancer using high-dose bolus interleukin 2. Jama 1994;271(12):907–913.

56. Rosenberg SA, Lotze MT, Muul LM, et al. A progress report on the treatment of 157 patients with advanced cancer using lymphokine-activated killer cells and interleukin-2 or high-dose interleukin-2 alone. N Engl J Med 1987;316(15):889–897.

57. Grimm EA, Smid CM, Lee JJ, Tseng CH, Eton O, Buzaid AC. Unexpected cytokines in serum of malignant melanoma patients during sequential biochemotherapy. Clin Cancer Res 2000;6(10): 3895–3903.

58. Leaman DW, Chawla-Sarkar M, Jacobs B, et al. Novel growth and death related interferon-stimulated genes (ISGs) in melanoma: greater potency of IFN-beta compared with IFN-alpha2. J Interferon Cytokine Res 2003;23(12):745–756.

59. Leaman DW, Chawla-Sarkar M, Vyas K, et al. Identification of X-linked inhibitor of apoptosis-associated factor-1 as an interferon-stimulated gene that augments TRAIL Apo2L-induced apoptosis. J Biol Chem 2002;277(32):28,504–28,511.

60. Morton DL, Foshag LJ, Hoon DS, et al. Prolongation of survival in metastatic melanoma after active specific immunotherapy with a new polyvalent melanoma vaccine. Ann Surg 1992;216(4):463–482.

61. Morton DL, Hsueh EC, Essner R, et al. Prolonged survival of patients receiving active immunotherapy with Canvaxin therapeutic polyvalent vaccine after complete resection of melanoma metastatic to regional lymph nodes. Ann Surg 2002;236(4):438–448; discussion 448–449.

62. DiFronzo LA, Gupta RK, Essner R, et al. Enhanced humoral immune response correlates with improved disease-free and overall survival in American Joint Committee on Cancer stage II melanoma patients receiving adjuvant polyvalent vaccine. J Clin Oncol 2002;20(15):3242–3248.

63. Hsueh EC, Essner R, Foshag LJ, et al. Prolonged survival after complete resection of disseminated melanoma and active immunotherapy with a therapeutic cancer vaccine. J Clin Oncol 2002;20(23): 4549–4554.

64. Hoon DS, Okamoto T, Wang HJ, et al. Is the survival of melanoma patients receiving polyvalent melanoma cell vaccine linked to the human leukocyte antigen phenotype of patients? J Clin Oncol 1998;16(4):1430–1437.

65. Sosman JA, Unger JM, Liu PY, et al. Adjuvant immunotherapy of resected, intermediate-thickness, node-negative melanoma with an allogeneic tumor vaccine: impact of HLA class I antigen expression on outcome. J Clin Oncol 2002;20(8):2067–2075.

66. Tsioulias GJ, Gupta RK, Tisman G, et al. Serum TA90 antigen-antibody complex as a surrogate marker for the efficacy of a polyvalent allogeneic whole-cell vaccine (CancerVax) in melanoma. Ann Surg Oncol 2001;8(3):198–203.

67. Wallack MK, Bash JA, Leftheriotis E, et al. Positive relationship of clinical and serologic responses to vaccinia melanoma oncolysate. Arch Surg 1987;122(12):1460–1463.

68. Wallack MK, Sivanandham M, Balch CM, et al. A phase III randomized, double-blind multi-institutional trial of vaccinia melanoma oncolysate-active specific immunotherapy for patients with stage II melanoma. Cancer 1995;75(1):34–42.

69. Wallack MK, Sivanandham M, Ditaranto K, et al. Increased survival of patients treated with a vaccinia melanoma oncolysate vaccine: second interim analysis of data from a phase III, multi-institutional trial. Ann Surg 1997;226(2):198–206.

70. Wallack MK, Sivanandham M, Balch CM, et al. Surgical adjuvant active specific immunotherapy for patients with stage III melanoma: the final analysis of data from a phase III, randomized, double-blind, multicenter vaccinia melanoma oncolysate trial. J Am Coll Surg 1998;187(1):69–77; discussion 77–79.

71. Kim EM, Sivanandham M, Stavropoulos CI, Bartolucci AA, Wallack MK. Overview analysis of adjuvant therapies for melanoma—a special reference to results from vaccinia melanoma oncolysate adjuvant therapy trials. Surg Oncol 2001;10(1–2):53–59.

72. Sosman JA, Sondak VK. Melacine: an allogeneic melanoma tumor cell lysate vaccine. Expert Rev Vaccines 2003;2(3):353–368.

73. Wang RF. Human tumor antigens: implications for cancer vaccine development. J Mol Med 1999;77(9):640–655.

74. Rosenberg SA. Development of cancer immunotherapies based on identification of the genes encoding cancer regression antigens. J Natl Cancer Inst 1996;88(22):1635–1644.

75. Jefford M, Maraskovsky E, Cebon J, Davis ID. The use of dendritic cells in cancer therapy. Lancet Oncol 2001;2(6):343–353.

76. Rosenberg SA, Yang JC, Restifo NP. Cancer immunotherapy: moving beyond current vaccines. Nat Med 2004;10(9):909–915.

77. Dudley ME, Ngo LT, Westwood J, Wunderlich JR, Rosenberg SA. T-cell clones from melanoma patients immunized against an anchor-modified gp100 peptide display discordant effector phenotypes. Cancer J 2000;6(2):69–77.

78. Mukherji B, Chakraborty NG, Yamasaki S, et al. Induction of antigen-specific cytolytic T cells in situ in human melanoma by immunization with synthetic peptide-pulsed autologous antigen presenting cells. Proc Natl Acad Sci USA 1995;92(17):8078–8082.

79. Riker A, Cormier J, Panelli M, et al. Immune selection after antigen-specific immunotherapy of melanoma. Surgery 1999;126(2):112–120.

80. Shimizu K, Kuriyama H, Kjaergaard J, Lee W, Tanaka H, Shu S. Comparative analysis of antigen loading strategies of dendritic cells for tumor immunotherapy. J Immunother 2004;27(4):265–272.

81. Parkhurst MR, DePan C, Riley JP, Rosenberg SA, Shu S. Hybrids of dendritic cells and tumor cells generated by electrofusion simultaneously present immunodominant epitopes from multiple human tumor-associated antigens in the context of MHC class I and class II molecules. J Immunol 2003;170(10):5317–5325.

82. Vaquerano JE, Cadbury P, Treseler P, Sagebiel R, Leong SP. Regression of in-transit melanoma of the scalp with intralesional recombinant human granulocyte-macrophage colony-stimulating factor. Arch Dermatol 1999;135(10):1276–1277.

83. Leong SP, Enders-Zohr P, Zhou YM, et al. Recombinant human granulocyte macrophage-colony stimulating factor (rhGM-CSF) and autologous melanoma vaccine mediate tumor regression in patients with metastatic melanoma. J Immunother 1999;22(2):166–174.

84. Mahvi DM, Shi FS, Yang NS, et al. Immunization by particle-mediated transfer of the granulocyte-macrophage colony-stimulating factor gene into autologous tumor cells in melanoma or sarcoma patients: report of a phase I/IB study. Hum Gene Ther 2002;13(14):1711–1721.

85. Wakimoto H, Abe J, Tsunoda R, Aoyagi M, Hirakawa K, Hamada H. Intensified antitumor immunity by a cancer vaccine that produces granulocyte-macrophage colony-stimulating factor plus interleukin 4. Cancer Res 1996;56(8):1828–1833.

86. Zorn E, Hercend T. A MAGE-6-encoded peptide is recognized by expanded lymphocytes infiltrating a spontaneously regressing human primary melanoma lesion. Eur J Immunol 1999;29(2):602–607.

87. Seiter S, Monsurro V, Nielsen MB, et al. Frequency of MART-1/MelanA and gp100/PMel17-specific T cells in tumor metastases and cultured tumor-infiltrating lymphocytes. J Immunother 2002; 25(3):252–263.

88. Dudley ME, Wunderlich JR, Shelton TE, Even J, Rosenberg SA. Generation of tumor-infiltrating lymphocyte cultures for use in adoptive transfer therapy for melanoma patients. J Immunother 2003;26(4):332–342.

89. Dudley ME, Wunderlich JR, Robbins PF, et al. Cancer regression and autoimmunity in patients after clonal repopulation with antitumor lymphocytes. Science 2002;298(5594):850–854.

90. Dudley ME, Wunderlich JR, Yang JC, et al. A phase I study of nonmyeloablative chemotherapy and adoptive transfer of autologous tumor antigen-specific T lymphocytes in patients with metastatic melanoma. J Immunother 2002;25(3):243–251.

91. Rosenberg SA, Dudley ME. Cancer regression in patients with metastatic melanoma after the transfer of autologous antitumor lymphocytes. Proc Natl Acad Sci USA 2004;101(suppl 2):14,639–14,645.

92. Dudley ME, Wunderlich J, Nishimura MI, et al. Adoptive transfer of cloned melanoma-reactive T lymphocytes for the treatment of patients with metastatic melanoma. J Immunother 2001;24(4): 363–373.

93. Yoshizawa H, Chang AE, Shu S. Specific adoptive immunotherapy mediated by tumor draining lymph node cells sequentially activated with anti-CD3 and IL-2. J Immunol 1991;147(2):729–737.
94. Kagamu H, Touhalisky JE, Plautz GE, Krauss JC, Shu S. Isolation based on L-selectin expression of immune effector T cells derived from tumor-draining lymph nodes. Cancer Res 1996;56(19): 4338–4342.
95. Kim JA, Rao P, Graor H, Rothchild K, O'Keefe C, Maciejewski JP. CDR3 spectratyping identifies clonal expansion within T-cell subpopulations that demonstrate therapeutic antitumor activity. Surgery 2004;136(2):295–302.
96. Meijer SL, Dols A, Hu HM, et al. Reduced L-selectin (CD62LLow) expression identifies tumor-specific type 1 T cells from lymph nodes draining an autologous tumor cell vaccine. Cell Immunol 2004;227(2):93–102.

37

Future Perspectives

Vincent J. Hearing and Stanley P. L. Leong

Cancers arise from their normal cellular counterparts, and, in this regard, malignant melanoma is no exception. Within this book, we have traced the origins of melanoblast precursors, their differentiation to melanocytes, the regulation of their physiological functions, and the pathways by which they become malignant and eventually metastasize. We are grateful to all authors who have made this book the first of its kind to trace the biology of melanocytes and their subsequent development to melanoma, and which details the current state of knowledge of mechanisms that underlie those processes. Melanoma is a highly aggressive cancer and with even small increments in Breslow thickness (measured in millimeters), the clinical behavior of the tumor rapidly worsens from a relatively curable disease to a highly aggressive and fatal disease. In contrast, breast and colon cancers develop more aggressive behaviors only with significantly higher tumor burden, for example, a T2 lesion is 2 cm in breast cancer, and, often, several centimeters are noted in primary colon cancers before they become overtly aggressive. Based on relatively small size increments, slight changes in cell volume can substantially affect the clinical behavior of melanoma.

In most instances (>95% of cases), melanoma is represented by a cutaneous distribution and, therefore, careful surveillance and awareness of any atypical lesions on the skin will allow clinicians to identify earlier stages of lesions to prevent progression or advancement of melanoma to a more aggressive stage. A very challenging question is why the white population is most affected by melanoma. Does this result from intrinsic genetic differences between different racial groups that are reflected by different levels of pigmentation that might explain the different incidences of melanoma in different racial populations? If that is the case, what are the genes responsible for such differences? The nagging question of whether melanoma forms as a result of the effects of ultraviolet radiation on melanocytes also needs further investigation. If that is the case, are melanocytes from the white population more vulnerable to such processes of carcinogenesis? Perhaps epidemiological studies can answer the question of whether white populations living in northern Europe with relatively lower levels of sun exposure will have lower incidences of melanoma than whites who have migrated to areas with higher exposure to ultraviolet radiation *(1)*. The role of ultraviolet radiation in the carcinogenesis of melanoma also needs to be further defined. Although multiple melanomas may

From: *From Melanocytes to Melanoma: The Progression to Malignancy*
Edited by: V. J. Hearing and S. P. L. Leong © Humana Press Inc., Totowa, NJ

occasionally occur in an individual, the majority of patients present with only one site of melanoma. The obvious question that arises is why a certain site gives rise to melanoma, whereas other sites in the same patient remain undisturbed. It is known that anatomical sites influence the outcome of a patient, for example head and neck melanomas appear to be more aggressive *(2)*. Is the distribution of melanomas in the head/neck or in the extremities/trunk a random or nonrandom process?

The chapters in this book detail the current state of our knowledge about biochemical and molecular events that occur in melanocytes and in melanoma cells, the stepwise progression in the transformation of melanocytes to malignant melanoma, and eventually in the metastasis of the tumor (*see* Fig. 1 in Chapters 10 and 15 for schematics of this sequence). However, there are still many gaps in our understanding of these complex processes. The challenges for future studies will be to define the precise molecular mechanisms involved in each step. Once such mechanisms are understood, potential approaches and therapies can be devised, either to divert or halt such progression and/ or to prevent the subsequent progression of the tumor to its more aggressive form.

The issue of lymphatic metastasis through lymphatic channels vs systemic dissemination through vascular channels also needs to be further explored. Are the two different modes of metastasis a reflection of the intrinsic biology of melanoma? Can it be that certain melanomas with specific molecular features will initially spread through lymphatic channels to sentinel lymph nodes and then later disseminate through the vascular system, as in the incubator hypothesis? On the other hand, do molecular markers exist that can define melanoma cells at primary sites that will disseminate through the vascular system simultaneously, as in the marker hypothesis (*see* Chapter 23)? Are these two processes clonally or epigenetically determined?

This book has summarized the latest findings in the development and differentiation of melanocytes and their progression to malignant melanoma. It is clear that we are still faced with a number of important but unanswered questions that should be resolved in the years to come, which should lead to a better understanding of the mechanisms involved in the progression from normal melanocytes to malignant melanoma. The ultimate goal is not only to study the basic biology of such progression but also, hopefully, when the mechanisms involved have been elucidated, to develop strategies for the precise and effective clinical diagnosis and treatment of malignant melanoma. It is also our hope that clinicians will soon be able to test new hypotheses developed in research laboratories and to then report those clinical observations to basic research scientists, which will allow further characterization of mechanisms involved in the transformation of melanocytes to melanoma.

REFERENCES

1. Gilchrest BA, Eller MS, Geller AC, Yaar M. The pathogenesis of melanoma induced by ultraviolet radiation. N Engl J Med 1999;340:1341–1348.
2. Balch CM, Soong S-J, Shaw HM. An analysis of prognostic factors in 8500 patients with cutaneous melanoma. In: Balch CM, Houghton AN, Sober AJ, Soong S-J, eds. Cutaneous Melanoma. J. B. Lippincott, Philadelphia, PA: 1992, p. 165.

INDEX